Diagnosis and Treatment of Soft Tissue Tumors

Harzem Özger • Franklin H. Sim • Ajay Puri
Levent Eralp
Editors

Diagnosis and Treatment of Soft Tissue Tumors

Changes, Challenges and Strategies

Springer

Editors
Harzem Özger
Department of Orthopedics and Traumatology
Istanbul University, Istanbul Medical Faculty
Istanbul, Türkiye

Franklin H. Sim
Department of Orthopaedic Surgery
Mayo Clinic
Rochester, MN, USA

Ajay Puri
Department of Surgical Oncology
Tata Memorial Hospital
Mumbai, Maharashtra, India

Levent Eralp
Department of Orthopedics and Traumatology
Istanbul University, Istanbul Medical Faculty
Istanbul, Türkiye

ISBN 978-3-031-77060-9 ISBN 978-3-031-77061-6 (eBook)
https://doi.org/10.1007/978-3-031-77061-6

This Springer imprint is published by the registered company Springer Nature Switzerland AG
The registered company address is: Gewerbestrasse 11, 6330 Cham, Switzerland

Foreword

This book is essential reading for anyone involved in the diagnosis or management of patients with soft tissue sarcomas. It fills a large gap in the world literature with sensible, practical advice from a multitude of world authorities in the fields of radiology, pathology, surgery, and oncology.

This book highlights the current state of knowledge but also identifies the dilemmas clinicians face in everyday practice and gives practical, sensible solutions to many of these challenges.

The chapters are arranged in a sensible order, starting with investigation and diagnosis and leading through to staging, management (both oncological and surgical), reconstruction, and finally, dealing with complications (and how to avoid them) and assessment of outcomes.

The second part of this book presents a series of case studies with many ingenious solutions to challenging cases, all of which contain an important lesson or message that can be used more generally.

This book is a pleasure to read and is generally consistent, although there is still a variance in the descriptions of margins of excision (should they be classified by distance or as R0, R1, R2 or wide, marginal, and intralesional?). Several excellent chapters deal with this and succinctly point out the benefits and limitations of the current systems.

One thing that stands out throughout this book is the wide variety of behaviour exhibited by different soft tissue sarcomas and the need to treat every different patient with a soft tissue sarcoma individually. The field of soft tissue sarcoma management is becoming increasingly complex with neoadjuvant therapy now staking an increasing claim to be of benefit and management within an experienced multidisciplinary team is essential for a good outcome. This team should involve a wide range of surgical skills for optimum outcomes, particularly when tumours involve multiple organs.

The amount of wisdom imparted in this book is huge and represents many years of experience from the authors—this book is an essential reference for anyone involved in the management of patients with soft tissue sarcomas.

Former Consultant Orthopaedic Oncologist
Royal Orthopaedic Hospital
Birmingham UK
rob.grimer@btopenworld.com

Rob Grimer

The foreword was inadvertently missed and the book was published. It has now been included and can be found in the book's front matter.

Preface

Soft tissue masses—"lumps and bumps"—are one of the most frequent entities physicians encounter. While the overwhelming majority of soft tissue masses are benign and may be observed or undergo simple excision, a small but significant percentage will have aggressive or malignant behavior and require distinct evaluation and treatment protocols for proper management.

The goal of *Diagnosis and Treatment of Soft Tissue Tumors: Changes, Challenges, and Strategies* is to address the wide variety of clinical presentations of different soft tissue tumors. Soft tissue tumors are not a single disease, and we seek to provide expert guidance on the recognition, evaluation, and treatment of this broad spectrum of conditions.

The work is presented in two parts: The first part covers the principles of soft tissue tumor evaluation and treatment and the second part presents case examples from expert clinicians around the world to highlight the application of these principles in practice and to understand pitfalls that treating physicians may encounter.

We hope that this book will serve as a useful guide for all physicians who treat patients with soft tissue tumors from diagnosis (radiologists and pathologists) to treatments (medical and radiation oncologists, oncologic surgeons, and reconstructive surgeons) and other individuals who may encounter these conditions in clinical practice.

Istanbul, Türkiye — Harzem Özger
Rochester, MN, USA — Franklin H. Sim
Mumbai, India — Ajay Puri
Istanbul, Türkiye — Levent Eralp

Contents

Part I

Overview of Current Applied Knowledge

1 The Classification of Soft Tissue Tumors: Historical Aspects and Recent Advances

Andrew L. Folpe

1.1 Introduction

Although attempts to categorize and classify soft tissue tumors date back to antiquity [1], Dr. Arthur Purdy Stout's 1953 Armed Forces Institute of Pathology (AFIP) fascicle on *Tumors of the Soft Tissues* is generally considered to represent the first widely accepted classification system in the "modern" era [2] (Table 1.1). As detailed in Table 1.1, Stout's system classified soft tissue tumors as either "benign" or "malignant," and then further subdivided these lesions based on their light microscopic appearance with hematoxylin and eosin staining. Thus, tumors having a predominantly fibrous appearance were classified as "fibromatoses" and "fibrosarcomas," tumors composed of fat as "lipomatoses" and "liposarcomas," and so forth. Although this classification includes lesions we no longer consider neoplastic (e.g., ganglion, xanthoma diabeticorum, fat necrosis) or of soft tissue origin (e.g., benign and malignant mesothelial and hematolymphoid tumors), the structure and principles of Stout's classification can still be recognized in more recent classification systems, including the first (1969) World Health Organization (WHO) Histologic Typing of Soft Tissue Tumors [3] (Table 1.2) and the most recent (2020) WHO Classification of Soft Tissue Tumors [4] (Table 1.3).

The 1969 WHO Histologic Typing of Soft Tissue Tumors, spearheaded by Dr. Franz Enzinger of the AFIP, represented the first multinational, consensus classification system for these rare tumors. The overall structure of the 1969 WHO classification was generally similar to Stout's, although increased emphasis was placed on "histogenesis" or "cell of origin," rather than simply microscopic appearance. Thus, tumors were divided first by tissue type (e.g., fibrous, fat, smooth muscle) and then into "benign," "borderline" and "malignant categories." For the first time, however, it was acknowledged that the histogenesis of some tumors might be difficult or even impossible to determine, with significant numbers of tumors classified as having "Disputed or Uncertain Histogenesis," including granular cell tumor (formerly known as "granular cell myoblastoma" and considered a tumor of muscle origin) and alveolar soft part sarcoma (formerly thought of as the malignant counterpart of "granular cell myoblastoma"). The creation of a "borderline" category of soft tissue tumors was another important conceptual advance, acknowledging for the first time that the biological behavior of a subset of mesenchymal neoplasms might not be easily labeled as simply "benign" or "malignant" (e.g., desmoid fibromatosis, dermatofibrosarcoma protuberans).

Despite these changes, it is likely that Dr. Stout would have felt quite comfortable with the 1969 WHO classification, recognizing it as an expansion and refinement of his own work, and fundamentally grounded in morphology. Whether Stout would have recognized our current (2020) WHO classification is much more open to question. As detailed in Table 1.3, our current classification system for soft tissue tumors has massively expanded, encompassing many entities unknown in Stout's era and employing new terminology for some established entities. Additionally, this classification includes many newer entities defined not by morphology alone, but by a synthesis of morphology, immunophenotype, and molecular genetic features (or even in some cases by genetics alone). Furthermore, Stout would likely have been surprised to find important entities of his time, such as fibrosarcoma and hemangiopericytoma, to have largely or completely vanished from our current diagnostic lexicon.

It is of course impossible to cover all the changes in the classification of soft tissue tumors that have taken place between 1953 and the present. This chapter will explore some of these changes, using former or current entities such as hemangiopericytoma, fibrosarcoma, liposarcoma, CD34-positive fibroblastic tumor, soft tissue angiofibroma, *EWSR1::PATZ1* sarcoma and *CIC*-rearranged sarcoma to illustrate the ways in which the classification of soft tissue tumors has evolved, and continues to evolve.

A. L. Folpe (✉)
Laboratory Medicine and Pathology, Mayo Clinic, Rochester, MN, USA
e-mail: folpe.andrew@mayo.edu

H. Özger et al. (eds.), *Diagnosis and Treatment of Soft Tissue Tumors*, https://doi.org/10.1007/978-3-031-77061-6_1

Table 1.1 Dr. Arthur Purdy Stout's classification of tumors of the soft tissues (1953) (modified from Reference [2])

Benign tumors and tumor-like proliferations	Category	Included entities
	Fibromatoses	Fibroma durum Fibroma molle Non-metastasizing fibrosarcomas Desmoid tumor Keloid Cicatricial fibromatosis Palmar and plantar fibromatosis Penile fibromatosis Fibromatosis colli Progressive myositis fibrosa Irradiation fibromatosis
	Myxomatoses	Ganglion Localized myxedema
	Xanthomatoses	Xanthoma diabeticorum Multiple xanthomatous giant cell tumors Xanthelasma Fibrous xanthoma Sclerosing hemangioma Xanthogranuloma Giant cell tumor Eosinophilic granuloma Histiocytoma Fat necrosis
	Lipomatoses	Lipoma Multiple lipomas Multiple symmetrical lipomatosis Lipoma dolorosa Lipoma arborescens Myelolipoma Myxolipoma Hibernoma
	Benign Tumors of Muscle	Leiomyoma Rhabdomyoma Granular cell myoblastoma
	Benign Angiomatoses	Capillary hemangioma Cavernous hemangioma Capillary hemangioma, granuloma-type Venous hemangioma Benign (infantile) hemangioendothelioma Benign hemangiopericytoma Glomus tumor Cirsoid aneurysm Venous racemose aneurysm Diffuse angiomatosis Lymphangioma
	Other Benign Tumors	Osteoma Osteochondroma Chondroma Myositis ossificans Benign synovioma Mixed tumor Benign mesenchymoma Benign mesothelioma of the genital tract Benign solitary fibroma mesothelioma Benign diffuse fibrous mesothelioma Blue nevus
Malignant tumors of the soft tissues	**Category**	**Included entities**
	Fibrosarcoma	Dermatofibrosarcoma protuberans of Hoffman Progressive and recurring dermatofibroma of Darier

(continued)

Table 1.1 (continued)

	Liposarcoma	Differentiated liposarcoma Undifferentiated liposarcoma
	Malignant tumors of muscle	Leiomyosarcoma Rhabdomyosarcoma Malignant granular cell myoblastoma
	Angiosarcomatoses	Malignant hemangioendothelioma Malignant hemangiopericytoma Kaposi's sarcoma Lymphangiosarcoma
	Malignant lymphoid and reticuloendothelial tumors	Lymphosarcoma Reticulum cell sarcoma Mycosis fungoides Plasma cell tumor
	Myxoid tumors	Myxoma
	Other malignant tumors	Osteogenic sarcoma Chondrosarcoma Synovial sarcoma Malignant mesenchymoma Malignant mesothelioma Melanosarcoma

Table 1.2 The 1969 World Health Organization histologic typing of soft tissue tumors (modified from Reference [3])

Tissue Type	Benign	Borderline	Malignant
Fibrous	"Fibroma durum" "Fibroma molle" (fibrolipoma) Dermatofibroma Elastofibroma	Fibromatoses • Intra- and extra-abdominal desmoid fibromatosis • Keloid • Palmar/plantar/penile/irradiation fibromatosis • Fibromatosis colli • Nasopharyngeal angiofibroma • Congenital generalized fibromatosis Dermatofibrosarcoma protuberans	Fibrosarcoma
Fat	Lipoma Intramuscular lipoma Hibernoma Renal angiomyolipoma Myelolipoma Lipoblastoma Diffuse lipomatosis		Liposarcoma • "Predominantly well-differentiated" • "Predominantly myxoid" • "Predominantly round-cell" • "Predominantly pleomorphic" • Mixed
Smooth muscle	Leiomyoma Angiomyoma Epithelioid leiomyoma/leiomyoblastoma		Leiomyosarcoma
Skeletal muscle	Rhabdomyoma		Rhabdomyosarcoma • "Predominantly embryonal" • "Predominantly alveolar" • "Predominantly pleomorphic" • Mixed
Blood vessels	"Benign hemangioendothelioma" Capillary hemangioma Cavernous hemangioma Venous hemangioma Intramuscular hemangioma "Systemic hemangiomatosis" "Hemangiomatosis with or without congenital arteriovenous fistula" Benign hemangiopericytoma Glomus tumor Angiomyoma Pyogenic granuloma		Malignant hemangioendothelioma (angiosarcoma) Malignant hemangiopericytoma

(continued)

Table 1.2 (continued)

Tissue Type	Benign	Borderline	Malignant
Lymph vessels	Lymphangioma Lymphangiomyoma Systemic lymphangiomatosis		Malignant lymphangioendothelioma (lymphangiosarcoma)
Synovial tissues	"Benign synovioma"		Synovial sarcoma ("malignant synovioma")
Peripheral nerve	Traumatic neuroma Neurofibroma Neurilemoma (schwannoma) Neurofibromatosis		Malignant schwannoma (neurofibrosarcoma) Peripheral primitive neuroectodermal tumor
Tumors of pluripotent mesenchyme	Mesenchymoma		Malignant Mesenchymoma
Tumors of vestigial embryonic structures	Chordoma		Malignant Chordoma
Tumors of disputed or uncertain histogenesis	Granular cell tumor Chondroma of soft parts Osteoma of soft parts Nasal glioma Pacinian tumor Adenomatoid tumor of genital tract Myxoma Melanotic progonoma (melanotic neuroectodermal tumor of infancy)		Alveolar soft part sarcoma Malignant granular cell tumor Chondrosarcoma of soft parts Osteosarcoma of soft parts Malignant giant cell tumor of soft parts Malignant fibroxanthoma (malignant fibrous histiocytoma) Kaposi's sarcoma Clear cell sarcoma of tendons and aponeuroses
Non-neoplastic or questionably neoplastic lesion of soft tissue	Nodular tenosynovitis (giant cell tumor of tendon sheath) Fibrous histiocytoma Atypical fibroxanthoma Xanthoma Juvenile xanthogranuloma Retroperitoneal xanthogranuloma		

Comment: For brevity, tumors derived from mesothelial tissues, sympathetic ganglia, paraganglionic structures, and extragonadal germ cells have been omitted from this modified table, as they are no longer classified as soft tissue tumors

Table 1.3 The 2020 World Health Organization classification of soft tissue tumors (reproduced with permission from reference [4])

Tissue type	Benign	Borderline/intermediate	Malignant
Adipocytic	Lipoma • Intramuscular lipoma • Chondrolipoma Lipomatosis • Diffuse lipomatosis • Multiple symmetrical lipomatosis • Pelvic lipomatosis • Steroid lipomatosis • HIV lipodystrophy Lipomatosis of nerve Lipoblastomatosis • Localized (lipoblastoma) • Diffuse Angiolipoma Myolipoma Chondroid lipoma Spindle cell lipoma Atypical spindle cell/pleomorphic lipomatous tumor Hibernoma	Atypical lipomatous tumor	Liposarcoma, well-differentiated • Lipoma-like • Inflammatory • Sclerosing Dedifferentiated liposarcoma Myxoid liposarcoma Pleomorphic liposarcoma Myxoid pleomorphic liposarcoma

(continued)

Table 1.3 (continued)

Tissue type	Benign	Borderline/intermediate	Malignant
Fibroblastic and myofibroblastic	Nodular fasciitis • Intravascular fasciitis • Cranial fasciitis Proliferative fasciitis Proliferative myositis Myositis ossificans Ischemic fasciitis Elastofibroma Fibrous hamartoma of infancy Fibromatosis colli Juvenile hyaline fibromatosis Fibroma of tendon sheath Desmoplastic fibroblastoma Myofibroblastoma Calcifying aponeurotic fibroma EWSR1::SMAD3-positive fibroblastic tumor Angiomyofibroblastoma Cellular angiofibroma Angiofibroma of soft tissue Nuchal fibroma Gardner fibroma Acral fibromyxoma	Locally aggressive • Palmar/plantar fibromatoses • Desmoid-type fibromatosis • Lipofibromatosis • Giant cell fibroblastoma Rarely metastasizing • Dermatofibrosarcoma protuberans • Fibrosarcomatous dermatofibrosarcoma protuberans • Solitary fibrous tumor • Inflammatory myofibroblastic tumor • Myofibroblastic sarcoma • Superficial CD34-positive fibroblastic tumor • Myxoinflammatory fibroblastic sarcoma • Infantine fibrosarcoma	Adult-type fibrosarcoma Myxofibrosarcoma Low-grade fibromyxoid sarcoma Sclerosing epithelioid fibrosarcoma
So-called fibrohistiocytic	Tenosynovial giant cell tumor Deep fibrous histiocytoma	Plexiform fibrohistiocytic tumor Giant cell tumor of soft parts	Malignant tenosynovial giant cell tumor
Vascular	Hemangioma Intramuscular hemangioma Arteriovenous hemangioma Venous hemangioma Epithelioid hemangioma Lymphangioma Cystic lymphangioma Acquired tufted angioma	Locally aggressive • Kaposiform hemangioendothelioma Rarely metastasizing • Retiform hemangioendothelioma • Composite hemangioendothelioma • Kaposi sarcoma • Pseudomyogenic hemangioendothelioma	Epithelioid hemangioendothelioma • With *WWTR1-CAMTA1* fusion. • With *YAP1-TFE3* fusion. Angiosarcoma
Pericytic (perivascular)	Glomus tumor Myopericytoma Angioleiomyoma		Malignant glomus tumor
Smooth muscle	Leiomyoma	Smooth muscle tumor of uncertain malignant potential	Leiomyosarcoma
Skeletal muscle	Rhabdomyoma • Fetal • Adult • Genital		Embryonal rhabdomyosarcoma Alveolar rhabdomyosarcoma Pleomorphic rhabdomyosarcoma Spindle cell rhabdomyosarcoma • Congenital with *VGLL2/NCOA2/CITED2* rearrangements • MYOD1-mutant spindle cell/sclerosing • Spindled and epithelioid with *TFCP2/NCOA2* rearrangements
Gastrointestinal stromal tumors	Low risk	Intermediate risk	High risk
Chondro-osseous	Chondroma		Extraskeletal osteosarcoma

(continued)

Table 1.3 (continued)

Tissue type	Benign	Borderline/intermediate	Malignant
Peripheral nerve	Schwannoma • Ancient • Cellular • Plexiform • Epithelioid • Microcystic/reticular Neurofibroma • Ancient • Cellular • Atypical • Plexiform Perineurioma • Reticular • Sclerosing Granular cell tumor Nerve sheath myxoma Solitary circumscribed neuroma Meningioma Neuromuscular choristoma Hybrid nerve sheath tumor		Malignant peripheral nerve sheath tumor Melanotic malignant peripheral nerve sheath tumor Malignant granular cell tumor Malignant perineurioma
Uncertain differentiation	Myxoma Aggressive angiomyxoma Pleomorphic hyalinizing angiectatic tumor Phosphaturic mesenchymal tumor Perivascular epithelioid cell tumor Angiomyolipoma	Locally aggressive • Hemosiderotic fibrolipomatous tumor • Epithelioid angiomyolipoma Rarely metastasizing • Atypical fibroxanthoma • Angiomatoid fibrous histiocytoma • Ossifying fibromyxoid tumor • Mixed tumor/myoepithelioma	Malignant phosphaturic mesenchymal tumor NTRK-rearranged spindle cell neoplasm Synovial sarcoma Epithelioid sarcoma Alveolar soft part sarcoma Clear cell sarcoma Extraskeletal myxoid chondrosarcoma Desmoplastic small round cell tumor Rhabdoid tumor Malignant perivascular epithelioid cell tumor Intimal sarcoma Malignant ossifying fibromyxoid tumor Myoepithelial carcinoma Undifferentiated spindle cell and pleomorphic sarcoma Undifferentiated round cell sarcoma Ewing sarcoma Round cell sarcoma with *EWSR1*-non-ETS fusions *CIC*-rearranged sarcoma Sarcomas with *BCOR* genetic alterations

1.2 Hemangiopericytoma: An Entity Vanishes

In 1942, Dr. Stout and Dr. Margaret Murray coined the term "hemangiopericytoma" to describe a small group of soft tissue tumors [5], thought to be derived from cells closely resembling the capillary pericytes described by Zimmermann in the German literature in 1923. Although Stout and Murray recognized hemangiopericytomas as distinct from glomus tumors, it is likely that most of the cases in this study would now be regarded as falling in the spectrum of myofibroma. A subsequent, larger series of "hemangiopericytomas," published by Stout alone in 1949, chiefly focused on tumors we would now label as solitary fibrous tumors, noting for the first time meningeal involvement, locally aggressive growth and metastases [6]. An additional series, published by Stout in 1956, further distinguished hemangiopericytoma from glomus tumors [7].

In 1976, Enzinger and Smith published a series of 106 hemangiopericytomas, keeping Stout's name, but signifi-

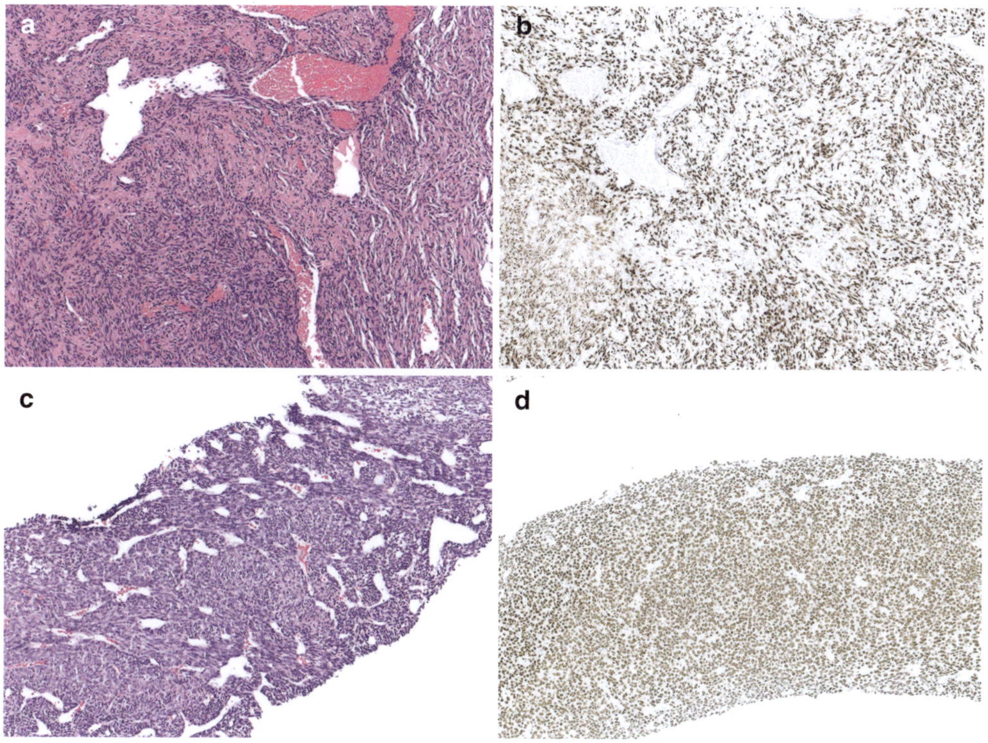

Fig. 1.1 (**a**) Most tumors previously classified as "hemangiopericytoma" are now regarded as examples of solitary fibrous tumor. Note the branching, "staghorn" vascular pattern thought at one time to be specific for "hemangiopericytoma." (**b**) STAT6 expression in solitary fibrous tumor, confirming the underlying *NAB2::STAT6* fusion specific to this entity. (**c**) Poorly differentiated synovial sarcoma, a well-known mimic of "malignant hemangiopericytoma." Numerous branching blood vessels are prominent. (**d**) Nuclear expression of SS18-SSX fusion protein in poorly differentiated synovial sarcoma

cantly modifying its morphologic definition to that of a tumor characterized by the presence of branching, "staghorn" vessels, often with perivascular hyalinization and abundant interstitial collagen, surrounded by small round to slightly spindled cells, and displaying no obvious light microscopic features of differentiation [8]. Furthermore, it was emphasized that it was a diagnosis of exclusion, to be rigorously distinguished from other tumors that might show a prominent branching vascular pattern, in particular high-grade synovial sarcomas. Enzinger and Smith also attempted, for the first time to define criteria that might distinguish clinically benign from clinically malignant hemangiopericytomas.

Over the next two decades, hemangiopericytoma became an increasingly controversial entity, as reproducibility was often poor for this "diagnosis of exclusion," true microvascular pericytic differentiation could not be shown by electron microscopy, and expression of pericyte-associate markers, such as actins, was absent by immunohistochemistry [9]. Increasing discomfort with the term "hemangiopericytoma" coincided with the recognition that tumors identical to solitary fibrous tumor of the pleura might also occur in the soft tissues [10], and it has subsequently become clear that the morphologic and immunohistochemical features of hemangiopericytoma and solitary fibrous tumor are essentially identical, with classical hemangiopericytoma representing a more cellular and less heavily collagenized variant. It is now known that identical *NAB2::STAT6* fusions and nuclear STAT6 expression are present in tumors classified as hemangiopericytoma and solitary fibrous tumor in all anatomic locations, including the meninges [11] (Figs. 1.1a, b). Thus, the term "hemangiopericytoma" is not part of the most recent WHO classification. In addition to solitary fibrous tumor, lesions previously classified as hemangiopericytoma are now considered to represent glomus tumor, myopericytomas, myofibromas, phosphaturic mesenchymal tumors, and poorly differentiated synovial sarcomas (Figs. 1.1c, d), among others [4].

1.3 Fibrosarcoma: A Single Entity Transforms into Multiple Entities

Whereas our abandonment of the term "hemangiopericytoma" represents chiefly "name changing" (owing to the recognition that these lesions were unrelated to true pericytes), the marked decrease in the diagnosis of "fibrosarcoma" since Stout's time is an outstanding example of how careful morphologic, immunohistochemical, and genetic study has resulted in important changes in our understanding and classification of soft tissue tumors.

At one time, fibrosarcoma was by far the most common adult soft tissue sarcoma, accounting for roughly two-thirds of all sarcomas seen at Mayo Clinic between 1910 and 1930 [12]. This view was challenged in 1948 by Stout, who emphasized that fibrosarcoma was a diagnosis of exclusion, to be distinguished from variants of liposarcoma, rhabdomyosarcoma, synovial sarcoma, malignant peripheral nerve sheath tumor, and desmoid fibromatosis [13]. The profound impact of this work is clearly illustrated in three subsequent Mayo Clinic series of fibrosarcoma. First, a retrospective review of 330 tumors diagnosed as "fibrosarcoma" between 1910 and 1968 showed over 33% to represent something else, with fibrosarcoma accounting for only 12% of soft tissue sarcomas seen during this time period [14]. A 1989 study from the same institution also reclassified the majority of putative fibrosarcomas as representing other entities [15], and a 2010 series of 163 "fibrosarcomas" from Mayo Clinic demonstrated over 80% to represent something else, when studied with modern immunohistochemical and molecular genetic tools [12]. It should come as no surprise then that the incidence of fibrosarcoma has declined dramatically over the past seven decades, with 2006 SEER data, for example, showing it to account for only 3.6% of soft tissue sarcomas [16]. Strictly defined fibrosarcomas likely account for <1% of adult soft tissue sarcomas [12].

What factors led to the striking decline in the relative incidence of fibrosarcoma? One, of course, was the reclassification during the 1970s and 1980s of many apparently undifferentiated sarcomas as "malignant fibrous histiocytoma" [17], and then the subsequent recognition that "malignant fibrous histiocytoma" itself represented a potpourri of poorly differentiated mesenchymal and nonmesenchymal tumors, rather than a discrete entity [18]. Equally important was the eventual recognition that desmoid fibromatosis, thought at one time to represent a form of fibrosarcoma, represent instead a genetically distinct, locally aggressive (but sometimes spontaneously regressing) fibroblastic tumor [19]. Furthermore, with the widespread use of immunohistochemical and molecular genetic testing, it has become apparent that many putative "fibrosarcomas" represent instead other tumor types, including monophasic synovial sarcoma, malignant solitary fibrous tumors, malignant peripheral nerve sheath tumor, spindle cell variants of rhabdomyosarcoma, angiosarcoma, epithelioid sarcoma, sarcomatoid carcinoma and melanoma.

It is also now understood that malignant fibroblastic neoplasms represent a variety of different entities, rather than simply "fibrosarcoma", and that these distinctions are important. A partial list of tumor types previously classified generically as "fibrosarcoma" encompasses several entities likely familiar to clinicians, including fibrosarcomatous dermatofibrosarcoma protuberans [20, 21], low-grade fibromyxoid sarcoma [22–24] (Fig. 1.2a), sclerosing epithelioid fibrosarcoma [25, 26], and myxofibrosarcoma [27–29] (Fig. 1.2b), as well as more recently described lesions such as *KMT2A* [30, 31] and *PRRX1/2*-rearranged fibroblastic tumors [32].

These new subcategories of fibrosarcoma are clinically and genetically distinctive, and not simply examples of "splitting for the sake of splitting". For example, fibrosarcomatous dermatofibrosarcoma protuberans are fusion-driven sarcomas harboring *COL1A1::PDGFB* fusions, and inhibition of PDGFB with tyrosine kinase inhibitors such as imatinib mesylate is increasingly important in the treatment of patients with unresectable or metastatic tumors of this type [33, 34]. Low-grade fibromyxoid sarcoma, a morphologically distinctive tumor characterized by *FUS/EWSR1::CREB3L2/CREB3L1* fusions, is characterized clinically by a distinct propensity for late metastases, warranting essentially indefinite clinical follow-up for the often-young patients with this disease [22, 24, 35]. Myxofibrosarcoma, usually a subcutaneous tumor in the extremity of older adults, grows in a strikingly infiltrative fashion often resulting in significant underestimation of tumor size, positive surgical margins and a high rate of local recurrence [36].

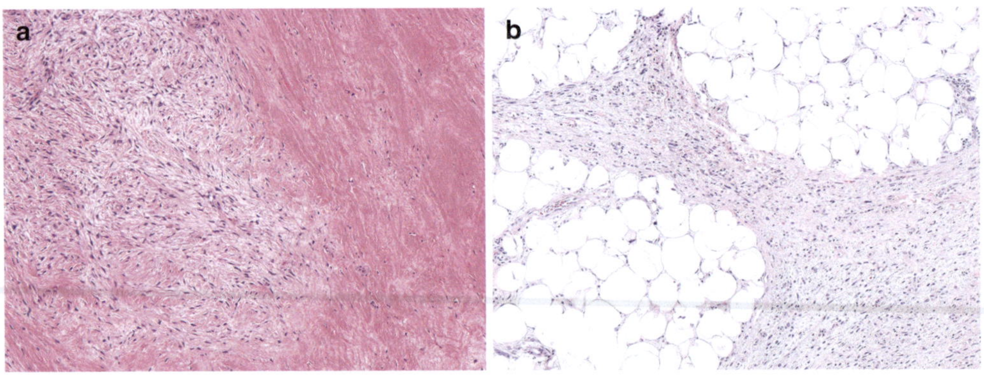

Fig. 1.2 (**a**) Low-grade fibromyxoid sarcoma, shown here, is a deceptively bland fibroblastic sarcoma with a propensity for very late metastases. (**b**) Despite similar names, myxofibrosarcoma (shown here) quite different from low-grade fibromyxoid sarcoma, usually occurring in the extremities of older patients, and having a very high risk for local recurrence

1.4 Liposarcoma: The Impact of Advances in Molecular Pathology on Classification

Liposarcomas represent the most common soft tissue sarcoma subtype [36]. Historically, the classification of liposarcomas, like all other types of soft tissue tumors, was based purely on morphology and was highly subjective. In 1944, Dr. Arthur Purdy Stout published the first well-known classification of liposarcomas, separating these tumors into (1) well-differentiated myxoid type, (2) poorly differentiated myxoid type, (3) round cell or adenoid type, and (4) mixed type [37]. This system was not widely accepted, however, with Stout himself classifying these tumors simply as "differentiated liposarcomas" and "undifferentiated liposarcomas" in his 1953 Armed Forces Institute of Pathology (AFIP) fascicle on Tumors of the Soft Tissues [2].

Our current classification of liposarcoma began to take shape in the early 1960s, with the publication of Enzinger and Winslow's landmark 1963 study, dividing liposarcomas into well-differentiated, myxoid, pleomorphic, and round cell types [38]. This was further refined by Evans, who recognized dedifferentiated liposarcoma, emphasized the kinship of myxoid and round cell liposarcoma, and proposed the classification of liposarcoma into well-differentiated, dedifferentiated, myxoid, round cell, pleomorphic, and mixed types [39]. This classification was embraced in Lattes' 1983 AFIP soft tissue fascicle [40] but was not universally accepted, with one then-contemporary textbook on soft tissue tumors sorting liposarcomas into well-differentiated, myxoid, lipoblastic, fibroblastic, and pleomorphic subtypes [1]. In the fourth edition of the WHO soft tissue and bone tumor classification, liposarcomas were subclassified as (1) atypical lipomatous tumor/ well-differentiated liposarcoma, (2) dedifferentiated liposarcoma, (3) myxoid liposarcoma (including round cell liposarcoma), (4) pleomorphic liposarcoma, and (5) mixed-type liposarcoma [41]. This classification has been modified in the fifth edition with the removal of "mixed-type liposarcoma," and the addition of a new liposarcoma subtype, myxoid pleomorphic liposarcoma [4]. It is important to appreciate that "atypical lipomatous tumor" is a synonym for "well-differentiated liposarcoma," used for identical tumors in the accessible soft tissues of the trunk and extremities. These different terms reflect the absent metastatic potential of this tumor in any location, and the much higher risk for local recurrence and progression to high-grade, dedifferentiated liposarcoma in locations such as the retroperitoneum, paratestis, and mediastinum [39, 42].

The current classification of liposarcoma reflects the numerous advances in our understanding of the molecular pathogenesis of adipocytic tumors made over the past 40 years. It is now understood that amplification of genes found on the long arm of chromosome 12, in particular *MDM2* and *CDK4*, underlie the pathogenesis of both well-differentiated and dedifferentiated liposarcoma [43], with additional genetic alterations driving progression towards dedifferentiated liposarcoma [44–46]. Similarly, identification of *MDM2* amplification in tumors previously classified as mixed-type liposarcoma with well-differentiated and pleomorphic liposarcoma-like components has shown them to represent instead unusual morphologic variants of dedifferentiated liposarcoma, containing pleomorphic lipoblasts ("homologous lipoblastic differentiation" [47, 48].

Similar advances have similarly improved our understanding and classification of myxoid liposarcoma (Fig. 1.3a). Although it was obvious on morphologic grounds alone that myxoid liposarcoma and its high-grade variant ("round cell liposarcoma") were closely related, identification of recurrent fusion events involving the *FUS* or less often *EWSR1* genes with the *DDIT3* gene confirmed these observations and gave us new tools for the study of these tumors [49–51]. For example, it is now understood that so-called "multifocal myxoid liposarcomas" represented instead metastatic disease involving soft tissue, bone, and pleura/

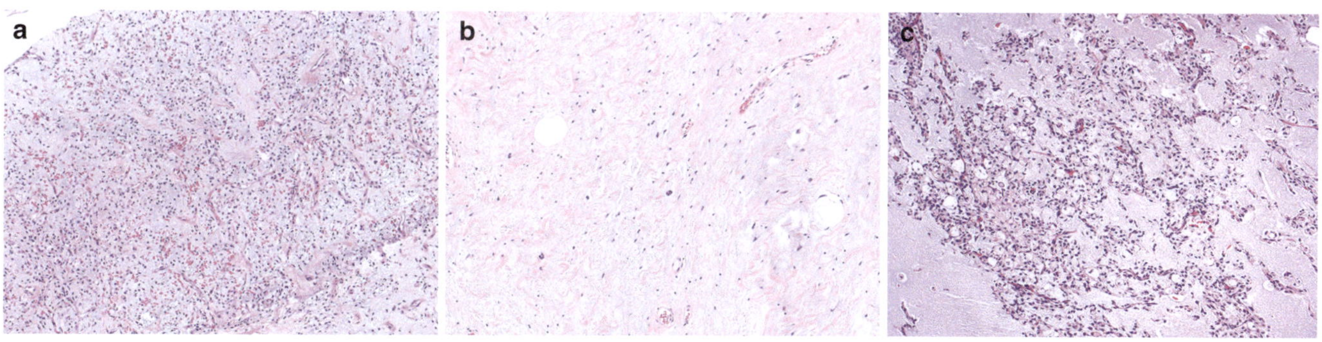

Fig. 1.3 (**a**) Conventional myxoid liposarcoma, of the type defined by *FUS/EWSR1::DDIT3* fusion. (**b**) Well-differentiated liposarcoma with myxoid change may be mistaken for true myxoid liposarcoma or for so-called "mixed-type" liposarcoma. Note the large, hyperchromatic cells, not seen in true myxoid liposarcoma. This tumor harbors *MDM2* amplification. (**c**) Myxoid pleomorphic liposarcoma is a highly aggressive form of liposarcoma which often occurs in children and in the mediastinum. These tumors are characterized genetically by massive loss of heterozygosity

peritoneum [52], and that myxoid liposarcomas essentially never occur in the retroperitoneum, representing instead metastases from extremity tumors [53]. It is also now clear that "mixed-type" liposarcomas of myxoid and well-differentiated type represent instead well-differentiated liposarcoma with extensive stromal myxoid change [51] (Fig. 1.3b).

Molecular genetics have had the least impact on the diagnosis and classification of pleomorphic liposarcoma, a tumor known to show changes similar to other pleomorphic sarcomas, with multiple non-specific chromosomal gains and losses [49, 50, 54, 55]. A small cell variant of pleomorphic liposarcoma may, however, be distinguished from high-grade myxoid liposarcoma, as it lacks the *FUS/EWSR::DDIT3* fusions seen in the latter entity [56]. Myxoid pleomorphic liposarcoma, the most recently described member of the liposarcoma family [57, 58], is characterized by widespread loss of heterozygosity and highly aggressive clinical behavior, clearly distinguishing it from conventional pleomorphic and myxoid liposarcomas [59] (Fig. 1.3c).

1.5 Superficial CD34-Positive Fibroblastic Tumor and Angiofibroma of Soft Tissue: New Morphologically Defined Entities Subsequently Shown to Harbor Characteristic Molecular Genetic Events

Although genetic study is increasingly important in the classification of soft tissue tumors, a considerable number of newly recognized entities were initially recognized by traditional morphologic study alone, and subsequently found to have characteristic genetic events [60, 61]. Two examples of this phenomenon are "superficial CD34-positive fibroblastic tumor" [62] and "angiofibroma of soft tissue" [63].

Superficial CD34-positive fibroblastic tumor was historically classified as "malignant fibrous histiocytoma"/"undifferentiated pleomorphic sarcoma," because of its striking nuclear pleomorphism, high cellularity, and absence of an apparent line of differentiation. However, in 2014 Carter and colleagues recognized the distinctive morphologic features of this rare tumor (abundant, eosinophilic, granular to "glassy" cytoplasm, marked nuclear pleomorphism, often in the form of elongated, multilobated nuclei, strikingly low mitotic activity, and diffuse CD34 expression, often in combination with more limited keratin immunoreactivity), as well as its indolent, very infrequently metastasizing clinical behavior [62] (Figs. 1.4a, b). Although there was initially some skepticism as to whether this truly represented a distinct entity, subsequent larger clinicopathologic series have confirmed these original observations [64], and superficial CD34-positive fibroblastic tumor is now classified by the WHO as a fibroblastic neoplasm of borderline malignancy [4]. Molecular genetic studies have shown most but not all cases to harbor rearrangements of the *PRDM10* gene, with downstream upregulation of CADM3 protein expression [64–68].

Angiofibroma of soft tissue is a recently described, benign soft tissue tumor, first reported by Marino-Enriquez and Fletcher in 2012 [63]. These cytologically bland fibroblastic neoplasms are most notable for their highly elaborate vasculature, somewhat resembling that seen in solitary fibrous tumors and myxoid liposarcoma, and they were likely previously misclassified as examples of "fibroma," "CD34-negative solitary fibrous tumor," "hemangiopericytoma," or "myxoma" (Fig. 1.5). They present as well-circumscribed, slowly growing, painless masses, often in the peri-articular soft tissues of the lower extremity. A subsequent molecular genetic study has confirmed that angiofibroma of soft tissue represents a discrete, new entity, characterized by the balanced translocation t(5;8), creating an *AHRR-NCOA2* fusion gene [69]. Variant *GTF2I-NCOA2* and *GAB1-ABL1* fusions may also rarely be found [70, 71].

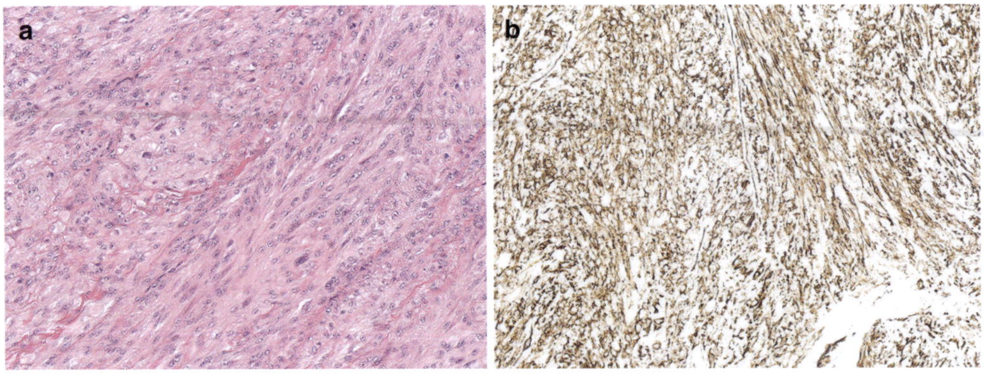

Fig. 1.4 (**a**) Superficial CD34-positive fibroblastic tumor is a recently described entity, previously misclassified as "malignant fibrous histiocytoma." Note the abundant, granular or glassy cytoplasm, the nuclear atypia, and the absence of mitotic figures. (**b**) Diffuse CD34 expression characterizes these rare, indolent neoplasms

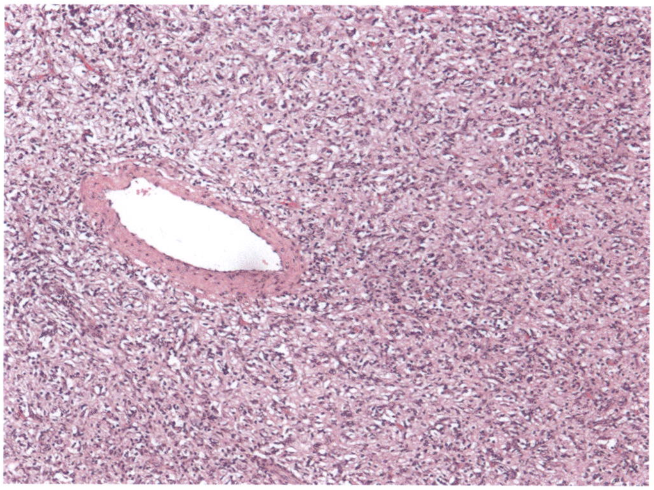

Fig. 1.5 Angiofibroma of soft tissue, another new entity, showing bland fibroblastic spindled cells and an elaborate capillary vasculature ("myxoid liposarcoma-like")

1.6 EWSR1::PATZ1 Sarcoma and CIC-Rearranged Sarcoma: New Entities Defined Chiefly by Molecular Genetics

Although traditional morphologic study with clinical correlation is still critical in the evolving classification of soft tissue tumors, the last decade has also seen the emergence of a new "class" of soft tissue tumors, fundamentally defined by their underlying molecular genetic events, rather than their morphologic features. Perhaps the best examples of this phenomenon are the new entities emerging from what was previously known as the "Ewing-like" family of primitive round-cell sarcomas [72].

Conventional Ewing sarcomas are characterized in the great majority of cases by fusions between the *EWSR1* gene and members of the ETS family of transcription factors, most often *FLI1* or *ERG* [73]. Indeed, round cell sarcomas harboring fusions between the *EWSR1* gene and genes other than ETS family members, (*EWSR1*-non-ETS) are not mentioned in the 2002 WHO classification of soft tissue and bone tumors. However, in the 2013 WHO classification, a new "umbrella" category of "Undifferentiated/Unclassified Sarcomas" was added, with subcategories including undifferentiated round cell sarcoma, undifferentiated spindle cell sarcoma, undifferentiated pleomorphic sarcoma, undifferentiated epithelioid sarcoma, and undifferentiated sarcoma, not otherwise specified [74]. Tumors grouped under the undifferentiated round or spindle cell sarcoma categories included those with *EWSR1*-non-ETS fusions (e.g., *EWSR1::PATZ1*, *EWSR1::POU5F1*, *EWSR1::NFATC2*), as well lesions harboring fusions involving the *CIC* or *BCOR* genes. Progress in the classification of these rare round cell tumors continued in the most recent WHO classification, with *CIC*-rearranged sarcomas and *BCOR*-altered sarcomas defined for the first time as discrete entities, and the *EWSR1*-non-ETS family of round cell sarcomas identified as another emerging group [4].

Sarcomas harboring fusion of *EWSR1* with the non-ETS gene *PATZ1* were first noted to form a potential entity in 2018 by Watson and co-workers, who found tumors harboring this fusion to cluster together by gene expression profiling, and apart from other *EWSR1*-rearranged sarcomas [75]. There have subsequently been several small series of these very rare tumors, and although they show some clinical, morphological and immunohistochemical variability, there appear to be enough common features such that they may be confidently regarded as representing a discrete entity [76–80]. These tumors have an equal sex distribution and may involve patients of any age. The trunk and abdomen are the most common sites of involvement.

Although *EWSR1::PATZ1* sarcomas were recognized genetically, rather than morphologically, they display relatively consistent morphologic features, including vaguely lobular growth, hyalinized to myxoid matrix, microcystic change, thick collagenous bands, prominent vasculature, and generally bland round to slightly spindled cells, with low mitotic activity [61] (Figs. 1.6a, b). Immunohistochemically, *EWSR1::PATZ1* sarcomas often express skeletal muscle markers, such as desmin and MyoD1, and are typically glial fibrillary acidic protein-positive. These tumors behave aggressively, with >50% of reported patients either presenting with metastatic disease or subsequently developing metastases; metastatic locations include the lung, pleura, pericardium, soft tissues, and lymph nodes.

CIC-rearranged sarcomas are the most frequent and best characterized subgroup of the Ewing-like round cell sarcomas. Fusions of the *CIC* gene with the *DUX4* gene are most common, with variant fusions involving *FOXO4, LEUTX, NUTM1*, and *NUTM2A* occurring in a small minority of cases [81, 82]. These sarcomas were first reported in 2006 by Kawamura-Saito and co-workers [83].

Again, as with *EWSR1::PATZ1* sarcomas, the morphologic and immunohistochemical features of *CIC*-rearranged sarcomas are sufficiently consistent such that they can be recognized as a discrete entity. Morphologically, *CIC*-rearranged sarcomas appear as moderately variable round-cell sarcomas, frequently with rhabdoid cells and prominent nucleoli. Stromal myxoid change is common and is a useful clue to diagnosis [81, 82] (Figs. 1.7a, b). By immunohistochemistry, these lesions typically express CD99, although in a less diffuse manner than does Ewing sarcoma, show strong nuclear WT1 expression, and are ETV4-positive [84].

CIC-rearranged sarcomas most often occur in older children and young adults and typically involve the deep soft tissue of the trunk, limbs, or head and neck region. Rare tumors may involve viscera or bone. The prognosis for CIC-

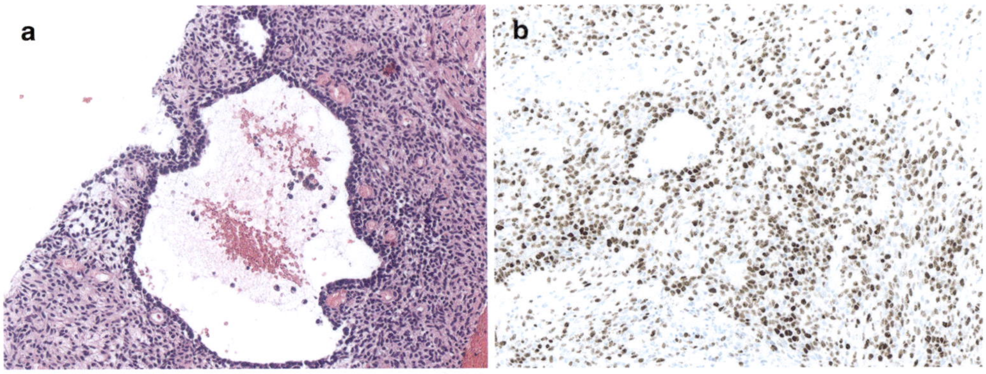

Fig. 1.6 (**a**) Sarcomas defined by *EWSR1::PATZ1* fusion display characteristic morphologic features, including formation of microcystic spaces, and represent a novel, molecularly-defined entity. (**b**) MYOD1 expression in *EWSR1::PATZ1* sarcoma

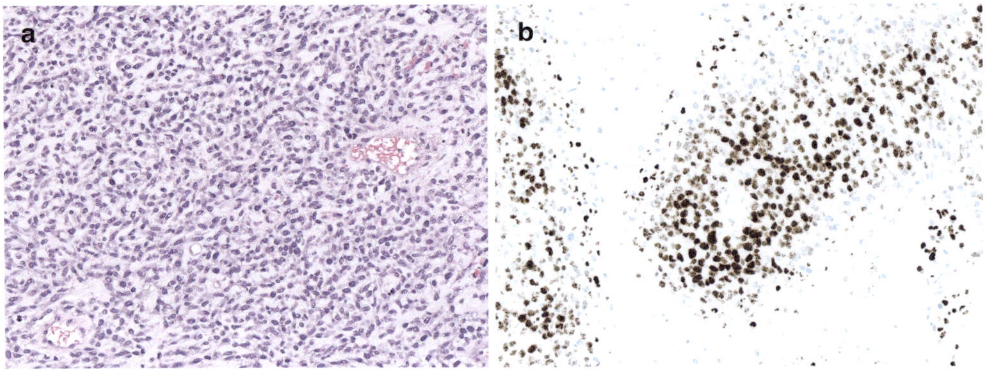

Fig. 1.7 (**a**) *CIC*-rearranged sarcoma, consisting of primitive round to spindled cells in a variably myxoid background. (**b**) Strong nuclear expression of WT1 is commonly seen in *CIC*-rearranged sarcomas and helps to distinguish them from other "Ewing-like" round cell sarcomas

rearranged sarcomas is poor, with frequent lung metastases at presentation and a 5-year overall survival of roughly 50% [81, 82]. They do not seem to respond well to standard Ewing sarcoma chemotherapeutic protocols [85].

1.7 Future Directions: Will Soft Tissue Tumors Be Classified Solely on a Genetic Basis?

Although new morphologically defined soft tissue entities, such as perinephric myxoid pseudotumor of fat [86] and pseudoendocrine sarcoma [87] continue to be described, it is likely fair to state that the "glory years" of morphology-driven classification are behind us. This raises the obvious question of whether molecular genetics alone will someday serve as the basis for the classification of soft tissue tumors. The answer to this question is almost certainly "no." With the widespread use of next-generation sequencing techniques, it has become increasingly clear that identical molecular genetic events may occur in clinically and wholly dissimilar entities, the best example of which is the ever-enlarging family of tumors harboring fusion involving the *EWSR1* or *FUS* genes with the *ATF1* or *CREB1* genes. *EWSR1/FUS::ATF1/CREB1* fusions were first identified in clear cell sarcoma of soft parts, a relatively indolent malignant neoplasm showing melanocytic differentiation [88]. Not long afterward, identical fusion events were found in angiomatoid fibrous histiocytoma, a non-melanocytic mesenchymal tumor of borderline malignancy that most often occurs in children [89] (Fig. 1.8a). It is now known that *EWSR1/FUS::ATF1/CREB1* fusions may also be seen in a highly aggressive sarcoma of the gastrointestinal tract (and less often somatic soft tissue), malignant gastrointestinal neuroectodermal tumor [90, 91] (Fig. 1.8b), clear cell carcinomas of salivary origin [92], and unusual myxoid neoplasms of the lung and central nervous system [93, 94]. Similarly, *EWSR1::WT1* fusions, once thought to be specific to desmoplastic small round cell tumors [95], are now known to also occur in low-grade spindle cell tumors of the gynecologic tract [96].

It seems increasingly likely that most other molecular genetic events will be found to lack specificity for a single entity. Thus, the correct classification of soft tissue tumors will increasingly depend on the careful integration of clinical, morphologic and molecular genetic findings, rather than on any one of these factors alone. This is especially true as high-throughput molecular genetic techniques identify an ever-enlarging number of fusion events and mutations, the significance of which can only be apparent with long-term clinical follow-up. However, there can be little doubt that the classification of soft tissue tumors will continue to evolve, hopefully allowing us to treat patients with these rare diseases more rationally and effectively.

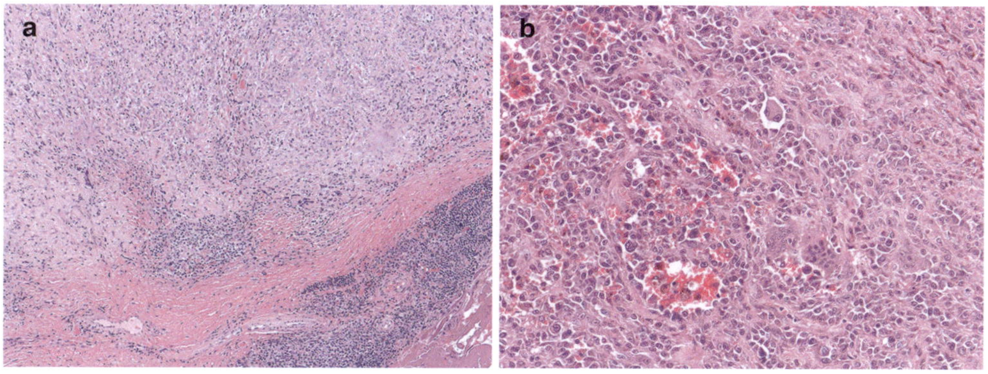

Fig. 1.8 (**a**) Angiomatoid fibrous histiocytoma, a mesenchymal tumor of borderline malignancy, harbors *EWSR1/FUS::ATF1/CREB1* gene fusions. (**b**) Identical gene fusions are seen in a wholly dissimilar, highly malignant tumor of the gastrointestinal tract and soft tissue, malignant gastrointestinal neuroectodermal tumor. Several other tumors also share this fusion event, emphasizing the need to integrate clinical, morphologic, immunohistochemical and molecular genetic findings in the classification of soft tissue tumors

References

1. Hajdu SI. Pathology of soft tissue tumors, vol. xi. Philadelphia: Lea & Febiger; 1979. p. 599.
2. Stout AP. Tumors of the soft tissues. Washington, DC: American Registry of Pathology; 1953.
3. Enzinger FM. Histological typing of soft tissue tumours. Geneva, Switzerland: World Health Organization; 1969.
4. Board TWCoTE, editor. Soft tissue and bone tumours. 5th ed. Lyon, France: International Agency for Research on Cancer; 2020.
5. Stout AP, Murray MR. Hemangiopericytoma: a vascular tumor featuring Zimmermann's Pericytes. Ann Surg. 1942;116(1):26–33.
6. Stout AP. Hemangiopericytoma; a study of 25 cases. Cancer. 1949;2(6):1027–54. illust
7. Stout AP. Tumors featuring pericytes; glomus tumor and hemangiopericytoma. Lab Investig. 1956;5(2):217–23.
8. Enzinger FM, Smith BH. Hemangiopericytoma. An analysis of 106 cases. Hum Pathol. 1976;7(1):61–82.
9. Folpe AL. "Hey! Whatever happened to hemangiopericytoma and fibrosarcoma?" An update on selected conceptual advances in soft tissue pathology which have occurred over the past 50 years. Hum Pathol. 2020;95:113–36.
10. Suster S, Nascimento AG, Miettinen M, Sickel JZ, Moran CA. Solitary fibrous tumors of soft tissue. A clinicopathologic and immunohistochemical study of 12 cases. Am J Surg Pathol. 1995;19(11):1257–66.
11. Armstrong SM, Demicco EG. What's new in fibroblastic tumors? Virchows Arch. 2020;476(1):41–55.
12. Bahrami A, Folpe AL. Adult-type fibrosarcoma: a reevaluation of 163 putative cases diagnosed at a single institution over a 48-year period. Am J Surg Pathol. 2010;34(10):1504–13.
13. Stout AP. Fibrosarcoma the malignant tumor of fibroblasts. Cancer. 1948;1(1):30–63.
14. Pritchard DJ, Soule EH, Taylor WF, Ivins JC. Fibrosarcoma—a clinicopathologic and statistical study of 199 tumors of the soft tissues of the extremities and trunk. Cancer. 1974;33(3):888–97.
15. Scott SM, Reiman HM, Pritchard DJ, Ilstrup DM. Soft tissue fibrosarcoma. A clinicopathologic study of 132 cases. Cancer. 1989;64(4):925–31.
16. Ng VY, Scharschmidt TJ, Mayerson JL, Fisher JL. Incidence and survival in sarcoma in the United States: a focus on musculoskeletal lesions. Anticancer Res. 2013;33(6):2597–604.
17. Weiss SW, Enzinger FM. Malignant fibrous histiocytoma: an analysis of 200 cases. Cancer. 1978;41(6):2250–66.
18. Fletcher CD. Pleomorphic malignant fibrous histiocytoma: fact or fiction? A critical reappraisal based on 159 tumors diagnosed as pleomorphic sarcoma. Am J Surg Pathol. 1992;16(3):213–28.
19. Folpe AL. Fibrosarcoma: a review and update. Histopathology. 2014;64(1):12–25.
20. Goldblum JR, Reith JD, Weiss SW. Sarcomas arising in dermatofibrosarcoma protuberans: a reappraisal of biologic behavior in eighteen cases treated by wide local excision with extended clinical follow up. Am J Surg Pathol. 2000;24(8):1125–30.
21. Swaby MG, Evans HL, Fletcher CD, Prieto VG, Patel KU, Lev DC, et al. Dermatofibrosarcoma protuberans with unusual sarcomatous transformation: a series of 4 cases with molecular confirmation. Am J Dermatopathol. 2011;33(4):354–60.
22. Evans HL. Low-grade fibromyxoid sarcoma: a clinicopathologic study of 33 cases with long-term follow-up. Am J Surg Pathol. 2011;35(10):1450–62.
23. Evans HL. Low-grade fibromyxoid sarcoma. A report of 12 cases. Am J Surg Pathol. 1993;17(6):595–600.
24. Guillou L, Benhattar J, Gengler C, Gallagher G, Ranchere-Vince D, Collin F, et al. Translocation-positive low-grade fibromyxoid sarcoma: clinicopathologic and molecular analysis of a series expanding the morphologic spectrum and suggesting potential relationship to sclerosing epithelioid fibrosarcoma: a study from the French Sarcoma Group. Am J Surg Pathol. 2007;31(9):1387–402.
25. Antonescu CR, Rosenblum MK, Pereira P, Nascimento AG, Woodruff JM. Sclerosing epithelioid fibrosarcoma: a study of 16 cases and confirmation of a clinicopathologically distinct tumor. Am J Surg Pathol. 2001;25(6):699–709.
26. Warmke LM, Meis JM. Sclerosing epithelioid fibrosarcoma: a distinct sarcoma with aggressive features. Am J Surg Pathol. 2021;45(3):317–28.
27. Mentzel T, Calonje E, Wadden C, Camplejohn RS, Beham A, Smith MA, et al. Myxofibrosarcoma. Clinicopathologic analysis of 75 cases with emphasis on the low-grade variant. Am J Surg Pathol. 1996;20(4):391–405.
28. Merck C, Angervall L, Kindblom LG, Oden A. Myxofibrosarcoma. A malignant soft tissue tumor of fibroblastic-histiocytic origin. A clinicopathologic and prognostic study of 110 cases using multivariate analysis. Acta Pathol Microbiol Immunol Scand Suppl. 1983;282:1–40.
29. Kindblom LG, Merck C, Svendsen P. Myxofibrosarcoma: a pathologico-anatomical, microangiographic and angiographic correlative study of eight cases. Br J Radiol. 1977;50(600):876–87.
30. Kao YC, Lee JC, Zhang L, Sung YS, Swanson D, Hsieh TH, et al. Recurrent YAP1 and KMT2A gene rearrangements in a subset of

MUC4-negative sclerosing epithelioid fibrosarcoma. Am J Surg Pathol. 2020;44(3):368–77.
31. Massoth LR, Hung YP, Nardi V, Nielsen GP, Hasserjian RP, Louissaint A Jr, et al. Pan-sarcoma genomic analysis of KMT2A rearrangements reveals distinct subtypes defined by YAP1-KMT2A-YAP1 and VIM-KMT2A fusions. Mod Pathol. 2020;33(11):2307–17.
32. Dermawan JK, Azzato EM, Jebastin Thangaiah J, Gjorgova-Gjeorgievski S, Rubin BP, Folpe AL, et al. PRRX1-NCOA1-rearranged fibroblastic tumour: a clinicopathological, immunohistochemical and molecular genetic study of six cases of a potentially under-recognised, distinctive mesenchymal tumour. Histopathology. 2021;79(6):997–1003.
33. Lim SX, Ramaiya A, Levell NJ, Venables ZC. Review of dermatofibrosarcoma protuberans. Clin Exp Dermatol. 2023;48(4):297–302.
34. Beaziz J, Battistella M, Delyon J, Farges C, Marco O, Pages C, et al. Long-term outcome of neoadjuvant tyrosine kinase inhibitors followed by complete surgery in locally advanced dermatofibrosarcoma protuberans. Cancers (Basel). 2021;13:9.
35. Mertens F, Fletcher CD, Antonescu CR, Coindre JM, Colecchia M, Domanski HA, et al. Clinicopathologic and molecular genetic characterization of low-grade fibromyxoid sarcoma, and cloning of a novel FUS/CREB3L1 fusion gene. Lab Investig. 2005;85(3):408–15.
36. Goldblum JR, Folpe AL, Weiss SW. Enzinger & Weiss's soft tissue tumors. 7th ed. Philadelphia: Elsevier; 2019. pages cm
37. Stout AP. Liposarcoma-the malignant tumor of lipoblasts. Ann Surg. 1944;119(1):86–107.
38. Enzinger FM, Winslow DJ. Liposarcoma. A study of 103 cases. Virchows Arch Pathol Anat Physiol Klin Med. 1962;335:367–88.
39. Evans HL. Liposarcoma: a study of 55 cases with a reassessment of its classification. Am J Surg Pathol. 1979;3(6):507–23.
40. Lattes R, Stout AP, Armed Forces Institute of Pathology (U.S.), Universities Associated for Research and Education in Pathology. Tumors of the soft tissues. Rev. ed, vol. v. Washington, D.C.: Armed Forces Institute of Pathology under the auspices of Universities Associated for Research and Education in Pathology For sale by the Armed Forces Institute of Pathology; 1982. p. 264.
41. Fletcher CD. The evolving classification of soft tissue tumours: an update based on the new WHO classification. Histopathology. 2006;48(1):3–12.
42. Azumi N, Curtis J, Kempson RL, Hendrickson MR. Atypical and malignant neoplasms showing lipomatous differentiation. A study of 111 cases. Am J Surg Pathol. 1987;11(3):161–83.
43. Creytens D. What's new in adipocytic neoplasia? Virchows Arch. 2020;476(1):29–39.
44. Traweek RS, Cope BM, Roland CL, Keung EZ, Nassif EF, Erstad DJ. Targeting the MDM2-p53 pathway in dedifferentiated liposarcoma. Front Oncol. 2022;12:1006959.
45. Cassinelli G, Pasquali S, Lanzi C. Beyond targeting amplified MDM2 and CDK4 in well differentiated and dedifferentiated liposarcomas: from promise and clinical applications towards identification of progression drivers. Front Oncol. 2022;12:965261.
46. Thway K. What's new in adipocytic neoplasia? Histopathology. 2022;80(1):76–97.
47. Boland JM, Weiss SW, Oliveira AM, Erickson-Johnson ML, Folpe AL. Liposarcomas with mixed well-differentiated and pleomorphic features: a clinicopathologic study of 12 cases. Am J Surg Pathol. 2010;34(6):837–43.
48. Marino-Enriquez A, Fletcher CD, Dal Cin P, Hornick JL. Dedifferentiated liposarcoma with "homologous" lipoblastic (pleomorphic liposarcoma-like) differentiation: clinicopathologic and molecular analysis of a series suggesting revised diagnostic criteria. Am J Surg Pathol. 2010;34(8):1122–31.
49. Tallini G, Akerman M, Dal Cin P, De Wever I, Fletcher CD, Mandahl N, et al. Combined morphologic and karyotypic study of 28 myxoid liposarcomas. Implications for a revised morphologic typing, (a report from the CHAMP Group). Am J Surg Pathol. 1996;20(9):1047–55.
50. Fletcher CD, Akerman M, Dal Cin P, de Wever I, Mandahl N, Mertens F, et al. Correlation between clinicopathological features and karyotype in lipomatous tumors. A report of 178 cases from the chromosomes and morphology (CHAMP) collaborative study group. Am J Pathol. 1996;148(2):623–30.
51. Antonescu CR, Elahi A, Humphrey M, Lui MY, Healey JH, Brennan MF, et al. Specificity of TLS-CHOP rearrangement for classic myxoid/round cell liposarcoma: absence in predominantly myxoid well-differentiated liposarcomas. J Mol Diagn. 2000;2(3):132–8.
52. Antonescu CR, Elahi A, Healey JH, Brennan MF, Lui MY, Lewis J, et al. Monoclonality of multifocal myxoid liposarcoma: confirmation by analysis of TLS-CHOP or EWS-CHOP rearrangements. Clin Cancer Res. 2000;6(7):2788–93.
53. de Vreeze RS, de Jong D, Tielen IH, Ruijter HJ, Nederlof PM, Haas RL, et al. Primary retroperitoneal myxoid/round cell liposarcoma is a nonexisting disease: an immunohistochemical and molecular biological analysis. Mod Pathol. 2009;22(2):223–31.
54. Anderson WJ, Jo VY. Pleomorphic liposarcoma: Updates and current differential diagnosis. Semin Diagn Pathol. 2019;36(2):122–8.
55. Mertens F, Fletcher CD, Dal Cin P, De Wever I, Mandahl N, Mitelman F, et al. Cytogenetic analysis of 46 pleomorphic soft tissue sarcomas and correlation with morphologic and clinical features: a report of the CHAMP Study Group. Chromosomes and MorPhology. Genes Chromosomes Cancer. 1998;22(1):16–25.
56. Meis-Kindblom JM, Sjogren H, Kindblom LG, Peydro-Mellquist A, Roijer E, Aman P, et al. Cytogenetic and molecular genetic analyses of liposarcoma and its soft tissue simulators: recognition of new variants and differential diagnosis. Virchows Arch. 2001;439(2):141–51.
57. Creytens D, Folpe AL, Koelsche C, Mentzel T, Ferdinande L, van Gorp JM, et al. Myxoid pleomorphic liposarcoma-a clinicopathologic, immunohistochemical, molecular genetic and epigenetic study of 12 cases, suggesting a possible relationship with conventional pleomorphic liposarcoma. Mod Pathol. 2021;34(11):2043–9.
58. Alaggio R, Coffin CM, Weiss SW, Bridge JA, Issakov J, Oliveira AM, et al. Liposarcomas in young patients: a study of 82 cases occurring in patients younger than 22 years of age. Am J Surg Pathol. 2009;33(5):645–58.
59. Dermawan JK, Hwang S, Wexler L, Tap WD, Singer S, Vanderbilt CM, et al. Myxoid pleomorphic liposarcoma is distinguished from other liposarcomas by widespread loss of heterozygosity and significantly worse overall survival: a genomic and clinicopathologic study. Mod Pathol. 2022;35(11):1644–55.
60. Kallen ME, Hornick JL. The 2020 WHO classification: what's new in soft tissue tumor pathology? Am J Surg Pathol. 2021;45(1):e1–e23.
61. Folpe AL. 'I Can't Keep Up!': an update on advances in soft tissue pathology occurring after the publication of the 2020 World Health Organization classification of soft tissue and bone tumours. Histopathology. 2022;80(1):54–75.
62. Carter JM, Weiss SW, Linos K, DiCaudo DJ, Folpe AL. Superficial CD34-positive fibroblastic tumor: report of 18 cases of a distinctive low-grade mesenchymal neoplasm of intermediate (borderline) malignancy. Mod Pathol. 2014;27(2):294–302.
63. Marino-Enriquez A, Fletcher CD. Angiofibroma of soft tissue: clinicopathologic characterization of a distinctive benign fibrovascular neoplasm in a series of 37 cases. Am J Surg Pathol. 2012;36(4):500–8.
64. Anderson WJ, Mertens F, Marino-Enriquez A, Hornick JL, Fletcher CDM. Superficial CD34-positive fibroblastic tumor: a clinicopathologic, immunohistochemical, and molecular study of 59 cases. Am J Surg Pathol. 2022;46(10):1329–39.
65. Zhao M, Yin X, He H, Fan Y, Ru G, Meng X. Recurrent PRDM10 fusions in superficial CD34-positive fibroblastic tumors : a clinico-

pathologic and molecular study of 10 additional cases of an emerging novel entity. Am J Clin Pathol. 2023;159(4):367–78.
66. Puls F, Carter JM, Pillay N, McCulloch TA, Sumathi VP, Rissler P, et al. Overlapping morphological, immunohistochemical and genetic features of superficial CD34-positive fibroblastic tumor and PRDM10-rearranged soft tissue tumor. Mod Pathol. 2022;35(6):767–76.
67. Perret R, Michal M, Carr RA, Velasco V, Svajdler M, Karanian M, et al. Superficial CD34-positive fibroblastic tumor and PRDM10-rearranged soft tissue tumor are overlapping entities: a comprehensive study of 20 cases. Histopathology. 2021;79(5):810–25.
68. Puls F, Pillay N, Fagman H, Palin-Masreliez A, Amary F, Hansson M, et al. PRDM10-rearranged soft tissue tumor: a clinicopathologic study of 9 cases. Am J Surg Pathol. 2019;43(4):504–13.
69. Jin Y, Moller E, Nord KH, Mandahl N, Von Steyern FV, Domanski HA, et al. Fusion of the AHRR and NCOA2 genes through a recurrent translocation t(5;8)(p15;q13) in soft tissue angiofibroma results in upregulation of aryl hydrocarbon receptor target genes. Genes Chromosomes Cancer. 2012;51(5):510–20.
70. Agaimy A, Perret R, Demicco EG, Gross J, Liu YJ, Azmani R, et al. GAB1::ABL1 fusions define a distinctive soft tissue neoplasm, with variable perineurial differentiation, and a predilection for children and young adults. Genes Chromosomes Cancer. 2023;62(8):449–59.
71. Panagopoulos I, Gorunova L, Andersen K, Tafjord S, Lund-Iversen M, Lobmaier I, et al. Recurrent fusion of the GRB2 associated binding protein 1 (GAB1) gene with ABL proto-oncogene 1 (ABL1) in benign pediatric soft tissue tumors. Cancer Genomics Proteomics. 2020;17(5):499–508.
72. Kallen ME, Hornick JL. From the ashes of "Ewing-like" sarcoma: a contemporary update of the classification, immunohistochemistry, and molecular genetics of round cell sarcomas. Semin Diagn Pathol. 2022;39(1):29–37.
73. Arvand A, Denny CT. Biology of EWS/ETS fusions in Ewing's family tumors. Oncogene. 2001;20(40):5747–54.
74. Fletcher CDM, World Health Organization, International Agency for Research on Cancer. WHO classification of tumours of soft tissue and bone. 4th ed. Lyon: IARC Press; 2013. p. 468.
75. Watson S, Perrin V, Guillemot D, Reynaud S, Coindre JM, Karanian M, et al. Transcriptomic definition of molecular subgroups of small round cell sarcomas. J Pathol. 2018;245(1):29–40.
76. Bridge JA, Sumegi J, Druta M, Bui MM, Henderson-Jackson E, Linos K, et al. Clinical, pathological, and genomic features of EWSR1-PATZ1 fusion sarcoma. Mod Pathol. 2019;32(11):1593–604.
77. Chougule A, Taylor MS, Nardi V, Chebib I, Cote GM, Choy E, et al. Spindle and round cell sarcoma with EWSR1-PATZ1 gene fusion: a sarcoma with polyphenotypic differentiation. Am J Surg Pathol. 2019;43(2):220–8.
78. Michal M, Rubin BP, Agaimy A, Kosemehmetoglu K, Rudzinski ER, Linos K, et al. EWSR1-PATZ1-rearranged sarcoma: a report of nine cases of spindle and round cell neoplasms with predilection for thoracoabdominal soft tissues and frequent expression of neural and skeletal muscle markers. Mod Pathol. 2021;34(4):770–85.
79. Ngo C, Khneisser P, Kanaan C, Valent A, Dumont S, Adam J, et al. EWSR1-PATZ1 fusion sarcoma - a new case report and review of the literature. Ann Pathol. 2021;41(2):207–11.
80. Siegfried A, Rousseau A, Maurage CA, Pericart S, Nicaise Y, Escudie F, et al. EWSR1-PATZ1 gene fusion may define a new glioneuronal tumor entity. Brain Pathol. 2019;29(1):53–62.
81. Antonescu CR, Owosho AA, Zhang L, Chen S, Deniz K, Huryn JM, et al. Sarcomas with CIC-rearrangements are a distinct pathologic entity with aggressive outcome: a clinicopathologic and molecular study of 115 cases. Am J Surg Pathol. 2017;41(7):941–9.
82. Le Loarer F, Baud J, Azmani R, Michot A, Karanian M, Pissaloux D. Advances in the classification of round cell sarcomas. Histopathology. 2022;80(1):33–53.
83. Kawamura-Saito M, Yamazaki Y, Kaneko K, Kawaguchi N, Kanda H, Mukai H, et al. Fusion between CIC and DUX4 up-regulates PEA3 family genes in Ewing-like sarcomas with t(4;19)(q35;q13) translocation. Hum Mol Genet. 2006;15(13):2125–37.
84. Hung YP, Fletcher CD, Hornick JL. Evaluation of ETV4 and WT1 expression in CIC-rearranged sarcomas and histologic mimics. Mod Pathol. 2016;29(11):1324–34.
85. Palmerini E, Gambarotti M, Italiano A, Nathenson MJ, Ratan R, Dileo P, et al. A global collaboRAtive study of CIC-rearranged, BCOR::CCNB3-rearranged and other ultra-rare unclassified undifferentiated small round cell sarcomas (GRACefUl). Eur J Cancer. 2023;183:11–23.
86. Dashti NK, Fritchie KJ, Folpe AL. Perinephric myxoid pseudotumor of fat: a distinctive pseudoneoplasm most often associated with non-neoplastic renal disease. Hum Pathol. 2019;87:37–43.
87. Papke DJ Jr, Dickson BC, Sholl L, Fletcher CDM. Pseudoendocrine sarcoma: clinicopathologic analysis of 23 cases of a distinctive soft tissue neoplasm with metastatic potential, recurrent CTNNB1 mutations, and a predilection for truncal locations. Am J Surg Pathol. 2022;46(1):33–43.
88. Meis-Kindblom JM. Clear cell sarcoma of tendons and aponeuroses: a historical perspective and tribute to the man behind the entity. Adv Anat Pathol. 2006;13(6):286–92.
89. Rossi S, Szuhai K, Ijszenga M, Tanke HJ, Zanatta L, Sciot R, et al. EWSR1-CREB1 and EWSR1-ATF1 fusion genes in angiomatoid fibrous histiocytoma. Clin Cancer Res. 2007;13(24):7322–8.
90. Ulici V, Hornick JL, Davis JL, Mehrotra S, Meis JM, Halling KC, et al. Extraenteric malignant gastrointestinal neuroectodermal tumor-A clinicopathologic and molecular genetic study of 11 cases. Mod Pathol. 2023;36(7):100160.
91. Stockman DL, Miettinen M, Suster S, Spagnolo D, Dominguez-Malagon H, Hornick JL, et al. Malignant gastrointestinal neuroectodermal tumor: clinicopathologic, immunohistochemical, ultrastructural, and molecular analysis of 16 cases with a reappraisal of clear cell sarcoma-like tumors of the gastrointestinal tract. Am J Surg Pathol. 2012;36(6):857–68.
92. Antonescu CR, Katabi N, Zhang L, Sung YS, Seethala RR, Jordan RC, et al. EWSR1-ATF1 fusion is a novel and consistent finding in hyalinizing clear-cell carcinoma of salivary gland. Genes Chromosomes Cancer. 2011;50(7):559–70.
93. Thway K, Nicholson AG, Lawson K, Gonzalez D, Rice A, Balzer B, et al. Primary pulmonary myxoid sarcoma with EWSR1-CREB1 fusion: a new tumor entity. Am J Surg Pathol. 2011;35(11):1722–32.
94. Domingo RA, Vivas-Buitrago T, Jentoft M, Quinones-Hinojosa A. Intracranial myxoid mesenchymal tumor/myxoid subtype angiomatous fibrous histiocytoma: diagnostic and prognostic challenges. Neurosurgery. 2020;88(1):E114–E22.
95. Ladanyi M, Gerald W. Fusion of the EWS and WT1 genes in the desmoplastic small round cell tumor. Cancer Res. 1994;54(11):2837–40.
96. Schoolmeester JK, Folpe AL, Nair AA, Halling K, Sutton BC, Landers E, et al. EWSR1-WT1 gene fusions in neoplasms other than desmoplastic small round cell tumor: a report of three unusual tumors involving the female genital tract and review of the literature. Mod Pathol. 2021;34(10):1912–20.

General Considerations in Magnetic Resonance Imaging of Soft-Tissue Tumors

2

Paolo Spinnato

2.1 Introduction

Magnetic Resonance Imaging (MRI) is a key element in the evaluation of soft-tissue tumors (STT), with different aims in several phases of the diagnostic flowchart. MRI is an accurate and complete imaging tool for the radiological assessment of a suspected or known STT. It is able to confirm the clinical suspect, define lesions' architectural features, intrinsic characteristics, dimensions, and surrounding tissue involvement, and, most importantly, offer indications for eventual additional diagnostic evaluations.

The conventional MRI study should be performed with a standard protocol including the following sequences at least in two planes:

- T1 weighted (with and without fat suppression).
- T2 weighted.
- Fluid-sensitive sequence (usually one among Short Thau Inversion Recovery –STIR- and T2 weighted with fat suppression).
- Contrast-enhanced T1 weighted (with fat suppression—better if implemented with subtracted reconstructions after and before contrast media intravenous injection). Dynamic acquisitions after contrast media injection may offer additional information.
- Diffusion Weighted Imaging (DWI).

2.1.1 Initial Imaging Assessment and Diagnostic Flowchart in Soft-Tissue Masses: The Role of MRI among the Other Radiological Examinations

After an accurate clinical assessment, imaging tools are essential in evaluating soft-tissue lumps. Imaging of soft-tissue masses has changed dramatically over the last decades, together with the continuous innovations of diagnostic radiology. Despite new technological advancements achieved in diagnostic imaging, the American College of Radiology Appropriateness Committee still recommends that Conventional Radiography (CR) should be performed as the first imaging tool in the assessment of soft-tissue lumps. Additionally, it has been recommended that for clearly superficial masses ultrasound (US) examination should be preferred as the first step, avoiding the use of CR [1, 2].

The first fundamental aim of diagnostic imaging is represented by the confirmation of a clinically suspected soft-tissue mass, and, subsequently its characterization, including indications for further investigations when needed.

Indeed, CR reveals positive findings in more than 60% of musculoskeletal soft-tissue neoplasms, confirming the presence of a mass, detecting the presence of calcifications, and/or areas with fat content, as well as cortical bone erosion [1, 3]. Moreover, CR may reveal that a clinically suspected soft-tissue neoplasm is actually a bone tumor with an extra-osseous soft-tissue involvement [4]. On the other hand, both negative and positive CR findings need to be further deepened with MRI or alternatively contrast-enhanced CT as second choice in patients with contraindications. Indeed, for deep soft-tissue masses after CR, the MRI examination is the suggested imaging tool, and its application at this step is preferred to the US [1, 5]. If the MRI features are clearly referable to one of the most common benign deep tumors or tumors-like conditions (namely ganglion cyst, ossificans myositis, elastofibroma dorsi), no further examinations are needed (Fig. 2.1). In addition, even a deep benign nervous tumor (schwannoma/neurinoma) can be recognized with MRI, and followed up over time (Fig. 2.2). On the contrary, if no features of the most common benign deep-seated mass are appreciable, further examinations are needed with evaluation in the sarcoma referral center considering core needle biopsy.

In the initial imaging workup of superficial lumps, the US examination has a proven high diagnostic performance. A group of soft-tissue lesions that can be easily recognized by

P. Spinnato (✉)
Diagnostic and Interventional Radiology,
IRCCS Istituto Ortopedico Rizzoli, Bologna, Italy
e-mail: paolo.spinnato1982@gmail.com

H. Özger et al. (eds.), *Diagnosis and Treatment of Soft Tissue Tumors*, https://doi.org/10.1007/978-3-031-77061-6_2

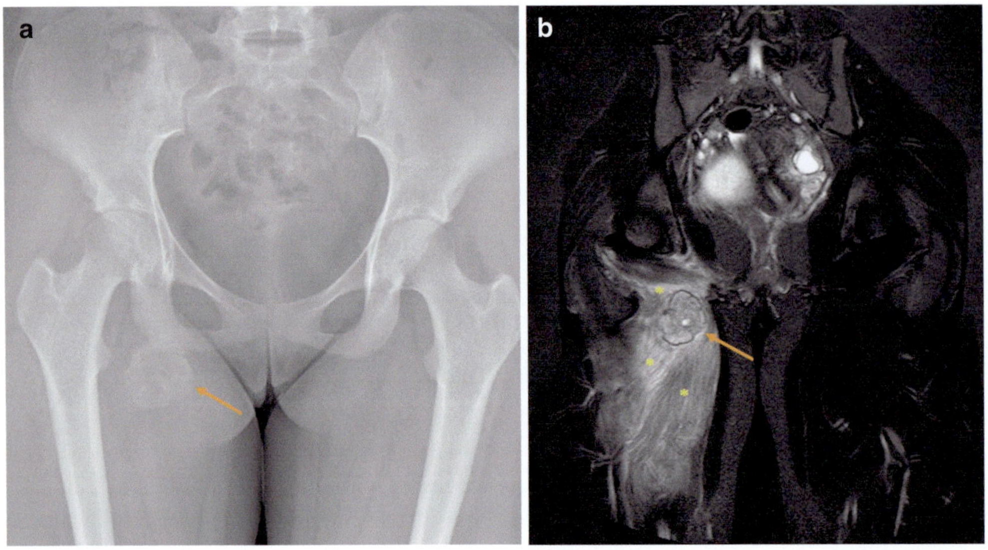

Fig. 2.1 (Panel **a**) Conventional radiography of a 15-year-old girl with a painful soft-tissue lump in the medial proximal aspect of the right thigh, confirmed the presence of a mass (4 cm) with thin peripheral calcifications (arrow). (Panel **b**) MRI coronal STIR sequence confirmed the presence of a mass with thin peripheral calcifications, deeply seated in the abductor region of the right thigh (arrow). Strong and widely diffuse edema of the surrounding tissue was also present (asterisks). Clinical-radiological features were consistent with myositis ossificans and a MRI follow-up was suggested

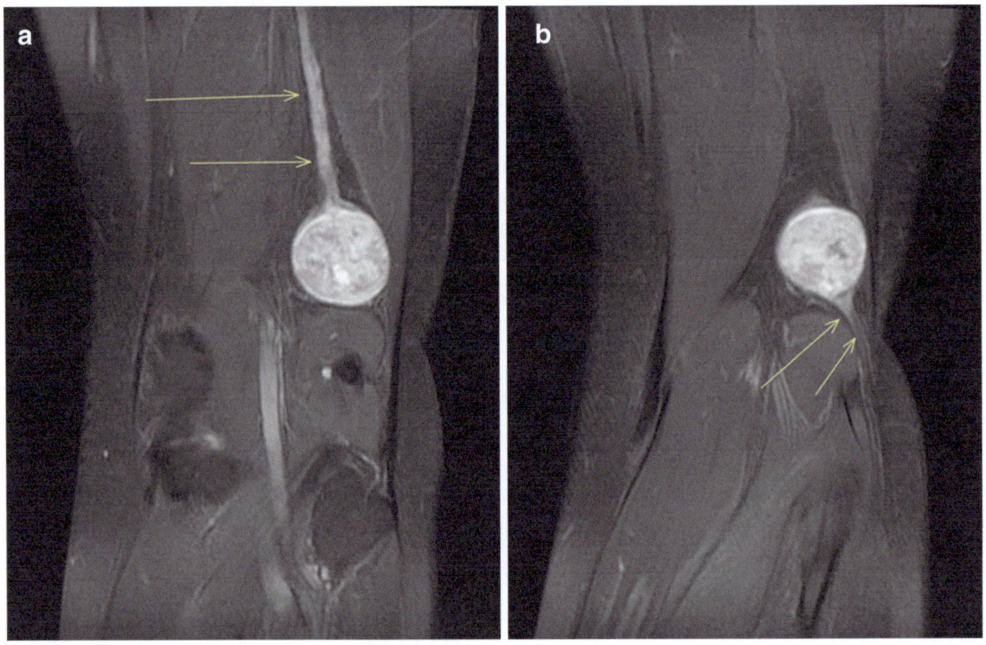

Fig. 2.2 MRI (Coronal T2-weighted with fat suppression Panel **a** and **b**) study in a 53-year-old woman with a painful small lump in the lateral aspect of the left knee. The study revealed a hyperintense well-defined mass (maximum diameter 2.5 cm) in connection with a tail-like edematous and thickened neural structure (arrows): external popliteal sciatic nerve. The MRI features are consistent with the diagnosis of a benign neurogenic tumor (possible schwannoma), and an MRI surveillance over time has been suggested

the US when they are superficially located above the investing fascia. Particularly, lipoma, epidermal inclusion cyst (epidermoid cyst), peripheral nerve-sheet tumors, ganglion cyst, and vascular malformation/hemangioma can be recognized in the US, and no further examinations are needed [2, 6, 7]. If classical US features of the above-mentioned lesions are not recognized, further examinations (MRI and/or biopsy) are needed, regardless of the lesions' size [2, 6, 7].

Regarding the initial imaging workup of fat-containing tumors, consensus guidelines have been recently provided by a multidisciplinary panel of experts [8]. The authors suggest that superficial adipocytic tumors without imaging features of malignancies and with a maximum diameter < 10 cm, should be evaluated with follow-up controls only. On the contrary, when the maximum diameter exceeds 10 cm, evaluation in a sarcoma referral center is needed, even without any imaging features of malignancy. If imaging signs of malignancy are detectable (heterogeneity within the adipocytic tissue) in superficial lesions, a referral to specialized centers is suggested if the diameter exceeds 3 cm. On the other hand, when the adipocytic tumor is deeply located an evaluation by sarcoma experts is

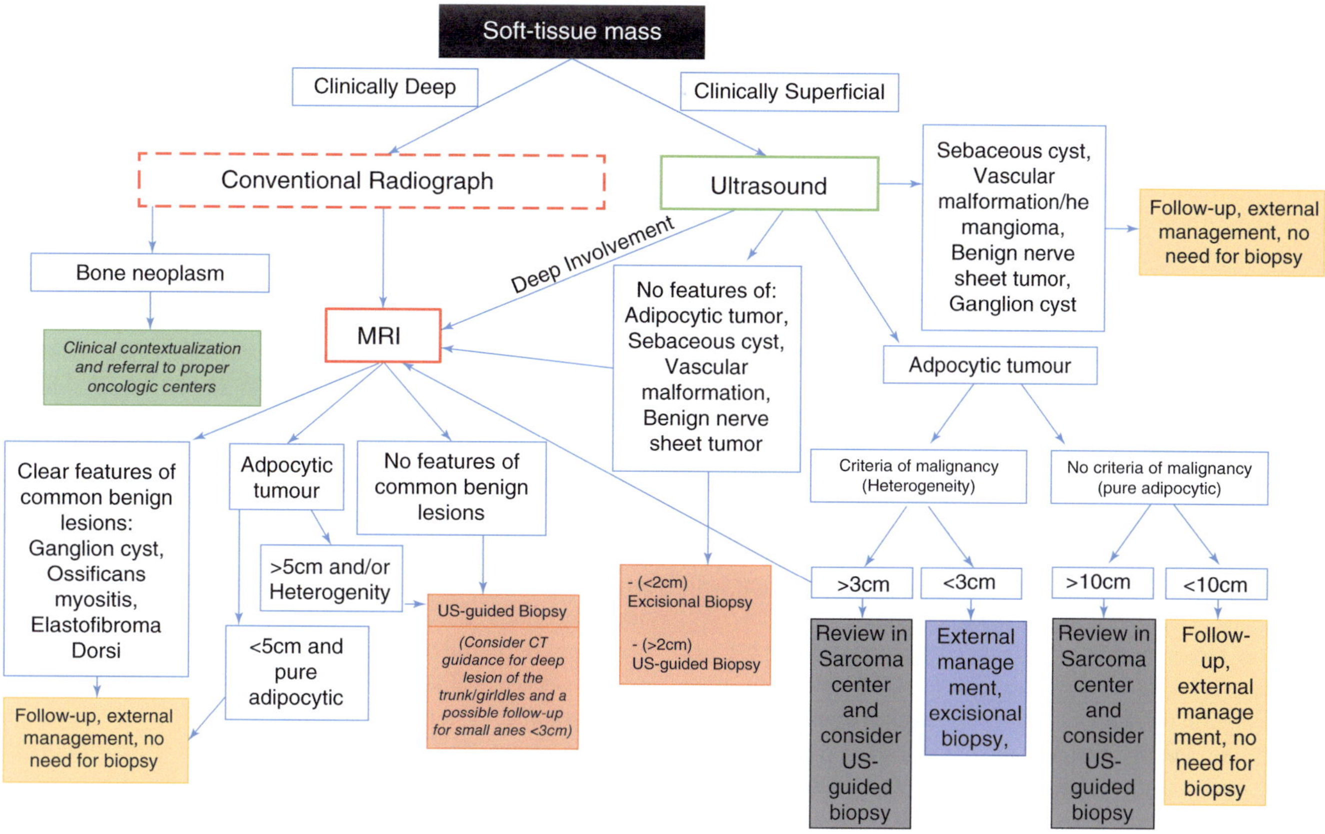

Fig. 2.3 Diagnostic imaging Flowchart for deep and superficial soft-tissue masses

suggested if the maximum diameter exceeds 5 cm. Moreover, if the location of the lesion is within the mediastinum, abdomen, or spermatic cord, an evaluation in sarcoma centers is always suggested [8].

For the initial histopathological examination of a soft-tissue tumor, US-guided percutaneous core needle biopsy is nowadays the preferred tool for all the deep lesions of the extremities and superficial mass greater than 2 cm in maximum diameter [9]. The addition of intratumoral vascularization evaluation with color-Doppler and/or contrast-enhanced ultrasound (CEUS) during US-guided biopsy for the needle approach planning, may improve the results of the biopsy specimen, particularly avoiding large necrotic areas within the sample.

CT-guided biopsy should be preferred to US guidance for deep lesions located in the trunk, and when a predominant osseous involvement is detected [10]. Excisional biopsy is recommended for small (<2 cm) superficially located neoplasms.

A biopsy is needed for deeply seated soft-tissue masses smaller than 3 cm, undetermined at MRI, but a follow-up control should also be considered, according to the patient's age, clinical conditions, lesion location, and physicians' experience. The speed of growth of these neoplasms should be accurately taken into account as a key element in the follow-up management of these patients, more than the 'static diameter' alone. Indeed, the speed of growth is associated with aggressive behaviors in soft-tissue sarcomas (complex genomic, increased mitosis) [11].

Interestingly, a recent large research on 579 deep-seated soft-tissue masses revealed that the radiologist was confident in 75% of cases with the US only. They conclude that the US should be effectively used instead of MRI even for deep-seated tumor characterization [12]. Large series also considering different radiologists' experiences are needed.

According to the above-mentioned guidelines, recent research, and current indications we summarized in a practical flow-chart the recommended imaging workup for deep and superficial soft-tissue masses, highlighting the role of MRI (Fig. 2.3).

2.2 Soft-Tissue Sarcoma: Baseline MRI Assessment and Staging

Soft-tissue sarcomas (STS) are a rare and heterogeneous group of malignancies representing only 1% of cancers in adult age.

The biological and clinical behaviors of STS may significantly vary according to different histotypes and histologic grades. The recommended histologic grade for STS is based on the French Federation of Cancer Centers (FNCLCC) system. This grading system is based on three factors: tumor necrosis, differentiation (taking into account the histologic type), and mitotic count. The FNLCC grading system is subdivided into three categories: low (I), intermediate (II), and high (III) grades.

When the diagnosis of STS is made, proper staging in sarcoma referral centers is needed.

Since surgical removal with wide resection margins is the cornerstone of STS treatment, an accurate imaging assessment is mandatory to plan the interventional procedure. Contrast-enhanced MRI is the gold standard tool for this aim and by far the most sensitive and accurate imaging modality to correctly plan the surgical resection [13]. Radiologists and surgeons should discuss the study performed in detail in order to understand the intrinsic characteristics of the lesion, its boundaries, and surrounding structures' involvement with the goal of a wide margins resection [13].

Loco-regional contrast-enhanced MRI and chest CT are recommended for all STS subtypes [14]. Moreover, in some specific subtypes, other additional examinations are needed at baseline. For example, in patients affected by high-grade (round-cells count > 5%) myxoid round-cells liposarcoma, one of the most common liposarcoma subtypes, an imaging assessment of the whole spine is recommended due to the possibility of metastatic disease within the vertebral column. Additionally, other rare STS subtypes require the inclusion of the abdomen in the baseline imaging workup. Nonetheless, nowadays, the request for more personalized medicine and the metastatic pattern of several STS subtypes, suggest that local and distant limited staging should be insufficient for several patients, and whole-body examinations such as PET or whole-body MRI could add a significant value [15]. At this aim, (FDG) PET-CT can be a valid tool to offer a whole-body assessment in a single step, offering also additional information in regards to patient prognosis as well as a baseline analysis helpful for the subsequent treatments responses' assessment [15, 16]. Recent research also revealed that the application of (FGD) PET-CT at staging for both bone and soft-tissue sarcomas offers additional information adding a slight non-significant delay in time to treatment [17].

2.2.1 Conventional MRI: Features Related to Prognosis

Conventional contrast-enhanced MRI is the key element in the local staging of STS. Planning surgery, evaluating tumor margins, and identifying critical peritumoral structures including arteries and nerves are the main objectives of the investigation. Nonetheless, baseline MRI is a valid tool in offering prognostic information that may help in the treatment strategy of STS. The assessment of these features is experience-dependent, mainly performed by radiologists who work in a sarcoma referral center. There are several MRI features related to poor prognosis in all STS subtypes, including tumor dimensions, surrounding tissues, growth patterns, and intrinsic tumoral features [18–20].

Tumor's dimension has been for decades the main data taken into account for prognosis in STS baseline MRI [21, 22]. Nowadays, even if the size (diameters and/or volume) of the main mass is still the key prognostic element for all solid malignancies including STS, several other features can be extrapolated from MRI to improve patients' prognostication [18, 19, 20, 22]. Some of these features can be detected in all STS subtypes, while others are important in some specific STS subtypes. Moreover, These MRI features can be divided into internal features, and surrounding tissue/marginal features. The first internal feature is necrosis. Necrosis can be easily assessed on contrast-enhanced MRI as areas without any enhancement after gadolinium contrast media intravenous injections; the necrotic areas are usually located in the central part of the mass (Fig. 2.4). As mentioned above, necrosis is one of the items evaluated in the FNCLCC histologic grading system. As a direct result of this, signs of necrosis detected on baseline MRI are associated with high-grade STS (grade III) and poor prognosis [19, 20]. Another

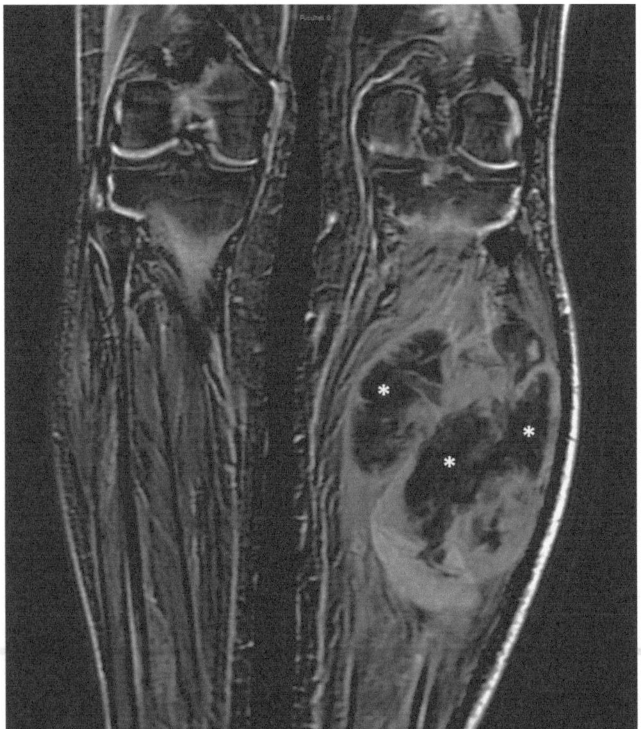

Fig. 2.4 MRI (Subtracted reconstruction: Coronal T1 weighted fat suppressed contrast-enhanced sequence—Coronal T1 weighted fat suppressed unenhanced sequence) of a 71 years old female affected by a high-grade (III) extra-skeletal osteostarcoma of the left calf. The study revealed large central areas without contrast enhancement (asterisks) consistent with wide internal necrosis

internal feature is the signal intensity inhomogeneity in more than 50% of tumor volume, depicted on T2 weighted sequences. This feature has been recognized as a predictor of poor prognosis and high grades (II-III) in all STS subtypes. Moreover, in a series focused on myxoid round-cell liposarcoma, including 35 baseline MRIs, it was associated with an increased risk of distant metastases [19–22].

The concomitant presence of two MRI features among necrosis, peritumoral enhancement, and signal intensity inhomogeneity on T2 weighted sequences increases the risk of distant metastases (hazard ratio, 4.5; $P = 0.01$) (Fig. 2.5) [19].

The MRI growth pattern of STS, namely pushing type, focally infiltrative, and diffusively infiltrative (Fig. 2.6), is associated with prognosis as well. Indeed, infiltrative patterns express signs of marginal infiltrations being associated with an increased risk of local recurrence after excision.

Other features are related to tumor margins and surrounding tissue. Above all, peritumoral enhancement, defined as a pathologic area of contrast enhancement outside the tumor borders, is a well-recognized sign of gross marginal infiltration; association with high histological grades (II–III), and reduced overall survival. In addition, the involvement of major vascular bundles (tumor-vascular contact or vascular encasement by the mass) depicted on MRI, is associated with an increased risk of local recurrence after excision in all STS subtypes [23].

Several other peculiar MRI features are associated with poor prognosis only in some STS subtypes. The most recognized and known of these features is the so-called 'tail sign' a curvilinear projection from the tumor usually along the fascial plane [24]; this sign is strongly associated with increased risk of local recurrence after excision in both myxofibrosarcoma and undifferentiated pleomorphic sarcoma [25, 26]. The recognition of this sign in preoperative

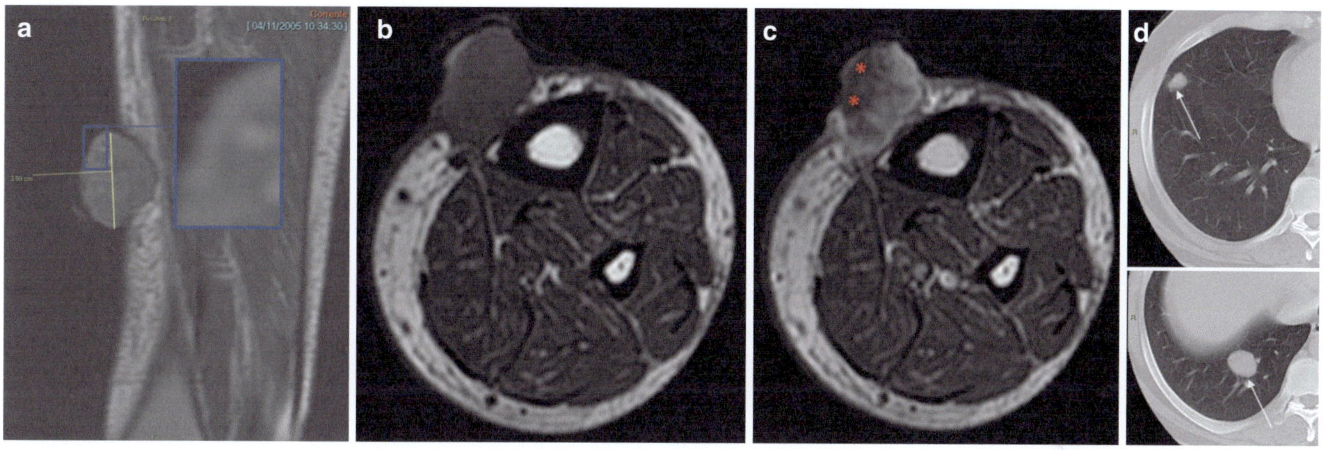

Fig. 2.5 Contrast-enhanced MRI in a 39-year-old man affected by superficially located spindle cell sarcoma of the leg ulcerating the skin (Panel **a**—T2w sequence, Panel **b**—T1w sequence, Panel **c** T1w sequence after gadolinium injection). Concomitant presence of signal intensity inhomogeneity on T2 weighted sequence (Panel **a**—square blue rectangle, enlargement), and intratumoral necrosis (Panel **c** - asterisks) are detected. Lung metastases were diagnosed at baseline CT staging (Panel **d** - arrows)

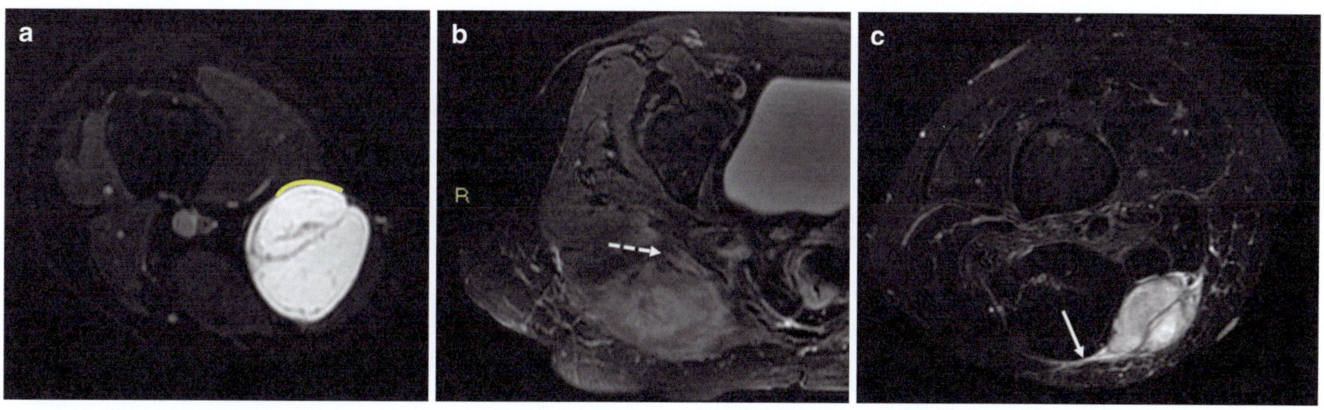

Fig. 2.6 T2 weighted with fat suppression in three cases of soft-tissue sarcoma. (Panel **a**) pushing type growth pattern in a low-grade (I) myxoid round cell liposarcoma of the thigh: well-defined margins can be depicted (curvilinear line). (Panel **b**) diffuse infiltrative growth pattern in a case of alveolar soft-part sarcoma of the hip girdle: hill-defined margins can be detected (dotted arrow). (Panel **c**) focally infiltrative growth pattern in a case of myxofibrosarcoma of the thigh: focal infiltration can be detected with the peculiar 'tail sign' appearance (arrow)

MRI should be taken into account for surgical planning, and margins of excision must be accurately planned in order to include the whole tail. Generally, all the MRI signs associated with infiltrative patterns recommend wider margins of resection for STS.

The water-like appearance of the lesion on fluid-sensitive sequences, an MRI sign related to high myxoid matrix content (increased water content), has been associated with an increased risk of local recurrence after myxofibrosarcoma excision as well [26, 27].

In patients affected by synovial sarcoma the presence of large cystic-hemorrhagic necrotic areas is associated with an increased risk of distant metastases and reduced overall survival [18, 28]. This sign could be associated with two other features in MRI of synovial sarcomas, with the simultaneous presence of three different signal intensities within the tumor on T2w sequences (fibrotic areas with low signal intensity, cellular elements with intermediate intensity, and cystic-hemorrhagic necrotic areas with high intensity): the so-called MRI 'triple-sign' [29]. These large cystic-hemorrhagic necrotic areas may also resemble a 'bowl of grapes'; a feature frequently encountered on MRI of synovial sarcomas [28, 29].

In patients affected by myxoid round-cell liposarcoma, the prevalence of adipose component within the tumor is associated with an increased risk of distant metastases and decreased overall survival [30].

Table 2.1 summarizes all the above-mentioned MRI features related to prognosis in STS.

2.2.2 Quantitative MRI and Future Perspectives

MRI offers important prognostic quantitative information at baseline assessment. Above all, diffusion-weighted sequences (DWI) were demonstrated to offer quantitative values that correlate with FNLCC histological grades. Particularly, it is known that hyper-cellularity demonstrates low diffusion apparent coefficient (ADC) and it is associated with high histological grades (III) in STS. ADC_{mean} = 0.90–1.39 × 10–3 mm^2 s^{-1} and ADC_{min} = 0.59–0.91 × 10–3 mm^2 s^{-1} are reported in high grades STS (FNLCC = 3) [20, 31]. Importantly, it must be taken into account that myxoid stroma and chondroid tumors naturally exhibit high ADC values due to the high intratumoral water content (Fig. 2.7).

Few studies are focused on MRI dynamic contrast enhancement in STS. The available data on this topic suggest that high histological grades (FNLCC = 3) showed a higher value of Ktrans [the transfer constant from the plasma to the interstitium (>0.163 min^{-1})] [20, 32].

Table 2.1 Conventional MRI Features associated with prognosis in STS

MRI finding	Significance	Prognostic relevance	Applicable in the following histotypes
Peritumoral enhancement	Margins infiltrations	– Association with high (II–III) histological grades – Reduced overall survival	All histotypes
Infiltrative growing pattern	Margins infiltrations	– Reduced disease-free survival	All histotypes
Involvement of major vascular bundles	Vascular infiltration/tumor-vascular contact	– Increased risk of local recurrence after surgical excision	All histotypes
Tail sign	Gross infiltrations	– Increased risk of local recurrence after excision – Increased risk of distant metastases	Myxofibrosarcoma, Undifferentiated pleomorphic sarcoma
Signal intensity heterogeneity	Altered tissue differentiation	– High histological grades – Reduced overall survival – Increased risk of distant metastases	All histotypes
Signs of necrosis	Altered vascularization, rapid proliferation	– High histological grades – Reduced overall survival – Increased risk of distant metastases	All histotypes
Hemorrhage—Cystic-like areas	Altered vascularization, rapid proliferation, bleeding	– Reduced overall survival – Increased risk of distant metastases	Synovial Sarcoma
High adipocytic content	Prevalence of fat tumoral content	– Reduced overall survival – Increased risk of distant metastases	Myxoid round-cells liposarcoma
Water-like appearance	Prevalence of myxoid matrix content	– Increased risk of local recurrence	Myxofibrosarcoma

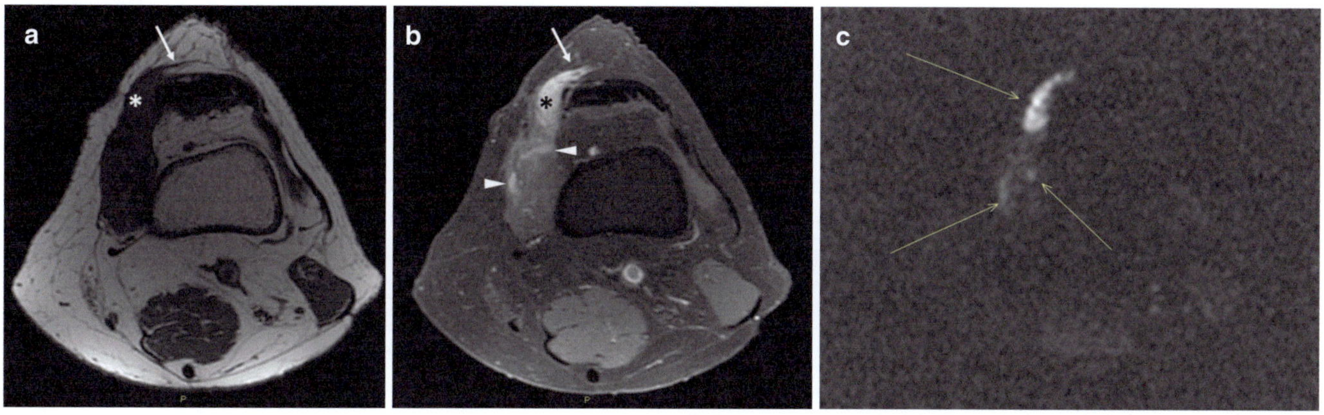

Fig. 2.7 MRI (Panel **a**: T1 weighted—Panel **b**: contrast-enhanced T1 weighted—Panel **c**: Diffusion Weighted images) of a 53-year-old woman with myxofibrosarcoma recurrence (asterisks) after excision. 'Tail sign' can be detected (Arrow), as well as areas of peritumoral enhancement (arrowheads). The Apparent Diffusion Coefficients (ADC) were very high, higher than the normal muscle, due to the high myxoid matrix content rich in water molecules

Table 2.2 Summary of quantitative MRI features associated with prognosis in soft-tissue sarcomas (STS)

Quantitative MRI features	Significance	Clinical/prognostic associations	Cut-off	STS subtypes
Low Apparent Diffusion Coefficient (ADC)	Hyper cellularity	– High histological grade	$ADC_{mean} = 0.90–1.39 \times 10^{-3}$ mm^2 s^{-1} (Grade III) $ADC_{min} = 0.59–0.91 \times 10^{-3}$ mm^2 s^{-1} (Grade III)	All histological subtypes (Subtypes with high myxoid or chondroid matrix content may differ for higher mean and min ADC)
Dynamic contrast enhancement (DCE)	Evaluation of intra-tumoral enhancement over time after i.v. contrast injection. K^{trans} = the transfer constant from the plasma to the interstitium (in min^{-1})	– High histological grade	$K^{trans} > 0.163$ min^{-1} (Grade III)	All histological subtypes
Radiomics Features (RFs) Applied on MRI	Several different Imaging Features extracted from MRI studies	– High histological grade – Risk of distant metastases – Lower overall survival	NA	All histological subtypes

In the future, the combination of the accurate morphological STS depiction offered by MRI with the biological-metabolic data obtained by (FGD)-PET is a very promising option [33]. Indeed, the use of (FDG)-PET in STS has continuously increased over the years. At baseline, this tool permits to offering of whole-body imaging staging together with relevant prognostic features, as well as a starting point for future post-treatment evaluations. This examination provides a quantitative assessment of tumor metabolic activity measured in standard uptake values (SUV). Particularly, SUV values are able to predict the risk of distant metastases (SUV > 6–7 g mL^{-1}) and are well associated with high grades (SUV > 5.2–6 g.mL^{-1} in FNLCC = 2/3) [20]. Novel PET-MRI clinical applications are promising tools in this field, merging the multiparametric potential of MRI with the metabolic quantification of PET. Preliminary researches suggest the extent of this application in the future, particularly in children also according to radiant dose reduction in comparison with classic PET-CT assessment [33].

The application of radiomics to MRI is another interesting research application, not yet completely applicable in clinical practice, but with great potential in the future. MRI-based radiomics analyses have yet been proved by recent research to offer prognostic information at baseline, as well as to predict the response to treatments (delta radiomics pre-post treatments) [34, 35].

Table 2.2 summarizes the main quantitative MRI features related to prognosis in STS.

2.3 Treatment Response Assessment and Follow-Up

The response evaluation criteria in solid tumors (RECIST v1.1), general criteria not unique to STS and to the neoadjuvant treatment provided to STS patients, are used as the standard in clinical practice and trials, and mainly performed on MRI studies.

Although the RECIST v1.1 criteria are repeatable and generally simple to use, they are only applicable to locally progressed STS with a single quantifiable lesion.

Actually, because dimensional fluctuation occurs after the formation of necrosis, fibrosis, and changes in tumor vascularization and metabolism, the diagnosis of response or progression is sometimes delayed. Hence, the majority of locally progressed STS are categorized by RECIST v1.1 as stable illnesses. Choi and modified Choi criteria, rely on changes in unidimensional measurements and contrast enhancement compared to the baseline or to the nadir, and can be applied to contrast-enhanced MR studies [14].

The lack of standardized acquisition protocols and methodology to measure DWI and DCE-MRI metrics, heterogeneous histologic types, a lack of a definition for a histologic response, and multicentric collaborations between radiological centers prevent changes in DWI and DCE-MRI metrics from being validated in clinical practice as response biomarkers despite these intriguing trends [14]. However, they can still be used to modify the conclusion of radiological reports in cases of stable disease with early indications of response (increase in ADC, decrease in Ktrans, and AUC) or progression (decrease in ADC, increase in Ktrans, and AUC), or in cases of dimensional progression brought on by necrosis brought on by treatment.

Due to contentious findings in retrospective research, the methods for local follow-up are under discussion.

In a cohort of 174 STS patients, local recurrences were clinically recognized in 30 out of 31 cases, whereas just one patient benefited from MRI, according to Rothermundt et al. [36]. Moreover, Labarre et al. demonstrated that routine follow-up MRI produced plenty of false positives. In contrast, MRI appeared more effective in the Park et al. investigation since it identified local relapses in 60% of all cases of their series that were missed by ultrasonography or clinical examination. Moreover, local relapses were identified by MRI earlier and with smaller size (2.3 cm versus 4 cm) (15.5 months versus 20 months).

2.4 Conclusion

MRI is the best imaging modality to evaluate soft-tissue tumors in different phases of the diagnostic flowchart. MRI is a key diagnostic element in undetermined soft-tissue mass, for the recognition of clearly benign conditions versus lesions that need further examinations, particularly for deeply located masses.

When a diagnosis of STS is made, MRI is the most accurate imaging tool to plan surgery and provide baseline evaluation offering several prognostic information. Even in follow-up controls and treatment response evaluation, MRI is the radiologic modality of choice.

In the future, the implementation of quantitative MRI and the possible association with metabolic examinations (PET-MRI) could improve the quality of the imaging assessment with the goal of more personalized care.

References

1. Kransdorf MJ, Murphey MD. Imaging of soft-tissue musculoskeletal masses: fundamental concepts. Radiographics. 2016;36(6):1931–48. https://doi.org/10.1148/rg.2016160084.
2. Hung EH, Griffith JF, Ng AW, Lee RK, Lau DT, Leung JC. Ultrasound of musculoskeletal soft-tissue tumors superficial to the investing fascia. AJR Am J Roentgenol. 2014;202(6):W532–W40. https://doi.org/10.2214/AJR.13.11457.
3. Gartner L, Pearce CJ, Saifuddin A. The role of the plain radiograph in the characterisation of soft tissue tumours. Skeletal Radiol. 2009;38(6):549–58. https://doi.org/10.1007/s00256-008-0513-9. Epub 2008 Jun 20
4. Bancroft LW, Pettis C, Wasyliw C. Imaging of benign soft tissue tumors. Semin Musculoskelet Radiol. 2013;17(2):156–67. https://doi.org/10.1055/s-0033-1343071. Epub 2013 May 14
5. Noebauer-Huhmann IM, Weber MA, Lalam RK, Trattnig S, Bohndorf K, Vanhoenacker F, Tagliafico A, van Rijswijk C, Vilanova JC, Afonso PD, Breitenseher M, Beggs I, Robinson P, de Jonge MC, Krestan C, Bloem JL. Soft tissue tumors in adults: ESSR-approved guidelines for diagnostic imaging. Semin Musculoskelet Radiol. 2015;19(5):475–82. https://doi.org/10.1055/s-0035-1569251. Epub 2015 Dec 22. Erratum in: Semin Musculoskelet Radiol. 2015 Dec;19(5):e1
6. Jacobson JA, Middleton WD, Allison SJ, Dahiya N, Lee KS, Levine BD, Lucas DR, Murphey MD, Nazarian LN, Siegel GW, Wagner JM. Ultrasonography of superficial soft-tissue masses: society of radiologists in ultrasound consensus conference statement. Radiology. 2022;304(1):18–30. https://doi.org/10.1148/radiol.211101. Epub 2022 Apr 12
7. Rimondi E, Mavrogenis AF, Errani C, Calabrò T, Bazzocchi A, Facchini G, Donatiello S, Spinnato P, Vanel D, Albisinni U, Pelotti P. Biopsy is not necessary for the diagnosis of soft tissue hemangiomas. Radiol Med. 2018;123(7):538–44. https://doi.org/10.1007/s11547-018-0862-y. Epub 2018 Feb 23
8. Moulin B, Messiou C, Crombe A, Kind M, Hohenberger P, Rutkowski P, van Houdt WJ, Strauss D, Gronchi A, Bonvalot S. Diagnosis strategy of adipocytic soft-tissue tumors in adults: a consensus from European experts. Eur J Surg Oncol. 2022;48(3):518–25. https://doi.org/10.1016/j.ejso.2021.10.009. Epub 2021 Oct 18
9. Roland CL. Soft tissue tumors of the extremity. Surg Clin North Am. 2020;100(3):669–80. https://doi.org/10.1016/j.suc.2020.02.015. Epub 2020 Apr 13
10. Traina F, Errani C, Toscano A, Pungetti C, Fabbri D, Mazzotti A, Donati D, Faldini C. Current concepts in the biopsy of musculoskeletal tumors. J Bone Joint Surg Am. 2015;97(1):e7.
11. Crombé A, Fadli D, Spinnato P, Michot A, Cousin S, Le Loarer F, Kind M. Natural speed of growth of untreated soft-tissue sar-

comas: a dimension-based imaging analysis. Eur J Radiol. 2022;146:110082. https://doi.org/10.1016/j.ejrad.2021.110082. Epub 2021 Dec 1
12. Griffith JF, Yip SWY, Hung EHY, Fong RCW, Leung J, Ng AWH, Tong CSL, Lee RKL. Accuracy of ultrasound in the characterisation of deep soft tissue masses: a prospective study. Eur Radiol. 2020;30(11):5894–903. https://doi.org/10.1007/s00330-020-07002-5. Epub 2020 Jun 26
13. Sambri A, Caldari E, Fiore M, Zucchini R, Giannini C, Pirini MG, Spinnato P, Cappelli A, Donati DM, De Paolis M. Margin assessment in soft tissue sarcomas: review of the literature. Cancers (Basel). 2021;13(7):1687. https://doi.org/10.3390/cancers13071687. PMID: 33918457; PMCID: PMC8038240
14. Crombé A, Kind M, Fadli D, Miceli M, Linck PA, Bianchi G, Sambri A, Spinnato P. Soft-tissue sarcoma in adults: imaging appearances, pitfalls and diagnostic algorithms. Diagn Interv Imaging. 2022. :S2211-5684(22)00241-8. Epub ahead of print; https://doi.org/10.1016/j.diii.2022.12.001.
15. Visgauss JD, Wilson DA, Perrin DL, Colglazier R, French R, Mattei JC, Griffin AM, Wunder JS, Ferguson PC. Staging and surveillance of myxoid liposarcoma: follow-up assessment and the metastatic pattern of 169 patients suggests inadequacy of current practice standards. Ann Surg Oncol. 2021;28(12):7903–11. https://doi.org/10.1245/s10434-021-10091-1. Epub 2021 May 7
16. Gabriel M, Rubello D. 18F-FDG PET-CT in soft tissue sarcomas: staging, restaging, and prognostic value? Nucl Med Commun. 2016;37(1):3–8. https://doi.org/10.1097/MNM.0000000000000407.
17. Elmanzalawy A, Vali R, Chavhan GB, Gupta AA, Omarkhail Y, Amirabadi A, Shammas A. The impact of 18F-FDG PET on initial staging and therapy planning of pediatric soft-tissue sarcoma patients. Pediatr Radiol. 2020;50(2):252–60. https://doi.org/10.1007/s00247-019-04530-1. Epub 2019 Oct 18
18. Scalas G, Parmeggiani A, Martella C, Tuzzato G, Bianchi G, Facchini G, Clinca R, Spinnato P. Magnetic resonance imaging of soft tissue sarcoma: features related to prognosis. Eur J Orthop Surg Traumatol. 2021;31(8):1567–75. https://doi.org/10.1007/s00590-021-03003-2. Epub 2021 May 29
19. Crombé A, Marcellin PJ, Buy X, Stoeckle E, Brouste V, Italiano A, Le Loarer F, Kind M. Soft-tissue sarcomas: assessment of MRI features correlating with histologic grade and patient outcome. Radiology. 2019;291(3):710–21. https://doi.org/10.1148/radiol.2019181659. Epub 2019 Apr 9
20. Crombé A, Matcuk GR, Fadli D, Sambri A, Patel DB, Paioli A, Kind M, Spinnato P. Role of imaging in initial prognostication of locally advanced soft tissue sarcomas. Acad Radiol. 2023;30(2):322–40. https://doi.org/10.1016/j.acra.2022.04.003. Epub 2022 May 6
21. D'Agostino V, Ponti F, Martella C, Miceli M, Sambri A, De Paolis M, Donati DM, Bianchi G, Longhi A, Crombé A, Spinnato P. Dimensional assessment on baseline MRI of soft-tissue sarcomas: longest diameter, sum and product of diameters, and volume-which is the best measurement method to predict patients' outcomes? Radiol Med. 2024. https://doi.org/10.1007/s11547-024-01895-8. Epub ahead of print. PMID: 39424744.
22. Crombé A, Le Loarer F, Sitbon M, Italiano A, Stoeckle E, Buy X, Kind M. Can radiomics improve the prediction of metastatic relapse of myxoid/round cell liposarcomas? Eur Radiol. 2020;30(5):2413–24. https://doi.org/10.1007/s00330-019-06562-5. Epub 2020 Jan 17
23. Sambri A, Caldari E, Montanari A, Fiore M, Cevolani L, Ponti F, D'Agostino V, Bianchi G, Miceli M, Spinnato P, De Paolis M, Donati DM. Vascular proximity increases the risk of local recurrence in soft-tissue sarcomas of the thigh-a retrospective MRI study. Cancers (Basel). 2021;13(24):6325. https://doi.org/10.3390/cancers13246325. PMID: 34944944; PMCID: PMC8699708
24. Spinnato P, Clinca R. MRI tail sign in soft-tissue sarcoma. Radiology. 2021;299(2):276. https://doi.org/10.1148/radiol.2021203877. Epub 2021 Mar 16
25. Imanishi J, Slavin J, Pianta M, Jackett L, Ngan SY, Tanaka T, Charoenlap C, Bella DIC, Choong PF. Tail of superficial myxofibrosarcoma and undifferentiated pleomorphic sarcoma after preoperative radiotherapy. Anticancer Res. 2016;36(5):2339–44.
26. Spinnato P, Clinca R, Vara G, Cesari M, Ponti F, Facchini G, Longhi A, Donati DM, Bianchi G, Sambri A. MRI features as prognostic factors in myxofibrosarcoma: proposal of MRI grading system. Acad Radiol. 2021;28(11):1524–9. https://doi.org/10.1016/j.acra.2020.08.018. Epub 2020 Sep 11. PMID: 32928636
27. Spinnato P, Sambri A, Fujiwara T, Ceccarelli L, Clinca R, Medellin MR, Paolis M, Donati DM, Bianchi G. Myxofibrosarcoma: clinical and prognostic value of MRI features. Curr Med Imaging. 2021;17(2):217–24. https://doi.org/10.2174/1573405616999200729152135.
28. Fiore M, Sambri A, Spinnato P, Zucchini R, Giannini C, Caldari E, Pirini MG, De Paolis M. The biology of synovial sarcoma: state-of-the-art and future perspectives. Curr Treat Options in Oncol. 2021;22(12):109. https://doi.org/10.1007/s11864-021-00914-4. PMID: 34687366; PMCID: PMC8541977
29. Baheti AD, Tirumani SH, Sewatkar R, Shinagare AB, Hornick JL, Ramaiya NH, Jagannathan JP. Imaging features of primary and metastatic extremity synovial sarcoma: a single institute experience of 78 patients. Br J Radiol. 2015;88(1046):20140608. https://doi.org/10.1259/bjr.20140608. Epub 2014 Nov 28. PMID: 25431890; PMCID: PMC4614246
30. Crombe A, Sitbon M, Stoeckle E, Italiano A, Buy X, Le Loarer F, Kind M. Magnetic resonance imaging assessment of chemotherapy-related adipocytic maturation in myxoid/round cell liposarcomas: specificity and prognostic value. Br J Radiol. 2020;93(1110):20190794. https://doi.org/10.1259/bjr.20190794. Epub 2020 Mar 6
31. Chhabra A, Ashikyan O, Slepicka C, Dettori N, Hwang H, Callan A, Sharma RR, Xi Y. Conventional MR and diffusion-weighted imaging of musculoskeletal soft tissue malignancy: correlation with histologic grading. Eur Radiol. 2019;29(8):4485–94. https://doi.org/10.1007/s00330-018-5845-9. Epub 2018 Dec 3
32. Li X, Wang Q, Dou Y, Zhang Y, Tao J, Yang L, Wang S. Soft tissue sarcoma: can dynamic contrast-enhanced (DCE) MRI be used to predict the histological grade? Skeletal Radiol. 2020;49(11):1829–38. https://doi.org/10.1007/s00256-020-03491-z. Epub 2020 Jun 10
33. Qi J, Thakrar PD, Browning MB, Vo N, Kumbhar SS. Clinical utilization of whole-body PET/MRI in childhood sarcoma. Pediatr Radiol. 2021;51(3):471–9. https://doi.org/10.1007/s00247-020-04834-7. Epub 2020 Oct 11
34. Fields BKK, Demirjian NL, Cen SY, Varghese BA, Hwang DH, Lei X, Desai B, Duddalwar V, Matcuk GR Jr. Predicting soft tissue sarcoma response to neoadjuvant chemotherapy using an MRI-Based Delta-Radiomics approach. Mol Imaging Biol. 2023; https://doi.org/10.1007/s11307-023-01803-y. Epub ahead of print. PMID: 36695966
35. Crombé A, Bertolo F, Fadli D, Kind M, Le Loarer F, Perret R, Chaire V, Spinnato P, Lucchesi C, Italiano A. Distinct patterns of the natural evolution of soft tissue sarcomas on pre-treatment MRIs captured with delta-radiomics correlate with gene expression profiles. Eur Radiol. 2023;33(2):1205–18. https://doi.org/10.1007/s00330-022-09104-8. Epub 2022 Aug 27
36. Rothermundt C, Whelan JS, Dileo P, Strauss SJ, Coleman J, Briggs TW, Haile SR, Seddon BM. What is the role of routine follow-up for localised limb soft tissue sarcomas? A retrospective analysis of 174 patients. Br J Cancer. 2014;110(10):2420–6. https://doi.org/10.1038/bjc.2014.200. Epub 2014 Apr 15. PMID: 24736584; PMCID: PMC4021531

3 MRI Assessment of Surgical Margins, Residual Tumors and Recurring Lesions

Nicolò Gennaro

3.1 Introduction

As shown in the previous chapter, MRI is the most accurate imaging modality to describe tumor characteristics in a multi-parametric manner, including both anatomical (spin-echo sequences) and functional information (DWI, DCE-MRI, etc.). High-field, high-quality MRI (1.5–3.0 T) is now available in all reference centers dealing with the diagnosis and treatment of soft tissue sarcoma. MRI provides a baseline study to guide tumor biopsy and allow surgical approaches aimed at wide-margin resections. In fact, an adequate preoperative assessment of both the tumor size and the peritumoral space reduces the likelihood of positive margin resections, which are associated with a higher risk of local tumor relapse, the development of distant metastases, and tumor-associated mortality [1]. Due to its exquisite contrast resolution of soft tissue, MRI is also the imaging modality of choice for postoperative follow-up, allowing postoperative changes to be distinguished from recurrent or residual tumors. In addition to morphological sequences, advanced imaging sequences help radiologists early detect tumor relapses, making a considerable impact on patient survival. In this chapter, we will discuss postoperative imaging of soft tissue sarcomas. We will also review the follow-up strategies and report the diagnostic performance of MRI according to the latest literature. To fully understand the pathologic findings, we will start first by briefly reviewing the etiopathogenesis and epidemiology of local recurrence, along with the normal appearance of soft tissue postoperative changes.

N. Gennaro (✉)
Radiology Department, Feinberg School of Medicine – Northwestern University, Chicago, IL, USA
e-mail: nicolo.gennaro@northwestern.edu

3.2 The Concept of Surgical Margins from a Radiological Perspective

The risk of local recurrence is intrinsically associated with the extent of surgical margins, which should theoretically be planned as wide as possible while limiting functional loss [1–3].

Given the importance of achieving adequate surgical margins, it is imperative that preoperative imaging properly assesses the extent of the tumor and its relationships with the surrounding structures. Thus, the radiologist needs to familiarize himself with the concept of surgical compartments and how it affects surgical planning. An anatomic compartment is represented by an anatomical structure or space whose boundaries are either bone, fascia, connective septa, articular cartilage, joint capsule, ligaments, tendon or tendon sheaths [4]. The skin, the subcutaneous tissue, the muscle compartments, the periosseous space, the bone, and the joints represent the five basic compartments. When a tumor or the peritumoral reactive zone (which is represented by peritumoral tissue visualized either as pseudocapsule or edema at MRI) invades a nearby compartment, it is referred to as extra-compartmental and is at higher risk of local and distant spread. The first to introduce the concept of the anatomical compartment into a staging system for sarcoma was Enneking et al., with the Enneking/MSTS evaluation criteria in 1980 [5]. They described four types of surgical margins: *curative wide* (>5 cm from the tumor-reactive zone), *wide margin* (<5 cm from tumor surface, being named adequate if >2 cm outside the reactive zone), *marginal margin* (within the tumor-reactive zone), and *intralesional margin* (macroscopic tumor left in place). Kawaguchi et al. further proposed an evaluation system to differentiate surgical margins according to the barrier theory, which takes not only the quantity of healthy tissue around the tumor but also the quality of it [6]. Accordingly, a *thick barrier* (strong membranous tissue with a white tendinous luster, iliotibial band, presacral fascia, joint capsule, pediatric periosteum) is the equivalent of 3-cm thickness of normal tissue, and a *thin barrier* (weaker membranous tissue

H. Özger et al. (eds.), *Diagnosis and Treatment of Soft Tissue Tumors*, https://doi.org/10.1007/978-3-031-77061-6_3

of muscle fascia, periosteum of an adult, vessel sheath, and epineurium) is the equivalent of 2-cm thickness of normal tissue. The growth plate may be either a thick or thin barrier, depending on age (in infant and young patients it is considered a thick one). Joint cartilage is considered the equivalent of a 5-cm thickness of normal tissue. Keeping these considerations in mind, the radiologist should carefully identify those structures on MRI to present them in a multidisciplinary tumor board to discuss surgical planning.

MRI is considered the best modality for local staging, as it allows accurate assessment of the anatomical compartments involved by the tumor. An infiltrative pattern along fascial planes ("tail sign") is typically found in myxofibrosarcoma and undifferentiated pleomorphic sarcoma (UPS) and is commonly associated with extra-compartmental growth [7] and tumor satellites (Fig. 3.1). Another finding that needs to be included in the radiological report is the extension through different anatomic compartments of peritumoral edema or peritumoral enhancing tissue [8], which has been associated with a higher risk of local recurrence [8].

Currently, there is no specific preoperative evaluation method to evaluate surgical margins. However, a novel method of designing an accurate surgical margin before operations for malignant bone and soft tissue tumors has been recently described by Hao et al. using a CT- and MRI-based augmented reality technique [9]. Once the tumor volume is segmented, the ideal surgical margins can be visualized and discussed, potentially improving the quality of the surgical planning.

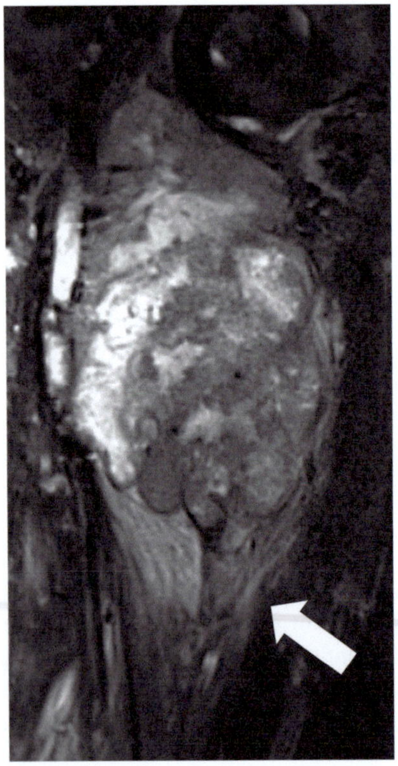

Fig. 3.1 Sagittal T2FS image of an undifferentiated pleomorphic sarcoma (UPS). Note the tail sign in the lower extremity of the tumor (arrow)

It is important to remember that for low-grade STS a narrower surgical margin (>2 mm) is considered adequate and that the ideal surgical margins vary depending on the specific histotypes [10].

3.3 Local Recurrence in Soft Tissue Sarcoma

Both intrinsic and extrinsic factors contribute to recurrent disease. Intrinsic patient and tumor characteristics include the biological aggressiveness of the tumor (FNCLCC grade), the age of the patient, the size of the tumor, and the anatomical location—especially the depth within the soft tissues. Grade III sarcoma are at the highest risk of local recurrence, as well as those sarcoma considered high-grade by definition (MPNST, rhabdomyosarcoma, Ewing sarcoma, clear cell sarcoma, alveolar sarcoma, epithelioid sarcoma). High-grade STS with a high risk of local recurrence are angiosarcoma, leiomyosarcoma, myxofibrosarcoma or UPS. Extrinsic factors are related to the quality of treatment received—in particular the adequacy of resection margins, contamination of the operative bed with friable/ruptured tumors, or specific surgical techniques (i.e. piecemeal resections). Soft tissue sarcoma are aggressive tumors that tend to recur locally, even if radical resection has been performed with free margins. This happens in up to 10–20% of cases (Figs. 3.2, 3.3 and 3.4). Local recurrences are higher in truncal, retroperitoneal and head and neck sarcomas, due to the technical challenge in achieving a radical resection. Positive margins after resection increase by up to six times the risk of local recurrence. Recurrence can occur after several years, and can either be located in the surgical bed or in deeper plans. Overall, the risk of local recurrence ranges from 6.5–8.5% after 2 years to 25–32% after 10 years [3]. The risk of local recurrence can be lowered when a multidisciplinary team cooperates to achieve wide resections to chase oncologic radicality [11]. Planned surgical resections significantly decrease the risk of recurrence, and that is why a comprehensive imaging assessment and multidisciplinary discussion before surgery are important. Late tumor recurrence can also be observed along the biopsy needle path due to tumor seeding. Finally, neoadjuvant/adjuvant therapies (chemo/radiation) can also reduce the risk of local recurrence [12]. Although it is not proven that neoadjuvant chemotherapy improves local tumor control, adjuvant/neoadjuvant radiotherapy does, at least in extremity sarcomas [13]. In the case of positive margins after a previous resection, revision surgery is always warranted regardless of the imaging appearance, as MR imaging might be unreliable

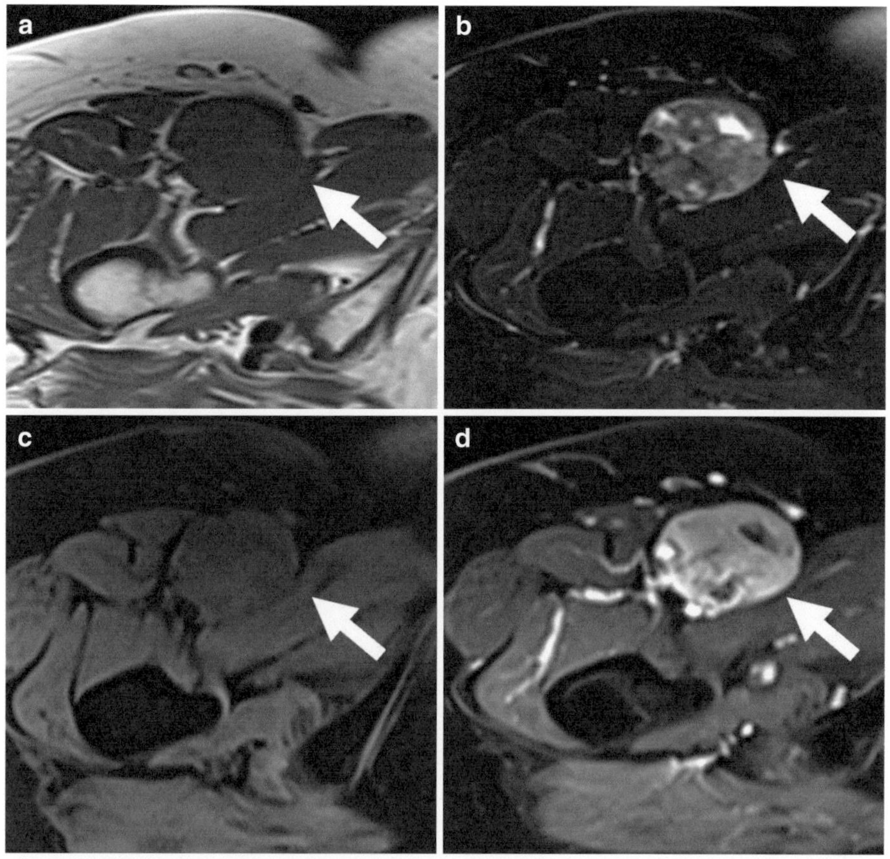

Fig. 3.2 70-year-old female patient. She presented with deep venous thrombosis and pulmonary embolism secondary to a 5.5 cm mass in the upper right thigh, consistent with G2 leiomyosarcoma. The mass shows intermediate T1 (**a**) and T1FS (**c**) signal intensity, necrotic/cystic internal areas on T2FS (**b**), and enhancing solid nodular tissue on T1FS after gadolinium (**d**). The lesion arose distal to the right saphenofemoral junction (arrows), between the right great saphenous vein and the right femoral vein. Radical resection of the mass with en-bloc resection of the right common femoral vein and sartorius transposition flap and veno-venous bypass with cryopreserved femoral-popliteal artery interposition graft in the femoral vein was planned. Negative proximal and distant surgical margins were achieved

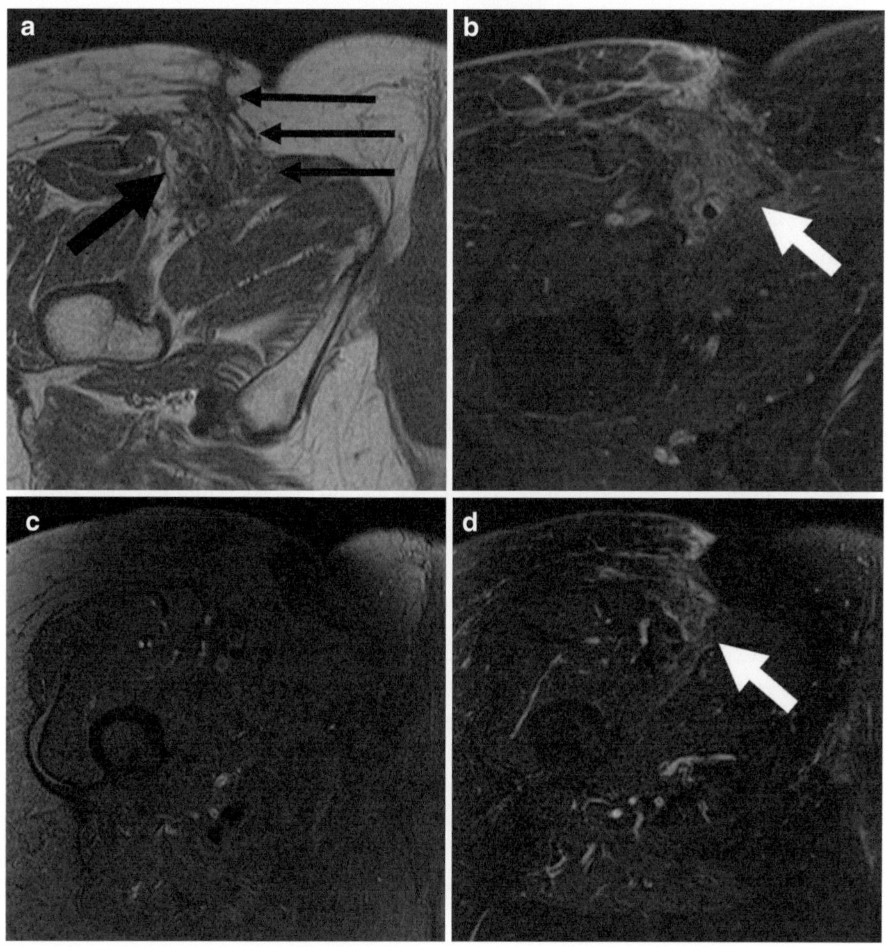

Fig. 3.3 The previously seen mass along the right femoral vessels is no longer visualized. There is no distortion of the subcutaneous fat with an intermediate T1 signal extending obliquely from the lateral hip to the medial proximal to mid-thigh, consistent with scarring (**a**, thin black arrows). The distorted subcutaneous soft tissues also demonstrate poorly defined edema on T2FS (**b**), isointense signal to muscle on T1FS (**c**), and enhancement on Gd-T1FS (**d**), none of which is nodular. The underlying muscle fibers are tethered in the region of the groin with similar, poorly defined signal areas in the overlying soft tissues at the level of the femoral vessels (thick black arrow, **a**). Findings are consistent with normal postoperative changes

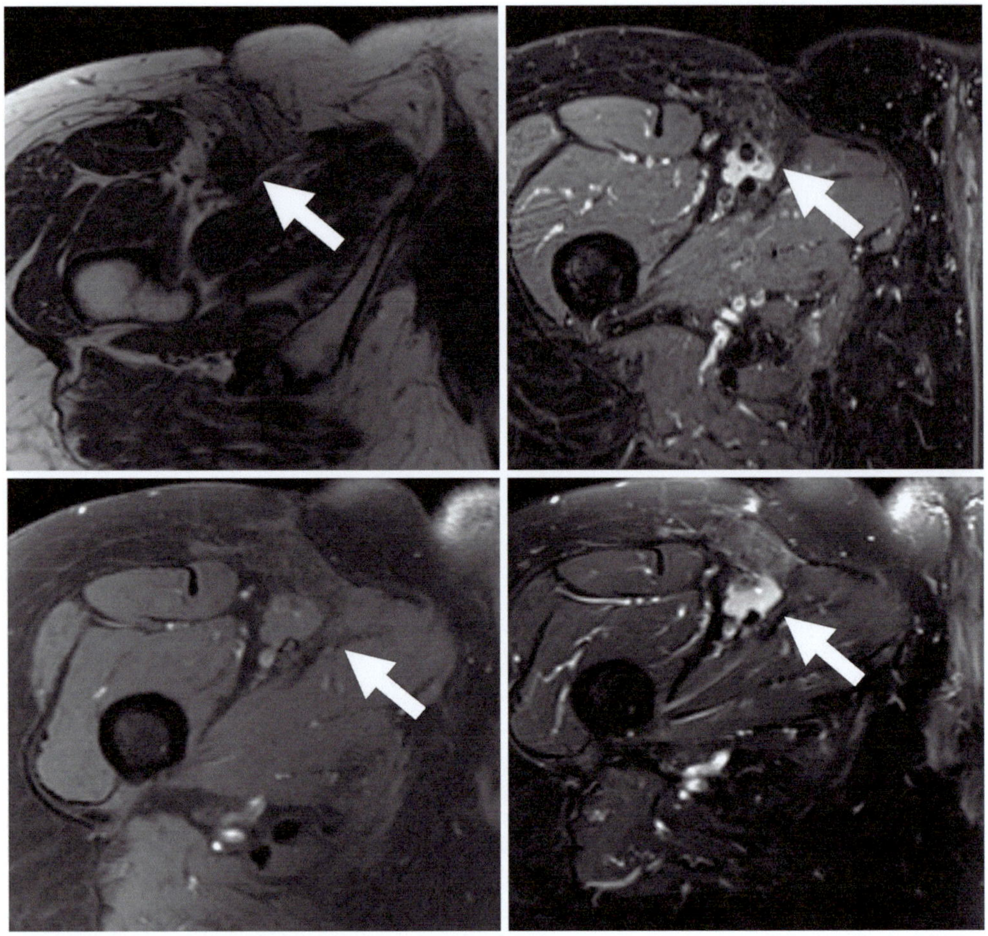

Fig. 3.4 There is a new 2 cm-nodular enhancing soft tissue lesion, partially encasing the right femoral artery. Signal intensity reminds us of the original lesion on all sequences. The sciatic nerve is distant from the mass. The mass is abutting the femoral nerve with suspicion of involvement (think black arrow). There is normal osseous alignment and marrow signal. Postsurgical changes are seen in the rectus femoris, with fatty atrophy and mild intramuscular edema. Radiotherapy was recommended in this case

in detecting microscopic disease [14, 15]. Still, preoperative MRI is always recommended to plan the revision surgery to identify vital structures and describe tumor margins in case of macroscopic residual disease, or to identify the most likely areas of residual tumors in case of microscopic residual disease. Due to its exquisite contrast resolution for soft tissues, MRI is also the imaging modality of choice for postoperative follow-up, allowing postoperative changes to be distinguished from recurrent or residual tumors. In addition to morphological sequences, advanced imaging sequences help radiologists in such a delicate task. DCE-MRI and DWI are advanced imaging techniques available in many reference centers that improve the detection of local recurrence and will be discussed later in this chapter [16, 17].

3.4 Postoperative Changes: Nonpathological Findings

Postoperative MRI evaluation requires a systematic approach to understanding normal anatomy and discriminating pathological from nonpathological findings. For a proper MRI assessment of the surgical bed, comprehensive information about the patient's clinical history, the type, and timing of the surgical resection need to be available, along with the report of any neoadjuvant or postoperative treatments the patient may have received (i.e. chemo and/or radiation therapy). The histopathology of the original tumor and access to previous imaging is critical, as the recurrent/residual tumor usually resembles the original one. Most of the tissue expected to be found in the surgical bed is reactive/inflammation and granulation tissue, but postoperative images are also important to identify potential complications, such as fatty necrosis/atrophy, local bursitis, cellulitis, abscess or osteomyelitis, neuroma, hematoma or heterotopic ossification.

If the patient receives radiation therapy, radiation-induced changes are time-dependent and usually appear as diffuse edema throughout the soft tissues within the radiation field (Fig. 3.6). Soft tissue edema or lymphoedema is usually most evident in the subcutaneous fat plane and can extend through the muscle fascias, where it usually persists longer than in the fat or muscle up to several years [8] (Fig. 3.6). After RT, subcutaneous fat within the radiation field tends to increase in thickness, whether the muscle tends to atrophy.

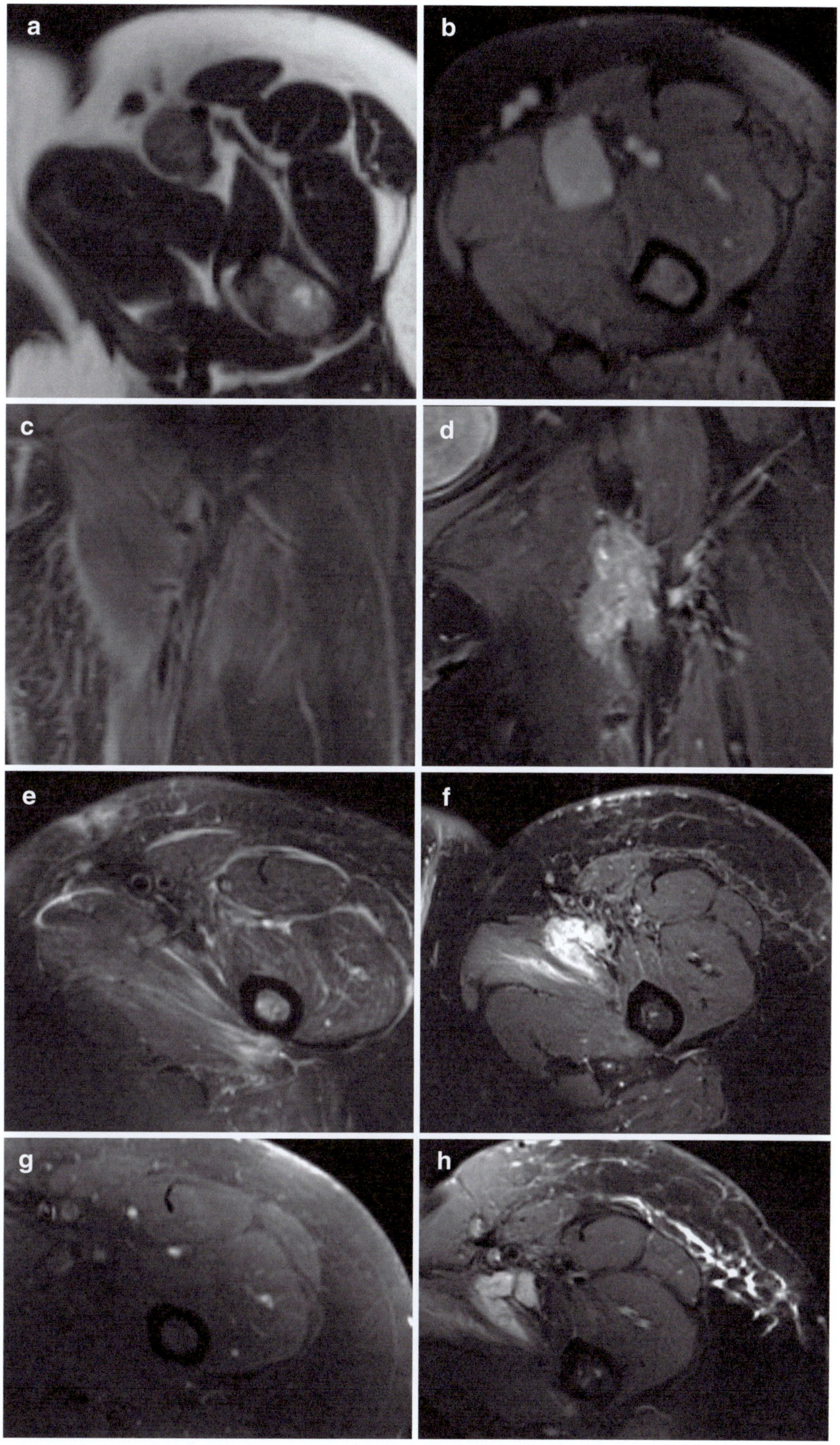

Fig. 3.5 30-year-old woman with a 10 cm-solid lesion in her left lower extremity, diagnosed with grade III undifferentiated spindle cell sarcoma. The lesion was slightly hyperintense on T2 (**a**) and strongly enhancing on Gd-T1FS (**b**). She was treated with femoral vein/artery endarterectomy and excision of the mass with reconstruction. Postsurgical study reveals scarring around the femoral artery, diffuse fascial and intramuscular edema on T2FS (**e**) and no enhancing nodular tissue on Gd-T1FS (**c**, axial plane; **g**, coronal plane). She further underwent adjuvant radiotherapy (60–65 Gy over 6 weeks) and systemic therapy. However, after 3 years she developed local recurrence, strongly hyperintense on T2FS (**f**) and enhancing on Gd-T1FS (**h**, axial plane; **d**, coronal plane). Interestingly, her first presentation was deep venous thrombosis and saddle pulmonary embolism, like the case shown in Figs. 3.1, 3.2 and 3.3

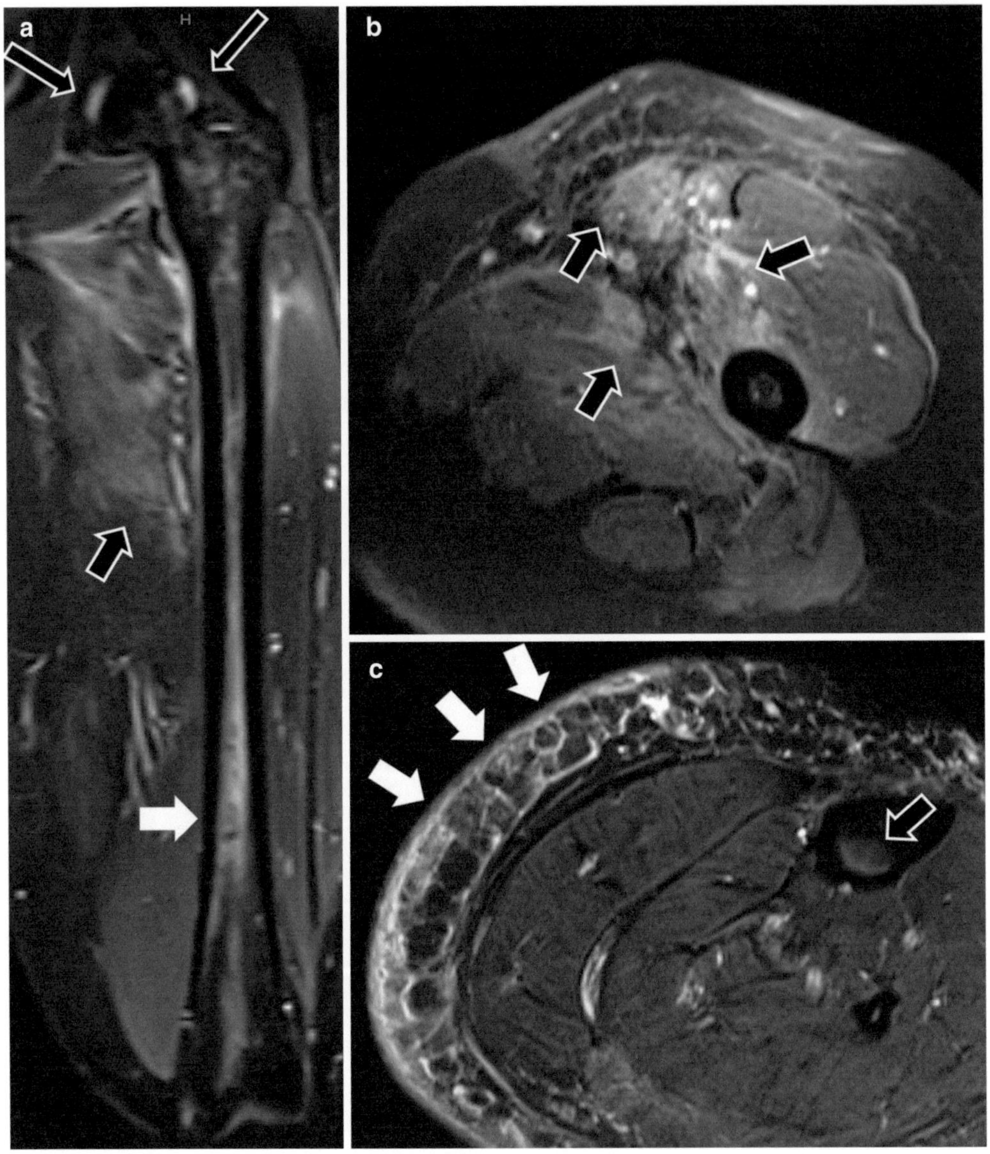

Fig. 3.6 Same case of Fig. 3.5. (**a**) Sagittal T2FS showing bone marrow edema (white arrow) due to radiation osteitis, along with intramuscular edema in the surgical bed (black arrow). Note the mild hip effusion (black thin arrows) and the bone marrow T2FS hyperintensity consistent with radiation osteitis (white arrow) (**b**) Strongly enhancing muscular tissue on Gd-T1FS consistent with postsurgical myositis (arrows) close to the surgical bed, characterized by architectural distortion due to scarring (**c**) Subcutaneous lymphedema is shown on T2FS after radiation therapy and surgery (white arrows)

RT-induced edema usually increases up to 18 months after radiation therapy, and it can take years to disappear [18]. It is better highlighted on fat-suppressed T2-weighted images or STIR images, which are more sensitive than T2-weighted fast spin-echo images in the detection of subtle fluid hyperintensity (Figs. 3.6 and 3.7). Similar to radiation therapy, chemotherapy may cause soft tissue edema-like signal-intensity changes on long-echo sequences [8]. Ill-defined bone marrow edema-like changes in signal intensity can be either associated with radiation-induced osteitis or fatty replacement due to the cytotoxic effect of radiation therapy or chemotherapy (Fig. 3.6). Postsurgical scarring and fibrotic tissue usually exhibit enhancement in the early phase of the postsurgical period (2–4 weeks), and then gradually fade. Scarring contraction is frequent in the last phase of the postsurgical period (months to years) [8] when the tissue presents a low-intensity signal on T1-T2-weighted images. Granulation tissue often represents a challenge in the differentiation between tumor recurrence/residual tumors and is characterized by intermediate signal intensity with moderate enhancement after contrast administration. Low signal-intensity areas after surgery are usually considered postoperative changes, including heterotopic ossifications [10], but tumor calcifications and fibrotic components can also theoretically be found in residual/recurrent lesions.

Postsurgical seromas are usually surrounded by mild edema and are typically found in the lower extremities. They have a taller-than-larger shape characterizes them with well-defined T2 hyperintense/T1w-hypo-intense areas and a thin rim enhancement after contrast administration. However, blood products can be found within them and influence their MR signal accordingly. In this case, T1-w hyperintense components can be found due to the presence of hemorrhagic breakdown products (extracellular meta-hemoglobin). In a

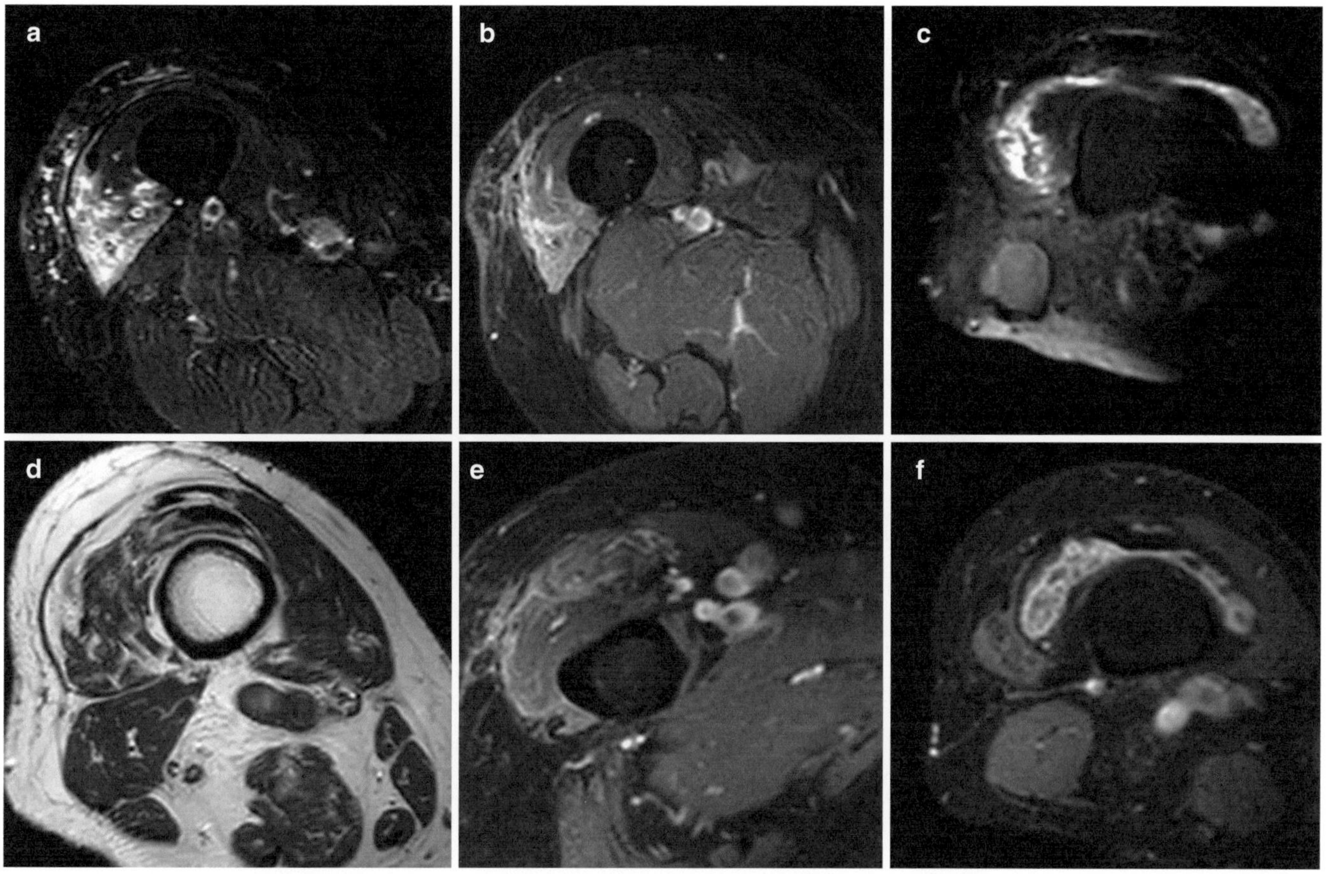

Fig. 3.7 Intramuscular edema is shown after surgical resection and neoadjuvant radiotherapy on T2FS (**a**) Moderate enhancement is seen on T1 after gadolinium at the myotendinous junction (**b**) in the vastus lateralis, while postsurgical scarring without nodular enhancement is seen at the site of resection (**e**). Fatty atrophy is seen in the vastus lateralis on T1 (**d**). Synovial hypertrophy is common after locoregional surgery, hyperintense on T2FS (**c**) with strong contrast enhancement on Gd-T1FS (**f**)

retrospective study on 175 patients, Lantos et al. described that 40% of the fluid collections had heterogeneous fluid signal intensity, 60% had septa, 16% had signal intensity consistent with blood products, 31% did not have a thin rim, and 88% had rim enhancement [19]. A nodule within postoperative fluid collection generally does not represent tumor recurrence, and a short-interval follow-up MRI is recommended rather than an immediate biopsy (Fig. 3.8).

Lymphoceles have similar imaging features to seromas, which occur more often in the pelvis and in the retroperitoneum. In the first weeks after surgery, local hematomas are frequent, and they tend to organize over time with a wide spectrum of MRI appearance according to the solid and cystic components and their maturation. They can have a mass effect and a peripheral rim of contrast enhancement, but, as seromas, they do not enhance internally. Resolution of seroma is variable, but they are usually reabsorbed within 3–18 months. The so-called muscle texture sign on T1-weighted sequences (whether the muscle texture sign is preserved) can help discriminate postoperative changes from viable tumor areas [20]. It is important to be aware that myocutaneous flaps can be used for complex reconstructive surgery. They appear T2-hyperintense with mild contrast-enhancement and can have T1-hyperintense components due to fatty atrophy. Tissue edema usually disappears progressively from the site of surgical resection, leaving space for the formation of fibrotic streaks that will lose their signal intensity progressively on both T1 and T2-weighted images.

Unfortunately, it is not rare for soft tissue sarcomas to undergo unplanned procedures without proper local staging, as a benign soft tissue tumor is expected (i.e. lipoma or ganglion). In this case, the lack of preoperative imaging represents a real challenge for the radiologist, as no information on the original tumor extent and morphology is available.

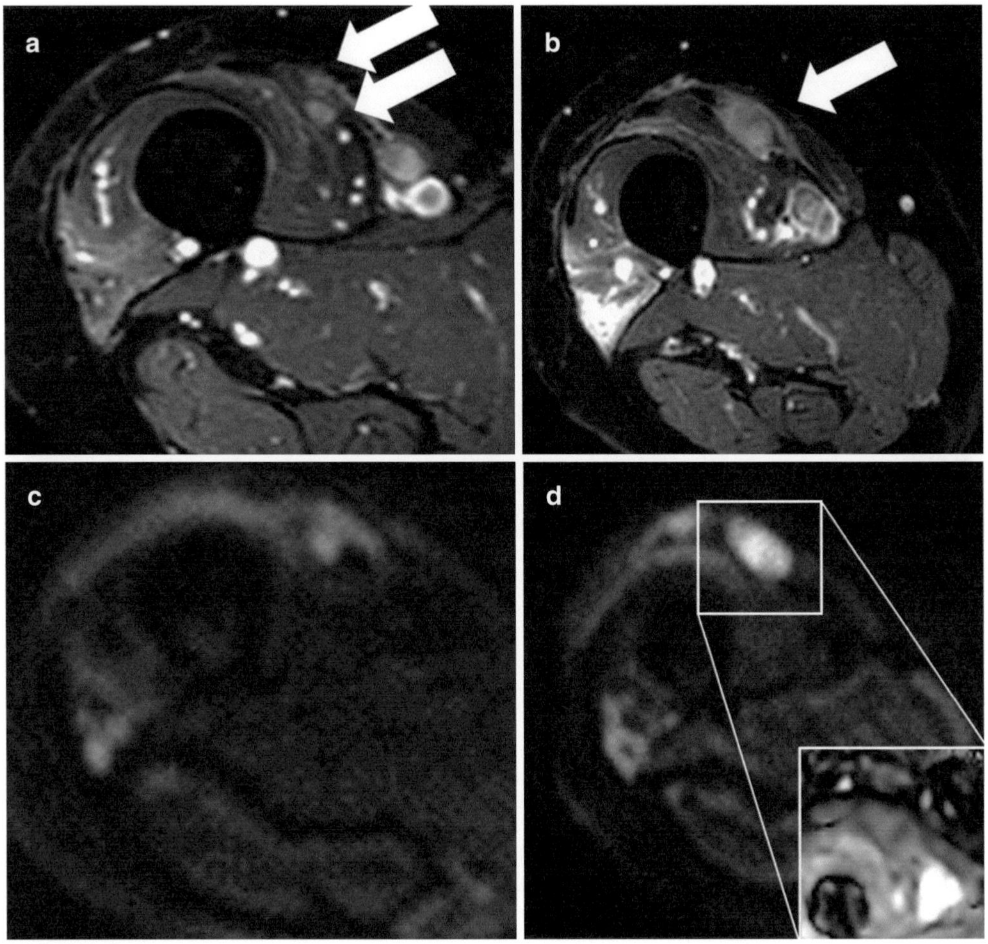

Fig. 3.8 Same patient of Fig. 3.6. 2-year follow-up Gd-T1FS axial image of two nodular enhancing lesions (arrows) in the vastus medialis (**a**) suspicious for local recurrence. DWI ($b = 100$) shows signal restriction (**c**), consistent with malignant tissue. The patient refused further treatment, and 6 months later Gd-T1FS showed a dimensional increase of the lesion (**b**), with restricted DWI signal and low ADC values (**d**)

3.5 Recurrent or Residual Tumor: Distinctive Features

A typical recurrent/residual soft tissue sarcoma is usually seen as intermediate-to-high signal-intensity discrete nodular mass on fat-saturated (or STIR) T2-weighted images, with low signal intensity on T1-weighted images (Fig. 3.5). It causes a mass-like replacement of normal muscle texture and creates a mass effect on the surrounding structures, as opposed to post-therapeutic strikes caused either by radiation therapy or chemotherapy, which retract surrounding structures rather than compress them. However, it can be challenging to distinguish postoperative inflammatory changes from recurrent or viable tumors, especially during the first 3–6 months. For example, local relapse of myxoid sarcomas can erroneously be diagnosed as seroma, particularly if the radiologist is not aware of the MR morphology of the original lesion and its inherent high signal intensity on T2-weighted images. Moreover, only minimal lace-like enhancement may be appreciated in sarcomas with myxoid content. Also, for this reason, preoperative imaging should always be available for comparison when assessing for postoperative recurrence. Inflammatory changes can also present as a nodular lesion, especially if there is a fibrotic component. DCE-MRI is a game-changer in this setting, as it identifies viable tumor areas as an early, conspicuous enhancement with a steep slope in the dynamic SI curve (Fig. 3.9). Benign entities such as pigmented villonodular synovitis (PVNS), nodular fasciitis (also called pseudosarcomatous fasciitis or infiltrative fasciitis), and fibromatosis can also present such enhancement characteristics, but they are usually of low signal intensity on T2-weighted images. Conversely, postoperative reactive and inflammatory changes are usually present with a slow, moderate and late enhancement curve on DCE-MRI. Subtraction imaging can be of valuable help, as it improves detection of recurrent tumors and increases lesion conspicuity. DWI is another key player to complement the interpretation of morphologic and dynamic sequences. DWI has been shown to provide 93.3% sensitivity and 92.5% specificity (b-1000 values, cut off 2 × 103 s/mm^2) [21]. However, DWI may present some interpretation caveats in the detection of local recurrence and residual tumors. Hematoma usually restricts the diffusion of water molecules, creating false positives on DWI. Conversely, myxoid liposarcoma and myxofibrosarcoma contain myxoid areas that allow diffusion of water molecules, creating false nega-

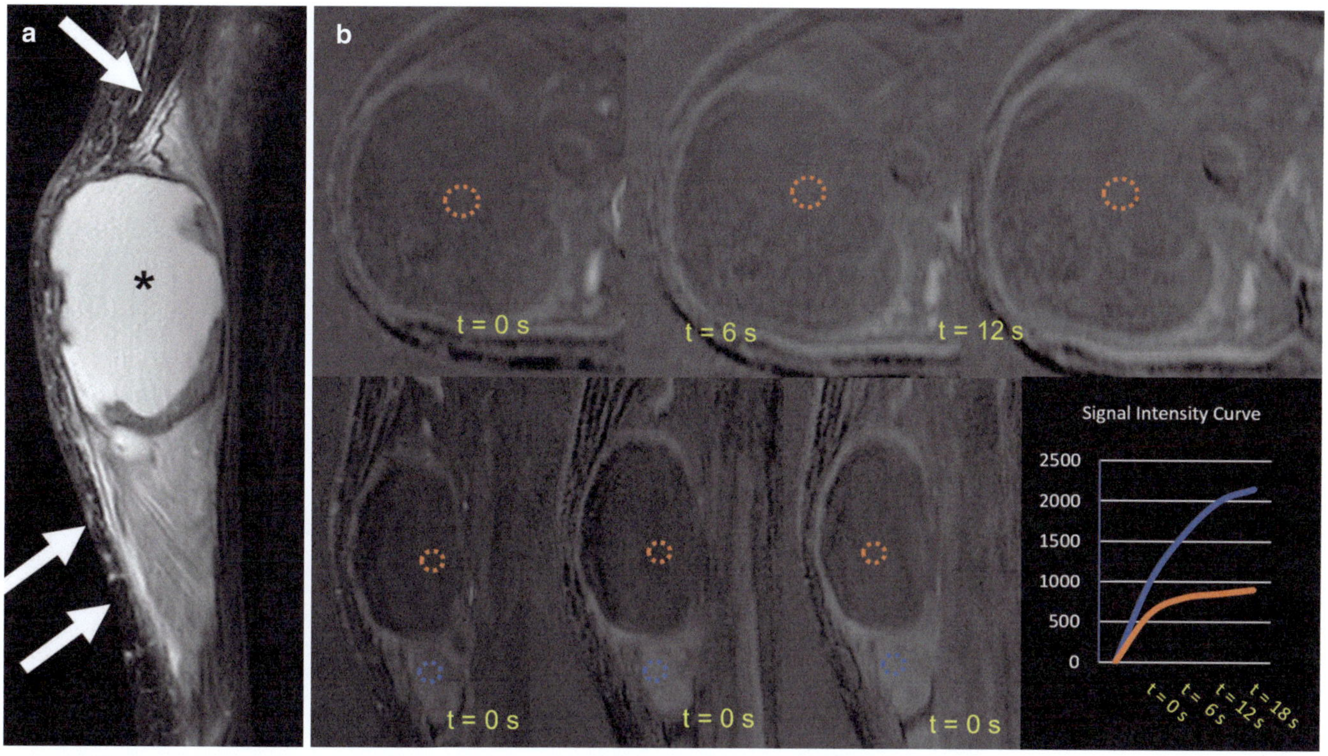

Fig. 3.9 T2FS sagittal image of a voluminous tumor in the anterior right lower thigh, consistent with local recurrence of a previously treated dedifferentiated liposarcoma of the right thigh. The intense muscular edema (**a**, arrows) is secondary to recent radiation therapy (V-MAT, 50Gy), as well as the high amount of necrotic tissue (**a**, asterisk) DCE-MRI (**b**) shows on subtraction Gd-T1FS different patterns of contrast enhancement in the necrotic habitat (orange line) and in the nodular residual tumor in the lower part of the lesion (blue line). The patient then underwent radical surgical resection

tives on DWI, with a high-intensity signal on the ADC map (Fig. 3.10). Such local recurrences may thus be misinterpreted as postoperative fluid collection or overlooked. Again, reviewing the characteristics of the original tumor and spotting solid nodules within the myxoid areas can prevent erroneous interpretations. Another characteristic of recurrent myxofibrosarcoma is that it can present as a tapering, tail-like margin growing along the deep fascia enveloping the underlying muscle. Recurrent UPS can also present as plaque-like “tails”, instead of the classical nodular appearance of tumor recurrence [21, 22].

Radiation-induced sarcomas have a different histologic composition than the patients’ original treated tumors. They grow within the field of previous radiation therapy treatment, therefore, MRI characteristics widely differ [23]. High-grade undifferentiated pleomorphic sarcoma (UPS) is the most common post-radiation sarcoma of the soft tissues. Extraskeletal osteosarcoma and fibrosarcoma follow, representing 13% and 11% of cases, respectively. Conversely, osteosarcoma is the most common radiation-induced malignancy that affects bone, accounting for approximately 60% of cases, followed by UPS (20%).

In the case of limb salvage procedures with reconstruction, myocutaneous flap placement, or amputation, MRI requires metal reduction techniques in the imaging algorithm. After positioning allografts, most recurrent tumors are found in the soft tissues of the surgical bed, and more rarely in the native bone adjacent to the host-al-graft junction. Recurrence in the allograft is unlikely due to its avascularity [24]. They are usually of higher histological grade compared to the original, reflecting an increased biological aggressiveness. Amputation does not prevent local recurrences. Proton MR spectroscopy is a noninvasive tool with the potential in the characterization of lesion composition and malignant activity. Both single-voxel and multivoxel MR spectroscopy are feasible with 3-T MRI. Fayad and colleagues found that choline signal-to-noise ratios were statistically different for malignant and benign lesions (11.7 vs 2.3, p = 0.04), as performed with a surface coil [25].

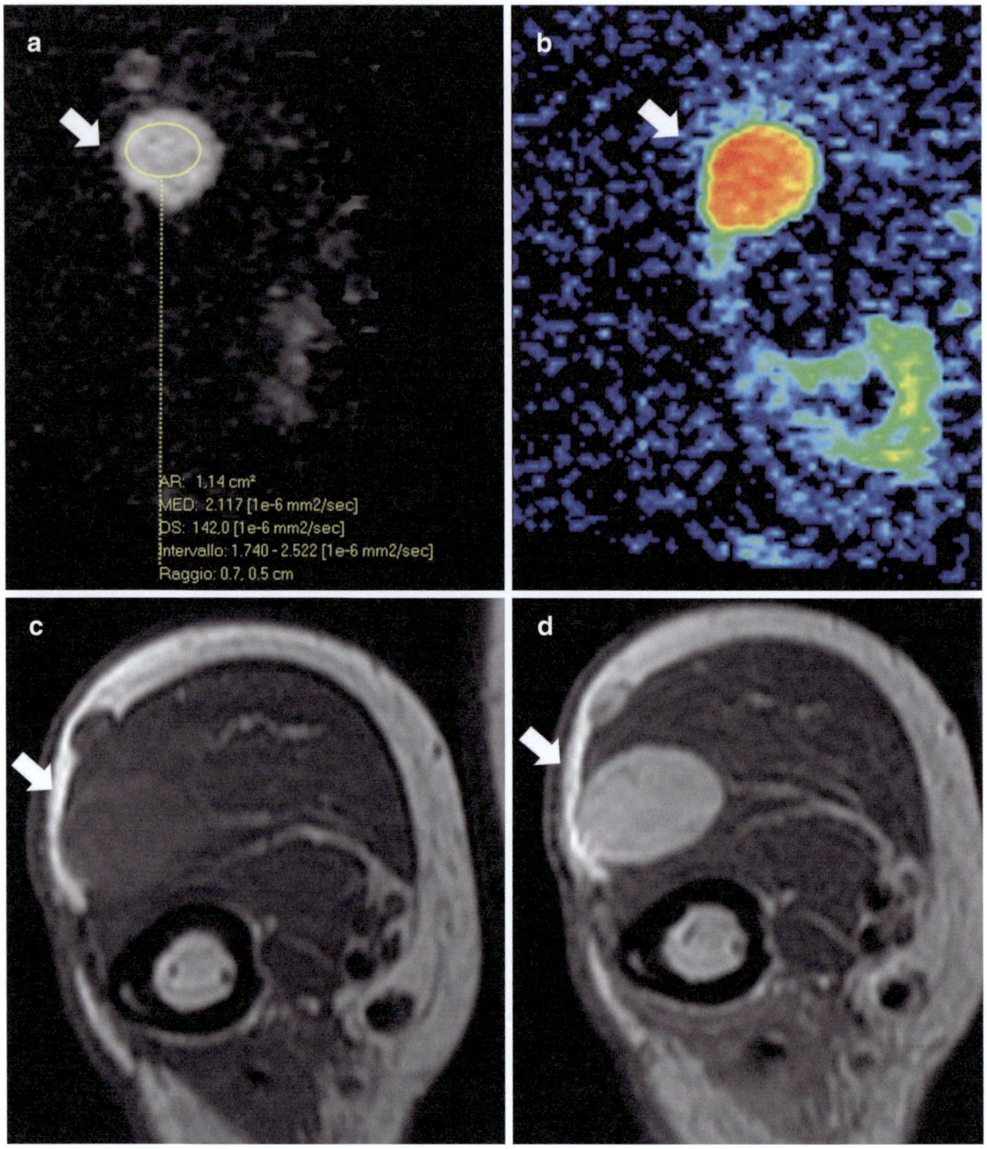

Fig. 3.10 Recurrence of myxofibrosarcoma of the upper right extremity. ADC map (**a**, **b**) shows high signal intensity due to the high content of the myxoid matrix. The lesion appears slightly hyperintense on T1 (**c**) and strongly hyperintense on T2 (**d**)

3.6 Diagnostic Performance of MRI

MRI has been reported to have excellent diagnostic accuracy in the detection of residual or recurrent disease, with a sensitivity and specificity as high as 98% and 90%, respectively [26–28]. However, the reported diagnostic performance of MRI in the detection of recurrent or residual tumors is heterogeneous across the radiologic literature, as it depends on the tumor site and the diagnostic protocols used. According to a recent systematic review, MRI provides a mean sensitivity and specificity of 71.7% and 79.3% for the identification of residual disease, and 87.9% and 85.9%, for local recurrence, respectively [28]. The diagnostic accuracy decreases in subcutaneous lesions and after surgery with radiation therapy, compared to intramuscular lesions and surgery alone. For example, in a retrospective study on soft tissue sarcoma of the hand surgically re-treated after initial marginal excision, the diagnostic accuracy of MRI was generally lower. The sensitivity of MRI in detecting residual soft tissue sarcoma of the hand was 60%, and the specificity was 78%, whereas for detecting gross residual disease, the sensitivity was 89% and the specificity was 79%. The inclusion of DCE-MRI and DWI in the MRI diagnostic protocol [16] can increase diagnostic accuracy, as well as PET [29–31]. It is important to remember that most local recurrences in the extremities are first detected during clinical follow-ups or by the patient itself [15, 16], but MRI can detect early local recurrences when still clinically silent [26, 32]. A recent meta-analysis of 19 studies assessing the usefulness of imaging follow-up in the detection of local recurrence and its impact on survival surveillance on survival concluded that high-field MRI surveillance detects clinically occult local recurrences (Fig. 3.11) or deep-seated lesions, with positive impact on patient survival in several studies [33].

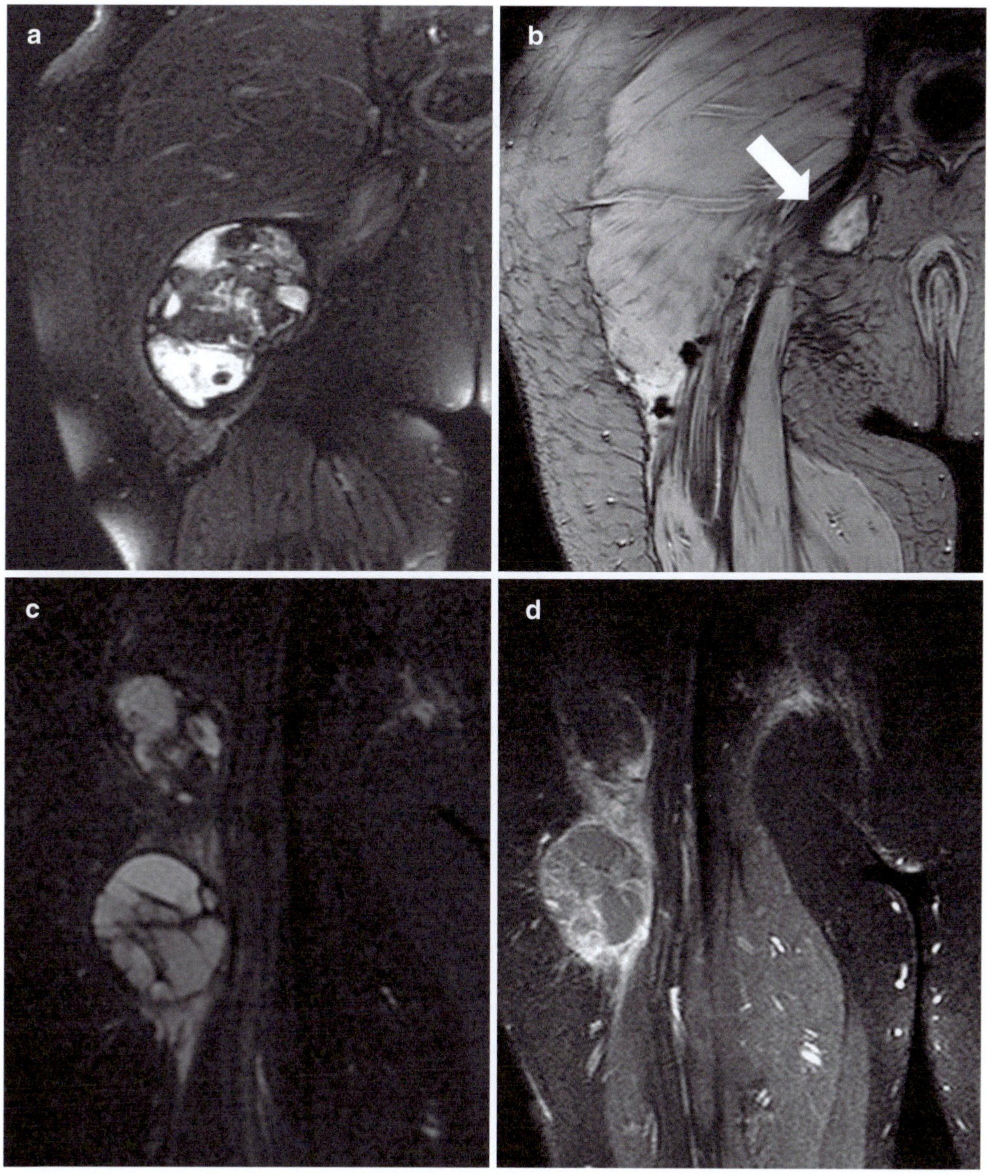

Fig. 3.11 Coronal T2FS image shows an inhomogeneous mass within the right gluteus with pseudocapsule and mild perilesional edema, clinically undetectable (**a**). The lesion was consistent with high-grade UPS. After 9 months, a 3-cm nodular enhancing lesion is found within the resection bed (GdT1FS, arrow, **b**). After neoadjuvant chemo-radiotherapy, the mass shows cystic changes (coronal T2FS, **c**) with solid peripheral nodular tissue and intralesional septa (coronal Gd-T1FS, **d**)

3.7 Follow-up Guidelines

No evidence-based follow-up schedules are available for surgically treated soft tissue sarcomas, nor many publications regarding the cost-effectiveness of follow-up strategies are available [34]. A paradigm for postoperative imaging is that it should not be performed until at least 6–8 weeks after the initial surgery, as in the immediate postoperative period inflammatory changes would hinder relevant imaging findings. Considering that around 70% of local recurrences occur within 2–3 years after surgery, the European Society of Medical Oncology (ESMO) and the European Society of Musculoskeletal Radiology (ESSR) recommend that intermediate or high-grade sarcomas undergo an MRI of the original tumor site every 3–4 months in the first 2–3 years, then every 6 months up to the fifth year, and once a year up to the tenth year. In selected cases, ultrasound has been proposed as an alternative to MRI in the follow-up of extremity soft tissue sarcomas with similar diagnostic performance [35].

3.8 Conclusion

MRI is currently the best imaging modality radiologists can count on for the diagnostic assessment, local staging, and follow-up of STS. The complexity of the imaging findings requires high-quality protocols and specific expertise available in reference centers. The increasing availability of advanced MRI is providing better diagnostic accuracy in the identification of both local recurrence and residual tumors, making an impact on patient survival. As a critical element of the multidisciplinary sarcoma expertise, imaging provides a continuous assessment of sarcoma patients throughout the therapeutic journey. The radiologist involved in sarcoma care should be intimately involved in the multidisciplinary discussion to understand the unique needs of this family of tumors to help guide patient management [36].

Acknowledgments Courtesy of Northwestern Memorial Hospital, Chicago, USA[1]: Figs. 3.1, 3.2, 3.3, 3.4, 3.5 and 3.6; Courtesy of Ente Ospedaliero Cantonale (EOC), Switzerland[2]: Figs. 3.7, 3.8 and 3.9; Courtesy of Rizzoli Orthopedic Institute, Bologna, Italy[3]: Fig. 3.10; Courtesy of Humanitas Research Hospital, Rozzano, Italy[4]: Fig. 3.11. The author thanks Dr. Ali Serhali[1], Meghana Karri[1], Prof. Yury Velichko[1], Dr. Claudia Corraliza, Dr. Giovanni Zancan[2], Dr. Marco Curti[2], Prof. Filippo Del Grande[2], Dr. Paolo Spinnato[3], Dr. Andrea Marrari[3], Dr. Luca Balzarini[4], Dr. Alexia F. Bertuzzi[4], Dr. Maria S. Grimaudo[4], Dr. Silvio Romano[4] for their support and expertise.

References

1. Potter BK, Hwang PF, Forsberg JA, et al. Impact of margin status and local recurrence on soft-tissue sarcoma outcomes. J Bone Joint Surg Am. 2013;9520:e151.
2. Jang WY, Kim H-S, Han I. Impact of surgical margin on survival in extremity soft tissue sarcoma: a systematic review and meta-analysis. Medicine (Baltimore). 2021;1003:e24124.
3. Harati K, Goertz O, Pieper A, et al. Soft tissue sarcomas of the extremities: surgical margins can be close as long as the resected tumor has no ink on it. Oncologist. 2017;2211:1400–10.
4. Anderson MW, Temple HT, Dussault RG, et al. Compartmental anatomy: relevance to staging and biopsy of musculoskeletal tumors. AJR Am J Roentgenol. 1999;1736:1663–71.
5. Enneking WF, Spanier SS, Goodman MA. A system for the surgical staging of musculoskeletal sarcoma. Clin Orthop Relat Res. 1980;153:106–20.
6. Kawaguchi N, Matumoto S, Manabe J. New method of evaluating the surgical margin and safety margin for musculoskeletal sarcoma, analysed on the basis of 457 surgical cases. J Cancer Res Clin Oncol. 1995;1219–10:555–63.
7. Nakamura T, Matsumine A, Matsubara T, et al. Infiltrative tumor growth patterns on magnetic resonance imaging associated with systemic inflammation and oncological outcome in patients with high-grade soft-tissue sarcoma. PLoS One. 2017;127:e0181787.
8. Crombé A, Le Loarer F, Stoeckle E, et al. MRI assessment of surrounding tissues in soft-tissue sarcoma during neoadjuvant chemotherapy can help predicting response and prognosis. Eur J Radiol. 2018;109:178–87.
9. Hao Y, Yang C, He J. The accurate surgical margin before surgery for malignant musculoskeletal tumors: a retrospective study. Am J Transl Res. 2018;108:2324–34.
10. Wittenberg S, Paraskevaidis M, Jarosch A, et al. Surgical margins in soft tissue sarcoma management and corresponding local and systemic recurrence rates: a retrospective study covering 11 years and 169 patients in a single institution. Life (Basel). 2022;12(11):1694.
11. Cariboni U, Gennaro N, Costa F, et al. Multi-step combined upfront surgery for locally advanced paravertebral sarcoma: a case report. Front Surg. 2021;8:664089.
12. Gennaro N, Reijers S, Bruining A, et al. Imaging response evaluation after neoadjuvant treatment in soft tissue sarcomas: where do we stand? Crit Rev Oncol Hematol. 2021;160:103309.
13. Smith HG, Memos N, Thomas JM, et al. Patterns of disease relapse in primary extremity soft-tissue sarcoma. Br J Surg. 2016;10311:1487–96.
14. Kaste SC, Hill A, Conley L, et al. Magnetic resonance imaging after incomplete resection of soft tissue sarcoma. Clin Orthop Relat Res. 2002;397:204–11.
15. Siebenrock KA, Hertel R, Ganz R. Unexpected resection of soft-tissue sarcoma. More mutilating surgery, higher local recurrence rates, and obscure prognosis as consequences of improper surgery. Arch Orthop Trauma Surg. 2000;1201–2:65–9.
16. Del Grande F, Subhawong T, Weber K, et al. Detection of soft-tissue sarcoma recurrence: added value of functional MR imaging techniques at 3.0 T. Radiology. 2014;2712:499–511.
17. Fayad LM, Jacobs MA, Wang X, et al. Musculoskeletal tumors: how to use anatomic, functional, and metabolic MR techniques. Radiology. 2012;2652:340–56.
18. Richardson ML, Zink-Brody GC, Patten RM, et al. MR characterization of post-irradiation soft tissue edema. Skeletal Radiol. 1996;256:537–43.
19. Lantos JE, Hwang S, Panicek DM. Benign mural nodules within fluid collections at MRI after soft-tissue sarcoma resection. AJR Am J Roentgenol. 2014;2026:1297–302.
20. Biondetti PR, Ehman RL. Soft-tissue sarcomas: use of textural patterns in skeletal muscle as a diagnostic feature in postoperative MR imaging. Radiology. 1992;1833:845–8.
21. Aktas E, Arikan SM, Ardıç F, et al. The importance of diffusion apparent diffusion coefficient values in the evaluation of soft tissue sarcomas after treatment. Pol J Radiol. 2021;86:e291–7.
22. Alpert JS, Boland P, Hameed M, et al. Undifferentiated pleomorphic sarcoma: indolent, tail-like recurrence of a high-grade tumor. Skeletal Radiol. 2018;471:141–4.
23. Lewis JJ, Leung D, Heslin M, et al. Association of local recurrence with subsequent survival in extremity soft tissue sarcoma. J Clin Oncol. 1997;152:646–52.
24. Kattapuram TM, Ozhathil DK, Hornicek FJ, et al. Imaging of pseudoneoplastic masses associated with allografts. Skeletal Radiol. 2007;36(8):747–53.
25. Fayad LM, Barker PB, Jacobs MA, et al. Characterization of musculoskeletal lesions on 3-T proton MR spectroscopy. AJR Am J Roentgenol. 2007;1886:1513–20.
26. Park JW, Yoo HJ, Kim H-S, et al. MRI surveillance for local recurrence in extremity soft tissue sarcoma. Eur J Surg Oncol. 2019;452:268–74.
27. England P, Hong Z, Rhea L, et al. Does advanced imaging have a role in detecting local recurrence of soft-tissue sarcoma? Clin Orthop Relat Res. 2020;47812:2812–20.
28. Pennington Z, Ahmed AK, Cottrill E, et al. Systematic review on the utility of magnetic resonance imaging for operative management and follow-up for primary sarcoma-lessons from extremity sarcomas. Ann Transl Med. 2019;710:225.
29. Erfanian Y, Grueneisen J, Kirchner J, et al. Integrated 18F-FDG PET/MRI compared to MRI alone for identification of local recurrences of soft tissue sarcomas: a comparison trial. Eur J Nucl Med Mol Imaging. 2017;4411:1823–31.
30. Park S-Y, Chung HW, Chae SY, et al. Comparison of MRI and PET-CT in detecting the loco-regional recurrence of soft tissue sarcomas during surveillance. Skeletal Radiol. 2016;4510:1375–84.
31. Gennaro N, Marrari A, Renne SL, et al. Multimodality imaging of adult rhabdomyosarcoma: the added value of hybrid imaging. Br J Radiol. 2020;931112:20200250.
32. Hovgaard TB, Nymark T, Skov O, et al. Follow-up after initial surgical treatment of soft tissue sarcomas in the extremities and trunk wall. Acta Oncol. 2017;567:1004–12.
33. Gorelik N, Paruthikunnan S, Uppal A, et al. Usefulness of MRI-based local surveillance after surgical treatment of musculoskeletal

soft-tissue sarcomas: a systematic review and meta-analysis. AJR Am J Roentgenol. 2023;
34. George A, Grimer RJ, James J, SL. Could routine magnetic resonance imaging detect local recurrence of musculoskeletal sarcomas earlier? A cost-effectiveness study. Indian J Orthop. 2018;521:81–6.
35. Bignotti B, Rossi F, Signori A, et al. Magnetic resonance imaging or ultrasound in localized intermediate- or high-risk soft tissue tumors of the extremities (MUSTT): final results of a prospective comparative trial. Diagnostics (Basel). 2022:122.
36. Gennaro N, Marrari A, Bertuzzi AF, et al. The radiologist empowerment through virtual multidisciplinary tumor boards: the commitment of oncologic care during COVID-19 pandemic. Clin Imaging. 2021;70:49–50.

4 Future Perspectives: Metabolic Imaging, Theranostics, and Radiomics

Jeffrey J. Peterson, Alexander D. Weston, and Fatemeh Ataei

4.1 Introduction

The last decade has provided us with small glimpses into novel futuristic approaches to diagnose and treat soft-tissue sarcomas. New innovative metabolic imaging pathways are emerging allowing interdisciplinary oncology teams to branch out from the traditional anatomic imaging modalities with more exotic imaging methods targeting specific cell receptors or tumor markers. Molecular imaging techniques continue to develop and emerge, permitting real-time, in vivo detection of physiological processes on the molecular level. These techniques allow measurement of regional radiotracer concentrations which enables quantification of physiological processes that can aid in the diagnosis of disease, monitoring disease progression, and the evaluation of responses to the therapeutic interventions.

In parallel to the growth of molecular imaging, theranostics are now being developed and utilized to provide precision medical therapies to target specific malignancies with focused treatment sparing surrounding normal tissues. Theranostics denotes the coupling of diagnostic biomarkers with therapeutic agents that share a specific target in diseased cells or tissues. This is typically achieved by seeking out the expression of specific targets of disease such as cell surface receptors or membrane transporters, and subsequently utilizing specifically designed agents to deliver ionizing radiation to the tissues that express those targets [1]. These techniques have the potential to provide a significant leap forward in the therapeutic approach to soft-tissue tumors and substantially improve treatment outcomes.

Advancements in the field of radiomics are beginning to provide pioneering approaches to mine imaging data to provide improved diagnosis, prognostication, and clinical decision support for soft-tissue sarcomas. Radiomics is evolving as a multidisciplinary field, involving physicians and data and imaging scientists performing tumor segmentation, image preprocessing, feature extraction, model development, and validation. These applications permit classification tasks that compute the probability of a case belonging to a specific category, such as benign versus malignant, tumor stage, or the presence or absence of metastases. Radiomics can also allow the prediction of clinical outcomes such as disease-free interval or overall survival. Practical approaches for implementing a radiomic workflow into routine practice continue to evolve and promise to play an increasing role in clinical decision-making.

The previous decade has seen the introduction and continued expansion of the roles of metabolic imaging, radiomics, and theranostics in clinical practice and it appears these techniques will continue to mature over the coming years. These emerging technologies have great promise and hold the potential to revolutionize and transform how we diagnose and treat malignancies. This chapter seeks to highlight these budding and evolving technologies and specifically discuss their relevance to the future care and management of soft-tissue sarcomas.

4.2 Metabolic Imaging

Imaging plays a key role in the diagnosis, staging, and restaging of soft-tissue sarcomas. Traditionally, anatomic imaging modalities such as computed tomography (CT) and MR have provided the backbone for the detection and characterization of soft-tissue tumors as well as clinical decision-making. Morphology, size, and tissue characteristics have been the important determinants of treatment strategies. More recently, however, novel physiologic and metabolic approaches to imaging soft-tissue lesions have emerged. These techniques allow specific cell receptors and tumor markers to be identified and localized. Most of these developing techniques utilize Positron Emission Tomography (PET) to specifically detect and quantify tracers targeting enzymes, antibodies, or

J. J. Peterson (✉) · A. D. Weston · F. Ataei
Department of Radiology, Mayo Clinic, Jacksonville, FL, USA
e-mail: Peterson.Jeffrey@mayo.edu; Weston.Alexander@mayo.edu; Fatemeh.Ataei@myLRH.org

H. Özger et al. (eds.), *Diagnosis and Treatment of Soft Tissue Tumors*, https://doi.org/10.1007/978-3-031-77061-6_4

surface markers allowing more precise depiction and characterization of specific types of soft-tissue neoplasms.

PET is a molecular imaging technique that utilizes radioisotopes that undergo positron emission decay. Positrons are emitted from the unstable radionuclide and interact with an electron in the surrounding tissues, resulting in an annihilation reaction with subsequent release of two, 511-keV photons in opposite directions (Fig. 4.1). A sophisticated ring detector surrounding the patient detects the coincident photons and registers the interaction in the image [2] (Fig. 4.2). PET scanners are typically paired with computed tomography (CT) systems which offer precise correlation between the anatomic information provided by the CT and the metabolic information provided by the PET. The CT also provides essential data for attenuation correction [2, 3]. More recently MR systems have been coupled with PET scanners to provide anatomic imaging correlation and attenuation correction. MR inherently allows improved soft-tissue contrast and tissue characterization when compared to CT. Availability of PET/MR units is gradually growing but currently, access to PET/MR is not nearly as widespread as access to PET/CT [4].

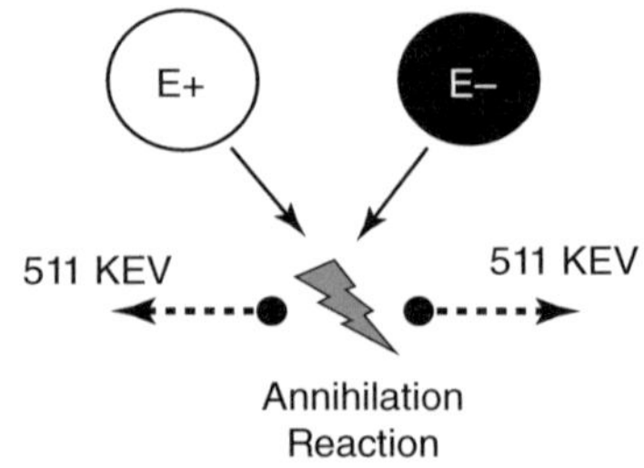

Fig. 4.1 Positron emission tomography. The positively charged positron is emitted from an unstable radionuclide and subsequently interacts with a negatively charged electron in the surrounding tissues resulting in an annihilation reaction. The annihilation reaction produces two 511 keV photons, which are emitted exactly 180 degrees apart in opposite directions

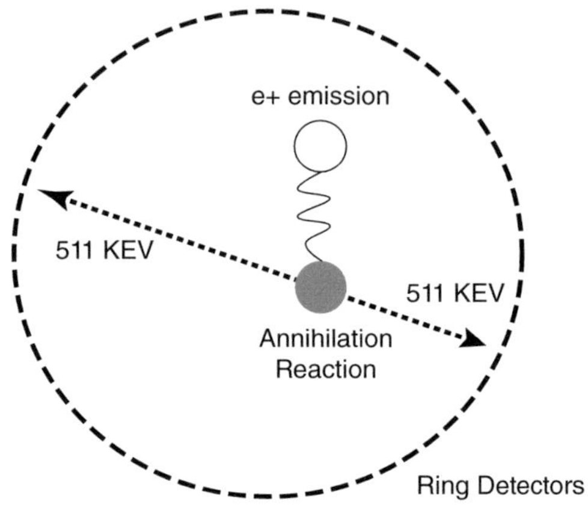

Fig. 4.2 PET scanner. A sophisticated ring of detector surrounding the gantry of the PET scanner. A positron is emitted from the radiopharmaceutical administered to the patient. The positron subsequently interacts with an electron causing an annihilation reaction. The detectors distinguish the coincident photons produced and register the interaction on the image

4.2.1 Molecular Imaging Radiotracers

PET provides a functional imaging technique that uses radioactive elements to identify and measure various metabolic processes and physiological activities including blood flow, regional chemical composition, and absorption. Different radiopharmaceuticals have been developed for various imaging purposes depending on the processes within the body that are targeted for assessment. Currently, Fluorine-18, Oxygen-15, Nitrogen-13, and Galium-68 are the PET radiotracers most accessible for medical imaging; however, Fluorine-18 is undoubtedly the most frequently employed. The most common F-18 radiopharmaceutical currently utilized with PET imaging is Fluorine-18 2-Fluoro-2-Deoxyglucose or F-18 FDG.

F-18 FDG in vivo behaves like glucose and provides a method of quantifying glucose metabolism. In the cell, FDG is phosphorylated by hexokinase, to 18F-FDG-phosphate. Unlike the metabolites of glucose (glucose-6-phosphate), 18F-FDG-phospate is not a substrate for glucose-6-phosphatase or fructose-6-phosphatase. The radioactive tracer is therefore trapped in the cell which allows for subsequent detection and quantification with PET imaging [2]. With PET imaging, the degree and amount of radiotracer accumulation reflects underlying glucose metabolism. High-grade malignancies tend to have higher rates of glycolysis than low-grade malignancies and benign lesions. Therefore, high-grade malignancies tend to have greater FDG accumulation than low-grade or benign lesions [2]. In addition, FDG accumulation within the cell is mediated by the glucose-transporter family (GLUT) which is localized in the cell membrane and regulates glucose uptake within the cell. Two subtypes, GLUT 1 and GLUT 3 are overexpressed on the cell membrane of tumor cells leading to greater glucose concentration within the tumor [5].

F-18 FDG PET can be useful for the identification and characterization of soft-tissue tumors. Soft-tissue sarcomas typically depict higher rates of glycolysis than surrounding tissues and can therefore be detected and quantified. The primary roles for FDG PET imaging for soft-tissue sarcoma include staging, restaging, and monitoring response to therapy as most lesions utilize glucose in sufficient quantities to reliably identify sites of residual or recurrent tumor as well as sites of distant tumor involvement [2, 6–11] (Fig. 4.3).

4.2.2 Indications for Molecular Imaging

Currently, FDG PET has only a limited role in the diagnosis of soft-tissue sarcomas and no role in screening for these types of malignancies. FDG PET lacks specificity for

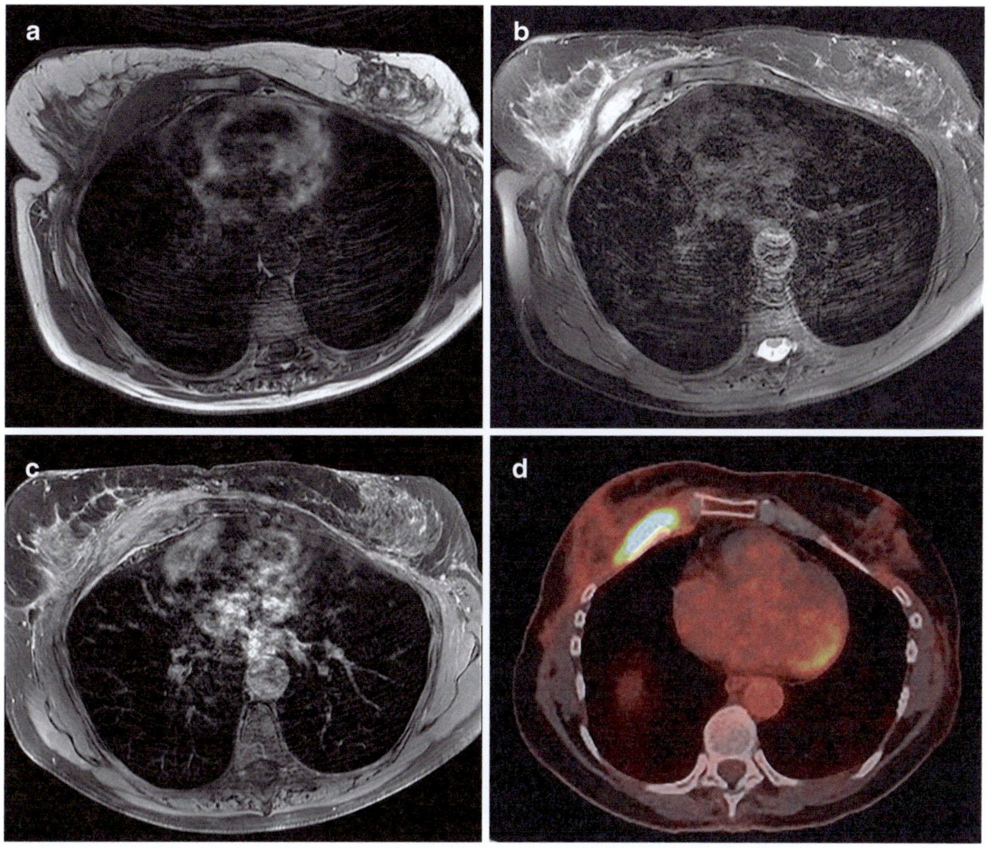

Fig. 4.3 65-year-old female with biopsy-proven undifferentiated pleomorphic sarcoma involving the right chest wall. T1-weighted (**a**), T2-weighed (**b**), and post-contrast (**c**) MR images depict an ill-defined soft tissue mass involving the right anterior chest wall with the invasion of the adjacent anterior right 4th rib. F18 FDG PET (**d**) depicts marked uptake within the tumor indicating significantly increased rates of glycolysis that surrounding tissues. This allows a precise depiction of the margins of the lesion and the degree of involvement of the chest wall

diagnosing soft-tissue lesions and conventional anatomic imaging combined with biopsy remains the mainstay technique for diagnosis of soft-tissue sarcomas [2, 7, 8, 11]. Imaging with these conventional methods reveals the morphological properties of the lesion such as tumor size and extent, tumor margins, and involvement of adjacent structures [2, 12–14]. MR imaging, in particular, can be of great utility in diagnosing certain types of soft-tissue sarcomas by evaluating the physical characteristics of the tumor assessed by the signal intensity of the lesion on various MR sequences. FDG PET imaging is good but not perfect in discriminating between benign and malignant soft-tissue tumors. Unfortunately, specificity has proven to be a concern when using PET for the diagnosis of soft-tissue masses as a wide variety of benign lesions (including nodular fascitis, tenosynovial giant cell tumor, peripheral nerve sheath tumors, etc.) can depict significant uptake. In addition, infectious and inflammatory conditions also depict significant FDG accumulation [2, 14–16]. The problem with specificity could be overcome if future radiotracers with tumor markers for specific soft-tissue sarcomas could be developed. There are several novel peptide and antibody antigen-based molecular imaging probes specifically targeting cancers including breast, prostate, ovary, and others under investigation and there is hope that breakthrough may occur in this area of study [17].

An area where molecular and metabolic imaging techniques are currently being utilized and proving very efficacious is for the staging and restaging of soft-tissue sarcomas. Staging of soft-tissue sarcomas involves the detection of additional sites of tumor involvement or metastatic disease prior to initial therapy but after confirmation of malignancy. Restaging entails imaging following the completion of therapy, to detect additional sites of tumor involvement or to evaluate the extent of recurrent or residual disease [2, 13]. Staging and restaging require accurate evaluation of both the original tumor site/s as well as assessment for local and distant metastatic disease [2, 9]. Soft-tissue sarcomas arise from mesenchymal tissues and have the potential to spread directly to involve the surrounding tissues or hematogenously disseminate, most frequently to the lungs [12] (Fig. 4.4). Prompt detection and localization of both local and distant spread of disease allows timely initiation of appropriate treatment options and improve the prognosis of patients with newly diagnosed soft-tissue sarcomas [2, 18, 19].

Determination of the presence and extent of distant metastatic disease can also help define the prognosis for patients with soft-tissue malignancies [2, 19]. FDG PET avidity has been shown to correlate with both the histologic grade of soft-tissue tumors as well as the overall prognosis for patients with soft-tissue sarcomas. Reyes Males et al. in 2021 studied 83 patients with soft-tissue sarcomas and demonstrated

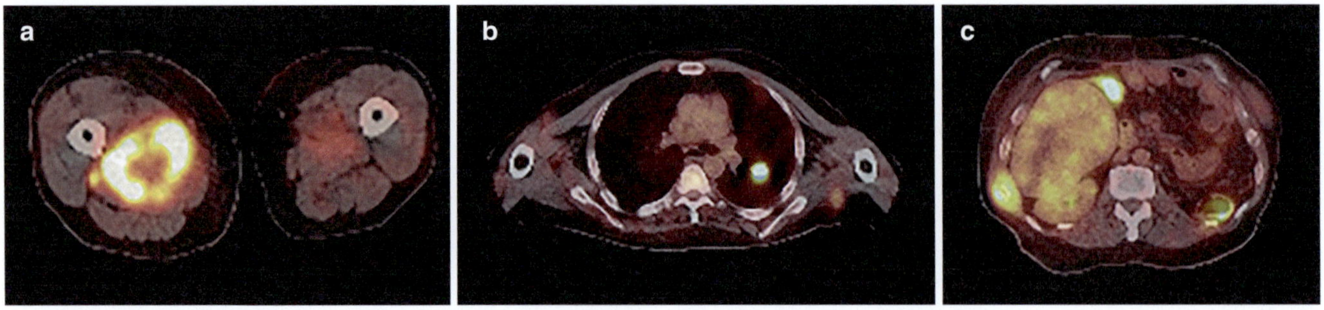

Fig. 4.4 51-year-old male with leiomyosarcoma of the right thigh. Staging F18 FDG PET depicts marked increased radiotracer accumulation in the primary tumor in the right thigh (**a**). Note the diminished activity centrally within the lesion corresponding to central necrosis seen with anatomic imaging. Staging FDG PET also depicts evidence of distant metastatic disease at the time of presentation with a large pulmonary metastasis in the left lung showing markedly increased radiotracer accumulation (**b**). There is also osseous metastatic disease with a hypermetabolic focus within a destructive lesion in the right 8th rib (**c**)

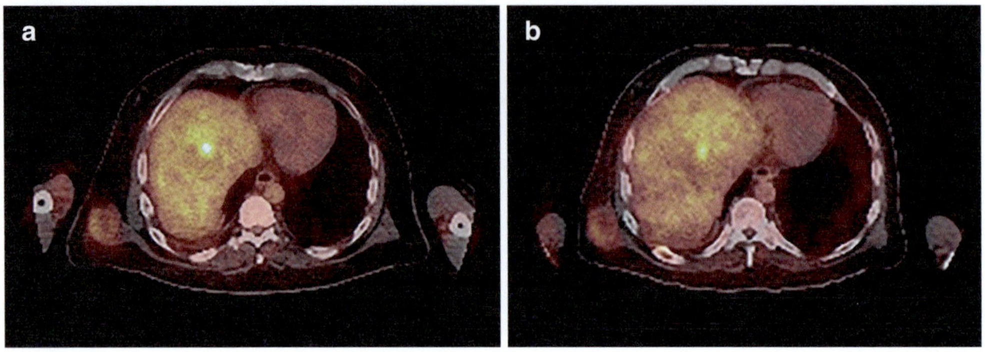

Fig. 4.5 62-year-old male patient with metastatic leiomyosarcoma involving the IVC. Staging F18 FDG PET depicts a focus of metastatic disease within the central portion of the liver (**a**). The patient was treated with neoadjuvant chemotherapy and follow up restaging FDG PET depicts partial response to therapy with decreased size and metabolic activity within the hepatic metastatic focus (**b**)

Standard Uptake Values (SUV) were useful in discriminating high-grade STS from low-grade lesions and that SUVs were predictors of overall survival [5]. Benz and colleagues reviewed 120 soft-tissue sarcoma patients had found a significant relationship between grade 3 soft-tissue sarcomas and a maximum standard uptake value of 6.6 g/mL [8]. Sambri and colleagues in a study of 50 patients with soft-tissue sarcomas found better overall survival and local recurrence rates for patients with soft-tissue sarcomas depicting SUV values less than 10.3 [20].

FDG PET has some particular advantages for staging and restaging of soft-tissue sarcomas. PET has the capability of providing whole-body assessment for the presence of distant metastatic disease and can also provide a method of characterization of the primary tumor and surrounding tissues [2]. PET/CT has high spatial resolution and provides whole-body multiplanar capability, able to obtain tomographic images providing great anatomic and morphologic detail. It provides assessment of both the osseous and soft-tissue structures, allowing identification of foci of pulmonary, nodal or other sites of soft-tissue tumor involvement in addition to skeletal metastases [2, 13]. It has been estimated that approximately 40% to 60% of patients with soft-tissue sarcomas will develop local or distant recurrence, and FDG PET can accurately detect and assess these sites providing invaluable information for developing a therapeutic strategy [2, 9, 18, 21].

Another potential indication in which molecular imaging is being currently investigated is for monitoring response to therapy of soft-tissue sarcomas. Neoadjuvant chemotherapy has gained favor for treating certain types of soft-tissue sarcomas. Following these treatments, it can be challenging to differentiate viable from nonviable tumor on post therapeutic anatomical imaging such as CT and MRI [2, 22]. FDG PET has shown the ability to provide a noninvasive method to assess response to therapy in patients with soft-tissue sarcoma [2, 18, 21–24]. FDG PET permits measurement of the internal glucose metabolism of the tumor which in turn allows differentiation of viable and nonviable tissue within the lesion which can provide evidence of the efficacy of prior treatments [2, 8, 22] (Fig. 4.5). In 2009, Benz and colleagues studied 50 patients with soft-tissue sarcomas undergoing neoadjuvant chemotherapy and demonstrated a 35% reduction in glucose metabolism assessed with PET provided a sensitive indicator of histopathologic tumor response [8]. This knowledge can furnish critical data which may dictate changes in the therapy if the desired response is not achieved [23, 24]. It can provide decisive evidence to aid in opting to continue effective therapy or discontinue ineffective treatments.

4.2.3 Future Developments in Molecular Imaging

Future development of even more specific peptide and antibody antigen based molecular imaging probes will be the next step in the evolution of PET imaging for staging and restaging soft-tissue sarcomas. FDG provides a sensitive but somewhat nonspecific whole-body evaluation, able to depict areas of focally increased glucose metabolism. Specific tracers however targeting biomolecules or other specific interactions related to the tumor could deliver much more specific means of evaluating for both local and distant disease.

As previously mentioned, there are a number of radiotracers that can be utilized for molecular imaging purposes. A majority of currently utilized radiotracers are created with a cyclotron. A cyclotron is a type of particle accelerator which repeatedly propels a beam of charged particles (specifically protons) in a circular path. Medical radioisotopes are created by bombarding non-radioactive materials or stable isotopes with protons. When the proton beam interacts with the stable isotopes, a nuclear reaction occurs, making the stable isotopes radioactive isotopes or radioisotopes. For radiotracers such as F-18 FDG with long half-lives the cyclotron may need to be located on site and doses can be brought to medical facilities from a remote cyclotron. Unfortunately, most radioisotopes have short halve lives and require a cyclotron on site. Cyclotrons are currently quite expensive and complicated machines however the cost is gradually improving, and a greater number of medical facilities are gaining access to cyclotrons for radioisotope production.

There are a few radiotracers other than FDG PET that have shown some potential for future use in imaging of soft-tissue sarcomas. One such tracer is F18-F-DOPA. F-DOPA is a cyclotron produced amino-acid radiotracer which has been highly studied for the diagnosis, staging, and restaging of gliomas in the brain. It seems that it may also be effective at imaging soft-tissue tumors. The cellular transport mechanism of amino-acid radiotracers is active, and uptake appears to be correlated with the histologic grade of the tumor (Fig. 4.6). This is due to the increased transport of amino acids into tumor cells via an overexpression of the amino-acid transport system L (LAT 1 and LAT 2). F-DOPA has a 110-minute half-life and is therefore more clinically applicable than other amino-acid radiotracers with much shorter half-lives [25]. Early trials are underway to determine the utility and efficacy of F-DOPA in the clinical management of soft-tissue sarcoma.

Another potential radiotracer for imaging soft-tissue tumors is F-18 Fluoromisonidazole (18F-FMISO). FMISO is a radiotracer with a 50-min half-life which has been studied to provide a noninvasive investigation of tumor hypoxia. Hypoxia is a feature of solid tumors that is often closely associated with radiotherapy and chemotherapy resistance. It can also be associated with greater propensity for metastatic disease and worse overall prognosis. FMSIS could provide a way to assess hypoxia in soft-tissue sarcomas and assist in selecting appropriate treatment options [26].

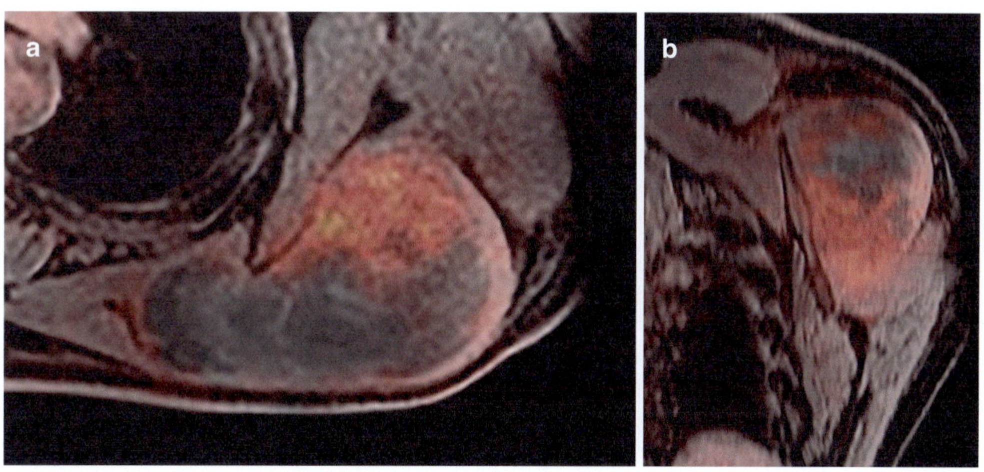

Fig. 4.6 52 year-old male patient with newly diagnosed Myxofibrosarcoma. Axial (**a**) and coronal (**b**) imaging from a staging F18-DOPA examination shows focal radiotracer accumulation in the primary tumor with now uptake elsewhere to suggest local or distant metastatic disease. The low level and sporadic uptake in the primary lesion reflects the prominent myxoid components and necrosis within the primary tumor confirmed histologically following resection

4.3 Theranostics

Modern Oncology focuses on individualized therapy to reduce the side effects and increase therapy success and compliance. The theranostic approach, a form of personalized medicine, combines diagnostic biomarkers with therapeutic agents that share specific molecular targets in malignant cells or tissues. It integrates both diagnostic imaging and therapy by utilizing the same molecule or at least very similar molecules, radiolabeled differently or delivered in different dosages [27]. This approach most commonly utilizes nuclear medicine techniques with radioactive agents utilized to image targets such as specific cell membrane transporters or surface receptors followed by specific radioactive agents administered to deliver ionizing radiation to tissues that express the specific target receptors. Theranostics allows for custom treatment plans based on the uniqueness of every individual tumor thus resulting in right drug for the right patient at the right time.

The first step with theranostics is to image the patient with a non-therapeutic radiolabeled tracer to identify if there are potential targets for treatment and to predict if a patient will benefit from a particular treatment by subsequently delivering therapeutic dosages of the desired radiopharmaceuticals. This step dramatic improves patient selection for treatment of malignancies. Patients who demonstrate appropriate targets can have customized treatment plans developed to specifically target the malignancy and minimize exposure to non-diseased tissues. Patients without significant targets for the given treatment avoid futile treatments and are spared the cost and potential side effects and risks associated with therapies. This allows more appropriate patient pre-selection to specifically target therapies which have proved to have acceptable safety profiles and efficacy [28].

The type of emission of a radionuclide determines its imaging or therapeutic application. Gamma (γ)-ray emitters like technetium-99 m (^{99m}Tc, $T_{1/2}$ = 6.0 h) and iodine-123 (^{123}I, $T_{1/2}$ = 13.2 h), as well as positron (β+) emitters such as gallium-68 (^{68}Ga, $T_{1/2}$ = 1.13 h), fluorine-18 (^{18}F, $T_{1/2}$ = 109.6 min) and copper-64 (^{64}Cu, $T_{1/2}$ = 12.7 h) are generally used for diagnostic purposes using SPECT and PET imaging respectively. Radionuclide therapies mainly utilize two major forms of particulate radiation, α-emitters and β-emitters. α-emitters and β-emitters both induce DNA damage and subsequent cell death by emitting high-energy particles. α-emitters have higher energy and greater mass and include such isotopes as bismuth-213 (^{213}Bi, $T_{1/2}$ = 46 min) and actinium-225 (^{225}Ac, $T_{1/2}$ = 9.9 days). β-emitters are more commonly utilized and include such isotopes as lutetium-177 (^{177}Lu, $T_{1/2}$ = 6.7 days) and iodine-131 (^{131}I, $T_{1/2}$ = 8.0 days).

4.3.1 Current and Potential Uses of Theranostics

The first widely utilized theranostic radiopharmaceutical was radioactive iodine, which proved remarkably successful at treating benign and malignant thyroid diseases [29]. Radioisotopes of sodium iodide, in particular, iodine-131 (^{131}I), are taken up in follicular cells in the thyroid. Thus, radioiodine therapy is an established highly successful technique to target specific thyroid malignancies with little effect to the rest of the body. This technique is widely utilized today, and in many cases, has proven to be the modality of choice for treatment of patients with differentiated thyroid cancer.

In recent years, labeling of somatostatin analogs with various isotopes has been employed for the treatment & management of neuroendocrine tumors (NETs). Somatostatin analogs bind to somatostatin receptors on the neuroendocrine tumors cell membrane and can then be used to deliver ionizing radiation specifically to the targeted tumor cells. The recent NETTER-1 trial confirmed the efficacy of the ^{177}Lu-DOTATATE therapy in neuroendocrine tumors, which led to its approval in the United States and later in Europe.

Theranostic techniques have recently been introduced for treatment of various forms of prostate cancer. Metastatic castration-resistant prostate cancer cells reveal high prostate-specific membrane antigen (PSMA) expression [30]. Therapeutic techniques can specifically seek out the PSMA receptors on malignant cells and deliver targeted therapy to the malignancy. The VISION Clinical Trials have shown ^{177}Lu-PSMA-617 therapy can prolong progression-free survival and overall survival when added to standard care in patients with advanced PSMA-positive metastatic castration-resistant prostate cancer [31, 32].

4.3.2 Potential Uses of Theranostics for Soft-Tissue Sarcoma

Tumor endothelial marker 1 (TEM1) is a tumor vascular marker with significant diagnostic and therapeutic potential in the treatment of soft-tissue sarcoma. TEM1, or endosialin, is a transmembrane glycoprotein that belongs to the C-type lectin receptor superfamily [33]. TEM1 reveals broad expression during the embryonal phase, but it gets silenced in normal tissues of adults. TEM1 re-expression has been documented in solid tumors, including sarcomas and carcinomas [34]. TEM1 overexpression in malignant tumors has been demonstrated to be associated with aggressive tumor behavior and ultimately poor patient prognosis [35]. Preclinical studies reveal that TEM1 is a safe and potentially very favorable target for future forms of cancer therapy [36]. In 2014, Li and colleagues studied Antibody-based tumor vascular theranostics targeting endosialin/TEM1 in a new mouse tumor vascular model [37]. This study significantly accelerated the development of novel theranostics targeting tumor vasculature. It appears promising that a theranostic approach for TEM1-expressing soft-tissue sarcomas may be possible [34] and several studies are currently underway.

In one such study in 2020, Delage and colleagues performed a preclinical study to radiolabel a novel anti-TEM1 fusion protein antibody (1C1m-Fc) with ^{177}Lu, for use specifically in soft-tissue sarcomas [38]. The study confirmed that ^{177}Lu-1C1m-Fc has promising performance for a theranostic approach for soft-tissue sarcomas. In 2021, the same group performed another study to define a favorable radiopharmaceutical companion for theranostic applications. They selected ^{64}Cu to radiolabel the fusion protein antibody. The study aimed to determine if ^{64}Cu-1C1m-Fc can be considered for TEM1 PET imaging and to predict the dosimetry of the ^{177}Lu-1C1m-Fc companion therapy [39]. This investigation revealed that ^{64} Cu-1C1m-Fc could be used for imaging TEM1 expression with high-resolution PET images. It also helped to select patients who could be candidates for ^{177}Lu-1C1m-Fc therapy. Regarding these recent studies, 1C1m-Fc radiolabeled with ^{64}Cu and ^{177} Lu-1C1m-Fc would be a potential theranostic pair for imaging and therapeutic use in soft-tissue sarcoma, respectively. The next step will be the future development of human dosimetry extrapolation studies for treatment safety assessment in patients for radiolabeled compounds targeting TEM1.

4.4 Radiomics

Radiomics is an emerging technique in the field of data science and artificial intelligence research. The term *radiomics* refers to a method of extracting features from medical images which quantify shape and texture patterns present in the image [40–42]. It is applicable to both CT and MRI imaging, although the two modalities present unique challenges and opportunities. The term is loosely borrowed from *genomics,* and shares similarities in the involved bioinformatics techniques, and in the ability to capture unseen information related to the underlying biology. Radiomics can be considered an extension of existing quantitative scoring systems such as LI-RADS in hepatocellular carcinoma and BI-RADS for breast lesions, however, in addition to capturing size and shape information, radiomics captures first-order and second-orders statistics and texture features [43].

Early breakthroughs of radiomics showed promise in predicting tumor aggressiveness and patient survival for several types of malignancy. Coroller et al. in 2015, successfully utilized radiomics to predict distant metastases in patients with lung cancer [44]. In that same year, Wibmer and colleagues used radiomic techniques in patients with prostate lesions seen with MR to effectively differentiate benign from malignant lesions [45]. Levner and colleagues were able to successfully utilize radiomics to prospectively predict chemotherapy effectiveness with glioblastoma based off MR tumor textural patterns [46]. This application of radiomic texture analysis used to predict genetic characteristics of tumors is particularly exciting and this evolving technique has been termed *radiogenomics.*

The field of radiomics has evolved significantly since its inception and has benefited immensely from efforts to standardize techniques for feature extraction to simplify analysis and ensure reproducible research. In the Python programming language, most studies leverage the *PyRadiomics* library for feature extraction [47]. The *PyRadiomics* library extracts a standard set of 1500 features which are divided into eight distinct classes of features, including first-order statistics, shape-based features, second-order statistics, and texture analysis. This provides the basis of radiomics.

4.4.1 Potential Uses of Radiomics

Radiomics have demonstrated usefulness for the prediction of a variety of patient outcomes in oncology. Many studies have demonstrated that the inclusion of radiomics features improves prediction of treatment response over conventional clinical techniques [48]. For example, in esophageal cancer [49, 50], radiomics features have also been shown to be predictive of metastatic potential [51], for determining true progression versus treatment effect in metastatic brain lesions [52], and for characterizing the underlying genetic makeup of the lesion [53]. They have also shown utility for prognostication, and to provide information related to staging [54].

An important aspect of evaluating a radiomics approach is to understand what the features may reveal about the underlying tumor biology. Radiomics analysis begins with segmentation of the lesion, which may be performed manually or by an AI algorithm with physician oversight. The features are extracted from voxels which are "masked" by the segmentation. Radiomics typically quantify shape features (either 2D or 3D) such as pixel surface area, sphericity, and perimeter-to-surface ratio which inform lesion morphology. First-order features capture the intensity distribution of voxels included in the lesion mask. In addition, first-order features also capture characteristics such as total energy, entropy, and the tenth and 90th percentile heterogeneity of lesion voxels. Features such as skewness and kurtosis capture of the distribution of voxels is also a first-order feature. Finally, texture features are divided into several classes such as Gray-Level Co-occurrence Matrix which quantify clusters of voxels that have a similar intensity (e.g., homogenous regions of the image), Gray-Level Run Length Matrix which quantify lines of consecutive voxels that have the same intensity (e.g., voxels contained in highly organized, striated muscle will have a high run length matrix value), and Gray-Level Dependence Matrix which captures the number of connected voxels within a correlated region.

Radiomics features vary in their complexity and clarity, although some features have an intuitive meaning that can be clearly understood. For example, a low sphericity value may indicate a lesion which is poorly circumscribed, and a high kurtosis value may indicate increased perfusion on a contrast-enhanced image. Unfortunately, many other textural features, however, are more difficult to understand and may not define characteristics which can be readily perceived by the naked eye [42].

4.4.2 Potential Uses of Radiomics for Soft-Tissue Sarcoma

Just as in other classes of neoplasm, the application of radiomics has several promising uses in the diagnosis and treatment of soft-tissue sarcoma. Individual results vary considerably, but overall, the use of radiomics in the context of soft-tissue sarcoma has similar prognostic performance to the use of radiomics for other cancer types, such as hepatocellular carcinoma and lung cancer, which are more widely documented in the literature [55]. Spraker and colleagues in 2019 found that radiomic features could accurately predict overall survival in patients with soft-tissue sarcoma [56]. Several additional studies are underway to further elucidate the efficacy of diverse radiomics features for predicting clinical behavior of soft-tissue sarcoma and the effectiveness of various treatments.

A review by Gitto et al. identified several broad applications of radiomics to the evaluation of soft-tissue sarcoma, including discrimination of malignant from benign tumors (n = 14 publications), tumor grading (n = 10), histopathological discrimination (n = 4), chemotherapy and/or radiotherapy treatment response (n = 8), and overall survival (n = 12) [57]. The authors specifically mention the utility of a publicly available dataset of 51 MR exams with both T1w and T2w fat-suppressed images of histologically proven soft-tissue sarcomas that are available through The Cancer Imaging Archive (TCIA) which is an NIH resource (link: https://doi.org/10.7937/K9/TCIA.2015.7GO2GSKS) [58]. Gitto and colleagues identified that 6% of all studies concerning soft-tissue sarcoma have leveraged this dataset [57].

Several challenges specific to the treatment of soft-tissue sarcoma can potentially be addressed with the use of radiomics. Although RECIST criteria is the gold-standard for quantitative assessment of treatment response, in many cases soft-tissue sarcomas may not significantly shrink with treatment. Groups have also reported that other common, qualitative radiologic markers such as edema, necrosis, and infiltration may also have limited diagnostic performance with an accuracy ranging from 0.5–0.75 [56]. The hope is that radiomic analysis may better capture more subtle features of soft-tissue sarcomas such as fibrotic and necrotic processes, infarction, or dedifferentiation which may affect radiomic heterogeneity measurements of the tumor.

4.4.3 Recent Scientific Data

Several illustrative examples of the use of radiomics for soft-tissue sarcoma have been recently published. Li et al. demonstrated the ability of a "radiomics risk score" to differentiate between benign and malignant soft-tissue sarcomas. This was derived via logistic regression from a subset of 10 texture features (GLCM features) [59]. Li et al.'s model had a predictive area under the receiver-operating characteristic curve (AUROC) of 0.76 (confidence interval (CI): 0.69–0.83) which improved to 0.84 (CI: 0.78–0.90) with the inclusion of clinical data to the radiomics features.

Peeken et al. used least-absolute shrinkage and selection operation for feature selection, paired with logistic regression to predict the histopathology grade of soft-tissue sarcomas from T1w and fat-suppressed T2w MR exams. Their final method selected 13 features from 2609 and achieved an AUROC performance of 0.84. A model trained solely on clinical parameters in contrast was proven not to provide predictive information related to histologic grade [60]. Xu et al. utilized a similar approach, also in an effort to predict the histopathology grade of soft-tissue sarcoma from radiomics features derived from T1w and fat-suppressed T2w MR exams. Their method also identified LASSO as the optimal approach from 11 options and selected Random Forest from seven options (77 total experiments). The final classifier had an AUROC of 0.92 (CI: 0.84–0.99) [22]. Giraudo et al. predicted the risk of metastatic spread from soft-tissue sarcoma with apparent-diffusion coefficient (ADC) diffusion-weighted MRI sequences and identified a single feature (Imc1) as predictive of metastasis with an accuracy of 0.76 [61]. All three of these approaches reinforce the importance of strict feature selection criteria to prevent overfitting from too many radiomics features.

Most publications involve tumor-specific outcomes such as benign/malignant classification or histopathologic grade, however, prediction of treatment response and overall survival are more difficult to ascertain from tumor-specific imaging. For example, Giraudo et al. failed to predict overall survival even though they were able to accurately predict metastatic spread [61]. Spraker et al. did however successfully predict 3-year survival from a combination of three texture features, tumor volume, age, and tumor grade. The final model (which also employed LASSO for feature selection) had a concordance index (c-index) value of 0.78 (CI: 0.66–0.88).

4.4.4 Challenges to the Radiomics Approach

Several challenges have emerged in applying a radiomics approach to soft-tissue sarcoma. These mainly focus on the topic of reproducibility. Radiomics feature extraction is dependent on the precise parameters of the MRI sequence being performed. For example, a feature set derived from ADC diffusion-weighed MR imaging [61] would not be applicable to T1w or T2w sequences [60, 62]. In addition, even slight differences between individual MR or CT scanners may affect feature extraction. As such, cross-site validation studies are rarely performed [56]. Reproducibility proving limited to specific sequences performed on a single individual scanner has proven to be a challenge to the overall clinical utility of radiomics.

Another challenge to the applicability of radiomics is related to the extraction of features. Feature reproducibility is also highly dependent on the steps of extraction. Tumor segmentation is most important in this regard, however, other factors such as the normalization and bin settings are significant as well. Many of these concerns have been largely addressed with the ISBI standard and the publicly available PyRadiomics package [47], but challenges in this realm remain. In addition, proper modeling requires the use of strict feature selection criteria to reduce hundreds or thousands of features, which are often highly correlated, to just a handful of features. This step is necessary to prevent overfitting with too much data. Studies prove that if segmentation and image preprocessing are properly performed, radiomics features are reproducible, but challenges remain in this regard [63]. Radiomics has a promising future for oncology but the field is just in its infancy. Much future study and investigation will be necessary to bring the field of radiomics from preclinical research to clinical practice.

4.5 Conclusion

Molecular imaging and theranostics have provided us with a means to combine the disciplines of molecular biology, medical imaging technology, and oncologic therapy. Radiomics has the potential to provide invaluable information extracted from subtle textural details far beyond what the human eye can see. These leaps forward in technology, imaging, and therapeutic techniques have delivered tremendous progress in healthcare practice and herald a significant leap forward in diagnosis, surveillance and treatment outcomes for malignancy [3]. New radiotracers, radiomic systems, and theranostic techniques continue to be developed and numerous studies are underway to assess the utility of these approaches in the diagnosis and treatment of malignant soft-tissue lesions. Growth in the field of molecular imaging, theranostics, and radiomics remains strong and will continue into the foreseeable future.

References

1. Marin JFG, Nunes RF, Coutinho AM, Zaniboni EC, Costa LB, Barbosa FG, Queiroz MA, Cerri GG, Buchpiguel CA. Theranostics in nuclear medicine: emerging and re-emerging integrated imaging and therapies in the era of precision oncology. Radiographics. 2020;40(6):1715–40.
2. Peterson JJ, Kransdorf MJ, O'Connor MI. Diagnosis of occult bone metastases: positron emission tomography. Clin Orthop Relat Res. 2003;415(Suppl):S120–S8.
3. Dash A, Chakravarty R. Radionuclide generators: the prospect of availing PET radiotracers to meet current clinical needs and future research demands. Am J Nucl Med Mol Imaging. 2019;9(1):30–66.
4. Schuler MK, Richter S, Beuthien-Baumann B, Platzek I, Kotzerke J, Van den Hoff J, Ehninger G, Reichardt P. PET/MRI imaging in high-risk sarcoma: first findings and solving clinical problems. Case Rep Oncol Med. 2013;793927. Epub 2013 Jul 1
5. Reyes Marlés RH, Navarro Fernández JL, García-Sandoval JPP, Medina FS, Salem LM, Esteban LF, Gutiérrez JFC, Sánchez MIC, Merino GR, Valderas MAC. Clinical value of baseline 18F-FDG PET/CT in soft tissue sarcomas. Eur J Hybrid Imaging. 2021;5(1):16.
6. Charest M, Hickeson M, Lisbona R, Novales-Diaz JA, Derbekyan V, Turcotte RE. FDG PET/CT imaging in primary osseous and soft tissue sarcomas: a retrospective review of 212 cases. Eur J Nucl Med Mol Imaging. 2009;36:1944–51.
7. Bestic JM, Peterson JJ, Bancroft LW. Use of FDG PET in staging, restaging, and assessment of therapy response in Ewing sarcoma. Radiographics. 2009;29(5):1487–500.
8. Benz MR, Czernin J, Allen-Aurbach MS, Tap WD, Dry SM, Elashoff D, Chow K, Evilevitch V, Eckardt JJ, Phelps ME. FDG PET/CT imaging predicts histopathologic treatment responses after the initial cycle of neoadjuvant chemotherapy in high-grade soft-tissue sarcomas. Clin Cancer Res. 2009;15(8):2856–63.
9. Piperkova E, Mikhaeil M, Mouasavi A, Libes R, Viejo-Rullan LH, Rosen G, Abdel-Dayem H. Impact of PET and CT in PET/CT studies for staging and evaluating treatment response in bone and soft tissue sarcomas. Clin Nucl Med. 2009;34(3):146–50.
10. Iagaru A, Masamed R, Chawla SP, Menendez LR, Fedenko A, Conti PS. F-18 FDG PET and PET/CT evaluation of response to chemotherapy in bone and soft tissue sarcomas. Clin Nucl Med. 2008;33(1):8–13.
11. Katal S, Gholamrezanezhad A, Kessler M, Olyaei M, Jadvar H. PET in the diagnostic management of soft tissue sarcomas of musculoskeletal origin. PET Clin. 2018;13(4):609–21.
12. Ho YY. Review of non-positron emission tomography functional imaging or primary musculoskeletal tumours: beyond the humble bone scan. Australas Radiol. 2005;49:445–59.
13. Peterson JJ. F-18 FDG-PET for detection of osseous metastatic disease and staging, restaging, and monitoring response to therapy of musculoskeletal tumors. Semin Musculoskelet Radiol. 2007;11(3):246–60.
14. Ioannidis JPA, Lau J. 18F-FDG PET for the diagnosis and grading of soft-tissue sarcoma: a meta-analysis. J Nucl Med. 2003;44(5):717–24.
15. Aoki J, Watanabe H, Shinozaki T, Takagishi K, Ishijima H, Oya N, Sato N, Inoue T, Endo K. FDG PET of primary benign and malignant bone tumors: standardized uptake value in 52 lesions. Radiology. 2001;219:774–7.
16. Goodin GS, Shulkin BL, Kaufman RA, McCarville MB. PET/CT characterization of fibroosseous defects in children:18F-FDG uptake can mimic metastatic disease. AJR. 2006;187:1124–8.
17. Deutscher SL. Phage display in molecular imaging and diagnosis of cancer. Chem Rev. 2010;110(5):3196–211.

18. El-Zeftawy H, Heiba SI, Jana S, Rosen G, Salem S, Santiago JF, Abdel-Dayem HM. Role of repeated F-18 fluorodeoxyglucose imaging in management of patients with bone and soft tissue sarcoma. Cancer Biother Radiopharm. 2001;16:37–46.
19. Volker T, Denecke T, Steffen I, Misch D, Schonberger S, Plotkin M, Ruf J, Furth C, Stover B, Hautzel G, Henze G, Amthauer H. Positron emission tomography for staging of pediatric sarcoma patients: results of a prospective multicenter trial. J Clin Oncol. 2007;25(34):5435–41.
20. Sambri A, Bianchi G, Longhi A, Righi A, Donati DM, Nanni C, Fanti S, Errani C. The role of 18F-FDG PET/CT in soft tissue sarcoma. Nucl Med Commun. 2019;40(6):626–31.
21. Jadvar H, Gamie S, Romanna L, Conti PS. Musculoskeletal system. Semin Nucl Med. 2004;34(4):254–61.
22. Bradella MA, Caputo GR, Steinbach LS. Value of FDG positron emission tomography in conjunction with MR imaging for evaluating therapy response in patients with musculoskeletal sarcomas. AJR. 2002;179(5):1145–50.
23. Hawkins DS, Rajendran JG, Conrad EU III, Bruckner JD, Eary JF. Evaluation of chemotherapy response in pediatric bone sarcomas by [F-18]-fluorodeoxy-d-glucose positron emission tomography. Am Cancer Soc. 2002;94(12):3277–84.
24. Hawkins DS, Rajendran JG, Conrad EU III, Bruckner JD, Eary JF. Evaluation of chemotherapy response in pediatric bone sarcoma by [f-18]-fluorodeoxy-d-glucose positron emission tomography. Cancer. 2002;94(12):3277–84.
25. Somme F, Bender L, Namer IJ, Noël G, Bund C. Usefulness of 18F-FDOPA PET for the management of primary brain tumors: a systematic review of the literature. Cancer Imaging. 2020;20(1):70.
26. Vallières M, Serban M, Benzyane I, Ahmed Z, Xing S, El Naqa I, Levesque IR, Seuntjens J, Freeman CR. Investigating the role of functional imaging in the management of soft-tissue sarcomas of the extremities. Phys Imaging Radiat Oncol. 2018;19(6):53–60.
27. Shrivastava S, et al. A review on theranostics: an approach to targeted diagnosis and therapy. Asian J Pharm Res Dev. 2019;7(2):63–9.
28. Vogenberg FR, Barash CI, Pursel M. Personalized medicine: part 1: evolution and development into theranostics. P T. 2010;35(10):560.
29. Hertz B. A tribute to Dr. Saul Hertz: the discovery of the medical uses of radioiodine. World J Nucl Med. 2019;18(01):8–12.
30. Minner S, et al. High level PSMA expression is associated with early PSA recurrence in surgically treated prostate cancer. Prostate. 2011;71(3):281–8.
31. Langbein T, Weber WA, Eiber M. Future of theranostics: an outlook on precision oncology in nuclear medicine. J Nucl Med. 2019;60(Supplement 2):13S.
32. Sartor O, et al. Lutetium-177–PSMA-617 for metastatic castration-resistant prostate cancer. N Engl J Med. 2021;385(12):1091–103.
33. Bagley RG, et al. Endosialin/TEM 1/CD248 is a pericyte marker of embryonic and tumor neovascularization. Microvasc Res. 2008;76(3):180–8.
34. Rouleau C, et al. Endosialin protein expression and therapeutic target potential in human solid tumors: sarcoma versus carcinoma. Clin Cancer Res. 2008;14(22):7223–36.
35. Davies G, et al. Levels of expression of endothelial markers specific to tumour-associated endothelial cells and their correlation with prognosis in patients with breast cancer. Clin Exp Metastasis. 2004;21:31–7.
36. Rouleau C, et al. Anti-endosialin antibody–drug conjugate: potential in sarcoma and other malignancies anti-Endosialin ADC. Mol Cancer Ther. 2015;14(9):2081–9.
37. Li C, et al. Antibody-based tumor vascular theranostics targeting endosialin/TEM1 in a new mouse tumor vascular model. Cancer Biol Ther. 2014;15(4):443–51.
38. Delage JA, et al. 177Lu radiolabeling and pre-clinical theranostic study of 1C1m-Fc: an anti-TEM-1 scFv-Fc fusion protein in soft tissue sarcoma. EJNMMI Res. 2020;10(1):98.
39. Delage JA, et al. Copper-64-labeled 1C1m-Fc, a new tool for TEM-1 PET imaging and prediction of Lutetium-177-labeled 1C1m-Fc therapy efficacy and safety. Cancers. 2021;13(23):5936.
40. Lambin P, et al. Radiomics: extracting more information from medical images using advanced feature analysis. Eur J Cancer. 2012;48(4):441–6.
41. Kumar V, et al. Radiomics: the process and the challenges. Magn Reson Imaging. 2012;30(9):1234–48.
42. Gillies RJ, Kinahan PE, Hricak H. Radiomics: images are more than pictures, they are data. Radiology. 2016;278(2):563–77.
43. Parekh VS, Jacobs MA. Multiparametric radiomics methods for breast cancer tissue characterization using radiological imaging. Breast Cancer Res Treat. 2020;180:407–21.
44. Aerts HJ, et al. Decoding tumour phenotype by noninvasive imaging using a quantitative radiomics approach. Nat Commun. 2014;5(1):4006.
45. Wibmer A, et al. Haralick texture analysis of prostate MRI: utility for differentiating non-cancerous prostate from prostate cancer and differentiating prostate cancers with different Gleason scores. Eur Radiol. 2015;25:2840–50.
46. Levner I, et al. Predicting MGMT methylation status of glioblastomas from MRI texture. in Medical image computing and computer-assisted intervention–MICCAI 2009: 12th International Conference, London, UK, September 20–24, 2009, Proceedings, Part II 12. 2009. Springer.
47. Van Griethuysen JJ, et al. Computational radiomics system to decode the radiographic phenotype. Cancer Res. 2017;77(21):e104–7.
48. Yip SS, Aerts HJ. Applications and limitations of radiomics. Phys Med Biol. 2016;61(13):R150.
49. Tixier F, et al. Intratumor heterogeneity characterized by textural features on baseline 18F-FDG PET images predicts response to concomitant radiochemotherapy in esophageal cancer. J Nucl Med. 2011;52(3):369–78.
50. Hatt M, et al. 18F-FDG PET uptake characterization through texture analysis: investigating the complementary nature of heterogeneity and functional tumor volume in a multi–cancer site patient cohort. J Nucl Med. 2015;56(1):38–44.
51. Coroller TP, et al. CT-based radiomic signature predicts distant metastasis in lung adenocarcinoma. Radiother Oncol. 2015;114(3):345–50.
52. Peng L, et al. Distinguishing true progression from radionecrosis after stereotactic radiation therapy for brain metastases with machine learning and radiomics. Int J Radiat Oncol Biol Phys. 2018;102(4):1236–43.
53. Gutman DA, et al. Somatic mutations associated with MRI-derived volumetric features in glioblastoma. Neuroradiology. 2015;57:1227–37.
54. Huang P, et al. Added value of computer-aided CT image features for early lung cancer diagnosis with small pulmonary nodules: a matched case-control study. Radiology. 2018;286(1):286–95.
55. Fanciullo C, et al. Radiomics of musculoskeletal sarcomas: a narrative review. J Imaging. 2022;8(2):45.
56. Spraker MB, et al. MRI radiomic features are independently associated with overall survival in soft tissue sarcoma. Adv Radiat Oncol. 2019;4(2):413–21.
57. Gitto S, et al. CT and MRI radiomics of bone and soft-tissue sarcomas: a systematic review of reproducibility and validation strategies. Insights Imaging. 2021;12(1):1–14.
58. Vallières M, et al. A radiomics model from joint FDG-PET and MRI texture features for the prediction of lung metastases in soft-tissue sarcomas of the extremities. Phys Med Biol. 2015;60(14):5471.
59. Li L, et al. Radiomics of MRI scans enables differentiation of benign from malignant soft tissue sarcoma. , American Society of Clinical Oncology 2022.
60. Peeken JC, et al. Tumor grading of soft tissue sarcomas using MRI-based radiomics. EBioMedicine. 2019;48:332–40.

61. Giraudo C, et al. Tumor cellularity beyond the visible in soft tissue sarcomas: results of an ADC-based, single center, and preliminary radiomics study. Front Oncol. 2022:5474.
62. Xu W, et al. Soft tissue sarcoma: preoperative MRI-based radiomics and machine learning may be accurate predictors of histopathologic grade. Am J Roentgenol. 2020;215(4):963–9.
63. Thrussell I, et al. Radiomic features from diffusion-weighted MR of retroperitoneal soft-tissue sarcomas are repeatable and exhibit change after radiotherapy. Front Oncol. 2022:3427.

The Role of Whole-Body Magnetic Resonance Imaging in Soft Tissue Tumors

5

Nefise Cagla Tarhan and Ercan Karaarslan

5.1 Whole-Body Magnetic Resonance Imaging in Soft Tissue Tumors

Magnetic resonance imaging (MRI) is the preferred imaging modality in the characterization of incidentally found soft tissue tumors with physical examination or ultrasound and also for preoperative staging of biopsy-proven malignant soft tissue tumors [1]. Dedicated regional MRI is used for lesion location, extension, size, morphological characteristics and surrounding alterations (Fig. 5.1). In patients with histologically proven sarcoma, whole-body staging is mandatory for further treatment options [1]. On ESSR (European Society of Skeletal Radiology) guidelines, the recommended imaging protocols are unenhanced chest computed tomography (CT) for lung metastases, regional abdominal and pelvic MRI or CT, brain and spine MRI for metastases to these sites and positron emission tomography (PET) scan for osseous metastases. In the initial staging and follow-up of these patients, the role of PET/CT and PET/MRI is still regarded as controversial because, in a small number of patients, they were shown to cause upstaging. While some groups do not recommend these imaging techniques for routine use; in many other centers, systematic evaluation is always used before treatment [2]. In patients with the diagnosis of soft tissue sarcoma, a 10-year follow-up is usually done after the initial diagnosis. Follow-up intervals are changed according to the grade of the tumor, with shorter intervals initially like 3–4 months in patients with higher-grade tumors. There is debate regarding whether follow-up examination should be performed regularly or only in symptomatic patients, but in ESSR guidelines, routine follow-up is recommended [3]. Dedicated MRI including contrast-enhanced sequences and diffusion-weighted imaging (DWI) is considered the method of choice for local follow-up [4–6].

Whole-body MRI (WB-MRI) has gained much interest in recent years with the development of new imaging methods and the advantage of fast imaging sequences. It has been mainly used in oncology, especially in metastatic bone disease, systemic infection evaluation such as pyrexia of unknown origin, recently in multifocal evaluation of rheumatologic diseases, and for screening of otherwise healthy high-risk patients or patients with cancer predisposition syndromes [7]. In recent years, this method has gained popularity for health checkups in healthy asymptomatic subjects [8]. There are well-established imaging modalities for follow-up of diagnosed soft tissue tumors like CT, bone scintigraphy and PET-CT. The main advantage of WB-MRI over other multisystemic imaging modalities is the lack of radiation. This becomes especially important in the follow-up of pediatric patients with serial examinations throughout the cancer therapy that will cause cumulative exposure to ionizing radiation [7]. In younger patients with repeated imaging modalities having ionizing radiation may lead to the development of new cancers [9].

Recent advanced techniques allowed faster imaging protocols and free-breathing imaging, especially in children with a high field-of-view coverage. In addition to anatomical imaging of the tumor and metastatic disease, DWI and contrast-enhanced imaging give information about tissue characteristics during follow-up of these patients [10].

In examining the patients, there are a few variations in coverage of patients. The most commonly used one covers the head, neck, thorax, abdomen and proximal part of the lower extremities. Some institutions do not include the neck or the proximal lower extremities.

N. C. Tarhan · E. Karaarslan (✉)
Department of Radiology, School of Medicine, Acibadem Mehmet Ali Aydinlar University, Istanbul, Turkey
e-mail: ercan.karaarslan@acibadem.com

H. Özger et al. (eds.), *Diagnosis and Treatment of Soft Tissue Tumors*, https://doi.org/10.1007/978-3-031-77061-6_5

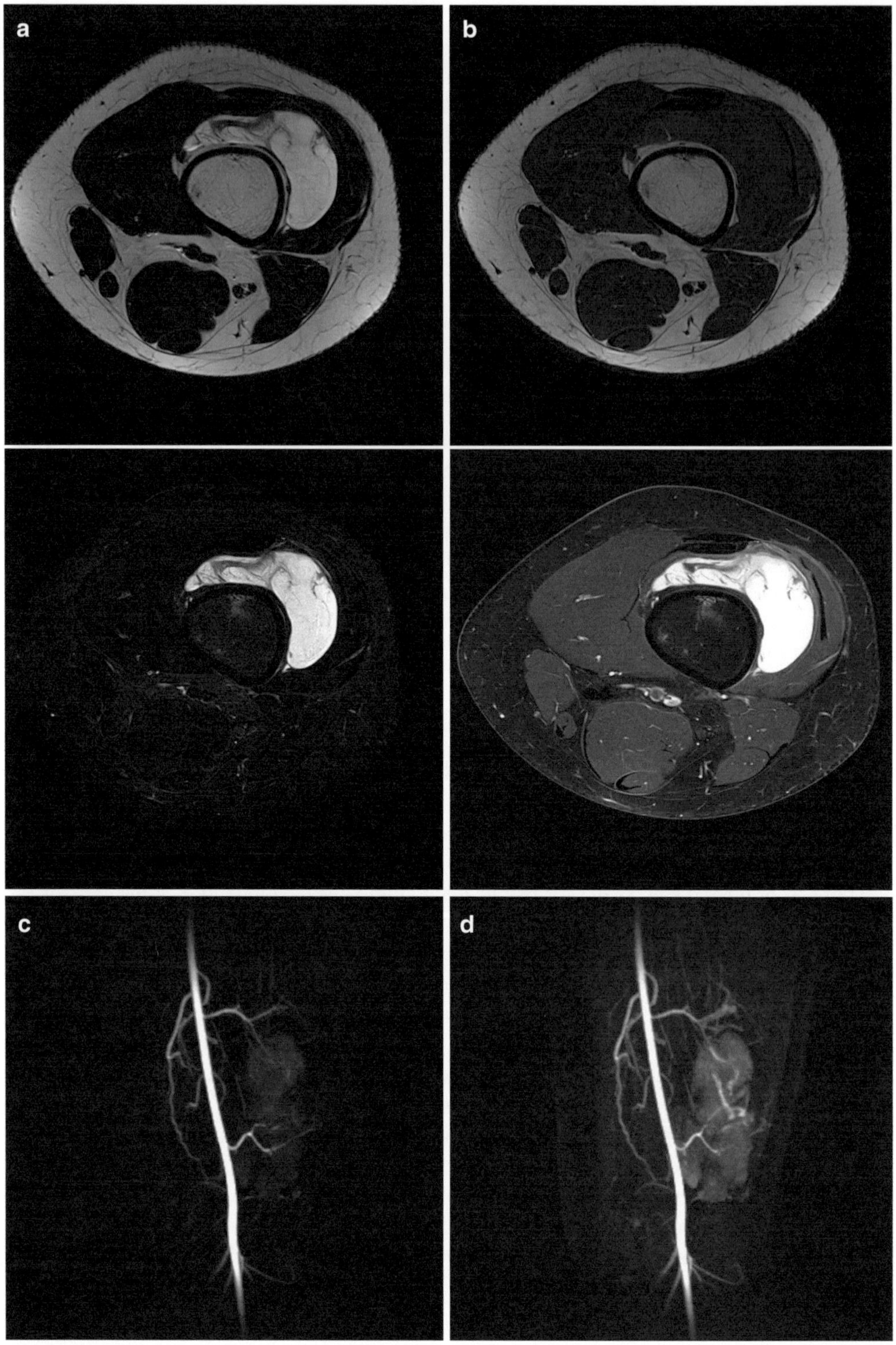

Fig. 5.1 34-year-old female with a soft tissue lesion in left knee histopathologically diagnosed as myxoid liposarcoma. A dedicated high-resolution MRI of the left knee was performed, which showed a well-defined soft tissue mass on T2-weighted and STIR axial images (**a**). The mass appeared hyperintense and heterogeneous, and there was no signal indicating the presence of fat. On pre-contrast T1-weighted and post-contrast fat saturated T1-weighted images (**b**) prominent enhancement is noted. On 4D TWIST MR Angiography early and late arterial phase images (**c**, **d**), the mass shows prominent and early avid enhancement

5.2 Whole-Body MRI Technical Considerations

Until the late 1990s, MRI was a limited, segmental imaging technique. With the advent of multiple receiver coils and table movement, this technique was transformed into a full-body imaging modality [11]. The introduction of DWI with its high sensitivity in detecting new malignant lesions and monitoring response to therapy in cancer patients brought this new method to the forefront of cancer imaging. This imaging technique when used has led to more efficient WB-MRI [12]. Further developments in especially abdominal imaging with parallel imaging techniques and obtaining high-quality images in shorter times made it possible to scan the whole body in acceptable time periods like less than 60 minutes [13–15]. New MRI acceleration methods using deep learning and novel reconstruction algorithms can reduce scanning times while maintaining high image quality.

The most significant developments that enable WB-MRI are parallel imaging, simultaneous multi-slice sequences, compressed sensing, DWI and moving table.

Parallel imaging is a recently introduced technique with simultaneous data acquisition via multiple receiver coil elements of the phased-array coils in new MRI scanners [16]. Multiple receiver coils acquire the data simultaneously from multiple regions. The use of parallel imaging shortens acquisition times of especially the abdominal sequences (which affect WB-MRI widely) without losing quality and spatial resolution [17], and sensitivity to motion artifacts have been decreased largely [13, 14, 18].

Simultaneous multi-slice sequence (SMS) is another new step after parallel imaging. SMS imaging goes beyond parallel imaging by stimulating several slices simultaneously and then spatially encoding their signals in a simultaneous way [19]. SMS offers the primary benefit of reducing scan times. Theoretically, the imaging speed can be increased by a factor equivalent to the number of slices that are stimulated at the same time, which is usually around 2 to 4 times faster. SMS acquisition also decreases the scan times when applied to DWI. It is possible to perform accelerated free-breathing DWI, especially of the abdomen and pelvis using simultaneous multi-slice acquisition, while still preserving the quality of the diagnostic image [20].

Compressed sensing is another newly introduced technique for fast acquisition, based on compression of medical images without losing essential information and degradation of image quality. It can be combined with parallel imaging to accelerate the image acquisition usually greater than four times in especially abdominal applications that makes possible to obtain sequences in less than 10 s.

In patients having problems of breath holding, high-temporal resolution of the breath-hold sequences becomes problem-solving. Compressed sensing is also used in dynamic imaging with high-temporal resolution. In patients who cannot hold their breaths at all, free-breathing T1-weighted dynamic imaging is also possible with the new techniques [16]. They are especially useful in sedated patients or patients who are unable to hold their breath. T2-weighted images can also be acquired within a suitable time period and with sufficient spatial resolution using compressed sensing and SMS technology [16]. By utilizing respiratory gating or navigator sequences, higher-quality images can be obtained for patients who are either unable to hold their breath or are sedated during the imaging procedure.

Novel imaging sequences utilize a different combination of data sampling techniques such as compressed sensing, golden-angle radial k-space filling, parallel imaging, and partial k-space filling to acquire free-breathing and faster sequences, which could be advantageous for imaging in pediatric patients [21].

DWI is a type of imaging that relies on the concept of reduced Brownian motion or hindered diffusion of water molecules in tissues with higher cell membranes as a result of increased cellularity [22]. Various levels of diffusion-weighting can be distinguished by a "*b*-value", which is determined by the strength and timing of the gradient. Typical protocols incorporate both low (50–100 s/mm^2) and high (600 and 1000 s/mm^2) *b*-values [23]. DWI is the essential component of WB-MRI in recent practice, especially in patients with follow-up of soft tissue tumors particularly in malignancies. DWI can detect small malignant lesions with high cellularity. Besides enhancing the visibility of small malignant lesions, DWI has the potential to perform functional tissue characterization, supplementing the anatomical evaluation [7]. Another important feature of DWI is that it does not require contrast for imaging and generates PET-like images without radiation. Furthermore, the SMS technique has enhanced DWI by decreasing scanning times by over 50% and minimizing artifacts associated with respiratory and motion-related movements. It is also possible to use compressed sensing in combination with DWI to achieve a higher temporal resolution [21].

With the recent software updates of different companies, artificial intelligence image enhancers are in use namely Deep Resolve Boost (Siemens) or Deep Learning Reconstruction (GE) for denoising in accelerated T2 and short-tau inversion recovery (STIR) sequences, which in turn decrease scan times with better resolution images.

5.3 Hardware

WB-MRI can be performed using high-strength MRI machines like 1.5 T or 3.0 T units. Until the common usage of multi-transmitter coils, 1.5 T machines were preferred for WB-MRI which requires a larger field-of-view because geometrical distortions and broken spine artifacts were more prominent in higher field strength units. With the advent of multi-transmitter coil technology, 3.0 T machines are used more often with lesser negligible artifacts. The latest MRI machines that feature high-quality amplitude and slew-rate gradients (with minimum values of 45 mT/m and 200 mT/m per second respectively) have a better Signal-to-Noise ratio (SNR). This is because they allow for higher bandwidths and quicker repetition times/echo times. By adjusting the number of averages for each acquired "*b*" value and shortening the k-space filling readouts, the effects of respiratory and cardiac motion are minimal, and therefore, gating is usually not needed [24]. In some instances, gating can be done for thorax and abdomen sections. For patients with metal endoprostheses, it is recommended to use a 1.5 T MRI rather than a 3 T MRI as it produces fewer artifacts [25].

The examination is done with the use of a moving table and dedicated multichannel and multi-element coils including a dedicated head and neck coil, body coils, phased-array in-table spine coil, and flexible lower extremity coils [7]. Images are acquired starting from the head, with the help of a moving table; and progress downward through the body, systematically capturing all the segments with an optimal field-of-view. The primary reason for using a moving table in WB-MRI is to bring the part of the body examined to the isocenter of the magnet, thereby producing higher-resolution images. This results in consecutive stacks of high-resolution images with 20–50 cm fields of view. The number of static body sections obtained depends on the height of the patient being examined. Later, all the obtained body parts are merged using reconstruction software [26].

5.4 Imaging Protocol

For a routine WB-MRI examination, no preparation is needed, except for a few hours of fasting to reduce the artifacts secondary to intestinal movements. Typically, the patient is positioned lying flat on their back with arms at their sides or over the trunk and legs in a straight position to be able to cover the whole extremities with a single peripheral lower extremity coil. In some cases, particularly for children, sedation or general anesthesia may be necessary during the scan [25]. This is especially important for children with recurrent malignant soft tissue tumors, as both whole-body MRI for detecting metastases and imaging of the original site can be performed during a single session while the child is under general anesthesia.

Usually, in routine imaging protocols, WB-MRI covers the area from the top of the head to the upper calf. However, it can be extended to cover the whole body from head to feet in certain scenarios, such as during screening of high-risk populations, when evaluating diseases that affect the long bones, or when investigating soft tissue disease in melanoma patients; similar to what is done in PET-CT [25]. When evaluating patients with soft tissue tumors, the coverage area for WB-MRI may be determined based on the location of the primary tumor. If the tumor is in the distal extremities, particularly in children, these areas should be included in the scan to examine the primary site along with the rest of the body. It is also important to include all extremities to rule out the presence of bone metastases (Fig. 5.2).

In the WB-MRI of patients with soft tissue tumors, morphological sequences (consisting of T1-weighted and T2-weighted images) should be combined with functional imaging techniques such as DWI and contrast-enhanced imaging.

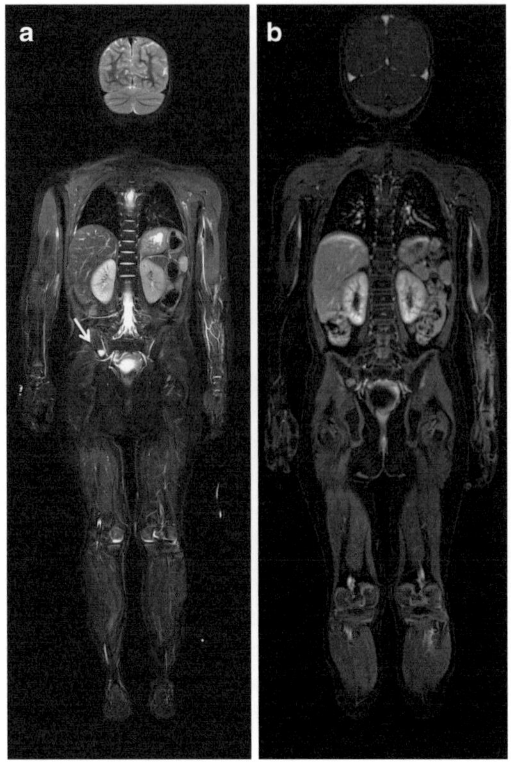

Fig. 5.2 4-year-old girl who had previous surgery for rhabdomyosarcoma in her left arm with a follow-up whole-body MRI obtained thoroughly including all the extremities to rule out any bone metastases. It showed a nodular lesion on her right iliac bone, which appeared hyperintense on the STIR sequence in the coronal plane (**a**). The lesion was also shown to have diffuse enhancement on the post-contrast T1-weighted VIBE sequence (**b**). The lesion was newly appearing indicating a solitary metastasis

5.4.1 Anatomical Sequences

Anatomical sequences are T1-weighted and T2-weighted images. Classically fast spin-echo imaging has been used for both T1 and T2-weighting. Recently, studies have shown the usefulness of WB-Dixon imaging. Dixon sequences are becoming more popular for detecting bone lesions in cancer patients due to their ability to provide high-quality images in a shorter time compared to traditional spin-echo images [20]. 2D T1-weighted images are obtained in a **coronal plane** to cover a larger area (usually 20–50 cm per station) in a shorter time.

Lately, the 3D T1 sequence has been developed as a potential replacement for various anatomical T1-weighted protocols used in bone and lymph node staging of cancer patients. This new sequence offers millimeter resolution, improved image quality, and can be reconstructed in any plane, compared to the previously used 2D sequences. They also offer good fat suppression especially in obese patients [27] (Fig. 5.3).

For T2-weighting, the most widely used sequence is the STIR sequence in the coronal plane [7, 28]. For fat suppres-

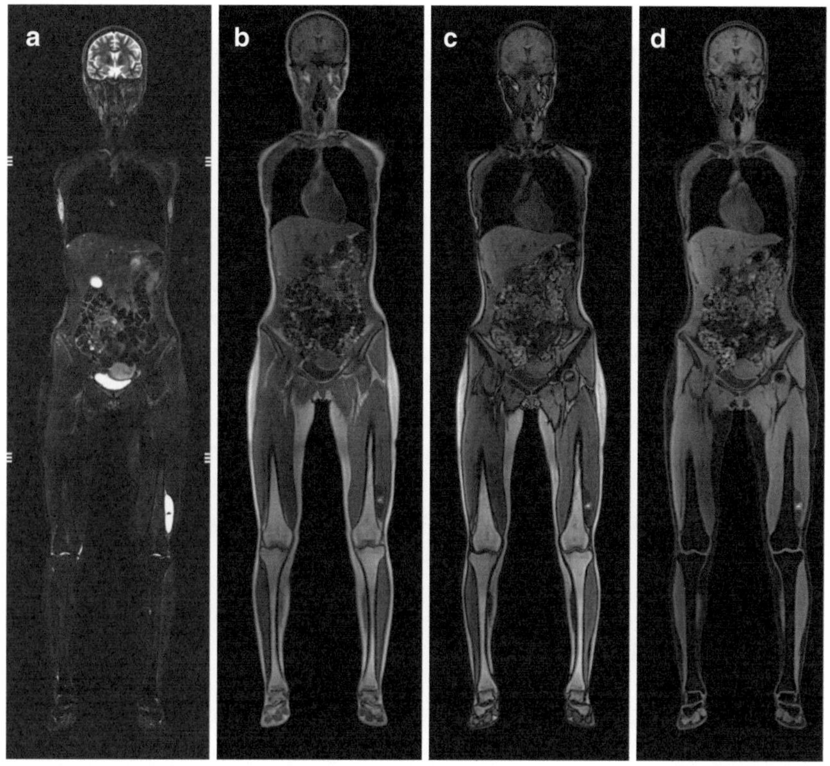

Fig. 5.3 34-year-old patient with a soft tissue sarcoma in left thigh. Whole-body MRI performed revealed an isolated soft tissue mass in the left thigh on coronal STIR (**a**), VIBE Dixon T1-weighted (**b**), out of phase (**c**) and water images (**d**). The lesion had a hyperintense area in the center consistent with hemorrhage on T1-weighted images, which could have been a result of a recent biopsy procedure

sion, STIR sequences are preferred over other fat-suppressing techniques since they cover a large anatomic area with more homogenous suppression [29]. Most diseased tissues contain high amounts of protein, resulting in high signal intensity on STIR images. Additionally, fat suppression in STIR images is stronger and more uniform compared to T2-weighted, fat-saturated images [28].

T1-weighted images are mostly used for a detailed view of the anatomy and for the detection of bone marrow lesions together with STIR images and DWI [7, 28]. Since STIR sequences are insensitive to sclerotic marrow lesions, Dixon-based T1-weighted images are preferred [30]. Dixon imaging is capable of achieving consistent suppression of fat throughout a wide field of view. Dixon images are commonly used for anatomical correlation of DWI, and for assessing the presence of bone metastases, and also T1-weighted contrast-enhanced imaging is done to evaluate solid-enhancing lesions [29]. For patients who are at high risk of bone metastases, a sagittal STIR scan of the entire spine may also be performed as an optional sequence [24].

5.4.2 Functional Sequences

DWI, a sensitive imaging technique to tissue cellularity and cell viability, is emerging as the core sequence in WB-MRI protocols in patients with cancer. Good image quality can be achieved on most modern MR systems. Diffusion-weighted WB imaging with background body signal suppression is a specialized DWI technique commonly used in WB-MRI scans. It features a free-breathing axial acquisition, low and high b-values and suppression of fat using either a presaturation pulse or STIR-based sequence. A single-shot DW echo-planar image is recommended for use in WB-MRI examinations. It should be obtained with at least two *b*-values to calculate the corresponding apparent diffusion coefficient (ADC) maps. Axially acquired images are then reconstructed into coronal planes for multiplanar viewing combined with other pulse sequences. They are also converted to negative gray-scale formats to give the appearance of PET images [31]. The low *b*-value gives a T2-weighted image with minimized perfusion effects and provides anatomical information [26, 32]. On high b-value images, lesions show increased signal intensity relative to background when active viable tumors with high cellularity are present. The combination of DWI with the T1-weighted and T2-weighted images gives more information about the exact anatomic site of the lesion detected. DWI also allows measurement of ADC values, which helps in diagnosing viable tumors and monitoring the response to treatment. The ADC value is measured in units of $\mu m^2/s$ [25, 33]. DWI has also been shown to be more effective in detecting bone metastases and muscle swelling compared to STIR images [34, 35]. DWI can be performed while the patient is breathing freely and in WB-MRI, DWI requires long acquisition times, usually around 10 to 15 minutes, in order to capture images of a large portion of the body. The combined use of the simultaneous multi-slice method and denoising, deep learning algorithm has resulted in enhancement in DWI, including reduced scan time to 6–8 minutes and fewer artifacts.

5.4.3 Contrast-Enhanced Sequences

Contrast-enhanced sequences should be used for improving the detection, characterization and staging of lesions in lung, liver, brain, and bone [36]. However, contrast administration is not routinely used in whole-body MRI because it lengthens the examination time for regular asymptomatic patients who are undergoing checkup screening [8, 37]. DWI can reduce the need for contrast-enhanced imaging in whole-body MRI scans, making the process less complex and invasive.

5.5 Image Interpretation

Typically, coronal plane T1-weighted (either 2D or 3D) and STIR images are obtained serially as mentioned above and all the obtained images of each sequence are later combined digitally to create a complete whole-body image for ease of analysis. Coronal acquisition is preferred as it leads to extensive coverage in a shorter imaging time [21]. Coronal plane has lower sensitivity for lesions of skull, spine, sternum and ribs [7, 30]. DWI is obtained in axial plane and later converted to coronal reformatted images to match the coronal planes of T1-weighted and STIR images. By using an inverted gray scale for displaying the image on DWI, the regions of restricted diffusion will appear as dark areas against a regular white background simulating PET images [38].

Axial DWI and additional fat-suppressed T2-weighted axial scans of the body are particularly useful in the detection of retroperitoneal lymph nodes or solid organ lesions. They are also helpful when evaluating detected lesions from another plane both anatomically and functionally, increasing the sensitivity for lesion detection [7]. DWI especially has gained prominence for detecting bone lesions in areas difficult to study on anatomic images such as ribs or the thoracic girdle, as well as for identifying visceral lesions, including lymph nodes, peritoneal nodules, and other internal abnormalities [39]. The ability of DWI to screen all organs in the body makes it the method of choice for whole-body staging in metastatic disease [26]. With this high sensitivity, it has lower specificity because increased signal intensity on DWI can also be observed in benign bone lesions like hemangiomas, fractures, inflammation or focal-diffuse bone marrow hyperplasia. ADC maps are helpful here to differentiate T2-shine through in benign lesions and diffusion restriction in malignant ones. Other factors that cause false-positive findings are treatment with granulocyte colony stimulating factors and the higher marrow cellularity in younger patients [40]. Evaluation of lesions together with T1-weighted and STIR sequences also have added value in decision-making [41].

T1-weighted images are especially important in evaluation of fat-containing tumors such as liposarcoma. T1-weighted images are particularly useful for identifying the presence of intra-lesional fat and its relationship with adjacent musculature, bones, and neurovascular structures, which is well-recognized in these patients [29].

Metastases to the bone are observed in 30–75% of individuals with malignant tumors, with the highest incidence noted in cases of prostate and breast cancer [42]. Bone metastases are the second most common distant site after lungs in soft tissue sarcomas. As many as 10% of individuals with soft tissue tumors may develop skeletal metastasis following a mean duration of 21.3 months [43]. Several studies have demonstrated that WB-MRI exhibits greater or at least comparable diagnostic accuracy than traditional bone scintigraphy in identifying osseous metastases even in younger patients with highly cellular hematopoietic marrow [44]. It only showed low sensitivity in patients with lesions in the ribs. In sclerotic osseous metastatic disease, STIR sequences show low sensitivity but the combinations of all three sequences (DWI, STIR and Dixon T1-weighted) improve lesion visibility [45]. Detection of lung metastases would be a challenge and the main limitation of WB-MRI especially if the lesions are small. Even though newer studies, mostly in adults, have demonstrated excellent MRI sensitivity in detecting nodules greater than 5 to 6 mm, CT is still the preferred diagnostic method for detecting lung metastases [46]. Using DWI sequences enhances the visibility of lesions in the lungs and improves the detection of metastatic lesions, especially in primary tumors, such as soft tissue sarcomas, with a high potential for lung metastasis. A low-dose chest CT without contrast can be added to the imaging protocol, particularly for these types of tumors. DW images can be evaluated together with the CT images if there's any nodular lesion of suspicion. Lesions in the lungs and lymph nodes can be better detected with PET/CT, while whole-body MR imaging with DWI is more effective for detecting lesions in the bones and liver [47, 48].

In patients with soft tissue tumors, contrast-enhanced sequences can play an important role, especially in children where imaging is done to assess both the recurrence of the primary site and the possibility of metastasis [26] (Fig. 5.4).

Contrast-enhanced imaging is also important to evaluate sclerotic bone lesions. Bone sclerosis affects DWI and ADC values. Sclerotic lesions as they pass a threshold of sclerosis do not show diffusion changes of malignant lesions but lower the ADC values much more than osteolytic metastases [49].

DWI MRI provides the opportunity for non-invasive evaluation of treatment effectiveness by measuring changes in overall tumor burden in the body as seen on high-b-value WB images and changes in ADC values of specific lesions. A noticeable increase in ADC values has been observed in various types of tumors, including bone metastases, when they respond to treatment [12, 50–52] (Fig. 5.5).

WB-MRI has emerged as a crucial imaging tool for patients with neurofibromatosis, which are genetic disorders that are linked to an increased risk of developing various types of peripheral nerve sheath tumors (PNST). Type I neurofibromatosis is characterized by the presence of plexiform neurofibromas, while multiple schwannomas are the most commonly observed type of tumor in type II neurofibromatosis. The primary concern associated with PNST is their potential to undergo malignant transformation, leading to a decrease in the life expectancy of individuals with NF1 and NF2. Malignant transformation of PNST has been associated with tumor sizes greater than 5 cm, so it is important to follow the tumor measurements [53, 54]. STIR images are mainly used in these patients. On STIR images these lesions exhibit high signal and follow the natural pathways of the peripheral nerves while growing (Fig. 5.6). DWI is used mainly to differentiate lesions with malignant transformation [55, 56]. DWI shows great potential in detecting these tumors in children, as they are typically small, circular, and easily identifiable through DWI [57].

WB-MRI is also valuable for assessing lymphovascular malformations, as these tumors can be widespread and affect multiple areas such as bones, soft tissues, and internal organs. It can be challenging to evaluate these complex cases using only one imaging technique. The combination of specific imaging characteristics seen on T1 and STIR MRI images, along with dynamic contrast-enhanced MR angiography, allows for a definitive diagnosis of lymphovascular malformations. This approach also enables differentiation between low-flow and high-flow malformations [58–60].

Assessing patients following treatment is another significant consideration in dealing with soft tissue tumors and metastases. Imaging is an important part of evaluation in these patients to show regression of primary lesion and the metastases. Assessing bone metastases has been an exception for evaluation of tumor regression due to the limitations of available techniques; particularly bone scintigraphy, which has reduced sensitivity and potential false-positive lesions [61]. The use of whole-body MR imaging seems to be highly beneficial in this context.

On anatomical sequences, the size and number of lesions are evaluated primarily. Contrast-enhanced images are also helpful to evaluate the dimensions and intensity of contrast-enhancement. The extent of response is also measured by analyzing the tumor burden on "functional images" using DWI, and by measuring the changes in ADC values in each followed lesion. Low ADC values are associated with the presence of viable tumors, while an increase in ADC values on subsequent examinations indicates a positive response to treatment. Bone metastases can also be evaluated with anatomical and DW images [62].

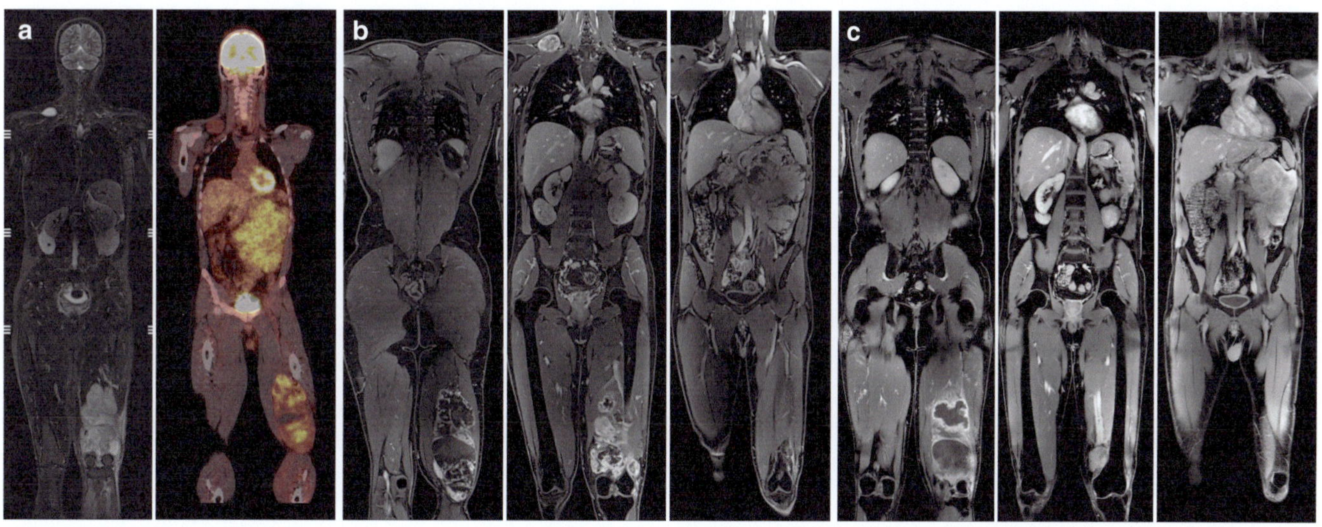

Fig. 5.4 32-year-old male patient who was diagnosed with liposarcoma. A whole-body MRI was performed, which revealed a large soft tissue tumor in the patient's left distal thigh with necrotic components. Additionally, on coronal STIR sequence there were solitary hyperintense lesions located below both kidneys and a nodular mass in the patient's right supraclavicular region. The PET-CT fused image showed increased tracer uptake in the mass located on the left side of the patient's abdomen and the mass in the left thigh. However, the right supraclavicular mass had minimal uptake (**a**). On T1-weighted post-contrast whole-body images, the mass in the left thigh demonstrated contrast-enhancement with necrotic components, while the other metastatic lesions showed diffuse contrast-enhancement (**b**). Follow-up WB-MRI, 3 months after treatment revealed a decrease in the size of all the lesions, and the intraabdominal mass showed less enhancement. The supraclavicular mass did not show any enhancement, which is compatible with necrosis (**c**)

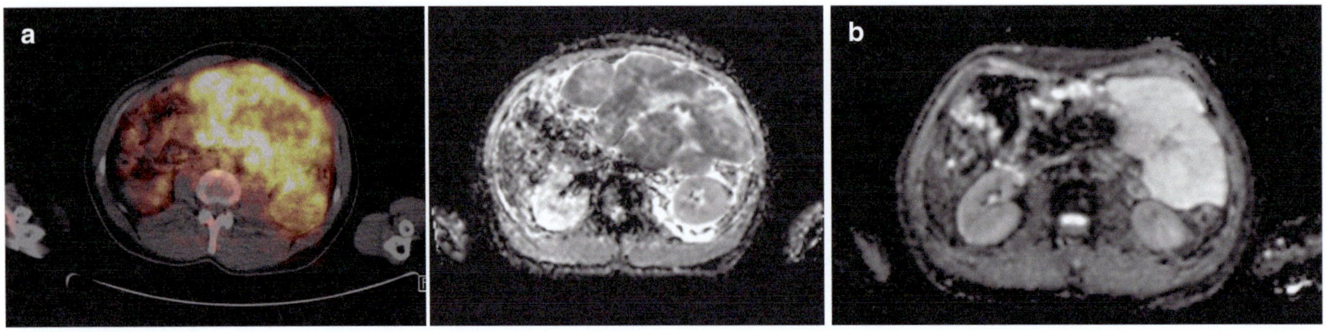

Fig. 5.5 The same patient in Fig. 5.4. There is a large intraabdominal mass showing increased tracer uptake on FDG-PET-CT fused image. On axial ADC maps of DWI, the mass showed hypointensity indicating diffusion restriction (**a**). 6 months after treatment, on follow-up DWI, ADC maps on axial plane revealed decrease in the size of mass with increased intensity implying decrease in diffusion restriction (**b**)

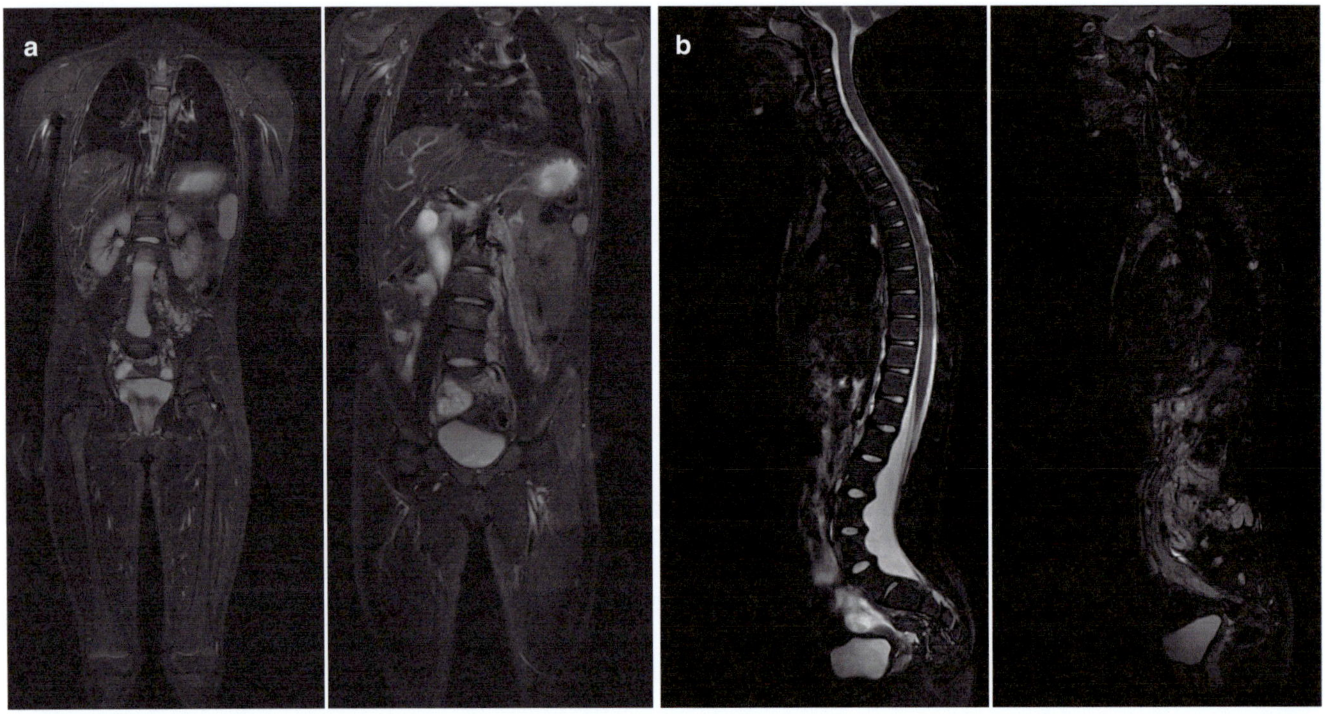

Fig. 5.6 8-year-old girl with the diagnosis of neurofibromatosis type I. On WB-MRI, coronal deep learning boost STIR images (magnified); multiple small dimension neurofibromas are noted along the upper and lower extremity nerve courses (**a**). On sagittal STIR images dural ectasia findings are noted (**b**)

References

1. Weber M-A, Lalam R, Trattnig S, Bohndorf K, Vanhoenacker F, Tagliafico A, et al. Soft tissue tumors in adults: ESSR approved guidelines for diagnostic imaging. Semin Musculoskelet Radiol. 2015;19(05):475–82.
2. Roberge D, Vakilian S, Alabed YZ, Turcotte RE, Freeman CR, Hickeson M. FDG PET/CT in initial staging of adult soft-tissue sarcoma. Sarcoma. 2012;2012:960194.
3. Roberts CC, Kransdorf MJ, Beaman FD, Adler RS, Amini B, Appel M, et al. ACR appropriateness criteria follow-up of malignant or aggressive musculoskeletal tumors. J Am Coll Radiol. 2016;13(4):389–400.
4. Verstraete KL, Lang P. Bone and soft tissue tumors: the role of contrast agents for MR imaging. Eur J Radiol. 2000;34(3):229–46.
5. Vanel D, Shapeero LG, Tardivon A, Western A, Guinebretière JM. Dynamic contrast-enhanced MRI with subtraction of aggressive soft tissue tumors after resection. Skeletal Radiol. 1998;27(9):505–10.
6. Del Grande F, Subhawong T, Weber K, Aro M, Mugera C, Fayad LM. Detection of soft-tissue sarcoma recurrence: added value of functional MR imaging techniques at 3.0 T. Radiology. 2014;271(2):499–511.
7. Gottumukkala RV, Gee MS, Hampilos PJ, Greer M-LC. Current and emerging roles of whole-body MRI in evaluation of pediatric cancer patients. Radiographics. 2019;39(2):516–34.
8. Ulus S, Suleyman E, Aksoy Ozcan U, Karaarslan E. Whole-Body MRI screening in asymptomatic subjects; preliminary experience and long-term follow-up findings. Pol J Radiol. 2016;81:407–14.
9. Brenner DJ, Shuryak I, Einstein AJ. Impact of reduced patient life expectancy on potential cancer risks from radiologic imaging. Radiology. 2011;261(1):193–8.
10. Guimarães MD, Noschang J, Teixeira SR, Santos MK, Lederman HM, Tostes V, Kundra V, Oliveira AD, Hochhegger B, Marchiori E.

Whole-body MRI in pediatric patients with cancer. Cancer Imaging. 2017;17:1.
11. Summers P, Saia G, Colombo A, Pricolo P, Zugni F, Alessi S, et al. Whole-body magnetic resonance imaging: technique, guidelines and key applications. Ecancermedicalscience. 2021;15:1164.
12. PadhaniAR LG, Mu-Koh D, Chenevert TL, Thoeny HC, Takahara T, et al. Diffusion-weighted magnetic resonance imaging as a cancer biomarker: consensus and recommendations. Neoplasia. 2009;11(2):102–25.
13. Pruessmann KP, Weiger M, Scheidegger MB, Boesiger P. SENSE: sensitivity encoding for fast MRI. Magn Reson Med. 1999;42(5):952–62.
14. Griswold MA, Jakob PM, Heidemann RM, Nittka M, Jellus V, Wang J, et al. Generalized autocalibrating partially parallel acquisitions (GRAPPA). Magn Reson Med. 2002;47(6):1202–10.
15. Katscher U, Börnert P, Leussler C, van den Brink JS. Transmit SENSE. Magn Reson Med. 2002;49(1):144–50.
16. Yoon JH, Nickel MD, Peeters JM, Lee JM. Rapid imaging: recent advances in abdominal MRI for reducing acquisition time and its clinical applications. Korean J Radiol. 2019;20(12):1597–615.
17. Glockner JF, Hu HH, Stanley DW, Angelos L, King K. Parallel MR imaging: a user's guide. Radiographics. 2005;25(5):1279–97.
18. Breuer FA, Blaimer M, Mueller MF, Seiberlich N, Heidemann RM, Griswold MA, et al. Controlled aliasing in volumetric parallel imaging (2D CAIPIRINHA). Magn Reson Med. 2006;55:549–56.
19. Larkman DJ, Hajnal JV, Herlihy AH, Coutts GA, Young IR, Ehnholm G. Use of multicoil arrays for separation of signal from multiple slices simultaneously excited. J Magn Reson Imaging. 2001;13(2):313–7.
20. Obele CC, Glielmi C, Ream J, Doshi A, Campbell N, Zhang HC, et al. Simultaneous multislice accelerated free-breathing diffusion-weighted imaging of the liver at 3T. Abdom Imaging. 2015;40(7):2323–30.
21. Kraus MS, Coblentz AC, Deshpande VS, Peeters JM, Itriago-Leon PM, Chavhan GB. State-of-the-art magnetic resonance imaging sequences for pediatric body imaging. Pediatr Radiol. 2022; [Internet] Available from: https://pubmed.ncbi.nlm.nih.gov/36255456/
22. Fayad LM, Jacobs MA, Wang X, Carrino JA, Bluemke DA. Musculoskeletal tumors: how to use anatomic, functional, and metabolic MR techniques. Radiology. 2012;265:340–56.
23. Messiou C, Hillengass J, Delorme S, Lecouvet FE, Moulopoulos LA, Collins DJ, et al. Guidelines for acquisition, interpretation, and reporting of whole-body MRI in myeloma: myeloma response assessment and diagnosis system (MY-RADS). Radiology. 2019;291:5–13.
24. Bezerra ROF, Recchimuzzi DZ, dos Santos Mota MM, Garcia MRT, de Menezes MR, Mazo PE, et al. Whole-Body magnetic resonance imaging in the oncology setting. J Comput Assist Tomogr. 2019;43(1):66–75.
25. Tunariu N, Blackledge M, Messiou C, Petralia G, Padhani A, Curcean S, et al. What's new for clinical Whole-body MRI (WB-MRI) in the 21st century. Br J Radiol. 2020;93(1115):20200562.
26. Lecouvet FE, Whole-Body MR. Imaging: musculoskeletal applications. Radiology. 2016;279(2):345–65.
27. Pasoglou V, Michoux N, Peeters F, Larbi A, Tombal B, Selleslagh T, et al. Whole-body 3D T1-weighted MR imaging in patients with prostate cancer: feasibility and evaluation in screening for metastatic disease. Radiology. 2015;275:155–66.
28. Nievelstein RAJ, Littooij AS. Whole-body MRI in paediatric oncology. Radiol Med. 2015;121(5):442–53.
29. Vicentini JRT, Bredella MA. Whole body imaging in musculoskeletal oncology: when, why, and how. Skeletal Radiol. 2023;52:281–95.
30. Morone M, Bali MA, Tunariu N, Messiou C, Blackledge M, Grazioli L, et al. Whole-body MRI: current applications in oncology. Am J Roentgenol. 2017;209(6):W336–W49.
31. Mürtz P, Kaschner M, Träber F, et al. Diffusion-weighted whole-body MRI with background body signal suppression: technical improvements at 3.0 T. J Magn Reson Imaging. 2012;35:456–61.
32. Padhani AR, Koh D-M, Collins DJ. Whole-body diffusion-weighted MR imaging in cancer: current status and research directions. Radiology. 2011;261:700–18.
33. Pasoglou V, Michoux N, Larbi A, Van Nieuwenhove S, Lecouvet F. Whole Body MRI and oncology: recent major advances. Br J Radiol. 2018;91(1090):20170664.
34. Pearce T, Philip S, Brown J, Koh DM, Burn PR. Bone metastases from prostate, breast and multiple myeloma: differences in lesion conspicuity at short-tau inversion recovery and diffusion-weighted MRI. Br J Radiol. 2012;85:1102–6.
35. Faruch M, Garcia AI, Del Amo M, Pomes J, Isern J, González SP, et al. Diffusion-weighted magnetic resonance imaging is useful for assessing inflammatory myopathies. Muscle Nerve. 2019;59:555–60.
36. Dutoit JC, Vanderkerken MA, Verstraete KL. Value of whole-body MRI and dynamic contrast enhanced MRI in the diagnosis, follow-up and evaluation of disease activity and extent in multiple myeloma. Eur J Radiol. 2013;82:1444–52.
37. Basar Y, Alis D, Tekcan Sanli DE, Akbas T, Karaarslan E. Whole-body MRI for preventive health screening: management strategies and clinical implications. Eur J Radiol. 2021;137:109584.
38. Koh D-M, Blackledge M, Padhani AR, Takahara T, Kwee TC, Leach MO, et al. Whole-body diffusion-weighted MRI: tips, tricks, and pitfalls. Am J Roentgenol. 2012;199(2):252–62.
39. Lecouvet FE, El Mouedden J, Collette L, et al. Can whole-body magnetic resonance imaging with diffusion-weighted imaging replace Tc-99m bone scanning and computed tomography for single-step detection of metastases in patients with highrisk prostate cancer?. Eur Urol. 2012;62(1):68–75.
40. Winfield JM, Blackledge MD, Tunariu N, Koh D-M, Messiou C. Whole-body MRI: a practical guide for imaging patients with malignant bone disease. Clin Radiol. 2021;76:715–27.
41. Larbi A, Omoumi P, Pasoglou V, Michoux N, Triqueneaux P, Tombal B, et al. Whole-body MRI to assess bone involvement in prostate cancer and multiple myeloma: comparison of the diagnostic accuracies of the T1, short tau inversion recovery (STIR), and high b-values diffusion-weighted imaging (DWI) sequences. Eur Radiol. 2019;29:4503–13.
42. Jiang W, Rixiati Y, Zhao B, Li Y, Tang C, Liu J. Incidence, prevalence, and outcomes of systemic malignancy with bone metastases. J Orthop Surg. 2020;28(2):230949902091598.
43. Pretell-Mazzini J, Seldon CS, D'Amato G, Subhawong TK. Musculoskeletal metastasis from soft-tissue sarcomas: a review of the literature. J Am Acad Orthop Surg. 2022;30(11):493–503.
44. Daldrup-Link HE, Henning T, Link TM. MR imaging of therapy-induced changes of bone marrow. Eur Radiol. 2007;17(3):743–61.
45. Mirowitz SA, Apicella P, Reinus WR, Hammerman AM. MR imaging of bone marrow lesions: relative conspicuousness on T1-weighted, fat-suppressed T2-weighted, and STIR images. Am J Roentgenol. 1994;162(1):215–21.
46. Heye T, Ley S, Heussel CP, et al. Detection and size of pulmonary lesions: how accurate is MRI? A prospective comparison of CT and MRI. Acta Radiol. 2012;53:153–60.
47. Antoch G, Vogt FM, Freudenberg LS, et al. Whole-body dual-modality PET/CT and whole-body MRI for tumor staging in oncology. JAMA. 2003;290(24):3199–206.
48. Schmidt GP, Baur-Melnyk A, Haug A, et al. Comprehensive imaging of tumor recurrence in breast cancer patients using whole-body MRI at 1.5 and 3 T compared to FDG-PET-CT. Eur J Radiol. 2008;65(1):47–58.

49. Bashir U, Tunariu N, Collins DJ, Bianchini D, Zivi A, Koh DM. Negative relationship between CT attenuation values and ADC values in densely sclerotic bone metastases from prostate cancer. In: Radiological Society of North America scientific assembly and annual meeting program. Oak Brook, Ill: Radiological Society of North America; 2013. p. 198.
50. Padhani AR, Makris A, Gall P, Collins DJ, Tunariu N, de Bono JS. Therapy monitoring of skeletal metastases with whole-body diffusion MRI. J Magn Reson Imaging. 2014;39(5):1049–78.
51. Giles SL, Messiou C, Collins DJ, et al. Whole-body diffusion-weighted MR imaging for assessment of treatment response in myeloma. Radiology. 2014;271(3):785–94.
52. Messiou C, Collins DJ, Giles S, de Bono JS, Bianchini D, de Souza NM. Assessing response in bone metastases in prostate cancer with diffusion weighted MRI. Eur Radiol. 2011;21(10):2169–77.
53. Cai W, Kassarjian A, Bredella MA, Harris GJ, Yoshida H, Mautner VF, et al. Tumor burden in patients with neurofibromatosis types 1 and 2 and schwannomatosis: determination on whole-body MR images. Radiology. 2009;250:665–73.
54. Ahlawat S, Blakeley JO, Langmead S, Belzberg AJ, Fayad LM. Current status and recommendations for imaging in neurofibromatosis type 1, neurofibromatosis type 2, and schwannomatosis. Skeletal Radiol. 2020;49:199–219.
55. Demehri S, Belzberg A, Blakeley J, Fayad LM. Conventional and functional MR imaging of peripheral nerve sheath tumors: initial experience. Am J Neuroradiol. 2014;35:1615–20.
56. Derlin T, Tornquist K, Münster S, Apostolova I, Hagel C, Friedrich RE, et al. Comparative effectiveness of 18F-FDG PET/CT versus whole-body MRI for detection of malignant peripheral nerve sheath tumors in neurofibromatosis type 1. Clin Nucl Med. 2013;38:e19–25.
57. Petralia G, Padhani AR. Whole-body magnetic resonance imaging in oncology. Magn Reson Imaging Clin N Am. 2018;26(4):495–507.
58. Atkin KL, Ditchfield MR. The role of whole-body MRI in pediatric oncology. J Pediatr Hematol Oncol. 2014;36(5):342–52.
59. Ley S, Ley-Zaporozhan J, Schenk J-P, et al. Whole-body MRI in the pediatric patient. Eur J Radiol. 2009;70:442–51.
60. Ohgiya Y, Hashimoto T, Gokan T, et al. Dynamic MRI for distinguishing high-flow from low-flow peripheral vascular malformations. Am J Roentgenol. 2005;185:1131–7.
61. Therasse P, Arbuck SG, Eisenhauer EA, et al. New guidelines to evaluate the response to treatment in solid tumors. European Organization for Research and Treatment of Cancer, National Cancer Institute of the United States, National Cancer Institute of Canada. J Natl Cancer Inst. 2000;92(3):205–16.
62. Blackledge MD, Collins DJ, Tunariu N, et al. Assessment of treatment response by total tumor volume and global apparent diffusion coefficient using diffusion-weighted MRI in patients with metastatic bone disease: a feasibility study. PLoS One. 2014;9(4):e91779.

Histopathologic Challenges in the Diagnostic Stage

6

A. H. G. Cleven and P. C. W. Hogendoorn

Soft tissue tumours are rare, and sarcomas account for less than 1% of all malignancies. Since many different soft tissue tumours exist with overlapping clinicopathological features, diagnostic decision-making can be challenging. Diagnosis relies upon a complex and integrated combination of clinical features (age, gender, site and size of tumour, hereditary context), imaging studies (superficial or deep-located, primary soft tissue or bone, including epiphysis, metaphysis, or diaphysis) [1], microscopic morphology (with representative biopsy material), immunohistochemistry, and molecular genetics [2]. When these prerequisites of appropriate clinical practice and radiology are met, the histopathological classification process begins [3].

Soft tissue tumours are classified according to the *WHO Classification of Tumours, 5th Edition. Soft tissue and Bone Tumours*, which serve as a guide to clarify diagnoses in a multidisciplinary team composed of pathologists, radiologists, surgeons, and medical oncologists [4]. The WHO classification is organized following the main assumed lineage groups of mesenchymal tumours, including adipocytic tumours, fibroblastic and myofibroblastic tumours, fibrohistiocytic tumours, vascular tumours, muscle tumours, peripheral nerve sheath tumours, tumours of uncertain differentiation and undifferentiated small round cell sarcomas of soft tissue.

In this chapter, we describe the histopathological differential diagnosis of common soft tissue tumours, integrating morphological, immunohistochemical, and genetic features for a final diagnosis.

6.1 Adipocytic Tumours

Lipomas are the most common benign adipocytic tumour, and most of them do not pass medical attention. However, approximately 20% of all sarcomas compromise atypical and malignant adipocytic tumours with four major liposarcoma subtypes, including atypical lipomatous tumour (ALT) (location in the extremities)/well-differentiated liposarcoma (location in the retroperitoneum), dedifferentiated liposarcoma, myxoid liposarcoma, and pleomorphic liposarcoma [5].

Clinical presentation such as age (young versus older patient) and localization (superficial versus deep seeded localization/retroperitoneum) is important for the differential diagnoses since certain adipocytic tumours are very common in young patients and uncommon in older patients, for example, lipoblastomas. Other adipocytic tumours—for example, lipomas or myxoid liposarcomas—do not primarily occur in the retroperitoneum [6].

The morphology of benign and malignant adipocytic tumours may show overlapping morphology, and especially with scarce biopsy material, additional immunohistochemistry or even genetic testing is mandatory. Lipomas with reactive changes may harbour fat cells that look like lipoblasts, which is a key morphological cell feature of ALT/well-differentiated liposarcoma (Fig. 6.1a). In contrast to lipomas, ALT/well-differentiated liposarcoma harbours *MDM2* gene amplification. Using immunohistochemistry, MDM2-positive nuclear staining in lesional cells favours the diagnosis of ALT/well-differentiated liposarcoma (Fig. 6.1b). ALT/well-differentiated liposarcoma may progress to a dedifferentiated liposarcoma (frequently seen in retroperitoneum) characterized by morphology with high-grade spindle cell proliferation with a lack of lipoblasts (Fig. 6.1c, d) and therefore difficult to distinguish from morphological mimickers

A. H. G. Cleven
Department of Pathology and Medical Biology, University Medical Center Groningen, University of Groningen, Groningen, The Netherlands

Department of Pathology, Leiden University Medical Center, Leiden, The Netherlands
e-mail: a.h.g.cleven@umcg.nl

P. C. W. Hogendoorn (✉)
Department of Pathology, Leiden University Medical Center, Leiden, The Netherlands

Department of Pathology, Vrije Universiteit Brussel (VUB)/Universitair Ziekenhuis Brussel (UZ Brussel), Brussels, Belgium
e-mail: pancras.hogendoorn@vub.be

H. Özger et al. (eds.), *Diagnosis and Treatment of Soft Tissue Tumors*, https://doi.org/10.1007/978-3-031-77061-6_6

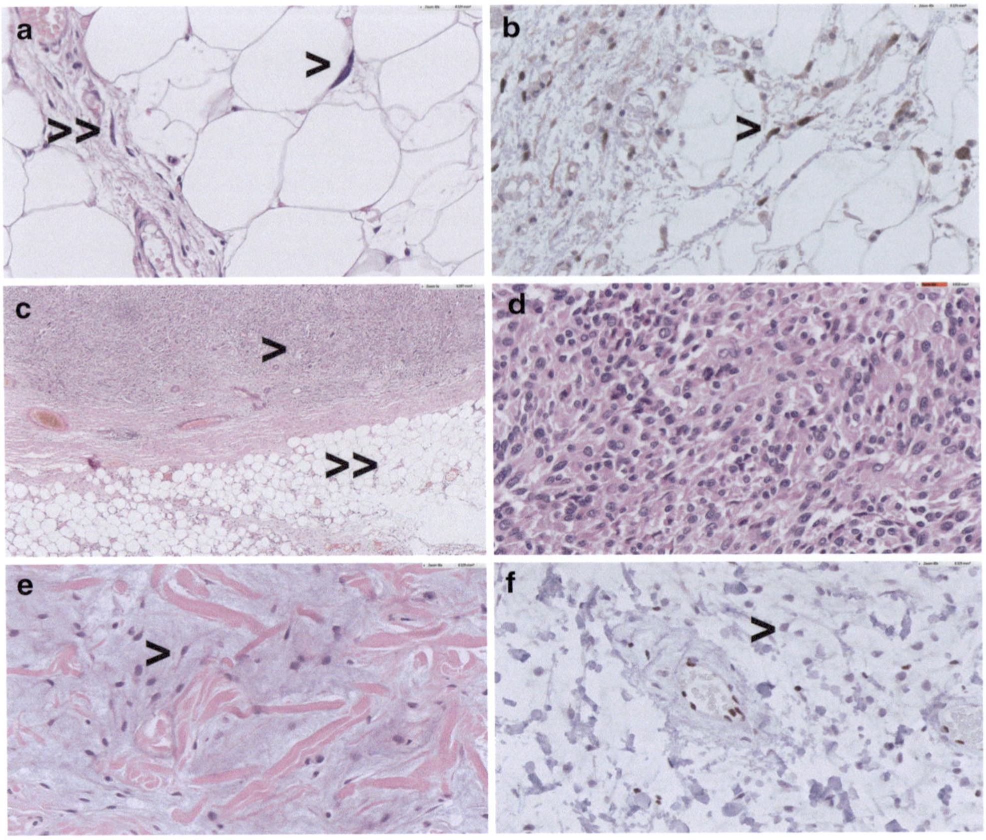

Fig. 6.1 Morphological and immunohistochemical findings in adipocytic tumours. (**a**) Atypical lipomatous tumour/well-differentiated liposarcoma with variation in adipocytic size, scattered lipoblasts (black arrow head) and atypical hyperchromatic stromal cells (double black arrow head) in a fibrous stroma. (**b**) MDM2 nuclear positivity in lipoblasts and atypical hyperchromatic stromal cells (black arrow head) in an atypical lipomatous tumour/well-differentiated liposarcoma. (**c**) Dedifferentiated liposarcoma with abrupt transition from well-differentiated liposarcoma (double black arrow head) to high-grade non-lipogenic sarcoma (black arrow head). (**d**) Pleomorphic hyperchromatic tumour cells in a dedifferentiated liposarcoma. (**e**) Bland spindle cells (black arrow head) with ropey collagen in a myxoid background in an example of spindle cell lipoma. (**f**) Loss of RB1 (black arrow head) in neoplastic cells of a spindle cell lipoma

such as pleomorphic liposarcoma or undifferentiated sarcoma of the soft tissue. MDM2 immunohistochemistry with diffuse positive staining fits with the diagnosis of dedifferentiated liposarcomas, and in cases with uncertain MDM2 staining results, Fluorescence in Situ Hybridization (FISH) may be used to determine the amplification of *MDM2* for a final diagnosis.

Besides lipomas, spindle cell/pleomorphic lipomas are common benign adipocytic tumours with a preference to occur in the subcutis of the posterior neck, back, and shoulders. These tumours are characterized by CD34 positive spindle cells in a ropey collagen-rich background with loss of RB1 and occasionally with lipoblast but without the atypical spindle cells seen in ALT/well-differentiated liposarcoma and negative for MDM2 staining (Fig. 6.1e, f).

Myxoid liposarcoma is an example of a malignant adipocytic tumour located in the deep soft tissue of the extremities in adults with a characteristic morphology composed of a blend of immature-appearing spindle cells in a myxoid background with scattered lipoblasts and a chicken wire vascular network. Molecular testing for *DDIT3(CHOP)*-involved gene fusions may be used for a definitive diagnosis in clinically and morphologically challenging cases.

6.2 Fibroblastic and Myofibroblastic Tumours

Nodular fasciitis is a relatively common self-limiting mesenchymal neoplasm that occurs in all ages but more often in young adults. Any anatomic site can be involved, but it typically develops on the surface of the fascia and extends into the subcutis. A (minor) trauma is often reported.

Although nodular fasciitis is self-limiting, clinical presentation and radiological features can be very suspicious for malignancy. At low-power microscopy, nodular fasciitis appears very atypical with high cellularity and myxoid changes and a typical infiltrative border. Mitotic figures may be plentiful, but nodular fasciitis is composed of plump spindle-shaped cells lacking nuclear atypia (Fig. 6.2a). The

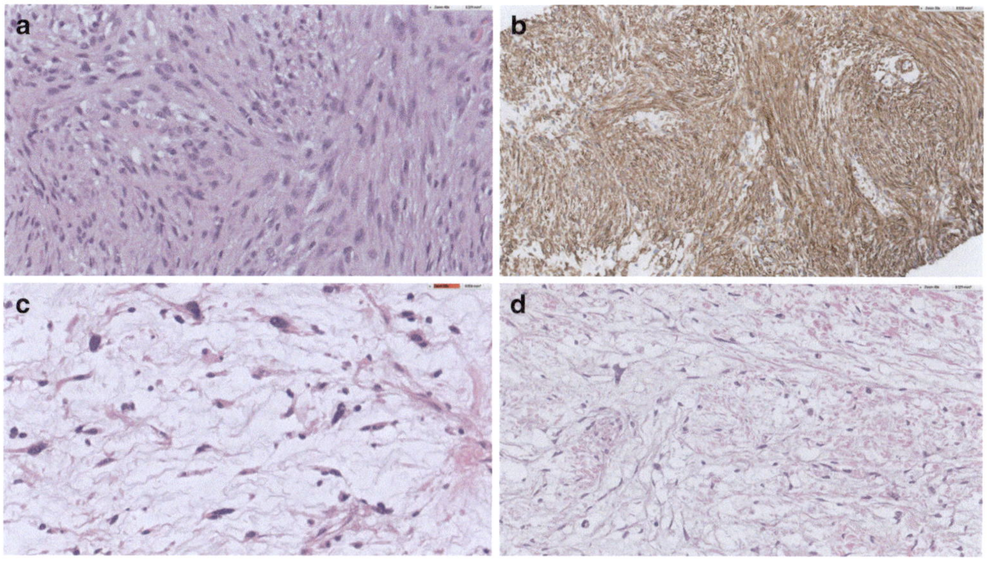

Fig. 6.2 Morphological and immunohistochemical findings in fibroblastic tumours. (**a**) Cellular proliferation in nodular fasciitis composed of plump spindle-shaped cells, strongly positive for myofibroblastic marker SMACT (**b**). (**c**) Myxofibrosarcoma with atypical hyperchromatic spindle cells in a myxoid background. (**d**) Liposarcoma with overlapping morphological features with myxofibrosarcoma

neoplastic cells in nodular fasciitis do show myofibroblastic differentiation using immunohistochemistry (Fig. 6.2b). Desmoid-type fibromatosis may mimic nodular fasciitis although desmoid-type fibromatosis does not show the characteristic tissue culture-like appearance seen in nodular fasciitis. *USP6* gene fusion detection using FISH or next-generation sequencing may be used to confirm the diagnosis of nodular fasciitis. In contrast to nodular fasciitis, desmoid-type fibromatosis lacks *USP6* gene fusions and is characterized by activating mutations in *CTNNB1* leading to nuclear beta-catenin accumulation, which can be determined using immunohistochemistry.

Myxofibrosarcoma is an example of a malignant fibroblastic neoplasm and also the most common sarcoma in elderly patients, typically located superficially in the soft tissue of the limbs [7–9]. Myxofibrosarcomas have a multinodular and highly infiltrative growth, a myxoid matrix, atypical hyperchromatic fibroblastic cells, and curvilinear blood vessels (Fig. 6.2c, d). No specific immunohistochemistry is available for myxofibrosarcomas.

Solely based on morphology, low-grade myxofibrosarcomas are difficult to distinguish from myxomas (benign) [10]. Myxomas are located in deep soft tissue of the thigh most often in middle-aged patients and harbour *GNAS* mutations, which can be used as a molecular marker to distinguish myxoma from low-grade myxofibrosarcoma.

High-grade myxofibrosarcomas are difficult to distinguish from pleomorphic, undifferentiated sarcoma of the soft tissue based on biopsy material. Both entities are comprised of a cellular pleomorphic spindle cell proliferation with a heterogenous amount of myxoid stroma in the background. There are no specific immunohistochemical stainings or genetic aberrations to distinguish both entities. However, if myxoid stroma is prominent, one should favour the diagnosis of myxofibrosarcoma, and recent genetic studies suggest that high-grade myxofibrosarcomas and pleomorphic undifferentiated sarcoma of the soft tissue represent a spectrum of the same disease.

Furthermore, dedifferentiated liposarcoma may show a morphology with a close resemblance to high-grade myxofibrosarcoma. Apart from a preferred anatomic location, with dedifferentiated liposarcomas in the retroperitoneum and myxofibrosarcomas in the limbs, using MDM2 immunohistochemistry or MDM2 FISH, both entities can be distinguished from each other.

6.3 Fibrohistiocytic Tumours

Tenosynovial giant cell tumour (TSGCT) is a mesenchymal tumour often arising in the vicinity of the synovium of joints, predominantly in the hands (localized) or knees (diffuse) [11]. These tumours have specific radiological features and are usually divided according to their site (intra- or extra-articular) and growth pattern (localized or diffuse). If the clinical radiological presentation fits with TSGCT, the diagnosis is relatively simple for a pathologist. In the case of a TSGCT, the morphology will show a variable amount of sclerosis with sheets of histiocyte-like cells admixed with osteoclast-type giant cells and foamy macrophages with scattered larger mononuclear cells containing a peripheral rim of haemosiderin. This typical morphology is not seen in chronic synovitis or a synovial haemangioma which may be a differential diagnosis based on the clinical presentation. Although TSGCT harbours *CSF1* gene fusions, based on the typical clinical radiological and morphological features in most cases, genetic testing is not necessary for a final diagnosis of TSGCT.

Fibrous histiocytoma also known as dermatofibroma is a frequently seen example of a fibrohistiocytic tumour with a broad age range and anatomic location. However, dermal skin localization or subcutis is essential for the correct diagnosis of fibrous histiocytoma. Many morphological variants are described in the WHO especially deep-located cellular and aneurysmal variants of fibrous histiocytoma are associated with a higher incidence for local recurrences. A pathognomonic morphological feature for the diagnosis of fibrous histiocytoma and its variants (including atypical fibrous histiocytoma) is the entrapment of pre-existent collagen by the lesional fibrohistiocytic cells at the periphery of the lesion. Immunohistochemistry is apart from rare subtypes like angiomatoid fibrous histiocytoma (Desmin positivity) or epithelioid fibrous histiocytoma (ALK positivity) non-specific in the case of fibrous histiocytoma. Several gene fusions are described in fibrous histiocytoma variants involving the genes *EWSR1* (angiomatoid fibrous histiocytoma) [12], *ALK* (epithelioid fibrous histiocytoma), *PRKCB,* and *LAMTOR1* (deep fibrous histiocytoma and aneurysmal fibrous histiocytoma).

6.4 Vascular Tumours

Benign vascular tumours are subdivided into tumours and malformations with clinical and specific genetic features. Haemangiomas are vascular tumours that arise as a result of cellular proliferation. It represents one of the most common soft tissue tumours in general and is the most common tumour during infancy and childhood. In contrast, vascular malformations are developmental abnormalities. Despite these definitions, haemangiomas and vascular malformations show overlapping histological features, which makes it sometimes difficult to distinguish from each other.

Superficial location in the head and neck region is the preferred localization for haemangiomas but they may also occur in organs for example the liver. Since haemangiomas are typically composed of small vessels lined by flattened epithelial cells (Fig. 6.3a) and malignant vascular tumours are very rare in children, the diagnosis is relatively simple for a pathologist in representative biopsy or excision material in the correct clinical setting. In adult patients, especially if only scarce biopsy material is available, benign vascular tumours are sometimes difficult to distinguish from intermediate (Kaposi sarcoma) or malignant vascular tumours (epithelioid haemangioendothelioma & angiosarcoma).

Kaposi sarcoma predominantly occurs in elderly men or HIV-affected patients and is associated with HHV8 infection. If there is a clinical suspicion for Kaposi sarcoma, a pathologist should test for HHV8 positive staining in the laesional endothelial cells to distinguish Kaposi sarcoma from a benign vascular or intermediate vascular tumour (Fig. 6.3b).

At the other end of the spectrum especially radiotherapy associated angiosarcoma (often located in the breast after radiotherapy for breast carcinoma) can be difficult to distinguish from atypical vascular proliferations, which are also radiotherapy associated. A combination of overt atypia and MYC nuclear positive staining (indicative for *MYC* amplification) should direct in the diagnosis of a radiotherapy associated angiosarcoma (Fig. 6.3c, d).

Epithelioid haemangioendothelioma (EHE) is an example of a malignant vascular tumour with a *WWTR1-CAMTA1* gene fusion in more than 90% of cases, which can be used as a diagnostic marker to distinguish EHE from angiosarcoma.

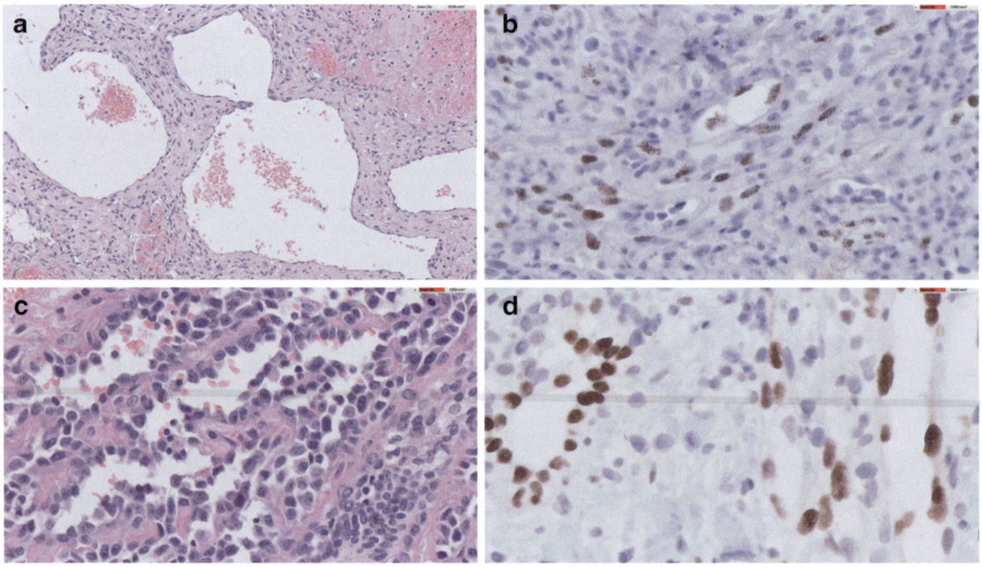

Fig. 6.3 Morphological and immunohistochemical findings in vascular tumours. (**a**) Vascular channels in a regular pattern with flat endothelial cells in an example of haemangioma. (**b**) HHV8 expression in endothelial cells in Kaposi sarcoma. (**c**) Atypical vascular spaces with atypical enlarged endothelial cells in an angiosarcoma. (**d**) Expression of C-MYC in endothelial cells of a radiotherapy-associated angiosarcoma

6.5 Muscle Tumours

Leiomyoma is a benign smooth muscle tumour that occurs in the deep somatic soft tissue, retroperitoneum or in the skin. The morphology is relatively straightforward with eosinophilic spindle cells arranged in fascicles without overt atypia or mitotic activity positive for at least two of three smooth muscle IHC markers (SMACT, Desmin or Caldesmon) .

If atypia and/or mitotic figures are observed in a leiomyomatous neoplasm located in the deep somatic soft tissue or in the retroperitoneum, a leiomyosarcoma is the preferred diagnosis (Fig. 6.4a). It is important to realize that leiomyomatous neoplasms primary in the uterus are differently graded compared to the soft tissue or bone leiomyomatous neoplasm.

Rabdomyosarcoma is a malignant neoplasm composed of a monomorphic population showing skeletal muscle differentiation with a peak incidence in young patients. Pending on the subtype of rabdomyosarcoma (RMS) with a unique diagnostic genetic aberration (Alveolar RMS (*PAX* involved gene fusions), spindle cell RMS (*MYOD1* mutation) [13] or spindle cell sclerosing RMS (*TFCP2* involved gene fusions)) [14] the morphology differs in percentage of rabdomyoblasts among a malignant appearing spindle cell proliferation (Fig. 6.4b). Genetic testing is mandatory for diagnosing the correct subtype of RMS, which has therapeutic consequences.

6.6 Peripheral Nerve Sheath Tumours

Schwannoma is a common benign slow-growing nerve sheath tumour composed of Schwann cells located in the peripheral nerves in the skin and subcutaneous tissue. Spinal, central nervous system and visceral locations are very rare. The morphology of schwannomas is typical with cellular Antoni-A areas and loose myxoid Antoni-B areas with diffuse positive staining for S100 in the laesional Schwann cells (Fig. 6.5a, b). Ancient schwannoma is a subtype with degenerative atypia that may be a pitfall if not distinguished from melanoma based on extensive staining for melanocytic markers such as Melan-A and HMB-45.

Neurofibroma is the most common benign peripheral nerve sheath tumour, commonly located in the skin and composed not only of Schwann cells like schwannomas but also fibroblasts, mast cells and axons. The majority of neurofibromas occur sporadically and less often in the context of neurofibromatosis type-1 (NF1).

Neurofibroma frequently shows the morphology of loose myxoid stroma intermixed with Schwann cells and fibroblast without atypia or mitotic activity (Fig. 6.5c, d). However, in patients with NF1, neurofibromas may show higher cellularity and atypia, causing difficulty to distinguish neurofibroma from atypical neurofibroma/atypical neurofibromatous neo-

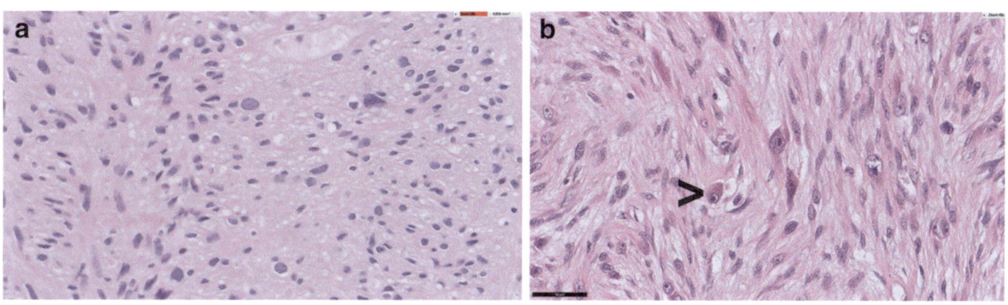

Fig. 6.4 Morphological findings in muscle tumours. (**a**) Fascicles of atypical spindle cells with enlarged hyperchromatic nuclei in a leiomyosarcoma. (**b**) Scattered rabdomyoblasts (black arrow head) with eccentric eosinophilic cytoplasm in an example of rabdomyosarcoma

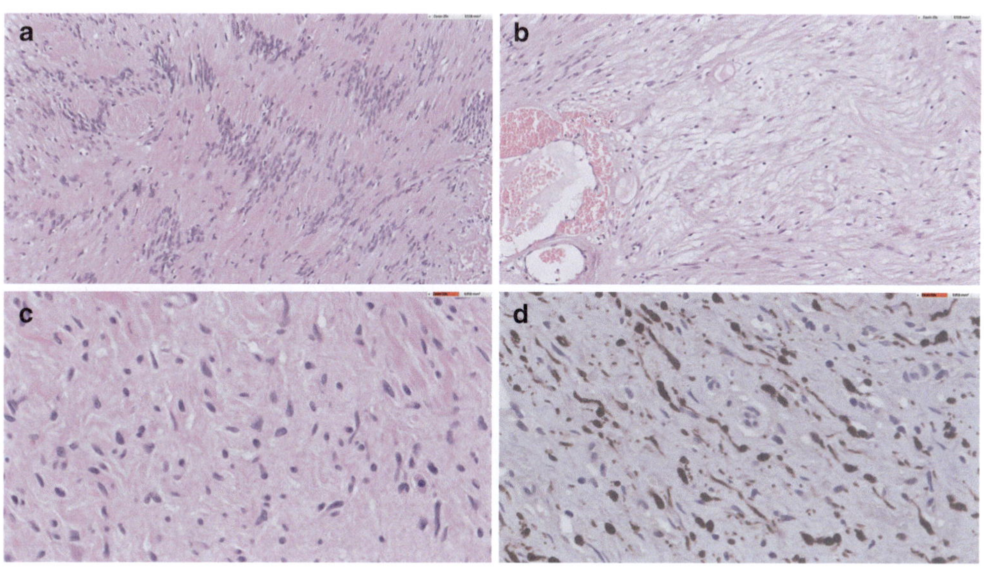

Fig. 6.5 Morphological and immunohistochemical findings in peripheral nerve sheath tumours. (**a**) Cellular Antoni-A area with so called Verocay bodies with palisaded spindle cells typical in schwannoma. (**b**) Myxoid low cellularity called Antoni-B area in a schwannoma. (**c**) Neurofibroma composed of Schwann cells admixed with fibroblastic cells in a myxoid background with S100 positivity in Schwann cells (**d**)

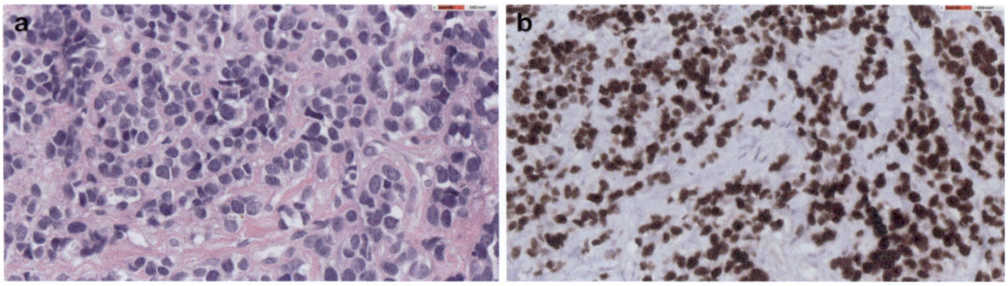

Fig. 6.6 Morphological and immunohistochemical findings in Ewing sarcoma. (**a**) Round tumour cells with hyperchromatic nuclei and almost no cytoplasm positive for the Ewing Sarcoma marker NKX2.2 (**b**)

plasm of uncertain biological potential (ANNUBP) or even low-grade malignant peripheral nerve sheath tumours (MPNST). Especially plexiform neurofibromas in patients with NF1 have an increased risk of progressing to ANNUBP or MPNST. Representative tumour material is crucial to distinguish neurofibromas from ANNUBP based on the amount of cellularity, atypia and mitotic figures. Loss of H3K27me3 is a characteristic feature of MPNSTs, which is used as a diagnostic marker for this malignant subtype of peripheral nerve sheath tumour [15].

6.7 Undifferentiated Small Round Cell Sarcomas of Soft Tissue

Round cell sarcomas represent a subgroup of sarcomas frequently seen in children and young adults that are associated with structural re-arrangements that generate fusion genes that can be used as a diagnostic tool. Solely based on morphology, a round cell sarcoma is difficult to distinguish from carcinoma, lymphoma, or melanoma, and a broad panel of immunohistochemistry should be used to differentiate between these entities [16]. The final diagnostic tool is testing for recurrent gene fusions, including *EWSR1* (Ewing sarcoma), *CIC* (*CIC*-rearranged sarcoma) [17], *BCOR* (sarcoma with *BCOR* genetic alterations) or *NFATC2* re-arrangements [18] (Fig. 6.6a, b).

6.8 Conclusion and Discussion

While soft tissue tumours are rare and there is a large spectrum of overlapping morphologies, most guidelines ask for diagnostic expert opinion or discussion within an experienced multidisciplinary team before therapeutic steps are taken. This has led to the centralisation of care for these patients, which on the one hand is beneficial for the patients but, on the other hand, makes it difficult for the non-specialised pathologist harder and harder to get any experience. In this regard, it should be stimulated to have regional centres for diagnosis and treatment that reach out to the community for diagnostic services as well as educational services in order to create an optimal setting for diagnostics.

In sum, the challenges in the diagnostic stage are in a wide range. Clinical and radiological information are very helpful, and the pathologist can do his job well when appropriate information and material is given. A famous remark by a well-known pathologist: the smaller the biopsy, the less clinical information and the more they want to know from me. (F. Eulderink; Pathological aphorisms).

References

1. van Rijswijk CS, Kunz P, Hogendoorn PC, Taminiau AH, Doornbos J, Bloem JL. Diffusion-weighted MRI in the characterization of soft-tissue tumors. J Magn Reson Imaging. 2002;15(3):302–7.
2. Hogendoorn PC, Collin F, Daugaard S, Dei Tos AP, Fisher C, Schneider U, et al. Changing concepts in the pathological basis of soft tissue and bone sarcoma treatment. Eur J Cancer. 2004;40(11):1644–54.
3. Jansen-Landheer ML, Krijnen P, Oostindier MJ, Kloosterman-Boele WM, Noordijk EM, Nooij MA, et al. Improved diagnosis and treatment of soft tissue sarcoma patients after implementation of national guidelines: a population-based study. Eur J Surg Oncol. 2009;35(12):1326–32.
4. Soft tissue and bone tumours. In: WHO classification of tumours editorial board, editors. WHO Classification of tumours IARC; 2020. p. 338–498.
5. Creytens D. What's new in adipocytic neoplasia? Virchows Arch. 2020;476(1):29–39.
6. Van Roggen JF, Hogendoorn PC. Soft tissue tumours of the retroperitoneum. Sarcoma. 2000;4(1–2):17–26.
7. Willems SM, van Remoortere A, van Zeijl R, Deelder AM, McDonnell LA, Hogendoorn PC. Imaging mass spectrometry of myxoid sarcomas identifies proteins and lipids specific to tumour type and grade, and reveals biochemical intratumour heterogeneity. J Pathol. 2010;222(4):400–9.
8. Jones EA, van Remoortere A, van Zeijl RJ, Hogendoorn PC, Bovee JV, Deelder AM, et al. Multiple statistical analysis techniques corroborate intratumor heterogeneity in imaging mass spectrometry datasets of myxofibrosarcoma. PLoS One. 2011;6(9):e24913.
9. Willems SM, Debiec-Rychter M, Szuhai K, Hogendoorn PC, Sciot R. Local recurrence of myxofibrosarcoma is associated with increase in tumour grade and cytogenetic aberrations, suggesting a multistep tumour progression model. Mod Pathol. 2006;19(3):407–16.
10. Graadt van Roggen JF, Hogendoorn PC, Fletcher CD. Myxoid tumours of soft tissue. Histopathology. 1999;35(4):291–312.
11. van der Heijden L, Gibbons CL, Dijkstra PD, Kroep JR, van Rijswijk CS, Nout RA, et al. The management of diffuse-type giant cell tumour (pigmented villonodular synovitis) and giant cell

tumour of tendon sheath (nodular tenosynovitis). J Bone Joint Surg Br. 2012;94(7):882–8.
12. Rossi S, Szuhai K, Ijszenga M, Tanke HJ, Zanatta L, Sciot R, et al. EWSR1-CREB1 and EWSR1-ATF1 fusion genes in angiomatoid fibrous histiocytoma. Clin Cancer Res. 2007;13(24):7322–8.
13. Szuhai K, de Jong D, Leung WY, Fletcher CD, Hogendoorn PC. Transactivating mutation of the MYOD1 gene is a frequent event in adult spindle cell rhabdomyosarcoma. J Pathol. 2014;232(3):300–7.
14. Le Loarer F, Cleven AHG, Bouvier C, Castex MP, Romagosa C, Moreau A, et al. A subset of epithelioid and spindle cell rhabdomyosarcomas is associated with TFCP2 fusions and common ALK upregulation. Mod Pathol. 2020;33(3):404–19.
15. Cleven AH, Sannaa GA, Briaire-de Bruijn I, Ingram DR, van de Rijn M, Rubin BP, et al. Loss of H3K27 tri-methylation is a diagnostic marker for malignant peripheral nerve sheath tumors and an indicator for an inferior survival. Mod Pathol. 2016;29(6):582–90.
16. Wang WL, Patel NR, Caragea M, Hogendoorn PC, Lopez-Terrada D, Hornick JL, et al. Expression of ERG, an Ets family transcription factor, identifies ERG-rearranged Ewing sarcoma. Mod Pathol. 2012;25(10):1378–83.
17. Kajtar B, Tornoczky T, Kalman E, Kuzsner J, Hogendoorn PC, Szuhai K. CD99-positive undifferentiated round cell sarcoma diagnosed on fine needle aspiration cytology, later found to harbour a CIC-DUX4 translocation: a recently described entity. Cytopathology. 2014;25(2):129–32.
18. Szuhai K, Ijszenga M, de Jong D, Karseladze A, Tanke HJ, Hogendoorn PC. The NFATc2 gene is involved in a novel cloned translocation in a Ewing sarcoma variant that couples its function in immunology to oncology. Clin Cancer Res. 2009;15(7):2259–68.

7 Histological Challenges in the Intra-operative Stage

Suk Wai Lam and Judith V. M. G. Bovée

7.1 Introduction

Intra-operative assessment in surgical pathology has been an ancillary tool to guide the surgeon in immediate decision-making during surgery. It encompasses both intra-operative gross examination, as well as microscopic consultation with rapid frozen sections. The latter is considered challenging, especially in case a pre-operative diagnosis is lacking. Without the possibility to use additional ancillary tests such as immunohistochemistry, it can be difficult to generate a differential diagnosis based on frozen sections because of limitations in morphology. Furthermore, shortcomings of frozen sections such as inferior quality of slides and sampling error due to tumor heterogeneity might hamper the diagnostic accuracy. In addition, soft tissue tumors represent a pathology subspecialty that is considered difficult by most pathologists due to the large amount of histological subtypes with overlapping morphology and their rarity. For these reasons, it is not always possible to distinguish benign from malignant using frozen sections. Despite these considerations, intra-operative tissue assessment of soft tissue tumors can be of additional value in certain cases. It needs to be emphasized that the main purpose of intra-operative consultation should be to guide surgical decision-making with regard to the extent of surgery, thus, the results of the frozen section should influence the course of the surgical procedure. The yield and quality of the frozen section can be increased by discussing the specific question preferably upfront with the pathologist, so that the answer will indeed guide the surgeon in decision-making. It should not be ordered routinely, as it is time-consuming and it might even hamper proper microscopical evaluation of permanent sections due to freezing artifacts or loss of tissue. Reasons for intra-operative pathological consultations are the determination of the presence and nature of a tumor, the evaluation of sample adequacy for diagnosis or special studies, and the assessment of surgical margins. These aspects will be discussed, together with the challenges and considerations of intra-operative consultations.

S. W. Lam · Judith V. M. G. Bovée (✉)
Department of Pathology, Leiden University Medical Center, Leiden, The Netherlands
e-mail: s.w.lam@lumc.nl; j.v.m.g.bovee@lumc.nl

7.2 Determining the Nature of a Lesion

Since obtaining the correct diagnosis plays a major role in the determination of optimal treatment, diagnostic biopsies are standardly obtained prior to surgery, after appropriate imaging assessment [1]. While in benign soft tissue tumors, an intralesional or marginal resection can be accepted, for intermediate locally aggressive and malignant soft tissue tumors excision with wide margins is standard of care [1]. Depending on tumor type, histological grade and tumor localization, neoadjuvant chemotherapy or radiotherapy prior to a wide resection can be considered after discussion of the results of the biopsy in a multidisciplinary team.

The golden standard for obtaining a primary diagnosis for soft tissue tumors is on permanent sections after the tissue has been fixated with formalin and embedded in paraffin. In addition to morphological evaluation of the tumor, ancillary tools such as immunohistochemistry and/or molecular analysis are often essential for definitive diagnosis. There usually is a turnaround time of several days, which increases when molecular testing is required. This is needed to achieve a high-quality diagnosis with as little uncertainty as possible. In contrast, when intra-operatively the pathologist is required to make a diagnosis of a tumor based on a frozen section, immunohistochemistry and molecular analysis are not possible, and the morphology is more difficult to evaluate as a consequence of the procedure (Fig. 7.1). Therefore, the diagnosis will be of lower quality with higher levels of uncertainty. This will remain until the tissue has been formalin-fixed and paraffin-embedded, and has been analyzed immunohistochemically and/or molecularly.

Since the clinical context can be highly variable, it is highly dependent on the specific question and the conse-

H. Özger et al. (eds.), *Diagnosis and Treatment of Soft Tissue Tumors*, https://doi.org/10.1007/978-3-031-77061-6_7

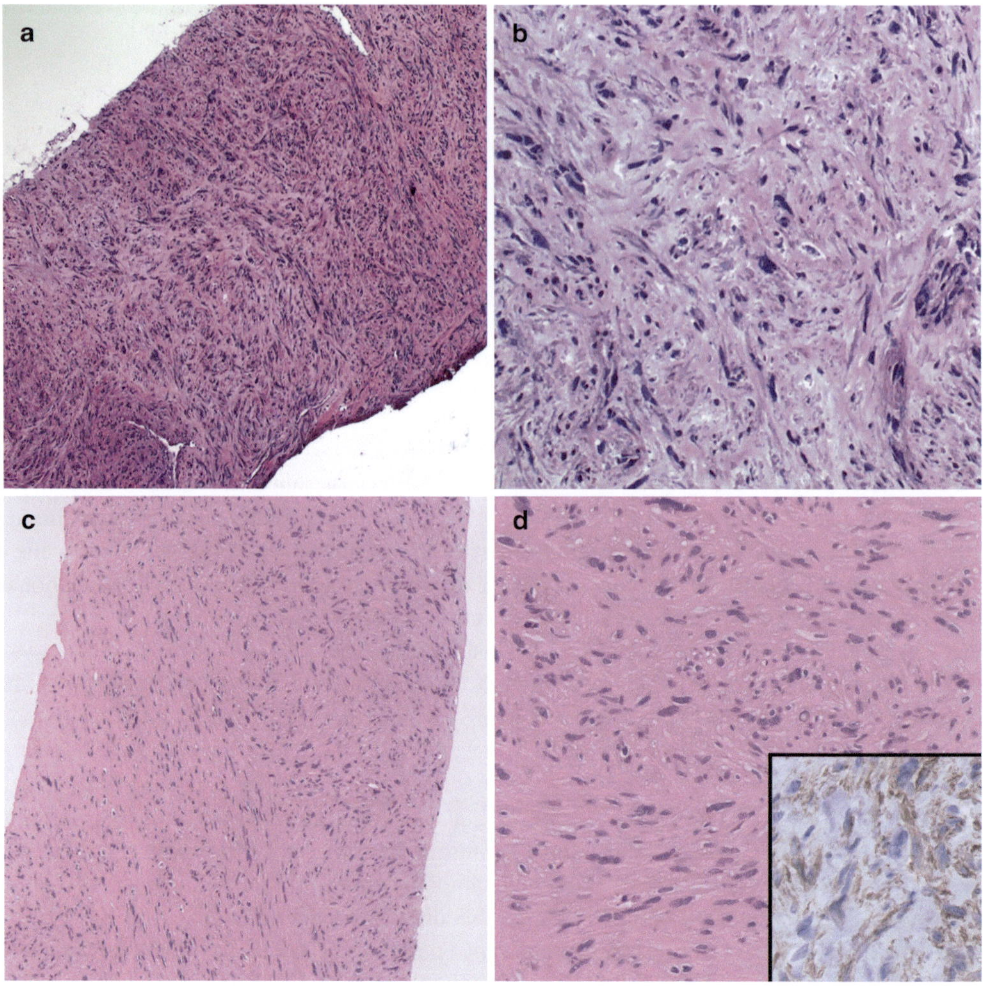

Fig. 7.1 Leiomyosarcoma (LMS). (**a**) Frozen section of a biopsy with an atypical cellular spindle cell tumor with a broad differential diagnosis. (**b**) On high magnification, some tumor cells contain large hyperchromatic nuclei, but other cellular details are difficult to evaluate on frozen sections. (**c**) Permanent section shows an atypical tumor with a fascicular growth pattern. Tumor cells have abundant eosinophilic cytoplasm, characteristic of LMS. (**d**) High magnification demonstrates tumor cells with broad, blunt-ended nuclei, which is also a feature of LMS. Immunohistochemistry for caldesmon, a smooth muscle marker, is positive, confirming the diagnosis of LMS (insert)

quences for surgery whether frozen section analysis to provide a provisional diagnosis of an unknown mass can have added value in intra-operative decision-making. For instance, if for some reason, the dignity of the tumor is unknown prior to surgery, and when an unequivocal diagnosis of a benign tumor can be made using an open biopsy on a frozen section, the tumor can be excised in one stage. This way, it will reduce medical costs and risks associated with anesthesia. However, discrepancies between the initial diagnosis of an intermediate or malignant tumor on permanent sections might lead to an inferior treatment regimen for these patients.

A valid reason for intra-operative pathology assessment is when an unexpected skip lesion is encountered during surgery. The resectability of the tumor or the extent of the surgery might be influenced by this finding. Therefore, the exact nature of the lesion needs to be clarified by frozen section analysis before continuing to evaluate whether and how to change the surgical strategy. Another indication for intra-operative consultation is when the surgeon encounters an abnormal lymph node that is not visible on pre-operative imaging. Although lymph node metastasis is relatively rare in sarcomas, few sarcoma types are associated with a higher risk of lymph node metastasis (i.e., synovial sarcoma, clear cell sarcoma, angiosarcoma, rhabdomyosarcoma and epithelioid sarcoma) [2, 3]. If a lymph node metastasis is confirmed by a frozen section, the surgeon might perform an additional lymphadenectomy in the same session, thereby avoiding a second surgery.

The accuracy of intra-operative frozen section analysis for diagnosis is widely studied in epithelial tumors, which stands in contrast to soft tissue tumors [4]. In several larger reports among various tumor types, the number of soft tissue tumors was limited (12% and 5.8% of all cases) [5, 6]. In these studies, an accurate frozen section diagnosis could be obtained in 94% of 133 and 96% of 581 bone and soft tissue cases [5, 6]. Of note, this was lower than the overall accuracy of 98% reported in a cohort of 10,000 frozen sections [6]. Other reports aiming at studying the diagnostic accuracy in soft tissue tumors specifically are sparse. In one study, a specific diagnosis could be obtained in 86% (73/85) of the musculoskeletal tumors [7], while the reported overall diagnostic accuracy in another study including 408 lesions was 95%. Lower accuracies were yielded in patients with adipocytic tumors (84%) and fibroblastic or myofibroblastic lesions

(87%) [8]. However, in the cohort of Golouh et al., an overall correct diagnosis was established in 84.2% of 57 patients, in which a specific diagnosis could only be made in approximately half of the cases. The diagnosis was deferred in 14% and mainly involved lipomatous tumors. Diagnosis on the frozen section was incorrect in one case (1.8%) [9].

Compared to epithelial tumors, the diagnostic accuracy in soft tissue tumors is lower, and obtaining a specific diagnosis on frozen sections is less often possible. As soft tissue tumors represent a broad scale of different tumor types with phenotypic overlap, combined with the limited exposure of these tumors in general hospitals, this contributes to the challenges of intra-operative frozen section analysis. One should understand that the diagnostic accuracy of frozen sections is highly dependent on the expertise of the pathologist. As is also the case for the evaluation of permanent slides, diagnosis of soft tissue frozen sections should be assigned to a well-trained pathologist specialized in soft tissue tumors to avoid incorrect diagnosis. Prior to the evaluation of frozen sections, the pathologist should be well-informed about the clinical presentation and history of the patient. Pathologists should be skilled in selecting representative material for frozen section analysis, as this might be a potential source of discrepant results between the frozen section and the permanent slides. In the case of lymph node evaluation or margin assessment, morphological comparison with the primary tumor is useful.

Occasionally, it is impossible to reach a definitive diagnosis on a frozen section in soft tissue tumor pathology as the distinction between benign and malignant purely based on morphology is difficult: for instance, nodular fasciitis can show high cellularity, nuclear atypia and increased mitotic rate worrisome for malignancy, while low-grade fibromyxoid sarcoma can be deceptively bland with low cellularity, no nuclear atypia and lack of mitoses and can be easily mistaken for a benign tumor or reactive change (Fig. 7.2). Therefore, when intra-operative frozen sections are considered to provide a primary diagnosis, the specific question within that specific clinical context should always be discussed directly between the surgeon and the pathologist, preferably upfront. Lastly, surgeons should be aware of the fact that technical issues might also contribute to an incorrect diagnosis, for example, if the diagnostic tissue is not present in the frozen section or not visible due to folding of slides, but is present in the corresponding permanent section.

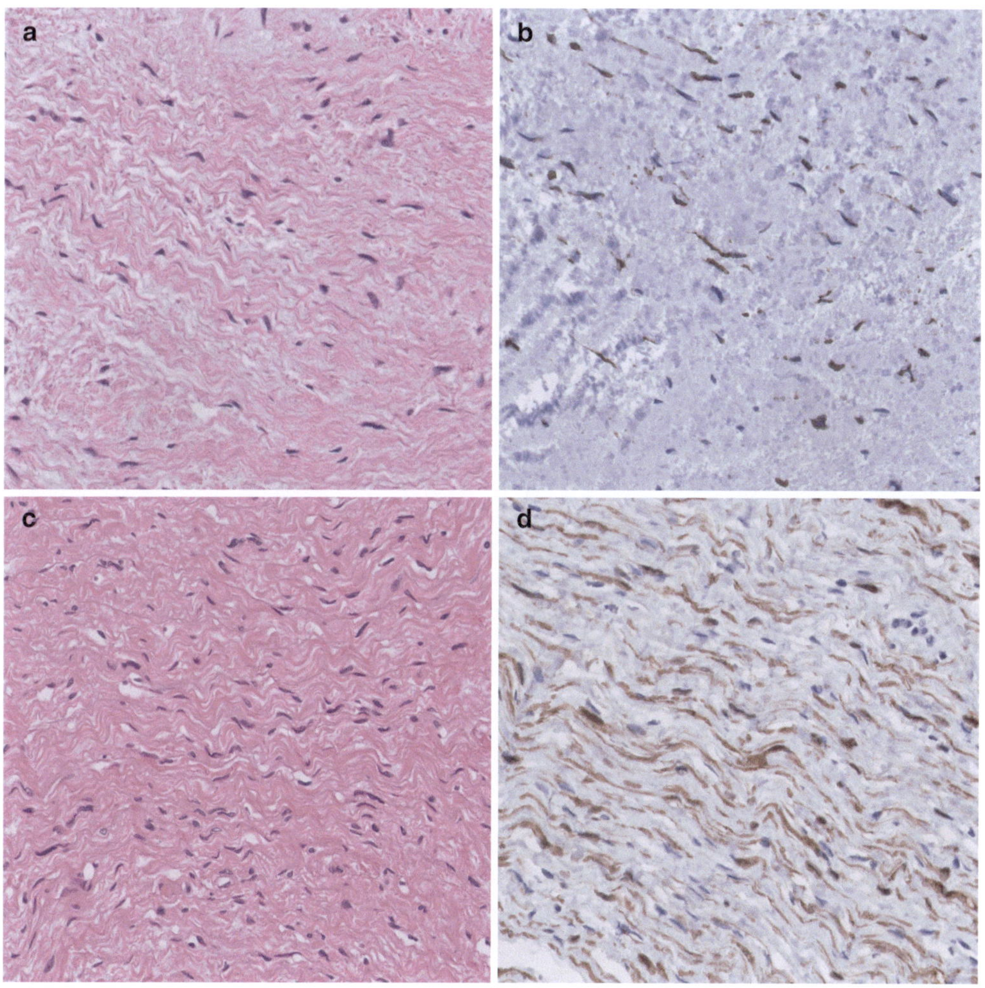

Fig. 7.2 (**a**) Low-grade fibromyxoid sarcoma (LGFMS) with deceptively bland tumor cells in a loose myxofibrous background. Some cells have buckled nuclei, resembling a neurofibroma. (**b**) immunohistochemistry shows strong nuclear staining for MUC4, a highly sensitive and specific marker for LGFMS. (**c**) Neurofibroma a with short to elongated spindle cells with buckled nuclei, arranged in a background of wavy collagen. Note the morphological resemblance between neurofibroma and LGFMS, illustrating the need of additional immunohistochemistry for differentiation, which cannot be performed during frozen section analysis. (**d**) S100 is positive in a subset of the tumor cells, confirming the diagnosis of neurofibroma

7.3 Adequacy of Tumor Sample

In some cases of open biopsy, frozen section analysis is requested to evaluate if the obtained material is representative and sufficient for making a diagnosis or sufficient for specific scientific studies. Obtaining adequate material in soft tissue tumors with extensive hemorrhage or necrosis can be problematic and in that case frozen section evaluation of (part of) the obtained material can be useful to avoid an extra procedure in case the material is insufficient. More material can be obtained in the same procedure if needed, preventing patients from returning for a second visit. The advantage of the frozen section to assess the representativity of the tumor is that material can immediately be preselected for microbacterial cultures or molecular analysis, based on the findings. However, image-guided biopsies with high accuracy are nowadays more routinely performed, thereby mostly replacing open biopsy procedures for assessing sampling adequacy [10]. In case the first attempt to obtain representative tissue with an image-guided biopsy fails, the frozen section could be considered when the procedure is repeated.

7.4 Margins Assessment

The quality of initial surgery is a well-established prognostic factor for local recurrence [11–13]. Obtaining adequate margins is of paramount importance in sarcoma surgery, although this has to be weighed against the maintenance of maximal function and preservation of vital structures. During routine pathological work-up, assessing surgical margins is usually performed on the definitive surgical specimen. Guidelines for standardized pathology reports of soft tissue tumors are provided by The International Collaboration for Cancer Reporting [14]. The specimen is orientated according to orienting sutures placed by the surgeon and measured in three dimensions. The margins of the specimen can be inked in multiple colors for orientation and to aid microscopical margin assessment, whereafter the specimen is cut and placed in a fixative solution. After fixation, the specimen is sliced and photographed and areas of interest are included according to macroscopic evaluation. After embedding in paraffin, sections are cut, stained with hematoxylin-eosin and microscopically examined. Traditionally, the Enneking classification system is mainly used for margin assessment. Margins are defined as intralesional, marginal, wide (tumor surrounded by a margin of healthy tissue) and radical (extra-compartmental en-bloc excision), relating the margin to the lesion, its reactive zone and anatomic compartment [15]. Over the years, other classification systems have been introduced. The residual tumor classification (R classification), combines the macroscopically and microscopically assessment of surgical margins [16]. The margin is considered as R0 if no tumor cells are present at the margin. If margins are only microscopically affected, the resection is classified as R1, while in R2 resections tumor contamination is already visible macroscopically. In the International Union against Cancer (UICC) classification, criteria for R0 resections are more stringent. A margin of at least 1 mm must be achieved for classification as R0 resection. As it is debatable which classification system is of the most prognostic value, the ESMO guideline advises using the R classification and additionally reporting the minimum distance to the tumor and the type of tissue between the tumor and the closest margin [1]. Of note, shrinkage due to fixation might lead to underestimation of margins [17].

The utility of intra-operative margin assessment of soft tissue tumors has not been examined thoroughly [9, 18], in contrast to for example breast-conserving surgery [19]. However, in certain cases, one might consider intra-operative consultation to evaluate tumor extent and tumor margins. Altogether with visual and tactile clues and intra-operative imaging, this might aid the surgeon in decision making. Gross evaluation of the specimen after thin slicing alone has limited value, unless the tumor is a well demarcated nodule and a rim of normal tissue appears after slicing. In other circumstances, areas close to the surgical margin can be sampled for frozen section analysis after the orientation of the specimen. Preferably, margins of interest are evaluated with sections perpendicular to the surgical margin. Some soft tissue tumors, such as myxofibrosarcoma, angiosarcoma, desmoid type fibromatosis or dermatofibrosarcoma protuberans, are notorious for their infiltrative growth with microscopic extensions that are far beyond what is visible macroscopically (Figs. 7.3 and 7.4). Occasionally, for these tumors, frozen sections can be obtained for microscopy [20, 21]. However, the distinction between desmoid-type fibromatosis or low-grade myxofibrosarcoma and reactive changes including scar tissue might be very difficult or sometimes impossible. In case of a positive margin, an additional resection might follow to obtain adequate surgical margins. However, local recurrence and survival rates remain unknown after these types of resections.

More literature is available for margin assessment using Mohs microsurgery in soft tissue tumors of the skin. Using this technique, the complete exterior surface of the excised tumor can be assessed using frozen sections. This method is mainly used in non-melanoma skin cancer, although this technique has also been used in a few cutaneous soft tissue tumors. In short, after resection of the specimen, the pieces of tissue are inked and mapped, frozen and cut using a cryostat. In contrast to vertical sections in a routine wide excision, horizontal frozen sections are used for examining margins in Mohs microsurgery. This allows examination of the whole bottom and sides of each specimen microscopically, instead of only portions of the margin. If needed, a

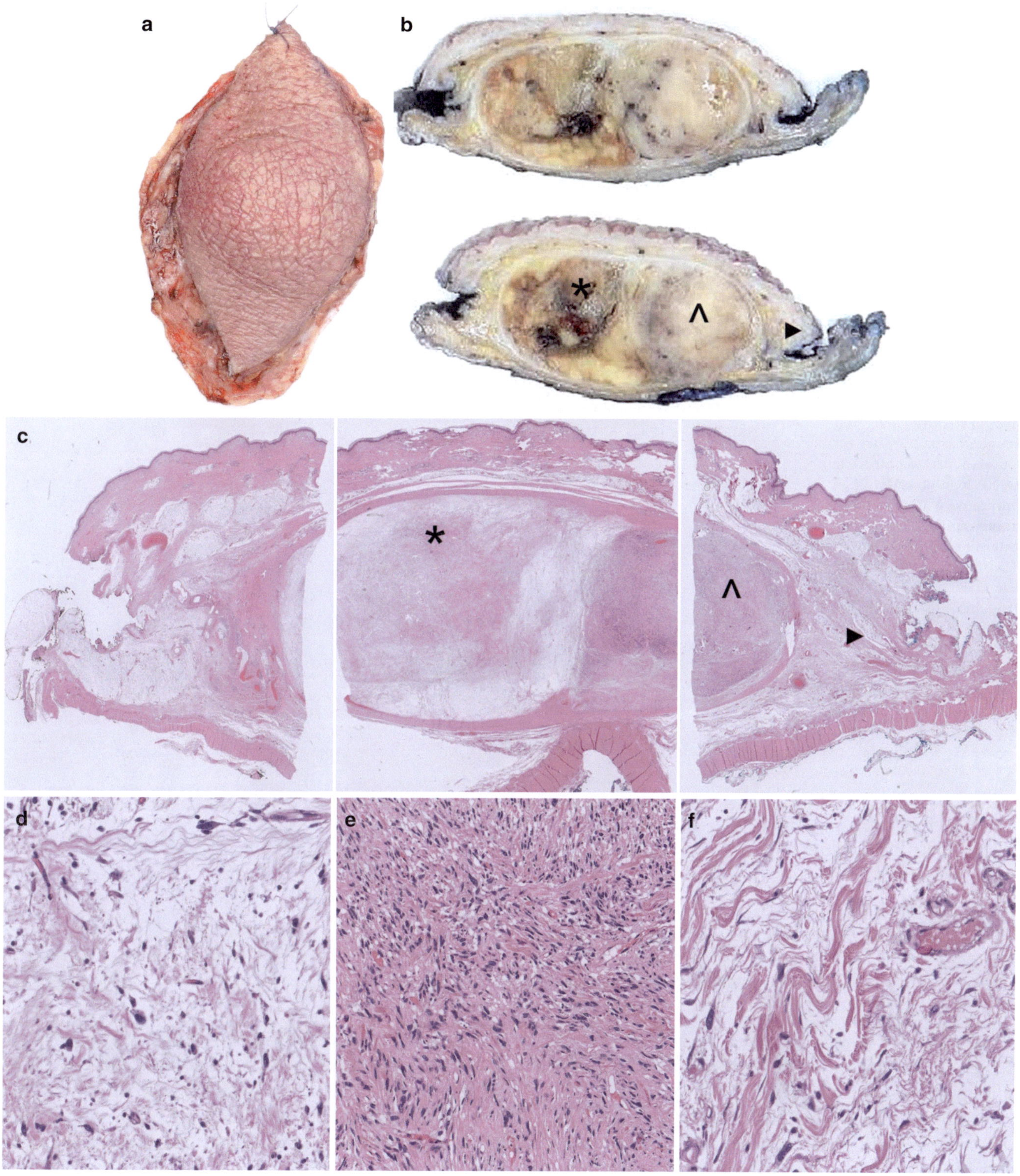

Fig. 7.3 Myxofibrosarcoma. (**a**) Fresh surgical specimen with a centrally located subcutaneous tumor. Note the suture placed by the surgeon for orientation. (**b**) Two representative sections of the tumor after formalin fixation. The tumor is encapsulated and has a heterogenous aspect with hemorrhage and glassy (*) and solid components (^). Resection margins toward the side (►) and bottom appear to be negative for tumor. Note that the surgical margins were inked in black and blue. (**c**) H&E staining of one representative section, divided into three, with myxoid (*) and solid (^) components. On low magnification, the area adjacent to the tumor bulk (►) seem to show some reactive changes with loose fibrosis. (**d**) On high magnification, the myxoid area (*) shows atypical spindled and stellate tumor cells with hyperchromatic nuclei in a loose myxoid background (*). (**e**) The solid component (^) is cellular with atypical spindle cells in a collagenous background. (**f**) In the area adjacent to the tumor (►) individual tumor cells are dispersed in a background of collagen fibers, illustrating the infiltrative growth pattern of myxofibrosarcoma growing beyond the estimated margins on gross evaluation

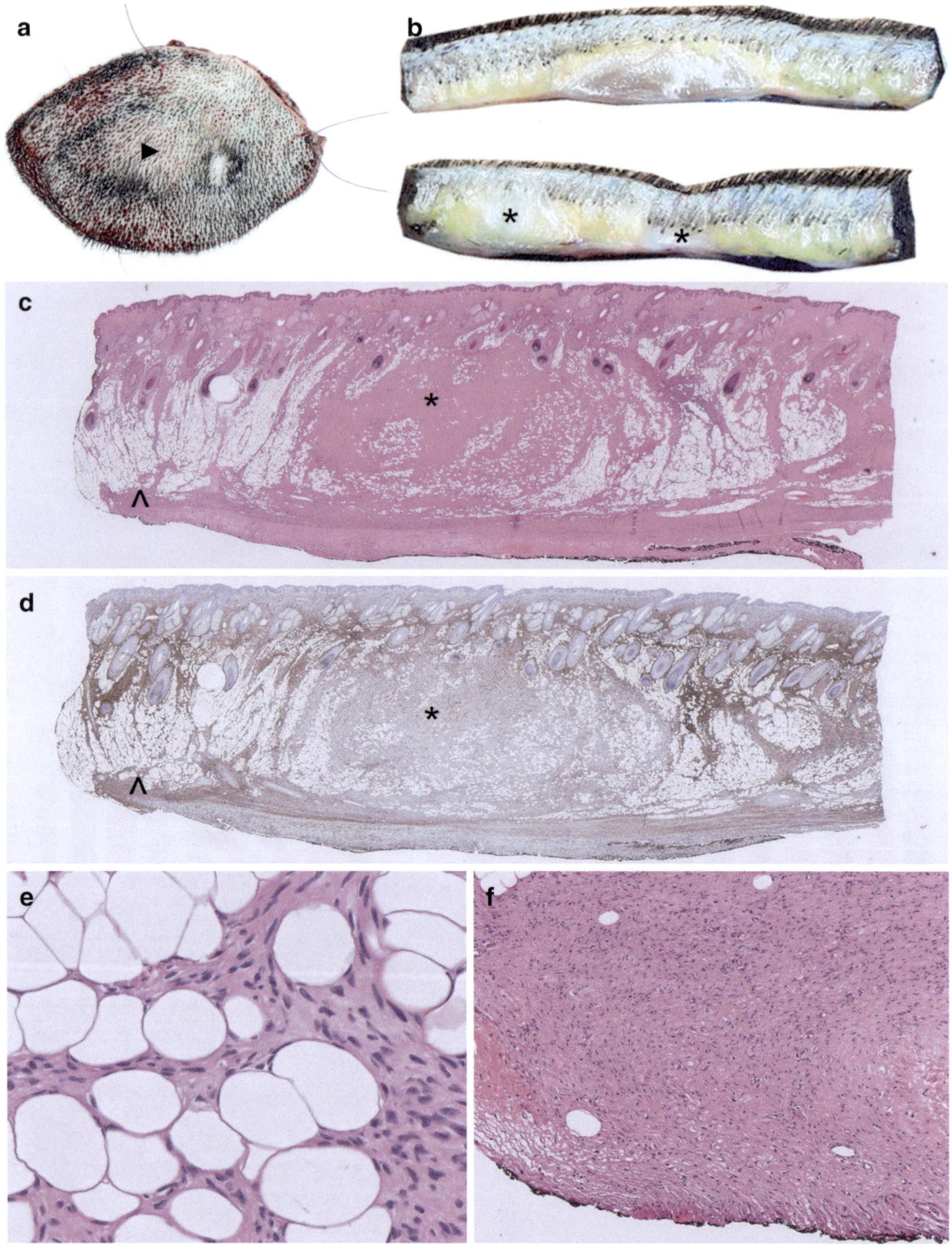

Fig. 7.4 Dermatofibrosarcoma protuberans (DFSP). (**a**) Skin excision of the head with a palpable mass (►). Note the pen marks of the estimated margins by palpation. (**b**) Sections of the specimen after fixation and slicing show a glassy mass in the upper lamel that appears to be well-circumscribed. However, in the lower lamel, multiple tumor foci (*) are visible. (**c**) H&E staining of the left half of the lower lamel. Low magnification shows the largeness of the tumor, growing far beyond the visible tumor mass (*) with tumor affecting the resection margin (^). (**d**) Immunohistochemistry for CD34, a marker positive in DFSP, highlights the infiltrative pattern of the tumor mass (*) and extensiveness of the tumor. The tumor reaches into the lateral excision margin (^). (**e**) High magnification of the tumor nodule demonstrates bland spindled tumor cells with a typical infiltrative honey combing growth pattern. (**f**) Tumor cells reach the inked resection margin

cyclic process of excision, mapping and microscopic evaluation can follow until no residual tumor is present, ultimately conserving the maximum amount of normal tissue [22].

Mohs microsurgery has been used as an alternative for conventional wide local excision in dermatofibrosarcoma protuberans. This is a superficial locally aggressive neoplasm with a typical honey combing infiltration of the subcutaneous fat (Fig. 7.4). Its diffuse growth pattern may lead to extension far beyond the clinically assessed margin with recurrence rates varying from 20%–50% in case of inadequate margins [23]. Several reports showed superior results in terms of cure rates after Mohs microsurgery [24–27]. A meta-analysis of 684 patients with DFSP comparing wide local excision to Mohs microsurgery revealed an overall recurrence rate of 9.1% and 2.7% in patients treated with wide local excision and Mohs microsurgery, respectively, in a median follow-up period of 5.3 years. In the head and neck zone, Mohs microsurgery also showed favorable recurrence rates as compared to wide local excision (23.4% and 38.2%) [28]. Additionally, primary closure was also more often possible after Mohs microsurgery than after wide local excision (73% vs 52%) [25] with greater preservation of healthy tissue and tumor clearance with smaller margins [27]. Similarly, a few case reports and series on Mohs microsurgery in atypical fibroxanthoma were published with favorable outcomes. This is a dermal-based tumor with uncertain differentiation arising in sun-exposed areas, that usually has a benign course after complete excision [23]. One retrospective cohort of 88 patients found recurrent disease in 2 of 23 patients after wide local excision, while none of the 65 patients treated with Mohs microsurgery had a local recurrence after follow-up of 5 years [29]. Another study revealed a recurrence rate of 6.9% in 29 patients after Mohs microsurgery. In certain cases, the clinician can decide to deviate from standard treatment to Mohs microsurgery. For example, Mohs microsurgery might serve as a good alternative in head and neck tumors due to the tissue-sparing nature. Ideally, treatment plans should be made after a multidisciplinary case discussion, where the advantages and disadvantages are considered. Importantly, it must be noted that the success rate is highly dependent on the quality and interpretation of frozen sections. Not only are surgeons required who are familiar with the Mohs microsurgery technique, but specially educated histotechnicians are necessary for cutting slides for frozen section analysis. Also, the pathologists evaluating the frozen sections should be familiar not only with the Mohs technique but also with the variable morphology of these superficial soft tissue lesions, which can have areas that may look deceptively benign. More specifically, detailed analysis of individual cells is difficult in frozen sections, so recognizing patterns becomes more imperative for pathologists. In addition, pathologists need to become more familiar with horizontal and tangential cuts, as the appearance of normal structures is different. Lastly, compared to routine excisions, Mohs microsurgery needs to be planned properly, is time-consuming and very labor intensive.

7.5 Conclusion

To conclude, intra-operative pathology assessment of soft tissue tumors is a procedure that is not performed on a routine basis for assessing surgical margins or for rendering a diagnosis. However, as it might help to guide the surgeon in decision-making during surgery, despite its limitations, it can be of added value at least in specific individual cases. As this depends on clinical context and the specific question to the pathologist this should therefore always be discussed upfront.

References

1. Gronchi A, Miah AB, Dei Tos AP, Abecassis N, Bajpai J, Bauer S, et al. Soft tissue and visceral sarcomas: ESMO-EURACAN-GENTURIS clinical practice guidelines for diagnosis, treatment and follow-up(☆). Ann Oncol. 2021;32(11):1348–65.
2. Basile G, Mattei JC, Alshaygy I, Griffin AM, Catton CN, Chung PW, et al. Curability of patients with lymph node metastases from extremity soft-tissue sarcoma. Cancer. 2020;126(23):5098–108.
3. Al-Refaie WB, Andtbacka RH, Ensor J, Pisters PW, Ellis TL, Shrout A, et al. Lymphadenectomy for isolated lymph node metastasis from extremity soft-tissue sarcomas. Cancer. 2008;112(8):1821–6.
4. Ferreiro JA, Myers JL, Bostwick DG. Accuracy of frozen section diagnosis in surgical pathology: review of a 1-year experience with 24,880 cases at Mayo Clinic Rochester. Mayo Clin Proc. 1995;70(12):1137–41.
5. Dalal BL, Malik AK, Datta BN. Frozen section diagnosis--a review of 1051 cases. Indian J Cancer. 1979;16(2):59–65.
6. Holaday WJ, Assor D. Ten thousand consecutive frozen sections. A retrospective study focusing on accuracy and quality control. Am J Clin Pathol. 1974;61(6):769–77.
7. Shah MS, Garg V, Kapoor SK, Dhaon BK, Gondal R. Fine-needle aspiration cytology, frozen section, and open biopsy: relative significance in diagnosis of musculoskeletal tumors. J Surg Orthop Adv. 2003;12(4):203–7.
8. Miwa S, Yamamoto N, Hayashi K, Takeuchi A, Igarashi K, Tada K, et al. Accuracy of histological grades from intraoperative frozen-section diagnoses of soft-tissue tumors. Int J Clin Oncol. 2020;25(12):2158–65.
9. Golouh R, Bracko M. Accuracy of frozen section diagnosis in soft tissue tumors. Mod Pathol. 1990;3(6):729–33.
10. Hau A, Kim I, Kattapuram S, Hornicek FJ, Rosenberg AE, Gebhardt MC, et al. Accuracy of CT-guided biopsies in 359 patients with musculoskeletal lesions. Skeletal Radiol. 2002;31(6):349–53.
11. Blay JY, Honoré C, Stoeckle E, Meeus P, Jafari M, Gouin F, et al. Surgery in reference centers improves survival of sarcoma patients: a nationwide study. Ann Oncol. 2019;30(7):1143–53.
12. Stoeckle E, Gardet H, Coindre JM, Kantor G, Bonichon F, Milbéo Y, et al. Prospective evaluation of quality of surgery in soft tissue sarcoma. Eur J Surg Oncol. 2006;32(10):1242–8.
13. Chandrasekar CR, Wafa H, Grimer RJ, Carter SR, Tillman RM, Abudu A. The effect of an unplanned excision of a soft-tissue sarcoma on prognosis. J Bone Joint Surg Br. 2008;90(2):203–8.
14. Dei Tos A, Agaimy A, Bovée J, Dickson B, Doyle L, Dry S, et al. Soft tissue sarcoma histopathology reporting guide–resection specimens. Sydney: International Collaboration on Cancer Reporting; 2021.
15. Enneking WF, Spanier SS, Goodman MA. A system for the surgical staging of musculoskeletal sarcoma. Clin Orthop Relat Res. 1980;153:106–20.
16. Beahrs OH, Henson DE, Hutter RV, Myers MH. Manual for staging of cancer. Am J Clin Oncol. 1988;11(6):686.
17. Fujiwara T, Kaneuchi Y, Tsuda Y, Stevenson J, Parry M, Jeys L. Low-grade soft-tissue sarcomas: what is an adequate margin for local disease control? Surg Oncol. 2020;35:303–8.
18. Sambri A, Caldari E, Fiore M, Zucchini R, Giannini C, Pirini MG, et al. Margin assessment in soft tissue sarcomas: review of the literature. Cancers (Basel). 2021;13(7):1687.
19. Fleming FJ, Hill AD, Mc Dermott EW, O'Doherty A, O'Higgins NJ, Quinn CM. Intraoperative margin assessment and re-excision rate in breast conserving surgery. Eur J Surg Oncol. 2004;30(3):233–7.
20. Dadrass F, Gusho C, Yang F, Culvern C, Bloom J, Fillingham Y, et al. A clinicopathologic examination of myxofibrosarcoma. Do surgical margins significantly affect local recurrence rates in this infiltrative sarcoma subtype? J Surg Oncol. 2021;123(2):489–96.
21. Endo M, Lin PP. Surgical margins in the management of extremity soft tissue sarcoma. Chin Clin Oncol. 2018;7(4):37.
22. Morgan MB, Hamill JR, Spencer JM. Atlas of Mohs and frozen section cutaneous pathology. 1st ed. New York: Springer; 2009.
23. WHO Classification of Tumours Editorial Board. Soft tissue and bone tumours. 5th ed. Lyon: International Agency Research on Cancer; 2020.
24. Gloster HM Jr, Harris KR, Roenigk RK. A comparison between Mohs micrographic surgery and wide surgical excision for the treat-

ment of dermatofibrosarcoma protuberans. J Am Acad Dermatol. 1996;35(1):82–7.
25. Lowe GC, Onajin O, Baum CL, Otley CC, Arpey CJ, Roenigk RK, et al. A comparison of Mohs micrographic surgery and wide local excision for treatment of dermatofibrosarcoma protuberans with long-term follow-up: the Mayo clinic experience. Dermatologic Surg. 2017;43(1):98–106.
26. Zehir A, Benayed R, Shah RH, Syed A, Middha S, Kim HR, et al. Mutational landscape of metastatic cancer revealed from prospective clinical sequencing of 10,000 patients. Nat Med. 2017;23(6):703–13.
27. Serra-Guillén C, Llombart B, Nagore E, Guillén C, Requena C, Traves V, et al. Mohs micrographic surgery in dermatofibrosarcoma protuberans allows tumour clearance with smaller margins and greater preservation of healthy tissue compared with conventional surgery: a study of 74 primary cases. Br J Dermatol. 2015;172(5):1303–7.
28. Malan M, Xuejingzi W, Quan SJ. The efficacy of Mohs micrographic surgery over the traditional wide local excision surgery in the cure of dermatofibrosarcoma protuberans. Pan Afr Med J. 2019;33:297.
29. Davis JL, Randle HW, Zalla MJ, Roenigk RK, Brodland DG. A comparison of Mohs micrographic surgery and wide excision for the treatment of atypical fibroxanthoma. Dermatologic Surg. 1997;23(2):105–10.

8 Histopathological Challenges in the Postoperative Stages

Bilge Bilgic

Soft tissue sarcomas are very rare tumours, occurring in approximately 1% of all malignancies.

Non-invasive approaches in tumor diagnosis are becoming more common day by day. Although these methods have many advantages for the patient and the surgeon, there are some limitations when it comes to soft tissue tumours. Soft tissue sarcomas are rare and they include more than 100 subtypes. In addition to this diversity, many tumours contain heterogeneity within themselves. These tumours, which usually have a large size, may have different patterns and grades within the same tumor, and not all these areas can be sampled with non-invasive trucut biopsies. When the diagnosis given in trucut biopsies is compared with the excision material, the diagnostic agreement is around 80–90% [1–6].

8.1 What Are the Causes of Microscopic Discrepancy Between Trucut Biopsy and Excision Material?

The main reason for the discrepancy is the heterogeneous nature of sarcomas. If tumor morphology is in question, what do we understand from heterogeneity? Heterogeneity is the coexistence of different morphology and patterns within the same tumor. A few examples can be given to understand this histological diversity. An example is the myxofibrosarcoma. This is a myxoid, spindle cell sarcoma. Not in all cases, but sometimes the tumor has low-grade as well as high-grade areas at the same time, in the same tumor (Fig. 8.1). Low-grade areas may have been sampled by the trucut biopsy and histopathological examination of the excision may show high-grade components. Another similar example is the myxoid liposarcoma; while classical myxoid liposarcoma morphology has been sampled in trucut biopsy, high-grade round cell areas may be encountered in excision (Fig. 8.2). Myxoid and round cell histology are two different faces of the same tumour with different biological behaviour; the round cell type has a worse prognosis.

Another example for diagnostic discordances can be observed in dedifferentiated sarcomas. Dedifferentiated sarcomas are composed of areas of original lower-grade tumour and a second component (Fig. 8.3), which exhibit completely different histology often having a higher grade and worse prognosis than the original tumour. A common example is the dedifferentiated liposarcoma which can develop on a preexisting well-differentiated liposarcoma but also de novo. This type of sarcoma contains areas of well-differentiated as well as dedifferentiated areas; the latter is completely different from the well-differentiated liposarcoma morphologically and they show mostly spindle cell and high-grade morphology [3, 7, 8].

Another type of tumour that can cause diagnostic error is the mesenchymal chondrosarcoma, a well-known biphasic tumour. This tumour has two different histologies consisting of cartilage and small round cell components

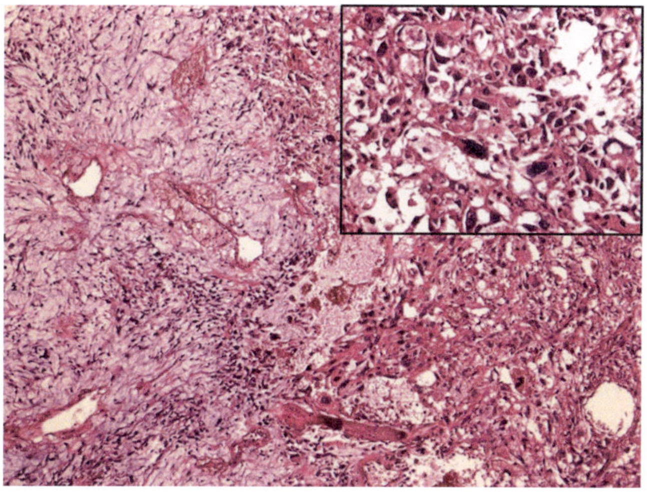

Fig. 8.1 A myxofibrosarcoma of lower grade (HEX100) on the left half of the figure shows focally anaplastic (insetx200) morphological changes

B. Bilgic (✉)
Department of Pathology, Istanbul Faculty of Medicine, Istanbul University, Istanbul, Türkiye
e-mail: bilge.bilgic@istanbul.edu.tr

H. Özger et al. (eds.), *Diagnosis and Treatment of Soft Tissue Tumors*, https://doi.org/10.1007/978-3-031-77061-6_8

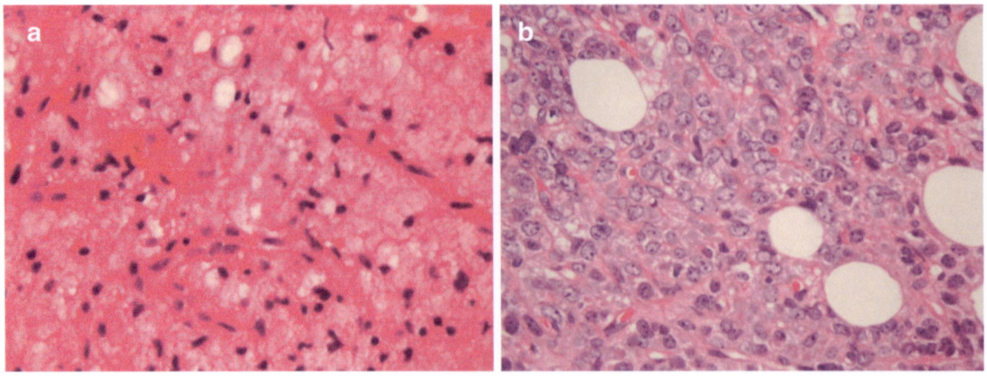

Fig. 8.2 Left myxoid liposarcoma (HEX100), Right round cell high-grade liposarcoma (HEX200)

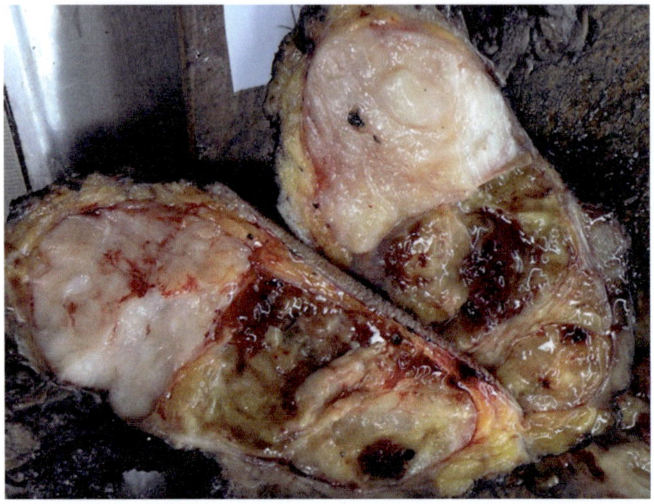

Fig. 8.3 Dediffrentiated liposarcoma; macroscopically two distinct areas in colour and consistency; lower yellowish areas reflect well differentiated liposarcoma, while the upper part shows the dedifferentiated component of the sarcoma

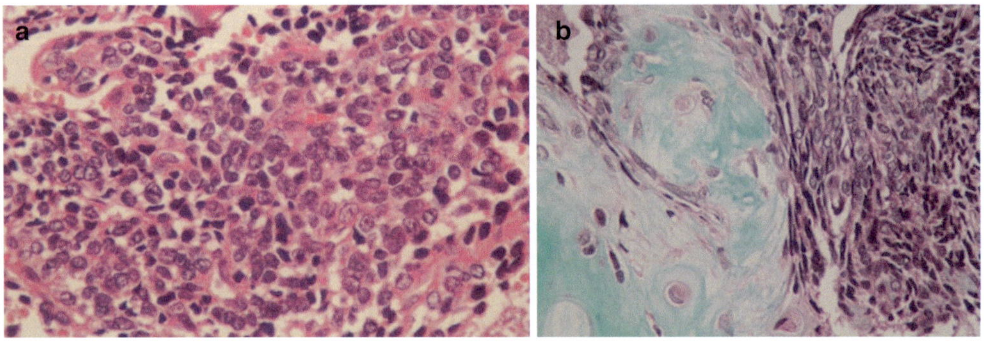

Fig. 8.4 Left round cell component (HEX200) right both chondroid and round cell components of mesenchymal chondrosarcoma (MTx200)

(Fig. 8.4). The predominant component often consists of round cell areas, and sometimes the diagnosis of round cell malignant tumour or even Ewing sarcoma can be made on the initial biopsy because of the misleading histological and immunohistochemical similarities. Histopathological examination of the excision reveals the chondroid component and finally mesenchymal chondrosarcoma can be diagnosed.

Sarcomas are malignant mesenchymal tumours that usually develop de novo. However, there are rare sarcomas that occur as a result of malignant transformation of benign tumours. The best known of these is the malignant peripheral nerve sheath tumour (Fig. 8.5) that may develop on neurofibromas. Although it is common in neurofibromatosis syndrome, it can also be seen independently. In a trucut biopsy, a diagnosis of benign nerve sheath tumour or neurofibroma can be made but the focus of transformation into sarcoma can be found in the excision material by observing increased cellularity, mitosis, pleomorphism, and often loss of S100 expression (Fig. 8.6).

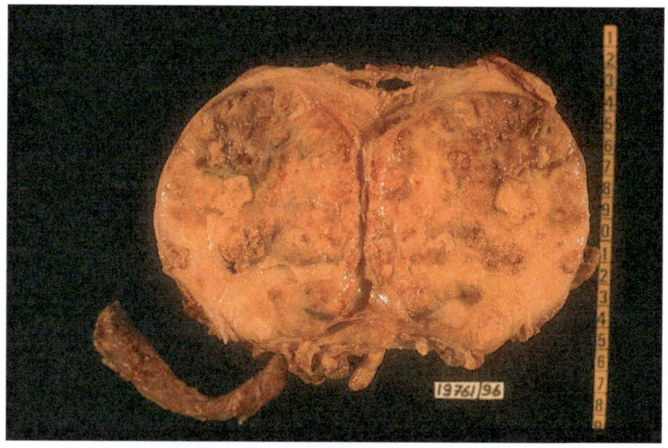

Fig. 8.5 Malignant peripheral nerve sheath tumor of sciatic nerve

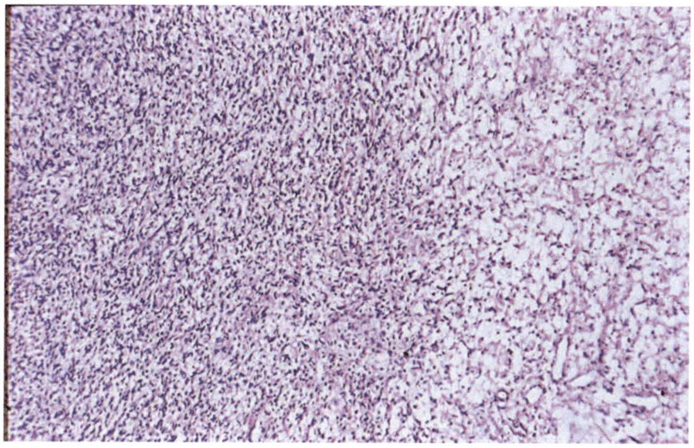

Fig. 8.6 Left half of the figure shows sarcomatous change in neurofibroma (HEX100)

8.2 Grading Challenges in Trucut Biopsies

In soft tissue sarcomas, one of the most important factors predicting the prognosis is the histopathological grade of the tumour. The most widely used system for determining the histological grade is the FNCLCC scoring system, as it is more detailed and practical to use [4, 9–11]. It has been shown to better reflect distant metastasis and tumour mortality than other grading systems. NCI scoring is an alternative method for grading.

FNCLCC grade is determined by the total score obtained from three different categories. These are the differentiation of the tumour, mitosis and finally the amount of necrosis. In the first category, the degree of differentiation of the tumour is evaluated. Trucut biopsies may not reflect the actual grade in some tumours due to heterogeneous morphology. Therefore, in trucut-small biopsies grading should be made with caution.

The second category is the number of mitosis. In recent years, the mitosis rate has been evaluated by the number of mitosis per mm^2, not by high power field (HPF) anymore. And finally, in the third category, the presence and rate of necrosis are determined [4, 10] and therefore the FNCLCC scoring should be made in pretreatment biopsies.

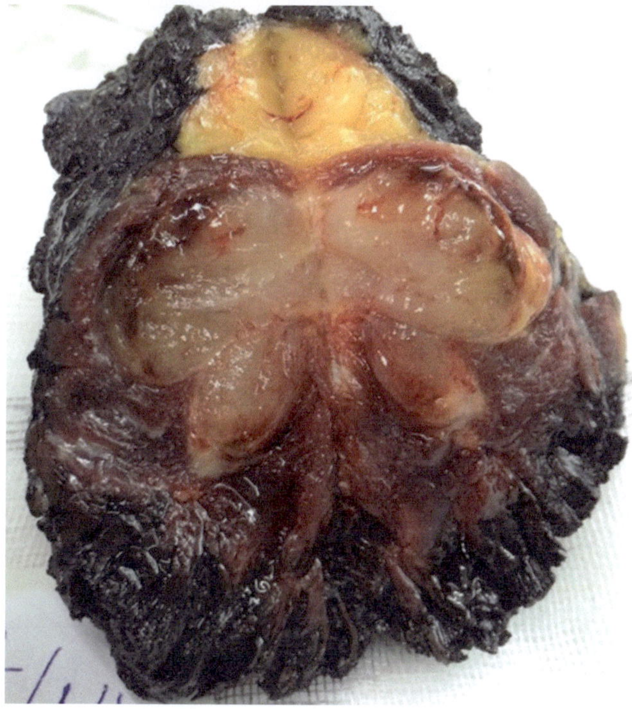

Fig. 8.7 Myxoid sarcoma excision, surface is covered with black ink

All these scores in three categories are added together and a final score is obtained.

One weakness of the FNCLCC system is that in some tumours, the grade obtained with the total score may not coincide with the behaviour of the tumour [1]. Examples include clear cell sarcoma, epithelioid sarcoma, and alveolar soft part sarcoma.

8.3 Evaluation of Surgical Margins

In addition to histological grade, another important prognostic factor for local recurrence and overall survival is the condition of the surgical margins [12–14]. These should be carefully evaluated macroscopically and then microscopically. Before the excision material is cut into slices, the outer

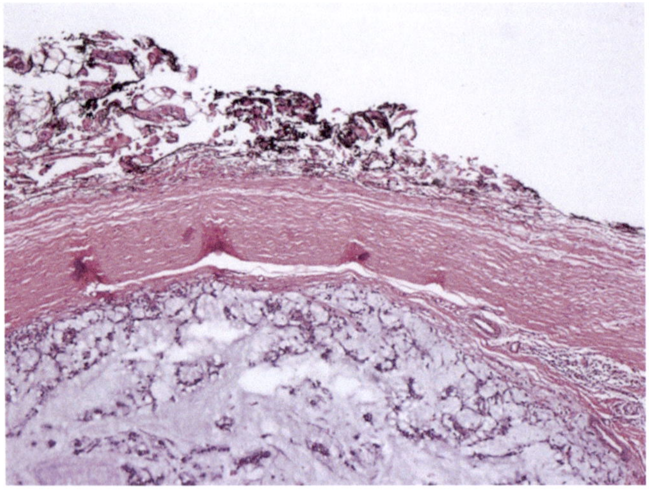

Fig. 8.8 Microscopically outside the capsule there is the stained surgical margin (HEX100)

surface is painted with ink (Fig. 8.7) using different colours. As a result of this staining, these stained borders are easily visible on microscopic examination (Fig. 8.8) and tumour-infiltrating borders are determined; if the surgical margins are negative, the surgical margin closest to the tumour is indicated in mm or cm. In large excision materials, when any surgical margin is positive, it must be specified which margin it is. Detection of this is only possible by finding orientation marks on the incoming material. If the tumour persists at the surgical margin, re-excision should be performed at this site to prevent recurrence; if this is not possible, radiotherapy can be applied. In order to perform re-excision or adjuvant treatment, it is necessary to specify in the pathology report which anatomical region the positive border corresponds to. The surgeon should mark the specimen topographically and also indicate important structures such as nerves, vessels, and periost. It is important for ease of application that this marking is standard for all excisions. A practical application is to mark the lateral part of the excision material with a long suture, and the superior part with a short suture (Fig. 8.9). In the biopsy submission form, it is necessary to specify how this marking is done [7, 11–14].

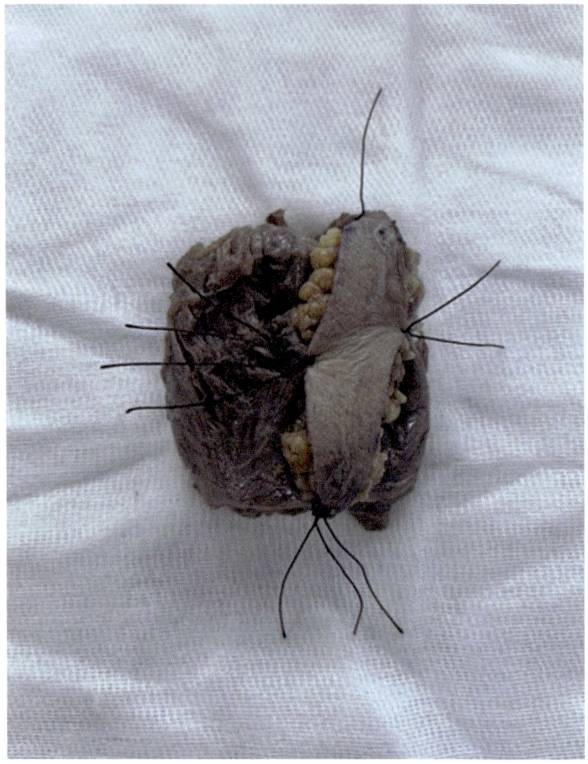

Fig. 8.9 Each direction of the excision is marked with different number of sutures

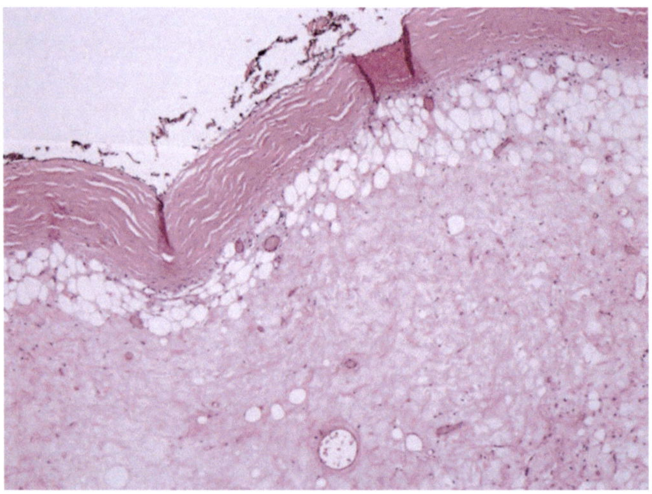

Fig. 8.10 Myxoid liposarcoma shows regresional changes and maturation after neoadjuvant therapy (HEX100)

8.4 Neoadjuvant Therapy and Its Effects on Histopathological Evaluation

Another important point to be considered in the excision material is the neoadjuvant therapy, which is applied preoperatively and may cause morphological changes compared to pretreatment biopsies. Neoadjuvant therapy, which has been widely used in many cancer types in recent years, is also used increasingly in soft tissue sarcomas. It is especially applied in high-grade, difficult-to-remove and large-scale tumours. The neoadjuvant therapies result in some morphological changes in tumour tissue. In addition to regression changes (Fig. 8.10) such as necrosis fibrosis, inflammation, haemorrhage and cystic changes, cellular changes are observed in tumoral cells. These include pyknosis, karyorrhexis, vacuolization as well as nuclear enlargement, hyperchromasia and cytoplasmic eosinophilia. Sometimes, it is difficult to decide, whether these bizarre-appearing cells with large, pleomorphic nuclei represent degenerative cells or are these viable tumour cells [15–17]. A macroscopic

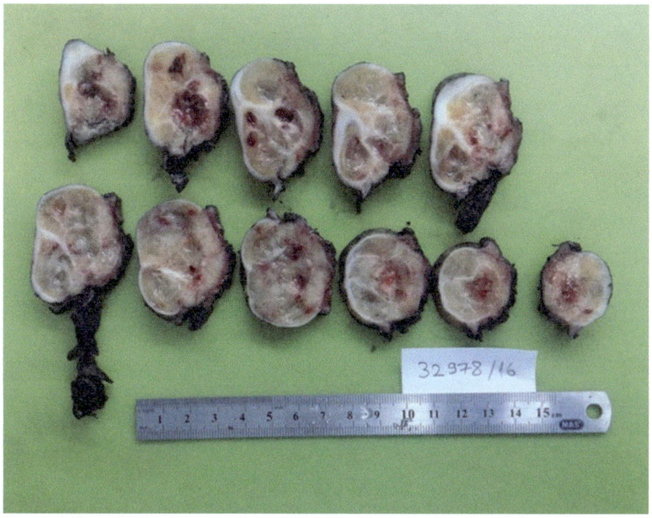

Fig. 8.11 Stained with ink on the surface and sliced at 1 cm intervals

description of the excision material should be made in detail; the macroscopical features including the three dimensions of the tumour, colour, consistency, cystic spaces, the amount of necrosis, and the distances to the surgical margins should be specified. The tumour surface is marked with permanent ink before cutting the specimen. If the orientation is not clear, the surgeon should be contacted [11, 13]. The excision material should be sliced at 1 cm intervals, with sections perpendicular to the larger diameter of the tumour (Fig. 8.11), and ideally, one section per centimetre of maximum dimension is recommended. Whenever possible, this sampling should be performed from areas that do not contain necrosis, and if there are areas with different macroscopical appearances such as colour, and consistency, all these should be sampled. It is advisable if convenient, to store fresh frozen tissue for future genomic studies, and this material can be used when new treatment methods are found. Molecular changes are used to provide most diagnostic information in soft tissue sarcomas.

8.5 Conclusion

In conclusion, soft tissue sarcomas may have different diagnoses in the excision material from the initial diagnosis in trucut material, due to heterogeneous histopathology within the same tumour. Considering which these tumours are and what we may encounter protects us from bad surprises.

Soft tissue sarcoma pathology report should include a well-defined macroscopy, tumour subtype, histological grade (FNCLCC), rate of necrosis, surgical margins, mitosis rate, immunohistochemical and molecular results if performed [3, 11, 18].

The pathologist should also write additional information about the tumour that she/he wants to convey to the clinician, an unusual finding than expected, and the features she/he deems important, as a comment.

Sufficient clinical information about the patient including radiological findings, previous history, former biopsies and an appropriately marked material are necessary for an optimal histopathological evaluation.

References

1. Grimer R, Judson I, Peake D, Seddon B. Guidelines for the management of soft tissue sarcomas. Sarcoma. 2010;6:Article ID 506182.: 15 pages.
2. Demetri GD, Antonia S, Benjamin RS, Bui MM, et al. Soft tissue sarcoma: clinical practice guidelines in oncology. J Natl Compr Cancer Netw. 2005 March;3(2):158–94.
3. Salvatore LR. Who, how and what of pathology of soft tissue sarcoma. Chin Clin Oncol. 2021;10(5):53.
4. Gamboa AC, Gronchi A, Cardona K. Soft-tissue sarcoma in adults: an update on the current state of histiotype-specific management in an era of personalized medicine. Ca Cancer J Clin. 2020;70:200–29.
5. Liegl-Atzwanger B. The role of pathology in sarcoma. Memo. 2020;13:159–63.
6. Baysal B, Anarat FB, Dogan MB, Zenginkinet T, Celik A, Toksoz AN, Sarı T, Ozkan K. Concordance of histopathological and radiological grading in soft tissue sarcomas. J Health Sci Med. 2022;5(5):1484–90.
7. Shan FY, Wu H, Zhong D, Ai D, Zreik R, Huang JH. Soft tissue tumors: molecular pathology and diagnosis. In: Advances in soft tissue tumors; 2022.
8. WHO Classification of Tumours Editorial Board. WHO classification of tumors. Soft tissue and bone tumors, vol. 3. 5th ed. Lyon: IARC; 2020.
9. Neuville A, Chibon F, Coindre JM. Grading of soft tissue sarcomas: from histological to molecular assessment. Pathology. 2014;46(2):113–20.
10. Coindre JM. Grading of soft tissue sarcomas. Review and updates. Arch Pathol Lab Med. 1993;130:1448–53.
11. Wardelmann E, Haas RL, Bove JVMG, Terrier P, Lazar A, et al. Evaluation of response after neoadjuvant treatment in soft tissue sarcomas; the European Organization for Research and Treatment of CancereSoft Tissue and Bone Sarcoma Group (EORTCeSTBSG) recommendations for pathological examination and reporting. Europ J Cancer. 2016;53:84–95.
12. Endo M, Lin PP. Surgical margins in the management of extremity soft tissue sarcoma. Chin Clin Oncol. 2018;7(4):37.
13. Stoeckle E, Coindre JM, Kind M, Kantor G, Bui BN. Evaluating surgery quality in soft tissue sarcoma. Treatment of bone and soft tissue sarcomas. Recent Results Cancer Res. 2009;179:229–42.
14. Shah C, Wang J, Mubako T, Fisher C, Thway K. Gross examination and reporting of soft tissue tumours: evaluation of compliance with the UK Royal College of Pathologists soft tissue sarcoma dataset. J Clin Pathol. 2016;69:761–6.
15. Sethi D, Sen R, Parshad S, Khetarpal S, et al. Histopathologic changes following neoadjuvant chemotherapy in various malignancies. Int J App Basic Med Res. 2012;2(2):111–6.
16. Roberge D, Skamene T, Nahal A, Turcotte RE, et al. Radiological and pathological response following preoperative radiotherapy for soft tissue sarcoma. Radiother Oncol. 2010;97(3):404–7.
17. Yoshinao O, Tanaka K, Hirose T, Hasegawa T, et al. Standardization of evaluation method and prognostic significance of histological response to preoperative chemotherapy in high-grade non-round cell soft tissue sarcomas. BMC Cancer. 2022;22(1):94.
18. Fisher C, Thway K. Dataset for histopathological reporting of soft tissue sarcoma; V6. London: The Royal College of Pathologists; 2022.

Staging of Soft Tissue Sarcomas

9

Michelle Ghert

9.1 Introduction and Current Soft-Tissue Sarcoma Staging Systems

Soft-tissue sarcomas are staged to determine the best treatment strategies and prognosis estimates. The American Joint Committee on Cancer (AJCC) system is currently used to stage tumors and direct treatment [1]. The staging process involves determining the size and location of the tumor, whether it has spread to nearby lymph nodes or other parts of the body, and the grade of the tumor [2]. The grade of the tumor is determined by examining the tumor cells histologically to assess cell morphology, necrosis, and mitosis [1]. Imaging techniques such as MRI and PET/CT scans are used to help stage soft-tissue sarcomas [3–5]. MRI is the favored modality for the evaluation of soft-tissue tumors, as it can clearly delineate tumor size in most cases [5]. PET/CT scans are used to determine the extent of distal metastasis [3, 4].

The AJCC has developed two staging systems for soft-tissue sarcoma: the previous seventh edition and the current eighth edition. The seventh edition was based on the TNM (Tumor, Node, Metastasis) system and was criticized for its inability to accurately predict patient outcomes. The eighth edition, released in 2018, is potentially a significant improvement over the previous edition. It separates soft-tissue sarcomas of the head and neck from those of other body sites, eliminated tumor depth in the categorization of 'T', and categorizes all node-positive diseases as Stage IV [6]. Studies have compared the prognostic implications of the seventh and eighth editions of the AJCC staging system for soft-tissue sarcoma and found that the eighth edition was a better predictor of survival for head and neck soft-tissue sarcomas than the seventh edition [7].

The AJCC current staging system consists of eight stages, ranging from IA to IVB [8]. Tumor size is classified as T1-T4, with T1 being the smallest and T4 being the largest (T1 </= 5 cm, T2 > 5 cm and </= 10 cm, T3 > 10 cm and </= 15 cm, and T4 > 15 cm). Lymph node involvement is classified as N0 or N1, with N1 indicating the presence of lymph node metastasis. Metastasis is classified as M0 or M1, with M1 indicating the presence of distant metastasis.

9.2 Nomograms

Despite its widespread use, the current staging system for soft-tissue sarcoma has limited discriminatory power between stages, and the methodological critiques of some studies argue that the eighth edition staging system does not improve prognostic accuracy compared with the prior seventh edition [9]. As an alternative, nomograms have several advantages over the AJCC TNM staging system for soft-tissue sarcoma prognosis prediction [6, 10], including:

1. *Incorporation of multiple risk factors*: Nomograms are predictive tools that incorporate multiple risk factors, such as patient age, tumor size, histologic grade, and treatment type, to calculate a patient's probability of a clinical event. In contrast, the TNM staging system relies on tumor size, nodal involvement, and metastasis to categorize patients into different stages.
2. *Granularity*: Nomograms can better account for the granularity of sarcomas, which have a wide spectrum of histologies and prognostic behaviors. They can be built for specific histologies, sites, or both, and can be personalized to each patient's unique characteristics.
3. *Recalibration*: Some new "dynamic" nomograms and prognostic tools have been developed, allowing sarcoma clinicians to "recalculate" a patient's prognosis by considering the time since primary surgery, the event history, and the potential time-dependent effect of covariates. This allows for prognosis prediction to be adapted and

M. Ghert (✉)
Department of Orthopaedcis, University of Maryland School of Medicine, Baltimore, MD, USA

Department of Surgery, Division of Orthopaedic Surgery, McMaster University, Hamilton, ON, Canada
e-mail: ghertm@mcmaster.ca; mghert@som.umaryland.edu

H. Özger et al. (eds.), *Diagnosis and Treatment of Soft Tissue Tumors*, https://doi.org/10.1007/978-3-031-77061-6_9

recalculated based on the occurrence (or not) of any event as time passes from the first computation. For example, Sarculator is a tool that is better at identifying patients with sarcoma at the highest risk of death than current staging systems [11].

Overall, nomograms provide a more personalized and accurate approach to prognosis prediction for soft-tissue sarcoma patients, which can help oncologists tailor individual treatments. While the TNM staging system is still widely used, nomograms are becoming increasingly important in the field of sarcoma research and clinical practice.

9.3 Future and Molecular Considerations

Beyond nomograms, further opportunities to improve soft-tissue sarcoma staging exist, particularly as molecular considerations become more apparent, and future evolution into an even more useful soft-tissue sarcoma staging system can be anticipated [12]. For example, a proposed new staging system for MDM2-amplified liposarcomas (well-differentiated and dedifferentiated subtypes) emphasizes retroperitoneal localization, degree of differentiation (histologic subtype), and presence of distant metastasis [13].

Molecular staging in soft-tissue sarcoma has several potential benefits, including:

1. *Improved prognostication*: Molecular staging can help identify underlying prognostic molecular features that may not be apparent based on clinical and pathological features alone. For example, the Complexity INdex in SARComas (CINSARC) gene expression signature has been shown to discriminate intermediate grade II patients with different prognoses [14].
2. *Tailored therapeutic strategies*: Accurate risk assessment is crucial to tailor therapeutic strategies and to identify high-risk patients who may benefit from perioperative chemotherapy. Molecular staging can help identify patients who are at high risk of developing metastases and who may benefit from more aggressive treatment [14].
3. *New therapeutic targets*: The advent of molecular pathology tools such as next-generation sequencing (NGS) has helped refine the classification of sarcomas and may help find new therapeutic targets. For example, a new group of soft-tissue sarcomas was described as harboring a distinct immunohistochemistry profile of S100 and CD34 co-expression and recurrent gene fusions involving RAF1, BRAF, or NTRK1/2 [15].
4. *Improved response to treatment*: Molecular staging can help identify patients who are likely to respond to specific treatments. For example, a sustained response to the mitogen-activated extracellular kinase (MEK) inhibitor trametinib was observed in a spindle cell sarcoma harboring a QKI-RAF1 gene fusion resistant to standard cytotoxic chemotherapy [15].
5. *More accurate staging*: Molecular staging can provide a more accurate assessment of the stage of the cancer, which can help guide treatment decisions. For example, the ability to clone the breakpoint region of the t(11;22) translocation in Ewing's sarcoma has allowed for molecular identification and detection of single tumor cells, opening a new era of diagnostic and staging possibilities [16].

Despite the potential benefits of molecular staging, it is not yet widely used in clinical practice, and more research is needed to determine its effectiveness in soft-tissue sarcoma [17].

9.4 Final Note: Liquid Biopsies

Over recent years, methods to detect, characterize, and monitor cancer through liquid biopsy have evolved rapidly. The analysis of circulating biomarkers in peripheral blood, such as circulating tumor cells (CTC) or circulating tumor DNA (ctDNA), could provide real-time information on tumor genetics, disease state, and extent of systemic disease. Although the first results in sarcomas are encouraging, there are technical challenges that need to be addressed for implementation in clinical practice [18]. Overall, the ability to assess tumor burden by systemic plasma analysis would be a significant step forward in the accurate staging of soft-tissue sarcoma and future and ongoing research will further elucidate the potential benefits of this approach [19].

References

1. Massarweh NN, Dickson PV, Anaya DA. Soft tissue sarcomas: staging principles and prognostic nomograms. J Surg Oncol. 2015;111(5):532–9. https://doi.org/10.1002/jso.23851.
2. Guedes A, Oliveira MB d R, Costa FM, de Melo AS. Updating on bone and soft tissue sarcomas staging. Rev Bras Ortop (Sao Paulo). 2021;56(4):411–8. https://doi.org/10.1055/s-0040-1710331.
3. Gabriel M, Rubello D. 18F-FDG PET-CT in soft tissue sarcomas: staging, restaging, and prognostic value? Nucl Med Commun. 2016;37(1):3–8. https://doi.org/10.1097/MNM.0000000000000407.
4. Annovazzi A, Rea S, Zoccali C, et al. Diagnostic and clinical impact of 18F-FDG PET/CT in staging and restaging soft-tissue sarcomas of the extremities and trunk: mono-institutional retrospective study of a sarcoma referral center. J Clin Med. 2020;9(8):2549. https://doi.org/10.3390/jcm9082549.
5. Walker EA, Song AJ, Murphey MD. Magnetic resonance imaging of soft-tissue masses. Semin Roentgenol. 2010;45(4):277–97. https://doi.org/10.1053/j.ro.2009.12.004.
6. Tseng WW, Pasquali S, Hu JS, Menendez LR, Gronchi A. Staging systems and nomograms in soft tissue sarcoma: outcome prediction by categorization or personalization? Chin Clin Oncol. 2019;8(S1):S12. https://doi.org/10.21037/cco.2019.01.05.

7. Ku JY, Roh JL, Cho KJ, et al. Risk factors for survival of head and neck soft tissue sarcomas: a comparison between 7th and 8th edition AJCC staging systems. Oral Oncol. 2020;106:104705. https://doi.org/10.1016/j.oraloncology.2020.104705.
8. Cates JMM. The AJCC 8th edition staging system for soft tissue sarcoma of the extremities or trunk: a cohort study of the SEER Database. J Natl Compr Cancer Netw. 2018;16(2):144–52. https://doi.org/10.6004/jnccn.2017.7042.
9. Yoon SS. The New American Joint Commission on cancer staging system for soft tissue sarcomas: splitting versus lumping. Ann Surg Oncol. 2018;25(5):1101–2. https://doi.org/10.1245/s10434-018-6419-4.
10. Danieli M, Gronchi A. Staging systems and nomograms for soft tissue sarcoma. Curr Oncol. 2023;30(4):3648–71. https://doi.org/10.3390/curroncol30040278.
11. Benjamin RS. There is more to soft tissue sarcomas than just grade and size. Cancer. 2022;128(1):28–9. https://doi.org/10.1002/cncr.33896.
12. Kotilingam D, Lev DC, Lazar AJF, Pollock RE. Staging soft tissue sarcoma: evolution and change. CA Cancer J Clin. 2006;56(5):282–91.; quiz 314–315. https://doi.org/10.3322/canjclin.56.5.282.
13. Tucci JJ, Dashti NK, Cates JMM. A proposed staging system for improved prognostication of MDM2-amplified liposarcoma. Am J Surg Pathol. 2021;45(1):101–7. https://doi.org/10.1097/PAS.0000000000001554.
14. Crombé A, Spalato-Ceruso M, Michot A, et al. Gene expression profiling improves prognostication by nomogram in patients with soft-tissue sarcomas. Cancer Commun (Lond). 2022;42(6):563–6. https://doi.org/10.1002/cac2.12268.
15. Panet F, Jung S, Alcindor T. Sustained response to the mitogen-activated extracellular kinase inhibitor trametinib in a spindle cell sarcoma harboring a QKI-RAF1 gene fusion. JCO Precis Oncol. 2022;6:e2100303. https://doi.org/10.1200/PO.21.00303.
16. Jürgens HF. Ewing's sarcoma and peripheral primitive neuroectodermal tumor. Curr Opin Oncol. 1994;6(4):391–6.
17. Devarakonda S, Govindan R. Biomarker-driven staging-are we there yet? JAMA Netw Open. 2019;2(12):e1917052. https://doi.org/10.1001/jamanetworkopen.2019.17052.
18. van der Laan P, van Houdt WJ, van den Broek D, Steeghs N, van der Graaf WTA. Liquid biopsies in sarcoma clinical practice: where do we stand? Biomedicines. 2021;9(10):1315. https://doi.org/10.3390/biomedicines9101315.
19. Namløs HM, Boye K, Moosavi SH, et al. Abstract A31: tracking the evolution of soft tissue sarcoma and GIST using liquid biopsies. Clin Cancer Res. 2020;26(11_Supplement):A31. https://doi.org/10.1158/1557-3265.LiqBiop20-A31.

10 Should Prediction Models Decide Treatment?

Ibtissam Acem and Michiel A. J. van de Sande

10.1 Introduction

The diagnosis and management of extremity soft-tissue sarcomas (eSTS) is often challenging due to their rarity, heterogeneous histology, and variable clinical behavior [2–4]. Treatment decisions should preferably be based on individual patients' risks of recurrence or metastasis and should be balanced with anticipated physical functioning and quality of life [5, 6]. This shared decision-making in the treatment of eSTS is facilitated by the development of accurate survival prediction models. One of the main benefits of outcome prediction models is that they can help clinicians identify patients who are at high risk of treatment failure or disease recurrence. This information can be used to guide treatment decisions, such as selecting more aggressive therapies or enrolling patients in clinical trials. Additionally, outcome prediction models can help patients better understand their prognosis and make informed decisions about their care.

There are various types of prediction models available to predict the outcome of sarcoma treatment, these include:

1. Staging systems: Staging systems are based on tumor characteristics such as tumor grade, size and location. They are used to predict the likelihood of survival. Conventional staging systems such as the American Joint Committee on Cancer (AJCC) TNM classification were historically widely used for the stratification of patients [7]. However, important prognostic patient and tumor-related factors such as age, histological subtype and treatment modalities are not incorporated in the TNM staging system.
2. Nomograms: Nomograms are graphical representations of statistical models that estimate the likelihood of a specific outcome or event based on the input of various variables. Nomograms have been developed for predicting overall survival and disease-specific survival in STS patients. Several nomograms based on the combination of clinicopathological factors, such as tumor size, histological grade, and depth, were developed to predict the overall survival of STS patients. Only a few have found their way into clinical use [8].
3. Online prediction applications: In the last decade, several new prognostic instruments such as online prediction applications for statistical sarcoma prognostication were published. In general, these tools generate individual probabilities of an event based on a combination of factors accounting for the fact that patients have multiple characteristics that vary simultaneously. This results in a more accurate individual prognosis which is easier to explain compared with conventional staging systems in cancer. Additionally, these tools are easier to use through applications on smartphones, more accurate in their prediction as they generate individual prognoses based on multiple characteristics, and provide more easily understood prognoses compared with conventional staging systems.

The value of modern prediction models in sarcoma can be seen in several ways:

Treatment decision-making: Prediction models can help clinicians make informed treatment decisions by providing information on the likely outcomes of different treatment options. For example, a prediction model may help a clinician decide whether a patient with a certain type of sarcoma would benefit from chemotherapy or surgery, or both. This could result in better-tailored treatment plans: With a better understanding of a patient's individual risk factors, physicians can develop more personalized treatment plans. This

This book chapter has been adapted from Acem I, van de Sande MAJ. Prediction tools for the personalized management of soft-tissue sarcomas of the extremity. The Bone & Joint Journal. 2022;104-B(9): 1011–6.

I. Acem · M. A. J. van de Sande (✉)
Department of Orthopaedic Oncology, Leiden University Medical Centre, ZA, Leiden, The Netherlands
e-mail: majvandesande@lumc.nl

H. Özger et al. (eds.), *Diagnosis and Treatment of Soft Tissue Tumors*, https://doi.org/10.1007/978-3-031-77061-6_10

may involve more aggressive treatment for high-risk patients or less invasive approaches for low-risk patients. It could also reduce side effects: By avoiding unnecessary treatments, patients may experience fewer side effects and better quality of life during and after treatment.

Clinical trial design: Prediction models can aid in the design of clinical trials by identifying patient subgroups that are likely to benefit from a specific treatment. This can lead to more efficient and targeted clinical trials and can help accelerate the development of new therapies for sarcoma [9, 10].

Risk stratification: Prediction models can help stratify patients into different risk categories based on the likelihood of experiencing certain outcomes. This can help identify patients who may require more intensive monitoring or more aggressive treatment.

Cost savings: By targeting treatment to those who are most likely to benefit, prediction models may help reduce overall healthcare costs. By identifying high-risk patients early, prediction models can also help reduce costs associated with the management of sarcoma patients. Early intervention can prevent the need for more costly treatments down the line.

In this chapter, we will briefly discuss the different treatment options in the management of eSTS and describe the role of prediction models in a shared decision-making process. We will describe the available prediction tools for eSTS, and facilitate clinicians and researchers with instruments to assess which prediction tool to use in the personalized management of eSTS.

10.2 Management of eSTS

Overall, the treatment of sarcoma in adult patients is often a combination of surgery, radiation therapy, and chemotherapy or targeted therapy. The goal of treatment is to remove the tumor and prevent its recurrence, while also minimizing the risk of side effects and maintaining the patient's quality of life. There are several clinical guidelines that have been developed for the management of eSTS [11, 12]. The multimodality treatment of eSTS should occur in a multidisciplinary team. Over the last decades clinical and epidemiological studies have demonstrated that treatment for STS in high-volume centers is associated with better oncological outcomes and improved functional results [6, 13–15].

10.2.1 Surgery and Radiotherapy

At present surgery with free surgical margins is the central pillar in the treatment of localized eSTS. (Neo)adjuvant radiotherapy (RTX) is often indicated in larger, deeply seeded, high-grade eSTS with a high risk of local relapse or microscopically positive surgical margins. Based on a multidisciplinary and global questionnaire the most important factors influencing the choice for RTX are (anticipated) microscopically positive surgical margins, high tumor grade, histological subtype, tumor size and location [16]. It has also been shown that a marginal resection after RTX may not compromise local control or overall survival over a wide resection without (neo)adjuvant radiation [17, 18]. Some studies even suggest that after an R1 excision (microscopic residual disease) or unplanned excision, re-excision may be postponed after multidisciplinary discussion until a local relapse occurs, without compromising overall survival or distant control [19, 20]. However, most clinical guidelines recommend systematic re-excision in case of incomplete surgical margins if R0 re-resection is feasible [11, 12].

10.2.2 Timing of Radiotherapy

To date, there is no clear preference concerning the timing of RTX. Local control rates and overall survival are described as comparable after neoadjuvant and adjuvant RTX around R0 resections [21–24]. Still, RTX is often offered postoperatively, as postoperative wound complications are less prevalent after adjuvant RTX. Neoadjuvant RTX however is correlated to less long-term morbidity such as fibrosis, joint stiffness and edema when compared with adjuvant RTX [21–24]. As postoperative or short-term complications are often manageable with modern wound care or prevented by plastic surgery for wound closure, RTX is offered preoperatively in many specialized sarcoma centers [11, 25].

10.2.3 Chemotherapy

(Neo)adjuvant chemotherapy (CTX) could be considered in patients with a high risk of developing distant metastasis (DM) or death. Some specialized sarcoma centers have incorporated CTX in their local treatment protocol but to date, perioperative CTX is not considered standard treatment in the management of primary eSTS. Guidelines have stated that CTX could be offered to a selected group of high-risk patients with chemo-sensitive tumors or in sensitive histological subtypes after multidisciplinary discussion [26–38].

Recent studies demonstrated a survival benefit for anthracycline and ifosfamide-based CTX in localized eSTS in a selected group of patients with a high risk for distant metastasis [37–39]. These high-risk patients were identified by two different prediction tools. These tools calculate 'individual' patient risks of death and DM based on patient, tumor and/or treatment characteristics [8, 40]. The aforementioned survey among sarcoma specialists showed that 81% of them would consider the use of a prediction tool to assess the indication for (neo)adjuvant chemotherapy in primary eSTS [16]. This underlines the recent trend of a patient-tailored approach in the management of eSTS.

10.3 Development of Prediction Tools for Personalized Prognosis

Recently, there has been a vast increase in the development and publication of prognostic tools in medicine. In the field of eSTS, several prognostic tools have been developed and made available to clinicians [8, 40–50]. A selective overview of published prediction tools for patients with primary STS is included in Table 10.1. Diagnostic models and histology-specific models are not included in this overview. Most prediction tools have differences in the inclusion criteria and included parameters. For example, the Memorial Sloan Kettering Cancer Center (MSKCC) nomogram is a widely used tool for predicting survival in patients with soft-tissue sarcoma. The MSKCC nomogram incorporates a number of clinical and pathological variables, such as age, tumor size, histologic grade, and presence of metastasis, to provide an estimate of 5-year overall survival [41]. Four tools only included STS located in the extremities while other studies included sarcomas of other sites [8, 40, 44, 50]. Some studies included patients with metastatic disease or local recurrence at presentation [43, 46–49]. One study combined bone and soft-tissue tumors in the prediction tool [48]. All prediction tools included sarcoma-specific survival (SSS) or overall survival (OS) as an outcome of the model [8, 40, 41, 43, 46–50], except from the nomogram of Cahlon et al. [44] Only four tools were externally validated [8, 40, 41, 43].

Two prediction tools, Sarculator and PERSARC, are different from the others as they also make use of dynamic predictions [51, 52]. Both dynamic tools were externally validated using coexisting datasets [52, 53]. Prediction tools usually predict the oncological outcomes towards a certain time point (e.g. 5-year OS) from the time of surgery. However, the prognosis of a patient will change as time and disease activity may proceed. For example, the longer a patient remains disease-free after surgery, the lower the chance of disease recurrence and the better the prognosis will be. In contrast to patients who eventually develop disease recurrence during follow-up. These patients will have a significantly worse prognosis. Dynamic predictions take these time-varying variables into account and can predict the prognosis at various time points during follow-up.

All prediction tools in eSTS include patient and tumor-specific parameters. Six out of ten studies included also treatment-related covariates in their nomogram [40, 44, 46, 48–50]. Besides these clinical predictors, the prognostic ability of various other factors such as gene expression profiles, radiomics, transcriptomics, proteomics and other (multi-)omics are widely investigated [54–60]. However, the assessment of the added value of these promising predictors and models, compared with the existing clinical prediction tools, and further external validation are warranted.

Patients in the data set, that was used for the careful model-building process, should preferably be comparable to other sarcoma patient populations to be applicable in broader clinical use. Secondly, a thorough assessment of how valid the predictions of a model are is always necessary. The performance of a model is often expressed by discrimination and calibration.

10.3.1 Discrimination

Discrimination of a prediction model describes how well the model can distinguish between patients who experienced an event from patients that did not. Discrimination is measured by the area under the curve (AUC) of a received operating curve (ROC), also known as the concordance index, Harrell's c-index or c-index. The ROC curve is a plot of the sensitivity (true positive rate) against the 1—specificity (false-positive rate) for different cut-off values of the probability of an outcome. Harrell's c-index for survival models is the probability that for all possible patient pairs, the patient with the shortest time-to-event has a higher predicted risk of the event. A c-index of 0.5 corresponds to a model that is no better than chance and a c-index of 1 corresponds to perfect discrimination (in this case the model could perfectly distinguish patients with a shorter time-to-event from the patient with a longer time-to-event).

10.3.2 Calibration

Calibration estimates how close the predicted risk based on the prediction tool is to the observed risk in the study population. Calibration could be assessed visually in a calibration plot in which the observed probability is plotted against the predicted probability. The 45-degree line in a calibration plot indicates perfect calibration (predicted and observed probability are equal). For survival data, the calibration plot is often reported for several clinically relevant time points.

Both discrimination and calibration are not intrinsic properties of a model. These measurements evaluate how well the model performs in a particular cohort. A good discriminative ability is important for risk stratification and identifying a high-risk subgroup, while a good calibration is important for informing patients about their prognosis and clinical decision-making.

Table 10.1 Overview of published prognostic tools for soft-tissue sarcoma (excl. Histology-specific tools)

Study (name)	Population at risk	Primary endpoint	Parameters	Dynamic prediction	Validation
Kattan et al., 2002, Mariani et al., 2005 (MSKSN) [41, 42]	Patients (>16 years of age) with primary, non-metastatic, STS treated with surgery	12-year SSS	Age, size (cat), grade, histological subtype, depth, site	No	External [61, 62]
Sampo et al., 2012 [43]	Patients (>16 years of age) with non-metastatic primary or locally recurrent eSTS or trunk wall STS	10-year SSS	Size (cat), grade, depth, site, necrosis, vascular invasion	No	External [43]
Cahlon et al., 2012 [44]	Patients (>16 years of age) with primary, non-metastatic, eSTS treated with limb-sparing surgery alone (excluding perioperative RTX and CTX)	3- and 5-year LR	Age (cat), size (cat), grade, histological subtype, margin	No	Internal [44]
Callegaro et al., 2016 (Sarculator) [8]	Patients (>18 years of age) with primary (non-recurrent and non-metastatic) eSTS operated with curative intent with macroscopically complete margins	5- and 10-year OS, 5- and 10-year DM	Age, size, grade, histological subtype	Yes [52]	External [8, 52, 62, 63]
Van Praag et al., 2017, Smolle et al., 2019 (PERSARC) [40, 45]	Patients (>18 years of age) with high-grade, primary (non-recurrent and non-metastatic) eSTS operated with curative intent	3-, 5- and 10-year OS, 3-, 5- and 10-year DM, 3-, 5- and 10-year LR	Age, size, grade, histological subtype, depth, margin, RTX	Yes [51]	External [45, 53]
Sekimizu et al., 2019 [46]	Patients (>18 years of age) with primary (N0M0 or N1M0), eSTS and trunk STS operated with curative intent	2-year LR, 2-year DM, and 2-year OS	Age (cat), size, grade, histological subtype, depth, site, margin, sex, nodal metastasis	No	Internal [46]
Zhang et al., 2019 [47]	Patients (>18 years of age) with primary STS surgically treated	3- and 5-year OS, 3- and 5-year SSS	Age (cat), size (cat), grade, histological subtype, sex, stage[a], marital status, insurance status	No	Internal [47][b]
Xu et al., 2020 [48]	Patients with bone and soft-tissue tumors (except from the heart)	3-month OS, 3-month SSS, 3-month non-SSS	Age (cat), grade, site, surgery, sex, stage[a], T-stage, brain metastasis, lung metastasis, laterality, race	No	No
Tu et al., 2021 [49]	Patients with primary STS	1-, 2-, and 3-year OS	Age (cat), size (cat), grade, histological subtype, surgery, RTX, CTX, lung metastasis	No	Internal [49][b]
De Sanctis., 2022 [50]	Patients (>18 years of age) with primary (non-recurrent and non-metastatic) eSTS operated with curative intent with macroscopically complete margins	5- and 10-year SSS, 2-, 5-, and 10-year LRFS, 2-. 5-, and 10-year DMFS	SSS: Age, sex, size, grade, histological subtype, margin LRFS: Age, size, grade, histological subtype, margin, anatomical site (upper/lower limb) DMFS: Sex, size, grade, histological subtype, margin	No	Internal [50]

STS soft-tissue sarcoma, *eSTS* soft-tissue sarcoma of the extremity, *cat* categorical, *SSS* sarcoma-specific survival, *OS* overall survival, *LR* local recurrence rate, *DM* distant metastasis rate, *LRFS* local recurrence-free survival, *DMFS* distant metastasis-free survival, *RTX* radiotherapy, *CTX* chemotherapy

[a]Stage includes localized, regional or distant disease

[b]In the paper stated as external validation, however, the validation cohort was a random split from the same source population (training and validation cohort both from SEER dataset), which is considered internal validation [64]

10.3.3 Internal Versus External Validation

The best assessment of model performance is in an external validation cohort. Validation is the process of assessing the model performance on different populations and the applicability (generalizability) to these populations. Most published prediction tools in eSTS are only validated internally [44, 46, 47, 49, 50]. Internal validation assesses validity for the setting where the training or development data originated from. It assesses the reproducibility of the model in the same underlying population. External validation assesses the validity in a fully independent cohort [64]. Poor external validation of a model may often be explained by inadequate model development, overfitting due to a relatively small sample size with many candidate predictors or a single center development cohort.

10.3.4 Model Update

Poor external validation may also be related to true differences between the development and validation cohort; differences could originate from within the patient population, but also from treatment preferences and follow-up strategies. Prediction tools should be updated for new settings (e.g., difference in time). This could be done by re-calibration, re-estimation of regression coefficients or model extension with new predictors. For example, one may argue that the accuracy of the predictions of a generic eSTS model in a patient with a malignant peripheral nerve sheath tumor (MPNST) of the extremity, would be less than based on an MPNST-specific prediction tool in which important MPNST-specific predictors, e.g., the presence of neurofibromatosis type 1 and rhabdomyoblastic differentiation (triton tumor), are incorporated [65]. A recent study showed that the discriminative ability of the Sarculator is less in MPNSTs compared with other histological subtypes, such as leiomyosarcomas (C-index: 0.66 vs 0.75, respectively) [63]. This could be a reason to update the Sarculator in the MPNST setting with additional important MPNST-specific predictors. For the extension of prediction tools, a trade-off between predictive value and usability or availability to assess the new predictor in clinical practice should be made. Several approaches for updating existing prediction models are described by E.W. Steyerberg [64].

10.4 Use of Prediction Tool for Personalized Care

Before the entrance of prediction tools in sarcoma care, patients with a larger than 5 cm, deep-seated, high-grade tumor, were considered 'high risk' patients [66]. However, the updated ESMO guideline of 2021 no longer uses this definition for high-risk patients and states that prognostic tools, such as Sarculator and PERSARC, could be used to identify high-risk patients, for example, the indication of (neo)adjuvant CTX [11]. Both prognostic tools are available as online applications that can be downloaded from the Apple App Store and Google Play Store.

10.4.1 Choice of Prediction Tool

Given the variety in eligibility criteria and the differences in the development and validation populations, it is difficult to compare the performance of the prediction tools based on their reported discriminative ability and other model performance measures. For the choice of which prediction tool to use in a clinical setting, one should assess whether the source population (development cohort) or the external validation cohort of the nomogram is comparable with its own patient population. Furthermore, the outcome of interest and relevance and availability of the used prognostic covariates in the model should guide the choice for prediction tool.

10.4.2 Decision Curve Analysis

Besides the applicability of the prediction tool in the physician's own patient population and the corresponding performance outcomes, the clinical usefulness should be assessed. This could be done with a decision curve analysis (DCA). In a DCA the net benefit of a prediction tool-assisted decision at different threshold probabilities is depicted and compared with the default decision of an intervention for all patients and an intervention for none of the patients. The net benefit is defined as the fraction of true positives subtracted by the fraction of false positives at a certain threshold probability, weighted by the relative harm of a false positive and a false negative result [67]. This weight corresponds to the harm (false positive) to benefit (false negative) - ratio [68]. For example, if we would accept 4 false positives for one true positive, this would correspond to a threshold probability of 20% and a harm-to-benefit ratio of 4, which means that missing a true positive is four times worse than having a false positive.

10.4.3 PERSARC for CTX Indication

In Fig. 10.1 the DCA of the PERSARC prediction tool is depicted in a multicenter cohort of patients with a high-grade eSTS as described by I. Acem et al. [37] As previously described, a majority of sarcoma specialists would consider the use of a prediction tool for the indication of (neo)adjuvant CTX [16]. This DCA illustrates that the PERSARC tool will be clinically useful for the indication of (neo)adjuvant CTX if physicians treat patients with eSTS with a predicted 5-year mortality between 6% and 45%. The threshold probability refers to the preference of a physician and reflects how physicians value different outcomes for their patients. If a physician is willing to offer (neo)adjuvant CTX for patients with a predicted 5-year mortality of less than 6% (5-year survival of more than 94%), the physician should treat all patients with (neo)adjuvant CTX and the prediction tool will not be clinically informative. If a physician is willing to treat patients only if they have a predicted 5-year mortality of more than 45% (5-year survival of less than 55%), the physi-

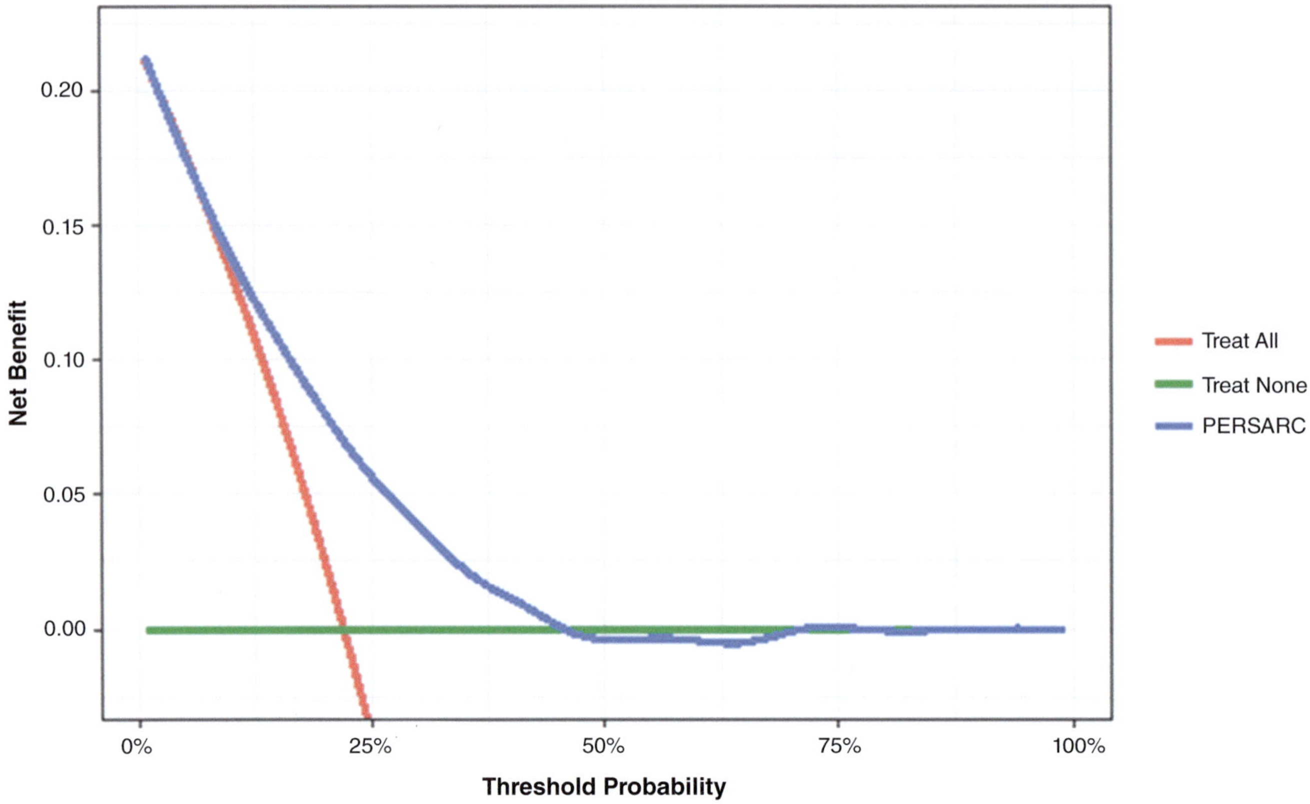

Fig. 10.1 Decision curve of the PERSARC prediction tool (Reproduced from Ref. [1] under the terms of the Creative Commons Attributions (CC BY 4.0) licence (https://creativecommons.org/licenses/by/4.0/), which permits unrestricted use, distribution, and reproduction in any medium or format, provided the original author and source are credited)

cian should treat none of the patients with (neo)adjuvant chemotherapy. Again, in this situation, the prediction tool will not be clinically informative. If the threshold probability of a physician lies within the range of 6% and 45%, taking the relative harm and benefit of (avoiding) treatment with (neo)adjuvant CTX into account, the PERSARC model is clinically useful. In the study of I. Acem et al. [37], the authors found a survival benefit for (neo)adjuvant anthracycline and ifosfamide-based CTX in a subgroup of patients with a 5-year predicted OS of ≤66% (5-year predicted mortality of 34%). This lies within the range of threshold probabilities in which the model is clinically useful.

10.4.4 Clinical Applications

Besides the use of prediction tools for the indication of (neo) adjuvant treatment, [37, 38] prediction tools provide an opportunity to tailor counseling and follow-up schedules.

Prediction tools could help physicians to inform their patients about their prognosis and to guide clinical decision-making. However, there is limited knowledge on patient comprehension, satisfaction and quality of life (QoL) with the use of prediction tools in the management of eSTS.

Furthermore, dynamic prognostic tools could be useful for tailoring follow-up regimens to the risk of tumor recurrence. The PERSARC group recently published a study in which conditional risks for LR and DM were predicted using flexible parametric competing risk regression models [45]. However, the optimal risk threshold upon which an individual patient needs to visit the outpatient clinic or undergo imaging should be further evaluated through for example (microsimulation) decision modeling for cost-effectiveness [69].

10.5 Conclusion and Future Perspectives

Prediction tools are important instruments for clinical decision-making in the modern world and facilitate the shift from a one-size-fits-all approach to patient-tailored management of eSTS. Prediction tools demonstrated to be valuable for the identification of high-risk patients that benefit from (neo)adjuvant anthracycline and ifosfamide-based CTX [37, 38]. Further development of existing tools with other promising predictors and re-calibration and re-estimation for different settings are warranted for a good application of the tools in clinical practice. For the extension of prediction tools, a trade-off between predictive value and the ability to obtain the predictor in clinical practice should be made, balancing precision and usability.

Disclosures No author has any form of disclosure.

References

1. Acem I, van de Sande MAJ. Prediction tools for the personalized management of soft-tissue sarcomas of the extremity. Bone Joint J. 2022;104-B(9):1011–6.
2. WHO Classification of TumoursEditorial Board. Soft tissue and bone tumours. 5th ed. Lyon: International Agency for Research on Cancer; 2020.
3. Siegel RL, Miller KD, Fuchs HE, Jemal A. Cancer statistics, 2021. CA Cancer J Clin. 2021;71(1):7–33.
4. Gatta G, Capocaccia R, Botta L, Mallone S, De Angelis R, Ardanaz E, et al. Burden and centralised treatment in Europe of rare tumours: results of RARECAREnet-a population-based study. Lancet Oncol. 2017;18(8):1022–39.
5. Stiller CA, Trama A, Serraino D, Rossi S, Navarro C, Chirlaque MD, et al. Descriptive epidemiology of sarcomas in Europe: report from the RARECARE project. Eur J Cancer. 2013;49(3):684–95.
6. Blay JY, Honoré C, Stoeckle E, Meeus P, Jafari M, Gouin F, et al. Surgery in reference centers improves survival of sarcoma patients: a nationwide study. Ann Oncol. 2019;30(7):1143–53.
7. American Joint Committee on Cancer. AJCC cancer staging manual. 8th ed. Chicago: Springer; 2017.
8. Callegaro D, Miceli R, Bonvalot S, Ferguson P, Strauss DC, Levy A, et al. Development and external validation of two nomograms to predict overall survival and occurrence of distant metastases in adults after surgical resection of localised soft-tissue sarcomas of the extremities: a retrospective analysis. Lancet Oncol. 2016;17(5):671–80.
9. Ferner RE, Gutmann DH. International consensus statement on malignant peripheral nerve sheath tumors in neurofibromatosis. Cancer Res. 2002;62(5):1573–7.
10. Vickers AJ, Kramer BS, Baker SG. Selecting patients for randomized trials: a systematic approach based on risk group. Trials. 2006;7:30.
11. Gronchi A, Miah AB, Dei Tos AP, Abecassis N, Bajpai J, Bauer S, et al. Soft tissue and visceral sarcomas: ESMO-EURACAN-GENTURIS clinical practice guidelines for diagnosis, treatment and follow-up. Ann Oncol. 2021;32(11):1348–65.
12. Von Mehren M, Kane JM, Agulnik M, Bui MM, Ganjoo KN, George S, et al. Soft tissue sarcoma, version 2.2018, NCCN clinical practice guidelines in oncology. J Natl Compr Canc Netw. 2018;16(5):536–63.
13. Vos M, Blaauwgeers HGT, Ho VKY, van Houdt WJ, van der Hage JA, Been LB, et al. Increased survival of non low-grade and deep-seated soft tissue sarcoma after surgical management in high-volume hospitals: a nationwide study from the Netherlands. Eur J Cancer. 2019;110:98–106.
14. Lazarides AL, Kerr DL, Nussbaum DP, Kreulen RT, Somarelli JA, Blazer DG 3rd, et al. Soft tissue sarcoma of the extremities: what is the value of treating at high-volume centers? Clin Orthop Relat Res. 2019;477(4):718–27.
15. Venigalla S, Nead KT, Sebro R, Guttmann DM, Sharma S, Simone CB 2nd, et al. Association between treatment at high-volume facilities and improved overall survival in soft tissue sarcomas. Int J Radiat Oncol Biol Phys. 2018;100(4):1004–15.
16. Acem I, Smit MM, Verhoef C, van Houdt WJ, Haas RL, van der Hage JA, et al. Management of Soft Tissue Sarcomas in extremities: variation in treatment recommendations and surveillance according to specialty and continent. Ann Surg Oncol. 2021;28(12):7923–36.
17. Dagan R, Indelicato DJ, McGee L, Morris CG, Kirwan JM, Knapik J, et al. The significance of a marginal excision after preoperative radiation therapy for soft tissue sarcoma of the extremity. Cancer. 2012;118(12):3199–207.
18. Gundle KR, Kafchinski L, Gupta S, Griffin AM, Dickson BC, Chung PW, et al. Analysis of margin classification Systems for Assessing the risk of local recurrence after soft tissue sarcoma resection. J Clin Oncol. 2018;36(7):704–9.
19. Danieli M, Barretta F, Fiore M, Radaelli S, Sangalli C, Barisella M, et al. Unplanned excision of extremity and trunk wall soft tissue sarcoma: to re-resect or not to re-resect? Ann Surg Oncol. 2021;28(8):4706–17.
20. Decanter G, Stoeckle E, Honore C, Meeus P, Mattei JC, Dubray-Longeras P, et al. Watch and wait approach for re-excision after unplanned yet macroscopically complete excision of extremity and superficial truncal soft tissue sarcoma is safe and does not affect metastatic risk or amputation rate. Ann Surg Oncol. 2019;26(11):3526–34.
21. Haas RL, Gronchi A, van de Sande MAJ, Baldini EH, Gelderblom H, Messiou C, et al. Perioperative management of extremity soft tissue sarcomas. J Clin Oncol. 2018;36(2):118–24.
22. O'Sullivan B, Davis AM, Turcotte R, Bell R, Catton C, Chabot P, et al. Preoperative versus postoperative radiotherapy in soft-tissue sarcoma of the limbs: a randomised trial. Lancet. 2002;359(9325):2235–41.
23. O'Sullivan B, Davis A, Turcotte R, Bell R, Wunder J, Catton C, et al. Five-year results of a randomized phase III trial of pre-operative vs post-operative radiotherapy in extremity soft tissue sarcoma. J Clin Oncol. 2004;22(14_suppl):9007.
24. Davis AM, O'Sullivan B, Turcotte R, Bell R, Catton C, Chabot P, et al. Late radiation morbidity following randomization to preoperative versus postoperative radiotherapy in extremity soft tissue sarcoma. Radiother Oncol. 2005;75(1):48–53.
25. Van Meekeren M, Fiocco M, Ho VKY, Bovée J, Gelderblom H, Haas RL. Patterns of perioperative treatment and survival of localized, resected, intermediate- or high-grade soft tissue sarcoma: a 2000-2017 Netherlands cancer registry database analysis. Sarcoma. 2021;2021:9976122.
26. Woll PJ, Reichardt P, Le Cesne A, Bonvalot S, Azzarelli A, Hoekstra HJ, et al. Adjuvant chemotherapy with doxorubicin, ifosfamide, and lenograstim for resected soft-tissue sarcoma (EORTC 62931): a multicentre randomised controlled trial. Lancet Oncol. 2012;13(10):1045–54.
27. Fakhrai N, Ebm C, Kostler WJ, Jantsch M, Abdolvahab F, Dominkus M, et al. Intensified adjuvant IFADIC chemotherapy in combination with radiotherapy versus radiotherapy alone for soft tissue sarcoma: long-term follow-up of a prospective randomized feasibility trial. Wien Klin Wochenschr. 2010;122(21–22):614–9.
28. Frustaci S, Gherlinzoni F, De Paoli A, Bonetti M, Azzarelli A, Comandone A, et al. Adjuvant chemotherapy for adult soft tissue sarcomas of the extremities and girdles: results of the Italian randomized cooperative trial. J Clin Oncol. 2001;19(5):1238–47.
29. Gortzak E, Azzarelli A, Buesa J, Bramwell VH, van Coevorden F, van Geel AN, et al. A randomised phase II study on neo-adjuvant chemotherapy for 'high-risk' adult soft-tissue sarcoma. Eur J Cancer. 2001;37(9):1096–103.
30. Petrioli R, Coratti A, Correale P, D'Aniello C, Grimaldi L, Tanzini G, et al. Adjuvant epirubicin with or without Ifosfamide for adult soft-tissue sarcoma. Am J Clin Oncol. 2002;25(5):468–73.
31. Zaidi MY, Ethun CG, Tran TB, Poultsides G, Grignol VP, Howard JH, et al. Assessing the role of neoadjuvant chemotherapy in primary high-risk truncal/extremity soft tissue sarcomas: an analysis of the multi-institutional U.S. sarcoma collaborative. Ann Surg Oncol. 2019;26(11):3542–9.

32. Callegaro D, Miceli R, Bonvalot S, Ferguson P, Strauss DC, Levy A, et al. Impact of perioperative chemotherapy and radiotherapy in patients with primary extremity soft tissue sarcoma: retrospective analysis across major histological subtypes and major reference centres. Eur J Cancer. 2018;105:19–27.
33. Mullen JT, Kobayashi W, Wang JJ, Harmon DC, Choy E, Hornicek FJ, et al. Long-term follow-up of patients treated with neoadjuvant chemotherapy and radiotherapy for large, extremity soft tissue sarcomas. Cancer. 2012;118(15):3758–65.
34. Pervaiz N, Colterjohn N, Farrokhyar F, Tozer R, Figueredo A, Ghert M. A systematic meta-analysis of randomized controlled trials of adjuvant chemotherapy for localized resectable soft-tissue sarcoma. Cancer. 2008;113(3):573–81.
35. Istl AC, Ruck JM, Morris CD, Levin AS, Meyer CF, Johnston FM. Call for improved design and reporting in soft tissue sarcoma studies: a systematic review and meta-analysis of chemotherapy and survival outcomes in resectable STS. J Surg Oncol. 2019;119(7):824–35.
36. Graham DS, van Dams R, Jackson NJ, Onyshchenko M, Eckardt MA, DiPardo BJ, et al. Chemotherapy and survival in patients with primary high-grade extremity and trunk soft tissue sarcoma. Cancers (Basel). 2020;12(9):2389.
37. Acem I, van Houdt WJ, Grünhagen DJ, van der Graaf WTA, Rueten-Budde AJ, Gelderblom H, et al. The role of perioperative chemotherapy in primary high-grade extremity soft tissue sarcoma: a risk-stratified analysis using PERSARC. Eur J Cancer. 2022;165:71–80.
38. Pasquali S, Pizzamiglio S, Touati N, Litiere S, Marreaud S, Kasper B, et al. The impact of chemotherapy on survival of patients with extremity and trunk wall soft tissue sarcoma: revisiting the results of the EORTC-STBSG 62931 randomised trial. Eur J Cancer. 2019;109:51–60.
39. Pasquali S, Palmerini E, Quagliuolo V, Martin-Broto J, Lopez-Pousa A, Grignani G, et al. Neoadjuvant chemotherapy in high-risk soft tissue sarcomas: a Sarculator-based risk stratification analysis of the ISG-STS 1001 randomized trial. Cancer. 2021;128:85.
40. van Praag VM, Rueten-Budde AJ, Jeys LM, Laitinen MK, Pollock R, Aston W, et al. A prediction model for treatment decisions in high-grade extremity soft-tissue sarcomas: personalised sarcoma care (PERSARC). Eur J Cancer. 2017;83:313–23.
41. Kattan MW, Leung DH, Brennan MF. Postoperative nomogram for 12-year sarcoma-specific death. J Clin Oncol. 2002;20(3):791–6.
42. Mariani L, Miceli R, Kattan MW, Brennan MF, Colecchia M, Fiore M, et al. Validation and adaptation of a nomogram for predicting the survival of patients with extremity soft tissue sarcoma using a three-grade system. Cancer. 2005;103(2):402–8.
43. Sampo M, Tarkkanen M, Tukiainen E, Popov P, Gustafson P, Lundin M, et al. A web-based prognostic tool for extremity and trunk wall soft tissue sarcomas and its external validation. Br J Cancer. 2012;106(6):1076–82.
44. Cahlon O, Brennan MF, Jia X, Qin LX, Singer S, Alektiar KM. A postoperative nomogram for local recurrence risk in extremity soft tissue sarcomas after limb-sparing surgery without adjuvant radiation. Ann Surg. 2012;255(2):343–7.
45. Smolle MA, Sande MV, Callegaro D, Wunder J, Hayes A, Leitner L, et al. Individualizing follow-up strategies in high-grade soft tissue sarcoma with flexible parametric competing risk regression models. Cancers (Basel). 2019;12(1):47.
46. Sekimizu M, Ogura K, Yasunaga H, Matsui H, Tanaka S, Inagaki K, et al. Development of nomograms for prognostication of patients with primary soft tissue sarcomas of the trunk and extremity: report from the bone and soft tissue tumor registry in Japan. BMC Cancer. 2019;19(1):657.
47. Zhang SL, Wang ZM, Wang WR, Wang X, Zhou YH. Novel nomograms individually predict the survival of patients with soft tissue sarcomas after surgery. Cancer Manag Res. 2019;11:3215–25.
48. Xu Y, Xu G, Wu H, Lin F, Mao M, Baklaushev VP, et al. The nomogram for early death in patients with bone and soft tissue tumors. J Cancer. 2020;11(18):5359–70.
49. Tu Q, Hu C, Zhang H, Kong M, Peng C, Song M, et al. Development and validation of novel nomograms for predicting specific distant metastatic sites and overall survival of patients with soft tissue sarcoma. Technol Cancer Res Treat. 2021;20:1533033821997828.
50. De Sanctis R, Zelic R, Santoro A. Nomograms predicting local and distant recurrence and disease-specific mortality for R0/R1 soft tissue sarcomas of the extremities. Front Oncol. 2022;12:941896.
51. Rueten-Budde AJ, van Praag VM, van de Sande MAJ, Fiocco M. Dynamic prediction of overall survival for patients with high-grade extremity soft tissue sarcoma. Surg Oncol. 2018;27(4):695–701.
52. Callegaro D, Miceli R, Bonvalot S, Ferguson PC, Strauss DC, van Praag VVM, et al. Development and external validation of a dynamic prognostic nomogram for primary extremity soft tissue sarcoma survivors. E Clin Med. 2019;17:100215.
53. Rueten-Budde AJ, van Praag VM, van de Sande MAJ, Fiocco M. External validation and adaptation of a dynamic prediction model for patients with high-grade extremity soft tissue sarcoma. J Surg Oncol. 2021;123(4):1050–6.
54. Chibon F, Lagarde P, Salas S, Pérot G, Brouste V, Tirode F, et al. Validated prediction of clinical outcome in sarcomas and multiple types of cancer on the basis of a gene expression signature related to genome complexity. Nat Med. 2010;16(7):781–7.
55. Chen S, Li N, Tang Y, Chen B, Fang H, Qi S, et al. Radiomics analysis of fat-saturated T2-weighted MRI sequences for the prediction of prognosis in soft tissue sarcoma of the extremities and trunk treated with neoadjuvant radiotherapy. Front Oncol. 2021;11:710649.
56. Tian L, Zhang D, Bao S, Nie P, Hao D, Liu Y, et al. Radiomics-based machine-learning method for prediction of distant metastasis from soft-tissue sarcomas. Clin Radiol. 2021;76(2):158.e19–e25.
57. Crombé A, Fadli D, Italiano A, Saut O, Buy X, Kind M. Systematic review of sarcomas radiomics studies: bridging the gap between concepts and clinical applications? Eur J Radiol. 2020;132:109283.
58. Bertucci F, De Nonneville A, Finetti P, Perrot D, Nilbert M, Italiano A, et al. The genomic grade index predicts postoperative clinical outcome in patients with soft-tissue sarcoma. Ann Oncol. 2018;29(2):459–65.
59. Zhang B, Yang L, Wang X, Fu D. Identification of a survival-related signature for sarcoma patients through integrated transcriptomic and proteomic profiling analyses. Gene. 2021;764:145105.
60. Song Y, Yang K, Sun T, Tang R. Development and validation of prognostic markers in sarcomas base on a multi-omics analysis. BMC Med Genet. 2021;14(1):31.
61. Eilber FC, Brennan MF, Eilber FR, Dry SM, Singer S, Kattan MW. Validation of the postoperative nomogram for 12-year sarcoma-specific mortality. Cancer. 2004;101(10):2270–5.
62. Squires MH, Ethun CG, Donahue EE, Benbow JH, Anderson CJ, Jagosky MH, et al. Extremity soft tissue sarcoma: a multi-institutional validation of prognostic nomograms. Ann Surg Oncol. 2022;29(5):3291–301.
63. Voss RK, Callegaro D, Chiang YJ, Fiore M, Miceli R, Keung EZ, et al. Sarculator is a good model to predict survival in resected extremity and trunk sarcomas in US patients. Ann Surg Oncol. 2022;29:4376.
64. Steyerberg EW. Clinical prediction models: a practical approach to development, validation, and updating. Cham: Springer; 2019.
65. Acem I, Martin E, van Houdt WJ, van de Sande MAJ, Grünhagen DJ, Verhoef C, et al. The association of metastasis pattern and management of metastatic disease with oncological outcomes in patients with malignant peripheral nerve sheath tumors: a multicenter cohort study. Cancers (Basel). 2021;13(20):5115.

66. Casali PG, Abecassis N, Aro HT, Bauer S, Biagini R, Bielack S, et al. Soft tissue and visceral sarcomas: ESMO-EURACAN Clinical Practice Guidelines for diagnosis, treatment and follow-up. Ann Oncol. 2018;29(Suppl 4):iv51–67.
67. Vickers AJ, Elkin EB. Decision curve analysis: a novel method for evaluating prediction models. Med Decis Mak. 2006;26(6):565–74.
68. Vickers AJ, van Calster B, Steyerberg EW. A simple, step-by-step guide to interpreting decision curve analysis. Diagn Progn Res. 2019;3:18.
69. Krijkamp EM, Alarid-Escudero F, Enns EA, Jalal HJ, Hunink MGM, Pechlivanoglou P. Microsimulation modeling for health decision sciences using R: a tutorial. Med Decis Mak. 2018;38(3):400–22.

Medical Oncological Treatment of Adult Patients with Soft Tissue Sarcoma

11

Emine Hatipoglu and Robin L. Jones

11.1 Localized Disease

Soft tissue sarcoma (STS) is a rare and heterogenous group of cancer that constitutes approximately 1% of all cancers. STS have a wide range of histological subtypes such as leiomyosarcoma, angiosarcoma, synovial sarcoma, rhabdomyosarcoma, and many others [1]. Systemic cancer treatment for localized disease in STS has been a topic of debate. Two large phase III clinical trials have analysed the clinical activity of doxorubicin-based adjuvant chemotherapy in localized high-grade soft tissue sarcoma patients. A total of 819 patients participated in the studies and had a median follow up for 8.2 years. In the EORTC 62771 study, patients were treated with the CYVADIC regimen (doxorubicin 50 mg/m^2 1 day, dacarbazine 400 mg/m^2, cyclophosphamide 500 mg/m^2, and vincristine 1.5 mg/m^2) while combination of doxorubicin 75 mg/m^2 and ifosfamide 5 g/m^2 was used in the EORTC 62931 study. There was no overall survival benefit with adjuvant chemotherapy in either of the studies [2]. In a different study with stage III STS patients, 338 patients were treated with local treatment and 336 patients received doxorubicin-based adjuvant chemotherapy in addition to local treatment. Follow up data showed that there was no long-term benefit from adjuvant chemotherapy although there was a small disease free survival benefit at 1 year [3].

Rhabdomyosarcoma is a STS that is seen both in children and adults and is one of the few STS subtypes where adjuvant systemic treatment has a role in treatment of localized disease. Embryonal subtype is the most common type and is mostly seen in children while alveolar rhabdomyosarcoma is seen in approximately 20% of the cases and is a very aggressive disease to treat. The standard of care treatment for localized rhabdomyosarcoma is combination treatment with vincrtistine, dactinomycin, and cyclophosphamide (VAC) and radiotherapy [4]. Recently, a multicentre, open-label, randomized, phase III clinical trial has shown that adding six cycles of vinorelbine (intravenous 25 mg/m^2 on days 1, 8, and 15) and cyclophosphamide (daily oral 25 mg/m^2, on days 1–28) as maintenance treatment to standard of care treatment leads to significantly better overall survival at 5 years (86.5%) compared to the arm without any maintenance treatment (73.7%) (HR 0.52, $p = 0.0097$) in patients with high risk rhabdomyosarcoma [5, 6].

Frustaci et al., evaluated the role of high-dose intensity adjuvant chemotherapy in patients with high-grade spindle cell sarcoma arising from extremities or girdles. Fifty-one patients were treated with surgery alone without any adjuvant chemotherapy and 53 patients were treated with five cycles of 4′-epidoxorubin 60 mg/m^2 on days 1 and 2 in combination with ifosfamide 1.8 g/m^2 from day 1 to day 5. The median disease free survival was better in the group treated with adjuvant chemotherapy (48 months) compared to the control group (16 months, $p = 0.04$). In addition, a significantly better overall survival was seen in the treated group (75 months) in comparison to the control group (46 months, $p = 0.03$) [7].

Role of neo-adjuvant chemotherapy in STS has also been an area of debate. Gortzak et al. have randomized patients with high risk STS to either surgery alone or neo-adjuvant doxorubicin (50 mg/m^2) in combination with ifosfamide (5 mg/m^2). Patients with involved surgical margins or recurrent disease were also treated with post-operative radiotherapy. The median follow up was 7.3 years. There was no significant difference in the 5 year disease free survival between the surgery alone arm (52%) and neo-adjuvant treatment arm (56%) ($p = 0.3548$). [8] In a different open-label, randomized, phase III multicentre clinical trial by Gronchi et al., patients with high risk STS (defined as size of 5 cm or above, deeply located, and high grade) were either randomized to standard of care chemotherapy or a chemotherapy tailored specifically to the histological subtype of the STS. In the standard of care chemotherapy arm, 145 patients were given a combination of epirubicin (60 mg/m^2 on days 1

E. Hatipoglu · R. L. Jones (✉)
Sarcoma Unit, Royal Marsden Hospital + Institute of Cancer Research, London, UK
e-mail: Emine.Hatipoglu@rmh.nhs.uk; robin.jones4@nhs.net

H. Özger et al. (eds.), *Diagnosis and Treatment of Soft Tissue Tumors*, https://doi.org/10.1007/978-3-031-77061-6_11

and 2) and ifosfamide (3 g/m^2 per day on days 1, 2, and 3) in 3 weekly cycles. In the second arm, 142 patients were given histotype specific chemotherapy. The histological subtypes and the chemotherapies given included leiomyosarcoma (gemcitabine 1800 mg/m^2 in combination with dacarbazine 500 mg/m^2 in two weekly cycles), undifferentiated pleomorphic sarcoma (gemcitabine 900 mg/m^2 on days 1 and 8 in combination with docetaxel 75 mg/m^2 on day 8 in three weekly cycles), high-grade myxoid liposarcoma (trabectedin 1·3 mg/m^2 in 3 weekly cycles), synovial sarcoma (high-dose ifosfamide 14 g/m^2 given over 14 days via an external infusion pump in 4 weekly cycles) and malignant peripheral nerve sheath tumour (etoposide 150 mg/m^2 per day in combination with intravenous ifosfamide 3 g/m^2 per day on days 1, 2, and 3 in 3 weekly cycles). The median follow up was 12.3 months and the projected disease free survival at 46 months was 62% in the standard of care neo-adjuvant chemotherapy arm and 38% in the histotype specific neo-adjuvant chemotherapy arm ($p = 0.004$, HR = 2.0). The findings suggest that chemotherapy specific to the histological subtypes does not give any benefit over standard of care chemotherapy in the neo-adjuvant setting in STS. However, the results seen in the standard of care chemotherapy arm suggest that neo-adjuvant chemotherapy might add benefit in term of disease free survival in STS [9].

11.2 Nomograms in STS

As discussed above, based on the clinical data published so far, it is very challenging to predict the clinical outcome and role of neo-adjuvant and adjuvant chemotherapy in patients with STS. Nomograms, which use computational modelling based on statistical data using the clinical and pathological characteristics of the patient and the tumour, can be useful in predicting the prognosis and risk stratifying STS patients [10]. The first nomogram in STS was published in 2002 with an aim to predict death and treatment related complications at 12 years from diagnosis. It used data from 2136 patients with different histological subtypes including leiomyosarcoma, synovial sarcoma, liposarcoma, and peripheral nerve sheet tumour. Factors that were taken into account while building the nomogram were age at the time of diagnosis, size and site of tumour as well as histological grade and subtype of the tumour. Validation of the nomogram against Kaplan-Meier and Cox regression analysis showed it can be reliably used in predicting the prognosis in STS [11]. This nomogram was validated using an external cohort consisting of 929 patients with localized STS who were treated in a different cancer centre. The concordance index was 0.76 and showed the nomograms had reliable prognostic function in the validation cohort [12]. Patients with localized retroperitoneal sarcoma were treated with neo-adjuvant chemotherapy (n = 55). Histopathological response (i.e necrosis) on the resected tumour was correlated with disease specific survival (DSS). Patients who had pathological necrosis of 95% or above were classified as responders. Following a median follow up 68 months, the DSS data collected was compared to the nomogram predicted DSS. The 5 year DSS was 47% and was similar to the predicted nomogram DSS (37%) without any significant difference ($p = 0.44$). On the other, the 5 year DSS for responders based on pathological response was higher in the observed values (83%) compared to the nomogram predicted values (39%) ($p = 0.018$). There was no significant difference in the observed and nomogram predicted value on the non-responders ($p = 0.51$) [13]. In addition, Canter et al. have developed a nomogram for synovial sarcoma patients who have been treated with curative intent surgery. They have taken into account variables such as age, size, site, bone and neurovascular invasion, surgical margin status and SYT-SSX fusion status. They have shown that size and site of disease were the two key factors in predicting the prognosis. It was also shown that the 3 year DSS was higher in the patients treated with neo-adjuvant anthracycline and ifosfamide combination chemotherapy (n = 59) compared to the patients who did not receive any chemotherapy (n = 196) [14]. These studies suggest that nomograms can have a role in risk stratifying patients while making decisions about peri-operative chemotherapy given the contradicting results about role of neo-adjuvant and adjuvant chemotherapy in STS.

11.3 Advanced Disease

11.3.1 Chemotherapy Regimes

11.3.1.1 Anthracycline-Based Therapy

Different types of chemotherapies including cyclophosphamide, vincristine, doxorubicin, and dimethyl triazeno imidazole carboxamide (DTIC) have been used both alone and in combination for treatment of advanced STS since the 1970s. Doxorubicin has formed the backbone of treatment of metastatic STS since then with response rates varying from 9% to 70% in depending on the histological subtype of STS. [15] Doxorubicin is an anthracycline chemotherapy that works by inhibiting DNA repair by the topoisomerase II enzyme [16].

The efficacy of doxorubicin treatment alone in metastatic STS was compared to cyclophosphamide, vincristine, doxorubicin, and dacarbazine (CYVADIC) and combination of doxorubicin and ifosfamide in a prospective randomized phase III trial in 663 patients with different histological subtypes of locally advanced or metastatic STS. Patients were allocated to either 75 mg/m^2 single agent doxorubicin (arm A), CYVADIC (cyclophosphamide 500 mg/m^2, vincristine 1.5 mg/m^2, doxorubicin 50 mg/m^2 and dacarbazine 750 mg/m^2) (arm B) or combination of doxorubicin (50 mg/m^2) and

24-h ifosfamide infusion (5 g/m^2) (arm C) in 3 weekly cycles. An overall response rate of 24% (95% confidence interval, 20.7–27.3%) was observed. However, there was no statistically significant difference in response rate (arm A, 23.3%; arm B, 28.4%; and arm C, 28.1%), remission duration (median, 46 weeks on arm A, 48 weeks on arm B, and 44 weeks on arm C), or overall survival (median, 52 weeks on arm A, 51 weeks on arm B, and 55 weeks on arm C) between the three arms of the study [17]. In a different phase III clinical trial, 262 patients with advanced STS were treated with either doxorubicin 80 mg/m^2 alone (arm A), combination of ifosfamide (7.5 g/m^2) and doxorubicin (60 mg/m^2) (arm B) or combination of mitomycin (8 mg/m^2), doxorubicin (40 mg/m^2), and cisplatin (60 mg/m^2) (arm C). Combination treatment with doxorubicin and ifosfamide was associated with a significantly higher tumour regression rate compared to single-agent doxorubicin ($p = 0.03$) but no difference was seen in the overall survival. In addition, a higher level of myelosuppression was seen in the combination group compared to the single-agent doxorubicin group [18]. Given the contradicting results from the previous studies, the randomized phase III clinical trial EORTC 62012 looked at the role of combination of intensified doxorubicin and ifosfamide versus doxorubicin alone in first-line treatment in locally advanced, unresectable and metastatic STS. In the first arm, 228 patients were given single-agent doxorubicin (75 mg/m^2 by intravenous bolus on day 1 or 72 h continuous intravenous infusion). In the second arm, 227 patients were given intensified doxorubicin (75 mg/m^2; 25 mg/m^2 per day, days 1–3) in combination with ifosfamide (10 g/m^2 over 4 days). The primary endpoint of the study was overall survival. Although there was no statistically significant difference in the overall survival in the single agent doxorubicin (12.8 months) and the doxorubicin and ifosfamide combination therapy group (14.3 months), a significantly higher median progression-free survival was seen in the doxorubicin and ifosfamide group (7·4 months) compared to the doxorubicin group (4·6 months, stratified log-rank test $p = 0{\cdot}003$). Higher levels of grade 3 and 4 myelosuppression were seen in the doxorubicin and ifosfamide combination treatment arm [19].

Ifosfamide is an alkylating agent and is an analogue of cyclophosphamide. Previously, it was shown to have activity in patients with both treatment naïve and previously treated STS. Myelosuppression, neurotoxicity in the form of confusion and hallucinations, and haematuria are associated with ifosfomide [20]. Alkylating agents other than ifosfamide have also been tried in combination with doxorubicin in patients with STS. Evofosfamide is a nitroimidazole prodrug of bromo-isophosphoramide mustard which is an alkylating cytotoxin. It becomes activated in hypoxic conditions and therefore is designed to specifically bind to tumour cells that survive in hypoxia. This intends to reduce the toxicity seen with other alkylating agents such as ifosfamide. The multicentre, open-label, randomized phase III clinical trial SARC021 looked at the efficacy of evofosfamide in combination with doxorubicin in 640 patients with locally advanced unresectable or metastatic STS. In one arm, 323 patients were randomized to receive doxorubicin alone (75 mg/m^2 via 3 weekly cycles for up to six cycles). In the second arm, 317 patients were given doxorubicin (same protocol as the single agent doxorubicin am) plus evofosfamide (300 mg/m^2 on days 1 and 8 in 3 weekly cycles for up to six cycles). There was no significant difference in the median overall survival between the doxorubicin and ifosfamide arm (18.4 months, 95% CI 15.6–22.1) and single-agent doxorubicin arm (19 months, 95% CI 16.2–22.4; $p = 0.527$). There was also no difference in survival in the histological subtype analysis. In terms of toxicity, a higher frequency of myelosuppression was seen in the combination therapy arm compared to the single-agent doxorubicin [21]. PICASSO III study is a placebo-controlled phase III clinical trial that looked at the efficacy of combining palifosfamide with doxorubicin in treatment naïve patients with metastatic STS. Palifosfamide is an active metabolite of ifosfamide that can exert antitumour activity without producing the metabolites that cause toxicity. 447 patients were involved in the study, 226 of which were given doxorubicin 75 mg/m^2 and palifosfamide 150 mg/m^2 on days 1–3 or doxorubicin and 221 patients were given doxorubicin 75 mg/m^2 and placebo every three weeks for up to six cycles. There was no significant difference in the PFS between the arm that received doxorubicin and palifosfamide (6.0 months) and doxorubicin and placebo (5.2 months) (hazard ratio, 0.86; 95% CI, 0.68–1.08; $P = 0.19$). Median overall survival was 15.9 months for doxorubicin and palifosfamide arm and 16.9 months for doxorubicin plus placebo arm with no significant difference between the two groups (hazard ratio, 1.05; 95% CI, 0.79–1.39; $P = 0.74$) [22].

Studies have shown that platelet-derived growth factor (PDGF) and PDGF receptor (PDGFR) play an important role in sarcoma pathophysiology. Therefore, a recombinant human immunoglobulin IgG1 monoclonal antibody called olaratumab has been developed. Olaratumab binds PFGFR α, blocks PDGF-AA and PDGF-BB and activated PDGF-CC. A phase 1b and phase II randomized clinical trial evaluated the role of adding olaratumab to doxorubicin in patients with locally advanced and metastatic STS patients. In one arm of the study, patients were given olaratumab (15 mg/kg) intravenously on day 1 and day 8 and doxorubicin (75 mg/m^2) in 3 weekly cycles for up to eight cycles. In the second arm, patients received doxorubicin alone (75 mg/m^2) in 3 weekly cycles for up to eight cycles. The phase II part of the study showed significantly better overall survival (26.5 months) in the olaratumab and doxorubicin arm compared to doxorubicin alone (14.7 months) (HR 0.46,

0.30–0.71, $p = 0.0003$) [23]. Based on this phase II study, the ANNOUNCE study which is a phase III double-blind clinical trial that studied the efficacy of olaratumab and doxorubicin combination therapy in advanced and metastatic STS. Patients were given olaratumab (20 mg/kg in cycle 1 followed by 15 mg/kg in the subsequent cycles) or placebo in combination with doxorubicin (75 mg/kg) for up to eight cycles. Contrary to the phase 2 study, combination treatment with olaratumab and doxorubicin did not give any overall survival benefit (20.4 months) compared to the doxorubicin and placebo group (19.7 months) (HR1.05, 95% CI 0.84–1.30, $p = 0.69$) [24].

11.3.1.2 Gemcitabine-Based Therapy

Gemcitabine is a cytosine arabinoside analogue and plays an important role in DNA synthesis. Gemcitabine is used in the treatment of different cancers including STS [25]. Phase II studies showed gemcitabine can be effective in patients with metastatic STS who have previously been treated with another line of chemotherapy such as doxorubicin [26, 27]. Following up on this data, the addition of docetaxel to gemcitabine in patients with metastatic STS was evaluated in a phase II clinical trial. In one arm, 73 patients were randomized to gemcitabine (900 mg/m^2 on days 1 and 8) and docetaxel (100 mg/m^2 on day 8) in 3 weekly cycles. In the second arm, 49 patients were given gemcitabine alone (1200 mg/m^2 days 1 and 8) in 3 weekly cycles. Combination of gemcitabine and docetaxel treatment had better median progression survival (6.2 months) and median overall survival (17.9 months) compared to gemcitabine alone (median progression-free survival of 3.0 months and overall survival of 11.5 months). Histological subtype analysis showed that patients with malignant fibrous histiocytoma/high-grade undifferentiated pleomorphic sarcoma and leiomyosarcoma had better responses to gemcitabine and docetaxel combination. In addition, non-haematological toxicities such as fatigue and myalgia were seen more frequently with combination treatment compared to gemcitabine alone [28]. In a different phase II clinical trial, 48 patients with unresectable uterine leiomyosarcoma who have progressed on the previous line of treatment were given gemcitabine (900 mg/m^2 on days 1 and 8) and docetaxel (100 mg/m^2 on day 8) in 3 weekly cycles. The median progression-free survival was 6.7 months, the overall survival was 14.7 months and 53% of the patients received an objective response rate which was an encouraging result in the second-line setting. [29] GeDDiS trial was a randomized phase III clinical trial that included 257 patients with locally advanced or metastatic STS. 128 patients were treated with gemcitabine (675 mg/m^2 on days 1 and 8) and docetaxel (75 mg/m^2 on day 8) in 3 weekly cycles and 129 patients were treated with doxorubicin 75 mg/m^2 every 3 weeks as first-line treatment. The median follow-up in the study was 22 months. There was no significant difference in the progression-free survival between the doxorubicin alone (23.3 weeks) and gemcitabine plus docetaxel (23.7 weeks) group. Similarly, at 24 weeks, the median overall survival was 86.8% in the doxorubicin arm and 82.6% in the gemcitabine and docetaxel arm. This suggested that doxorubicin should remain as first-line treatment for advanced or metastatic STS but gemcitabine and docetaxel can be used as second-line therapy [30].

Dacarbazine is another chemotherapy that has been used in treatments of STS. It has been shown that high-dose dacarbazine is active in patients with metastatic STS who have received previous lines of treatment [31]. Combining dacarbazine with gemcitabine in metastatic STS patients who have progressed on a previous line of treatment has been studied in a randomized, multicentre, phase II clinical trial. A total of 113 patients were involved in the study of whom 59 patients were given gemcitabine (1800 mg/m^2 followed by dacarbazine 500 mg/m^2 every 2 weeks) and 54 patients were given dacarbazine alone (1200 mg/m^2 every 3 weeks). The median progression-free survival was 4.2 months in the combination treatment arm and 2 months in the single agent dacarbazine arm (HR 0.58, 95% CI0.39–0.86, $p = 0.005$). The median overall survival was significantly better with gemcitabine and dacarbazine combination treatment (16.8 months) compared to dacarbazine alone (8.2 months) (HR 0.56, 95% CI 0.36–0.90, $p = 0.14$) [32]. This study suggests that gemcitabine and dacarbazine can be used for patients with metastatic STS who have progressed on previous lines of treatment.

11.3.1.3 Trabectedin-Based Therapy

Trabectedin is a chemotherapy that is derived from *Ecteinascidia turbinate* and works by causing double-stranded DNA breaks, downregulating the expression of FUS-CHOP and EWS-CHOP transcription factors as well as inhibiting the cytokine release from the monocytes and macrophages in the tumour microenvironment [33]. The use of trabectedin in metastatic STS has been investigated in several studies over the past years. One of the first studies that showed the activity of trabectedin in advanced soft tissue and bone sarcoma patients who have been treated with previous lines of treatment was a phase I trial which demonstrated response and disease stabilization with trabectedin [34]. Following up on these findings, a phase II clinical trial compared trabectedin to best supportive care in metastatic translocation-related STS patients who progressed in previous lines of treatment. 37 patients were treated with trabectedin (1·2 mg/m^2 given over 24 h in 3 weekly cycles) and 36 patients were randomized to best supportive care. The trabectedin treatment was well tolerated and was associated with significantly better median progression-free survival (5.6 months) compared to the best supportive arm (0.9 months) (HR 0.07, 95% CI 0.03–0.16, $p < 0.0001$). In addition, the three-month progression-free survival was 70.3% in the group treated with trabectedin while all the patients in the best supportive care group had progressive disease at three months [35]. This study suggests that trabectedin can be used for patients who have progressed on previous lines of treatment. Although beyond first-line treatment trabectedin has shown activity in advanced and metastatic STS, trabectedin was not as effective in the first-line setting. In the open-labelled randomized phase II clinical trial, 55 patients were treated with trabectedin 1.1 mg/m^2 in a 3-h infusion plus doxorubicin 60 mg/m^2 up to 6 cycles and 60 patients were treated with doxorubicin 75 mg/m^2 in the other arm in the first-line setting for advanced STS patients. The analysis demonstrated no significant difference in progression-free survival between the combination treatment arm (5.7 months) and the standard of care treatment with doxorubicin (5.5 months) (HR, 1.16; 95% CI, 0.79–1.71; $p = 0.45$) [36]. This study showed that although trabectedin can be used beyond first-line treatment, doxorubicin remains the first-line treatment for advanced STS. Demetri and his colleagues have compared the role of trabectedin to dacarbazine in patients with metastatic liposarcoma or leiomyosarcoma who have progressed on previous chemotherapy. In this multicentre randomized phase III clinical trial, 345 patients were randomized to trabectedin and 173 patients were randomized to dacarbazine. Trabectedin showed better disease control compared to dacarbazine with a 45% reduction in disease progression and death (HR 0.55, $p < 0.001$). This study supports the use of trabectedin in patients with metastatic liposarcoma or leiomyosarcoma after first-line treatment [37].

11.3.1.4 Eribulin-Based Therapy

Eribulin is a chemotherapy agent that works by inhibiting microtubule growth by binding to the beta subunit. This leads to cell death due to the irreversible arrest from the G2 to M phase of the cell cycle. It has been shown to be effective in the treatment of different cancer types in the advanced disease setting [38]. Eribulin was also shown to have activity in metastatic STS. Initially, a phase II clinical trial with 52 Japanese patients with advanced or metastatic STS was treated with eribulin mesylate (1.4 mg/m^2 on days 1 and 8 every 3 weeks). In addition to seeing a clinical activity with eribulin, patients with liposarcoma and leiomyosarcoma histological subtypes had significantly better progression-free survival and overall survival compared to the other histological subtypes in the study [39]. In light of this phase II study findings, in a randomized, open-label, multicentre phase III clinical trial patients with advanced liposarcoma and leimyosarcoma who have progressed on previous chemotherapy treatment were randomized to either eribulin mesylate (1.4 mg/m^2 on days 1 and 8 every 3 weeks) (228 patients) or dacarbazine (850 mg/m^2, 1000 mg/m^2 or 1200 mg/m^2 every 3 weeks depending on the centre) (224 patients) until disease progression. Significantly better overall survival was seen in the cohort treated with eribulin (13.5 months) compared to the group treated with dacarbazine (11.5 months) (HR 0.77, 95% CI 0.62–0.95, $p = 0.0169$). The most commonly seen toxicity associated with eribulin was myelosuppression [40]. This suggests that eribulin can be considered an important treatment option for liposarcoma and leimyosarcoma following progression on first-line treatment. Based on this phase III clinical trial, FDA has approved eribulin as second-line treatment for patients with unresectable or metastatic liposarcoma who have progressed on an anthracycline-containing chemotherapy treatment [41].

11.3.2 Targeted Therapies

11.3.2.1 Pazopanib

Pazopanib is a tyrosine kinase inhibitor that is used in treatment of different cancers. It works by inhibiting the endothelial growth factor (VEGF) receptors (VEGFR), platelet-derived growth factor receptor (PDGFR), and c-Kit tyrosine kinases. This impairs tumour angiogenesis and leads to tumour cell death [42]. Angiogenesis is an important oncogenic pathway in sarcoma, especially in higher grade STS. Therefore, the effectiveness of inhibiting angiogenic pathways in sarcoma has been studied. EORTC 62043 study evaluated the safety and efficacy of pazopanib in patients with intermediate to high-grade advanced STS who were ineligible for surgery, radiotherapy or chemotherapy or have progressed on one or two lines of cytotoxic treatment. 142 patients were given 800 mg pazopanib everyday. The treatment was well tolerated mainly with grade 1 to grade 2 toxicity and the common side effects included fatigue, hypertension, deranged liver enzymes and myelosuppression. Pazopanib showed efficacy in STS, especially in leiomyosarcoma and synovial sarcoma subtypes [43]. The PALETTE study which was a randomized, double-blind, placebo-controlled phase III clinical trial evaluated the efficacy of pazopanib in patients with non-adipocytic metastatic STS who have received no more than two previous lines of treatment. 246 patients were randomized to 800 mg of pazopanib treatment daily and 123 patients were randomized to placebo. Although the overall survival was similar in both arms, the progression-free survival was significantly better in the arm treated with pazopanib (4.6 months) compared to the placebo arm (1.6 months) (HR 0.31, 95% CI 0.24–0.40, $p < 0.0001$) [44]. This study provided evidence for using pazopanib in patients progressing following previous lines of chemotherapy.

11.3.2.2 NTRK Inhibitors

NTRK1, NTRK2 and NTRK3 genes encode for the tropomycin receptor kinase (Trk) receptors A, B and C. These proteins are important in neural signalling and development of the nervous system. Fusions in the *NTRK* genes lead to rearrangement of Trk proteins that activate oncogenic pathways. Consequently, *NTRK* fusions are associated with different types of cancer including colorectal cancer, lung adenocarcinoma, glioblastoma and sarcomas [45]. Phase I and phase II studies have evaluated the safety and efficacy of entrectinib which is an inhibitor of Trk A, B and C and patients with lung cancer, breast cancer, STS, pancreatic cancer, thyroid cancer and colorectal cancer were involved in the studies. Entrectinib had an acceptable safety profile with mainly grade 1 and 2 toxicity. The objective response rate was 57% and the median progression-free survival was 11 months which is a promising result [46]. Larotrectinib is another Trk inhibitor that was shown to be more effective in advanced STS patients with NTRK fusions compared to standard-of-care chemotherapy [47].

11.3.2.3 EZH2 Inhibitor

Epithelioid sarcoma is a rare and aggressive form of STS. Approximately 90% of the patients with epithelioid sarcoma have integrase interactor 1(INI 1) loss. INI1 is a tumour suppressor which encodes for a subunit of the SW1/SNF chromatin remodelling complex which plays an important role in the enhancer of zeste homolog (EZH2) downregulation. INI1 loss leads to upregulation of EZH2 which is critical in oncogenesis [48, 49]. Tazemetostat is a selective inhibitor of EZH2. The NCT01897571 was a first in human, open-label phase 1 trial with tazemetostat which demonstrated an acceptable safety profile for the drug as well as promising anti-tumour activity in several cancers including non-Hodgkin lymphoma and epithelioid sarcoma [50]. Following the results of this phase 1 trial, an international, open-label, phase 2 basket study showed a median progression-free survival of 5.5 months and a median overall survival of 19 months in the cohort with epithelioid sarcoma. In addition, it was seen that treatment naïve patients had better progression-free survival compared to patients who had previous lines of treatment [51]. This was an important study demonstrating the anti-tumour activity of tazemetostat in patients with epithelioid sarcoma.

11.3.2.4 Immunotherapy and Cellular Therapies

Immunotherapy with checkpoint blockade has revolutionized the treatment of cancer with durable responses in different types of cancer. However, this success has been limited in sarcoma. A combination of pembrolizumab (anti-PD-1 antibody) with axitinib (tyrosine kinase inhibitor targeting VEGF) was evaluated in patients with advanced or metastatic STS who had at least one line of prior treatment. 33 patients were involved in the study and the median overall survival was 18.7 months and the median progression-free survival was 6.9 months. Analysis of histological subtypes shows alveolar soft part sarcoma (ASPS) had significantly better progression-free survival (12.4 months) compared to the non-ASPS histological subtypes (3 months). In addition, duration of response was longer in the ASPS patients. This was an important finding in highlighting the potential activity of immunotherapy in ASPS patients [52]. Due to limited effective treatments available in ASPS and the promising results of immune checkpoint blockade therapy, immunotherapy was then approved for ASPS patients in the USA [53].

In addition, cellular therapy studies have shown promising results in synovial sarcoma which has poor clinical survival due to limited effective therapies. Up to 80% of the synovial sarcoma patients express the cancer antigen NY-ESO. Engineered HLA-A2 restricted high-affinity T cell receptor (TCR) targeting the NY-ESO-1/LAGE1a antigen has been used in treating 12 patients with metastatic synovial sarcoma who have progressed on previous lines of treatment. This study demonstrated the safety and feasibility of NY-ESO-1^{c259} T cell therapy in synovial sarcoma as well as showing promising clinical activity [54].

11.4 Conclusion

Systemic therapies for STS have evolved over the past years with a better understanding of different histological subtypes. Although the role of neo-adjuvant and adjuvant chemotherapy in localized disease is still debatable, most studies did not show any long-term benefit from chemotherapy. In addition, it was also shown that histotype-specific neo-adjuvant chemotherapy does not provide any additional clinical benefit. Given the contradictory results for the use of neo-adjuvant and adjuvant chemotherapy in STS, nomograms can have a role in risk stratifying patients to decide which cohort of patients will benefit from peri-operative chemotherapy.

In advanced and metastatic STS patients, doxorubicin with or without ifosfamide is used as first-line treatment. Gemcitabine-based treatment or trabectedin have been shown to be effective as a second-line treatment. Eribulin was also shown to be effective as second-line treatment in leiomyosarcoma and liposarcoma. Dacarbazine and pazopanib can also be used in advanced diseases beyond second-line treatment.

Targeted therapies also play an important role in the treatment of advanced and metastatic STS. NTRK inhibitors such as entrectinib can be used in patients with NTRK fusions. Tazemetostat is another targeted therapy that was proven to be effective in epithelioid sarcoma patients with INI1 loss.

More recently, there has been promising data supporting the role of immunotherapy and TCR-based cellular therapies in advanced or metastatic sarcoma. However, further studies are needed. In addition, despite the progress in STS treatment over the years, the progress is still limited. The small number of patients and large number of histological subtypes are limiting factors in running clinical trials in STS. However, a better understanding of the molecular characteristics of STS subtypes can help with developing more effective therapies.

References

1. Krikelis D, Judson I. Role of chemotherapy in the management of soft tissue sarcomas. Expert Rev Anticancer Ther. 2010;10:249–60.
2. Cesne AL, et al. Doxorubicin-based adjuvant chemotherapy in soft tissue sarcoma: pooled analysis of two STBSG-EORTC phase III clinical trials. Ann Oncol. 2014;25:2425–32.
3. Cormier JN, et al. Cohort analysis of patients with localized, high-risk, extremity soft tissue sarcoma treated at two cancer centers: chemotherapy-associated outcomes. J Clin Oncol. 2016;22:4567. https://doi.org/10.1200/JCO.2004.02.057.
4. Crist WM, et al. Intergroup rhabdomyosarcoma study-IV: results for patients with nonmetastatic disease. J Clin Oncol. 2016;19:3091. https://doi.org/10.1200/JCO.2001.19.12.3091.
5. Bisogno G, et al. Vinorelbine and continuous low-dose cyclophosphamide as maintenance chemotherapy in patients with high-risk rhabdomyosarcoma (RMS 2005): a multicentre, open-label, randomised, phase 3 trial. Lancet Oncol. 2019;20:1566–75.
6. Miwa S, et al. Recent advances and challenges in the treatment of rhabdomyosarcoma. Cancers. 2020;12:1758.
7. Frustaci S, et al. Adjuvant chemotherapy for adult soft tissue sarcomas of the extremities and girdles: results of the Italian randomized cooperative trial. J Clin Oncol Off J Am Soc Clin Oncol. 2001;19:1238–47.
8. Gortzak E, et al. A randomised phase II study on neo-adjuvant chemotherapy for 'high-risk' adult soft-tissue sarcoma. Eur J Cancer. 2001;37:1096–103.
9. Gronchi A, et al. Histotype-tailored neoadjuvant chemotherapy versus standard chemotherapy in patients with high-risk soft-tissue sarcomas (ISG-STS 1001): an international, open-label, randomised, controlled, phase 3, multicentre trial. Lancet Oncol. 2017;18:812–22.
10. Iasonos A, Schrag D, Raj GV, Panageas KS. How to build and interpret a nomogram for cancer prognosis. J Clin Oncol. 2008;26:1364–70.
11. Kattan MW, Leung DHY, Brennan MF. Postoperative nomogram for 12-year sarcoma-specific death. J Clin Oncol. 2002;20:791–6.
12. Eilber FC, et al. Validation of the postoperative nomogram for 12-year sarcoma-specific mortality. Cancer. 2004;101:2270–5.
13. Donahue TR, et al. Evaluation of neoadjuvant therapy and histopathologic response in primary, high-grade retroperitoneal sarcomas using the sarcoma nomogram. Cancer. 2010;116:3883–91.
14. Canter RJ, et al. A synovial sarcoma-specific preoperative nomogram supports a survival benefit to ifosfamide-based chemotherapy and improves risk stratification for patients. Clin Cancer Res. 2008;14:8191–7.
15. Pinedo HM, Kenis Y. Chemotherapy of advanced soft-tissue sarcomas in adults. Cancer Treat Rev. 1977;4:67–86.
16. Thorn CF, et al. Doxorubicin pathways: pharmacodynamics and adverse effects. Pharmacogenet Genomics. 2011;21:440–6.
17. Santoro A, et al. Doxorubicin versus CYVADIC versus doxorubicin plus ifosfamide in first-line treatment of advanced soft tissue sarcomas: a randomized study of the European Organization for Research and Treatment of Cancer Soft Tissue and Bone Sarcoma Group. J Clin Oncol Off J Am Soc Clin Oncol. 1995;13:1537–45.
18. Edmonson JH, et al. Randomized comparison of doxorubicin alone versus ifosfamide plus doxorubicin or mitomycin, doxorubicin, and cisplatin against advanced soft tissue sarcomas. J Clin Oncol. 1993;11:1269–75.
19. Judson I, et al. Doxorubicin alone versus intensified doxorubicin plus ifosfamide for first-line treatment of advanced or metastatic soft-tissue sarcoma: a randomised controlled phase 3 trial. Lancet Oncol. 2014;15:415–23.
20. Antman KH, Ryan L, Elias A, Sherman D, Grier HE. Response to ifosfamide and mesna: 124 previously treated patients with metastatic or unresectable sarcoma. J Clin Oncol Off J Am Soc Clin Oncol. 1989;7:126–31.
21. Tap WD, et al. Doxorubicin plus evofosfamide versus doxorubicin alone in locally advanced, unresectable or metastatic soft-tissue sarcoma (TH CR-406/SARC021): an international, multicentre, open-label, randomised phase 3 trial. Lancet Oncol. 2017;18:1089–103.
22. Ryan CW, et al. PICASSO III: a phase III, placebo-controlled study of doxorubicin with or without palifosfamide in patients with metastatic soft tissue sarcoma. J Clin Oncol Off J Am Soc Clin Oncol. 2016;34:3898–905.
23. Tap WD, et al. Olaratumab and doxorubicin versus doxorubicin alone for treatment of soft-tissue sarcoma: an open-label phase 1b and randomised phase 2 trial. Lancet Lond Engl. 2016;388:488–97.
24. Tap WD, et al. Effect of doxorubicin plus olaratumab vs doxorubicin plus placebo on survival in patients with advanced soft tissue sarcomas: the ANNOUNCE randomized clinical trial. JAMA. 2020;323:1266–76.
25. Mini E, Nobili S, Caciagli B, Landini I, Mazzei T. Cellular pharmacology of gemcitabine. Ann Oncol. 2006;17:v7–v12.
26. Späth-Schwalbe E, et al. Phase II trial of gemcitabine in patients with pretreated advanced soft tissue sarcomas. Anti-Cancer Drugs. 2000;11:325.
27. Okuno S, Ryan LM, Edmonson JH, Priebat DA, Blum RH. Phase II trial of gemcitabine in patients with advanced sarcomas (E1797). Cancer. 2003;97:1969–73.
28. Maki RG, et al. Randomized phase II study of gemcitabine and docetaxel compared with gemcitabine alone in patients with metastatic soft tissue sarcomas: results of sarcoma alliance for research through collaboration study 002 [corrected]. J Clin Oncol Off J Am Soc Clin Oncol. 2007;25:2755–63.
29. Hensley ML, et al. Fixed-dose rate gemcitabine plus docetaxel as second-line therapy for metastatic uterine leiomyosarcoma: a Gynecologic Oncology Group phase II study. Gynecol Oncol. 2008;109:323–8.
30. Seddon B, et al. Gemcitabine and docetaxel versus doxorubicin as first-line treatment in previously untreated advanced unresectable or metastatic soft-tissue sarcomas (GeDDiS): a randomised controlled phase 3 trial. Lancet Oncol. 2017;18:1397–410.
31. Buesa JM, et al. High-dose DTIC in advanced soft-tissue sarcomas in the adult. A phase II study of the E.O.R.T.C. Soft Tissue and Bone Sarcoma Group. Ann Oncol Off J Eur Soc Med Oncol. 1991;2:307–9.
32. Garcia del Muro X, et al. Randomized phase II study comparing gemcitabine plus dacarbazine versus dacarbazine alone in patients with previously treated soft tissue sarcoma: a Spanish Group for Research on Sarcomas Study. J Clin Oncol Off J Am Soc Clin Oncol. 2011;29:2528–33.
33. Gordon EM, Sankhala KK, Chawla N, Chawla SP. Trabectedin for soft tissue sarcoma: current status and future perspectives. Adv Ther. 2016;33:1055–71.
34. Delaloge S, et al. Ecteinascidin-743: a marine-derived compound in advanced, pretreated sarcoma patients--preliminary evidence of activity. J Clin Oncol Off J Am Soc Clin Oncol. 2001;19:1248–55.

35. Kawai A, et al. Trabectedin monotherapy after standard chemotherapy versus best supportive care in patients with advanced, translocation-related sarcoma: a randomised, open-label, phase 2 study. Lancet Oncol. 2015;16:406–16.
36. Martin-Broto J, et al. Randomized phase II study of trabectedin and doxorubicin compared with doxorubicin alone as first-line treatment in patients with advanced soft tissue sarcomas: a Spanish Group for Research on sarcoma study. J Clin Oncol Off J Am Soc Clin Oncol. 2016;34:2294–302.
37. Demetri GD, et al. Efficacy and safety of trabectedin or dacarbazine for metastatic liposarcoma or leiomyosarcoma after failure of conventional chemotherapy: results of a phase III randomized multicenter clinical trial. J Clin Oncol Off J Am Soc Clin Oncol. 2016;34:786–93.
38. Jain S, Vahdat LT. Eribulin Mesylate. Clin Cancer Res. 2011;17:6615–22.
39. Kawai A, et al. Phase 2 study of eribulin in patients with previously treated advanced or metastatic soft tissue sarcoma. Jpn J Clin Oncol. 2017;47:137–44.
40. Schöffski P, et al. Eribulin versus dacarbazine in previously treated patients with advanced liposarcoma or leiomyosarcoma: a randomised, open-label, multicentre, phase 3 trial. Lancet Lond Engl. 2016;387:1629–37.
41. Osgood CL, et al. FDA approval summary: eribulin for patients with unresectable or metastatic liposarcoma who have received a prior anthracycline-containing regimen. Clin Cancer Res Off J Am Assoc Cancer Res. 2017;23:6384–9.
42. Kumar R, et al. Pharmacokinetic-pharmacodynamic correlation from mouse to human with pazopanib, a multikinase angiogenesis inhibitor with potent antitumor and antiangiogenic activity. Mol Cancer Ther. 2007;6:2012–21.
43. Sleijfer S, et al. Pazopanib, a multikinase angiogenesis inhibitor, in patients with relapsed or refractory advanced soft tissue sarcoma: a phase II study from the European organisation for research and treatment of cancer-soft tissue and bone sarcoma group (EORTC study 62043). J Clin Oncol Off J Am Soc Clin Oncol. 2009;27:3126–32.
44. van der Graaf WTA, et al. Pazopanib for metastatic soft-tissue sarcoma (PALETTE): a randomised, double-blind, placebo-controlled phase 3 trial. Lancet Lond Engl. 2012;379:1879–86.
45. Amatu A, Sartore-Bianchi A, Siena S. NTRK gene fusions as novel targets of cancer therapy across multiple tumour types. ESMO Open. 2016;1:e000023.
46. Doebele RC, et al. Entrectinib in patients with advanced or metastatic NTRK fusion-positive solid tumours: integrated analysis of three phase 1-2 trials. Lancet Oncol. 2020;21:271–82.
47. Suh K, Carlson JJ, Xia F, Williamson T, Sullivan SD. The potential long-term comparative effectiveness of larotrectinib vs standard of care for treatment of metastatic TRK fusion thyroid cancer, colorectal cancer, and soft tissue sarcoma. J Manag Care Spec Pharm. 2022;28:622–30.
48. Modena P, et al. SMARCB1/INI1 tumor suppressor gene is frequently inactivated in epithelioid sarcomas. Cancer Res. 2005;65:4012–9.
49. Italiano A. Targeting epigenetics in sarcomas through EZH2 inhibition. J Hematol Oncol. 2020;13:33.
50. Italiano A, et al. Tazemetostat, an EZH2 inhibitor, in relapsed or refractory B-cell non-Hodgkin lymphoma and advanced solid tumours: a first-in-human, open-label, phase 1 study. Lancet Oncol. 2018;19:649–59.
51. Gounder M, et al. Tazemetostat in advanced epithelioid sarcoma with loss of INI1/SMARCB1: an international, open-label, phase 2 basket study. Lancet Oncol. 2020;21:1423–32.
52. Wilky BA, et al. Axitinib plus pembrolizumab in patients with advanced sarcomas including alveolar soft-part sarcoma: a single-centre, single-arm, phase 2 trial. Lancet Oncol. 2019;20:837–48.
53. Bergsma EJ, et al. Atezolizumab as the first systemic therapy approved for alveolar soft part sarcoma. Ann Pharmacother. 2023;58:407. https://doi.org/10.1177/10600280231187421.
54. D'Angelo SP, et al. Antitumor activity associated with prolonged persistence of adoptively transferred NY-ESO-1 c259T cells in synovial sarcoma. Cancer Discov. 2018;8:944–57.

Medical Oncological Treatment of the Pediatric Patient

12

Stefan S. Bielack, Monika Sparber-Sauer, and Claudia Blattmann

12.1 Introduction

Soft-tissue sarcomas in children and adolescents come in a wide variety of histologies, but also sites, sizes, and grades of malignancy. Awareness regarding their presentation and diagnostic guidelines among both primary care physicians as well as specialists must be increased to help diagnose such malignant tumors early [1]. Untreated or, depending on the individual situation, when treated by local therapy only, they often progress rapidly, metastasize, and have fatal outcomes. Other than in adults, however, the majority of these often highly aggressive tumors are amenable to systemic treatments [2, 3]. This chapter will review some of the most frequent soft-tissue sarcomas presented in the young. It will particularly attempt to put systemic therapies into perspective.

S. S. Bielack (✉)
Cooperative Osteosarcoma Study Group, Pädiatrie 5 (Onkologie, Hämatologie, Immunologie), Zentrum für Kinder-, Jugend- und Frauenmedizin, Stuttgart Cancer Center, Klinikum Stuttgart gKAöR—Olgahospital, Stuttgart, Germany

Klinik für Kinder- und Jugendmedizin, Pädiatrische Hämatologie und Onkologie, Universitätsklinikum Münster, Münster, Germany
e-mail: coss@klinikum-stuttgart.de

M. Sparber-Sauer
Cooperative Weichteilsarkom-Studiengruppe, Pädiatrie 5 (Onkologie, Hämatologie, Immunologie), Zentrum für Kinder-, Jugend- und Frauenmedizin, Stuttgart Cancer Center, Klinikum Stuttgart gKAöR – Olgahospital, Stuttgart, Germany

Medizinische Fakultät der Universität Tübingen, Tübingen, Germany

C. Blattmann
Cooperative Osteosarcoma Study Group, Pädiatrie 5 (Onkologie, Hämatologie, Immunologie), Zentrum für Kinder-, Jugend- und Frauenmedizin, Stuttgart Cancer Center, Klinikum Stuttgart gKAöR—Olgahospital, Stuttgart, Germany

Medizinische Fakultät der Universität Tübingen, Tübingen, Germany

12.2 Treatment Infrastructure

Therapy of soft-tissue sarcomas within collaborative infrastructures, if available, is clearly the current standard. Only by treating affected patients in this fashion can local and systemic treatments be performed according to up-to-date practices. Many European countries therefore register and treat their pediatric soft-tissue sarcomas within disease-specific study groups, for instance, the Cooperative Weichteilsarkom-Studiengruppe (CWS) or the equally multi-national European pediatric Soft-tissue Sarcoma Group (EpSSG). It might be considered medical malpractice not to register and treat eligible pediatric or adolescent patients within such cooperative infrastructures. This holds true regardless of the tumor's expected chemosensitivity and the projected treatment plan: It takes a multi-disciplinary discussion of every single individual case to decide whether systemic therapy should be part of this patient's treatment plan and to decide upon the sequence of therapeutic events.

Here, even the slightest mistake can be costly, as life itself may be at stake. Such deleterious mistakes can be minimized by involving relevant disciplines from the very start, even if not all of them will ultimately be required to carry out the actual therapeutic procedures.

12.3 Tumor Types and Basics of Staging

STS of the young are anything but a single disease, quite to the contrary. Multiple different histotypes [4] as well as various tumor stages require exquisite expertise of the treating multi-disciplinary team. STS are clinically divided into rhabdomyosarcomas (RMS), non-rhabdomyosarcoma STS (NRSTS), and rare tumors. Many entities may vary histologically between benign-intermediate and malignant. Certain NRSTS are called "adult type sarcoma" and different approaches are being used to unify treatments [2]. However, new molecular markers constantly define new entities and new systemic approaches are available. Innovative risk

H. Özger et al. (eds.), *Diagnosis and Treatment of Soft Tissue Tumors*, https://doi.org/10.1007/978-3-031-77061-6_12

stratification systems taking into account molecular markers are undoubtedly going to be established in the future.

Tumor-stage is commonly determined taking into account the patient's age and the tumor's histology, size, and resectability. In all classification systems, primary metastases, be they to lymph nodes or, even more so, to distant sites, define high-risk cohorts. The higher the tumor stage, the more urgent the requirement for systemic therapies in addition to surgery and/or radiotherapy. Nowadays, gene-fusion status and molecular markers need to be integrated into the risk stratification system. For instance, PAX-FOXO positive RMS seems more aggressive than fusion negative RMS and requires different treatment strategies. It should be self-evident that the diagnosis of a germ-cell tumor with STS elements should always be excluded, particularly if tumors affect the gonads.

12.4 Sequence of Therapeutic Procedures

After imaging according to the respective guidelines [5], biopsy is the next important step. Reference pathology of any suspected STS and its molecular analysis [6] are mandatory. Not all STS are sensitive to chemotherapy. For certain entities, treatment with innovative agents may be available. Therefore, all patients need to be treated in expert centers [7].

If preoperative systemic treatment is indicated, the sequence of therapeutic measures has to be discussed between all disciplines potentially involved in the local treatment and the responsible oncologist. Radiotherapy may be administered preoperatively, instead of surgery, or thereafter, depending on the tumor entity, the tumor location, the tumor size and certain protocols. Primary surgery is generally only indicated when a microscopically complete resection is feasible without relevant functional or cosmetic mutilation. Otherwise, in selected tumor types, a trial period of preoperative chemotherapy might be initiated.

12.5 STS-Types Observed in the Young

12.5.1 Rhabdomyosarcoma

12.5.1.1 Rhabdomyosarcoma Basics

Europe's interdisciplinary disease experts have recently agreed upon uniform imaging guidelines for RMS of the young [5]. The determination of the extent of local and systemic disease should follow these guidelines, as should imaging during follow-up.

Rhabdomyosarcoma is the most frequent subtype among pediatric soft-tissue sarcomas [8]. It has become a paradigm for the benefits of chemotherapy in selected tumor types. In the past, RMS was classified into alveolar or embryonal RMS based upon histology. Nowadays, the RMS-fusion status important: PAX3/7-FOXO defines the alveolar subtype. However, also here differences in outcome are well known. Of note, many novel gene fusions have been identified up to date. Hence, the so-called fusion negative RMS might in reality carry some very aggressive mutational abnormalities such as the MYOD1-fusion or others.

Rhabdomyosarcoma might be associated with certain tumor-predisposition syndromes. This involves the Li-Fraumeni syndrome in particular. The Costello-, Rubinstein-Taybi-, or DICER1- syndromes, just to name a few of many, may also be involved [9]. Genetic testing should therefore be offered to individuals affected by RMS [10, 11].

12.5.1.2 Treatment of RMS

Local therapy of rhabdomyosarcoma may incorporate surgery, radiotherapy, or both. Modern systemic treatment protocols continue to vary the intensity of systemic treatment according to certain risk factors such as the PAX-FOXO fusion status [12, 13]. Widely used active agents include vincristine, actinomycin D, and alkylators (cyclophosphamide or ifosfamide). The role of anthracyclines still remains to be defined. This is one of the main goals of the current European multi-national FaR-RMS study (EudraCT 2018-000515-24). It has become evident that maintenance therapy with low-dose chemotherapy is capable of further improving the prognosis after intensive chemotherapy is terminated [14, 15]. Maintenance chemotherapy is therefore the current standard for high-risk rhabdomyosarcoma.

The prognosis of multi-modally treated RMS is actually rather favorable with well over three-quarters of affected young individuals being cured [16, 17]. Certain molecularly defined subgroups might indeed need very little systemic treatment, as affected patients seem to carry a particularly favorable prognosis [18]. Therapeutic intensifications by additional agents as well as innovative drugs are being studied for others. The reader is referred to recent reviews for details [8, 19].

12.6 Certain NRSTS-Subtypes

12.6.1 Synovial Sarcoma (SyS)

Pediatric SyS mainly affects adolescents and then the extremities but may occur at any age and at any site. It usually carries the t(X;18) translocation of the ssx1, ssx2, or ssx4 genes on chromosome Xp11 and the syt-gene on chromosome 18q11 [20, 21].

For many years, a clear therapeutic distinction was made between SyS-patients being cared for in pediatric or adult institutions. Here, they received all-out systemic therapy based on rhabdomyosarcoma principles. There, patients received no systemic treatment at all, only local therapeutic measures were used. In recent years, the two treatment philosophies have begun to merge: Pediatricians have realized that some SyS patients, particularly those with small, localized tumors located in favorable sites, might be treated by local therapy alone [22]. Medical oncologists, on the other hand, have acknowledged that chemotherapy might benefit patients with higher-stage primaries. If receiving systemic therapy, affected patients are often treated with the same drugs as would be those with rhabdomyosarcoma [20, 21, 23].

SyS patients are at risk for very late recurrences. Tumor-directed follow-up must therefore be for years or, even better, decades.

12.6.2 Extraosseous Ewing Sarcoma (EES)

These malignancies are classified molecularly: They carry a translocation of a member of the TET-family (EWSR1, FUS) with a member of the ETS family (FLI1, ERG, ETV1, ETV4, FEV) [24]. Tumors characterized as peripheral primitive neuroectodermal tumors (pPNET) belong to the same family of malignancies genetically.

Important messages were learned from Ewing sarcomas arising in osseous sites, one of the most frequent bone tumors of the young: The tumor is chemosensitive, and its prognosis is fatal without chemotherapy. Its prognosis is far better when chemotherapy is part of the therapeutic armamentarium. Systemic chemotherapy should therefore always be administered [24]. The current, well-tested standard regimen in both Europe and North America is the dose-intensified VDC/IE protocol of vincristine, doxorubicin, and cyclophosphamide alternating with high doses of ifosfamide and etoposide [25, 26].

Ewing sarcomas of soft tissues, less frequent but equally malignant, should also receive appropriate systemic therapies. Its prognosis seems to be somewhat more favorable than with its osseous counterparts. Within CWS, such patients were treated with a somewhat less intensive chemotherapy regimen than common with osseous primaries but achieved very similar outcomes [27]. Therefore, the use of full-intensity Ewing chemotherapy has been questioned by some. The administration of multi-agent chemotherapy as such is out of the question.

Ewing sarcomas of the skin are extremely rare but may form a therapeutic and prognostic particularity. If such a tumor remains confined to the skin's upper layers, the exact role and composition of chemotherapy may be debated [28, 29].

Formerly deemed Ewing sarcomas on morphological grounds, several tumor types have recently been delineated from these as carrying distinct genetic alterations. These include sarcomas with BCOR or CIC rearrangements. Information about the best therapeutic approaches are limited [30, 31]. Within Europe, these STS are mostly treated according to NRSTS guidelines. New international protocols for these rare entities are required.

12.6.3 Undifferentiated Pleomorphic Sarcoma (UDS)

Sometimes, an STS is so poorly differentiated that it is impossible to define its histogenicity. Like any STS, these tumors express vimentin. The expression of other antigens remains inconclusive. The diagnosis of UDS is generally made by ruling out any other, identifiable sarcoma subtype. Treatment of pediatric UDS patients generally reflects rhabdomyosarcoma principles, including the use of adjuvant chemotherapy in all cases [32].

12.6.4 Desmoplastic Small Round Cell Tumor (DSRCT)

DSRCT is a very aggressive tumor with frequent metastases and an extremely poor prognosis [2, 33]. It mainly affects the abdomen or trunk of teenagers and is characterized by recurrent EWSR and WT1 fusions [3]. Local therapy may only be made feasible by adjuvant measures such as heated intraperitoneal chemoperfusion (HIPEC) [33]. While no systemic regimen has been proven more effective than others, there is a general consensus that very intensive combination chemotherapy in combination with aggressive local therapies is indicated if a cure is to be attempted [2, 3, 34].

12.6.5 Malignant Peripheral Nerve Sheet Tumor (MPNST)

Neurofibromatosis type 1 brings with it an increased risk of developing such tumors, also known as malignant Schwannoma [35]. Chemotherapy is notoriously ineffective. The tyrosine-kinase inhibitor selumetinib is active in the precursor lesion, plexiform neurofibroma [36]. This drug may also prove to be active in MPNST, but appropriate trials are lacking.

12.6.6 Malignant Rhabdoid Tumor (MRT)

MRT (also known as AT/RT (atypical teratoid/rhabdoid tumor) if arising in the brain) typically arises in early life [37]. The tumor may even present before or at birth. Genetically, it is characterized by mutations in the SMARCB1 or, rarely, SMARCA4 genes. Patients afflicted by this rare cancer should be collected in collaborative, preferentially international, disease-specific registries [38].

MRT is a highly aggressive tumor. It was long believed largely refractory to medical therapies. Recent results have, however, demonstrated that this tumor is clearly a candidate for intensive, multi-agent chemotherapy [39]. Vincristine, doxorubicin, cyclophosphamide, ifosfamide, and etoposide have been suggested as active [2]. With such systemic therapies and effective local measures, some 40–50% of affected patients may survive for at least 2 years.

12.6.7 Infantile Fibrosarcoma (IFS)

Infantile fibrosarcoma is a rare tumor of newborns and infants. Tumor growth may become apparent even before birth. Very importantly, it always carries one of several varying fusions involving the NTRK genes [40].

Surgical removal is the treatment of choice if the tumor is very small and resectable with microscopically complete margins causing no functional deficiencies. Patients may, however, be endangered by life-threatening symptoms of local tumor extension. In such situations, effective systemic treatments are direly required. Chemotherapy (vincristine/actinomycin D or vincristine/actinomycin D/cyclophosphamide) is the standard of care. In the case of progressive disease, metastatic disease, or local disease extension, treatment with the targeted tyrosine-kinase blocker larotrectinib is clearly indicated [41–43].

Some patients with IFS seem to be cured by larotrectinib alone. Weaning of the drug may hence be considered after a year or more of therapy. If the tumor recurs during such a weaning period, retreatment will often again be efficacious.

12.6.8 Alveolar Soft-Part Sarcoma (ASPS)

Similar by name only, this tumor is actually quite distinct from alveolar rhabdomyosarcoma. [3, 44]. Resection is the treatment of choice. Conventional chemotherapy is definitely not effective. Therapy with innovative agents such as the tyrosine-kinase inhibitors sunitinib, cediranib, or pazopanib seems much more promising [2, 45].

12.6.9 Clear Cell Sarcoma (CCS)

CCS is located in the tendons or aponeurotic tissues. It is rare in young patients. This is an aggressive tumor in which conventional chemotherapy is largely ineffective. Immunotherapy with checkpoint inhibitors might be a reasonable choice. Studies to better delineate their efficacy are underway [2].

12.6.10 Dermatofibrosarcoma Protuberans (DFSP)

DFSP, usually a low-grade malignancy, is most often characterized by COL1A1:PDGFB-translocations (NOUJAIM 2015). Resection with wide margins is the treatment of choice. Resection with functional deficiencies should be avoided. Treatment with a tyrosine-kinase inhibitor, e.g. imatinib, is the treatment of choice in locally challenging cases [46, 47].

12.7 Selected Rare Tumors

12.7.1 Pleuropulmonary Blastoma (PPB)

PPB is a rare pulmonary sarcoma of infancy and early childhood. It carries a significant risk of systemic spread. This is usually to the brain, liver, bone, or other organs. Approximately 40% of these tumors have a genetic basis, mostly the DICER1-syndrome. This syndrome also leads to an increased risk for other specific tumor types like medulloblastoma or thyroid cancer [48]. Patients and their young siblings should be enrolled in adequate surveillance protocols [49].

Adjuvant chemotherapy is often indicated. It is guided by local and systemic tumor extension. If chemotherapy is thus used, the chosen multi-drug regimen is based on rhabdomyosarcoma-protocols including anthracyclines. The probability of cure of adequately treated individuals is excellent in lower-stage tumors. Only around half of affected patients with higher-stage lesions survive despite adequate therapies [50–52].

12.7.2 Desmoid Type-Fibromatosis (DTF)

Desmoids, musculo-aponeurotic, fibroblastic, locally aggressive tumors of borderline malignancy, may occur sporadically or given the background of familial adenomatous polyposis. Even though not considered metastasizing, this tumor may become disabling or life-threatening due to local progression. It may, however, also remain stable without treatment. After initial imaging using magnetic-resonance imaging, the first approach is therefore a watch-and-wait strategy [2, 53]. Mutilating resection is very clearly not indicated without such a trial of observation.

The standard treatment of DTF is low-dose methotrexate and vinblastine [54, 55]. Response to therapy may require 6–12 months, so that significant patience may be required. In pediatric patients, no data on treatment with innovative agents is available so far. However, tyrosine-kinase inhibitors might well turn out to be an option [56].

12.7.3 Inflammatory Myofibroblastic Tumor (IMT)

IMT is a mesenchymal tumor of intermediate malignancy. It mainly arises in the lungs or abdomen of children or adolescents [57]. Genetically, it is characterized by fusions of the ALK gene with various partners or fusions involving the ROS1, PDGFRβ, RET, or NTRK genes [58]. Low-dose chemotherapy used against desmoid fibromatosis may be considered. In recent years, treatment with targeted tyrosine-kinase inhibitors has been gaining importance and is now considered common practice. The optimal approach to any individual tumor is the focus of current investigations [57].

12.8 Follow-Up After Intensive Treatment

All patients require disease-related follow-up as well as evaluations for late effects (of local and systemic therapies). European guidelines describing the latter are available for orientation [59, 60].

Appropriate disease-related follow-up varies considerably by histology, site, and stage of the tumor and other factors. Some STS histologies show a propensity for recurrences at uncommon sites, for instance, mammary or brain metastases in alveolar rhabdomyosarcoma. These risks need to be accounted for by individualized, evidence-based follow-up plans. Most STS histotypes do not recur later than 5 years after diagnosis, so the search for recurrences should be particularly frequent and intensive during this period. The possibility of late recurrences can, however, not be excluded. Alveolar soft-part sarcoma, synovial sarcoma, mesenchymal chondrosarcoma, and some others show a particular risk to recur late.

Modern chemotherapy can be exquisitly effective, even life-saving. On the downside, nothing comes without its cost, and that is clearly not only financial. Side effects of systemic therapy may be acute, like neutropenic fever, they may be late or very late, like anthracycline cardiotoxicity. They may affect many or even all patients, they may be uncommon. They may be temporarily or even permanently disabling. Secondary malignancies may arise in some patients, be they therapy-related, like osteosarcomas after radiotherapy or acute non-lymphocytic leukemia following chemotherapy, or related to genetic tumor-predisposition, particularly in the Li-Fraumeni syndrome [11]. All of these side effects require long-term, optimally life-long, qualified surveillance and treatment.

12.9 Systemic Treatment Options in Case of Progressive or Relapsed Soft-Tissue Sarcomas

First-line therapy has to be structured in a way that chances for cure are not carelessly endangered. Even if potentially curative therapeutic approaches are meticulously followed, however, the risk of recurrence is omnipresent. Progressive or relapsed soft-tissue sarcomas may affect the local site, be systemic, or be combined. The prognosis of such recurrences is generally much worse than the outlook was in the primary situation and the role of systemic chemotherapies has been far less well defined.

Inadequate local surgical or radiotherapeutic procedures may lead to locoregional recurrences. As a general rule, such locoregional failures cannot be salvaged by systemic second-line therapies. It is the surgeon and radiotherapist who must strive to avoid such locoregional mishaps in the first place.

The role of systemic therapies for systemic failures is actually quite limited. Patients in whom such therapies were indicated but not administered in the first line should, of course, receive them in case of recurrence. The decision of whether to again administer systemic therapies in patients who have already received such treatments at initial tumor presentation is unfortunately much more complex. Embryonal rhabdomyosarcoma may be an exception: These very chemosensitive tumors are often only treated with limited intensity at initial presentation, as their prognosis with such limited therapies can actually be quite favorable. In the unfortunate case of recurrence, an all-out systemic approach, now for instance including anthracyclines, seems mandatory. Cure may then still be a definitive possibility. Such cure, however, is - unfortunately - highly unlikely in recurrent synovial sarcoma or recurrent extraosseous Ewing sarcoma. Here, second-line chemotherapy may assist in delaying relentless tumor progression and hence prolonging the lifespan. The same may hold true for a variety of other, often less chemosensitive recurrent soft-tissue sarcomas.

In some well-defined tumor entities, novel approaches with immunologic or other innovative agents seems promising. Depending on the specific morphologically and molecularly defined tumor entity, second-line experimental systemic treatment, preferably within a phase II/III study, may thus be recommended. Local treatment, of course, will also depend on the specific disease entity and also on its location within the body. Any decision about whether treatment within a trial of an innovative agent should be attempted always requires a very focused discussion within the multi-disciplinary tumor board and, not less importantly, an informed decision-making process of the affected patient and her or his family.

12.10 Outlook into the Future

The overview above describes chemotherapy indications for STS-entities which were mainly defined on a purely morphological basis. The classification systems, mostly based upon only these aspects, are currently experiencing a true revolution. More and more, molecular characteristics are being introduced and might even replace morphology. Tumors that were formerly grouped together in classification systems that were based on morphological characteristics may then fall into completely new and distinct molecular groups. On the other hand, some tumors that might have been considered distinct entities are suddenly found to share the same genetic basis. It would be beyond the scope of this chapter to detail current studies and future prospects. The interested reader is pointed to recent papers describing these no less than revolutionary discoveries and developments [61, 62].

12.11 Conclusion

Soft-tissue sarcomas of the young may affect all parts of the body. They come in different histologies and molecular subtypes as well as in different shapes and sizes. These tumors are bound to present any treating team with truly multiple challenges. Systemic treatment is an essential part of therapy in a more or less well-defined subset of affected patients. The complexities of the disease require care by an experienced interdisciplinary team. Treatment should not be started before all involved disciplines have had their say about the kind and order of diagnostic and therapeutic events. With appropriate care, many affected young individuals may become long-term, disease-free survivors. Even those, however, will still live with their own, specific challenges and require life-long follow-up by experts.

Further progress is likely to require close collaboration within interdisciplinary and multi-institutional networks. Such collaborations are ongoing on the national, international, and even global levels. They may result in further progress in the fight against these challenging malignancies.

References

1. Hoshi M, Oebisu N, Iwai T, et al. Review of the referral documents of patients with malignant soft tissue tumors. Sci Rep. 2022;12:19527. https://doi.org/10.1038/s41598-022-24158-w.
2. Ferrari A, Spunt SL, Sparber-Sauer M, et al. Cotroversies and challenges in the management of paediatric non-rhabdomyosarcoma soft tissue sarcomas. Lancet Child Adolesc Health. 2022;6(4):221–3. https://doi.org/10.1016/S2352-4642(22)00036-0.
3. Ferrari A, Brennan B, Casanova M, et al. Pediatric Non-rhabdomyosarcoma soft tissue sarcomas: standard of care and treatment recommendations from the European Paediatric Soft Tissue Sarcoma Study Group (EpSSG). Cancer Manag Res. 2022;14:2885–902. https://doi.org/10.2147/CMAR.S368381.
4. WHO Classification of Tumours Editorial Board. Soft tissue and bone tumours, WHO Classification of Tumours, vol. 3. 5th ed. Lyon: International Agency for Research on Cancer; 2020.
5. van Ewijk R, Schoot RA, Sparber-Sauer M, et al. European guideline for imaging in paediatric and adolescent rhabdomyosarcoma – joint statement by the European Paediatric Soft Tissue Sarcoma Study Group, the Cooperative Weichteilsarkom Studiengruppe and the Oncology Task Force of the European Society of Paediatric Radiology. Pediatr Radiol. 2021 Sep;51(10):1940–51. https://doi.org/10.1007/s00247-021-05081-0.
6. Hettmer S, Linardic CM, Kelsey A, et al. Molecular testing of rhabdomyosarcoma in clinical trials to improve risk stratification and outcome: a consensus view from European Paediatric Soft Tissue Sarcoma Study Group, Children's Oncology Group and Cooperative Weichteilsarkom-Studiengruppe. Eur J Cancer. 2022;172:367–86. https://doi.org/10.1016/j.ejca.2022.05.036.
7. Collignon C, Carton M, Brisse HJ, et al. Soft tissue sarcoma in children, adolescents and young adults: outcomes according to compliance with international initial care guidelines. Eur J Surg Oncol. 2020;46(7):1277–86. https://doi.org/10.1016/j.ejso.2019.11.518.
8. Skapek SX, Ferrari A, Gupta A, et al. Rhabdomyosarcoma. Nat Rev Dis Primers. 2019;5(1):1. https://doi.org/10.1038/s41572-018-0051-2.
9. Martin-Giacalone BA, Weinstein PA, et al. Pediatric rhabdomyosarcoma: epidemiology and genetic susceptibility. J Clin Med. 2021;10(9):2028. https://doi.org/10.3390/jcm10092028.
10. Kratz CP, Villani A, Nichols KE, et al. Cancer surveillance for individuals with Li-Fraumeni syndrome. Eur J Hum Genet. 2020;28(11):1481–2. https://doi.org/10.1038/s41431-020-00709-5.
11. Li H, Sisoudiya SD, Martin-Giacalone BA, et al. Germline cancer predisposition variants in pediatric rhabdomyosarcoma: a report from the Children's Oncology Group. J Natl Cancer Inst. 2021;113(7):875–83. https://doi.org/10.1093/jnci/djaa204.
12. Chen C, Dorado Garcia H, Scheer M, et al. Current and future treatment strategies for rhabdomyosarcoma. Front Oncol. 2019;9:1458. https://doi.org/10.3389/fonc.2019.01458.
13. Gartrell J, Pappo A. Recent advances in understanding and managing pediatric rhabdomyosarcoma. F1000Res. 2020;9:F1000 Faculty Rev-685. https://doi.org/10.12688/f1000research.22451.1.
14. Klingebiel T, Boos J, Beske F, et al. Treatment of children with metastatic soft tissue sarcoma with oral maintenance compared to high dose chemotherapy: report of the HD CWS-96 trial. Pediatr Blood Cancer. 2008;50(4):739–45. https://doi.org/10.1002/pbc.21494.
15. Bisogno G, De Salvo GL, Bergeron C, et al. Vinorelbine and continuous low-dose cyclophosphamide as maintenance chemotherapy in patients with high-risk rhabdomyosarcoma (RMS 2005): a multicentre, open-label, randomised, phase 3 trial. Lancet Oncol. 2019;20(11):1566–75. https://doi.org/10.1016/S1470-2045(19)30617-5.
16. Oberlin O, Rey A, Brown KLB, et al. Prognostic factors for outcome in localized extremity rhabdomyosarcoma. Pooled analysis from four international cooperative groups. Pediatr Blood Cancer. 2015;62(12):2125–31. https://doi.org/10.1002/pbc.25684.
17. McEvoy MT, Siegel DA, Dai S, et al. Pediatric rhabdomyosarcoma incidence and survival in the United States: an assessment of 5656 cases, 2001–2017. Cancer Med. 2023;12(3):3644–56. https://doi.org/10.1002/cam4.5211.
18. Whittle S, Venkatramani R, Schönstein A, et al. Congenital spindle cell rhabdomyosarcoma: an international cooperative analysis. Eur J Cancer. 2022;168:56–64. https://doi.org/10.1016/j.ejca.2022.03.022.
19. Ingley KM, Cohen-Gogo S, Gupta AA. Systemic therapy in pediatric-type soft-tissue sarcoma. Curr Oncol. 2020;27(Suppl 1):6–16. https://doi.org/10.3747/co.27.5481.
20. Gazendam AM, Popovic S, Munir S, et al. Synovial sarcoma: a clinical review. Curr Oncol. 2021;28(3):1909–20. https://doi.org/10.3390/curroncol28030177.
21. Venkatramani R, Xue W, Randall RL, et al. Synovial sarcoma in children, adolescents, and young adults: a report from the Children's Oncology Group ARST0332 Study. J Clin Oncol. 2021;39(35):3927–37. https://doi.org/10.1200/JCO.21.01628.
22. Ferrari A, Chi YY, De Salvo GL, et al. Surgery alone is sufficient therapy for children and adolescents with low-risk synovial sarcoma: a joint analysis from the European Paediatric Soft Tissue Sarcoma Study Group and the Children's Oncology Group. Eur J Cancer. 2017;78:1–6. https://doi.org/10.1016/j.ejca.2017.03.003.

23. Scheer M, Vokuhl C, Bauer S, et al. The effect of adjuvant therapies on long-term outcome for primary resected synovial sarcoma in a series of mainly children and adolescents. J Cancer Res Clin Oncol. 2021;147(12):3735–47. https://doi.org/10.1007/s00432-021-03614-6.
24. Grünewald TGP, Cidre-Aranaz F, Surdez D, et al. Ewing sarcoma. Nat Rev Dis Primers. 2018;4(1):5. https://doi.org/10.1038/s41572-018-0003-x.
25. Womer RB, West DC, Krailo MD, et al. Randomized controlled trial of interval-compressed chemotherapy for the treatment of localized Ewing sarcoma: a report from the Children's Oncology Group. J Clin Oncol. 2012;30(33):4148–54. https://doi.org/10.1200/JCO.2011.41.5703.
26. Brennan B, Kirton L, Marec-Bérard P, et al. Comparison of two chemotherapy regimens in patients with newly diagnosed Ewing sarcoma (EE2012): an open-label, randomised, phase 3 trial. Lancet. 2022;400(10362):1513–21. https://doi.org/10.1016/S0140-6736(22)01790-1.
27. Koscielniak E, Sparber-Sauer M, Scheer M, et al. Extraskeletal Ewing sarcoma in children, adolescents, and young adults. An analysis of three prospective studies of the Cooperative Weichteilsarkomstudiengruppe (CWS). Pediatr Blood Cancer. 2021 Oct;68(10):e29145. https://doi.org/10.1002/pbc.29145.
28. Delaplace M, Lhommet C, de Pinieux G, et al. Primary cutaneous Ewing sarcoma: a systematic review focused on treatment and outcome. Br J Dermatol. 2012;166(4):721–6. https://doi.org/10.1111/j.1365-2133.2011.10743.x.
29. Di Giannatale A, Frezza AM, Le Deley MC, et al. Primary cutaneous and subcutaneous Ewing sarcoma. Pediatr Blood Cancer. 2015 Sep;62(9):1555–61. https://doi.org/10.1002/pbc.25535.
30. Lam SW, Silva TM, Bovée JVMG. New molecular entities of soft tissue and bone tumors. Curr Opin Oncol. 2022;34(4):354–61. https://doi.org/10.1097/CCO.0000000000000844.
31. Palmerini E, Gambarotti M, Italiano A, et al. A global collaboRAtive study of CIC-rearranged, BCOR::CCNB3-rearranged and other ultra-rare unclassified undifferentiated small round cell sarcomas (GRACefUl). Eur J Cancer. 2023;183:11–23. https://doi.org/10.1016/j.ejca.2023.01.003.
32. Graves L, Jeck WR, Grilley-Olson JE. A league of its own? Established and emerging therapies in undifferentiated pleomorphic sarcoma. Curr Treat Options Oncol. 2023;24(3):212–28. https://doi.org/10.1007/s11864-023-01054-7.
33. Mello CA, Batista Campos FA, Santos TG, et al. Desmoplastic small round cell tumor: a review of main molecular abnormalities and emerging therapy. Cancers (Basel). 2021;13(3):498. https://doi.org/10.3390/cancers13030498.
34. Scheer M, Vokuhl C, Blank B, et al. Desmoplastic small round cell tumors: multimodality treatment and new risk factors. Cancer Med. 2019 Feb;8(2):527–42. https://doi.org/10.1002/cam4.1940.
35. Hirbe AC, Gutmann DH. Neurofibromatosis type 1: a multidisciplinary approach to care. Lancet Neurol. 2014;13(8):834–43. https://doi.org/10.1016/S1474-4422(14)70063-8.
36. Gross AM, Wolters PL, Dombi E, et al. Selumetinib in children with inoperable plexiform neurofibromas. N Engl J Med. 2020;382(15):1430–42. https://doi.org/10.1056/NEJMoa1912735.
37. Nemes K, Johann PD, Steinbügl M, et al. Infants and newborns with atypical teratoid rhabdoid tumors (ATRT) and extracranial malignant rhabdoid tumors (eMRT) in the EU. Cancers (Basel). 2022;14(9):2185. https://doi.org/10.3390/cancers14092185.
38. Frühwald MC, Nemes K, Boztug H, et al. Current recommendations for clinical surveillance and genetic testing in rhabdoid tumor predisposition: a report from the SIOPE Host Genome Working Group. Fam Cancer. 2021;20(4):305–16. https://doi.org/10.1007/s10689-021-00229-1.
39. Nemes K, Johann PD, Tüchert S, et al. Current and emerging therapeutic approaches for extracranial malignant rhabdoid tumors. Cancer Manag Res. 2022 Feb;9(14):479–98. https://doi.org/10.2147/CMAR.S289544.
40. Lassen U. How I treat NTRK gene fusion-positive cancers. ESMO Open. 2019;4(Suppl 2):e000612. https://doi.org/10.1136/esmoopen-2019-000612.
41. Hong DS, DuBois SG, Kummar S, et al. Larotrectinib in patients with TRK fusion-positive solid tumours: a pooled analysis of three phase 1/2 clinical trials. Lancet Oncol. 2020;21(4):531–40. https://doi.org/10.1016/S1470-2045(19)30856-3.
42. Orbach D, Sparber-Sauer M, Laetsch TW, et al. Spotlight on the treatment of infantile fibrosarcoma in the era of neurotrophic tropomyosin receptor kinase inhibitors: International consensus and remaining controversies. Eur J Cancer. 2020;137:183–92. https://doi.org/10.1016/j.ejca.2020.06.028.
43. Blauel ER, Laetsch TW. The promise of TRK inhibitors in pediatric cancers with NTRK fusions. Cancer Genet. 2022;262–263:71–9. https://doi.org/10.1016/j.cancergen.2022.01.004.
44. Sparber-Sauer M, Seitz G, von Kalle T, et al. Alveolar soft-part sarcoma: primary metastatic disease and metastatic relapse occurring during long-term follow-up: treatment results of four Cooperative Weichteilsarkom Studiengruppe (CWS) trials and one registry. Pediatr Blood Cancer. 2018;65(12):e27405. https://doi.org/10.1002/pbc.27405. Epub 2018 Aug 19.PMID: 30124238.
45. Paoluzzi L, Maki RG. Diagnosis, prognosis, and treatment of alveolar soft-part sarcoma: a review. JAMA Oncol. 2019;5(2):254–60. https://doi.org/10.1001/jamaoncol.2018.4490.
46. Noujaim J, Thway K, Fisher C, et al. Dermatofibrosarcoma protuberans: from translocation to targeted therapy. Cancer Biol Med. 2015;12(4):375–84. https://doi.org/10.7497/j.issn.2095-3941.2015.006.
47. Krewer J, Rolle U, Koscielniak E, et al. Dermatofibrosarcoma protuberans in children and adolescents: primary and relapsed disease-experience of the Cooperative Weichteilsarkomstudiengruppe (CWS). J Surg Oncol. 2020;122(2):263–72. https://doi.org/10.1002/jso.25943.
48. Caroleo AM, De Ioris MA, Boccuto L, et al. DICER1 syndrome and cancer predisposition: from a rare pediatric tumor to lifetime risk. Front Oncol. 2021;10:614541. https://doi.org/10.3389/fonc.2020.614541.
49. Schultz KAP, Stewart DR, Kamihara J, et al. DICER1 tumor predisposition. 2014 Apr 24 [updated 2020 Apr 30]. In: Adam MP, Everman DB, Mirzaa GM, Pagon RA, Wallace SE, LJH B, Gripp KW, Amemiya A, editors. GeneReviews® [Internet]. Seattle (WA): University of Washington, Seattle; 1993–2023.
50. Bisogno G, Sarnacki S, Stachowicz-Stencel T, et al. Pleuropulmonary blastoma in children and adolescents: The EXPeRT/PARTNER diagnostic and therapeutic recommendations. Pediatr Blood Cancer. 2021;68(Suppl 4):e29045. https://doi.org/10.1002/pbc.29045.
51. Sparber-Sauer M, Tagarelli A, Seitz G, et al. Children with progressive and relapsed pleuropulmonary blastoma: a European collaborative analysis. Pediatr Blood Cancer. 2021;68(12):e29268. https://doi.org/10.1002/pbc.29268.
52. Mlika M, Anjum F, El Mezni F. Pleuropulmonary Blastoma. 2022 Jun 19. In: StatPearls [Internet]. Treasure Island: StatPearls Publishing; 2022.
53. Desmoid Tumor Working Group. The management of desmoid tumours: a joint global consensus-based guideline approach for adult and paediatric patients. Eur J Cancer. 2020;127:96–107. https://doi.org/10.1016/j.ejca.2019.11.013.
54. Orbach D, Brennan B, Bisogno G, et al. The EpSSG NRSTS 2005 treatment protocol for desmoid-type fibromatosis in children: an international prospective case series. Lancet Child Adolesc Health. 2017;1(4):284–92. https://doi.org/10.1016/S2352-4642(17)30045-7.

55. Sparber-Sauer M, Seitz G, von Kalle T, et al. Systemic therapy of aggressive fibromatosis in children and adolescents: Report of the Cooperative Weichteilsarkom Studiengruppe (CWS). Pediatr Blood Cancer. 2018 May;65(5):e26943. https://doi.org/10.1002/pbc.26943.
56. Sparber-Sauer M, Orbach D, Navid F, et al. Rationale for the use of tyrosine kinase inhibitors in the treatment of paediatric desmoid-type fibromatosis. Br J Cancer. 2021;124(10):1637–46. https://doi.org/10.1038/s41416-021-01320-1.
57. Gros L, Dei Tos AP, Jones RL, et al. Inflammatory myofibroblastic tumour: state of the art. Cancers (Basel). 2022;14(15):3662. https://doi.org/10.3390/cancers14153662.
58. Lovly CM, Gupta A, Lipson D, et al. Inflammatory Myofibroblastic Tumors harbor multiple potentially actionable kinase fusions. Cancer Discov. 2014;4(8):889–95. https://doi.org/10.1158/2159-8290.CD-14-0377.
59. Hilgendorf I, Bergelt C, Bokemeyer C, et al. Long-term follow-up of children, adolescents, and young adult cancer survivors. Oncol Res Treat. 2021;44(4):184–9. https://doi.org/10.1159/000514381.
60. Gronchi A, Miah AB, Dei Tos AP, et al. Soft tissue and visceral sarcomas: ESMO–EURACAN–GENTURIS Clinical Practice Guidelines for diagnosis, treatment and follow-up. Ann Oncol. 2021;32:1348–65. https://doi.org/10.1016/j.annonc.2021.07.006.
61. Koelsche C, Schrimpf D, Stichel D, et al. Sarcoma classification by DNA methylation profiling. Nat Commun. 2021;12:498. https://doi.org/10.1038/s41467-020-20603-4.
62. Pfister SM, Reyes-Múgica M, Chan JKC, et al. A summary of the inaugural WHO classification of pediatric tumors: transitioning from the optical into the molecular era. Cancer Discov. 2022;12(2):331–55. https://doi.org/10.1158/2159-8290.CD-21-1094.

13 Radiotherapy for Treatment of Adult Soft Tissue Sarcomas

Fulya Yaman Ağaoğlu

Soft tissue sarcomas (STS) are rare malignant mesenchymal tumors, less than 1% among the primary malignant tumors, and can occur in any organ or anatomic location of the body [1]. The STS are localized most frequently in the lower extremity (46.4%), in order of frequency trunk, retroperitoneal, and upper extremity [2]. The majority of extremity STS occur in the muscle groups of the extremities so are confined to the muscle compartment. This knowledge is useful for radiation oncologists for defining the compartments at risk. There are many histological subtypes and there have been different behaviors to treatments. About 65% of STS are high grade and 35% are low-grade. On the contrary, the historic belief of radioresistance of STS, high-grade STS have similar radiosensitivity to epithelial neoplasms [3]. Previous studies reported radiotherapy (RT) efficacy at limb-sparing surgery, especially for extremity STS [4, 5]. Assessment of risk factors for local recurrence is complex and incorporates multiple factors. These factors include surgical margin status, grade, tumor size, localization of the tumor, histopathologic subtype, extension of disease, and treatment modality. The curative treatment for localized STS is surgery with negative margins. Chemotherapy (CT) and RT, administered in adjuvant or neoadjuvant settings, have important roles in the multimodal management of STS. Intermediate or high grade, larger size (> 5 cm) sarcomas may have a high risk of local recurrence and developing metastases. Furthermore, wide local excision with a 5 cm margin in extremity sarcomas is also associated with a local recurrence rate of 20–25% [6–9]. Regarding these factors, the addition of RT (pre or postoperative) to surgery allows excellent local control with functional limb salvage. Surgery has been the main treatment for all STS. Despite wide surgical procedures, local recurrence still could be mortal and other treatment consequences were analyzed. One of the first trials reporting the role of RT at STS in 1981 showed similar results with conservative surgery and postoperative RT [5]. Rosenberg et al. randomized 43 patients to amputation or limb-sparing surgery with adjuvant external RT and both groups received adjuvant chemotherapy (CT) [4]. No differences in disease-free and overall survival at 5 years were observed with this prospective study. Yang et al. trial questioned the role of RT on limb-sparing surgery and showed that adjuvant RT significantly decreases the probability of local recurrence without influencing overall survival rates [10]. However, adjuvant RT efficacy on overall survival at 3 years (73% vs 63%, $p < 0.01$) has been reported in the retrospective study from the SEER database with 6960 patients treated for high-grade extremity STS [11]. To understand the role of RT, trials continue, and ensuing studies also reported RT significance on local control at STS patients with high-grade, large tumors, and close or positive surgical margins [12, 13].

Ultimately, the significant role of adjuvant RT (postoperative or preoperative or during operation) in the treatment of STS has been seen with the randomized clinical trials showing improved local control rates. Local control rates exceeding 85% in patients with extremity sarcomas were achieved with combined therapies. Limb-sparing surgery must be given with adjuvant RT for high-grade or large-size (>5 cm) sarcomas or borderline resectable tumors [10]. Whether an analysis to determine the group at whom RT can be omitted, concluded the similar control rates at patients with small (<5 cm), high grade, and negative margins STS, but even within this favorable group of patients, age and tumor location were determined significantly related with increased local recurrence [14]. So, the successful treatment of STS requires team experience. Before the initiation of therapy, all patients should be evaluated and managed by a multidisciplinary team with expertise and experience in sarcoma [15]. Both the European and North American guidelines suggest combining limb-sparing surgery and RT for high-grade or large extremity soft tissue sarcomas [15, 16].

Albertsmeier et al. reported a meta-analysis in 2018 including 16 studies that adjuvant RT in patients with local-

F. Y. Ağaoğlu (✉)
Department of Radiation Oncology, Acıbadem Atakent Hospital, Istanbul, Türkiye
e-mail: fulya.agaoglu@acibadem.com

H. Özger et al. (eds.), *Diagnosis and Treatment of Soft Tissue Tumors*, https://doi.org/10.1007/978-3-031-77061-6_13

Table 13.1 Preoperative vs. postoperative RT for extremity STS

	Advantages	Disadvantages
Preoperative RT	• Smaller irradiated volume • Resectability rate is higher (pseudo capsulated tumor) • Reduced dose (or time) RT • Lesser rate of late complication	• Postponing surgery • Surgical wound healing problems
Postoperative RT	• True histopathologic and staging evaluation • Less surgical healing problem	• Larger irradiated volume (including all surgical scars) • Necessity of surgical bed clips High late complication rate

ized and resectable STS might have improved overall survival rates [17]. Therefore RT is recommended for patients who have an increased risk of local recurrence after operation with STS of extremity, particularly if close or microscopically positive margins are anticipated or have occurred. Resection margin status is the major factor for predicting local recurrence. If the surgeon is planning safe but close margins, preoperative RT must be given. There is no difference in local control and overall survival in terms of preoperative or postoperative RT, but the acute and late toxicity profiles are observed different with these modalities [18–21]. Although preoperative RT causes higher wound complication rates, postoperative RT causes soft tissue fibrosis-related late effects [22]. So, an increase in rates of preferring pre- over postoperative RT for STS of the extremity especially has just been observed in recent years. In 2020 Yang et al. revealed a meta-analysis comparing local - overall survivals and acute late effects between preoperative and postoperative RT at STS patients [23]. In terms of oncological outcomes, no difference was observed. However, acute effects were seen at higher rates with preoperative RT, in consideration of a limited number of studies reporting adverse effects. The summary of the efficacy of RT practice is shown in Table 13.1.

For localized STS, if an unplanned excision were performed, oncologic tumor bed resection has to be planned for safe margins, and in this situation we know, that preoperative RT is superior to postoperative RT. However, we have to wait for the ongoing studies' results to understand the differences between pre- or postoperative RT schedules.

The role of routine adjuvant CT for localized, resectable STS remains controversial. Although CT is not standard, high-risk patients (high grade, deep localization, >10 cm) may benefit from CT and RT combination before surgery [24]. Especially for recurrent high-grade STS, neoadjuvant treatment decisions must be given with a multidisciplinary team.

13.1 Preoperative (Neoadjuvant) Radiotherapy for Soft Tissue Sarcomas

Preoperative RT, biologically, controls microscopic tumor margins and allows the sparing of critical organs and neurovascular structures. After preoperative RT, tumor shrinkage and pseudocapsulation with fibrotic tissue help the surgeon to achieve clear margins (Fig. 13.1). On the other hand, RT also has a potential reduction of the seeding of sarcoma cells during surgical resection (Fig. 13.2). As the result of all these information, preoperative RT becomes more preferable at specific STS clinics and academic centers.

Preoperative RT can be applied conventionally fractionated as 5–6 weeks in daily fractions of 1.8–2 Gy to a total dose of 50–50.4 Gy. Hypofractionation is treated with higher fraction doses and preferred frequently in recent years with some advantages radiobiologically. Tumors can be defined as radiosensitive or radioresistant according to their α/β rates in the radiobiology discipline and tumors with lower α/β ratios are expected to give more response to higher fraction doses. Recent trials for breast, prostate, and rectum cancer using hypofractionation resulted in similar even better control rates [25–27]. Kilic et al. reported preoperative RT results with a total dose of 28 Gy at a fraction dose of 3.5 Gy, 8 fraction, and in this retrospective trial, similar adverse effects had been observed [28]. Similarly, different regimes of hypofractionation at STS trials were reported in the last 20 years and a recent review by Roohani et al. in 2022 showed similar toxicity rates between conventional and hypofractionated regimes with comparable local control rates [29]. Different schemas for hypofractionation were observed at these trials and compared with normofractinated RT trial results listed in Table 13.2. The analysis resulted in favor of preoperative hypofractionated RT, however, they considered that the trials were retrospective or phase II and treatment had to be decided with attention. STS includes a large histology of tumors and the majority of them have lower α/β ratios. Also due to the shortened time of the treatment, better cost efficiency and logistic situations can be achieved and increased patient compliance with treatment is expected.

Randomized studies were conducted on this preoperative topic and they continue accruing patients. They will give the results of compared schemas of RT and also acute and late effects in the coming years. In a Dutch study, 14 fractions with 3 Gy per fraction schema are being compared with conventional RT schema preoperatively [42]. Mayo Clinic and M.D. Anderson Cancer Center trials compare 15 fractions, 2.85 Gy per fraction schemas with conventional in terms of oncologic results and also the quality of life for the first STS patients [43, 44].

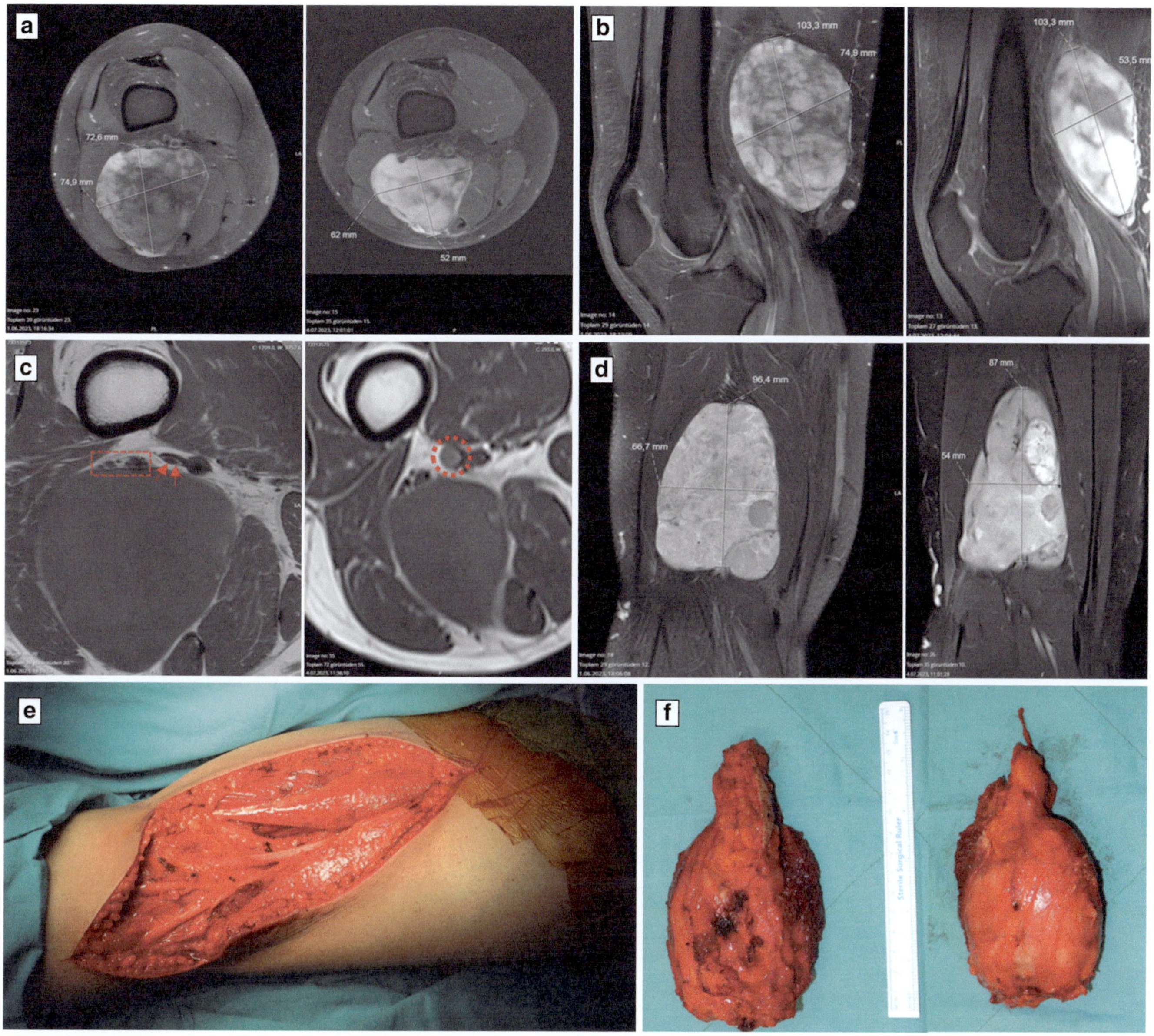

Fig. 13.1 Pre- and postradiotherapy MR images (**a–d**) demonstrate tumor shrinkage following hypofractionated radiotherapy in a deep-seated myxoid liposarcoma of the popliteal region. T1-weighted axial images in figure (**c**) show the tibial and fibular nerves (red-dashed rectangle) as well as popliteal vessels (red arrows show the popliteal vein) compressed by the tumor at presentation and the decompression (red-dashed circle shows the popliteal vein) following radiotherapy. Intraoperative images show the exposed tibial and fibular nerves in the resection site (**e**) and the superficial and deep aspects of the specimen (**f**). The nerves could be dissected from the tumor with marginal margins, as evidenced by the presence of only pseudocapsule on the deep aspect, thanks to preoperative radiotherapy. Popliteal vessels were spared with relative ease. Pathological examination yielded "R0" margins and 90% regressive changes

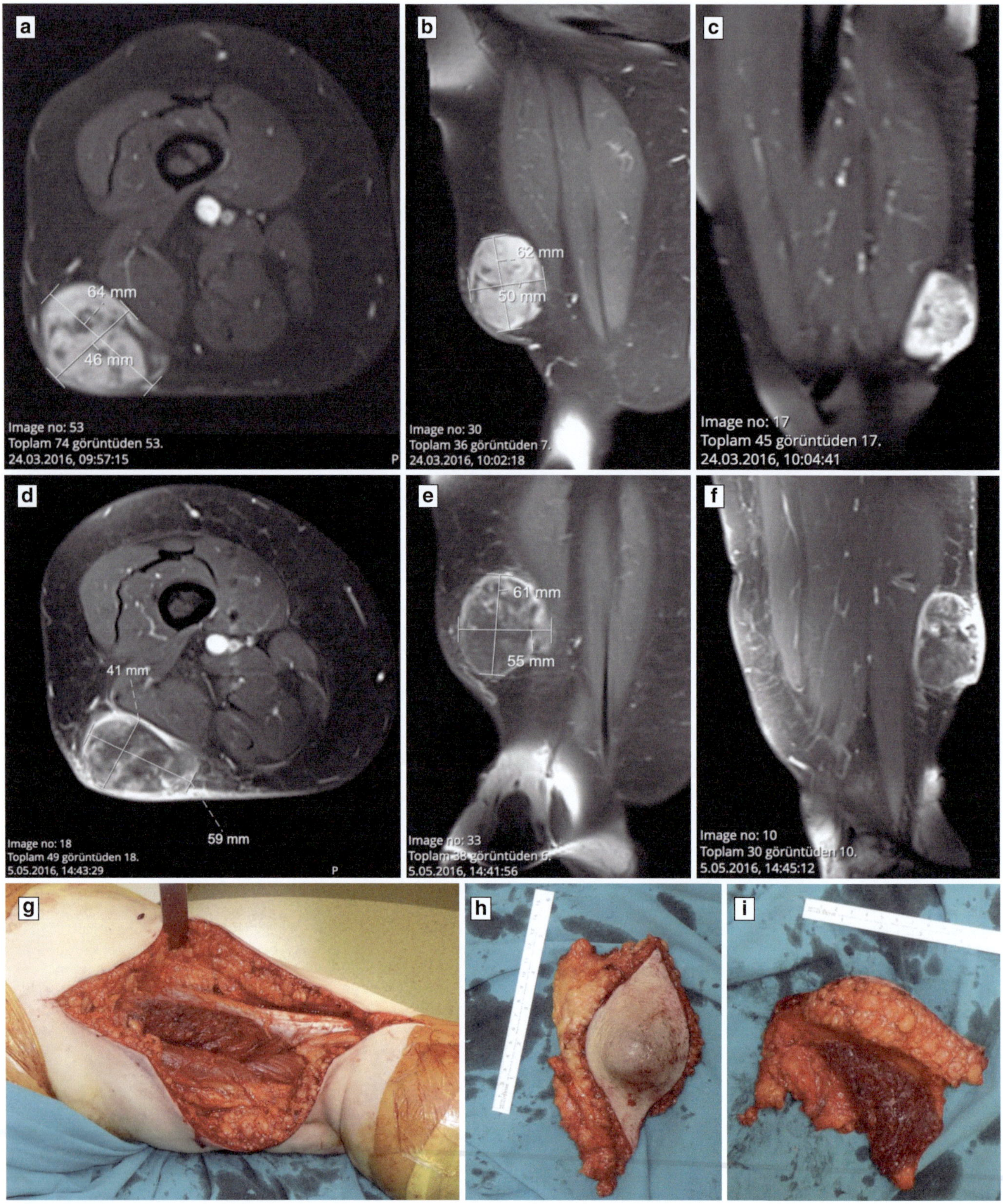

Fig. 13.2 MR images at presentation show a large (>5 cm) superficial high-grade pleomorphic sarcoma (**a**–**c**). While superficial and not adjacent to vital structures, the tumor is mostly surrounded by subcutaneous fat tissue, which is a permeable tumor barrier. Wide excision without causing unnecessary morbidity can be challenging when effective tumor barriers are not present. MR images after preoperative hypofractionated radiotherapy (**d**–f) demonstrate a marked decrease in contrast enhancement despite no decrease in tumor size. Intraoperative images show wide resection including parts of the overlying skin and underlying muscle (**g**–**i**). MR images at postoperative 3 years show no evidence of local disease (**j**–**l**)

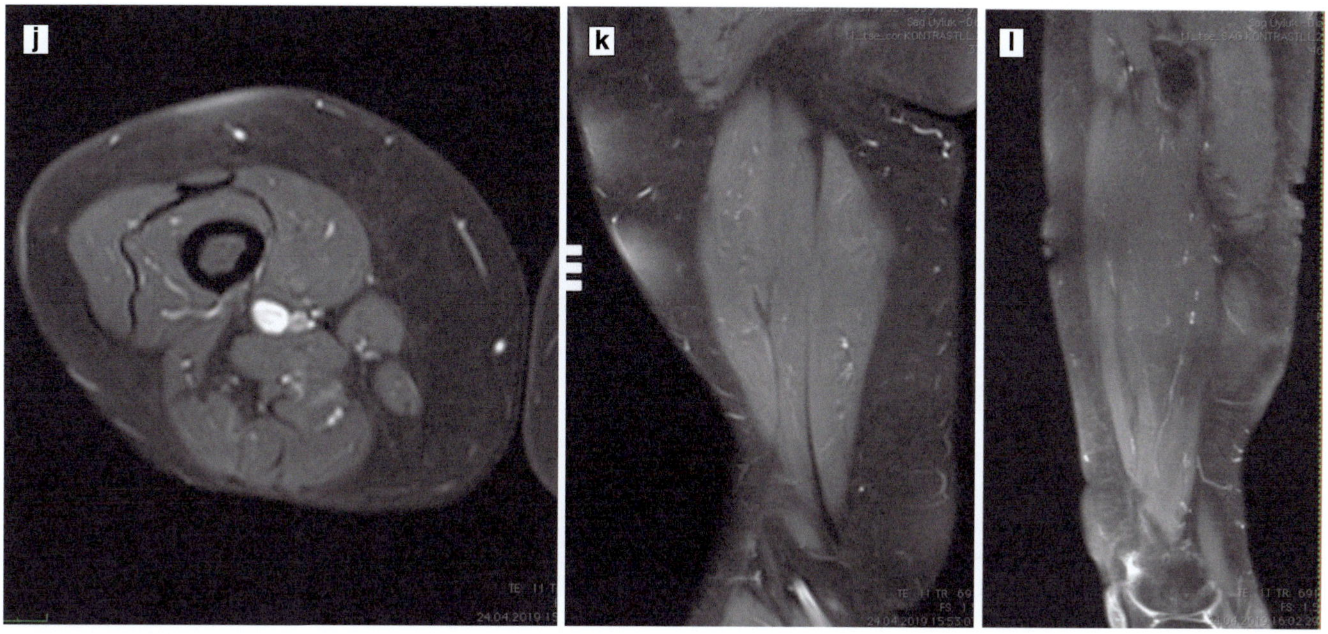

Fig. 13.2 (continued)

Table 13.2 Preoperative trials adapted from a systematic review by Roohani et al. [29] Reproduced under a Creative Commons Attribution 4.0 International License http://creativecommons.org/licenses/by/4.0/ which permits use, sharing, adaptation, distribution and reproduction in any medium or format, as long as you give appropriate credit to the original author(s) and the source, provide a link to the Creative Commons licence, and indicate if changes were made

Trials/year	Patient	Median tm	Fraction	Time to surgery	LRFS	OS
Koseła-Paterczyk et al./2021 [30]	311	10 cm	5 fr × 5 Gy/fr	2–4 days	N/A	63%
Spalek et al./2021 [31]	46	17.4 cm	5 fr × 5 Gy/fr	6–8 weeks	67%	53%
Leite et al./2021 [32]	25	14 cm	5 fr × 8 Gy/fr	8.6 weeks	85%	85%
Potkrajcic et al./2021 [33]	18	7.9 cm	5 fr × 5 Gy/fr	4.1 weeks	N/A	100%
Silva et al./2021 [34]	18	8.9 cm	5 fr × 5 Gy/fr	6 weeks	N/A	95%
Koseła-Paterczyk et al./2020 [35]	27	13 cm	5 fr × 5 Gy/fr	7 weeks	N/A	93%
Kalbasi et al./2020 [36]	50	24% >10 cm	5 fr × 6 Gy/fr	4 weeks	N/A	84%
Parsai et al./2020 [37]	16	43.8% >5 cm	5 fr × 5 Gy/fr, 5 fr × 6 Gy/fr	1 day	N/A	87.5%
Pennington et al./2018 [38]	116	47% >10 cm	8 fr × 3.5 Gy/fr	1–2 weeks	N/A	82%
Kubicek et al./2018 [39]	13	7.6 cm	5 fr × 7 Gy/fr	37 days	N/A	N/A
Kilic et al./2017 [28]	67	9.6 m	8 fr × 3.5 Gy/fr	2–3 weeks	65.7%	90%
Koseła-Paterczyk et al./2017 [40]	32	10.5 cm	53% 5 fr × 5 Gy/fr	3–7 days	N/A	68%
Koseła-Paterczyk et al./ 2014 [41]	272	8.5 cm	5 fr × 5 Gy/fr	3–7 days	N/A	72%

13.2 Postoperative (Adjuvant) Radiotherapy

Postoperative RT is the traditional RT schedule and RT implementation is decided due to final pathological report. The prognostic factors such as real tumor size, margin status, and grade can be determined with this report and adjuvant treatment decisions can be achieved due to evidence-based literature and a multidisciplinary team.

Therefore, the literature consists of many retrospective and randomized trials assessing the role of adjuvant RT, and knowledge of which patients have advantages of postoperative RT or RT and CT can be easier than preoperative concept. Nowadays, low-grade STS usually do not require adjuvant therapies. However, grade is not the only factor determining adjuvant therapies. So, large tumors, close or positive margins must be also evaluated for the decision. These situations are subject to limb-sparing surgeries, but if compartmental resection or amputation is practiced for the patient, adjuvant RT is not indicated for the wide surgical excision.

High or intermediate-grade STS usually occurs with the necessity of adjuvant RT. Both preoperative and postoperative RT are effective and safe for STS. Davis et al. observed similar long-term local and distant control rates between pre and postoperative RT groups in phase III randomized trial with 190 patients and slightly increased rates of late effects including fibrosis in the postoperative group [18, 22].

13.3 Radiation Therapy Techniques

Patients should be positioned to remove treated volume as much as possible as the other part of the body. However, extremity STS are preferred to be settled in the alpha-cradle devices, localization of STS being the major deterministic immobilization (Fig. 13.3).

The studies first investigating the role of RT at STS used conformal techniques some of them brachytherapy (BT) [14]. Treatment planning improved due to technological improvements and intensity-modulated RT (IMRT) or image-guided RT (IGRT) was started to be used in STS planning (Fig. 13.2). Recently, trials showed the advantages of modern techniques on the adverse effects of pre- or postoperative RT due to the ability to protect critical structures [45–47]. All target volumes, gross tumor volume (GTV), clinical target volume (CTV), and planning target volume (PTV), should be defined for the most appreciated planning for the patient. The Radiation Therapy Oncology Group (RTOG) reported a consensus for all these volumes, and these are widely accepted for STS treatment plans [48]. Also, magnetic resonance imaging (MRI) of patients should be used and fused with simulation computed tomography (CT) images.

Preoperative RT

- Conventional RT: 50–50.4 Gy external RT (1.8 Gy or 2 Gy per fraction)
- GTV: Tumor defined at T1-contrast enhanced MRI and delineated with a fusion of MRI and CT images
- CTV: GTV plus 3 cm margin longitudinally and 1.5 cm margin radially and recommendation of including the suspicious edema area at T2-weighted MRI
- PTV: CTV plus 1 cm margin uniformly
- To avoid lymphedema, at least a 1 cm strip of soft tissue in the circumference of the extremity should be spared
- To reduce bone fraction, all circumferential bone radiation should be avoided
- Hypofractionation should be evaluated due to the factors of STS and patient

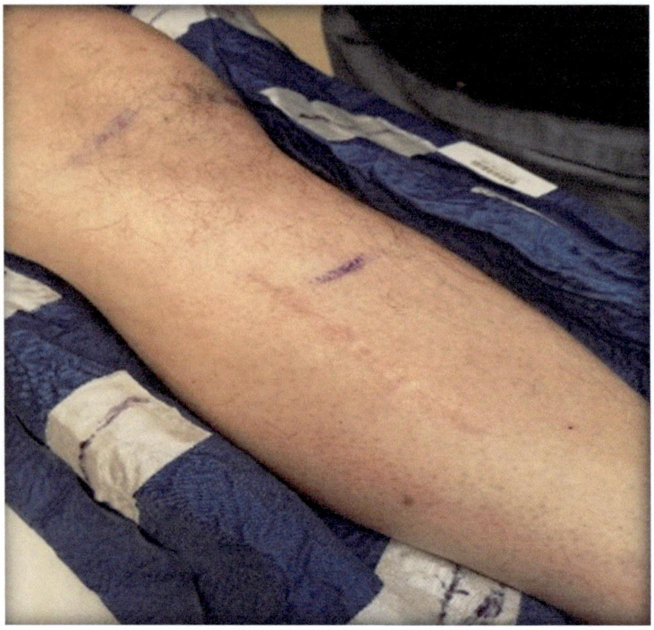

Fig. 13.3 Extremity stabilization with alpha-cradle device during radiotherapy

Postoperative RT

- Conventional RT: 60–66 Gy external RT (1.8 Gy or 2 Gy per fraction); 50 Gy may be followed with a boost dose of 10–16 Gy (due to margin status and grade)
- No GTV, but tumor bed, clips, incision scars, and drain sites should be contoured
- CTV: Tumor bed, including scars and drain sites, plus 1–1.5 cm longitudinally and 1 cm radially
- PTV: CTV plus 1 cm margin uniformly
- To avoid lymphedema, at least a 1 cm strip of soft tissue in the circumference of the extremity should be spared
- To reduce bone fraction, all circumferential bone radiation should be avoided
- Hypofractionation should be evaluated due to the factors of STS and patient (Fig. 13.4)

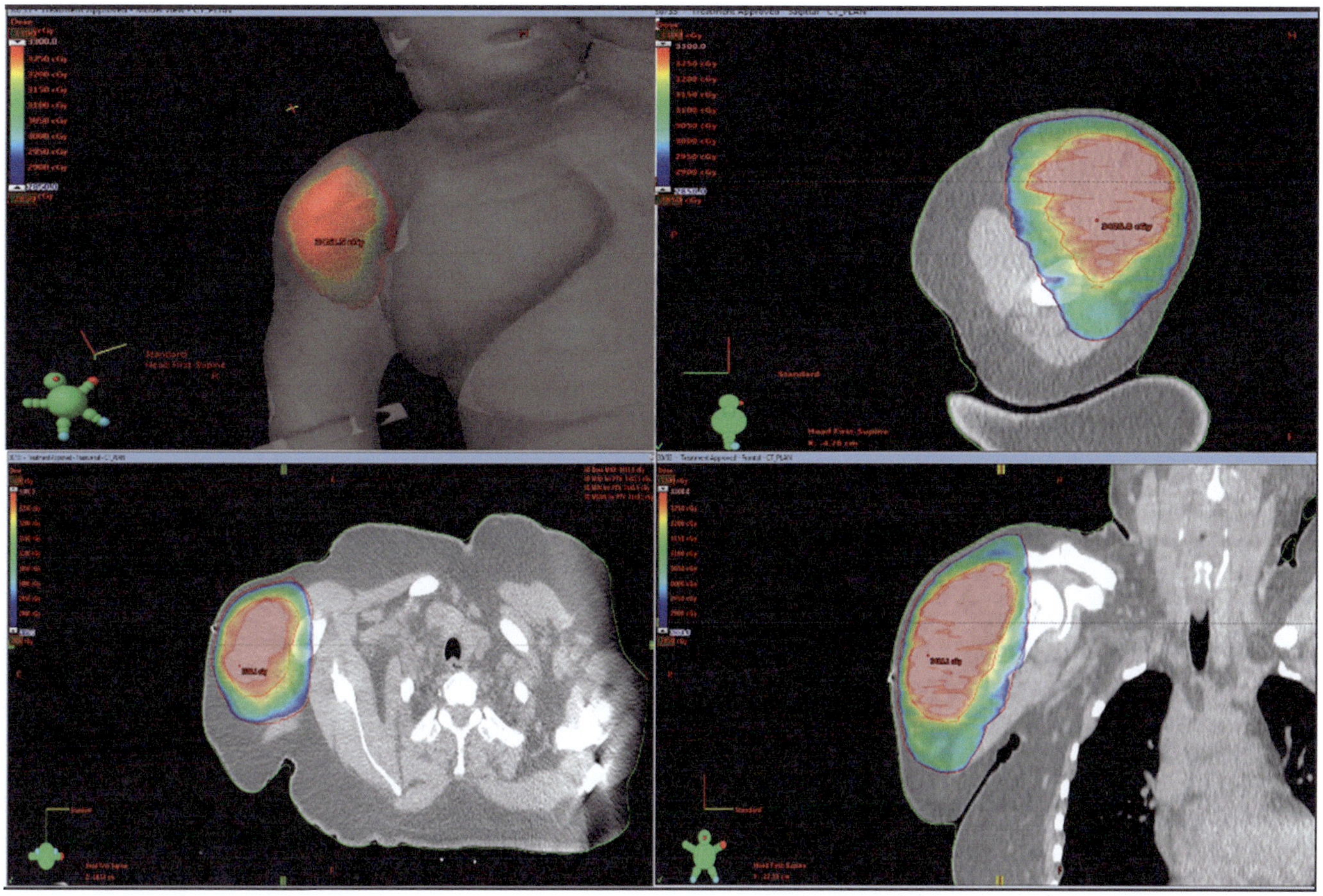

Fig. 13.4 Treatment planning with IMRT in STS of upper extremity demonstrating transverse, coronal, and sagittal CT sections and coverage of doses with color-wash technique

13.4 Conclusion

Surgery alone is limited to a low number of STS patients and RT may be applied in all patients expected to have increased local recurrence. The extent of most surgery can be reduced with the addition of RT as an adjuvant or neoadjuvant. Although studies on RT timing have not been concluded, we know the adverse effects of RT. RT should be applied preoperatively to facilitate limb-sparing surgery in the setting of bulky tumors, for which obtaining clear margins is difficult or impossible due to proximity to or invasion of neurovascular structures or facilitating, with pseudocapsule creation. Surgery time after RT differs in preoperative RT trials, so no optimal time can be determined. Fibrosis in soft tissues may increase the complications during surgery. It is recommended to proceed with surgery before fibrosis develops, which usually occurs after as much time as RT treatment. For adjuvant RT, completion of wound healing is important to start treatment. The recommended schedule to achieve local control is not to exceed 6 weeks postoperatively.

References

1. Lahat G, Lazar A, Lev D. Sarcoma epidemiology and etiology: potential environmental and genetic factors. Surg Clin N Am. 2008;88(3):451–81.
2. Lawrence W, Donegan WL, Natarajan N, et al. Adult soft tissue sarcomas. Ann Surg. 1987;205:349–59.
3. Ruka W, Taghian A, Gloloso D, et al. Comparison between the in vitro intrinsic radiation sensitivity of human soft tissue sarcoma and breast cancer cell lines. J Surg Oncol. 1996;61:290–4.
4. Rosenberg SA, Tepper J, Glatstein E, et al. The treatment of soft-tissue sarcomas of the extremities: prospective randomized evaluations of (1) limb-sparing surgery plus radiation therapy compared with amputation and (2) the role of adjuvant chemotherapy. Ann Surg. 1982;196(3):305–15.
5. Lindberg RD, Martin RG, Romsdahl MM, et al. Conservative surgery and postoperative radiotherapy in 300 adults with soft-tissue sarcomas. Cancer. 1981;47(10):2391–7.
6. Simon MA, Enneking WF. The management of soft-tissue sarcomas of the extremities. J Bone Joint Surg Am. 1976;58(3):317–27.
7. Suit HD, Mankin HJ, Wood WC, et al. Treatment of the patient with stage M0 soft tissue sarcoma. J Clin Oncol. 1988;6(5):854–62.
8. Tran LM, Mark R, Meier R, et al. Sarcomas of the head and neck. Prognostic factors and treatment strategies. Cancer. 1992;70(1):169–77.
9. Freedman AM, Reiman HM, Woods JE. Soft-tissue sarcomas of the head and neck. Am J Surg. 1989;158(4):367–72.

10. Yang JC, Chang AE, Baker AR, et al. Randomized prospective study of the benefit of adjuvant radiation therapy in the treatment of soft tissue sarcomas of the extremity. J Clin Oncol. 1998;16(1):197–203.
11. Koshy M, Rich SE, Mohiuddin MM. Improved survival with radiation therapy in high-grade soft tissue sarcomas of the extremities: a SEER analysis. Int J Radiat Oncol Biol Phys. 2010;77(1):203–9.
12. Toulmonde M, Le Cesne A, Mendiboure J, et al. Long-term recurrence of soft tissue sarcomas: prognostic factors and implications for prolonged follow-up. Cancer. 2014;120(19):3003–6.
13. Liebel SA, Tranbaugh RF, Wara WM, et al. Soft tissue sarcomas of the extremities: survival and patterns of failure with conservative surgery and postoperative irradiation compared to surgery alone. Cancer. 1982;50(6):1076–83.
14. Pisters PW, Harrison LB, Leung DH, et al. Long-term results of a prospective randomized trial of adjuvant brachytherapy in soft tissue sarcoma. J Clin Oncol. 1996;14(3):859–68.
15. The ESMO/European Sarcoma Network Working Group. Soft tissue and visceral sarcomas: ESMO clinical practice guidelines for diagnosis, treatment and follow up. Ann Oncol. 2014;25:102–12.
16. National Comprehensive Cancer Network. Soft tissue sarcoma version 2023.
17. Albertsmeier M, Rauch A, Roeder F, et al. External beam radiation therapy for Resectable soft tissue sarcoma: a systematic review and meta-analysis. Ann Surg Oncol. 2018;25:754–67.
18. O'Sullivan B, Davis AM, Turcotte R, et al. Preoperative versus postoperative radiotherapy in soft-tissue sarcoma of the limbs: a randomized trial. Lancet. 2002;359:2235–41.
19. Zagars GK, Ballo MT, Pisters PW, et al. Preoperative vs. postoperative radiation therapy for soft tissue sarcoma: a retrospective comparative evaluation of disease outcome. Int J Radiat Oncol Biol Phys. 2003;56:482–8.
20. Kuklo TR, Temple HT, Owens BD, et al. Preoperative versus postoperative radiation therapy for soft-tissue sarcomas. Am J Orthop (Belle Mead NJ). 2005;34:75–80.
21. Lazarev S, McGee H, Moshier E, et al. Preoperative vs postoperative radiation therapy in localized soft tissue sarcoma: nationwide patterns of care and trends in utilization. Pract Radiat Oncol. 2017;7:e507–e16.
22. Davis AM, O'Sullivan B, Turcotte R, et al. Late radiation morbidity following randomization to preoperative versus postoperative radiotherapy in extremity soft tissue sarcoma. Radither Oncol. 2005;75:48–3.
23. Yang X, Zhang L, Yang X, et al. Oncologic outcomes of pre- versus post-operative radiation in resectable soft-tissue sarcoma: a systematic review and meta-analysis. Radiat Oncol. 2020;15:158–65.
24. Anonymous. Adjuvant chemotherapy for localized resectable soft tissue sarcoma of adults: meta-analysis of individual data. Sarcoma Meta-analysis Collaboration. Lancet. 1997;350(9092):1647–54.
25. Whelan TJ, Pignol J-P, Levine MN, et al. Long-term results of hypofractionated radiation therapy for breast cancer. N Engl J Med. 2010;362(6):513–20.
26. Widmark A, Gunnlaugsson A, Beckman L, et al. Ultra-hypofractionated versus conventionally fractionated radiotherapy for prostate cancer: 5-year outcomes of the HYPO-RT-PC randomised, non-inferiority, phase 3 trial. Lancet. 2019;394(10196):385–95.
27. Haviland JS, Owen JR, Dewar JA, et al. The UK Standardisation of Breast Radiotherapy (START) trials of radiotherapy hypofractionation for treatment of early breast cancer: 10-year follow-up results of two randomised controlled trials. Lancet Oncol. 2013;14(11):1086–94.
28. Kılıç L, Ekenel M, Karabulut S, et al. Neoadjuvant sequential chemoradiotherapy versus radiotherapy alone for treatment of high-risk extremity soft tissue sarcoma: a single-institution experience. Contemp Oncol (Pozn). 2017;21(1):60–5.
29. Roohani S, Ehret F, Kobus M, et al. Preoperative hypofractionated radiotherapy for soft tissue sarcomas: a systematic review. Radiat Oncol. 2022;17:159–78.
30. Koseła-Paterczyk H, Teterycz P, Spałek MJ, et al. Efficacy and safety of hypofractionated preoperative radiotherapy for primary locally advanced soft tissue sarcomas of limbs or trunk wall. Cancers (Basel). 2021;13(12):2981.
31. Spałek MJ, Koseła-Paterczyk H, Borkowska A, et al. Combined preoperative hypofractionated radiotherapy with doxorubicin-ifosfamide chemotherapy in marginally resectable soft tissue sarcomas: results of a phase 2 clinical trial. Int J Radiat Oncol Biol Phys. 2021;110(4):1053–63.
32. Leite ETT, Munhoz RR, Camargo VP, et al. Neoadjuvant stereotactic ablative radiotherapy (SABR) for soft tissue sarcomas of the extremities. Radiother Oncol. 2021;161:222–9.
33. Potkrajcic V, Traub F, Hermes B, et al. Hypofractionated preoperative radiotherapy for high-risk soft tissue sarcomas in a geriatric patient population. Radiol Oncol. 2021;55(4):459–66.
34. Gobo Silva ML, Lopes de Mello CA, Aguiar Junior S, et al. Neoadjuvant hypofractionated radiotherapy and chemotherapy for extremity soft tissue sarcomas: safety, feasibility, and early oncologic outcomes of a phase 2 trial. Radiother Oncol. 2021;159:161–7.
35. Koseła-Paterczyk H, Spałek M, Borkowska A, et al. Hypofractionated radiotherapy in locally advanced myxoid liposarcomas of extremities or trunk wall: results of a single-arm prospective clinical trial. J Clin Med. 2020;9(8):2471.
36. Kalbasi A, Kamrava M, Chu FI, Telesca D, Van Dams R, Yang Y, et al. A phase II trial of 5-day neoadjuvant radiotherapy for patients with high-risk primary soft tissue sarcoma. Clin Cancer Res. 2020;26(8):1829–36.
37. Parsai S, Lawrenz J, Kilpatrick S, et al. Early outcomes of preoperative 5-fraction radiation therapy for soft tissue sarcoma followed by immediate surgical resection. Adv Radiat Oncol. 2020;5(6):1274–9.
38. Pennington JD, Eilber FC, Eilber FR, et al. Long-term outcomes with ifosfamide-based hypofractionated preoperative chemoradiotherapy for extremity soft tissue sarcomas. Am J Clin Oncol. 2018;41(12):1154–61.
39. Kubicek GJ, LaCouture T, Kaden M, et al. Preoperative radiosurgery for soft tissue sarcoma. Am J Clin Oncol. 2018;41(1):86–9.
40. Koseła-Paterczyk H, Szumera-Ciećkiewicz A, Szacht M, et al. Efficacy of neoadjuvant hypofractionated radiotherapy in patients with locally advanced myxoid liposarcoma. Eur J Surg Oncol. 2016;42(6):891–88.
41. Koseła-Paterczyk H, Szacht M, Morysiński T, et al. Preoperative hypofractionated radiotherapy in the treatment of localized soft tissue sarcomas. Eur J Surg Oncol. 2014;40(12):1641–7.
42. Short Course of Preoperative Radiotherapy in Head and Neck, Trunk and Extremity Soft Tissue Sarcomas; a Randomized Phase II Clinical Trial. ClinicalTrials.gov, The Netherlands Cancer Institute. ClinicalTrials.gov Identifier: NCT04425967.
43. Hypofractionated radiation therapy before surgery for the treatment of localized, resectable soft tissue sarcoma of the extremity and superficial trunk. https://ClinicalTrials.gov/show/NCT04562480.
44. Shorter course, hypofractionated pre-surgery radiation therapy in treating patients with localized, resectable soft tissue sarcoma of the extremity of superficial trunk.
45. Alektiar KM, Brennan MF, Healey JH, et al. Impact of intensity-modulated radiation therapy on local control in primary soft-tissue sarcoma of the extremity. J Clin Oncol. 2008;26:3440–4.
46. Alektiar KM, Brennan M, Singer S. Local control comparison of adjuvant brachytherapy to intensity-modulated radiotherapy in primary high-grade sarcoma of the extremity. Cancer. 2011;15:3229–34.
47. Folkert M, Singer S, Brennan MF, et al. Comparison of local recurrence with conventional and intensity-modulated radiation therapy for primary soft-tissue sarcomas of the extremity. J Clin Oncol. 2014;32:3236–41.
48. Wang D, Bosch W, Roberge D, et al. RTOG sarcoma radiation oncologists reach consensus on gross tumor volume and clinical target volume on computed tomographic images for preoperative radiotherapy of primary soft tissue sarcoma of extremity in Radiation Therapy Oncology Group studies. Int J Radiat Oncol Biol Phys. 2011;81(4):e525–8.

14 IORT and Brachytherapy for Extremity Soft Tissue Sarcoma

Brady S. Laughlin and Safia K. Ahmed

14.1 Intraoperative Electron Radiation Therapy (IOERT)

14.1.1 Introduction

Rosenberg et al. demonstrated overall survival between amputation and limb salvage surgery are equivalent for extremity sarcoma [1]. Since this seminal study, limb-sparing surgery and radiation have been the standard of care for high-risk extremity sarcoma. In the essential SR2 study, post-operative radiotherapy was demonstrated to lead to higher rates of fibrosis, edema, and worse function than preoperative radiation [2, 3]. This may be attributed to doses of 60 Gy or higher applied to large fields in the postoperative setting [4]. With preoperative radiotherapy, lower doses are directed toward smaller fields, thereby reducing late toxicity. However, this comes at the cost of double the rate of wound complications [2]. Intraoperative electron radiation therapy (IOERT) and brachytherapy provide a unique opportunity to deliver higher doses of radiation focally to areas considered at high risk for microscopic residual disease while limiting doses to adjacent structures. By boosting a smaller volume and excluding OARs (such as major nerves) from the radiation field, local control could be improved while potentially reducing late toxicity. IOERT and brachytherapy are often delivered in conjunction with preoperative radiation therapy. In this chapter, we describe the essential aspects of planning and delivering IOERT and brachytherapy.

14.1.2 Practical Aspects

Intraoperative radiotherapy allows for dose escalation to high-risk areas to achieve local control while allowing for reduced toxicity. This is accomplished by delivering a single high dose of radiation to areas deemed to be at higher risk for local recurrence by the orthopedic surgeon and radiation oncologist. The target is usually the tumor bed after gross total resection or areas concerning residual tumor or microscopic disease. Performing IOERT is a major interdisciplinary effort and therefore, should only be performed at sarcoma specialty centers. When considering the delivery of intraoperative radiotherapy, we consider using electrons. Electrons have a well-defined range, which means that they can be used to treat to a shallow depth. Variable electron energies can be used to deliver a uniform dose distribution to the desired target area. By keeping a radiation boost to superficial structures, toxicity can be minimized with this approach.

Practical aspects of IOERT delivery are as follows:

1. Typically, surgery and IOERT are performed in a dedicated, shielded operation room with an integrated linear accelerator or small mobile linac capable of delivering electrons (Fig. 14.1).
2. Prior to the delivery of IOERT, the surgeon and radiation oncologist assess the aim of the treatment and resection margin. The surgeon and radiation oncologist identify the target volume, which is considered to be the area at the highest risk for local recurrence. When the surgeon and radiation oncologist have decided upon an area of high risk, IOERT can be performed. Higher-risk areas often encompass bone and neurovasculature.
3. The team then considers shielding or moving uninvolved organs or structures, such as bone or nerve, so that acute or late toxicity can be reduced. Lead shields may be placed in front of normal tissue such as nerves or bone to reduce the amount of radiation dose received by them. A lead sheet may potentially reduce the dose to these structures by 50%. An applicator or cone of appropriate size is selected, and then positioned and attached to the operating room table [5]. There are different sizes and bevel angles to best fit into the surgical bed. Despite these options, the limited amount of cone sizes and bevel angles may make IOERT more challenging to deliver to an area

B. S. Laughlin · S. K. Ahmed (✉)
Department of Radiation Oncology, Mayo Clinic, Phoenix, AZ, USA
e-mail: Laughlin.Brady@mayo.edu; Ahmed.Safia@mayo.edu

H. Özger et al. (eds.), *Diagnosis and Treatment of Soft Tissue Tumors*, https://doi.org/10.1007/978-3-031-77061-6_14

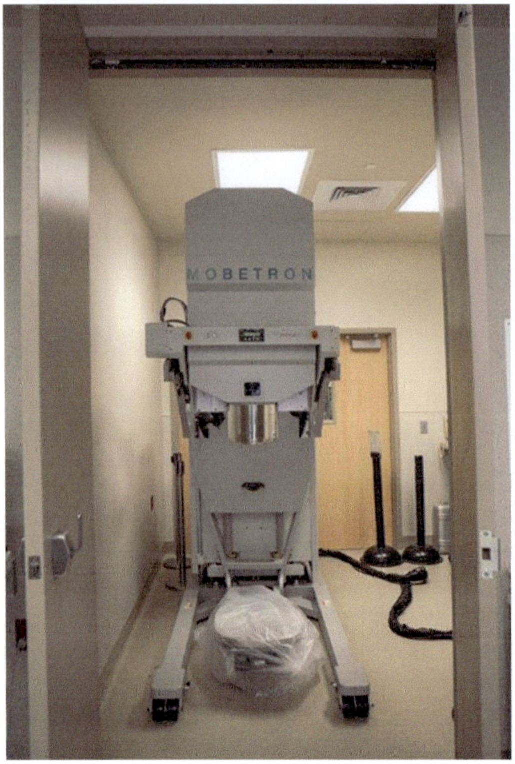

Fig. 14.1 IntraOp® Mobetron® for IOERT

that is particularly large and/or has an associated curvature/irregularly shaped. Before the delivery of radiation, the applicator axis is aligned with the linear accelerator (LINAC) axis. Most LINACs can deliver 4–12 MeV electrons, prescribed to the 90% isodose line.

4. The dose is selected according to a surgeon's suspicion regarding margin status. For suspected close margins, a dose of 10–12.5 Gy is administered. For microscopic positive margins, a dose of 12–15 Gy is administered. For gross residual disease, a dose of 16–20 Gy. It is recommended that the IOERT dose be limited to ≤12.5 Gy if major nerves need to be included. The radiation therapist or physicist together with the radiation oncologist are responsible for the delivery of the radiation. Treatment generally lasts 5–10 min.

Figure 14.2 demonstrates a case in which a linear accelerator is docked to the operating bed table, delivering IOERT to the tumor bed in the lower extremity following wide local excision of soft tissue sarcoma.

14.1.3 Literature

Retrospective studies provide the basis for the rationale of IOERT. As previously demonstrated in seminal trials in extremity sarcoma, higher doses in the postoperative setting

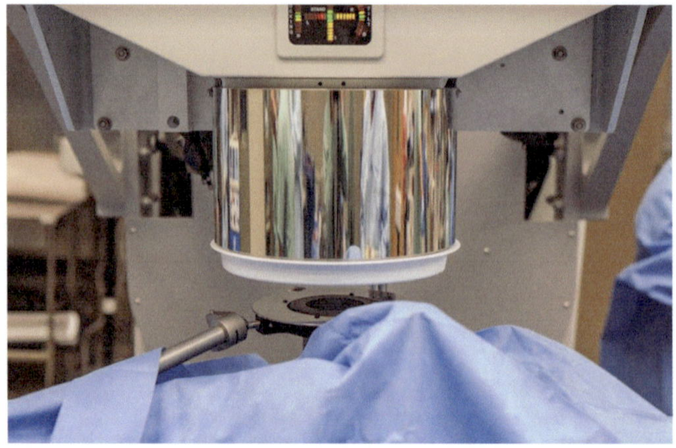

Fig. 14.2 The Mobetron linear accelerator is docked to the operating bed table, delivering IOERT to the tumor bed in the lower extremity following wide local excision of soft tissue sarcoma

are correlated with late toxicity, such as fibrosis, edema, and impaired joint function. These ultimately result in undesirable functional outcomes. A recent European Society for Radiation Oncology (ESTRO) reports guidelines for intraoperative radiation in treating soft tissue sarcoma [6].

Since intraoperative electron boost is targeted toward a small area deemed the highest risk for recurrence, toxicity can be reduced and function preserved by moving critical structures out of the field and treating only the necessary component of the tumor bed. When IOERT is used at limb salvage surgery following external beam radiation therapy (EBRT), local control can range from 82% to 97%, limb preservation rates from 81% to 100%, and functional outcomes of 59–100% [7–12]. The largest retrospective study contains 183 patients who underwent limb salvage surgery, IOERT, or pre- or post-operative EBRT. In this experience, Roeder reported a 5-year and 10-year local control of 86% and 84% [13]. Roeder reported a 5-year LC of 86% in a pooled analysis of multiple European centers. The 5-year OS in these studies ranged from 77% to 78% [14]. IOERT was delivered in a dedicated operating room with an integrated linear accelerator capable of delivering 6–18 MeV in these studies [13]. The target area was delineated by the surgeon and radiation oncologist. The median IOERT dose was 15 Gy (range 8–20 Gy), prescribed to the 90% isodose line [13]. If major nerves were included in the radiation field, the IOERT dose was restricted to 10–12 Gy [13]. Patients received EBRT either preoperatively (9%) or post-operatively (91%), receiving a median dose of 45 Gy (range 20–60 Gy).

When considering IORT, it is important to consider potential toxicity. Overall, late toxicity may be as high as 20% of cases of patients receiving IORT. Toxicity of combined external beam radiation and IORT includes late neuropathy, fracture, osteonecrosis, and lymphedema. Neuropathy may be considered as the most dose-limiting late toxicity when considering IORT. Neuropathy rates correspond to the length of nerve treatment and dose given during IOERT. Prospective analyses and retrospective series have demonstrated relatively low rates of neuropathy. In his prospective analysis, Roeder and colleagues reported neuropathy rates of 12% (all grades) with grade 3 toxicity of 3% [12]. Similarly, Azinovic et al. reported an 11% neuropathy rate in his series. Calvo et al. reported a 3% grade 3 neuropathy rate [8]. When major nerves are included in the field receiving IORT, neuropathy rates increase to 25%, which is demonstrated by a series published by Roeder [12] and Azinovic [11]. IOERT-related neuropathy is typically characterized by pain without weakness or sensory loss. When it occurs, it is often chronic. The pain may be severe but can be managed with medications such as gabapentin or pregabalin [15].

Despite potential long-term toxicity, limb preservation and functional outcomes are exceptional. High preservation rates and good function may be attributable to a small high dose volume. IORT approaches have had very high limb preservation rates (83–100%) and good functional outcomes (59–86%) [9–11, 14, 16, 17]. In their pooled analysis, Roeder et al. reported limb preservation and good functional outcomes in 95% and 81% of patients [14].

14.2 Brachytherapy

14.2.1 Introduction

Brachytherapy is a type of internal radiation treatment in which radioactive material sealed in needles, seeds, wires, or catheters is placed directly into the body in order to treat cancers. Brachytherapy is another treatment option to be considered in the treatment of extremity sarcoma. Whether used alone or in combination with EBRT as a radiation boost, brachytherapy can be used to improve local control and reduce toxicity. Advantages of brachytherapy include shortened treatment duration and direct placement of brachytherapy catheters over the tumor bed [18]. With rapid-dose fall-off, high doses can be delivered precisely to the area containing microscopic disease [19].

There are multiple techniques to deliver brachytherapy: high dose rate (HDR) implants, permanent/low dose rate (LDR) implants, pulsed dose rate (PDR), and intraoperative radiation delivered with HDR (IORT-HDR) [18, 20]. The most common technique for the use of brachytherapy is an HDR implant with a high-energy Ir-192 source, which can be delivered as an outpatient [18]. An HDR system contains three components: (1) the after loader, which contains the radioactive source Ir-192 and delivers treatment to the patient; (2) The control console, which enables the operator to deliver the treatment from the after loader remotely; (3) the planning workstation to plan the treatment. Temporary LDR implants were commonly used in the past. However, their use has decreased as LDR implants require inpatient hospital stays and increase staff exposure to radiation.

Brachytherapy should be considered as one of the following: (1) Monotherapy for patients with a low risk of recurrence or after local recurrence after previous EBRT. (2) Patients with a higher risk of local recurrence can be considered for brachytherapy boost [18]. Brachytherapy may be more advantageous to IOERT in certain situations such as boosting a large or irregularly shaped area that cannot be encompassed by IOERT cones. A disadvantage of brachytherapy is that there could be highly non-uniform dose distribution.

As monotherapy, the American Brachytherapy Society (ABS) recommends brachytherapy as monotherapy for patients with intermediate/high-grade sarcomas less than 10 cm with negative margins. The dose of radiation should be 45–50 Gy for LDR/PDR and 30–54 in 2–4.5 Gy fractions delivered twice daily at least 6 h apart for HDR. The NCCN guidelines support the use of 3.6 Gy delivered for 10 fractions [18].

The ABS recommends consideration of brachytherapy boost with EBRT in patients with intermediate/high-grade sarcomas greater than 10 cm, resected with negative margins, low-grade tumors greater than 5 cm which are deep, patients with tumors with close/positive margins, or patients with locally recurrent tumors not previously treated with radiation [18]. As a boost, options for dose include 15–25 Gy for LDR/PDR or 12–20 Gy in 2–4.5 Gy per fraction delivered twice daily at least 6 h apart for HDR [18].

14.2.2 Practical Aspects

If brachytherapy is being performed, the following should be considered.

1. The radiation oncologist and their team should be present with the orthopedic surgeon during the primary surgery.
2. Surgical clips may be placed after removal of the tumor to determine the clinical target volume.
3. Brachytherapy catheters are then placed intra-operatively. Hollow plastic flexible catheters may be placed using flexible steel needles. These needles are inserted through the skin over the tumor bed parallel or perpendicular to the incision line. This decision depends on the location and size of the tumor bed. The aimed distance between catheters is 1–1.5 cm. The catheters may extend 1–2 cm laterally and 2 cm craniocaudally to ensure adequate dose delivery of the target. Buttons/balls should be placed on both ends of the catheters.
4. The orthopedic surgeon and radiation oncologist must decide on the method of wound closure, whether it is

immediate or delayed. This decision should be made according to the orthopedic surgeon's assessment of a patient's risk for wound complications. If there is immediate closure, the catheters must be inspected after the closure of the skin to assess for kinking of the catheters and ensure that the catheters are parallel to each other.

5. If brachytherapy is performed post-operatively, a CT scan with or without contrast, should be performed to delineate the tumor bed by localizing the surgical clips. The placement of brachytherapy catheters is performed by the radiation oncologist utilizing the surgical note, pathological findings, and surgical clips. Generally, this procedure is performed utilizing regional anesthesia. Brachytherapy can be delivered as early as postoperative day 0 and days 2–4 [21].
6. During treatment, a radioactive source, traditionally ^{192}Ir, passes from the after loader through the catheters, thereby delivering a high radiation dose to the surgical bed. HDR treatment lasts about 10–20 min.

14.2.3 Literature

When brachytherapy is added to a local excision, brachytherapy can result in a significant improvement in local control. Memorial Sloan Kettering Cancer Center randomized 164 extremity soft tissue sarcoma patients to adjuvant brachytherapy or no further therapy after limb-sparing surgery [22, 23]. The 5-year local control was 82% and 69% in the brachytherapy and no brachytherapy arms (p = 0.04). Additionally, there was a statistically significant difference in local control with high-grade lesions with the addition of brachytherapy (89% vs. 66%, p = 0.0025) [23]. It is important to note that brachytherapy had no impact on local control for low-grade lesions.

The experience with brachytherapy in the management of extremity soft tissue sarcoma is associated with excellent oncologic and functional outcomes as well as toxicity profile. Local control rates may range from 71% to 100% and grade 3+ toxicity of 25–30% [18, 19, 24–33].

14.3 Re-irradiation

Approximately 20% of sarcomas recur locally [34]. The optimal management of locally recurrent sarcoma is unclear. Re-irradiation could potentially reduce subsequent recurrence. However, conservative salvage surgery and re-irradiation could potentially cause debilitating and severe complications that impact quality of life and function [21, 34–42]. Patients with recurrent sarcoma are challenging, as re-operation and re-irradiation are planned around factors of distorted anatomy, fibrosis, and ischemia.

In patients who have received prior radiation, brachytherapy or IOERT boost may reduce local recurrence. IOERT and brachytherapy can spare normal tissue receiving radiation. If a case is associated with higher risk, a free flap or rotational flap may be needed to maintain fresh tissue to preserve health and reduce the risk of toxicity [18, 39].

14.3.1 Practical Aspects

Recurrent extremity soft tissue sarcoma presents challenging cases, as patients with prior radiation may have local control and higher toxicity with treatment. When considering treatment approaches for patients with recurrent extremity sarcoma, IOERT and brachytherapy are viable considerations for this cohort of patients.

14.3.2 Risk Factors/Benefits

As previously described, toxicity is a limiting factor when considering re-irradiation and the use of IOERT and brachytherapy. Specifically, rates of wound complications and salvage amputations are quite high, greater than >50% in a number of series [34, 36, 38–41].

Brachytherapy is typically delivered immediately following wound closure. Alternatively, a delayed or staged reconstruction could be considered, in which a negative pressure wound closure acts as a temporary closure, which is kept in place during the course of brachytherapy [43]. By considering this approach, wound healing may be improved due to increased granulation tissue, decreased serous fluid, improved oxygenation, and blood flow to the tumor bed. Additionally, the brachytherapy catheters are removed from the final reconstruction.

References

1. Rosenberg SA, Tepper J, Glatstein E, Costa J, Baker A, Brennan M, DeMoss EV, Seipp C, Sindelar WF, Sugarbaker P, Wesley R. The treatment of soft-tissue sarcomas of the extremities: prospective randomized evaluations of (1) limb-sparing surgery plus radiation therapy compared with amputation and (2) the role of adjuvant chemotherapy. Ann Surg. 1982;196:305–15.
2. O'Sullivan B, Davis AM, Turcotte R, Bell R, Catton C, Chabot P, Wunder J, Kandel R, Goddard K, Sadura A, Pater J, Zee B. Preoperative versus postoperative radiotherapy in soft-tissue sarcoma of the limbs: a randomised trial. Lancet (London, England). 2002;359:2235–41.
3. Davis AM, O'Sullivan B, Turcotte R, Bell R, Catton C, Chabot P, Wunder J, Hammond A, Benk V, Kandel R, Goddard K, Freeman C, Sadura A, Zee B, Day A, Tu D, Pater J. Late radiation morbidity following randomization to preoperative versus postoperative radiotherapy in extremity soft tissue sarcoma. Radiother Oncol. 2005;75:48–53.

4. Stinson SF, Delaney TF, Greenberg J, Yang JC, Lampert MH, Hicks JE, Venzon D, White DE, Rosenberg SA, Glatstein EJ. Acute and long-term effects on limb function of combined modality limb sparing therapy for extremity soft tissue sarcoma. Int J Radiat Oncol Biol Phys. 1991;21:1493–9.
5. Roeder F, Krempien R. Intraoperative radiation therapy (IORT) in soft-tissue sarcoma. Radiat Oncol (London, England). 2017;12:20.
6. Roeder F, Morillo V, Saleh-Ebrahimi L, Calvo FA, Poortmans P, Ferrer Albiach C. Intraoperative radiation therapy (IORT) for soft tissue sarcoma—ESTRO IORT Task Force/ACROP recommendations. Radiother Oncol. 2020;150:293–302.
7. Carbó-Laso E, Sanz-Ruiz P, Calvo-Haro JA, Cuervo-Dehesa M, Pérez-Mañanes R, Mediavilla-Santos L, Sánchez-Pérez C, Álvarez-González A, Vaquero-Martín J. Intraoperative radiotherapy for extremity soft-tissue sarcomas: can long-term local control be achieved? Int J Clin Oncol. 2017;22:1094–102.
8. Calvo FA, Sole CV, Polo A, Cambeiro M, Montero A, Alvarez A, Cuervo M, San Julian M, Martinez-Monge R. Limb-sparing management with surgical resection, external-beam and intraoperative electron-beam radiation therapy boost for patients with primary soft tissue sarcoma of the extremity. Strahlenther Onkol. 2014;190:891–8.
9. Oertel S, Treiber M, Zahlten-Hinguranage A, Eichin S, Roeder F, Funk A, Hensley FW, Timke C, Niethammer AG, Huber PE. Intraoperative electron boost radiation followed by moderate doses of external beam radiotherapy in limb-sparing treatment of patients with extremity soft-tissue sarcoma. Int J Radiat Oncol Biol Phys. 2006;64:1416–23.
10. Kretzler A, Molls M, Gradinger R, Lukas P, Steinau H-U, Würschmidt F. Intraoperative radiotherapy of soft tissue sarcoma of the extremity. Strahlenther Onkol. 2004;180:365–70.
11. Azinovic I, Martinez Monge R, Aristu JJ, Salgado E, Villafranca E, Hidalgo OF, Amillo S, San Julian M, Villas C, Aramendía JM, Calvo FA. Intraoperative radiotherapy electron boost followed by moderate doses of external beam radiotherapy in resected soft-tissue sarcoma of the extremities. Radiother Oncol. 2003;67:331–7.
12. Roeder F, Lehner B, Schmitt T, Kasper B, Egerer G, Sedlaczek O, Grüllich C, Mechtersheimer G, Wuchter P, Hensley FW. Excellent local control with IOERT and postoperative EBRT in high grade extremity sarcoma: results from a subgroup analysis of a prospective trial. BMC Cancer. 2014;14:1–12.
13. Roeder F, Lehner B, Saleh-Ebrahimi L, Hensley FW, Ulrich A, Alldinger I, Mechtersheimer G, Huber PE, Krempien R, Bischof M, Debus J, Uhl M. Intraoperative electron radiation therapy combined with external beam radiation therapy and limb sparing surgery in extremity soft tissue sarcoma: a retrospective single center analysis of 183 cases. Radiother Oncol. 2016;119:22–9.
14. Roeder F, de Paoli A, Saleh-Ebrahimi L, Alldinger I, Bertola G, Boz G, Navarria F, Cuervo M, Uhl M, Alvarez A, Buechler M, Lehner B, Debus J, Calvo FA, Krempien R. Intraoperative electron radiation therapy combined with external beam radiation therapy after gross Total resection in extremity soft tissue sarcoma: a European pooled analysis. Ann Surg Oncol. 2018;25:3833–42.
15. Haddock MG. Intraoperative radiation therapy for colon and rectal cancers: a clinical review. Radiat Oncol. 2017;12:11.
16. Edmonson JH, Petersen IA, Shives TC, Mahoney MR, Rock MG, Haddock MG, Sim FH, Maples WJ, O'Connor MI, Gunderson LL, Foo ML, Pritchard DJ, Buckner JC, Stafford SL. Chemotherapy, irradiation, and surgery for function-preserving therapy of primary extremity soft tissue sarcomas: initial treatment with ifosfamide, mitomycin, doxorubicin, and cisplatin plus granulocyte macrophage-colony-stimulating factor. Cancer. 2002;94:786–92.
17. Llácer C, Delannes M, Minsat M, Stoeckle E, Votron L, Martel P, Bonnevialle P, Bui BN, Chevreau C, Kantor G. Low-dose intraoperative brachytherapy in soft tissue sarcomas involving neurovascular structure. Radiother Oncol. 2006;78:10–6.
18. Campbell SR, Shah C, Scott JG, Mesko N, Nystrom L, Kolar M, Largo AC, Kamrava M, Mourtada F, Naghavi AO, Harrison LB. American Brachytherapy Society (ABS) consensus statement for soft-tissue sarcoma brachytherapy. Brachytherapy. 2021;20:1200–18.
19. Manir KS, Basu A, Choudhury KB, Basu S, Ghosh K, Gangopadhyay S. Interstitial brachytherapy in soft tissue sarcoma: a 5 years institutional experience with Cobalt 60-based high-dose-rate brachytherapy system. J Contemp Brachytherapy. 2018;10:431–8.
20. Tom MC, Joshi N, Vicini F, Chang AJ, Hong TS, Showalter TN, Chao ST, Wolden S, Wu AJ, Martin D. The American Brachytherapy Society consensus statement on intraoperative radiation therapy. Brachytherapy. 2019;18:242–57.
21. Naghavi A, Gonzalez R, Scott J, Abuodeh Y, Echevarria M, Mullinax J, Ahmed K, Harrison L, Fernandez D. Staged reconstruction brachytherapy has lower overall cost in recurrent soft tissue sarcoma. Int J Radiat Oncol Biol Phys. 2016;96:E398–E9.
22. Harrison LB, Franzese F, Gaynor JJ, Brennan MF. Long-term results of a prospective randomized trial of adjuvant brachytherapy in the management of completely resected soft tissue sarcomas of the extremity and superficial trunk. Int J Radiat Oncol Biol Phys. 1993;27:259–65.
23. Pisters PW, Harrison LB, Leung DH, Woodruff JM, Casper ES, Brennan MF. Long-term results of a prospective randomized trial of adjuvant brachytherapy in soft tissue sarcoma. J Clin Oncol. 1996;14:859–68.
24. Alekhteyar KM, Leung DH, Brennan MF, Harrison LB. The effect of combined external beam radiotherapy and brachytherapy on local control and wound complications in patients with high-grade soft tissue sarcomas of the extremity with positive microscopic margin. Int J Radiat Oncol Biol Phys. 1996;36:321–4.
25. Pisters PW, Pollock RE, Lewis VO, Yasko AW, Cormier JN, Respondek PM, Feig BW, Hunt KK, Lin PP, Zagars G. Long-term results of prospective trial of surgery alone with selective use of radiation for patients with T1 extremity and trunk soft tissue sarcomas. Ann Surg. 2007;246:675–82.
26. Chaudhary AJ, Laskar S, Badhwar R. Interstitial brachytherapy in soft tissue sarcomas. Strahlenther Onkol. 1998;174:522–8.
27. Alektiar KM, Leung D, Zelefsky MJ, Healey JH, Brennan MF. Adjuvant brachytherapy for primary high-grade soft tissue sarcoma of the extremity. Ann Surg Oncol. 2002;9:48–56.
28. Lazzaro G, Lazzari R, Pelosi G, De Pas T, Mariani L, Mazzarol G, Sances D, Tosti G, Baldini F, Mosconi M. Pulsed dose-rate perioperative interstitial brachytherapy for soft tissue sarcomas of the extremities and skeletal muscles of the trunk. Ann Surg Oncol. 2005;12:935–42.
29. Laskar S, Bahl G, Puri A, Agarwal MG, Muckaden M, Patil N, Jambhekar N, Gupta S, Deshpande DD, Shrivastava SK. Perioperative interstitial brachytherapy for soft tissue sarcomas: prognostic factors and long-term results of 155 patients. Ann Surg Oncol. 2007;14:560–7.
30. Mierzwa ML, McCluskey CM, Barrett WL, Lowy A, Sussman J, Sorger J. Interstitial brachytherapy for soft tissue sarcoma: a single institution experience. Brachytherapy. 2007;6:298–303.
31. Petera J, Soumarová R, Růžičková J, Neumanová R, Dušek L, Sirák I, Mačingová Z, Paluska P, Kašaová L, Hodek M. Perioperative hyperfractionated high-dose rate brachytherapy for the treatment of soft tissue sarcomas: multicentric experience. Ann Surg Oncol. 2010;17:206–10.
32. Emory CL, Montgomery CO, Potter BK, Keisch ME, Conway SA. Early complications of high-dose-rate brachytherapy in soft tissue sarcoma: a comparison with traditional external-beam radiotherapy. Clin Orthop Relat Res. 2012;470:751–8.
33. Klein J, Ghasem A, Huntley S, Donaldson N, Keisch M, Conway S. Does an algorithmic approach to using brachytherapy and external beam radiation result in good function, local control rates, and

low morbidity in patients with extremity soft tissue sarcoma? Clin Orthop Relat Res. 2018;476:634.
34. Indelicato DJ, Meadows K, Gibbs CP Jr, Morris CG, Scarborough MT, Zlotecki RA. Effectiveness and morbidity associated with reirradiation in conservative salvage management of recurrent soft-tissue sarcoma. Int J Radiat Oncol Biol Phys. 2009;73:267–72.
35. Braschi EL, Kharod SM, Morris CG, Spiguel AR, Gibbs CP, Scarborough MT, Zlotecki RA. Reirradiation in conservative salvage of recurrent soft-tissue sarcoma: an analysis of treatment efficacy and toxicities. Am J Clin Oncol. 2021;44:624–8.
36. Torres MA, Ballo MT, Butler CE, Feig BW, Cormier JN, Lewis VO, Pollock RE, Pisters PW, Zagars GK. Management of locally recurrent soft-tissue sarcoma after prior surgery and radiation therapy. Int J Radiat Oncol Biol Phys. 2007;67:1124–9.
37. Moureau-Zabotto L, Thomas L, Bui BNG, Chevreau C, Stockle E, Martel P, Bonneviale P, Marques B, Coindre J-M, Kantor G, Matsuda T, Delannes M. Management of soft tissue sarcomas (STS) in first isolated local recurrence: a retrospective study of 83 cases. Radiother Oncol. 2004;73:313–9.
38. Nori D, Shupak K, Shiu M, Brennan M. Role of brachytherapy in recurrent extremity sarcoma in patients treated with prior surgery and irradiation. Int J Radiat Oncol Biol Phys. 1991;20:1229–33.
39. Pearlstone DB, Janjan NA, Feig BW, Yasko AW, Hunt KK, Pollock RE, Lawyer A, Horton J, Pisters P. Re-resection with brachytherapy for locally recurrent soft tissue sarcoma arising in a previously radiated field. Cancer J Sci Am. 1999;5:26–33.
40. Spierer MM, Alektiar KM, Zelefsky MJ, Brennan MF, Cordiero PG. Tolerance of tissue transfers to adjuvant radiation therapy in primary soft tissue sarcoma of the extremity. Int J Radiat Oncol Biol Phys. 2003;56:1112–6.
41. Arbeit JM, Hilaris B, Brennan M. Wound complications in the multimodality treatment of extremity and superficial truncal sarcomas. J Clin Oncol. 1987;5:480–8.
42. Catton C, Davis A, Bell R, O'Sullivan B, Fornasier V, Wunder J, McLean M. Soft tissue sarcoma of the extremity. Limb salvage after failure of combined conservative therapy. Radiother Oncol. 1996;41:209–14.
43. Heller L, Ballo MT, Cormier JN, Oates SD, Butler CE. Staged reconstruction for resection wounds in sarcoma patients treated with brachytherapy. Ann Plast Surg. 2008;60:58–63.

Classification from a Surgical Perspective

15

Harzem Özger and Buğra Alpan

Classification systems are essential in clinical decision-making as they provide a framework for understanding and categorizing various diseases and conditions. These systems allow clinicians to classify patients into distinct groups so that they can develop a more standardized approach towards correct evaluation and effective treatment of patients as well as providing more comprehensive answers about the predicted outcomes for the patients being treated. While pathological classification is a crucial aspect of surgical practice as it guides surgical decision-making, it refers to classifying diseases based on their underlying pathophysiology and histopathological features. As discussed thoroughly in Chap. 1, the modern pathological classification of soft tissue tumors by the WHO Classification of Tumours Editorial Board takes into consideration a wide variety of histologic (cellular morphology, tissue of origin, grading), immunohistochemical, molecular, and genetic properties. As our ability to investigate histopathological parameters, which were previously unavailable or scarcely available, increases, we might anticipate radical changes in pathological classification, resulting in the emergence of new categories and the omission of other entities. The continuous evolution of this classification system guarantees better insight into the diagnosis and treatment of these diseases, but this is also concerning for the clinician, who is trying to adapt to the pace of these changes. While they are closely related, classification from a surgical perspective differs from pathological classification. Defining the problem is the primary purpose of pathologic classification, whereas solving the problem is the primary goal from a surgical perspective.

Surgical classification of soft tissue tumors necessitates a clinical scenario-based approach, which encompasses the histopathologic diagnoses with all known clinical implications but also considers other important factors such as anatomic location, pathoanatomic features, stage of the disease, and temporal relation of relevant treatment methods. Although the classification is based on intended local treatment categories rather than specific diseases, characteristics of specific histopathologic diagnoses must be known to understand the context in which that local treatment category is preferred. Classification from a surgical point of view naturally includes non-surgical treatment modalities since a multidisciplinary approach, albeit supervised by an orthopedic oncologist, is essential to musculoskeletal tumor management. While the treating surgeon usually determines the surgical classification at presentation, the classification might change during treatment. Treatment strategies can be and typically are further individualized in daily practice according to demographic features, psychosocial factors, the multidisciplinary team's experience, and the capabilities of the treating institution. However, individualized decision-making is beyond the scope of surgical classification of soft tissue tumors [1, 2].

15.1 Curable Conditions

15.1.1 Curative Resection

This category comprises benign, intermediate, or malignant neoplasms and tumor-like conditions for which surgical treatment can provide a total cure with or without adjuvant methods. Specific histopathology and anatomic factors determine the extent of surgery and the need for and timing of additional treatment. It should be emphasized that even though the marginal status might vary according to the intended resection type, piecemeal resection is not acceptable, and en bloc resection is the rule for curative resection.

15.1.1.1 Marginal Resection

Removal of the tumor with marginal margins is adequate for a small subset of soft tissue tumors. Hence, resection must be

H. Özger (✉)
Department of Orthopedics and Traumatology,
Istanbul University, Istanbul Medical Faculty, Istanbul, Türkiye
e-mail: harzemo@yahoo.com

B. Alpan
Department of Orthopedics and Traumatology,
Acıbadem Mehmet Ali Aydınlar University, School of Medicine,
Istanbul, Türkiye
e-mail: bugra.alpan@acibadem.edu.tr

H. Özger et al. (eds.), *Diagnosis and Treatment of Soft Tissue Tumors*, https://doi.org/10.1007/978-3-031-77061-6_15

completed with an intact capsule or pseudocapsule (Fig. 15.1). This procedure is typically indicated in Enneking stage 1 (latent) or stage 2 (active) benign soft tissue tumors and tumor-like conditions, which have a low local recurrence rate [3–8]. The most common examples are:

- lipoma (subcutaneous, ≤5 cm),
- schwannoma,
- elastofibroma dorsi,
- intramuscular myxoma,
- fibroma of the tendon sheath,
- nodular fasciitis,
- ganglion cysts,
- traumatic/amputation neuroma,
- hemangioma (subcutaneous, ≤2 cm),
- glomus tumor,
- myositis ossificans (residual ossified symptomatic mass),
- organized hematoma,
- arthroplasty-related pseudotumor.

Most of these lesions can be diagnosed accurately with clinical and radiological findings alone, but a core-needle biopsy must nevertheless be performed if the findings are ambiguous. Despite nonaggressive benign histology, resection with more than marginal margins is encouraged depending on pathoanatomic features like gelatinous content prone to an eruption during dissection (e.g., myxoma), infiltrative ill-defined borders (e.g., nodular fasciitis) or peripheral pathologic venous connections (e.g., hemangioma).

Even though the predicted local recurrence rate is low in this category, a certain clinical and radiological follow-up period is recommended in light of the definitive pathology result.

15.1.1.2 Relative Wide Resection

Wide resection is also indicated in certain scenarios involving pathologies ranging from Enneking stage 2 (active) and 3 (aggressive) benign soft tissue tumors to intermediate lesions. However, wide resection in this category is nuanced in that sparing critical structures with marginal margins may be acceptable even if no margin-modifying adjuvant treatment was used. Dissection with "conventional" wide margins is still essential in other parts of the tumor, where the risk of morbidity is low, to optimize local control. The most common examples are:

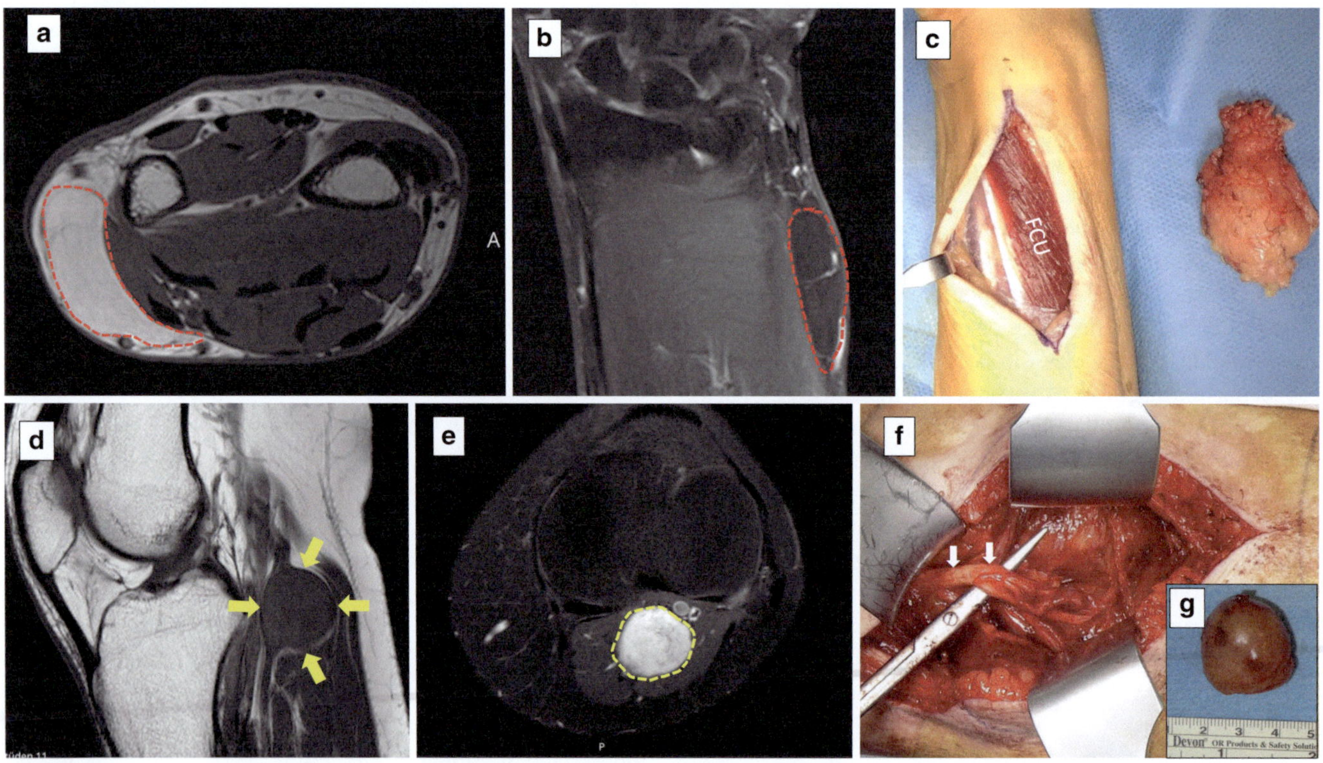

Fig. 15.1 Axial (T1) and coronal (fat-suppressed) MRI sections demonstrate a subcutaneous lipoma on the ulnar aspect of the wrist (**a** and **b**). The mass was painless, well-defined, and had a typical soft consistency in physical examination. Considering clinical and radiological characteristics, an excisional biopsy was performed with marginal margins. (**c**). Sagittal T1 weighted and axial fat-suppressed proton-density MRI sections of the knee demonstrate a well-circumscribed, globular soft tissue mass adjacent to the popliteal vascular bundle (**d** and **e**). The sagittal section shows tail-like projections on the proximal and distal poles of the lesion. The patient had paresthesia radiating from the calf to the plantar aspect of the foot, and a Tinel sign was present on the soft tissue mass. Marginal excision was performed with dissection of the lesion from the tibial nerve to confirm a presumed diagnosis of schwannoma (**f** and **g**). Curative resection was achieved in both cases

- well-differentiated liposarcoma (WDLS)/atypical lipomatous tumor (ALT),
- lipoma (deep-seated, retroperitoneal, intramuscular, >5 cm),
- synovial chondromatosis (embedded within or attached to synovium),
- localized-type tenosynovial giant cell tumor (TGCT),
- hemangioma (deep-seated, intramuscular, >2 cm, progression under observation),
- desmoid fibromatosis (progression under observation).

While these examples represent various histopathologic entities with different pathoanatomic features, the common ground for the surgical rationale is their ability to profoundly threaten the patient's quality of life and possibly limb rather than life. From a surgical perspective, there are tips and tricks regarding the resection of each of these tumors to maintain a standard of "**relative wide resection**." The surgeon must also know the potential consequences of inadequate local control.

Although WDLS/ALT can be distinguished from a large, deep-seated but nonaggressive lipoma based on the presence or absence of *MDM2* and *CDK4* gene amplification, this might not be reliable in limited tissue samples obtained by core-needle biopsy. Wide resection—whenever possible without unacceptable morbidity—should be the preferred strategy in any large, deep-seated lipomatous tumor of proximal extremities or the trunk (Fig. 15.2). In intramuscular lipomas, muscle fibers covering the surface of and passing through the tumor must be sacrificed, with particular care given to extensions along the longitudinal axis of fibers. On the other hand, less than wide surgical margins should be expected in specific anatomic locations, such as the retroperitoneum tumor, or with anatomical relations, such as a tumor compressing the sciatic nerve. An intact capsule or pseudocapsule will suffice for marginal safety in critical

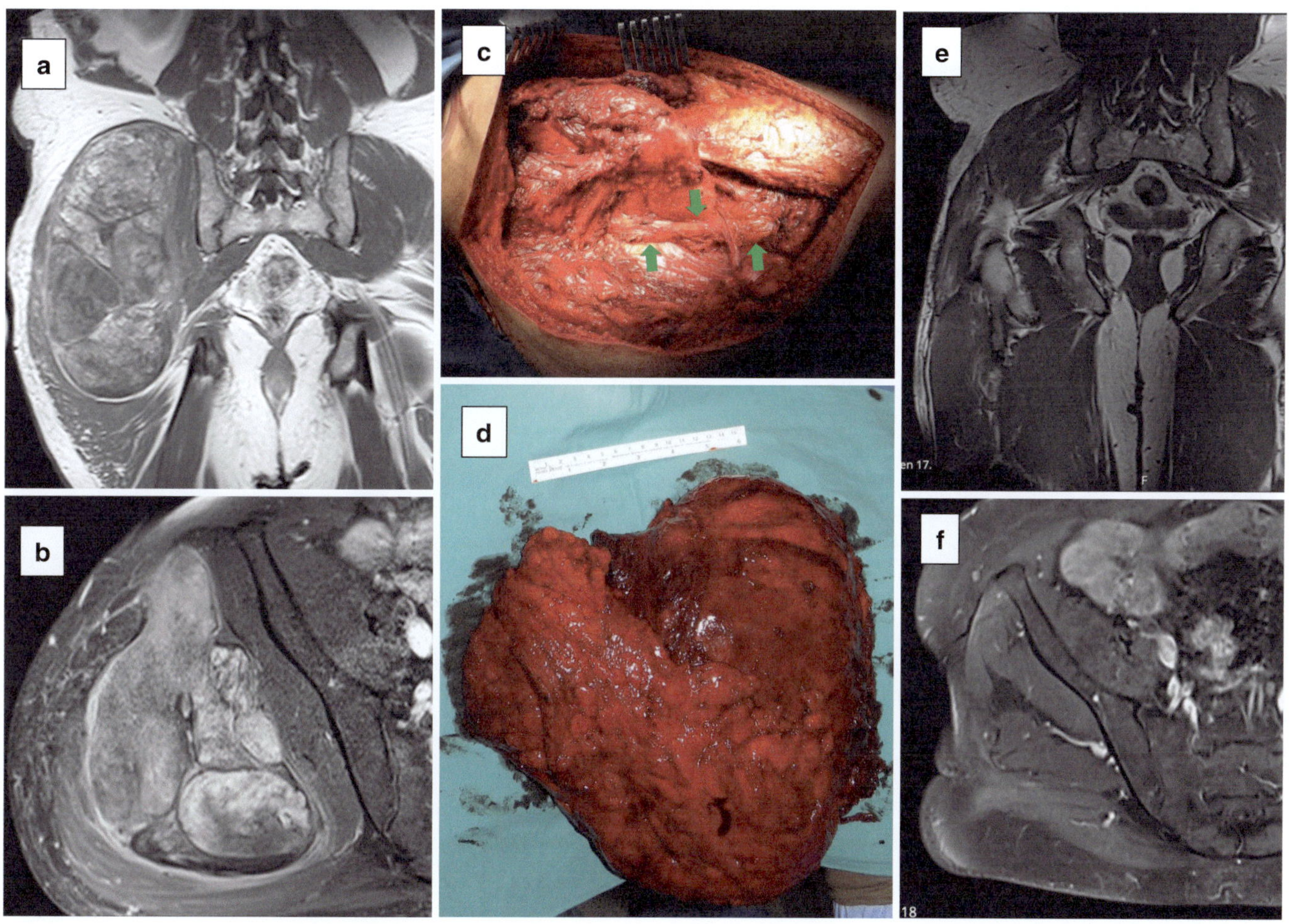

Fig. 15.2 Coronal T1 and axial fat-suppressed contrast-enhanced MR images show a giant, biopsy-confirmed, well-differentiated liposarcoma deeply seated in the right gluteal compartment (**a** and **b**). Relative wide resection was performed with curative intent and without any neoadjuvant treatment. The sciatic nerve (green block arrows) was preserved with marginal dissection on the deep aspect of the tumor (**c**). The superficial aspect of the tumor, on the other hand, was dissected with relatively wide margins by leaving some subcutaneous fat tissue and muscle fibers lying intact over the tumor (**d**). No adjuvant treatment was given. Local MR images at 30 months follow-up demonstrate no evidence of disease (**e** and **f**)

locations (Fig. 15.3). However, a non-encapsulated lipomatous neoplasm with lobules blending with the surrounding normal adipose tissue is always a serious challenge to the surgeon. It must be remembered that WDLS/ALT might rarely dedifferentiate and metastasize, usually because of local recurrence [3, 9].

While synovial chondromatosis might present with loose bodies, for which margins are irrelevant and a thorough collection of bodies from the joint cavity is enough, some lesions present as embedded in the synovial lining of the joint or as conglomerates adherent to intraarticular or periarticular structures. The latter forms must be removed with wide margins from where they are embedded or adherent since this is an intermediate pathology with rare but concerning potential to dedifferentiate into chondrosarcoma with local recurrence. Degenerative changes of articular surfaces should also be anticipated with multiple recurrences [3, 4].

Localized TGCT has an excellent chance of cure if widely excised with arthrotomy rather than the common practice of piecemeal excision with an arthroscopic shaver. The surgical margin on the intraarticular aspect of the lesion is usually covered with only synovial lining and cannot be modified. The lesion must be handled gently so as not to disrupt the thin synovial barrier and prevent tumor spillage into the joint cavity. On the other hand, the base or the pedicle of the lesion must be dissected with wide margins from intraarticular or periarticular structures like the synovia or Hoffa's fat pad. Since local recurrence might lead to joint degeneration with diffuse involvement and loss of another chance for curative resection, resection with adequate margins in index surgery is crucial [3, 4, 10].

Hemangiomas and desmoid fibromatoses are non-metastasizing benign soft tissue tumors (Enneking stage 2 and 3, respectively), for which an initial observation period is currently the standard approach to avoid unsatisfactory outcomes with an unnecessary intervention. Wide resection is indicated for both symptomatic hemangiomas and desmoid tumors, which show progression under observation, are likely to cause morbidity with further progression, and are amenable to resection without significant morbidity by the

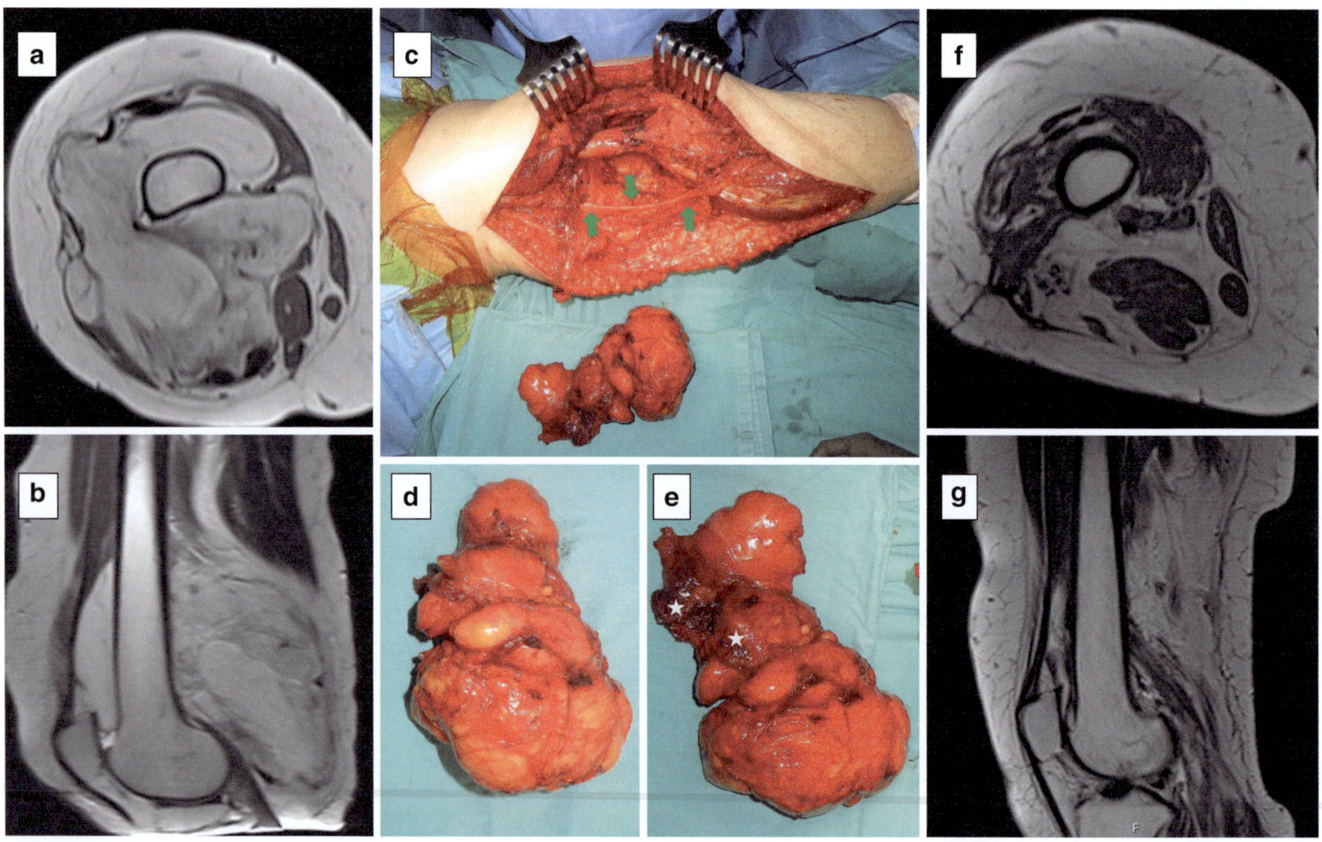

Fig. 15.3 Axial and sagittal T1-weighted MR images show a sizeable lipomatous neoplasm surrounding the distal femur 360° and having a predominantly homogenous signal characteristic (**a** and **b**). A trucut biopsy from a relatively heterogenous-appearing part of the tumor revealed fibrous changes but no sign of malignancy. The tumor was designated as an atypical lipoma, and surgical resection without any neoadjuvant treatment was indicated. Sciatic-nerve (green block arrows) sparing resection was performed with mostly marginal margins and intact capsules (**c** and **d**), while wider margins were achieved in some parts by leaving attached muscle and subcutaneous fat tissue (white stars) over the tumor (**e**). The patient did not receive any adjuvant treatment. Axial and sagittal MR images at 24 months show no local recurrence or residual tumor (**f** and **g**)

latest follow-up (Figs. 15.4 and 15.5). Pathologic peripheral vascular extensions (e.g., along muscle fibers), which are challenging to identify intraoperatively in hemangiomas and infiltrative borders with tumoral extension along fascial planes in desmoid tumors, usually make wide resection very challenging. Marginal dissection is acceptable to spare critical structures in both pathologies since preserving function is vital for quality of life, and local recurrence is not associated with survival. However, it must be remembered that local recurrences are associated with severe morbidity in both tumors [3, 4, 10–12].

15.1.1.3 Absolute Wide Resection

The classic concept of Enneking's tumor compartments suggests a reactive zone around the tumor beyond the capsule or pseudocapsule. While the definition of wide margins is debatable, it refers to tumor resection with an intact, healthy tissue envelope, which is presumed to include the reactive zone. The width of surgical margins can theoretically be quantified according to the barrier qualities of surrounding tissues. The surgical procedure can also be described as resection with "safe/adequate margins" due to the varying width of surgical margins (Fig. 15.6). This treatment category mainly involves low-grade soft tissue sarcomas, which are typically radio- and chemoresistant and, therefore, either do not benefit at all or insignificantly benefit from any adjuvant treatment. Consequently, local control depends on the quality of surgical treatment. The most common examples are:

- low-grade myxoid fibrosarcoma,
- malignant peripheral nerve sheath tumor,
- leiomyosarcoma,
- dermatofibrosarcoma protuberans (DFSP).

Wide resection is an absolute indication and cannot be compromised under any circumstance in this group [1–3, 13–16]. Without margin-modifying beneficial adjuvant modalities, the surgeon must be ready to sacrifice with an uncompromising resection and perform neurovascular, soft tissue, or osteoarticular reconstruction as necessary. Local control directly impacts the overall survival of non-metastatic patients in this category. It should also be remembered that while DFSP has an intermediate character with local aggressive behavior, its local recurrence might increase histological grade and the potential to metastasize.

15.1.1.4 Wide Resection with Modified Margins

This treatment category pertains to surgical treatment in the setting of high-grade soft tissue sarcomas. General tumor knowledge suggests that high-grade tumors benefit more from adjuvant treatment methods mainly due to their high vascularity and high mitotic activity. While the role of adjuvant treatment modalities has not been as established in soft tissue sarcomas as in osteosarcoma or Ewing's sarcoma, the consensus among orthopedic oncologists is that radiotherapy is essential for improved local control, chemotherapy is very effective in a few specific entities, and it has some contribution to overall survival in certain histologic subtypes and in

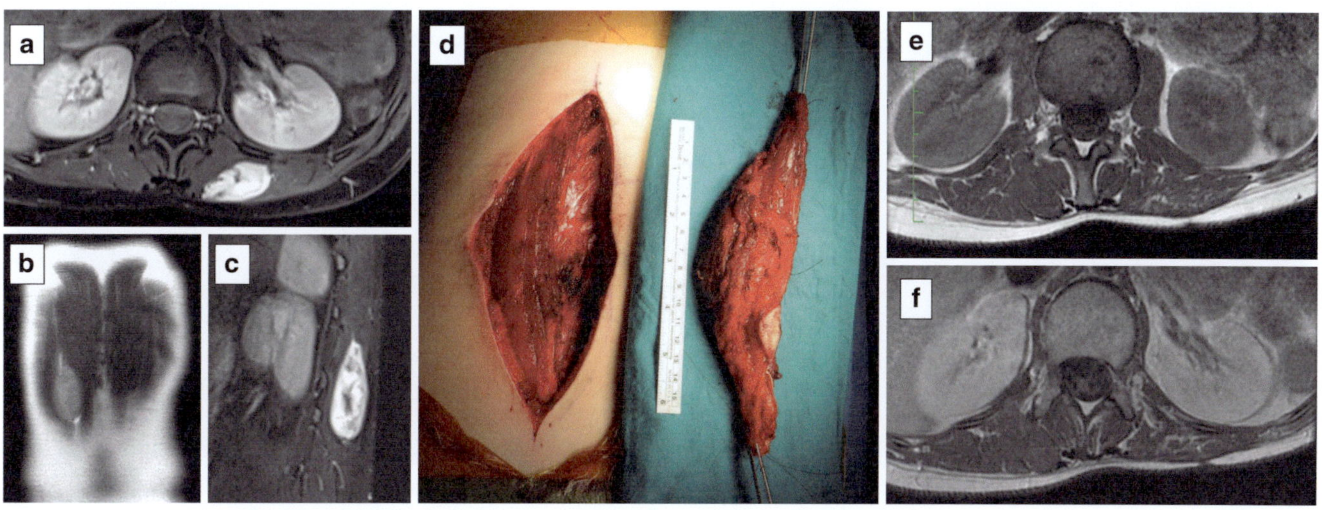

Fig. 15.4 Axial, coronal, and sagittal MRI sections show a soft tissue mass embedded in the paravertebral muscles (**a**–**c**). A core-needle biopsy of the lesion revealed a desmoid tumor. Considering the size and location of the lesion, resection without significant morbidity was deemed possible, but an initial observation period was planned. Due to slight progression under observation over three months, wide resection was indicated, and a curative intervention was attempted. Intraoperative photos show the resection site and the specimen following wide resection (**d**). The skin island includes the needle biopsy scar, while the rest of the tumor is covered with a healthy muscle envelope. MRI sections at 30 months postoperatively demonstrate no residual or recurrent lesion with a negligible reduction in subcutaneous fat tissue and paravertebral muscle mass (**e** and **f**). While wide resection is not an absolute indication for desmoid tumors and marginal margins are acceptable to preserve critical structures, wide margins are desirable for resection with curative intent

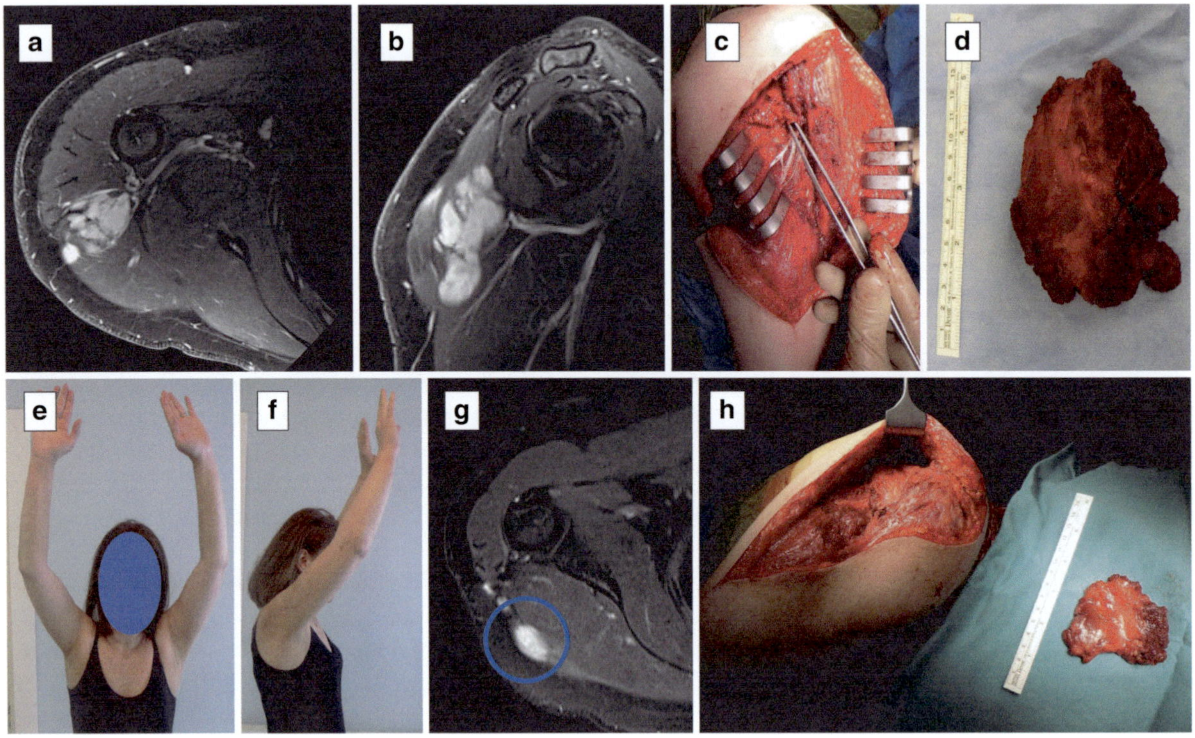

Fig. 15.5 Axial and sagittal MRI sections show a soft tissue mass inside the deltoid muscle and adjacent to the axillary nerve and posterior circumflex humeral vessels (**a** and **b**). A trucut biopsy of the lesion revealed a desmoid tumor. While the lesion was already painful and causing limitation of shoulder function, possible progression under observation was deemed unacceptable due to the risk of missing the window of opportunity to save the axillary nerve. Wide resection, including a portion of the deltoid muscle, was performed, and the lesion was dissected from the axillary nerve (**c** and **d**). While active shoulder elevation was successfully preserved following resection (**e** and **f**), local recurrence was observed at postoperative 12 months (**g**), and a re-resection with curative intent was performed (**h**)

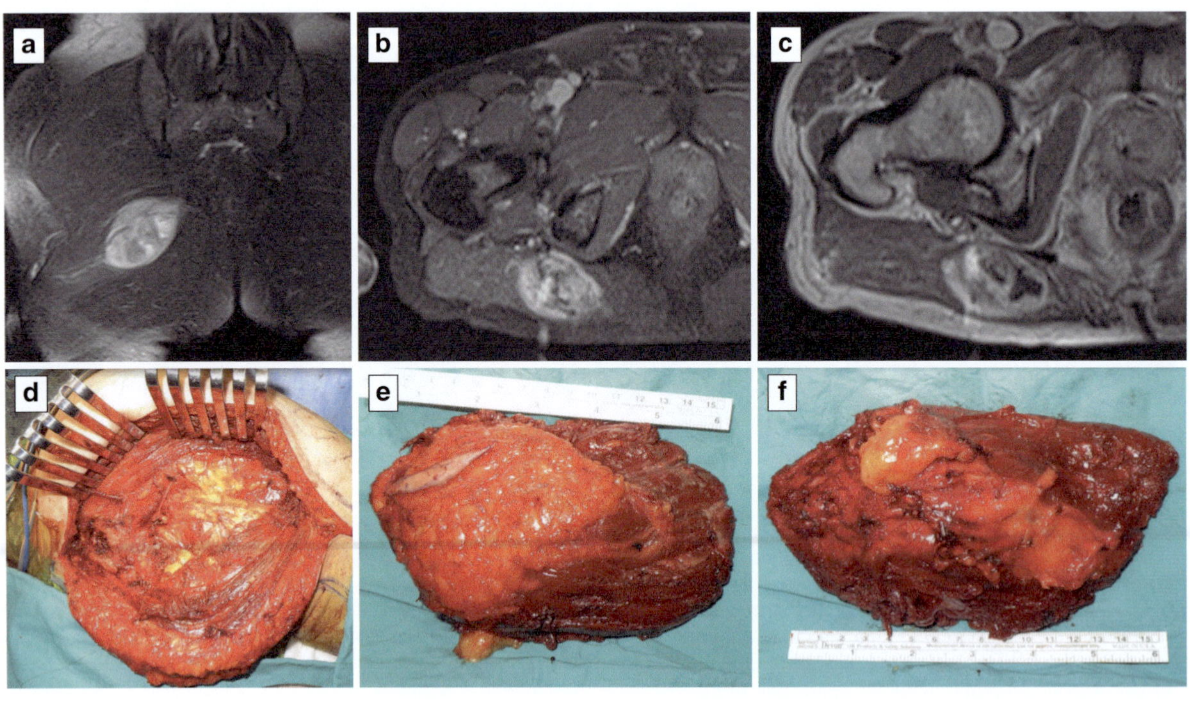

Fig. 15.6 Coronal and axial MR images of the right gluteal region of an 84-year-old male patient show a low-grade myxoid fibrosarcoma, which was confirmed with a core needle biopsy (**a–c**). Although the mass is seated close to the sciatic nerve, adjuvant treatment modalities can be considered ineffective for this pathology regarding margin modification, and wide resection is the only option. Fortunately, the T1 weighted contrast-enhanced axial image shows a dissection plane of fatty tissue (red arrows) so that the nerve can be spared with acceptable safety (**c**). Intraoperative images demonstrate the resection site and the superficial and deep aspects of the specimen, which have been removed with wide margins (**d–f**)

metastatic disease. Resection with "modified margins" denotes either resection following evident shrinkage of the tumor or, in case of neglectable shrinkage, with presumed marginal maturation and fortification by adjuvant modalities. While the components and the timing of margin modifying adjuvant treatment are determined primarily by specific histology, stage, and anatomic localization, there might be more than one reasonable treatment strategy for a given clinical scenario depending on patient-related factors or the treating center's capabilities and experience. Commonly encountered soft tissue pathologies such as undifferentiated pleomorphic sarcoma, synovial sarcoma, myxoid liposarcoma, epithelioid sarcoma, or clear cell sarcoma are often treated within the confines of wide resection with modified margins [15, 16]. In addition to adjuvant oncologic treatment modalities, advanced wound management with special surgical techniques must be considered in limb salvage using margin modification.

A. Neoadjuvant Radiotherapy and Wide Resection

Neoadjuvant radiotherapy and wide resection can be applied in all clinical scenarios involving high-grade soft tissue sarcomas, which:

- are non-metastatic or only have "lymph node metastasis,"
- are resectable with acceptable morbidity at presentation or,
- become resectable with acceptable morbidity following neoadjuvant radiotherapy (e.g., tumors, which are exulcerated and hemorrhagic at presentation).

While some specific histologic subtypes are known to benefit more frequently and in a more pronounced way from radiotherapy, this modality can also be utilized in large, deeply seated, low-grade tumors, which have infiltrative borders and are in contact with vital structures since, for the latter group, any attempt at "wide resection only" carries a high risk of local recurrence or is not compatible with functional limb salvage [15–18].

Neoadjuvant radiotherapy and wide resection are also often indicated for tumor bed resection in patients who present with positive surgical margins following inadvertent soft tissue sarcoma resection and in patients who present with local recurrence [19–21] (Fig. 15.7). However, the feasibility of neoadjuvant radiotherapy in the setting of local recurrence depends on the previous irradiation history of the anatomic site [18, 19].

Neoadjuvant radiotherapy offers the following advantages compared to adjuvant radiotherapy:

1. The total radiation dose is less.
2. The course of treatment is shorter.
3. A smaller volume is irradiated (Late radiation toxicity is less, and functional outcome is better).
4. Treatment planning targets the primary sarcoma.
5. Possible downstaging of borderline resectable extremity sarcomas facilitates limb salvage (Fig. 15.8).
6. Restaging is possible after neoadjuvant treatment but before wide resection.

Major disadvantages, on the other hand, are:

1. Increased incidence of postoperative wound complications, and.
2. Possibility of detecting distant metastases at the time of restaging before surgery, which could invalidate a curative resection attempt.

Based on high-level evidence regarding the advantages and disadvantages of neoadjuvant versus adjuvant radiotherapy, the National Comprehensive Cancer Network prefers neoadjuvant radiotherapy [16].

Wide Resection and Adjuvant Radiotherapy

Wide resection and adjuvant radiotherapy can be applied in the following clinical scenarios involving high-grade soft tissue sarcomas, which are:

- non-metastatic or only have "lymph node metastasis," and,
- resectable with acceptable morbidity at presentation.

While adjuvant radiotherapy can be acceptable in "R0" but close margins, it cannot compensate for R1 or R2 margins following intended curative resection, in which case a re-resection must be performed. Adjuvant radiotherapy can only be justified as a palliative rather than a curative method in cases of positive surgical margins.

Adjuvant radiotherapy offers the following advantages compared to adjuvant radiotherapy:

1. Definitive pathologic evaluation of the specimen, including unchanged histology and surgical margin status, is possible.
2. Postoperative wound complications are seen less.

Although there is high-level evidence in the literature regarding the oncologically safe use of this strategy in limb salvage, the "margin modifying" effect is controversial, at least in philosophical terms [15, 16].

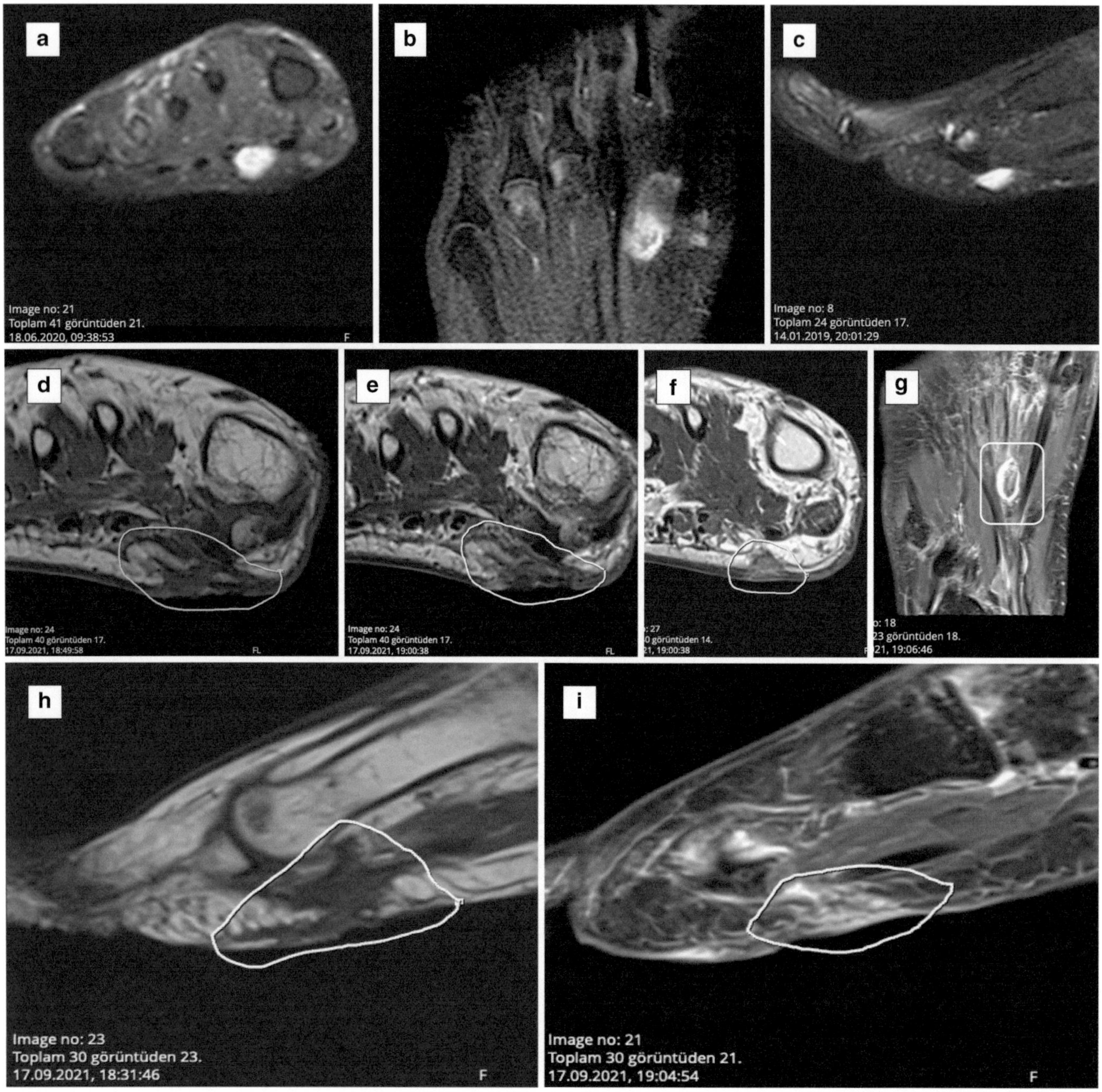

Fig. 15.7 Axial, coronal, and sagittal MR images show a soft tissue lesion in the medial plantar aspect of the forefoot in a 25-year-old female patient at presentation to another institution (**a**–**c**). The lesion was excised with positive margins with the presumption of Morton's neuroma, and the pathology was reported as synovial sarcoma. Axial T1, axial contrast-enhanced T1, and coronal fat-suppressed contrast-enhanced MR images demonstrate the contaminated region from the plantar skin to the flexor tendons and sesamoid bones as well as a more proximal, separate, nodular lesion between the flexor tendons, at presentation to the authors' clinic (**d**–**g**). A tumor bed resection was deemed mandatory due to positive margins in the unplanned index intervention. Although the primary lesion, hence the contaminated tissue volume, was not of considerable size, wide resection with "modified margins" was planned to limit the magnitude of morbidity in a compact anatomic site like the foot, where it is challenging to achieve proper wide margins while sparing function and cosmesis. Hypofractionated neoadjuvant radiotherapy was applied. Sagittal MR images demonstrate the consolidation of the contaminated volume following radiotherapy (**h**, **i**). Wide resection, including the incision scar, the underlying subcutaneous tissue, and the proximal separate nodule, sparing the flexor tendons and the sesamoid bones (**j**–**m**). Clinical images show excellent wound healing with plantigrade weight-bearing and normal function (**n**–**p**). Follow-up MR images at postoperative 22 months show no evidence of disease (**q**, **r**)

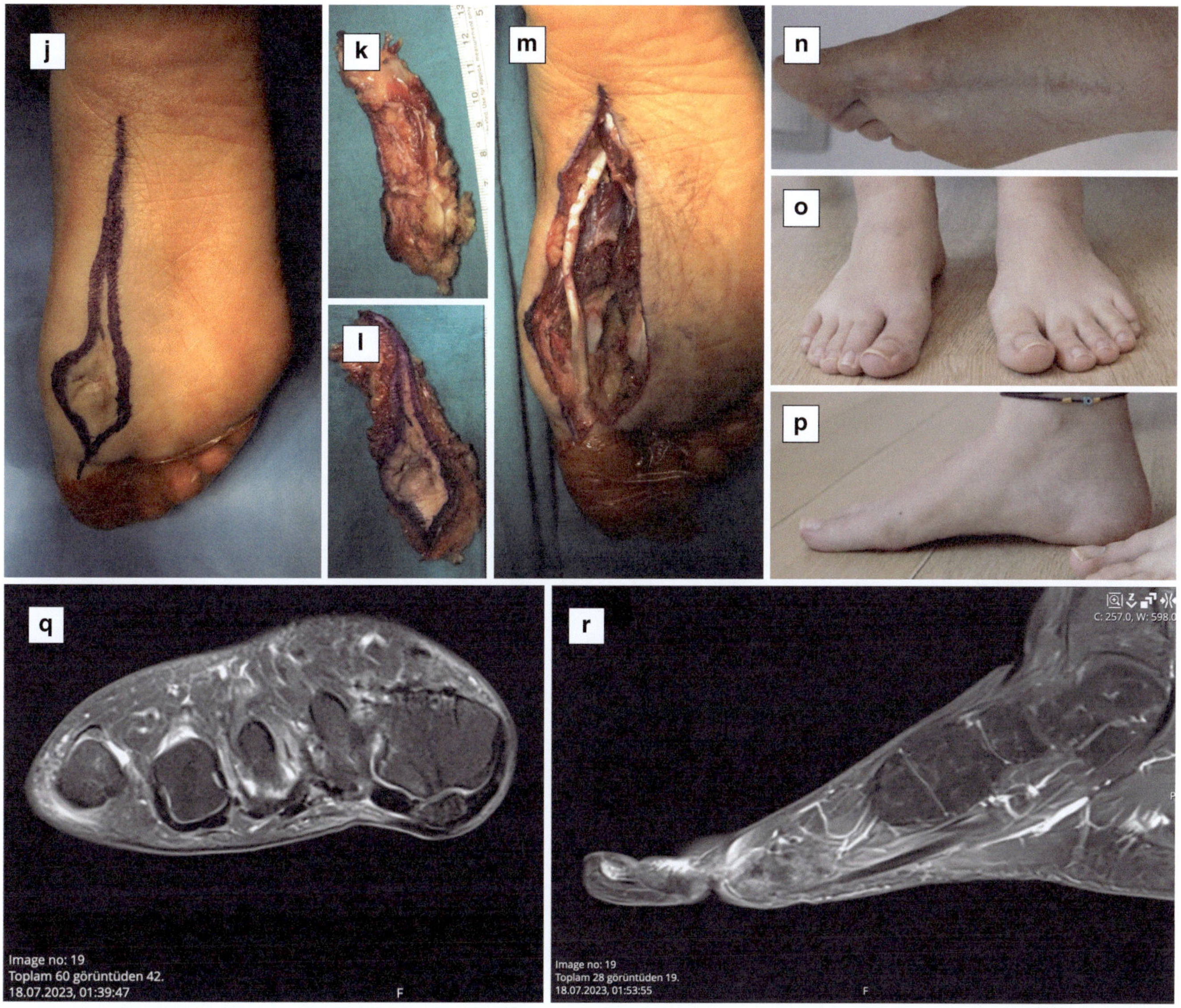

Fig. 15.7 (continued)

Wide Resection and Intraoperative Radiotherapy (IORT)/Brachytherapy

IORT or brachytherapy in combination with wide resection offers the advantages of increasing local control and sparing normal tissue, particularly in:

- small high-grade soft tissue sarcomas,
- frail and elderly patients, or,
- children.

IORT or brachytherapy can also modify "R1" or "close R0" margins following a planned marginal resection to spare critical structures. This is also a controversial approach, which should only be used in centers with sufficient experience with this modality [16, 22].

Neoadjuvant Concurrent Chemoradiotherapy and Wide Resection

This treatment strategy is the most relevant in the following clinical scenarios [16]:

- The presence of a specific histologic subtype in a high-grade soft tissue sarcoma is expected to benefit from neoadjuvant chemotherapy so that more pronounced tumor shrinkage can be achieved compared to neoadjuvant radiotherapy alone. Classic examples include the hypercellular (formerly round blue cell variant) subtype of myxoid liposarcoma or dedifferentiated liposarcoma [18].
- Limb salvage is intended for a non-metastatic high-grade soft tissue sarcoma with a high tumor burden (e.g.,

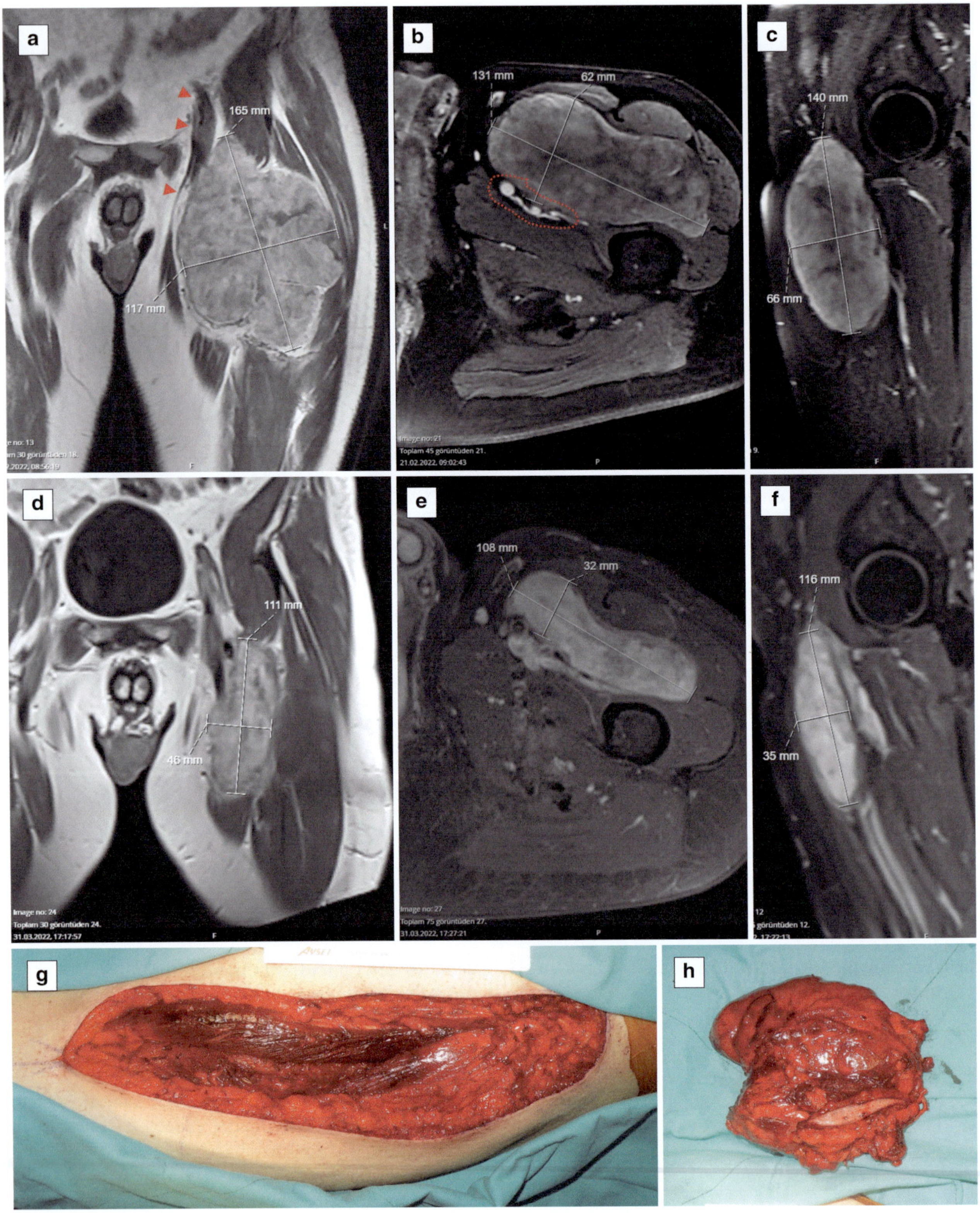

Fig. 15.8 MR images in the first row show myxoid liposarcoma in the anterior aspect of the left hip in a 54-year-old male patient (**a–c**). The tumor location is very critical as it is adjacent to and compressing the femoral neurovascular bundle; red arrows in the coronal image show the route of femoral vessels along the medial border of the mass, while the red-dashed freeform in the axial image shows the compressed vascular structures against the pectineus muscle. A curative resection was intended with modified margins due to the proximity of major neurovascular structures. The myxoid character of liposarcoma enabled radiotherapy as a beneficial neoadjuvant modality. MR images in the second row demonstrate the evident regression of tumor volume while the contrast enhancement was not affected (**d–f**). Nevertheless, wide resection with modified margins was achieved while sparing the femoral nerve and vessels (**g**, **h**). MR images at postoperative 15 months show no evidence of disease with spared and patent femoral vessels (green-dashed circles) (**i–n**)

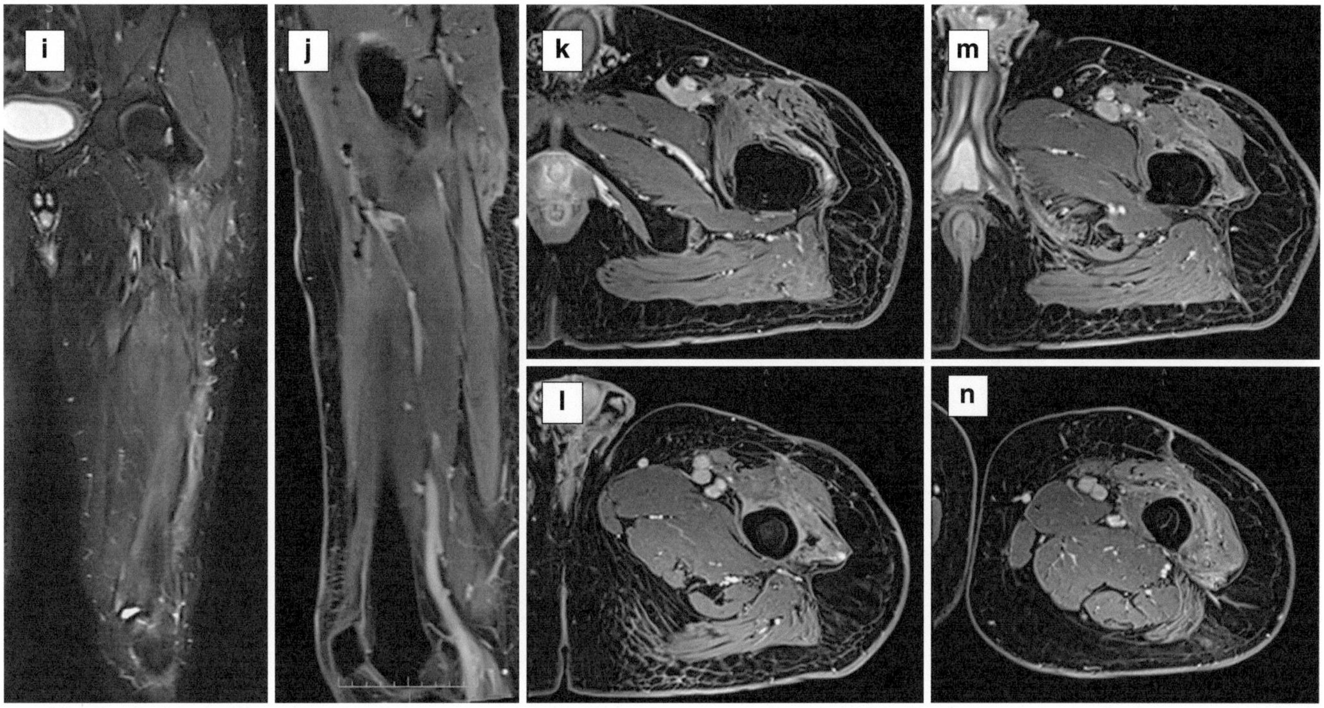

Fig. 15.8 (continued)

AJCC Stage IIIB), and systemic therapy, in addition to local treatment, is desired until the time of curative resection.

- Limb salvage is intended in the setting of high-grade soft tissue sarcoma, which is not resectable with acceptable morbidity. However, neoadjuvant radiotherapy alone is not predicted to make the tumor amenable to oncologically safe resection. Then, concurrent chemotherapy might augment the local treatment (Figs. 15.9 and 15.10).
- Limb salvage is intended in the setting of oligometastatic high-grade soft tissue sarcoma, where the metastases are also amenable to curative local treatment (e.g., pulmonary metastasectomy) and neoadjuvant radiotherapy is also indicated for the primary tumor.
- Non-pleomorphic rhabdomyosarcoma is a particularly chemosensitive group of tumors, and concurrent chemoradiotherapy might be applied as neoadjuvant treatment if neoadjuvant chemotherapy alone cannot make the tumor amenable to oncologically safe resection.

Neoadjuvant Chemotherapy and Wide Resection

This treatment strategy would be best employed in the following clinical settings:

- infantile fibrosarcoma, which is inoperable or unresectable with acceptable morbidity due to size or critical location [23, 24],
- low-risk, localized, non-pleomorphic rhabdomyosarcoma in a pediatric patient with excellent chemotherapy response, thus avoiding late toxicity associated with radiotherapy [16, 25] (Figs. 15.11 and 15.12).

Isolated Limb Perfusion Followed by Wide Resection

This less common treatment modality might be employed to facilitate limb salvage in the setting of high-grade soft tissue sarcoma, which is not resectable with acceptable morbidity at presentation. Depending on the treatment response, it might be combined with neoadjuvant radiotherapy. However, isolated limb perfusion must only be attempted at centers with sufficient experience with this modality [16, 26].

15.1.1.5 Amputation

Amputation is the last treatment option for curative resection, but it might be inevitable even in the most experienced centers [27, 28]. The most common indications are:

- as a life-saving measure in locally advanced unresectable soft tissue tumor, which is lethally hemorrhagic or causes severe sepsis,
- as a measure to increase the quality of life in locally advanced unresectable soft tissue tumor, which causes intractable pain and renders the extremity nonfunctional,
- locally advanced soft tissue sarcoma, which is either unresectable or not resectable with acceptable morbidity despite aggressive neoadjuvant treatment (Fig. 15.13).

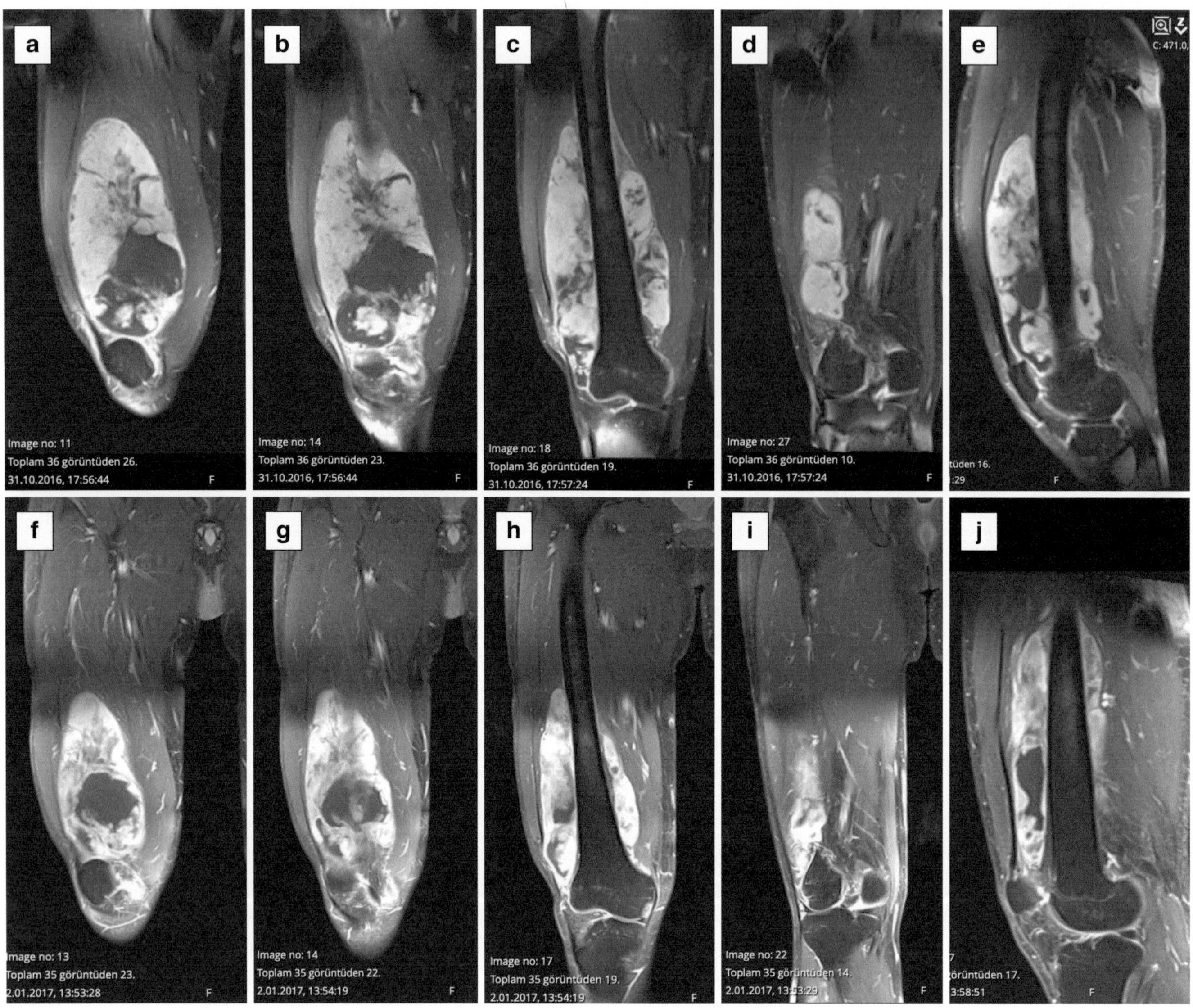

Fig. 15.9 Coronal and sagittal MR images of the right thigh show a myxoid liposarcoma almost encasing the distal two-thirds of the femur in a 27-year-old male patient (**a**–**e**). Function-preserving and femur-sparing limb salvage surgery was intended. While neoadjuvant radiotherapy is strongly indicated to facilitate surgery in myxoid liposarcoma, large tumor volume, extensive peripheral involvement of the femur, proximity to the knee joint, and the extensor mechanism necessitated reinforcement of the neoadjuvant treatment with chemotherapy to achieve the resection goals in this case. Coronal and sagittal MR images in the second row demonstrate moderate regression of the tumor following concurrent chemoradiotherapy (**f**–**j**). Wide resection was performed with extensive periosteal stripping and without prophylactic fixation (**k**–**m**). Axial, coronal, and sagittal MR images (**n**–**q**) at postoperative 5 years show no evidence of disease, while clinical images show excellent knee function (**r**–**t**)

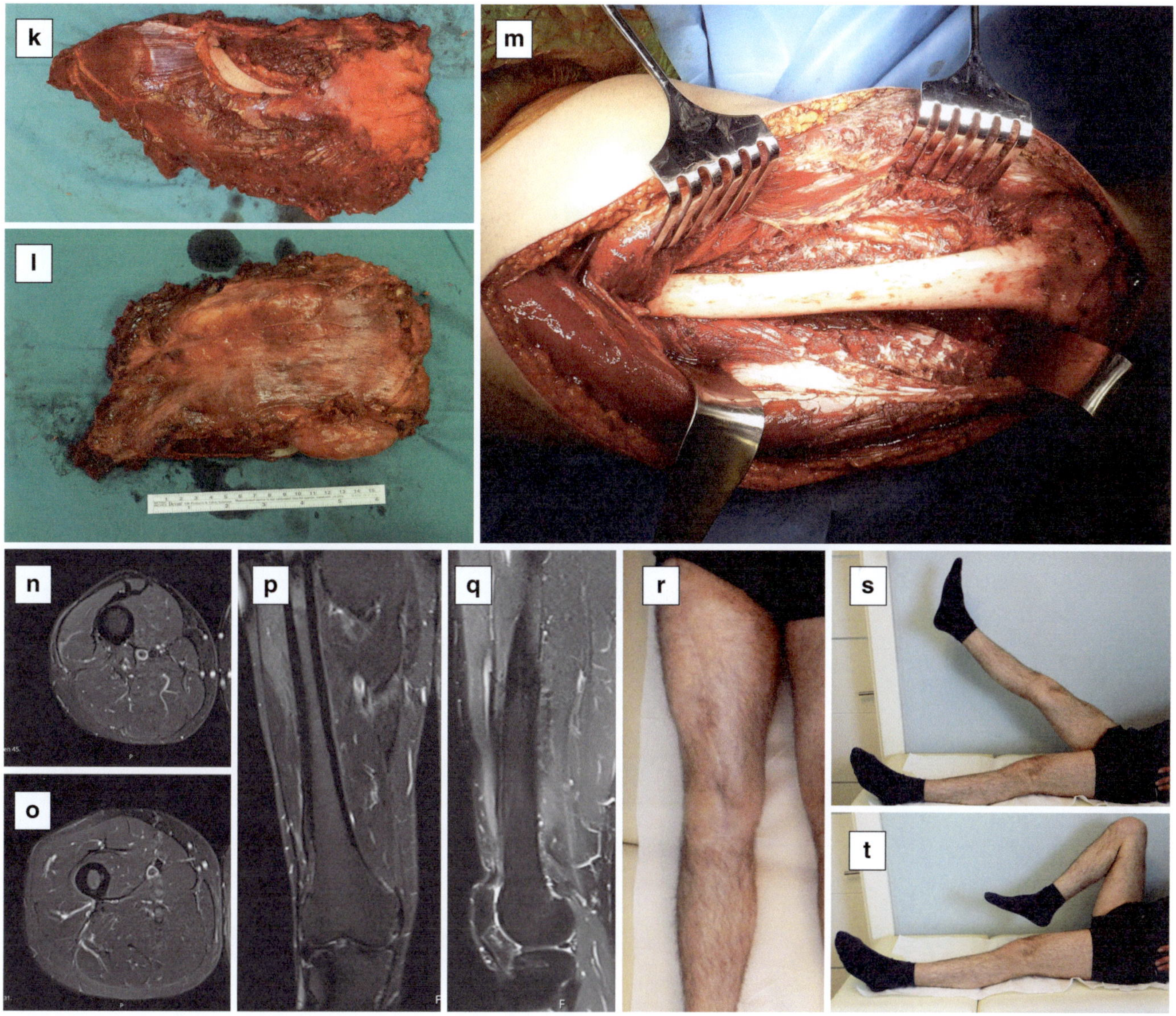

Fig. 15.9 (continued)

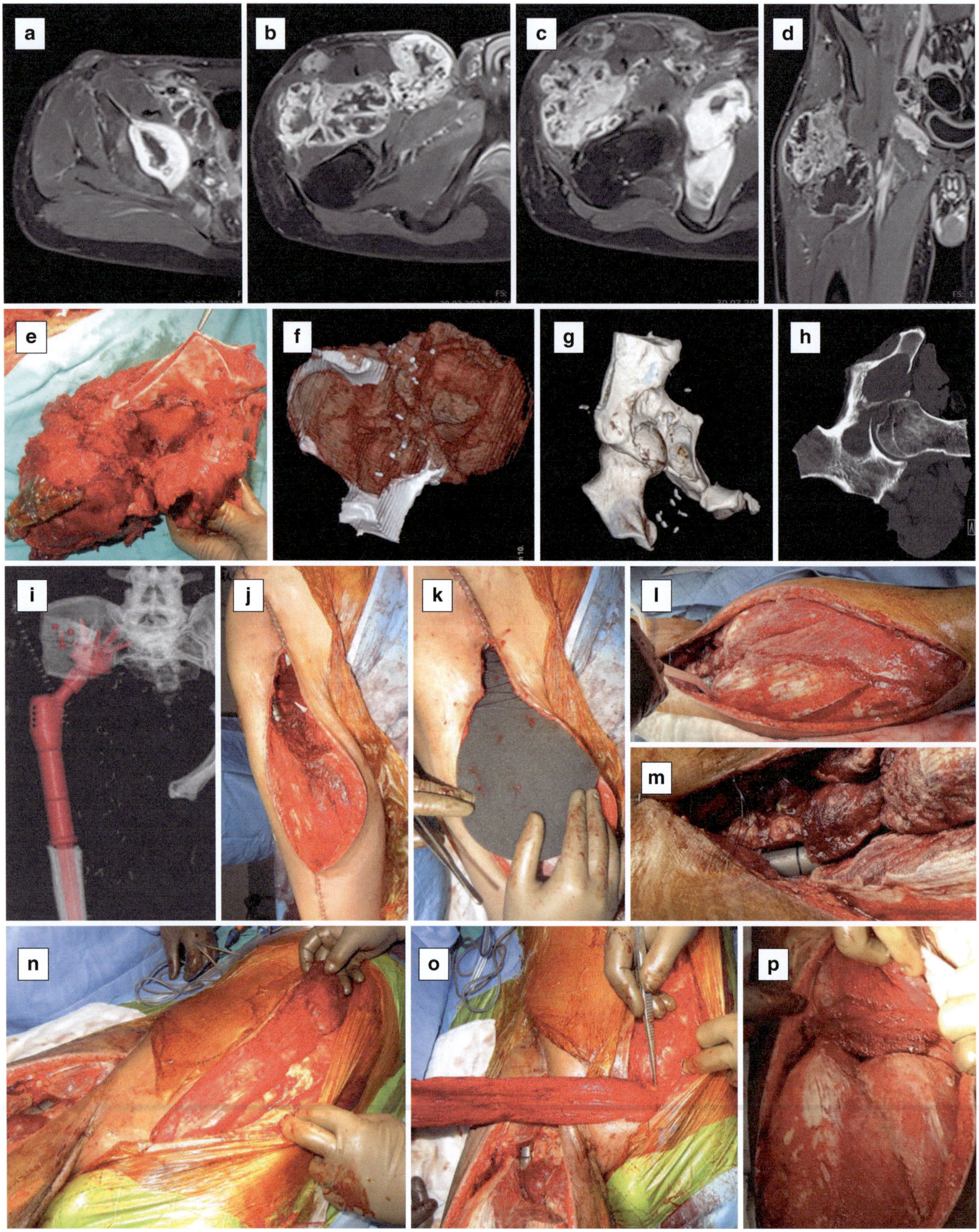

Fig. 15.10 (continued)

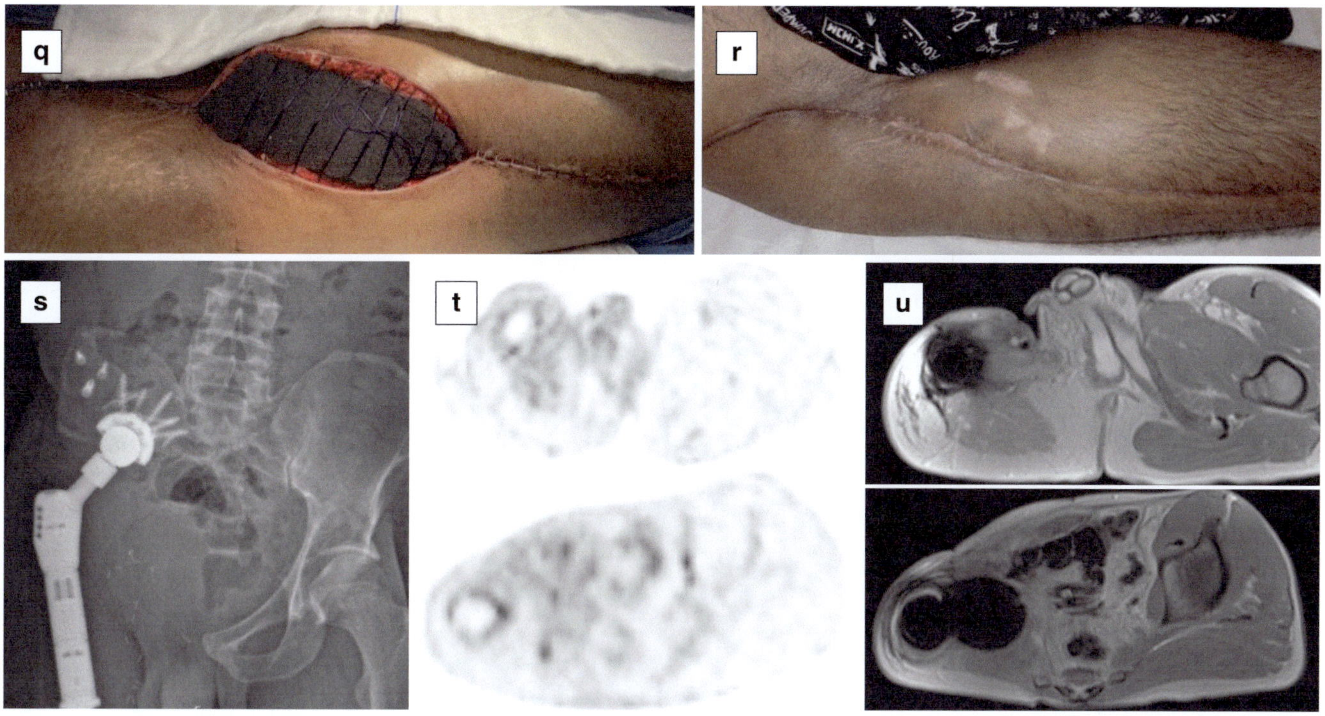

Fig. 15.10 MR images demonstrate extraskeletal myxoid chondrosarcoma with bone invasion in the right hip and inguinal region of a 22-year-old male patient (**a–d**). The patient presented with progression under two cycles of Ifosfamide/Mesna/Adriamicyn (IMA) chemotherapy, which was administered elsewhere, and the patient was subsequently offered amputation. External hemipelvectomy was an option due to the extensive involvement of the femoral neurovascular structures, soft tissues, and osteoarticular structures. However, it was not possible to guarantee local control even with external hemipelvectomy, and the patient refused ablative surgery. An Enneking and Durham type 2 + 3 wide internal hemipelvectomy, including extraarticular resection of the hip joint, ligation of the femoral vein, and megaprosthetic reconstruction of the hip joint and the proximal femur, was performed following margin modification with neoadjuvant concurrent chemoradiotherapy (cisplatin & 37.5 Gy in 15 fractions, equivalent to a total dose of 45 Gy) (**e-l**). Severe swelling of the whole lower extremity, as well as edema around the operation site, was anticipated due to ligation of the femoral vein combined with the adverse effect of neoadjuvant radiotherapy (**j**). Negative pressure wound treatment (NPWT) was applied for delayed closure and damage control (**k**). Massive swelling of the thigh anterior compartment muscles ensued within the first two postoperative days, as anticipated, and the megaprosthesis was exposed (**l**, **m**). A pedicled vertical rectus abdominus muscle (VRAM) flap was utilized to cover the exposed implant (**n-p**). The NPWT was continued for 5 weeks, over which the edema slowly subsided and delayed primary closure was achieved (**q**, **r**). The plain radiograph shows stable implant reconstruction at postoperative 12 months, while the PET scan and MR images show no evidence of local disease (**s–u**). This case exemplifies what can be classified as a candidate for curative resection utilizing modified wide margins and special reconstructive techniques

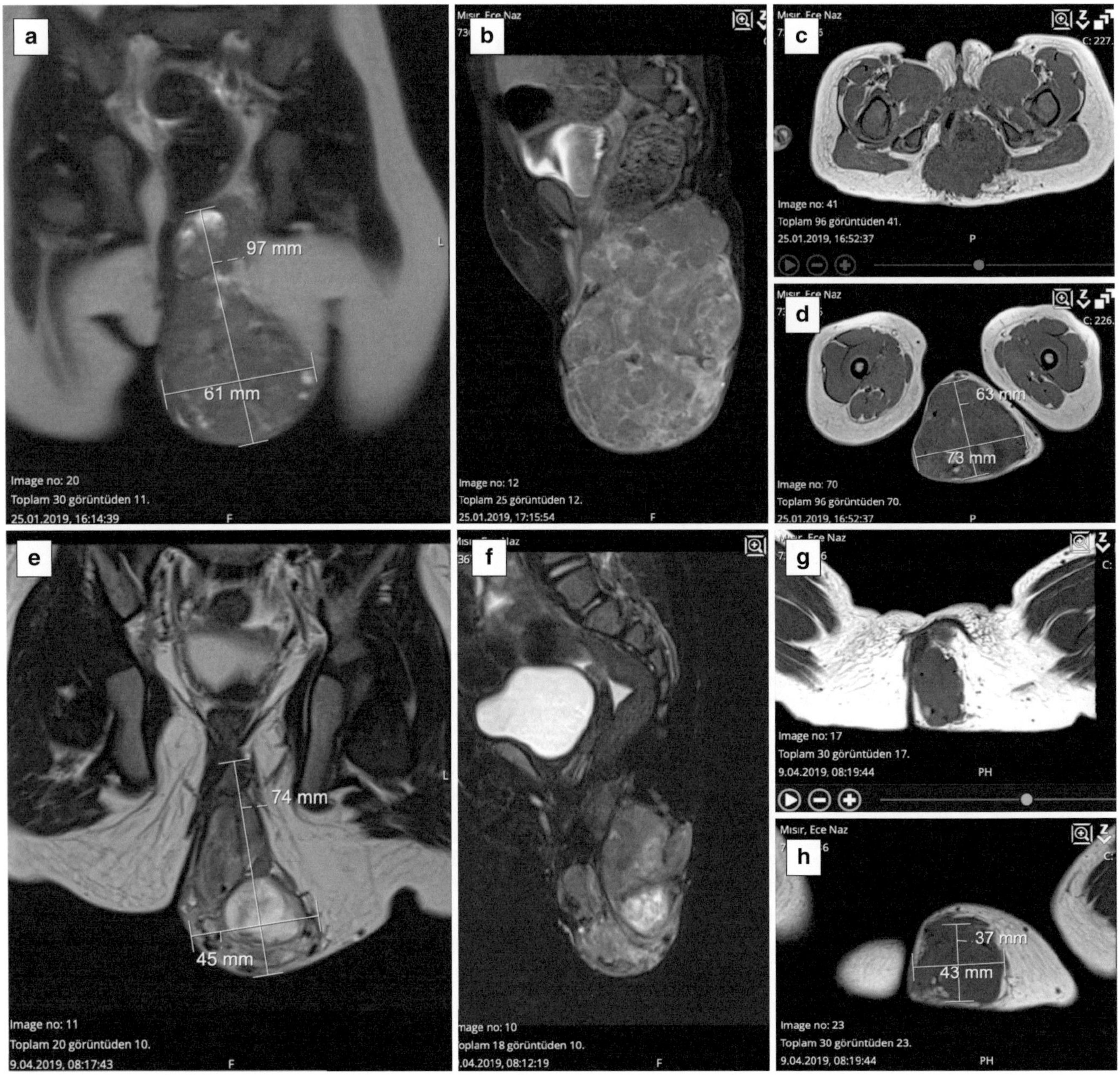

Fig. 15.11 Coronal, sagittal, and axial MR images show a large perineal soft tissue tumor in a 23-month-old female patient (**a**–**d**). Trucut biopsy yielded non-pleomorphic rhabdomyosarcoma. Sparing the vagina and the anal sphincter was only possible through resection with "modified margins." The patient underwent neoadjuvant chemotherapy (vincristine, actinomycin D, cyclophosphamide—VAC) for six cycles, and a significant size reduction was achieved (**e**–**h**). Intraoperative photos show wide resection with close margins (the green-dashed circle shows the anus while white arrows indicate the sphincter and anal canal), as demonstrated by the perineal skin flap reflected to the contralateral side (**i**–**k**). The patient subsequently received adjuvant chemotherapy. The follow-up MRI at postoperative 4 years shows no evidence of disease (**l**–**n**)

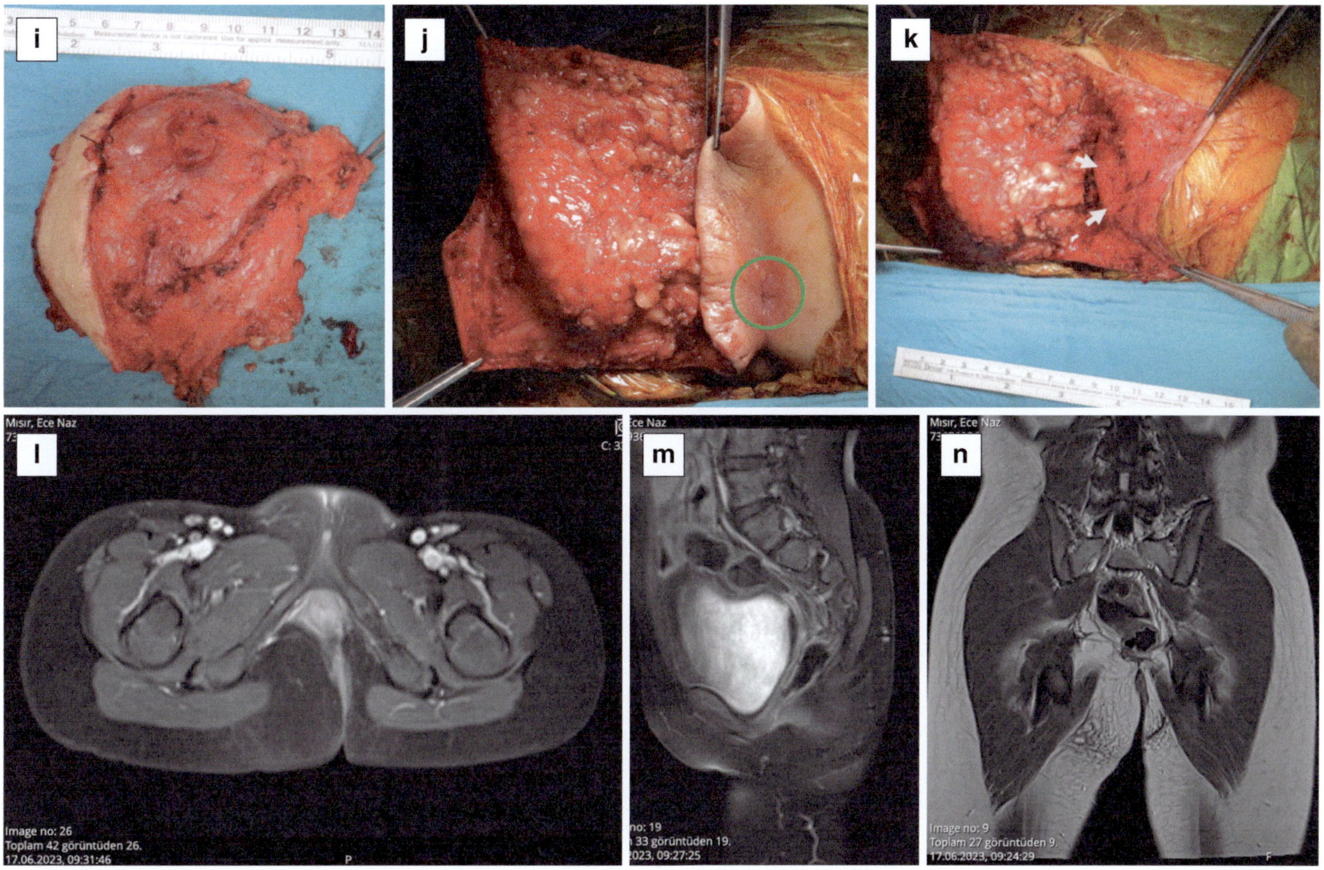

Fig. 15.11 (continued)

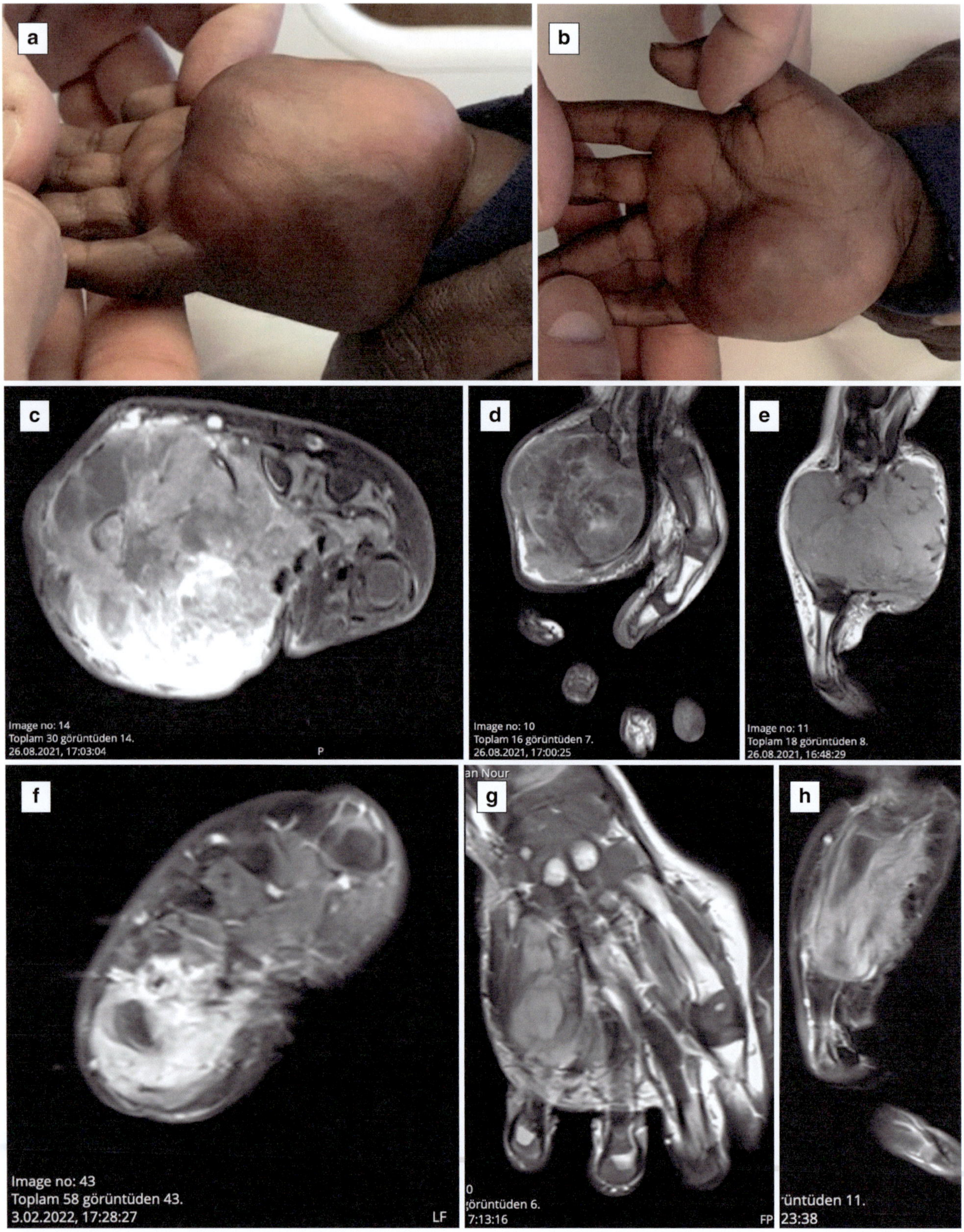

Fig. 15.12 Clinical images show a sizeable tumoral mass involving the ulnar half of the hand in a 22-month-old male patient (**a**, **b**). Axial, coronal, and sagittal MR images show that the tumor has completely engulfed the fifth metacarpal while the fourth metacarpal has been severely compressed (**c**–**e**). Trucut biopsy yielded a diagnosis of rhabdomyosarcoma. A significant reduction in tumor size was achieved with neoadjuvant chemotherapy (**f**–**h**), which facilitated limb salvage surgery with only fifth-ray amputation (**i**–**j**). Follow-up MR images at 13 months postoperatively show no evidence of disease despite close margins at resection, confirming the "margin-modifying" effect of neoadjuvant chemotherapy in rhabdomyosarcoma (**k**–**m**)

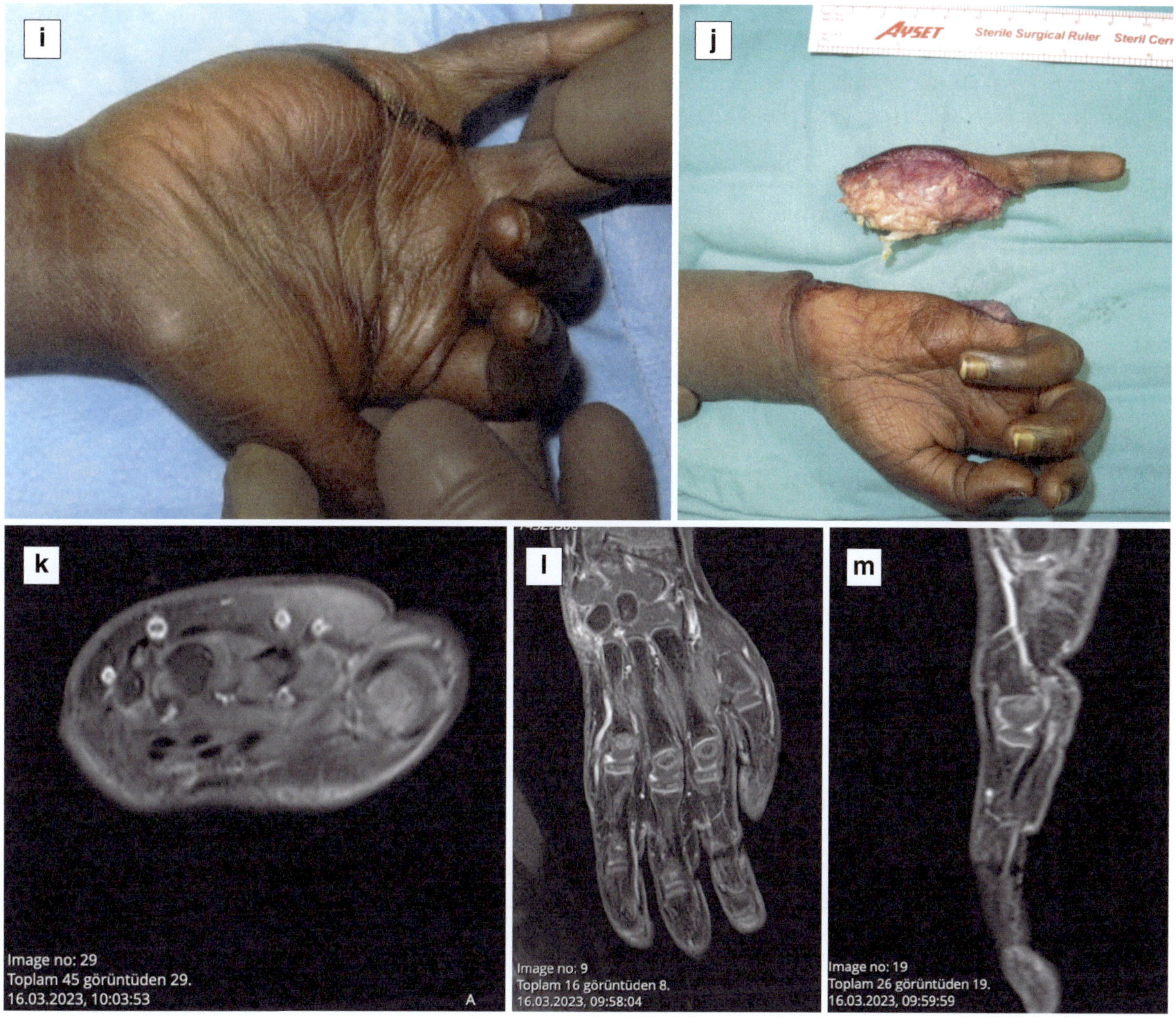

Fig. 15.12 (continued)

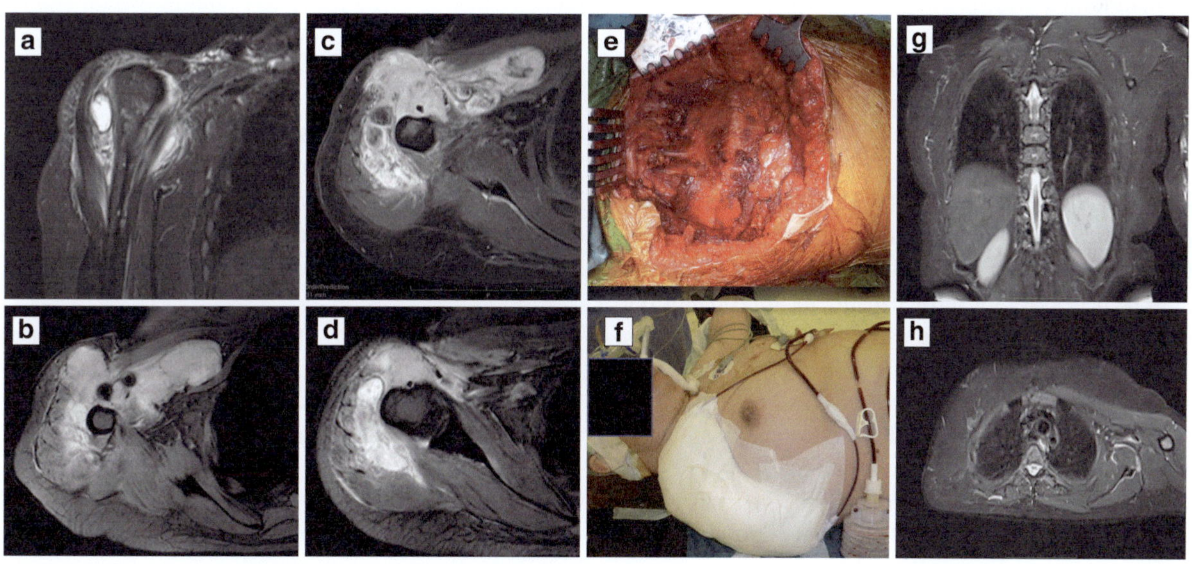

Fig. 15.13 Coronal and axial MR images show locally recurring low-grade myxoid fibrosarcoma with extensive involvement of the soft tissues and main neurovascular structures around the shoulder (**a**–**d**). Limb salvage was not considered feasible since the specific histology and the advanced local stage were incompatible with the "margin-modifying" effects of neoadjuvant treatment modalities like radiotherapy and chemotherapy. Thus, forequarter amputation with wide margins on the thoracic wall was the only safe treatment option (**e**–**f**). Coronal and axial MR images at postoperative 8 years demonstrate no local recurrence, and the patient is metastasis-free (**g**–**h**)

15.2 Incurable Conditions

While the primary goal of the orthopedic surgeon and the multidisciplinary team is always to cure the disease, some clinical scenarios associated with soft tissue tumors fall into the category of "Incurable Conditions" from a surgical perspective. The revised goal of the surgeon and the multidisciplinary team then becomes "managing" these incurable conditions instead of "hopelessly trying to cure" them. The management philosophy in this category requires the clinician to clearly understand what he/she is aiming at and communicate with the patient accordingly since the management strategy is based on:

- accepting and learning to live together with the pathology,
- maintenance of quality of life, and,
- improving patient survival.

Management of incurable conditions is possible through strategies ranging from observation only to multimodal conservative treatment and various forms of surgery.

15.2.1 Conservative Management

15.2.1.1 Observation

Observation might be the primary approach, particularly in benign soft tissue tumors with multiplicity or diffuse involvement throughout the body [3]:

- Multiple lipomas [29].
- Multiple hemangiomas (Mafucci syndrome) [30].
- Lymphangiomatosis [3].
- Neurofibromatosis (NF1/von Recklighausen disease) [3].
- Intramuscular myxomas in Mazabraud syndrome [3].
- Vascular malformations and hemihypertrophy syndromes [31].

It is advisable to map all lesions with appropriate imaging (e.g., whole-body MRI) for future reference. Most detectable lesions will only require continued surveillance, while resection might be necessary for those causing local problems due to compression of other structures or showing progression, which is suspicious for malignant transformation (e.g., from lipoma to liposarcoma or from neurofibroma to neurofibrosarcoma). However, surgeons should refrain from the removal of stable and asymptomatic lesions to avoid unnecessary morbidity. The patients, on the other hand, should be informed about the natural history of their disease and the importance of early detection regarding malignant transformation.

Another major pathology in the observation category is "desmoid fibromatosis." As our understanding of desmoid fibromatosis has evolved, observation of these lesions as a management strategy has become ever more critical. For newly diagnosed desmoid tumors, clinical scenarios where observation is indicated can be summarized as follows [11, 16, 32–34]:

1. The tumor is in an anatomic location, where progression would not be morbid.
   (a) If spontaneous regression is observed, then continued observation.
   (b) If stable, then continued observation.
   (c) If progression is observed, then reassessment of symptoms, functional impairment, and possible future morbidity to decide whether continued observation or surgical treatment.
2. The tumor is in an anatomic location, where progression would be morbid. The lesion is very closely monitored.
   (a) If spontaneous regression is observed, then continued observation.
   (b) If stable, then continued observation.
   (c) If progression is observed initially but the tumor remains stable during close monitorization, then continued observation.
   (d) If steady progression is observed, surgical treatment should be considered for resectable tumors.

Hemangiomas and lymphangiomas in anatomic locations such as hands and feet, where wide resection is not possible with acceptable morbidity and the risk of local recurrence is high, should also be best observed with a philosophy like that of desmoid tumors. Observation of desmoid tumors and non-resectable benign vascular neoplasms in all scenarios includes symptom management [1, 4, 35]. Recurrent, unresectable tenosynovial giant cell tumors, which can be managed symptomatically, are also mandatory candidates for observation (Fig. 15.14).

15.2.1.2 Medical Treatment

While almost all forms of medical treatment used for managing incurable conditions are administered by medical oncologists, not all medications are oncological in the conventional sense. Typical examples could be listed as:

- Sirolimus (immunosuppressant) for lymphangioma (Fig. 15.15).
- Propranolol (beta blocker) for hemangioma (Fig. 15.16).
- Meloxicam (non-steroidal anti-inflammatory) for desmoid tumors.

Systemic chemotherapy with conventional agents has long been the mainstay of palliative treatment in disseminated metastatic disease in soft tissue sarcomas (AJCC Stage IV) [16, 36, 37]. Conventional chemotherapy has also been a

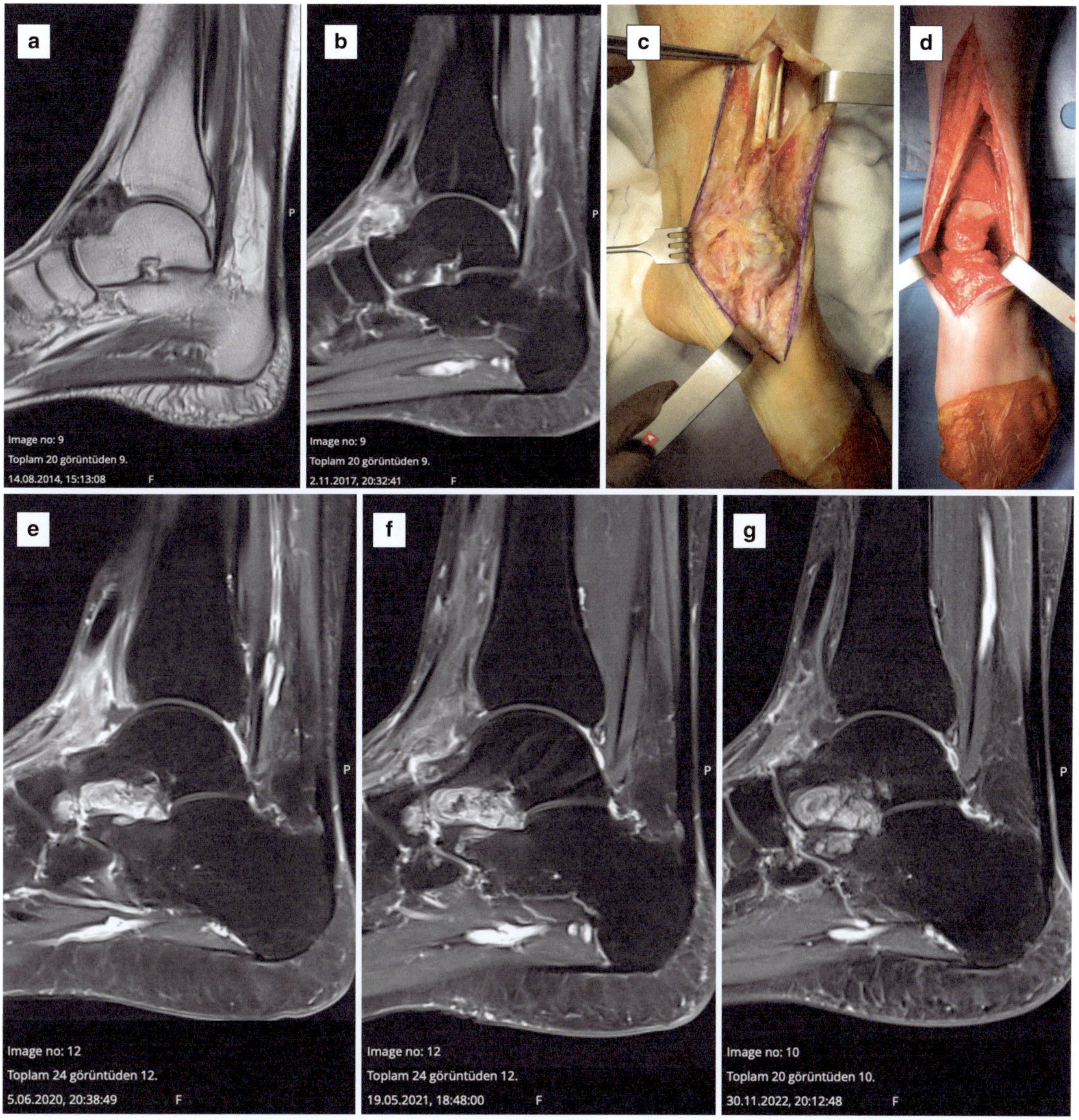

Fig. 15.14 Sagittal MR images demonstrate a tenosynovial giant cell tumor in the anterior aspect of the ankle at first presentation and at the time of first local recurrence following surgical resection (**a**, **b**). Intraoperative images show the recurring tumor and the resection site at the time of the third and last operation (**c**, **d**). However, the patient presented with a third recurrence involving the sinus tarsi, calcaneus, and navicular bone. A trucut biopsy was performed to rule out any malignancy. Any further resection was presumed not to have any meaningful impact on local control while deemed likely to cause severe morbidity since the patient maintained good function in daily activities despite slight discomfort and occasional swelling. The patient, who did not receive any further medical or surgical treatment, was observed for 3 years with a very gradual progression of the tumor (**e**–**g**) and is being considered for advanced medical treatment such as pexidartinib or imatinib

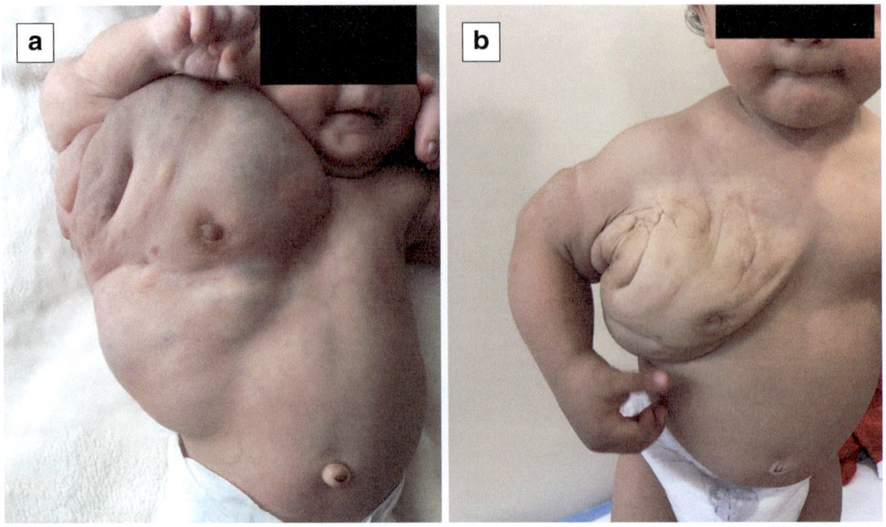

Fig. 15.15 Clinical image shows unresectable chest wall lymphangioma in a 2-month-old female patient (**a**). Since the condition was considered incurable for the foreseeable future, the patient was started on sirolimus and propranolol to achieve local control. The lesion shows dramatic shrinkage 1 year after the initiation of medical treatment (**b**). However, long-term follow-up with possible continued medical treatment, surgical and/or radiological intervention, and physiotherapy will be required. (Courtesy of Prof. Funda Çorapçıoğlu, Dept. of Pediatric Oncology, Acıbadem Maslak Hospital, Istanbul, Türkiye)

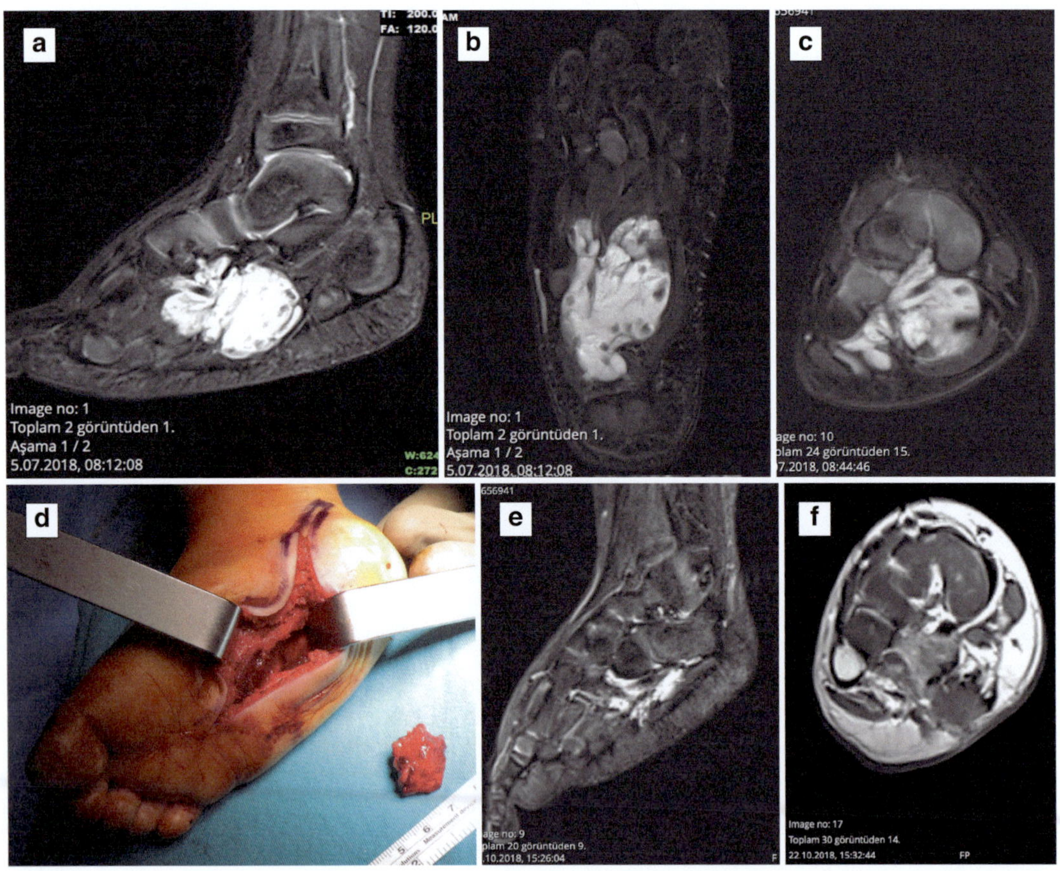

Fig. 15.16 Sagittal, coronal, and axial MR images at presentation show intramuscular hemangioma in the deep plantar aspect of the foot in a 20-month-old male patient with walking difficulty (**a**–**c**). Proper wide resection with curative intent was not considered to be compatible with functional limb salvage in such a young patient, especially for benign pathology. The intraoperative photo shows the resected specimen, which was resected with less-than-wide margins (**d**) and is smaller than preoperative MRI measurements due to emptying of the pooled blood. While the MRI at postoperative third month (**e**, **f**) shows a small residual/recurrent lesion, the patient is followed up with observation under oral propranolol treatment. MRI images at postoperative 45 months (**g**–**i**) show an asymptomatic and stable residual lesion, absence of any foot deformity, and good ambulation with plantigrade weight-bearing (**j**, **k**)

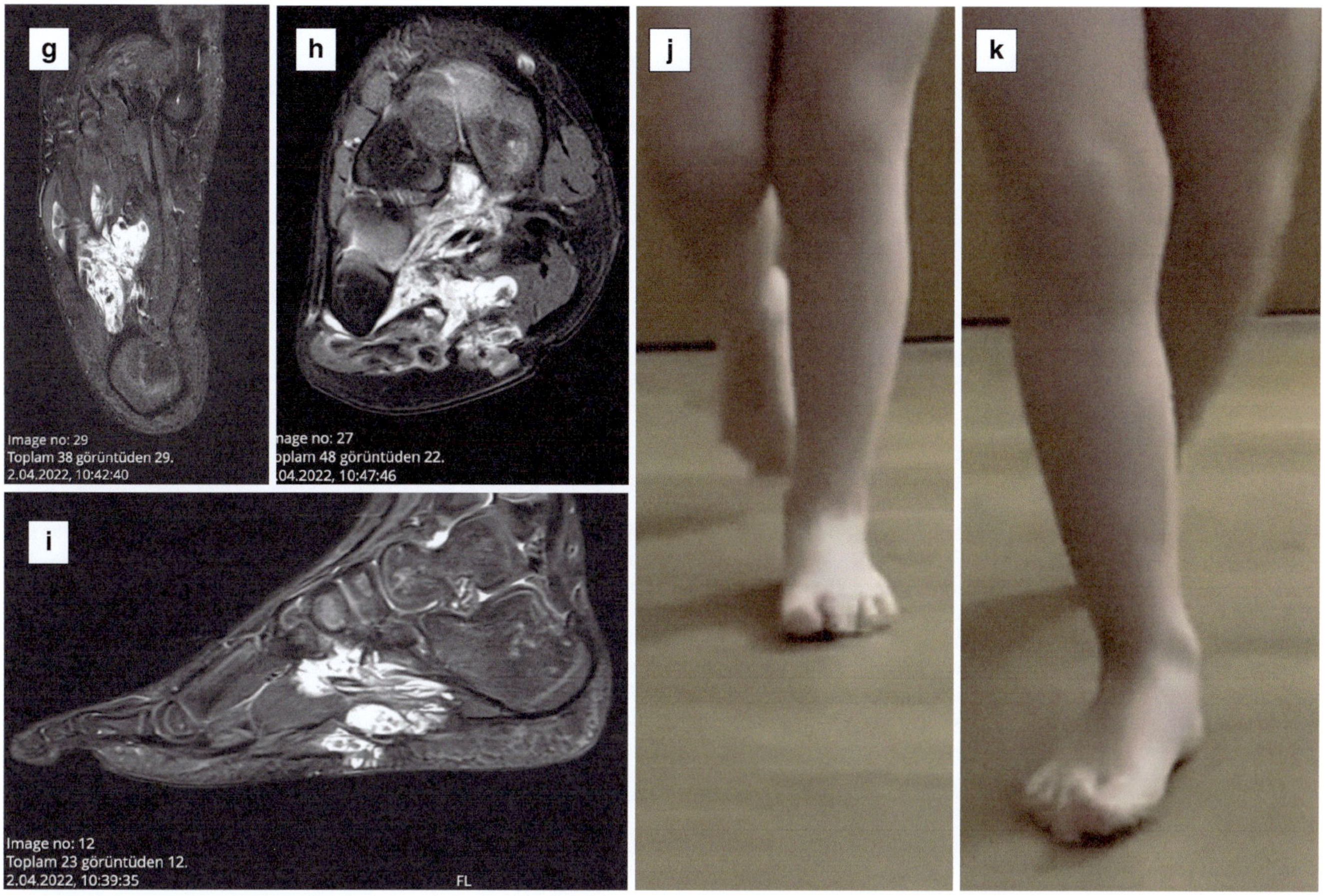

Fig. 15.16 (continued)

part of unresectable, progressive, and symptomatic desmoid tumors [16, 32].

Targeted therapies and immunotherapies are the most recent weapons of medical oncologists in managing surgically incurable benign and malignant conditions [2, 36] (Fig. 15.17). While trabectedin and pazopanib can be cited as the pioneering agents in advanced soft tissue sarcomas, imatinib and sorafenib are effective medications in advanced desmoid tumors, and pexidartinib is beneficial in recurrent and unresectable tenosynovial giant cell tumors [2, 16, 34, 36–45].

15.2.1.3 Radiotherapy

Different radiotherapy modalities are used prevalently and effectively in managing incurable conditions. While stereotactic body radiotherapy is the most precise form of conventional radiotherapy, proton beam or carbon-ion therapies are the most advanced radiotherapy modalities. The most common clinical scenarios are:

1. Palliation in disseminated metastatic disease in soft tissue sarcomas [44].
2. Palliation in unresectable, progressive, and symptomatic desmoid tumors [32, 34]. Radiotherapy has been shown to stop progression and even achieve regression in desmoid tumors (Fig. 15.18). However, the risk of malignant transformation to fibrosarcoma in the long term must be considered for young patients.

15.2.1.4 Interventional Radiology Procedures

Sclerotherapy and embolization can be used to treat symptomatic benign vascular pathologies, which are either unresectable or can only be resected with high morbidity [47]. On the other hand, metastases of soft tissue sarcomas can benefit from embolization and ablation (e.g., radiofrequency) procedures, both in terms of slowing disease progression and pain palliation.

15.2.1.5 Nuclear Medicine Interventions

A typical example of this kind of treatment would be the intraarticular application of Yttrium-90 in unresectable or recurrent diffuse-type tenosynovial giant cell tumors [48]. Theranostics is an advanced form of treatment administered by nuclear medicine specialists and is effective in metastatic soft tissue sarcomas in clinical trials [49, 50].

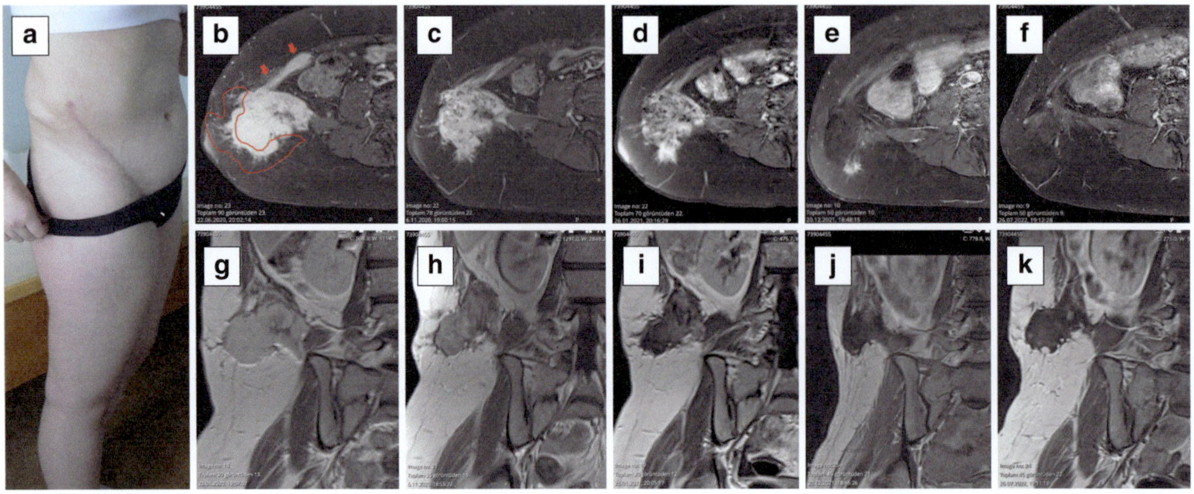

Fig. 15.17 Clinical image shows right ilioinguinal incision scar in a 13-year-old female patient who presented with a locally recurring desmoid tumor in the iliac crest region following resection in another institution (**a**). Fat-suppressed contrast-enhanced axial MR image at presentation shows infiltrative lesion borders (red dashed free-form) and a tail-like extension (red block arrows) toward the anterior abdominal wall (**b**–**f**). While curative-wide resection was theoretically possible, observation under medical treatment was planned to avoid unnecessary morbidity. Surgery and radiotherapy were reserved as salvage options in case of progression under treatment. Serial axial fat-suppressed and coronal T1-weighted contrast-enhanced MR images over a 2-year follow-up period, during which she received first pazopanib and subsequently sirolimus, demonstrate moderate shrinkage of the tumor with complete disappearance of contrast-enhancement (**g**–**k**). The patient continued medical treatment with an asymptomatic residual mass at the time of the last follow-up

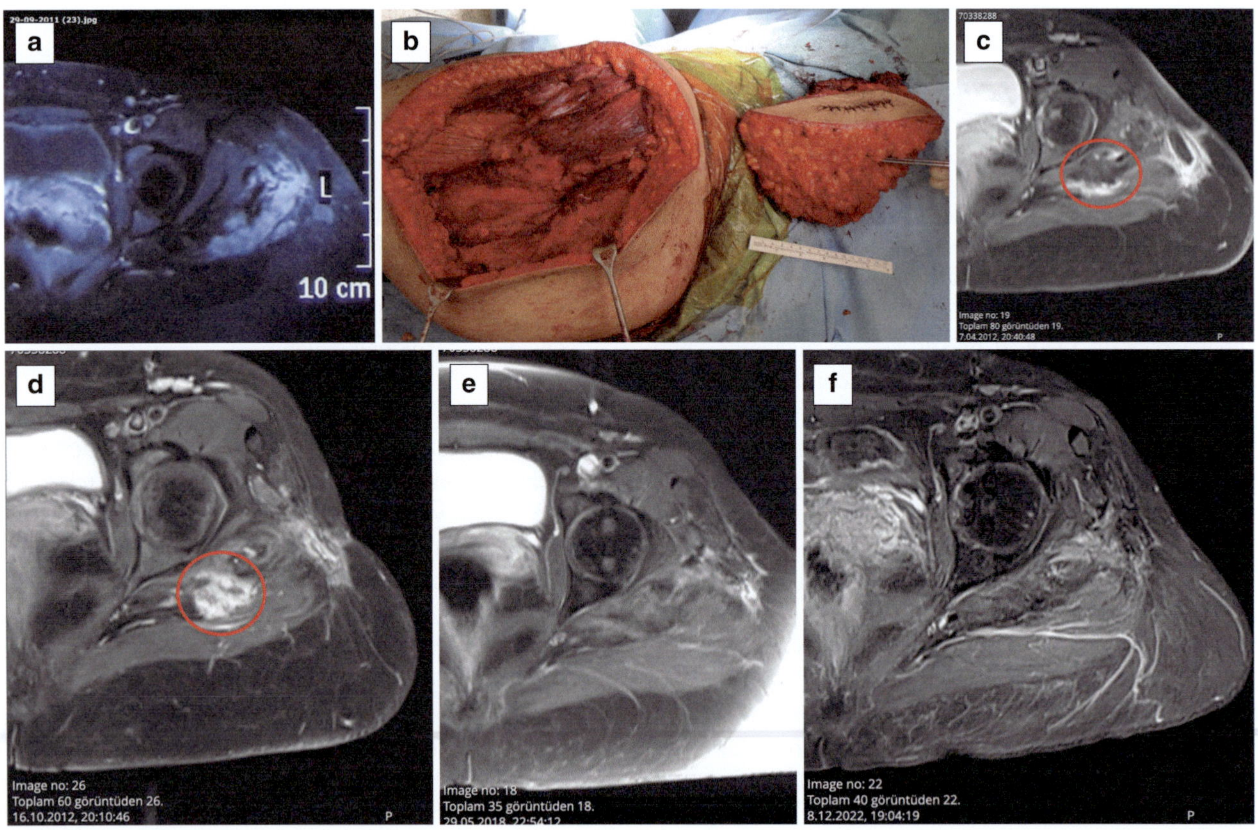

Fig. 15.18 Axial MR image shows a desmoid tumor in the gluteal region (**a**). The 30-year-old female patient presented following a "whoops procedure." While sciatic nerve sparing wide resection was performed (**b**), an asymptomatic local recurrence was observed within the first postoperative year (**c**). The recurring tumor was directly adherent to the sciatic nerve. Due to the unacceptable morbidity associated with the sciatic nerve, wide resection was not considered a reasonable option at this point. A brief observation period under tamoxifen treatment revealed gradual progression (**d**), and eventually, radiotherapy was administered to achieve complete regression of the tumor (**e**). At postoperative 10 years, the patient is still under surveillance without any complaints and with no evidence of disease (**f**)

15.2.2 Surgical Treatment

Even if curative resection of a soft tissue tumor is not possible, surgery aimed at improving the quality of life can be offered to patients in specific clinical scenarios:

15.2.2.1 Intralesional Resection or Debulking Surgery

This is usually performed for a symptomatic, progressive tumor that cannot be solely managed with conservative methods. Classic examples for this scenario can be listed as:

1. A recurrent and progressive desmoid tumor, which compresses the neurovascular structures and/or causes joint contracture [11, 16, 32–34] (Fig. 15.19). Removing as much tumor tissue as possible without causing unacceptable morbidity is the primary goal. While vascular resection and reconstruction might be acceptable if the tumor totally encases the vessels 360°, sacrification of major nerves is not acceptable since this would cause permanent disability. If possible, intralesional dissection of major nerves should be considered. Following such a palliative resection, the spared neurovascular structures can be protected by encasing them

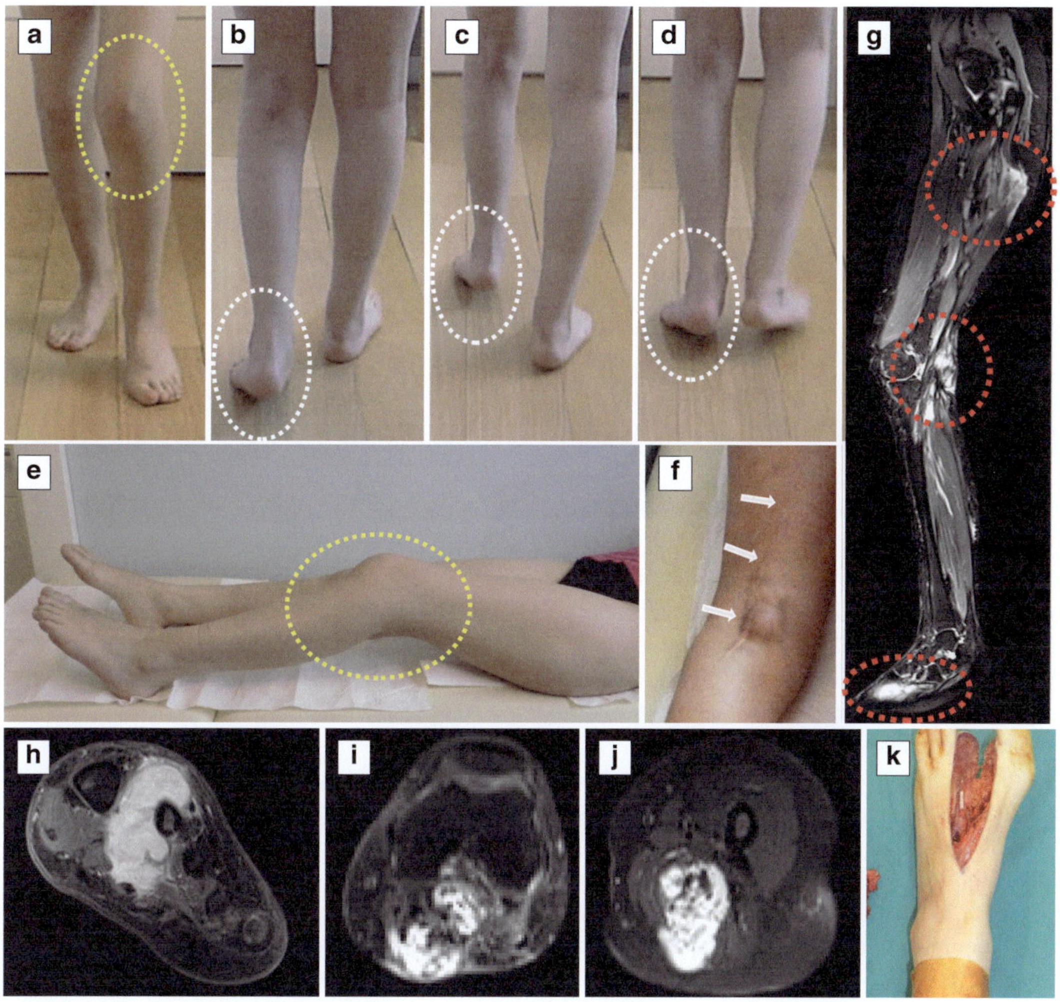

Fig. 15.19 Still images from a video show equinus deformity (white dashed ellipses in Figs. **b**, **c** and **d** mark the absence of heel contact at any point during ambulation), knee flexion contracture (yellow dashed ellipses in Figs. **a** and **e** exhibit knee contracture), and an incision scar extending from the posterior aspect of the thigh to the popliteal region (**f**) in the left lower extremity of a 23-year-old female patient, who presented to the authors' clinic with intractable pain and walking difficulty due to lack of plantigrade ambulation and restricted knee motion. Her history revealed that she had undergone several surgeries, conventional chemotherapy, and radiotherapy for desmoid tumor of the posterior thigh in other institutions. Sagittal MR images of the left lower extremity and axial images from respective levels show locally recurring lesions in the posterior proximal thigh and the popliteal region and a new lesion in her forefoot (**g**–**j**). Second-ray amputation of the left foot was performed (**k**) while a palliative resection was done for the posterior thigh and popliteal region, sparing the sciatic, tibial, and fibular nerves (**l** and **m**) to address the chronic pain associated with tumor compression of the sciatic nerve and to release the knee contracture. A proper wide resection was not considered a realistic goal, and the intervention was accepted as a debulking surgery. A synthetic vessel graft (green block arrows) was applied as an impenetrable sheath around the spared nerves to prevent invasion and to facilitate dissection of these critical structures in case of highly probable local recurrence of the desmoid tumor (**n**). Still images from a video of the patient at postoperative 2 years show the corrected knee contracture and ankle deformity, while the patient states that she is pain-free (O&P)

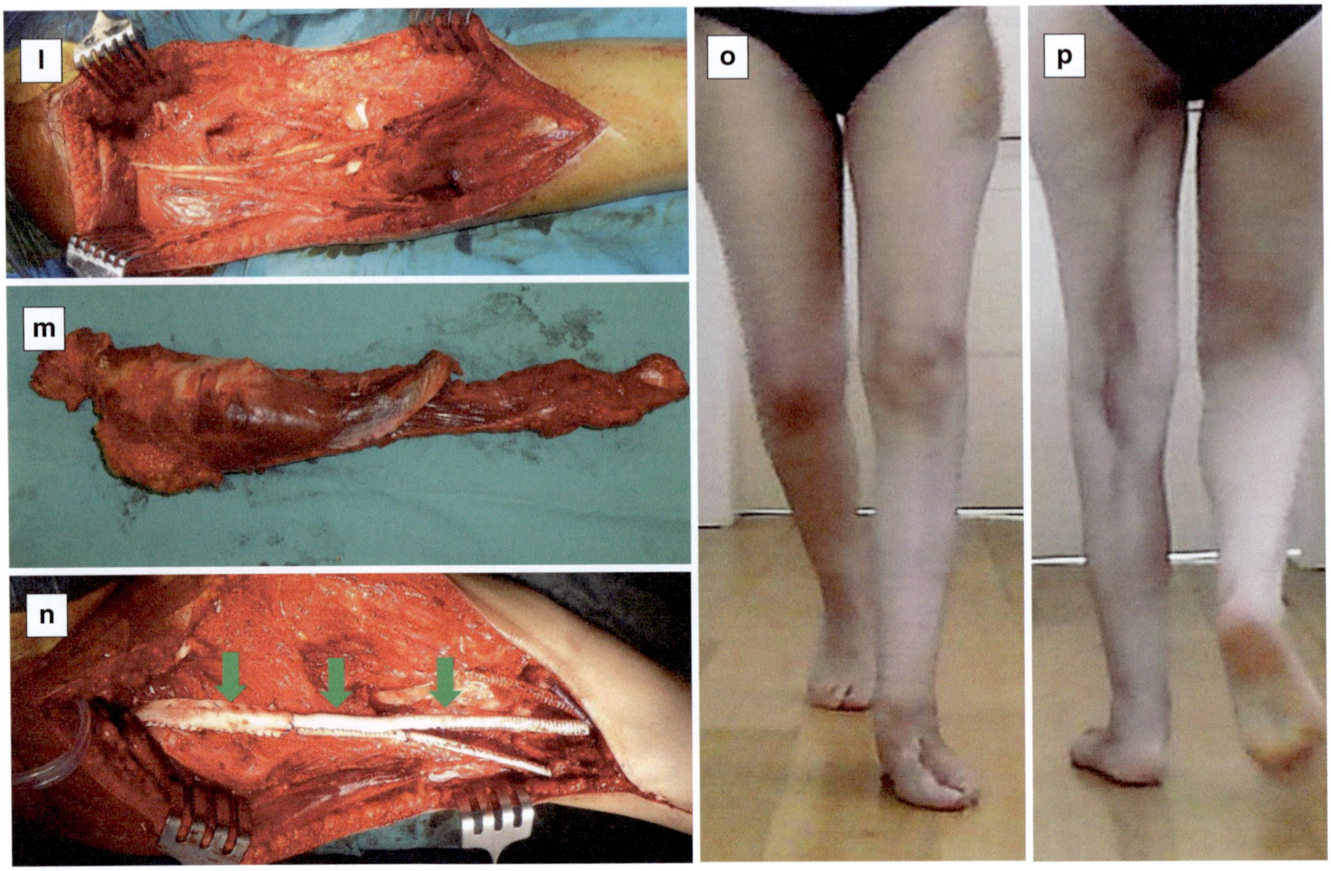

Fig. 15.19 (continued)

with synthetic vessel grafts so that when the highly probable local recurrence occurs, there will be a second chance to spare them with dissection [51]. Also, desmoid tumors spanning the joints should be removed to release contractures. This type of palliative surgery must be complemented primarily by medical treatment.

2. A primary or metastatic lesion with compression of neurovascular structures in an extremity causing severe pain and risk of limb ischemia, or compression of the spinal cord with risk of plegia, in the setting of an end-stage soft tissue sarcoma [2, 16, 52, 53]. This type of palliative surgery must be complemented with adjuvant treatment, especially palliative radiotherapy [46].
3. Recurrent or unresectable diffuse-type tenosynovial giant cell tumor [42, 44]. Open or arthroscopic total/subtotal synovectomy can be attempted. Medical treatment and intraarticular radioisotope injections can be used as adjuvant modalities.
4. A progressive neurofibroma (e.g., originating from the lumbosacral plexus and growing into the pelvis) that causes intractable pain or restricts mobility [54].
5. Intractable tumoral calcinosis is complicated by pain and other mass-related symptoms [55].
6. Severe lymphedema, which restricts mobility. Extensive debulking surgery of the skin and subcutaneous tissue can be performed to improve limb function [56]. Surgery must be followed by aggressive physical therapy and compressive measures.

15.3 Conclusion

Once the orthopedic oncologist, who is faced with a soft tissue tumor, has the answers to the elemental questions of "What is this tumor?" and "Where is it located?," the naturally following questions will be "What should be done with this tumor and how should it be done?". While everyday clinical scenarios almost always show up with twists not included in guidelines or algorithms, classifying these tumors from a general surgical perspective might help the surgeon better navigate the answers regarding what needs to be done and how. We must accept that the surgical classification is subject to change as histopathological classifications are updated and new evidence on the outcomes of a wide range of treatment modalities is reported.

References

1. Gronchi A, Colombo C, Raut CP. Surgical management of localized soft tissue tumors. Cancer. 2014;120:2638–48.
2. Gamboa AC, Gronchi A, Cardona K. Soft-tissue sarcoma in adults: an update on the current state of histiotype-specific management in an era of personalized medicine. CA Cancer J Clin. 2020;70(3):200–29.
3. WHO Classification of Tumours Editorial Board, editor. Soft tissue and bone tumours [Internet], vol. 3. 5th ed. Lyon: International Agency for Research on Cancer; 2020. [cited 2023 May 11]. Available from: https://publications.iarc.fr/588.
4. Erwteman AS, Balach T. Clinical evaluation and management of benign soft tissue tumors of the extremities. Cancer Treat Res. 2014;162:171–202.
5. Gambarotti M. Schwannoma (Neurilemoma, Neurinoma). In: Atlas of musculoskeletal tumors and tumorlike lesions. Cham: Springer; 2014. p. 337–9.
6. Fabbri N. Lipomas. In: Atlas of musculoskeletal tumors and tumor-like lesions. Cham: Springer; 2014. p. 291–4.
7. Rochwerger A, Mattei JC. Management of soft tissue tumors of the musculoskeletal system. Orthopaedic Traumatol: Surg Res. 2018;104:S9–17.
8. Colman MW, Lozano-Calderon S, Raskin KA, Hornicek FJ, Gebhardt M. Non-neoplastic soft tissue masses that mimic sarcoma. Orthop Clin N Am. 2014;45:245–55.
9. Choi KY, Jost E, Mack L, Bouchard-Fortier A. Surgical management of truncal and extremities atypical lipomatous tumors/well-differentiated liposarcoma: a systematic review of the literature. Am J Surg. 2020;219(5):823–7.
10. Thacker MM. Benign soft tissue tumors in children. Orthop Clin N Am. 2013;44:433–44.
11. Kasper B, Raut CP, Gronchi A. Desmoid tumors: to treat or not to treat, that is the question. Cancer. 2020;126:5213–21.
12. Bella GPB, Manivel JC, Thompson RC, Clohisy DR, Cheng EY. Intramuscular hemangioma: recurrence risk related to surgical margins. Clin Orthop Relat Res. 2007;459:186–91.
13. von Mehren M, Kane JM, Agulnik M, Bui MM, Carr-Ascher J, Choy E, et al. Soft Tissue Sarcoma, Version 2.2022, NCCN clinical practice guidelines in oncology. J Natl Compr Cancer Netw. 2022;20(7):815–33.
14. Gambarotti M. Malignant Schwannoma: malignant peripheral nerve sheath tumor. In: Atlas of musculoskeletal tumors and tumor-like lesions. Cham: Springer; 2014. p. 341–4.
15. von Mehren M, Randall RL, Benjamin RS, Boles S, Bui MM, Ganjoo KN, et al. Soft Tissue Sarcoma, Version 2.2018, NCCN clinical practice guidelines in oncology. J Natl Compr Cancer Netw. 2018;16(5):536–63.
16. NCCN Clinical Practice Guidelines in Oncology (NCCN Guidelines®) soft tissue sarcoma. Version 2.2021 — April 28, 2021 [Internet]. [cited 2023 May 11]. Available from: http://nccn.ir/Guidelines/Summary/sarcoma.html#pf23.
17. Allignet B, Meurgey A, Bouhamama A, Karanian M, Meeus P, Vaz G, et al. Impact of histological subtype on radiological and pathological response after neoadjuvant radiotherapy in soft tissue sarcoma. Eur J Surg Oncol. 2021;47(12):2995–3003.
18. Salduz A, Alpan B, Valiyev N, Özmen E, İribaş A, Ağaoğlu F, Bayram A, Bilgiç B, Özger H. Neoadjuvant radiotherapy for myxoid liposarcomas: oncologic outcomes and histopathologic correlations. Acta Orthop Traumatol Turc. 2017;51(5):355–61. https://doi.org/10.1016/j.aott.2017.03.009.
19. Özger H, Alpan B, Aycan OE, Valiyev N, Kir MÇ, Ağaoğlu F. Management of primary malignant bone and soft tissue tumors of foot and ankle: is it worth salvaging? J Surg Oncol. 2018;117(2):307–20. https://doi.org/10.1002/jso.24817.
20. Grimer R, Parry M, James S. Inadvertent excision of malignant soft tissue tumours. EFORT Open Rev. 2019;4(6):321–9.
21. Jones DA, Shideman C, Yuan J, Dusenbery K, Carlos Manivel J, Ogilvie C, et al. Management of unplanned excision for soft-tissue sarcoma with preoperative radiotherapy followed by definitive resection. Am J Clin Oncol. 2016;39(6):586–92.
22. Naghavi AO, Fernandez DC, Mesko N, Juloori A, Martinez A, Scott JG, et al. American Brachytherapy Society consensus statement for soft tissue sarcoma brachytherapy. Brachytherapy. 2017;16(3):466–89.
23. Thacker MM. Malignant soft tissue tumors in children. Orthop Clin N Am. 2013;44:657–67.
24. Brennan MF, Antonescu CR, Alektiar KM, Maki RG. Fibrosarcoma and its variants. In: Management of soft tissue sarcoma. Cham: Springer; 2016. p. 203–19.
25. Chen C, Dorado Garcia H, Scheer M, Henssen AG. Current and future treatment strategies for rhabdomyosarcoma. Front Oncol. 2019;9:1458.
26. Martin-Tellez KS, van Houdt WJ, van Coevorden F, Colombo C, Fiore M. Isolated limb perfusion for soft tissue sarcoma: current practices and future directions. A survey of experts and a review of literature. Cancer Treat Rev. 2020;88:102058.
27. Smith HG, Thomas JM, Smith MJF, Hayes AJ, Strauss DC. Major amputations for extremity soft-tissue sarcoma. Ann Surg Oncol. 2018;25(2):387–93.
28. Stevenson MG, Musters AH, Geertzen JHB, van Leeuwen BL, Hoekstra HJ, Been LB. Amputations for extremity soft tissue sarcoma in an era of limb salvage treatment: local control and survival. J Surg Oncol. 2018;117(3):434–42.
29. Goldblum JR, Folpe AL, Weiss SW. Benign lipomatous tumors. In: Enzinger and Weiss's soft tissue tumors. 7th ed. Philadelphia, PA: Elsevier; 2020. p. 476–519.
30. Prokopchuk O, Andres S, Becker K, Holzapfel K, Hartmann D, Friess H. Maffucci syndrome and neoplasms: a case report and review of the literature. BMC Res Notes. 2016;9(1):126.
31. Schook CC, Mulliken JB, Fishman SJ, Alomari AI, Grant FD, Greene AK. Differential diagnosis of lower extremity enlargement in pediatric patients referred with a diagnosis of lymphedema. Plast Reconstr Surg. 2011;127(4):1571–81.
32. Alman B, Attia S, Baumgarten C, Benson C, Blay JY, Bonvalot S, et al. The management of desmoid tumours: a joint global consensus-based guideline approach for adult and paediatric patients. Eur J. 2020;127:96–107.
33. Wirth L, Klein A, Baur-Melnyk A, Knösel T, Lindner LH, Roeder F, et al. Desmoid tumours of the extremity and trunk. A retrospective study of 44 patients. BMC Musculoskelet Disord. 2018;19(1):2.
34. Kasper B, Baumgarten C, Garcia J, Bonvalot S, Haas R, Haller F, et al. An update on the management of sporadic desmoid-type fibromatosis: a European Consensus Initiative between Sarcoma PAtients EuroNet (SPAEN) and European Organization for Research and Treatment of Cancer (EORTC)/Soft Tissue and Bone Sarcoma Group (STBSG). Ann Oncol. 2017;28:2399–408.
35. Jablecki J, Elsaftawy A, Kaczmarzyk J, Kaczmarzyk L. Surgical treatment of hemangiomas and arteriovenous malformations in upper extermity. Polski Przeglad Chirurgiczny/Pol J Surg. 2013;85(3):107–13.
36. McGovern Y, Zhou CD, Jones RL. Systemic therapy in metastatic or unresectable well-differentiated/dedifferentiated liposarcoma. Front Oncol. 2017;7:292.
37. Singhi EK, Moore DC, Muslimani A. Metastatic soft tissue sarcomas: a review of treatment and new pharmacotherapies. P T. 2018;43:410.
38. Hoang NT, Acevedo LA, Mann MJ, Tolani B. A review of soft-tissue sarcomas: translation of biological advances into treatment measures. Cancer Manag Res. 2018;10:1089–114.

39. Song HN, Kang MG, Park JR, Hwang JY, Kang JH, Lee WS, et al. Pembrolizumab for refractory metastatic myxofibrosarcoma: A case report. Cancer Res Treat. 2018;50(4):1458–61.
40. Dharmani C, Wang E, Salas M, McCabe C, Diggs A, Choi Y, et al. Turalio risk evaluation and mitigation strategy for treatment of tenosynovial giant cell tumor: framework and experience. Future Oncol. 2022;18:1595–607.
41. Stephan SR, Shallop B, Lackman R, Kim TWB, Mulcahey MK. Pigmented villonodular synovitis: a comprehensive review and proposed treatment algorithm. JBJS Rev. 2016;4:e3.
42. Healey JH, Bernthal NM, van de Sande M. Management of tenosynovial giant cell tumor: a neoplastic and inflammatory disease. J Am Acad Orthop Surg Glob Res Rev. 2020;4(11):e20.00028.
43. Tawbi HA, Burgess M, Bolejack V, Van Tine BA, Schuetze SM, Hu J, et al. Pembrolizumab in advanced soft-tissue sarcoma and bone sarcoma (SARC028): a multicentre, two-cohort, single-arm, open-label, phase 2 trial. Lancet Oncol. 2017;18(11):1493–501.
44. Grignani G, D'Ambrosio L, Pignochino Y, Palmerini E, Zucchetti M, Boccone P, et al. Trabectedin and olaparib in patients with advanced and non-resectable bone and soft-tissue sarcomas (TOMAS): an open-label, phase 1b study from the Italian Sarcoma Group. Lancet Oncol. 2018;19(10):1360–71.
45. Staals EL, Ferrari S, Donati DM, Palmerini E. Diffuse-type tenosynovial giant cell tumour: current treatment concepts and future perspectives. Eur J Cancer. 2016;63:34–40.
46. Gutkin PM, von Eyben R, Chin A, Donaldson SS, Oh J, Jiang A, et al. Local control outcomes using stereotactic body radiation therapy or surgical resection for metastatic sarcoma. Int J Radiat Oncol Biol Phys. 2022;114(4):771–9.
47. Dalili D, Isaac A, Bazzocchi A, Åström G, Bergh J, Lalam R, et al. Interventional techniques for bone and musculoskeletal soft tissue tumors: current practices and future directions-part I Stablation. Semin Musculoskelet Radiol. 2020;24(6):692–709.
48. Brennan MF, Antonescu CR, Alektiar KM, Maki RG. Mostly benign/rarely metastasizing. In: Management of soft tissue sarcoma. Cham: Springer; 2016. p. 355–67.
49. Gu B, Liu X, Wang S, Xu X, Liu X, Hu S, et al. Head-to-head evaluation of [18F]FDG and [68 Ga]Ga-DOTA-FAPI-04 PET/CT in recurrent soft tissue sarcoma. Eur J Nucl Med Mol Imaging. 2022;49(8):2889–901.
50. Delage JA, Faivre-Chauvet A, Fierle JK, Gnesin S, Schaefer N, Coukos G, et al. 177Lu radiolabeling and preclinical theranostic study of 1C1m-Fc: an anti-TEM-1 scFv-Fc fusion protein in soft tissue sarcoma. EJNMMI Res. 2020;10(1):98.
51. Ozger H. Preventing neurovascular invasion in desmoid tumors. Acta Orthop Traumatol Turc. 2013;47(4):286–90.
52. Smolle MA, van Praag VM, Posch F, Bergovec M, Leitner L, Friesenbichler J, et al. Surgery for metachronous metastasis of soft tissue sarcoma—a magnitude of benefit analysis using propensity score methods. Eur J Surg Oncol. 2019;45(2):242–8.
53. Krishnan CK, Kim HS, Park JW, Han I. Outcome after surgery for extremity soft tissue sarcoma in patients presenting with metastasis at diagnosis. Am J Clin Oncol. 2018;41(7):681–6.
54. Ikuta K, Nishida Y, Sakai T, Koike H, Ito K, Urakawa H, et al. Surgical treatment and complications of deep-seated nodular plexiform neurofibromas associated with neurofibromatosis type 1. J Clin Med. 2022;11(19):5695.
55. Campanacci M. Tumoral calcinosis. In: Bone and soft tissue tumors: clinical features, imaging, pathology and treatment. Vienna: Springer; 1999. p. 1257–63.
56. Cormier JN, Rourke L, Crosby M, Chang D, Armer J. The surgical treatment of lymphedema: a systematic review of the contemporary literature (2004–2010). Ann Surg Oncol. 2012;19(2):642–51.

The Concept of Surgical Margins from a Surgical Perspective

16

Ajay Puri

In the world of surgical oncology—Biology is King; selection of cases is Queen, and the technical details of surgical procedures are princes and princesses of the realm who frequently try to overthrow the powerful forces of the King and Queen, usually to no long-term avail, although with some temporary apparent victories.—Blake Cady, MD [1].

While overall outcomes are largely influenced by the inherent biology of the soft tissue sarcoma and the stage at presentation, improved local control can still be influenced by the surgeon by adequate/inadequate oncologic resection. A positive surgical margin after resection of an extremity soft tissue sarcoma is a well-documented risk factor for local recurrence. Hence, it is important to plan and execute surgery to achieve adequate surgical margins.

Sarcomas respect anatomical borders and local anatomical structures influence tumor growth by setting natural boundaries to spread. Anatomic compartments present natural barriers to occult tumor extension (Fig. 16.1). In soft tissues, the barriers are the major fascial septa and the tendinous origins and insertions of muscles. Sarcomas grow along the path of least resistance and initially extend within the compartment they arise from. At a later stage with advancing disease, they violate their compartmental barriers and become extra compartmental. Sarcomas are not enclosed by a true capsule but are generally surrounded by a pseudocapsule or reactive zone. High-grade sarcomas have a poorly defined reactive zone that may be locally infiltrated by microscopic tumor nodules leading to satellite lesions in the reactive zone and skip lesions at some distance from the tumor in the surrounding normal tissues. The principal goal of adequate oncologic "wide" resection is obtaining long term local control. It has been well demonstrated that the presence of soft tissue or dense regular connective tissue at the margins of resection is associated with a significantly decreased incidence of local recurrence compared to a margin composed of pseudocapsular tissue. Recognizing the potential of this reactive zone, satellite lesions and skip lesions to jeopardize local control even after a seemingly adequate resection is the key to reducing local

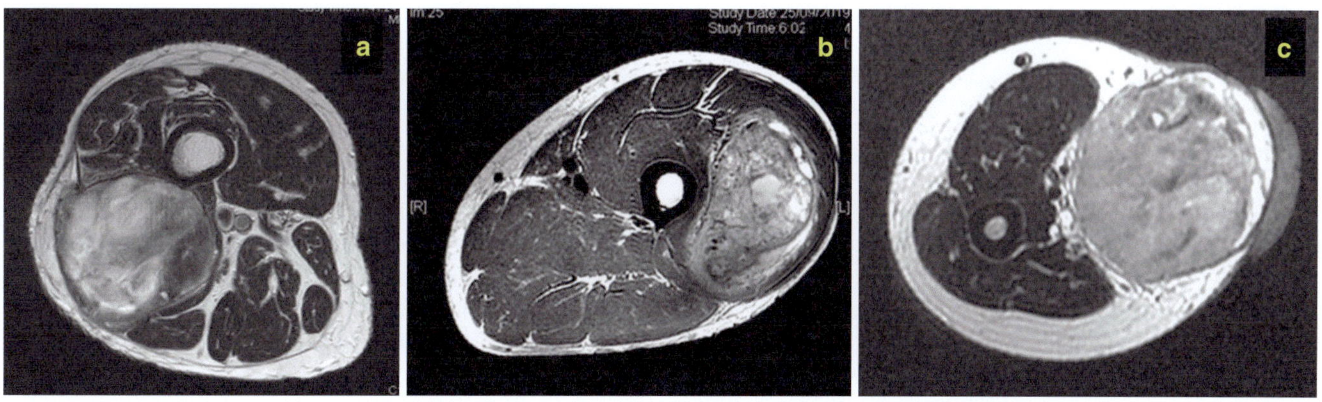

Fig. 16.1 Sarcomas respect anatomical borders and grow along the path of least resistance, initially restricting themselves to within the compartment they arise from. Naturally occurring tissue that has resistance against tumor invasion (fascia, septae) presents "oncologic" barriers to tumor spread—medial thigh (**a**), lateral thigh (**b**), medial arm (**c**)

A. Puri (✉)
Department of Surgical Oncology, Tata Memorial Hospital, Mumbai, Maharashtra, India
e-mail: docpuri@gmail.com

H. Özger et al. (eds.), *Diagnosis and Treatment of Soft Tissue Tumors*, https://doi.org/10.1007/978-3-031-77061-6_16

failure by including uninfiltrated surrounding normal tissue outside of the pseudocapsule in the surgical resection.

A simple system that uses a dichotomous terminology in which the presence or absence of tumor cells at the margin of the excised tissue specimen indicates positive or negative margins would not be representative of the various nuances that are now prevalent in planning and reporting margins. Based on the relationship of the dissection plane relative to the tumor and its pseudocapsule, Enneking described four types of surgical excisions [2] (Table 16.1).

Though inadequate surgical resection with involved margins has been demonstrated to be a poor prognostic factor by multiple authors, there is no consistent correlation between incremental margin width and local control. Authors have defined varying quantitative distances that would maximize the possibility of achieving tumor free margins. Current guidelines recommend resection with a negative surgical margin, with lack of consensus regarding the width of that margin or a standard definition of a negative margin. The surgeon also needs to balance the potential morbidity of including adjoining adjacent critical structures (major blood vessels, nerves, bony structures) while striving to achieve negative margins.

The circumferential margin assessment of the tumor is prone to imperfection because the soft tissue around the resected tumor tends to collapse and adopt its inherent shape when not under continuous tension. This results in discordance between the intraoperative perception of the surgeon and pathologic evaluation of the gross surgical margin [3]. Hence, it is best that resection specimens are delivered fresh at the earliest to the reporting pathologist with multiplanar orientation of the specimen by the surgeon. Marking the anticipated closest clinical margin with ink by the surgeon for focused pathologic assessment and interaction between the surgeon and pathologist can further help the accuracy of margin reporting. The use of frozen section analysis for margins is time consuming and technically challenging and is not commonly practiced.

Table 16.1 Types of surgical excision: Enneking

Margin	Surgical procedure	Result
Intralesional	Piecemeal debulking of the tumor or tumor excision in multiple bits	This leaves behind gross macroscopic disease
Marginal	The tumor is shelled out en bloc or through the pseudocapsule or reactive zone	This may leave residual "satellite" lesions in the vicinity of the tumor
Wide	En bloc excision within the same compartment with a cuff of normal tissue around the tumor	May occasionally leave lesions within the same compartment at a distance from the main tumor if these are not recognized pre operatively by imaging
Radical	Extracompartmental en bloc excision of the entire compartment	No residual local disease remains

While the concept of adequate "quantitative" margins is still relevant, the importance of adequate "qualitative" margins is equally important where native anatomy may not always permit conventionally adequate "quantitative" margins. The ability of different tissue types to resist penetration by the microscopic tumor cells outside of the sarcoma pseudocapsule varies. While fat and muscle are more readily invaded by tumor extension, fascia and periosteum offer better "oncologic" barriers.

Kawaguchi's concept of "barrier effects" has helped surgeons to better understand adequacy of resection margins and their co relation with local control [4]. Kawaguchi converted anatomical structures (any tissue that has resistance against tumor invasion like muscle fascia, joint capsule, tendon, tendon sheath, epineurium and vascular sheath) into definitive thickness of normal tissue and classified them as either a thick barrier or a thin barrier. For purposes of margin evaluation, a thick barrier was equivalent of 3 cm thickness of normal tissue, a thin barrier was considered to be 2 cm. By translating these barrier effects into concrete distance equivalents, oncologically safe surgery can be planned at sites where barriers exist by using margins less than those mandated by conventional quantitative true physical distance.

Before planning any intervention, appropriate imaging and a biopsy are essential investigations. The principles of biopsy should always be respected with all local imaging being completed prior to biopsy. A contrast-enhanced MRI is the preferred method for limb lesions because of its multiplanar imaging capability and excellent tissue contrast. MRI helps to evaluate the extent of the lesion, identify invasion of the compartments, plan the best route and area for biopsy (avoid necrotic areas) and delineate the relation of the tumor to the neurovascular bundle and adjacent anatomic landmarks. It helps categorize tumor margins as well defined (clear and sharp) or ill-defined with an infiltrative growth pattern. MRI can also identify the tail sign (a thick aponeurotic enhancement) characteristic of some tumors, differentiate between the tumor and peritumoral edema, and recognize peritumoral enhancement beyond the apparent tumor borders. These imaging indicators reflect a propensity to spread in surrounding tissues, thus sensitizing the surgeon to be cognizant of this while planning the planes of dissection when resecting the tumor. Occasionally, a CT scan may better delineate cortical erosion or a reactive periosteal reaction in lesions that closely abut the bone.

The entire biopsy tract needs to be excised at definitive surgery; hence, the position of biopsy incision is critical and must always be in the line of planned definitive surgery. A core needle biopsy is the method preferred by many surgeons.

The biopsy site must be clearly documented to enable easy identification for excision at definitive surgery.

Preoperative planning is vital. Adequate oncological resection with appropriate margins needs to be ensured with due consideration given to imaging studies, anatomic landmarks and the histopathology of the tumor. Resections may need to be tailored based on the proximity of anatomical structures and histologic subtype [5]. While in an atypical lipomatous tumor it may be acceptable to do a marginal resection (Fig. 16.2), a myxofibroma with an infiltrative growth pattern (tail sign) may require wider margins up to 3 cm or beyond.

Relatively few soft tissue sarcomas are able to penetrate cortical bone (Fig. 16.3). Unless there is clear invasion, extremity soft tissue sarcomas patients can be spared bone resection, and the periosteum is an adequate surgical margin for sarcoma excision (Fig. 16.4) [6].

Unless directly invaded or encased, an attempt can be made to preserve critical structures (such as major nerves and blood vessels). Dissection through the epineurium can often preserve the nerve while excision of a small section of adventitia may allow for vascular preservation (Fig. 16.5).

The American Joint Committee on Cancer (AJCC) residual tumor classification (R classification), is a commonly followed margin classification. R0 denotes the absence of any microscopic residual tumor after resection, R1 denotes microscopic residual tumor and R2 corresponds to macroscopic residual tumor [7]. In 2002, the Union Against Cancer (UICC) proposed an R + 1 mm classifica-

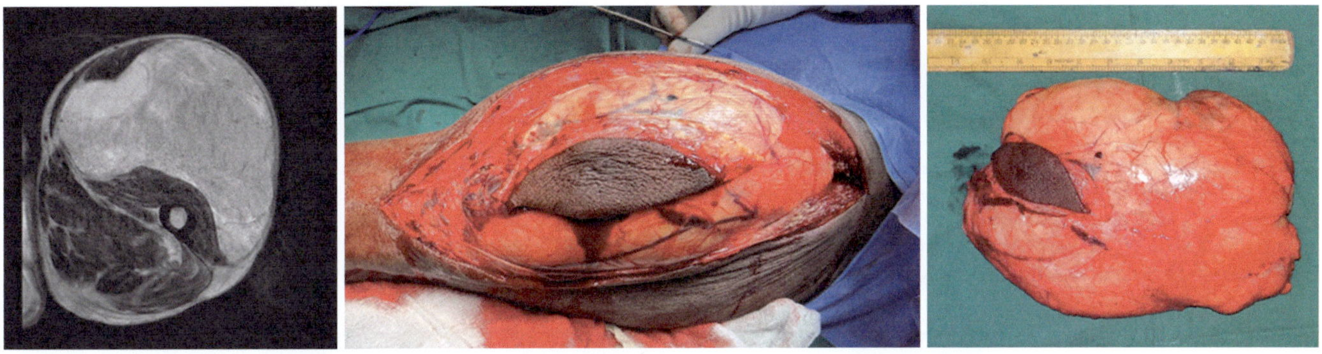

Fig. 16.2 An atypical lipomatous tumor excised with marginal margins

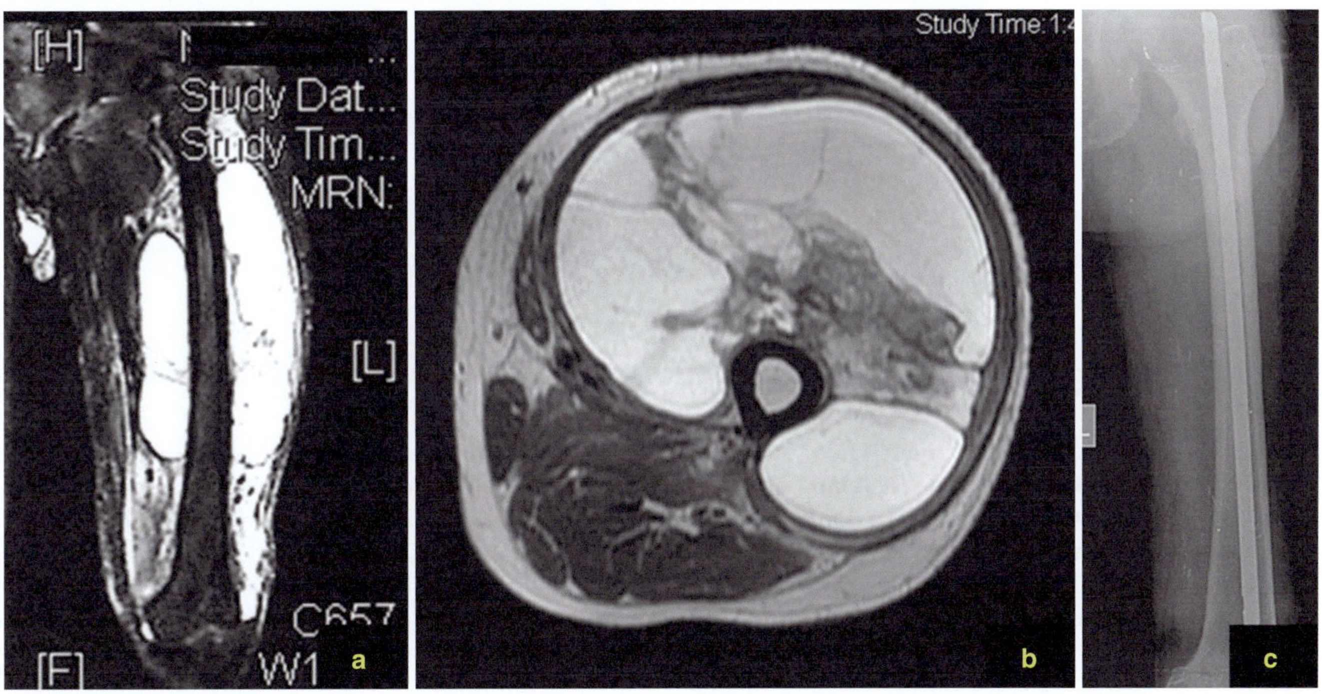

Fig. 16.3 In spite of near circumferential extent around the femur (**a** & **b**), there is no bony extension, enabling adequate oncologic surgical removal (subperiosteal) without bony resection. (**c**) A prophylactic intramedullary nail was inserted intraoperatively in view of extensive periosteal stripping and perioperative radiotherapy, radiograph at 5 years follow-up

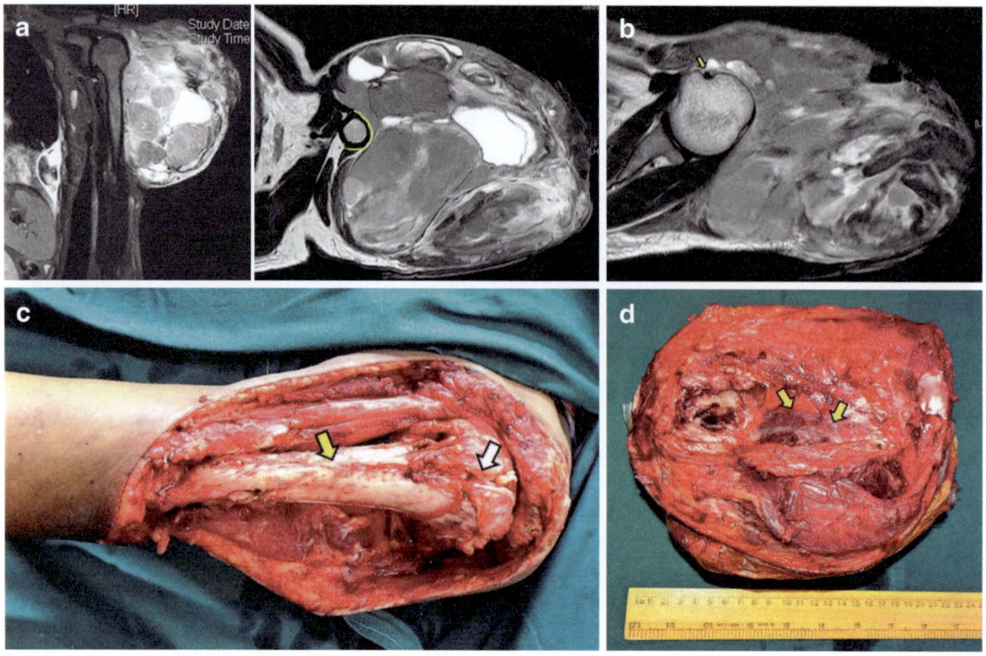

Fig. 16.4 (**a**) In spite of near circumferential extent around the upper humerus, there is no bony extension, enabling adequate oncologic surgical removal (subperiosteal) without bony resection—the yellow line depicts the plane of dissection (subperiosteal). (**b**) Near circumferential extent around the head of humerus; the biceps tendon (yellow arrow) is excised with the tumor to ensure adequate oncologic margins. (**c**) Intraoperative image showing the uninvolved cortical bone (yellow arrow) after subperiosteal resection; white arrow depicts the bicipital groove. (D) Periosteum (yellow arrows) excised with tumor enabling adequate oncologic surgical removal (subperiosteal)

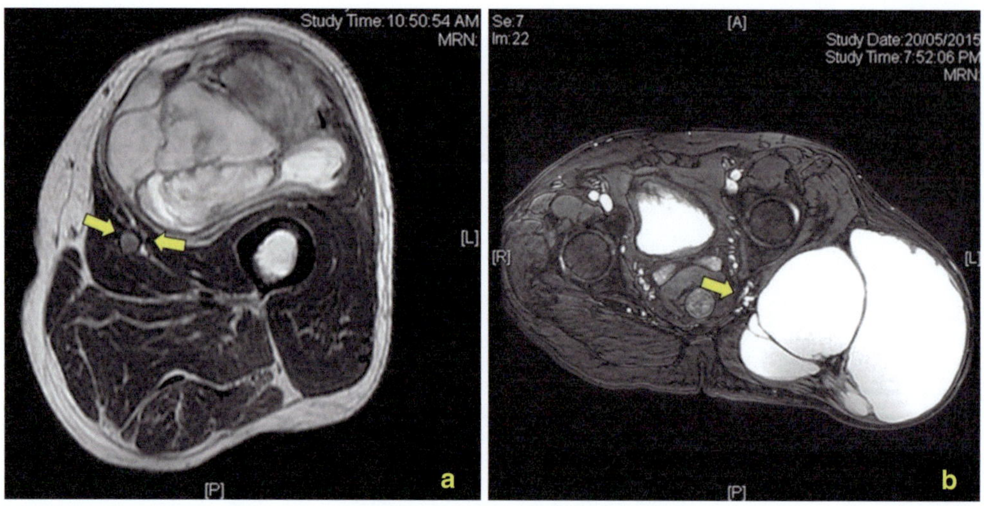

Fig. 16.5 Though "quantitative" margins may not be possible, "qualitative" barriers permit safe margins near femoral vessels (A) and sciatic nerve (B) enabling resection with limb salvage without neurovascular resection

tion [8]. For specimens to be considered microscopically negative (R0), there needed to be at least 1 mm of normal tissue between the tumor and the inked border, whereas specimens with tumor within 1 mm of the inked border were categorized as microscopically positive (R1). The Toronto Margin Context Classification (TMCC) in which positive margins are separated into planned close but positive at critical structures, positive after re-excision for inadequately excised tumors, and inadvertent positive margins demonstrated that negative margins achieved through resection of critical structures because of tumor invasion or encasement only slightly improved the 5-year rates of local recurrence-free survival compared to a planned close but ultimately positive margin along fixed critical structures such as bone or a major neurovascular bundle with the use of perioperative radiotherapy [9].

Gundle et al. compared the ability of different margin classification systems to determine local recurrence risk after soft tissue sarcoma resection [10]. Margins were determined by the conventional residual tumor (R) classification (in which microscopic tumor at inked margin defines R1), the R + 1 mm classification (in which microscopic tumor within

1 mm of ink defines R1), and the Toronto Margin Context Classification. R + 1 mm classification resulted in increased R1 margins. While it led to decreased local recurrence for R1 margins, it did not change local recurrence for R0. For TMCC, local recurrence rates for positive margins on critical structures were not different from R0. They concluded that the R classification identified three distinct risk levels for local recurrence in soft tissue sarcomas. As the R + 1 mm classification reduced local recurrence differences between R1 and R0, a negative but <1-mm margin may be adequate with multidisciplinary treatment. The TMCC helped to provide additional stratification of positive margins that may aid in surgical planning and patient education.

The use of radiotherapy can affect margins and their subsequent implications. While a negative margin is essential for optimizing local control, the absolute quantitative width of the negative margin may not significantly influence outcome in patients receiving perioperative radiotherapy. Radiation may help biologically "sterilize" microscopic extensions of tumor tissue and radiotherapy may thus decrease the risk of local recurrence with anticipated close/positive margins. Unlike radiotherapy, there are very limited clinical studies evaluating the effect of chemotherapy on rates of local recurrence and recommendations are not possible.

Matsumoto et al. described a surgical method, "in situ preparation," to avoid sacrifice of neurovascular bundles in close proximity to tumor [11]. The tumor and neurovascular structure were lifted en bloc from the surgical bed while preserving the continuity of the neurovascular structure and separated from the main surgical field by the use of a vinyl sheet (Fig. 16.6). The neurovascular structure was separated from the tumor by splitting the sheath and sterilized using additional intraoperative alcohol soaking without contaminating the surgical field by tumor cells. This ensured a safe surgical margin and good functional results.

In an innovative approach, Matsubara et al. used adjuvant photodynamic therapy with acridine orange, a photosensitizer, as neoadjuvant therapy to kill tumor cells and thereby reduce the surgical margin [12]. Patients with soft tissue sarcomas who underwent acridine orange therapy received intentional marginal or intralesional tumor excisions around the major nerves, vessels, or organs that were in close contact with the tumor and were important for the maintenance of limb function. They found similar overall survival and local recurrence rates in the acridine orange therapy group and the wide margin resection group. They thus demonstrated that acridine orange therapy can potentially reduce the surgical margin, thereby enabling normal surrounding tissue to be preserved by highlighting residual disease for further intraoperative removal during the same procedure after intentional marginal or intralesional tumor excisions.

Intraoperative tumor spillage and contamination can result in contamination of the entire surgical field with microscopic tumor cells. A possible "salvage" option would be to suture the defect in the tumor capsule, resect additional margin of normal tissue adjacent to the area of tumor violation and extensively irrigate the surgical field with sterile water or saline once the sarcoma is resected.

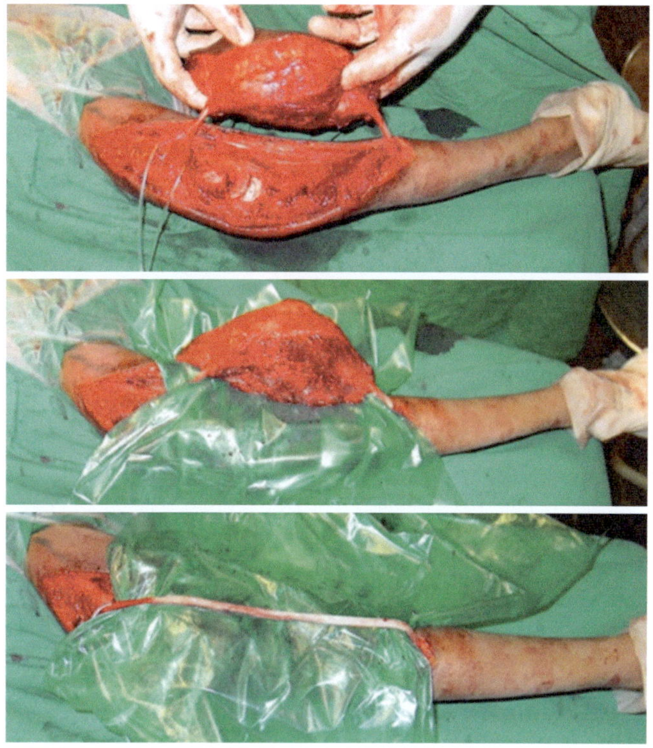

Fig. 16.6 In situ preparation to sterilize the margins around the sciatic nerve in close proximity to tumor

Amputation for an extremity sarcoma is an uncommon event in the modern era of multimodality therapy. Extensive multifocal tumor invasion, involvement of multiple critical structures, a potentially nonfunctional, severely painful extremity after sarcoma resection or multiple patient comorbidities that preclude complex surgery may be potential indications for an amputation.

The sarcoma community is yet to reach a consensus on the consistency of reporting margins after surgical resection in soft tissue sarcomas. While some prefer the use of quantitative values, others prefer qualitative determinants to denote adequacy of resection. All cases are best discussed at multidisciplinary tumor boards. Treatment decisions including those regarding surgical resection, subsequent morbidity, and functional impairment need to be tailored based on clinical characteristics, specific histotype behaviors, the proximity of adjacent critical structures, and informed discussions between the patient and the treating team.

The art of surgical oncology is to apply basic principles flexibly to the individual patient [1].

References

1. Cady B. Basic principles in surgical oncology. Arch Surg. 1997;132(4):338–46.
2. Enneking WF, Spanier SS, Goodman MA. A system for the surgical staging of musculoskeletal sarcoma. Clin Orthop Relat Res. 1980;153:106–20.
3. Cates MM, Cates JMM. Surgical resection margin classifications for high-grade pleomorphic soft tissue sarcomas of the extremity or trunk: definitions of adequate resection margins and recommendations for sampling margins from primary resection specimens. Modern Pathol. 2019;32(10):1421–33.
4. Kawaguchi N, Ahmed AR, Matsumoto S, Manabe J, Matsushita Y. The concept of curative margin in surgery for bone and soft tissue sarcoma. Clin Orthop Relat Res. 2004;419:165–72.
5. Cable MG, Randall RL. Extremity soft tissue sarcoma: tailoring resection to histologic subtype. Surg Oncol Clin N Am. 2016;25(4):677–95.
6. Lin PP, Pino ED, Normand AN, Deavers MT, Cannon CP, Ballo MT, et al. Periosteal margin in soft-tissue sarcoma. Cancer. 2007;109(3):598–602.
7. Tunn P-U, Kettelhack C, Dürr HR. Standardized approach to the treatment of adult soft tissue sarcoma of the extremities. In: Tunn P-U, editor. Treatment of bone and soft tissue sarcomas. Berlin/Heidelberg, Springer; 2009. p. 211–28.
8. Wittekind C, Compton CC, Greene FL, Sobin LH. TNM residual tumor classification revisited. Cancer. 2002;94(9):2511–6.
9. O'Donnell PW, Griffin AM, Eward WC, Sternheim A, Catton CN, Chung PW, et al. The effect of the setting of a positive surgical margin in soft tissue sarcoma. Cancer. 2014;120(18):2866–75.
10. Gundle KR, Kafchinski L, Gupta S, Griffin AM, Dickson BC, Chung PW, et al. Analysis of margin classification Systems for Assessing the risk of local recurrence after soft tissue sarcoma resection. J Clin Oncol. 2018;36(7):704–9.
11. Matsumoto S, Kawaguchi N, Manabe J, Matsushita Y. "In situ preparation": new surgical procedure indicated for soft-tissue sarcoma of a lower limb in close proximity to major neurovascular structures. Int J Clin Oncol. 2002;7(1):51–6.
12. Matsubara T, Kusuzaki K, Matsumine A, Nakamura T, Sudo A. Can a less radical surgery using photodynamic therapy with acridine orange be equal to a wide-margin resection? Clin Orthop Relat Res. 2013;471(3):792–802.

Is It Right, Safe, and Justified to Modulate the Margins?

17

Meshal K. Alfaraidy, Nicholas C. Eastley, Patrick Qi Wang, Anthony M. Griffin, Kim M. Tsoi, Jay S. Wunder, and Peter C. Ferguson

17.1 Introduction

The standard treatment of localised soft tissue sarcoma (STS) of the extremity is surgical excision with a margin of normal, uninvolved tissue surrounding it [1–4] to minimise local recurrence (LR) risk. The addition of radiation therapy has also aided in the shift to limb-salvage surgery as the mainstay of treatment without detrimentally impacting local recurrence, metastasis-free survival, and overall survival [5–7]. Surgical margin status has greater influence on local disease control than other factors like tumour grade, size, or depth [8]. Current guidelines, however, are inconsistent in their definition of a negative margin and in the quantitative assessment of that margin [9].

17.2 Different Classifications of Surgical Margin

To determine the adequacy of a resection, assess the need for adjuvant therapy and ascertain the risk of local relapse, evaluation of the surgical margin is crucial [10]. There are multiple classification systems for surgical margins in sarcoma. This can cause a problem in the field of sarcoma treatment as the definition can vary between clinicians and centres, making comparison of outcomes difficult [10]. The most commonly utilised classification systems include the Enneking classification, the R classification, the Union International Contre le Cancer (UICC) classification (R+1 mm classification), the Toronto Margin Context Classification (TMCC), dichotomous classification, and measurement of distance [10–12].

M. K. Alfaraidy (✉) · N. C. Eastley · P. Q. Wang · A. M. Griffin
K. M. Tsoi · J. S. Wunder · P. C. Ferguson
The University of Toronto Musculoskeletal Oncology Unit, Mount Sinai Hospital, Toronto, ON, Canada
e-mail: MKAlfaraidy@moh.gov.sa; Neastley@doctors.org.uk; patrick-qi.wang.med@ssss.gouv.qc.ca; Anthony.Griffin@sinaihealth.ca; Kim.Tsoi@sinaihealth.ca; Jay.Wunder@sinaihealth.ca; Peter.Ferguson@sinaihealth.ca

17.2.1 Enneking Classification (MSTS)

A system for the surgical staging of sarcoma was first proposed by Enneking et al. in 1980 [13]. The four categories of surgical margins in this classification system are intralesional, marginal, wide, and radical (compartmental). The relationship between the margin, the tumour and its pseudocapsule served as the basis for this classification system. O'Donnell et al. surmised that the pseudocapsule is composed of pre-existing connective tissue peripheral to the tumour that is compressed as the tumour expands, but it is also the product of active fibrogenesis caused by the tumour, possibly through growth factors, or as a result of tumour involution [14]. During the surgery, when the tumour's pseudocapsule is opened or violated and the dissection passes within the lesion, an intralesional margin is obtained. Macroscopic tumour tissue is left at the margins, and the exposed tissue planes become contaminated. Intralesional procedures are most commonly incisional diagnostic biopsies or "debulking" or "piecemeal" resections of the tumour. A marginal margin is when the tumour is removed through the pseudocapsule or "reactive zone" around the tumour. Microscopic residual tumour is a possibility with this type of resection. Marginal resections are usually performed as an excisional biopsy. Resection with marginal margins is sometimes necessary when the tumour is close to critical structures, including nerves, vessels, and bone. A wide margin is when the tumour is resected with surrounding healthy tissue outside the pseudocapsule but within the involved compartment. This is the mainstay of treatment for extremity soft tissue sarcoma [3]. A radical margin is when the entire anatomic compartment containing the tumour is resected.

The macroscopic findings made during surgery form the basis for much of Enneking's classification. The margin that is closest to the resection surface should be considered when assessing the margins. For example, if a wide margin resection is undertaken but the reactive zone is entered even in a small part, the margin for this resection is considered marginal. Trovik *et al.* modified the Enneking's criteria to report

H. Özger et al. (eds.), *Diagnosis and Treatment of Soft Tissue Tumors*, https://doi.org/10.1007/978-3-031-77061-6_17

adequate (radical or wide) or inadequate (marginal or intralesional) margins [15].

Because of its conceptual appeal and practical application in surgical planning, the Enneking classification system has been a popular method for evaluating surgical margin in soft tissue sarcoma. However, reproducibility can be a problem. Trovik et al. reported that disagreement of margin assessment, especially between wide and marginal margins, occurred in 23 of the 117 randomly selected cases (19.7%) [16].

17.2.2 R Classification (the Residual Tumour Classification)

The AJCC Manual for Staging of Cancer first adopted the R classification in the 3rd edition [17]. This classification system is based upon macroscopic as well as microscopic margin assessment after surgical resection. An R2 has gross tumour at the margin, an R1 resection has microscopic tumour at the margin, and an R0 margin has no tumour cells at the inked margin microscopically. These definitions of R2, R1, and R0 are clear and easily recognisable, which is leading to increasing use of the R classification over time [11].

17.2.3 UICC Classification (R+1 mm Classification)

The International Union Against Cancer (UICC) in recent years has evolved the R classification into the "R+1 mm" classification. The margins are classified as R2 being grossly positive, R1 being microscopically positive where the tumour is within 1 mm of the inked border under microscope, and R0 being microscopically negative where there is at least 1 mm of normal tissue between the tumour and the inked margin [18]. This is a more stringent requirement for R0 margin than that of the R classification. It remains controversial whether this is a better predictor of local recurrence in soft tissue sarcoma [19, 20]

17.2.4 Toronto Margin Context Classification (TMCC)

The TMCC divides margins into four categories: negative margins (R0 according to the R classification), unplanned positive margins, a planned close but with an ultimately positive microscopic margin along a critical structure, and a positive margin after a tumour bed re-excision in patients treated initially with a positive margin resection elsewhere (the whoops procedure) [20, 21]. Gundle et al. showed that the TMCC provides additional stratification of positive margins that may aid in surgical planning and patient education [20].

17.2.5 Dichotomous Classification (Positive or Negative)

The dichotomous classification, which only reports positive or negative margins, is used in some papers [22]. In the majority of papers, microscopically positive margins are reported as positive margins; however, the number of macroscopically positive cases included in the positive margin group is not always clear. This classification is not recommended for scientific publication because macroscopically and microscopically positive margins differ greatly. It is essential to specify whether positive margins mean macroscopically positive or microscopically positive for the purpose of clear communication [10].

17.2.6 Measurement of the Distance

The measurement of the distance between the edge of the tumour and the surface of the surgical resection is described in some papers [23, 24]. The effect of formalin's muscle shortening on the distance between the resection surface and the tumour could cause this method to have some drawbacks. A significant error in distance estimation is also caused by a change in shape brought about by improper fixation techniques. Distance is a continuous variable in data analysis, so its conversion to a categorical variable can be challenging due to the various papers' different cut-off values. The results of different studies can't be easily compared because of this [10].

17.2.7 Quality of the Margin

The appropriateness of the margin may be further impacted by anatomical factors like the tissue composition of the margin [13, 25], with dense regular connective tissue assumed to provide a more robust anatomic barrier to tumour cell infiltration. Some authors consider the intact fascia (which can be a millimetre thick) to be an adequate margin [26, 27]. Wide margins in the Enneking classification were further subclassified by Rydholm and Rooser [28] as wide-S (subcutaneous), wide-F (fascia), and wide-AM (areolar tissue and muscle). The local recurrence (LR) risk stratification offered by this subclassification had a 10% 5-year rate of LR with wide-S and wide-F margins and 30% with a wide-AM margin. The significance of margin quality has been rarely investigated, so the efficacy of these structures as a barrier is still debated [12].

17.2.8 Which Is Best?

When Cates et al. [29] compared the R classification, MSTS, and margin distance method, they found that none of them stood out as being clearly superior to the others. However, they noted that the dichotomised R system and MSTS classifications appear adequate in this clinical setting given the increased specificity and positive predictive value of a binary positive versus negative reporting system. By directly comparing three schemes (R, R+1, and TMCC classifications), Gundle et al. [20] came to the conclusion that the traditional R classification best determined the risk of local recurrence. However, TMCC provides additional stratification of positive margins that may help in surgical planning. R1 resections as per the UICC-classification identify more patients at high risk of LR than R1 resections in the R-classification, Kainhofer et al. [19].

It is challenging to compare study results because of the inconsistent sample size across studies as well as the lack of consistency in margin definition. As a result, there is a critical need for evidence-based standardisation with regard to resection margin status. Based on current evidence, none of the reported classifications can consistently and accurately predict the risk of recurrence in isolation [9, 10, 12].

17.3 Importance of Surgical Margins

17.3.1 Local Recurrence

Surgical margin is closely related to the risk of local recurrence risk [15, 19, 20, 23, 24, 30–32]. In one study that used the MSTS classification, the 5-year local recurrence rate was reported to be 11%, 5%, and 21% with radical (compartmental), wide, and marginal resection of the soft tissue sarcoma of the thigh, respectively [30]. The fact that local recurrence was higher in the radical margin than wide margin group highlights one of the weaknesses of this system. In this same study, surgical margin was shown to be an independent prognostic factor for local recurrence and there was a statistically significant difference between wide and marginal margins in local recurrence rates [30]. Looking at utilising the R classification, one study showed that the 5-year local recurrence rate was reported to be 9.5% for R0 resections and 36.7% for R1 margins [19], showing the risk of local recurrence can be estimated with the R classification.

It is still unclear whether the UICC (R+1 mm) classification is better at predicting local recurrence than the original R classification [10]. Harati et al. reported that achieving a negative margin is essential for optimising local control and survival, but the absolute quantitative width of the negative margin does not influence outcome [33]. The absolute value of the local recurrence rate and the difference in the local recurrence rate between R0 and R1 resections should be kept in mind when comparing the classification schemes. A low absolute value of the local recurrence rate following surgery alone with R0 margins may indicate that no additional adjuvant therapy (such as radiotherapy) is required. Adjuvant therapy should be considered when surgery with R1 margins has a significantly higher risk of local recurrence than R0 resection [10].

In a retrospective study of 2217 patients with non-metastatic axial and extremity soft tissue sarcoma treated with surgery and multidisciplinary modalities, Gundle et al. found that, according to the UICC classification, the 5-year local recurrence rate was 6%, 10%, and 38% in patients treated with R0, R1, and R2 margins, respectively. R0, R1, and R2 resections had local recurrence rates of 6%, 17%, and 38%, respectively, when their cohort was re-analysed using the R classification. R1 resection had a higher local recurrence rate in the R classification, whereas R0 resection had a rate that was nearly identical in both classifications. Because the UICC classification reduced the difference in local recurrence rate between R0 and R1, the authors concluded that the R classification is more useful in the clinical setting. The results suggested that a negative R0 margin with less than 1 mm width of the normal tissue might be adequate with adjuvant treatment [20].

The highest risk of local recurrence is associated with unexpected positive margins that do not affect critical structures but rather the soft tissues surrounding the excised soft tissue sarcoma as a result of surgical error or tumour extension beyond what is visible on cross-sectional imaging (i.e. Intralesional margins in MSTS system or R2 margins in UICC and AJCC systems) [20]. Close dissection for the preservation of major vessels, nerves, or bone, however, can also result in microscopically positive margins [21]. While unexpected positive margins showed the worst outcome for local recurrence, planned close but ultimately positive margins (R1) along critical structures is acceptable in particular in patients who receive preoperative radiotherapy [20, 34].

17.3.2 Overall Survival

In soft tissue sarcomas of the extremities, it has been consistently established that both macroscopic and microscopic positive surgical margins reduce local recurrence-free survival [23, 24, 31]. There is less agreement on the extent to which the surgical margin affects overall or disease-specific survival.

In a study of 2084 adult patients with localised primary soft tissue sarcoma, Stojadinovic et al. demonstrated that positive microscopic margins reduce both the disease-specific survival rate and the distant recurrence-free survival rate [35]. In contrast to this, Tanabe et al. observed that in 95 patients with extremity soft tissue sarcoma, negative surgical margins improved local disease control but had no positive effect on overall survival (5-year overall survival rate; 65% vs. 70% for negative and positive margins, respectively)

[36]. Bonvalot et al. had similar findings when they studied 531 patients with primary extremity soft tissue sarcoma and reported that the margin status had no correlation to overall survival [37].

With regards to the impact of margins on overall or disease-specific survival, based on the available literature, it is challenging to reach a definitive conclusion, and it is likely that additional research will be required in this area.

17.4 Radiation Therapy

Radiotherapy (RT) is being used with increasing frequency as part of a multimodal approach to the management of STS. In the past 20 years, technological advancements like intensity-modulated (IMRT), image-guided (IGRT), and stereotactic (SBRT) radiotherapy have improved patient care. They have permitted either dose escalation (with resulting improved efficacy) or toxicity reduction (with resulting improved functional outcome) [38].

Radiotherapy combined with surgery has been shown to have a positive effect on local tumour control, with local recurrence rates lower than 15% [39, 40]. Combined therapy is currently recommended in international guidelines [41]. Radiotherapy can be used in the setting of a planned close margin against a critical structure such as bone, nerves or vessels to aid in local tumour control [20, 21].

17.5 Peritumoral Oedema

Soft tissue sarcomas have a centrifugal manner of growth by compression of peripheral cells in parallel layers [42]. There frequently appears to be a pseudocapsule surrounding the tumour due to secondary adjacent normal tissue atrophy [42, 43]. A "reactive zone", which is distinguished by neovascularisation, oedema, and possibly satellite tumour cells, can exist outside the pseudocapsule [43]. This can be visualised as varying degrees of peritumoral T2-weighted signal changes on MR imaging [42, 44].

Based on the few reports, the existence of malignant cells within the oedematous perilesional area are variable, and true rates are still unknown [45]. In 3 out of 11 patients, Beltran et al. found biopsy-proven malignant cells in the oedematous area surrounding malignant musculoskeletal tumours [46]. Only one patient had massive oedema surrounding an osteosarcoma in a series of 41 tumours with peritumoral oedema that included osteosarcomas, Ewing's sarcomas, and soft tissue sarcomas [47]. Peritumoral oedema and microscopic tumour deposits are strongly correlated, according to White et al. [48]. In 10 patients in their series of 15 patients, tumour cells were discovered up to 4 cm away from the tumour margin or pseudocapsule. The tumour cells were found histologically in regions with corresponding high T2-weighted signal changes on MRI in 9 of the 10 cases with tumour beyond the primary tumour mass. The existence of satellite tumour cells in 9 out of 10 cases justified the inclusion of oedema in radiotherapy volumes, even though this was a small study and the potential for these satellite cells to develop and form an actual tumour was not studied and is still debatable [45]. Currently, the Radiation Therapy Oncology Group (RTOG) sarcoma panel agrees that radiation therapy should be contoured to include any suspect peritumoral oedema not included in the planned surgical margin, but the degree of inclusion is still up to clinical judgement [45, 49].

There remains a paucity of evidence with regards to the impact of satellite tumour cells in peritumoral oedema tails. Until this relationship is fully established, they should be taken into account for radiation therapy and multidisciplinary care.

17.6 Special Considerations

17.6.1 Infiltrative Soft Tissue Sarcomas

Some soft tissue sarcomas have a growth pattern that is highly infiltrative and invasive, which can be seen as the "tail sign" on an MRI [50]. The "tails" are curvilinear projections extending from the sarcoma's primary mass noted on T2-weighted and post-contrast MRI images [51]. Specifically subtypes such as myxofibrosarcoma (MFS) and undifferentiated pleomorphic sarcoma (UPS) commonly present with this infiltrative pattern [52–56]. Myxofibrosarcoma, which tends to spread on a fascial plane [57], has a risk of local recurrence estimated to be between 20% and 30% [57–59]. This is higher than other soft tissue sarcoma subtypes, even with negative margin resections [60]. Iwata et al. investigated the effects of infiltrative growth on the prognosis of patients with myxofibrosarcoma and undifferentiated pleomorphic sarcoma [53]. According to their protocol, invasive soft tissue sarcoma resection was planned to remove 2 to 3 cm from the edge of the tumour extension. The surgical margin was microscopically positive in 43 of the 89 patients (48%) despite efforts to remove a large margin, and the 5-year local recurrence-free survival rate was 81% [53].

According to Fujiwara et al. [61], neither the R-classification nor the R+1-classification was able to stratify the risk of LR in patients with negative margins in the cases of MFS and UPS, proving that these classification systems are insufficiently sensitive to determine what constitutes an adequate margin of resection for infiltrative STS. Fujiwara et al. [62] noted that a fascia/periosteum margin <10 mm was equivalent to any quality margin of tissue > 10 mm in terms of local recurrence risk. According to Goertz et al. [63], only the quality of surgical margins—not the margin width—had an impact on prognosis.

In cases of infiltrative soft tissue sarcomas, more than 3 cm of radial margin on MRI images may be necessary in the planning of the operation in order to achieve microscopically negative surgical margins. Such a wide resection raises the possibility of wound complications, the need for plastic surgery reconstruction, and functional morbidity. It is unclear and still up for debate what the ideal excision margin for these tumours should be [10, 12].

17.6.2 Myxoid Liposarcoma

Myxoid liposarcoma differs from other STS in a number of significant ways, including its predilection for non-pulmonary sites for metastasis [64, 65] and its higher radiation sensitivity compared to most other soft tissue sarcoma subtypes [7, 66, 67]. These tumours more reliably reduce in volume after preoperative RT compared to other soft tissue sarcomas [66, 68]. As they are commonly intermuscular lesions, when they do get smaller, they often remain separated from surrounding muscle, fascia and neurovascular structures by a thin pseudocapsule [69]. Given this response to radiotherapy, myxoid liposarcoma is typically treated with pre-operative radiation followed by resection. An adequate margin for this resection has been controversial with some reporting a goal of 1–3 cm margins surrounding the tumour given its frequent intermuscular location [67, 70].

Perrera et al. [69] reviewed the safety of a marginal resection of intermuscular myxoid liposarcomas after receiving neoadjuvant radiotherapy and showed that margin status had no association with local recurrence-free, metastasis-free, or overall survival. With their study they concluded that marginal resection of extremity intermuscular myxoid liposarcoma that has received radiation is safe and does not compromise oncologic control.

17.6.3 Hand Soft Tissue Sarcomas

Due to its complex anatomy and lack of reliable partitions like fascia to demarcate anatomic compartments, treating soft tissue sarcomas of the hand presents a challenge to surgeons. Significant functional loss could result from sacrificing tendons, blood vessels, and nerves in order to obtain adequate margins. The rate of positive margin after surgery is reported to range from 11.3% to 36.4%, and it is frequently challenging to obtain adequate margins in the resection of soft tissue sarcomas of the hand [71–73]. Macroscopic positive margin is strongly associated with local recurrence, as is the case with other anatomic sites in the extremities. For wide or marginal margins, the 5-year risk of local recurrence is 14%, and for intralesional margins, it is 80% [71]. Adjuvant radiotherapy can be used postoperatively in some cases when margins are close or microscopically positive, though radiotherapy does not completely mitigate the effects of positive margins [74]. It is important to note that radiotherapy for the hand is linked to a higher risk of complications and poorer outcome. Early side effects of radiotherapy to the hand include wound dehiscence and necrosis, and late side effects include ankylosis, joint contracture, adduction contracture, and osteitis [75, 76]. Preoperative radiotherapy, with its lower dose, may be preferred to help mitigate some of these effects.

Aggressive surgery aimed at negative margins with or without radiotherapy should be undertaken whenever possible. The surgeon should not refrain from performing ray amputations, especially of digits other than the thumb. Most authors have come to the conclusion that surgery combined with adjuvant radiotherapy is an acceptable course of treatment for patients with soft tissue sarcoma of the hand in situations where the margins will be close even with partial hand amputations [10, 77].

17.6.4 Foot Soft Tissue Sarcomas

The surgical considerations for the foot are somewhat similar to those for the hand due to the proximity of vital structures like nerves, vessels, and tendons as well as the lack of expendable muscle and other connective tissue. The functional loss of movement and sensation in the digits does not have the same functional significance as it does in the hand, which is one significant distinction. As a result, soft tissue resections in the foot may be more extensive than those in the hand. Even if the plantar arteries and nerves are sacrificed along with the tumour, patients with excellent perfusion and collateral blood flow can recover well from these resections. In the surgical management of soft tissue sarcomas of the foot, limb-salvage surgery with or without radiotherapy is regarded as an acceptable, mainstream procedure, associated with excellent local control and a positive functional outcome [77, 78]. In a retrospective study of 27 patients who underwent limb-sparing surgery for a soft tissue sarcoma of the foot or ankle, Cribb et al. found that all 27 survivors were able to wear regular shoes and that none needed a walking aid [79].

Due to the rarity of soft tissue sarcomas of the foot, these tumours are frequently removed by inexperienced surgeons during an unplanned procedure. Unplanned surgery for foot sarcomas had a high rate of local recurrence and a comparatively poor prognosis, which Nishimura et al. brought to light [80]. Modern prosthetics provide excellent function after below-knee amputation, so surgeons should not hesitate to perform it if the margins would be unacceptable for a limb-sparing procedure [10].

17.6.5 Atypical Lipomatous Tumor

One of the members of the adipocytic family of tumours is the atypical lipomatous tumour, which develops in the extremities. Although it has previously been referred to as "well-differentiated liposarcoma", this moniker does not seem appropriate in the extremities because it does not have the same prognosis as similar tumours arising in the retroperitoneum. It has no chance of metastasising when it develops in the extremities unless it undergoes dedifferentiation. This finding led to the term "atypical lipomatous tumour" being coined to describe lesions that appeared on the limbs and trunk and were amenable to surgery [81, 82]. Since recurrence of atypical lipomatous tumour after excision with a macroscopically clear margin is uncommon, resection should aim to cause the least amount of surgical morbidity possible. Even when the tumour microscopically approaches the inked margins, en bloc complete resection is typically sufficient to achieve long-term local control [83–85]. Radiation may be useful in cases with multiple recurrences to enhance disease control [86].

17.6.6 Soft Tissue Sarcomas After Unplanned Excision ("Whoops" Surgery)

Unplanned excision is the term used to describe the removal of a tumour without performing preoperative diagnostic tests and without the goal of obtaining microscopically negative margins [87]. Since soft tissue sarcomas occur infrequently enough that few clinicians have sufficient experience treating the disease, they are frequently treated by unplanned surgery [88]. The main issue with unintentional excision is the spread of tumour cells into the surgical site and the surrounding tissue. After an unplanned excision, macroscopic residual tumour is frequently present [89]. Therefore, it is not surprising that unplanned excisions, unless they are followed by tumour bed re-excision, are linked to a high risk of local recurrence [90]. The objective of re-resection surgery following an unplanned excision should be to remove the entire surgical bed, including skin incisions, surgical drains, and postoperative hematoma [91]. Transverse or oblique incisions at the unplanned excision may cause contamination of several or adjacent compartments, necessitating a much larger resection to achieve microscopically negative margins. Such situations frequently call for the reconstruction of soft tissue using a flap [10] and for adjuvant radiotherapy.

17.7 Periosteal Margin

Soft tissue sarcomas can occasionally develop close to bones and rest against the periosteal layer. In these situations, a careful MRI and/or CT scan evaluation of the presence of bone invasion is required. Extension into bone has reportedly been associated with a poor prognosis [92]. If there is obvious invasion into bone, resection of the tumour along with the adjacent bone should be undertaken. In one study with 50 cases of periosteal soft tissue sarcoma, only three cases (6%) had histopathologic evidence of true invasion into the bone [93]. In that study, 8 of the 50 patients (16%) developed a local recurrence in the soft tissues, but there was no statistically significant difference in the local recurrence rate between patients who had only the soft tissues removed and patients who also had the adjacent bone removed. The authors came to the conclusion that only a small percentage of soft tissue sarcomas can invade cortical bone and suggested composite bone and soft tissue resections for those tumours that clearly show evidence of bone invasion on imaging. According to the authors, the periosteum served as a solid barrier that was largely impermeable to soft tissue sarcoma. The majority of cases were thought to be adequately treated with wide resection, which included subperiosteal dissection using Bovie electrocautery and radiation therapy to the bone. There may be an increased risk of a late radiation-associated fracture of the bone in cases of extensive periosteal stripping and radiation to bone, which can be very challenging to heal [92, 93]. In some cases, prophylactic intramedullary fixation may be appropriate, especially in older women, patients receiving higher radiation doses, and patients with low bone mineral density. However, this is a contentious issue, and it has not yet been established that prophylactic nailing leads to better outcomes [10].

17.8 Planned Close Margins

Soft tissue sarcomas in the extremity can arise close to fixed critical structures such as major nerves, blood vessels or bone. Resection of these structures with the tumour can impart significant morbidity to patients. Patients with microscopic positive margins have been shown to have lower rates of local recurrence when the surgical excision is combined with adjuvant radiation therapy [25, 94, 95]. O'Donnell et al. noted that after planned close dissection to preserve critical structures, the 5-year local recurrence-free survival of 97% was obtained with microscopic negative margins and 85.4% with microscopic positive margins. Furthermore, negative margins achieved through resection of critical structures because of tumour invasion or encasement did not improve the local recurrence rate significantly compared to retention of those structures with a resultant positive margin [21]. They concluded that sparing adjacent critical structures is safe and contributes to improved functional outcomes. Gundle et al. reviewed 2217 patients with nonmetastatic extremity and truncal soft tissue sarcomas treated with surgical resection and multidisciplinary consideration of perioperative radiotherapy. They found that local recurrence rates for planned close but ultimately positive margins on critical structures were no different from negative margin resections (11% vs. 8%, $p = 0.18$) [20].

17.9 Conclusion

Obtaining local control of soft tissue sarcomas is dependent on adequate surgical resection. Risk of local recurrence can be predicted based on context of the margin as not all positive margins are "equal". Resection of critical structures with negative margins does not improve oncologic outcomes in terms of local recurrence or metastatic risk. Biologic aggressiveness inherent to an STS that invaded critical structure portends a worse overall prognosis, more so than the quality of the final margin [92, 96]

References

1. Wilson AN, Davis A, Bell RS, O'Sullivan B, Catton C, Madadi F, et al. Local control of soft tissue sarcoma of the extremity: the experience of a multidisciplinary sarcoma group with definitive surgery and radiotherapy. Eur J Cancer. 1994;30a(6):746–51.
2. Clark MA, Fisher C, Judson I, Thomas JM. Soft-tissue sarcomas in adults. N Engl J Med. 2005;353(7):701–11.
3. Casali PG, Jost L, Sleijfer S, Verweij J, Blay JY. Soft tissue sarcomas: ESMO clinical recommendations for diagnosis, treatment and follow-up. Ann Oncol. 2009;20(Suppl 4):132–6.
4. O'Sullivan B, Wylie J, Catton C, Gutierrez E, Swallow CJ, Wunder J, et al. The local management of soft tissue sarcoma. Semin Radiat Oncol. 1999;9(4):328–48.
5. Clark MA, Thomas JM. Major amputation for soft-tissue sarcoma. Br J Surg. 2003;90(1):102–7.
6. Stevenson MG, Musters AH, Geertzen JHB, van Leeuwen BL, Hoekstra HJ, Been LB. Amputations for extremity soft tissue sarcoma in an era of limb salvage treatment: Local control and survival. J Surg Oncol. 2018;117(3):434–42.
7. O'Sullivan B, Davis AM, Turcotte R, Bell R, Catton C, Chabot P, et al. Preoperative versus postoperative radiotherapy in soft-tissue sarcoma of the limbs: a randomised trial. Lancet. 2002;359(9325):2235–41.
8. Biau DJ, Ferguson PC, Chung P, Griffin AM, Catton CN, O'Sullivan B, et al. Local recurrence of localized soft tissue sarcoma: a new look at old predictors. Cancer. 2012;118(23):5867–77.
9. Kandel R, Coakley N, Werier J, Engel J, Ghert M, Verma S. Surgical margins and handling of soft-tissue sarcoma in extremities: a clinical practice guideline. Curr Oncol. 2013;20(3):e247–54.
10. Endo M, Lin PP. Surgical margins in the management of extremity soft tissue sarcoma. Chin Clin Oncol. 2018;7(4):37.
11. Hoang K, Gao Y, Miller BJ. The variability in surgical margin reporting in limb salvage surgery for sarcoma. Iowa Orthop J. 2015;35:181–6.
12. Sambri A, Caldari E, Fiore M, Zucchini R, Giannini C, Pirini MG, et al. Margin assessment in soft tissue sarcomas: review of the literature. Cancers (Basel). 2021;13(7):1687.
13. Enneking WF, Spanier SS, Goodman MA. A system for the surgical staging of musculoskeletal sarcoma. Clin Orthop Relat Res. 1980;153:106–20.
14. O'Donnell PW, Manivel JC, Cheng EY, Clohisy DR. Chemotherapy influences the pseudocapsule composition in soft tissue sarcomas. Clin Orthop Relat Res. 2014;472(3):849–55.
15. Trovik CS, Bauer HC, Alvegård TA, Anderson H, Blomqvist C, Berlin O, et al. Surgical margins, local recurrence and metastasis in soft tissue sarcomas: 559 surgically-treated patients from the Scandinavian Sarcoma Group Register. Eur J Cancer. 2000;36(6):710–6.
16. Trovik CS, Skjeldal S, Bauer H, Rydholm A, Jebsen N. Reliability of Margin Assessment after Surgery for Extremity Soft Tissue Sarcoma: The SSG Experience. Sarcoma. 2012;2012:290698.
17. Beahrs OH, Henson DE, Hutter RVP, Myers MH. Manual for staging of cancer, 3rd edition. Am J Clin Oncol. 1988;11(6):686.
18. Wittekind C, Compton CC, Greene FL, Sobin LH. TNM residual tumor classification revisited. Cancer. 2002;94(9):2511–6.
19. Kainhofer V, Smolle MA, Szkandera J, Liegl-Atzwanger B, Maurer-Ertl W, Gerger A, et al. The width of resection margins influences local recurrence in soft tissue sarcoma patients. Eur J Surg Oncol. 2016;42(6):899–906.
20. Gundle KR, Kafchinski L, Gupta S, Griffin AM, Dickson BC, Chung PW, et al. Analysis of margin classification systems for assessing the risk of local recurrence after soft tissue sarcoma resection. J Clin Oncol. 2018;36(7):704–9.
21. O'Donnell PW, Griffin AM, Eward WC, Sternheim A, Catton CN, Chung PW, et al. The effect of the setting of a positive surgical margin in soft tissue sarcoma. Cancer. 2014;120(18):2866–75.
22. Rodriguez-Galindo C, Shah N, McCarville MB, Billups CA, Neel MN, Rao BN, et al. Outcome after local recurrence of osteosarcoma: the St. Jude Children's Research Hospital experience (1970-2000). Cancer. 2004;100(9):1928–35.
23. Novais EN, Demiralp B, Alderete J, Larson MC, Rose PS, Sim FH. Do surgical margin and local recurrence influence survival in soft tissue sarcomas? Clin Orthop Relat Res. 2010;468(11):3003–11.
24. Dickinson IC, Whitwell DJ, Battistuta D, Thompson B, Strobel N, Duggal A, et al. Surgical margin and its influence on survival in soft tissue sarcoma. ANZ J Surg. 2006;76(3):104–9.
25. Gerrand CH, Wunder JS, Kandel RA, O'Sullivan B, Catton CN, Bell RS, et al. Classification of positive margins after resection of soft-tissue sarcoma of the limb predicts the risk of local recurrence. J Bone Joint Surg Br. 2001;83(8):1149–55.
26. Bell RS, O'Sullivan B, Liu FF, Powell J, Langer F, Fornasier VL, et al. The surgical margin in soft-tissue sarcoma. J Bone Joint Surg Am. 1989;71(3):370–5.
27. Casali PG, Blay JY. Soft tissue sarcomas: ESMO Clinical Practice Guidelines for diagnosis, treatment and follow-up. Ann Oncol. 2010;21(Suppl 5):v198–203.
28. Rydholm A, Rööser B. Surgical margins for soft-tissue sarcoma. J Bone Joint Surg Am. 1987;69(7):1074–8.
29. Cates VM, Cates JMM. Surgical resection margin classifications for high-grade pleomorphic soft tissue sarcomas of the extremity or trunk after neoadjuvant cytotoxic therapy. Am J Surg Pathol. 2019;43(6):844–50.
30. Vraa S, Keller J, Nielsen OS, Jurik AG, Jensen OM. Soft-tissue sarcoma of the thigh: surgical margin influences local recurrence but not survival in 152 patients. Acta Orthop Scand. 2001;72(1):72–7.
31. Gronchi A, Miceli R, Fiore M, Collini P, Lozza L, Grosso F, et al. Extremity soft tissue sarcoma: adding to the prognostic meaning of local failure. Ann Surg Oncol. 2007;14(5):1583–90.
32. Ahmad R, Jacobson A, Hornicek F, Haynes AB, Choy E, Cote G, et al. The width of the surgical margin does not influence outcomes in extremity and truncal soft tissue sarcoma treated with radiotherapy. Oncologist. 2016;21(10):1269–76.
33. Harati K, Goertz O, Pieper A, Daigeler A, Joneidi-Jafari H, Niggemann H, et al. Soft tissue sarcomas of the extremities: surgical margins can be close as long as the resected tumor has no ink on it. Oncologist. 2017;22(11):1400–10.

34. Biau DJ, Weiss KR, Bhumbra RS, Davidson D, Brown C, Griffin A, et al. Monitoring the adequacy of surgical margins after resection of bone and soft-tissue sarcoma. Ann Surg Oncol. 2013;20(6):1858–64.
35. Stojadinovic A, Leung DH, Hoos A, Jaques DP, Lewis JJ, Brennan MF. Analysis of the prognostic significance of microscopic margins in 2,084 localized primary adult soft tissue sarcomas. Ann Surg. 2002;235(3):424–34.
36. Tanabe KK, Pollock RE, Ellis LM, Murphy A, Sherman N, Romsdahl MM. Influence of surgical margins on outcome in patients with preoperatively irradiated extremity soft tissue sarcomas. Cancer. 1994;73(6):1652–9.
37. Bonvalot S, Levy A, Terrier P, Tzanis D, Bellefqih S, Le Cesne A, et al. Primary extremity soft tissue sarcomas: does local control impact survival? Ann Surg Oncol. 2017;24(1):194–201.
38. Cammelli S, Cortesi A, Buwenge M, Zamagni A, Ferioli M, Ghigi G, et al. The role of radiotherapy in adult soft tissues sarcoma of the extremities. Eur J Orthopaed Surg Traumatol. 2021;31(8):1583–96.
39. Yang JC, Chang AE, Baker AR, Sindelar WF, Danforth DN, Topalian SL, et al. Randomized prospective study of the benefit of adjuvant radiation therapy in the treatment of soft tissue sarcomas of the extremity. J Clin Oncol. 1998;16(1):197–203.
40. Pisters PW, Harrison LB, Leung DH, Woodruff JM, Casper ES, Brennan MF. Long-term results of a prospective randomized trial of adjuvant brachytherapy in soft tissue sarcoma. J Clin Oncol. 1996;14(3):859–68.
41. Casali PG, Bielack S, Abecassis N, Aro HT, Bauer S, Biagini R, et al. Bone sarcomas: ESMO-PaedCan-EURACAN Clinical Practice Guidelines for diagnosis, treatment and follow-up. Ann Oncol. 2018;29(Suppl 4):iv79–95.
42. Ilaslan H, Schils J, Nageotte W, Lietman SA, Sundaram M. Clinical presentation and imaging of bone and soft-tissue sarcomas. Cleve Clin J Med. 2010;77(Suppl 1):S2–7.
43. Enneking WF, Spanier SS, Malawer MM. The effect of the Anatomic setting on the results of surgical procedures for soft parts sarcoma of the thigh. Cancer. 1981;47(5):1005–22.
44. Kroon HM, Bloem JL, Holscher HC, van der Woude HJ, Reijnierse M, Taminiau AH. MR imaging of edema accompanying benign and malignant bone tumors. Skeletal Radiol. 1994;23(4):261–9.
45. Bahig H, Roberge D, Bosch W, Levin W, Petersen I, Haddock M, et al. Agreement among RTOG sarcoma radiation oncologists in contouring suspicious peritumoral edema for preoperative radiation therapy of soft tissue sarcoma of the extremity. Int J Radiat Oncol Biol Phys. 2013;86(2):298–303.
46. Beltran J, Simon DC, Katz W, Weis LD. Increased MR signal intensity in skeletal muscle adjacent to malignant tumors: pathologic correlation and clinical relevance. Radiology. 1987;162(1 Pt 1):251–5.
47. Hanna SL, Fletcher BD, Parham DM, Bugg MF. Muscle edema in musculoskeletal tumors: MR imaging characteristics and clinical significance. J Magn Reson Imaging. 1991;1(4):441–9.
48. White LM, Wunder JS, Bell RS, O'Sullivan B, Catton C, Ferguson P, et al. Histologic assessment of peritumoral edema in soft tissue sarcoma. Int J Radiat Oncol Biol Phys. 2005;61(5):1439–45.
49. Wang D, Bosch W, Roberge D, Finkelstein SE, Petersen I, Haddock M, et al. RTOG sarcoma radiation oncologists reach consensus on gross tumor volume and clinical target volume on computed tomographic images for preoperative radiotherapy of primary soft tissue sarcoma of extremity in Radiation Therapy Oncology Group studies. Int J Radiat Oncol Biol Phys. 2011;81(4):e525–8.
50. Yoo HJ, Hong SH, Kang Y, Choi JY, Moon KC, Kim HS, et al. MR imaging of myxofibrosarcoma and undifferentiated sarcoma with emphasis on tail sign; diagnostic and prognostic value. Eur Radiol. 2014;24(8):1749–57.
51. Lefkowitz RA, Landa J, Hwang S, Zabor EC, Moskowitz CS, Agaram NP, et al. Myxofibrosarcoma: prevalence and diagnostic value of the "tail sign" on magnetic resonance imaging. Skeletal Radiol. 2013;42(6):809–18.
52. Spinnato P, Clinca R, Vara G, Cesari M, Ponti F, Facchini G, et al. MRI features as prognostic factors in myxofibrosarcoma: proposal of MRI grading system. Acad Radiol. 2021;28(11):1524–9.
53. Iwata S, Araki A, Funatsu H, Yonemoto T, Kamoda H, Itami M, et al. Optimal surgical margin for infiltrative soft tissue sarcomas: Assessing the efficacy of excising beyond the infiltration. J Surg Oncol. 2018;118(3):525–31.
54. Sambri A, Spinnato P, Bazzocchi A, Tuzzato GM, Donati D, Bianchi G. Does pre-operative MRI predict the risk of local recurrence in primary myxofibrosarcoma of the extremities? Asia Pac J Clin Oncol. 2019;15(5):e181–e6.
55. Imanishi J, Slavin J, Pianta M, Jackett L, Ngan SY, Tanaka T, et al. Tail of superficial myxofibrosarcoma and undifferentiated pleomorphic sarcoma after preoperative radiotherapy. Anticancer Res. 2016;36(5):2339–44.
56. Sanfilippo R, Miceli R, Grosso F, Fiore M, Puma E, Pennacchioli E, et al. Myxofibrosarcoma: prognostic factors and survival in a series of patients treated at a single institution. Ann Surg Oncol. 2011;18(3):720–5.
57. Kikuta K, Kubota D, Yoshida A, Suzuki Y, Morioka H, Toyama Y, et al. An analysis of factors related to recurrence of myxofibrosarcoma. Jpn J Clin Oncol. 2013;43(11):1093–104.
58. Ghazala CG, Agni NR, Ragbir M, Dildey P, Lee D, Rankin KS, et al. Myxofibrosarcoma of the extremity and trunk: a multidisciplinary approach leads to good local rates of LOCAL control. Bone Joint J. 2016;98-b(12):1682–8.
59. Haglund KE, Raut CP, Nascimento AF, Wang Q, George S, Baldini EH. Recurrence patterns and survival for patients with intermediate- and high-grade myxofibrosarcoma. Int J Radiat Oncol Biol Phys. 2012;82(1):361–7.
60. Dadrass F, Gusho C, Yang F, Culvern C, Bloom J, Fillingham Y, et al. A clinicopathologic examination of myxofibrosarcoma. Do surgical margins significantly affect local recurrence rates in this infiltrative sarcoma subtype? J Surg Oncol. 2021;123(2):489–96.
61. Fujiwara T, Stevenson J, Parry M, Tsuda Y, Tsoi K, Jeys L. What is an adequate margin for infiltrative soft-tissue sarcomas? Eur J Surg Oncol. 2020;46(2):277–81.
62. Fujiwara T, Sumathi V, Parry M, Stevenson J, Tsuda Y, Kaneuchi Y, et al. The role of surgical margin quality in myxofibrosarcoma and undifferentiated pleomorphic sarcoma. Eur J Surg Oncol. 2021;47(7):1756–62.
63. Goertz O, Pieper A, Lohe LV, Stricker I, Dadras M, Behr B, et al. The impact of surgical margins and adjuvant radiotherapy in patients with undifferentiated pleomorphic sarcomas of the extremities: a single-institutional analysis of 192 patients. Cancers (Basel). 2020;12(2):362.
64. Gorelik N, Reddy SMV, Turcotte RE, Goulding K, Jung S, Alcindor T, et al. Early detection of metastases using whole-body MRI for initial staging and routine follow-up of myxoid liposarcoma. Skeletal Radiol. 2018;47(3):369–79.
65. Visgauss JD, Wilson DA, Perrin DL, Colglazier R, French R, Mattei J-C, et al. Staging and surveillance of myxoid liposarcoma: follow-up assessment and the metastatic pattern of 169 patients suggests inadequacy of current practice standards. Ann Surg Oncol. 2021;28(12):7903–11.
66. Chung PWM, Deheshi BM, Ferguson PC, Wunder JS, Griffin AM, Catton CN, et al. Radiosensitivity translates into excellent local control in extremity myxoid liposarcoma. Cancer. 2009;115(14):3254–61.
67. Guadagnolo BA, Zagars GK, Ballo MT, Patel SR, Lewis VO, Benjamin RS, et al. Excellent local control rates and distinctive patterns of failure in myxoid liposarcoma treated with conservation surgery and radiotherapy. Int J Radiation Oncol Biol Phys. 2008;70(3):760–5.

68. Engström K, Bergh P, Cederlund C-G, Hultborn R, Willen H, Åman P, et al. Irradiation of myxoid/round cell liposarcoma induces volume reduction and lipoma-like morphology. Acta Oncologica. 2007;46(6):838–45.
69. Perera JR, AlFaraidy M, Ibe I, Aoude A, Acem I, van de Sande MAJ, et al. Intermuscular extremity myxoid liposarcoma can be managed by marginal resection following neoadjuvant radiotherapy. Eur J Surg Oncol. 2023;49(2):362–7.
70. Zagars GK, Goswitz MS, Pollack A. Liposarcoma: Outcome and prognostic factors following conservation surgery and radiation therapy. Int J Radiation Oncol Biol Phys. 1996;36(2):311–9.
71. Pradhan A, Cheung YC, Grimer RJ, Peake D, Al-Muderis OA, Thomas JM, et al. Soft-tissue sarcomas of the hand: oncological outcome and prognostic factors. J Bone Joint Surg Br. 2008;90(2):209–14.
72. Brien EW, Terek RM, Geer RJ, Caldwell G, Brennan MF, Healey JH. Treatment of soft-tissue sarcomas of the hand. J Bone Joint Surg Am. 1995;77(4):564–71.
73. Puhaindran ME, Rohde RS, Chou J, Morris CD, Athanasian EA. Clinical outcomes for patients with soft tissue sarcoma of the hand. Cancer. 2011;117(1):175–9.
74. Lin PP, Guzel VB, Pisters PW, Zagars GK, Weber KL, Feig BW, et al. Surgical management of soft tissue sarcomas of the hand and foot. Cancer. 2002;95(4):852–61.
75. Bray PW, Bell RS, Bowen CV, Davis A, O'Sullivan B. Limb salvage surgery and adjuvant radiotherapy for soft tissue sarcomas of the forearm and hand. J Hand Surg Am. 1997;22(3):495–503.
76. Rohde RS, Puhaindran ME, Morris CD, Alektiar KM, Schupak KD, Healey JH, et al. Complications of radiation therapy to the hand after soft tissue sarcoma surgery. J Hand Surg Am. 2010;35(11):1858–63.
77. Talbert ML, Zagars GK, Sherman NE, Romsdahl MM. Conservative surgery and radiation therapy for soft tissue sarcoma of the wrist, hand, ankle, and foot. Cancer. 1990;66(12):2482–91.
78. Colterjohn NR, Davis AM, O'Sullivan B, Catton CN, Wunder JS, Bell RS. Functional outcome in limb-salvage surgery for soft tissue tumours of the foot and ankle. Sarcoma. 1997;1(2):67–74.
79. Cribb GL, Loo SC, Dickinson I. Limb salvage for soft-tissue sarcomas of the foot and ankle. J Bone Joint Surg Br. 2010;92(3):424–9.
80. Nishimura A, Matsumine A, Asanuma K, Matsubara T, Nakamura T, Uchida A, et al. The adverse effect of an unplanned surgical excision of foot soft tissue sarcoma. World J Surg Oncol. 2011;9:160.
81. Evans HL, Soule EH, Winkelmann RK. Atypical lipoma, atypical intramuscular lipoma, and well differentiated retroperitoneal liposarcoma: a reappraisal of 30 cases formerly classified as well differentiated liposarcoma. Cancer. 1979;43(2):574–84.
82. Dei Tos A. Atypical lipomatous tumour/well differentiated liposarcoma. In: Fletcher CDM, Unni KK, Mertens F, editors. Pathology and genetics of tumours of soft tissue and bone. Lyon: IARC Press; 2002.
83. Mussi CE, Daolio P, Cimino M, Giardina F, De Sanctis R, Morenghi E, et al. Atypical lipomatous tumors: should they be treated like other sarcoma or not? Surgical consideration from a bi-institutional experience. Ann Surg Oncol. 2014;21(13):4090–7.
84. Errani C, Cocchi S, Ali N, Chehrassan M, Righi A, Gambarotti M, et al. Recurrence after marginal excision for atypical lipomatous tumors versus lipomas of the extremities. Orthopedics. 2016;39(4):e610–4.
85. Rauh J, Klein A, Baur-Melnyk A, Knösel T, Lindner L, Roeder F, et al. The role of surgical margins in atypical Lipomatous Tumours of the extremities. BMC Musculoskelet Disord. 2018;19(1):152.
86. Bishop AJ, Zagars GK, Torres KE, Hunt KK, Cormier JN, Feig BW, et al. Combined modality management of retroperitoneal sarcomas: a single-institution series of 121 patients. Int J Radiat Oncol Biol Phys. 2015;93(1):158–65.
87. Noria S, Davis A, Kandel R, Levesque J, O'Sullivan B, Wunder J, et al. Residual disease following unplanned excision of soft-tissue sarcoma of an extremity. J Bone Joint Surg Am. 1996;78(5):650–5.
88. Randall RL, Bruckner JD, Papenhausen MD, Thurman T, Conrad EU 3rd. Errors in diagnosis and margin determination of soft-tissue sarcomas initially treated at non-tertiary centers. Orthopedics. 2004;27(2):209–12.
89. Giuliano AE, Eilber FR. The rationale for planned reoperation after unplanned total excision of soft-tissue sarcomas. J Clin Oncol. 1985;3(10):1344–8.
90. Morii T, Yabe H, Morioka H, Anazawa U, Suzuki Y, Toyama Y. Clinical significance of additional wide resection for unplanned resection of high grade soft tissue sarcoma. Open Orthop J. 2008;2:126–9.
91. Pretell-Mazzini J, Barton MD Jr, Conway SA, Temple HT. Unplanned excision of soft-tissue sarcomas: current concepts for management and prognosis. J Bone Joint Surg Am. 2015;97(7):597–603.
92. Ferguson PC, Griffin AM, O'Sullivan B, Catton CN, Davis AM, Murji A, et al. Bone invasion in extremity soft-tissue sarcoma: impact on disease outcomes. Cancer. 2006;106(12):2692–700.
93. Lin PP, Pino ED, Normand AN, Deavers MT, Cannon CP, Ballo MT, et al. Periosteal margin in soft-tissue sarcoma. Cancer. 2007;109(3):598–602.
94. Dagan R, Indelicato DJ, McGee L, Morris CG, Kirwan JM, Knapik J, et al. The significance of a marginal excision after preoperative radiation therapy for soft tissue sarcoma of the extremity. Cancer. 2012;118(12):3199–207.
95. King DM, Hackbarth DA, Kirkpatrick A. Extremity soft tissue sarcoma resections: how wide do you need to be? Clin Orthop Relat Res. 2012;470(3):692–9.
96. Panicek DM, Go SD, Healey JH, Leung DH, Brennan MF, Lewis JJ. Soft-tissue sarcoma involving bone or neurovascular structures: MR imaging prognostic factors. Radiology. 1997;205(3):871–5.

Surgical Strategy in Primary, Relapse, and "Whoops" Cases

18

Maria Danieli and Alessandro Gronchi

18.1 General Principles

Curative intent surgery serves as the standard and exclusive potentially curative modality for treating extremity soft tissue sarcomas (ESTS). It involves performing a wide excision, which encompasses the removal of the tumor along with a surrounding cuff of healthy tissue in order to achieve negative margins and minimize the presence of residual microsatellites and tumor surface contamination. The importance of obtaining negative margins is underscored by the fact that positive margins are a critical determinant of local failure and even mortality in cases of local relapse (LR), particularly in critical anatomical locations.

The concept of a "safe margin" remains a contentious issue and it is acknowledged that no universal definition exists. Tailored evaluations on a case-by-case basis are required, incorporating tumor-related factors (biological traits, tumor location, tumor history) and patient-specific factors including quality of life and preferences. The presence of a multidisciplinary team comprising oncologists, radiologists, radiotherapists, and pathologists contributes significantly to optimizing outcomes and refining diagnostic and therapeutic pathways [1]. Accurate pathological diagnosis is a pivotal step, particularly for histologically complex cases, requiring close collaboration between the surgeon and pathologist. The surgeon should orient the tumor specimen with sutures and work closely with the pathologist to ensure the correct orientation and an adequate tissue sampling. In addition, since sarcomas ideally arise in any site of the body, the availability of other specialized surgeons such as neurosurgeons, orthopedics, or plastic surgeons may be of crucial importance for counseling or technical help when approaching tumors located at sites of relevance.

M. Danieli · A. Gronchi (✉)
Department of Surgery, Fondazione IRCCS Istituto Nazionale dei Tumori, Milan, Italy
e-mail: alessandro.gronchi@istitutotumori.mi.it

18.2 Addressing Adequate Margins

The extent of healthy tissue that should be excised around the tumor to achieve an "adequate" margin continues to be a topic of ongoing debate. Unlike epithelial tumors, a single definition of an adequate margin isn't universally applicable due to variations in histology, location, treatment, and patient characteristics. Nonetheless, several key considerations emerge: (1) Positive margins significantly impact local outcomes, and even mortality in critical sites; (2) Some experts consider a surgical margin of <1 mm as microscopically positive, but when multidisciplinary treatment is administered, a margin of <1 mm might still be considered adequate [2]; (3) Planned close but ultimately positive margins following multidisciplinary treatment within a referral center can yield outcomes comparable to negative margins, whereas intratumoral margins or positive margins after inadequate initial excision do not [3, 4]. A deeper discussion about factors concurring in margin evaluation is presented in the following paragraphs.

18.2.1 Tumor Depth Relative to Fascia

Tumors situated below or involving the investing fascia are categorized as deep, whereas those located above the fascia without any involvement are classified as superficial. When a tumor infiltrates the fascia, it retains its classification as a deep tumor, irrespective of its predominant location in the subcutaneous tissue. For tumors with a superficial component, regardless of fascial plane involvement, a skin paddle covering the superficial portion should be resected. In cases of substantial tissue loss, options such as skin grafts or flaps can be considered. Conversely, in deep tumors without an extension into the superficial layers, the resection of a skin paddle isn't necessary, and the investing fascia can serve as an appropriate superficial margin. Even in superficial tumors without any fascial involvement, it is important to include the fascia as deep margin [5]. There are instances

H. Özger et al. (eds.), *Diagnosis and Treatment of Soft Tissue Tumors*, https://doi.org/10.1007/978-3-031-77061-6_18

where achieving an adequate margin might be challenging or require sacrificing a limb or part of it. In such scenarios, factors like the administration of medical or locoregional treatments and patient prognosis should be carefully weighed when deciding on the aggressiveness of the surgical strategy.

18.2.2 Presence of a Biologic Barrier

Muscular fascia, vascular adventitia, periosteum, and epineurium can function as "biologic barriers" due to the lower likelihood of tumor infiltration into these tissues. Recent evidence highlights that patients exhibiting focal positive margins near critical structures (such as bone, nerves, or vessels) who undergo a planned close excision to preserve these structures, but ultimately exhibit microscopically positive margins upon final pathological examination, do not display a heightened risk of local recurrence compared to patients in whom these critical structures are excised [3, 4]. Consequently, in cases where bone, nerves, or vessels are only tangentially involved, their complete removal may not be necessary for achieving equivalent local control rates. The elimination of periosteum, epineurium, and vascular adventitia might suffice, especially when accompanied by perioperative treatments (Fig. 18.1). Conversely, when these structures are markedly invaded, en-bloc removal with the tumor is recommended, followed by reconstruction [5]. Notably, in situations involving nerve reconstruction, opting for preoperative radiotherapy is advisable to avert damage to the reconstructed nerve.

18.2.3 Use of Perioperative Treatments

The prognostic significance of a positive margin can be counteracted through the utilization of perioperative treatments. Perioperative radiotherapy has been extensively proven to diminish the occurrence of local recurrence, particularly in high-risk patients [6–8]. However, the influence of the timing of radiotherapy delivery on local control remains somewhat uncertain.

In a retrospective study encompassing 317 patients with nonmetastatic ESTS treated with preoperative radiotherapy and limb-sparing surgery, cases where marginal excision followed preoperative radiotherapy exhibited comparable local control and amputation-free survival rates to those undergoing wide/radical margin resections [9]. Another investigation by Gronchi et al. examined the impact of surgical quality in a cohort participating in a prospective randomized study on preoperative chemotherapy in localized high-risk STS. The findings revealed that among high-risk sarcoma patients undergoing marginal resections, those who were pretreated

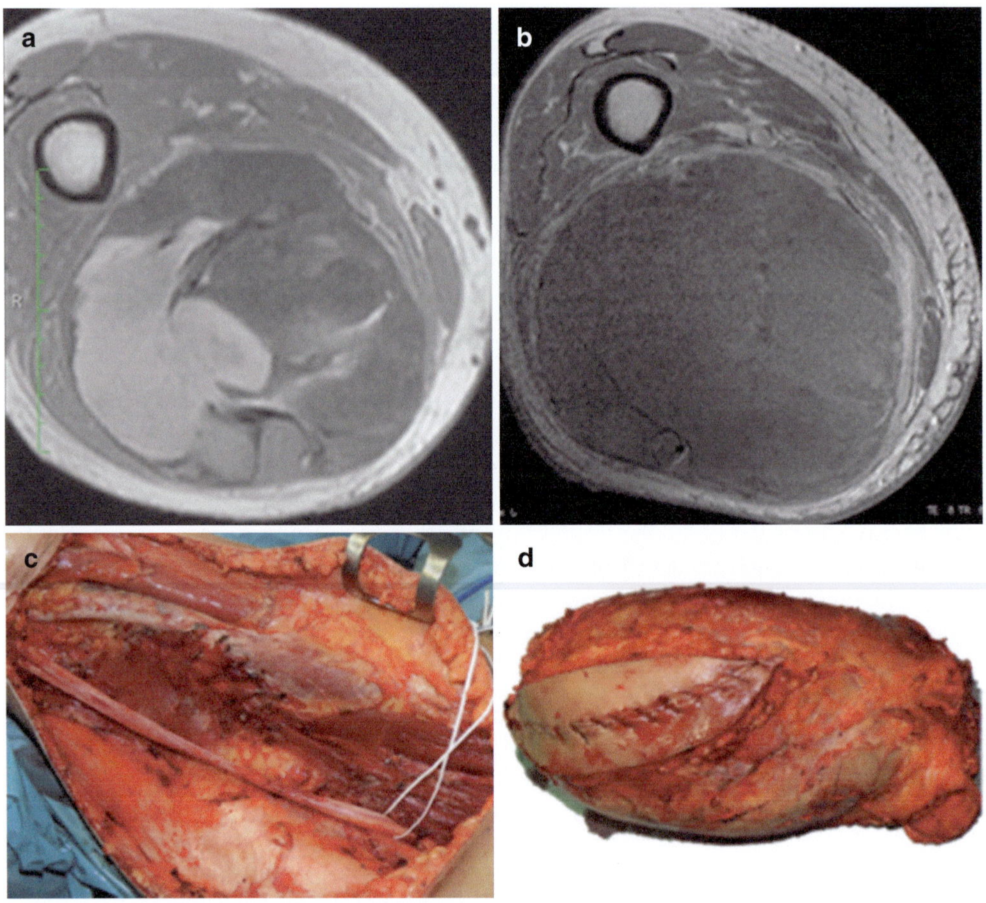

Fig. 18.1 Axial magnetic resonance image of an undifferentiated pleomorphic sarcoma grade 3 of the posterior aspect of the right high in close proximity to the ischiatic nerve (arrows) before (**a**) and after (**b**) radiotherapy to a total dose of 50 Gy. Intraoperative images demonstrating en bloc tumor resection together with perineurium and a close margin on the ischiatic nerve (**c** and **d**)

with chemotherapy-radiotherapy had a cumulative incidence of local recurrence akin to patients achieving R0 margins, a trend not observed in patients who solely received preoperative chemotherapy [10].

Collectively, these studies hint that in scenarios involving anticipated close or positive margins, preoperative radiotherapy might offer an advantage by potentially mitigating the negative prognostic impact of such margins. This concept is mirrored in the increased utilization of preoperative radiotherapy over recent years [11].

18.2.4 Histology

Soft tissue sarcomas encompass over 70 histologic entities, each characterized by distinct behaviors, recurrence patterns, and responses to treatment. Nomograms provide valuable tools for understanding tumor heterogeneity, considering various patient and tumor-related factors and their interactions for risk assessment [12–15]. In general, we strongly encourage the use of available nomograms by clinicians as a guide for treatment planning (Fig. 18.2). An online and app

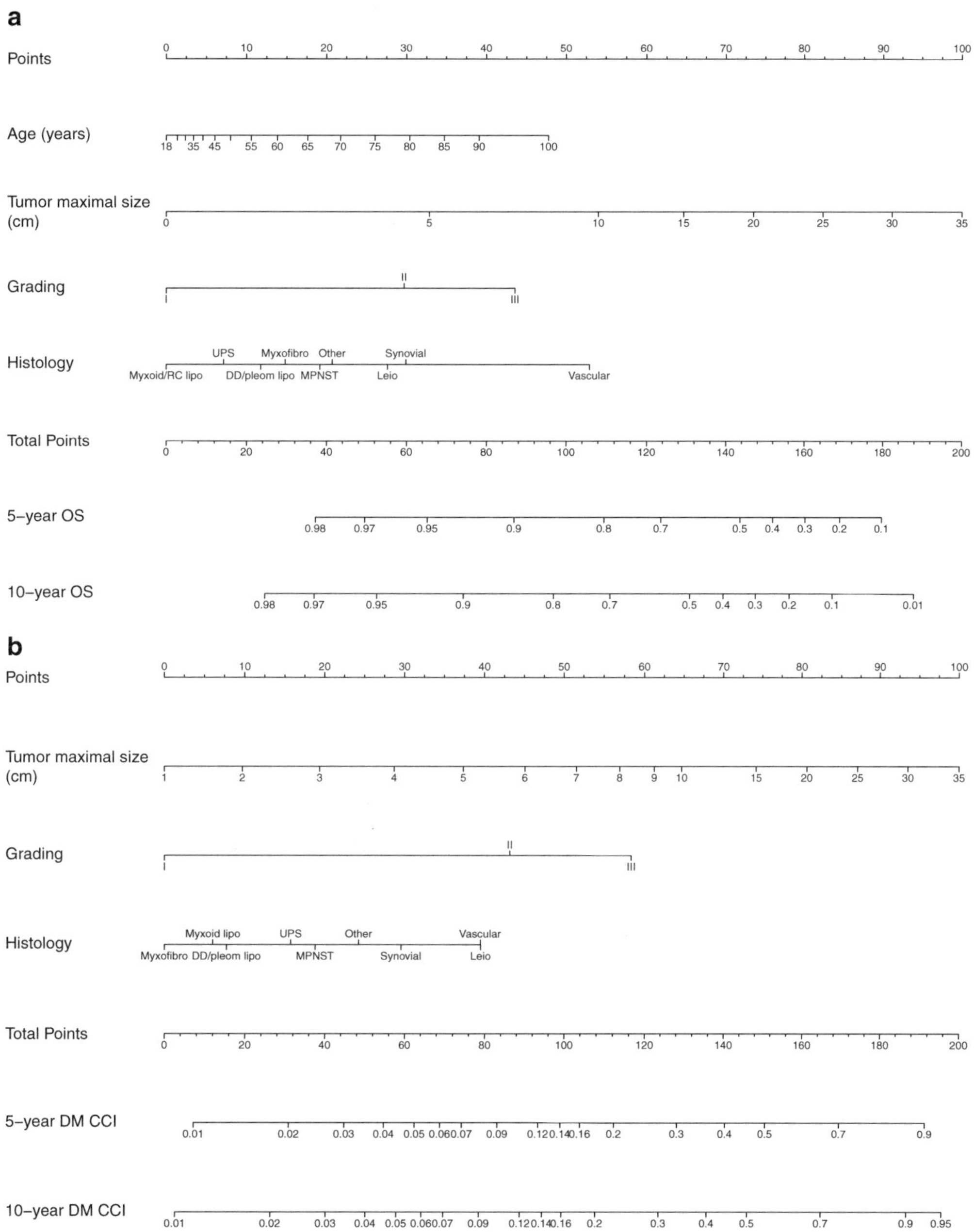

Fig. 18.2 Nomograms for the calculation of the 5-year and 10-year probability of overall survival (**a**) and the crude cumulative incidence of developing distant metastases (**b**) after surgical resection of a primary soft tissue sarcoma of the extremities on the basis of patient-related and tumor-related covariates. DD/pleom lipo indicates dedifferentiated/pleomorphic liposarcoma; Leio, leiomyosarcoma; MPNST, malignant peripheral nerve sheath tumor; Myxofibro, myxofibrosarcoma; Myxoid lipo, myxoid liposarcoma; UPS, undifferentiated pleomorphic sarcoma (Reprinted with permission from Ref. [19] (License Number 5617651334459))

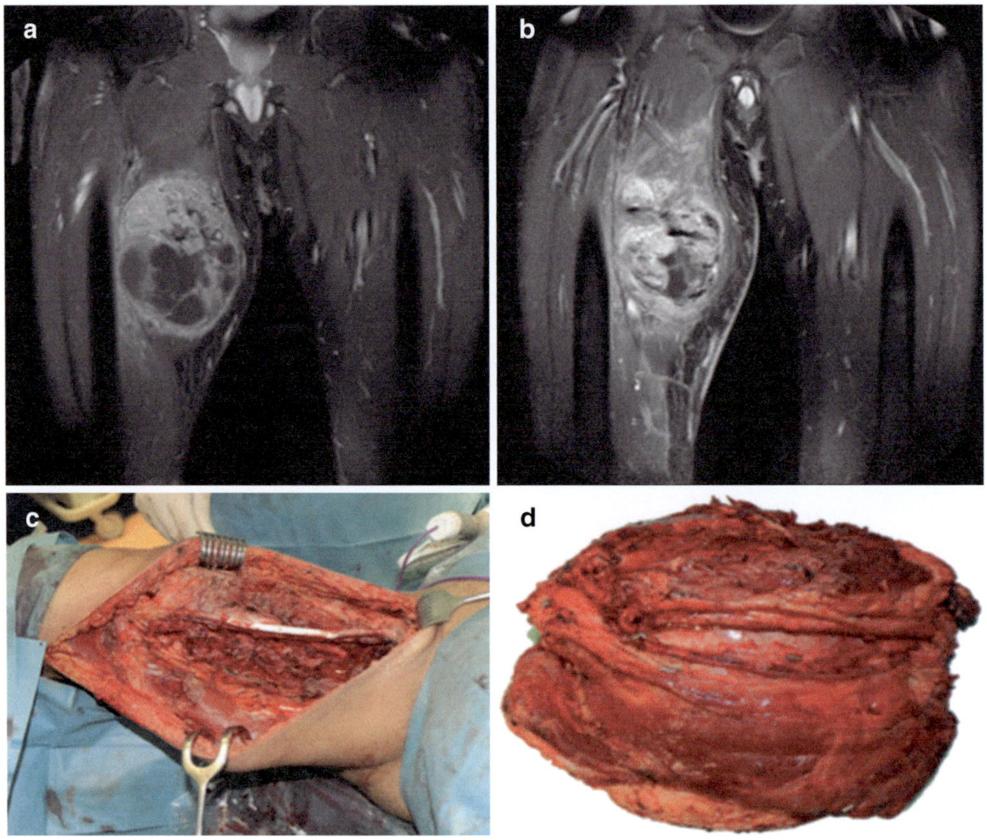

Fig. 18.3 Coronal magnetic resonance image of an undifferentiated pleomorphic sarcoma grade 3 of the medial aspect of the left high with close proximity/infiltration of the superficial femoral artery before (**a**) and after (**b**) 3 cycles of chemotherapy with Epirubicin-Ifosfamide. Intraoperative images display the wide excision of the tumor en bloc with the involved tract of the superficial femoral artery and its reconstruction with a 6 mm diameter PDTE prosthesis (**c** and **d**)

version is also available for the nomogram by Callegaro et al. [16]. Specific surgical strategies for some histologic subtypes will be discussed at the end of this chapter.

18.3 Plastic, Neurovascular, and Tendinous Reconstruction

When aiming for curative surgery, it is not uncommon to face the challenge of excising substantial portions of soft tissues or resecting vital structures like nerves, vessels, or tendons when they are visibly invaded by tumors (Fig. 18.3). In contrast to vascular and tendinous reconstruction, nerve reconstructions are complex procedures with relatively high failure rates and extended functional recovery periods. In such cases, selecting the appropriate plastic reconstruction approach should be guided by prognosis estimates using nomograms. For aggressive tumors with unfavorable outcomes, opting for simpler, less morbid reconstructions with swift functional recovery might be advisable, while complex reconstructions can be pursued in cases with better prognoses.

18.4 Re-Excision in Unplanned Surgery

Between 20% and 60% of patients diagnosed with ESTS who present at a Sarcoma Center have previously undergone unplanned surgery at non-referral centers. Re-excision subsequent to unplanned surgery can significantly improve the prognosis for these patients, both in terms of overall survival (OS) and reduced risk of metastasis, even for those with high-risk sarcomas [17–19]. However, re-excision comes with increased morbidity and a higher risk of functional impairment, which consequently strains healthcare resources. In absence of visible residual disease on magnetic resonance imaging (MRI), re-excision becomes even more challenging, as it is not guided by the presence of a visible mass. Additionally, pathology often does not reveal residual disease in more than half of cases.

For these reasons some authors have questioned the need for systematic re-excision in patients without visible tumors on MRI. Research by Bonvalot et al. in 2017 suggested that while the presence of residual disease in re-excision specimens correlated with a higher risk of local recurrence (LR), it did not necessarily lead to higher metastatic risk or worse survival [20]. Moreover, in a retrospective study by the same group, patients who did not undergo re-excision (intentionally or because RT was preferred due to poor performance status) had comparable overall survival and metastatic relapse-free survival to those who did undergo primary excision or re-excision after unplanned surgery. Interestingly, this study found that radiotherapy was associated with a lower LR incidence, especially in patients who were not re-excised or were re-excised at non-referral centers [21]. A 2021 retrospective analysis by Istituto Nazionale dei Tumori (INT, Milan) also showed that re-excision after unplanned

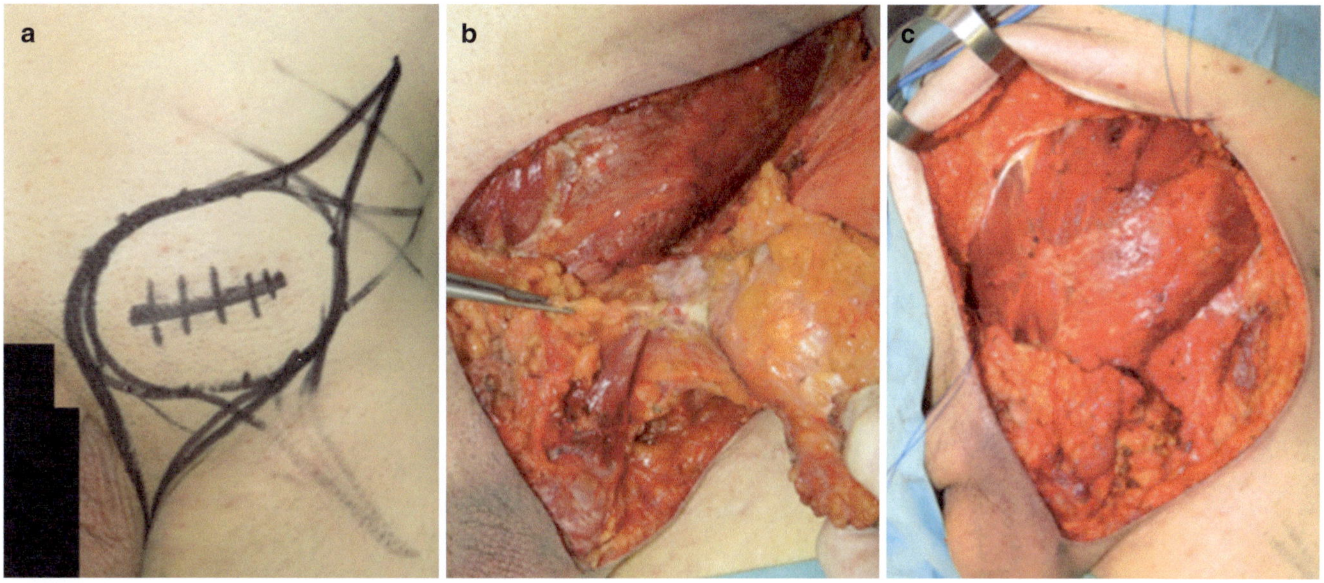

Fig. 18.4 Preoperative (**a**) and intraoperative (**b** and **c**) images of a wide re-excision in a patient who underwent marginal unplanned surgery for myxoid liposarcoma grade 3 of the left groin. Despite the absence of clinical and radiological evidence of disease, re-excision to include scar tissue is still recommended for critical sites

surgery increased the risk of LR for ESTS patients, but this did not directly translate into higher risks of distant spread or lower OS. Similarly, in patients who underwent re-excision after macroscopically complete UE, the presence of microscopic residual tumor was associated with a significantly higher risk of LR, but not with a higher risk of DM or lower OS [22].

These observations suggest that local relapse might not be the primary cause of metastatic spread and associated increased mortality. Instead, a local relapse might reflect the tumor's biological aggressiveness and histology, factors that directly determine the overall prognosis of the patient.

Taken together, these findings support the "watch and wait" approach endorsed by the French group for carefully selected patients with macroscopically complete unplanned surgery, where re-excision is postponed until LR occurs. While this approach appears safe based on current evidence, the impact of delaying broader excision at recurrence on final survival remains uncertain. A case-by-case, multidisciplinary assessment remains crucial for patient selection. However, for tumors located in critical sites, where local relapse could lead to patient death, re-excision remains the standard treatment even without visible residual disease (Fig. 18.4).

18.5 Surgery in Locally Recurrent Disease

The occurrence of local recurrence in ESTS can range from 5% to 15% within a 10-year period, influenced by various tumor, treatment, and patient-related factors [11].

A dynamic nomogram has recently been developed to predict 5-year overall survival in the initial 3 years of follow-up for primary ESTS patients [12]. This tool permits a recalculation of patient prognosis, accounting for local recurrence or distant metastasis, time since primary surgery, and the potential time-dependent effects of covariates. This nomogram proves valuable when deciding on the surgical strategy for locally relapsed tumors. If the prognosis indicates low survival, prioritizing limb preservation and patient quality of life becomes essential. Conversely, when prognosis is more favorable, amputation might be considered to maximize chances of cure.

18.6 Isolated Limb Perfusion

Isolated limb perfusion (ILP) involves infusing high doses of chemotherapeutic agents under mild hyperthermia into a limb or limb region after surgically isolating the vascular peduncle from the systemic circulation.

While ILP mitigates systemic toxicity, its minimal systemic distribution also implies limited systemic control of metastasis.

ILP is primarily indicated to enable conversion to limb-sparing procedures in patients who would otherwise require primary or secondary amputations. This includes cases with multifocal presentation or recurrence, locally advanced tumors invading neurovascular bundles, bones, or cases where radical resections are unfeasible based on clinical and imaging assessments [23] (Fig. 18.5). ILP may also be considered for patients who do not respond to preoperative chemo-radiotherapy.

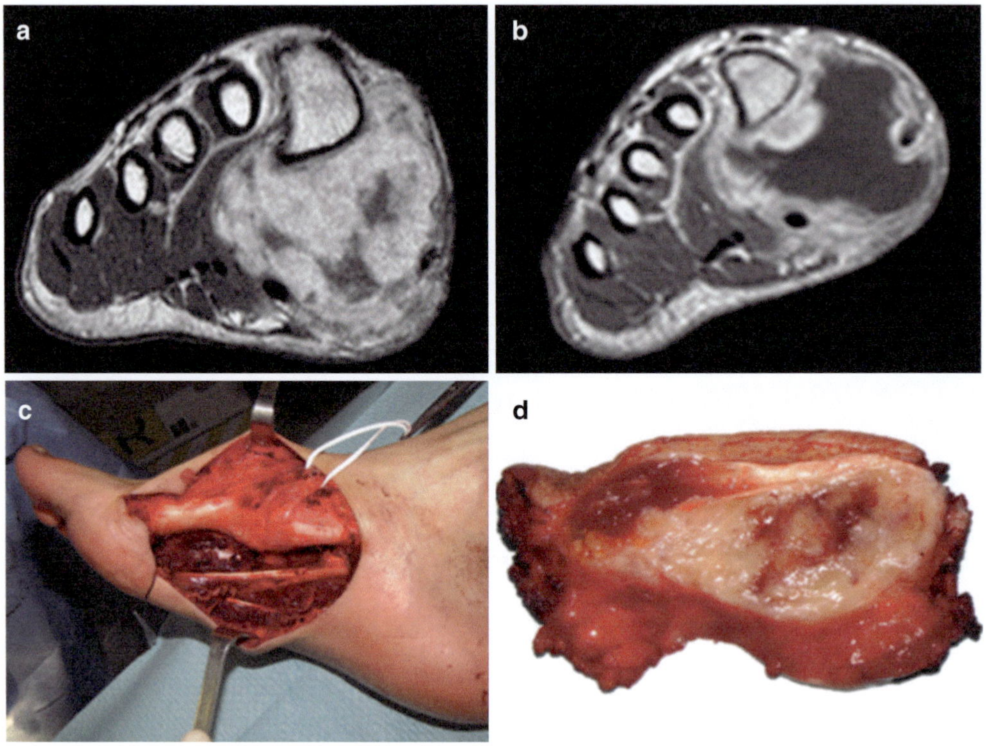

Fig. 18.5 Axial view magnetic resonance image of a malignant myoepithelioma of the left foot before (**a**) and after isolated limb perfusion (**b**). Surgical excision of the tumor involved the removal of the first metatarsal bone along with periosteum (**c** and **d**)

18.7 Histology-Specific Surgical Strategies

18.7.1 Well-Differentiated Liposarcoma of the Extremity

Well-differentiated liposarcoma (WDLPS) typically presents as an indolent and painless mass most frequently arising in the extremities. WDLPS is difficult to differentiate radiologically from a benign lipoma and is characterized by a low rate of local recurrence with almost absent metastatic potential. However, a dedifferentiated component within a WD tumor may be encountered in 1–2% of cases, or dedifferentiation may occur in locally recurrent diseases, resulting in a significantly adverse outcome [24].

In entirely WDLPS, excellent outcomes are achieved through surgical intervention alone, with LR incidence reaching 0% at 5 years in patients treated at referral centers. Given its indolent behavior even in case of recurrence, limited negative margins or even positive margins are considered acceptable, especially when functional preservation or cosmetic outcomes are of concern [25, 26].

Consequently, in select cases, the "watch and wait" approach, previously discussed, can be deemed a safe option. Notably, some authors recently proposed an active surveillance strategy for primary WDLPS patients, given an assessment of the natural history in which only a minority required surgery due to symptomatology or tumor growth [27].

Conversely, in primary WDLPS with a DD component or in recurrent WDLPS, surgical excision remains pivotal. This involves either a wider margin resection, if feasible, or adjunctive radiation therapy to optimize local control, as LR emerges as the most prevalent event post-surgery.

18.7.2 Myxoid Liposarcoma

Among liposarcoma subtypes, myxoid liposarcoma (MLPS) is the most common entity observed in the extremities, particularly in younger patients. It can be categorized into classic/low-grade and cellular/high-grade variants. The notable chemosensitivity and radiosensitivity of MLPS makes the preoperative utilization of either or both treatments a crucial tool, especially when dealing with tumors situated adjacent to vital structures like nerves, tendons, or vessels [28–31].

The heightened radiosensitivity of MLPS provided the rationale for the Dose Reduction of Preoperative Radiotherapy in Myxoid Liposarcomas (DOREMY) trial. This prospective, single-group, phase 2 multicentric nonrandomized controlled trial administered a lower dose (36 Gy) of radiation therapy followed by surgery to 77 patients with localized MLPS of the extremity and trunk [32]. When compared to historical data involving a traditional neoadjuvant dose of 50 Gy, the experimental data showed comparable outcomes and a more favorable toxic effect profile favoring the lower dose regimen.

A recent multicentric retrospective study revealed no association between margin status and outcome (local recurrence-free, metastasis-free, and overall survival) in patients with intermuscular MLPS who received preoperative radiation therapy [33]. Thus, when preoperative RT is administered, marginal resection can be deemed safe without compromising oncologic control (Fig. 18.6).

In addition to its heightened response to standard first-line chemotherapy regimens involving anthracycline +/− ifosfamide, MLPS also demonstrates sensitivity to trabectedin [34, 35]. Notably, a randomized trial comparing anthracycline and ifosfamide with "histotype-tailored" chemotherapy for high-risk STS revealed that the histotype-tailored chemotherapy with trabectedin in MLPS was the only regimen showing results comparable to those achieved with anthracycline and ifosfamide treatment. This led to the inception of an international, open-label, phase 2 nonrandomized clinical trial involving 46 patients with MLPS treated with trabectedin plus preoperative radiation therapy at a total dose of 45 Gy [36]. These findings suggest that this combination therapy was well tolerated and exhibited effectiveness in terms of pathologic response, thereby positioning trabectedin plus radiotherapy as a viable option from a tolerability standpoint.

18.7.3 Dermatofibrosarcoma Protuberans

Dermatofibrosarcoma protuberans (DFSP) is a superficial tumor most frequently arising in middle-aged adults. In approximately 90–95% of cases, it exhibits minimal metastatic potential and slow growth, yet it possesses a propensity to extend beyond evident macroscopic margins, contributing to its strong tendency for local recurrence. Nevertheless, an aggressive variant comprising 5–10% of cases poses a significant risk of both local and distant recurrence [37, 38].

For the more common variant, wide-margin surgery remains the cornerstone of treatment, obviating the need for adjuvant therapy in cases with adequate margins. Due to its infiltrative growth pattern, performing a wide local excision with the goal of attaining a radial margin of 3 cm and a deep fascial margin effectively minimizes the risk of local recurrence. However, plastic surgery reconstruction is frequently required in these patients. Since DFSP primarily affects superficial tissues, excising deep muscles is generally unnecessary. Unfortunately, intraoperative frozen sections are unreliable due to potential artifact generation caused by surrounding fat. Given its relatively indolent behavior, acceptance of positive margins might be considered for aesthetic reasons, and a broader resection could be deferred until recurrence manifests. Furthermore, in cases requiring reconstruction, a tissue expander might be introduced prior to resection in order to facilitate the attainment of an adequate flap for reconstruction.

Conversely, aggressive variants should be managed like conventional sarcomas, necessitating wide-margin resections that encompass the deep muscle tissue adjacent to the

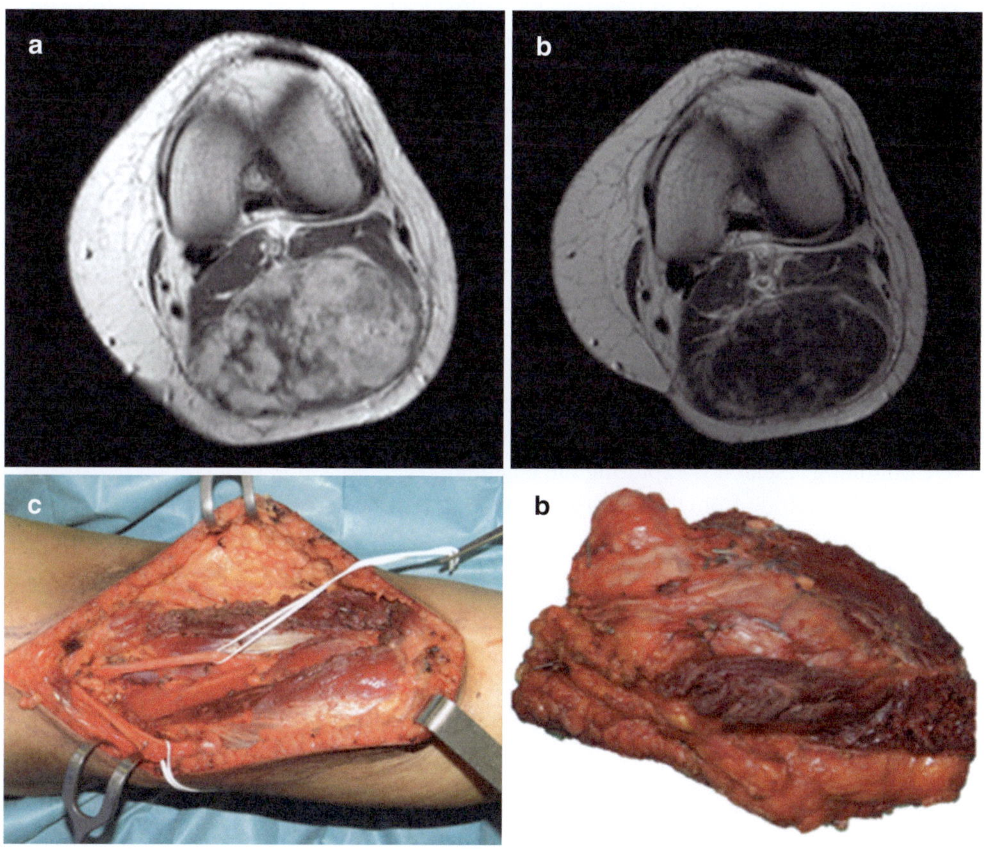

Fig. 18.6 Axial magnetic resonance image of a myxoid liposarcoma grade 3 of the left popliteal region before (**a**) and after (**b**) 3 cycles of chemotherapy with Trabectedin plus radiotherapy for a total dose of 45 Gy. Intraoperative images showing wide excision of the tumor. The superficial branch of the common peroneal nerve was infiltrated and resected en block with the tumor while the deep branch of the peroneal nerve (inferior white lace) and the posterior tibial nerve (superior white lace) has been dissected through the subperineurial plane (**c** and **d**). At pathological analysis, positive margins were found on the perineurium with the closest free margin being at 0.5 mm from the tumor. No adjuvant therapy was administered

tumor. Radiotherapy is generally not recommended for these variants, while Imatinib finds utility in cases of local advancement or metastasis [39, 40]. Importantly, neoadjuvant Imatinib-induced tumor shrinkage does not permit more conservative resection, as the original tumor extent remains unaltered. In the context of locally advanced tumors, the administration of adjuvant Imatinib while employing a tissue expander may help constrain local growth.

18.7.4 Myxofibrosarcoma

Myxofibrosarcoma (MFS) is one of the most frequent histologic subtypes of ESTS and is generally diagnosed in the elderly. When located superficially or along fascial planes, these tumors tend to infiltrate the subcutaneous adipose tissue and the fascia, extending several centimeters beyond the palpable mass's confines.

The typical radiological marker of this infiltration is represented by "tails," visible at MRI, that branch off from the gross tumor. In cases where MFS is located intramuscularly, the extent of infiltration may be limited by anatomical barriers. Nevertheless, this histological variant displays a tendency overcome such barriers, which is mirrored by the relatively high rate of positive margins (around 20% in high volume centers series) resulting in a high incidence of local recurrence [41]. Consequently, surgical excision should encompass a breadth of 2–4 cm beyond the palpable mass, encompassing the tumor-associated "tails" identified through MRI. Plastic reconstruction of soft tissue losses as well as critical structures is often required. Furthermore, the possibility exists to conduct surgical excision of the tumor, subsequently applying vacuum-assisted closure (VAC) therapy within the resection site, while deferring the definitive reconstruction to a second surgical intervention guided by the definitive pathological report. This two-step approach enables margins optimization in case of positivity [42].

MFS shows a very good response to adjuvant RT, and its preoperative use in case of planned positive margins or in large, high-grade, deep tumors is robustly recommended to enhance the attainment of favorable local control rates [43, 44]. Continuing research is exploring the potential synergistic outcomes resulting from the strategic interaction between radiotherapy and immune checkpoint inhibitors. This therapeutic approach is currently being investigated in the context of both myxofibrosarcoma (MFS) and undifferentiated pleomorphic sarcoma (UPS) [45–47].

18.7.5 Radiation-Induced Sarcoma

Radiation-induced sarcoma encompasses a spectrum of distinct histologic types, most frequently including UPS, angiosarcoma, and malignant peripheral nerve sheath tumor (MPNST). These tumors, in addition to sharing specific histologic characteristics, exhibit an aggressively formidable behavior characterized by a pronounced propensity for local recurrence and an overall poor prognosis. Surgical management of these tumors is intricate due to the challenge of distinguishing between healthy tissue invaded by the tumor and tissue damaged by prior radiation exposure.

Moreover, these tumors often present as multifocal entities within the irradiated field. Consequently, the surgical imperative involves executing the broadest feasible excision, a maneuver that frequently mandates subsequent plastic reconstruction. Systemic chemotherapy and reirradiation (with caution) might be considered.

18.7.6 Malignant Peripheral Nerve Sheath Tumors

MPNST commonly originate in young and middle-aged adults, emerging from major peripheral nerves. Roughly half of these tumors occur within the context of neurofibromatosis type I, while the remaining cases arise sporadically or as a consequence of previous radiation therapy. MPNSTs carry an unfavorable prognosis marked by a heightened risk of local failure and the potential for metastatic dissemination. The cornerstone of therapeutic intervention remains surgical resection, characterized by the pursuit of wide margins, with a recommended minimum of 4 cm of macroscopically unaffected nerve tissue when feasible.

Intraoperative frozen sections can help in discerning clean margins during surgery. Adjuvant chemotherapy and radiation therapy might contribute to outcome improvement, although the decision to administer the latter should be weighed carefully, taking into account the elevated risk of radiation-induced sarcomas [48–50].

18.8 Conclusions

In summary, centralizing patient care within high-volume reference centers is a crucial step. This ensures the application of a comprehensive, multidisciplinary strategy that significantly improves outcomes for individuals dealing with the rarity of ESTS. Modern surgical approaches prioritize both limb and function preservation, aiming to minimize excision extent while safeguarding the patient's prognosis.

The primary objective of curative intent surgery for ESTS is achieving wide excision with negative margins to enhance local disease control. However, surgical management and assessing margin adequacy require comprehensive consideration of various factors, including patient quality of life and the intricate tumor heterogeneity related to different site and histologic subtypes. In selected cases, in fact, accepting microscopically positive margins does not necessarily jeopardize patient prognosis. Conversely, aiming at resection margins of maximal extent is crucial for malignancies characterized by infiltrative growth patterns.

Prognostic evaluation through the employment of available nomograms plays a fundamental role in helping clinicians tailor personalized treatment strategies and in assisting surgeon decision-making, giving a rationale for the calibration of surgical excision aggressiveness and the complexity of subsequent reconstructions.

In cases of unplanned excisions, re-excision is mandatory when macroscopic residual tumor is identified through MRI. Conversely, in selected patients with microscopically positive margins without postoperative macroscopic residual disease evident on imaging, a cautious "watch and wait" approach emerges as a viable consideration.

References

1. Blay JY, Soibinet P, Penel N, Bompas E, Duffaud F, Stoeckle E, Mir O, Adam J, Chevreau C, Bonvalot S, Rios M, Kerbrat P, Cupissol D, Anract P, Gouin F, Kurtz JE, Lebbe C, Isambert N, Bertucci F, Toumonde M, Thyss A, Piperno-Neumann S, Dubray-Longeras P, Meeus P, Ducimetière F, Giraud A, Coindre JM, Ray-Coquard I, Italiano A, Le Cesne A. Improved survival using specialized multidisciplinary board in sarcoma patients. Ann Oncol. 2017;28(11):2852–9. https://doi.org/10.1093/annonc/mdx484. PMID: 29117335; PMCID: PMC5834019.
2. Kainhofer V, Smolle MA, Szkandera J, Liegl-Atzwanger B, Maurer-Ertl W, Gerger A, Riedl J, Leithner A. The width of resection margins influences local recurrence in soft tissue sarcoma patients. Eur J Surg Oncol. 2016;42(6):899–906. https://doi.org/10.1016/j.ejso.2016.03.026. Epub 2016 Apr 12. PMID: 27107792.
3. O'Donnell PW, Griffin AM, Eward WC, Sternheim A, Catton CN, Chung PW, O'Sullivan B, Ferguson PC, Wunder JS. The effect of the setting of a positive surgical margin in soft tissue sarcoma. Cancer. 2014;120(18):2866–75. https://doi.org/10.1002/cncr.28793. Epub 2014 Jun 3. PMID: 24894656.
4. Kawaguchi N, Ahmed AR, Matsumoto S, Manabe J, Matsushita Y. The concept of curative margin in surgery for bone and soft tissue sarcoma. Clin Orthop Relat Res. 2004;419:165–72. https://doi.org/10.1097/00003086-200402000-00027. PMID: 15021149.
5. Gronchi A, Raut CP. Management of soft tissue sarcoma. In: Current surgical therapy. 13th ed. Elsevier; 2020. p. 825–40.
6. Beane JD, Yang JC, White D, Steinberg SM, Rosenberg SA, Rudloff U. Efficacy of adjuvant radiation therapy in the treatment of soft tissue sarcoma of the extremity: 20-year follow-up of a randomized prospective trial. Ann Surg Oncol. 2014;21(8):2484–9. https://doi.org/10.1245/s10434-014-3732-4. Epub 2014 Apr 23. PMID: 24756814; PMCID: PMC6293463.
7. Yang JC, Chang AE, Baker AR, Sindelar WF, Danforth DN, Topalian SL, DeLaney T, Glatstein E, Steinberg SM, Merino MJ, Rosenberg SA. Randomized prospective study of the benefit of adjuvant radiation therapy in the treatment of soft tissue sarcomas of the extremity. J Clin Oncol. 1998;16(1):197–203. https://doi.org/10.1200/JCO.1998.16.1.197. PMID: 9440743.
8. Callegaro D, Miceli R, Bonvalot S, Ferguson P, Strauss DC, Levy A, Griffin A, Hayes AJ, Stacchiotti S, Le Pèchoux C, Smith MJ, Fiore M, Dei Tos AP, Smith HG, Catton C, Casali PG, Wunder JS, Gronchi A. Impact of perioperative chemotherapy and radiotherapy in patients with primary extremity soft tissue sarcoma: retrospective analysis across major histological subtypes and major reference centres. Eur J Cancer. 2018;105:19–27. https://doi.org/10.1016/j.ejca.2018.09.028. Epub 2018 Oct 29. PMID: 30384013.
9. Dagan R, Indelicato DJ, McGee L, Morris CG, Kirwan JM, Knapik J, Reith J, Scarborough MT, Gibbs CP, Marcus RB Jr, Zlotecki RA. The significance of a marginal excision after preoperative radiation therapy for soft tissue sarcoma of the extremity. Cancer. 2012;118(12):3199–207. https://doi.org/10.1002/cncr.26489. Epub 2011 Oct 21. PMID: 22020375.
10. Gronchi A, Verderio P, De Paoli A, Ferraro A, Tendero O, Majò J, Martin J, Comandone A, Grignani G, Pizzamiglio S, Quagliuolo V, Picci P, Frustaci S, Dei Tos AP, Palassini E, Stacchiotti S, Ferrari S, Fiore M, Casali PG. Quality of surgery and neoadjuvant combined therapy in the ISG-GEIS trial on soft tissue sarcomas of limbs and trunk wall. Ann Oncol. 2013;24(3):817–23. https://doi.org/10.1093/annonc/mds501. Epub 2012 Oct 30. PMID: 23110811.
11. Danieli M, Barretta F, Fiore M, Radaelli S, Sangalli C, Barisella M, Stacchiotti S, Palassini E, Miceli R, Frezza AM, Callegaro D, Casali PG, Gronchi A. Refining the approach to patients with primary soft tissue sarcoma of the extremities and trunk wall: outcome improvement over time at a single institution. Ann Surg Oncol. 2022;29(5):3274–86. https://doi.org/10.1245/s10434-021-11189-2. Epub 2022 Jan 8. PMID: 35000087.
12. Callegaro D, Miceli R, Bonvalot S, Ferguson PC, Strauss DC, van Praag VVM, Levy A, Griffin AM, Hayes AJ, Stacchiotti S, Pèchoux CL, Smith MJ, Fiore M, Tos APD, Smith HG, Catton C, Szkandera J, Leithner A, van de Sande MAJ, Casali PG, Wunder JS, Gronchi A. Development and external validation of a dynamic prognostic nomogram for primary extremity soft tissue sarcoma survivors. E Clin Med. 2019;22(17):100215. https://doi.org/10.1016/j.eclinm.2019.11.008. PMID: 31891146; PMCID: PMC6933187.
13. Callegaro D, Miceli R, Bonvalot S, Ferguson P, Strauss DC, Levy A, Griffin A, Hayes AJ, Stacchiotti S, Pechoux CL, Smith MJ, Fiore M, Dei Tos AP, Smith HG, Mariani L, Wunder JS, Pollock RE, Casali PG, Gronchi A. Development and external validation of two nomograms to predict overall survival and occurrence of distant metastases in adults after surgical resection of localised soft-tissue sarcomas of the extremities: a retrospective analysis. Lancet Oncol. 2016;17(5):671–80. https://doi.org/10.1016/S1470-2045(16)00010-3. Epub 2016 Apr 5. PMID: 27068860.
14. van Praag VM, Rueten-Budde AJ, Jeys LM, Laitinen MK, Pollock R, Aston W, van der Hage JA, Dijkstra PDS, Ferguson PC, Griffin AM, Willeumier JJ, Wunder JS, van de Sande MAJ, Fiocco M. A prediction model for treatment decisions in high-grade extremity soft-tissue sarcomas: personalised sarcoma care (PERSARC). Eur J Cancer. 2017;83:313–23. https://doi.org/10.1016/j.ejca.2017.06.032. Epub 2017 Aug 8. PMID: 28797949.
15. Rueten-Budde AJ, van Praag VM, PERSARC Study Group, van de Sande MAJ, Fiocco M. Dynamic prediction of overall survival for patients with high-grade extremity soft tissue sarcoma. Surg Oncol. 2018;27(4):695–701. https://doi.org/10.1016/j.suronc.2018.09.003. Epub 2018 Sep 7. PMID: 30449495.
16. Digital Forest srl. https://play.google.com/store/apps/details?id=it.digitalforest.sarculator&pcampaignid=web_share or https://apps.apple.com/it/app/sarculator/id1052119173. Accessed August 28, 2023.
17. Fiore M, Casali PG, Miceli R, Mariani L, Bertulli R, Lozza L, Collini P, Olmi P, Mussi C, Gronchi A. Prognostic effect of re-excision in adult soft tissue sarcoma of the extremity. Ann Surg Oncol. 2006;13(1):110–7. https://doi.org/10.1245/ASO.2006.03.030. Epub 2006 Jan 1. PMID: 16372156.
18. Traub F, Griffin AM, Wunder JS, Ferguson PC. Influence of unplanned excisions on the outcomes of patients with stage III extremity soft-tissue sarcoma. Cancer. 2018;124(19):3868–75. https://doi.org/10.1002/cncr.31648. Epub 2018 Oct 15. PMID: 30321451.

19. Smolle MA, Tunn PU, Goldenitsch E, Posch F, Szkandera J, Bergovec M, Liegl-Atzwanger B, Leithner A. The prognostic impact of unplanned excisions in a cohort of 728 soft tissue sarcoma patients: a multicentre study. Ann Surg Oncol. 2017;24(6):1596–605. https://doi.org/10.1245/s10434-017-5776-8. Epub 2017 Jan 20. PMID: 28108827; PMCID: PMC5413518.
20. Bonvalot S, Levy A, Terrier P, Tzanis D, Bellefqih S, Le Cesne A, Le Péchoux C. Primary extremity soft tissue sarcomas: does local control impact survival? Ann Surg Oncol. 2017;24(1):194–201. https://doi.org/10.1245/s10434-016-5462-2. Epub 2016 Aug 4. PMID: 27491785.
21. Decanter G, Stoeckle E, Honore C, Meeus P, Mattei JC, Dubray-Longeras P, Ferron G, Carrere S, Causeret S, Guilloit JM, Fau M, Rosset P, Machiavello JC, Delhorme JB, Regenet N, Gouin F, Blay JY, Coindre JM, Penel N, Bonvalot S. Watch and wait approach for re-excision after unplanned yet macroscopically complete excision of extremity and superficial truncal soft tissue sarcoma is safe and does not affect metastatic risk or amputation rate. Ann Surg Oncol. 2019;26(11):3526–34. https://doi.org/10.1245/s10434-019-07494-6. Epub 2019 Jul 23. PMID: 31338771.
22. Danieli M, Barretta F, Fiore M, Radaelli S, Sangalli C, Barisella M, Stacchiotti S, Palassini E, Miceli R, Callegaro D, Casali PG, Gronchi A. Unplanned excision of extremity and trunk wall soft tissue sarcoma: to re-resect or not to re-resect? Ann Surg Oncol. 2021;28(8):4706–17. https://doi.org/10.1245/s10434-020-09564-6. Epub 2021 Jan 28. PMID: 33511543.
23. Martin-Tellez KS, van Houdt WJ, van Coevorden F, Colombo C, Fiore M. Isolated limb perfusion for soft tissue sarcoma: current practices and future directions. A survey of experts and a review of literature. Cancer Treat Rev. 2020;88:102058. https://doi.org/10.1016/j.ctrv.2020.102058. Epub 2020 Jun 19. PMID: 32619864.
24. Tseng WW, Barretta F, Baia M, Barisella M, Radaelli S, Callegaro D, Yoon DH, Fiore M, Gronchi A. Dedifferentiation within well-differentiated liposarcoma of the extremity or trunk: implications for clinical management. J Surg Oncol. 2021;124(5):838–45. https://doi.org/10.1002/jso.26590. Epub 2021 Jul 13. PMID: 34254688.
25. Olson CR, Suarez-Kelly LP, Ethun CG, Shelby RD, Yu PY, Hughes TM, Palettas M, Tran TB, Poultsides G, Tseng J, Roggin KK, Chouliaras K, Votanopoulos K, Krasnick BA, Fields RC, King DM, Bedi M, Pollock RE, Grignol VP, Cardona K, Howard JH. Resection status does not impact recurrence in well-differentiated Liposarcoma of the extremity. Am Surg. 2021;87(11):1752–9. https://doi.org/10.1177/00031348211054536. Epub 2021 Nov 10. PMID: 34758653.
26. Choi KY, Jost E, Mack L, Bouchard-Fortier A. Surgical management of truncal and extremities atypical lipomatous tumors/well-differentiated liposarcoma: a systematic review of the literature. Am J Surg. 2020;219(5):823–7. https://doi.org/10.1016/j.amjsurg.2020.01.046. Epub 2020 Jan 28. PMID: 32029218.
27. Vos M, Grünhagen DJ, Koseła-Paterczyk H, Rutkowski P, Sleijfer S, Verhoef C. Natural history of well-differentiated liposarcoma of the extremity compared to patients treated with surgery. Surg Oncol. 2019;29:84–9. https://doi.org/10.1016/j.suronc.2019.04.004. Epub 2019 Apr 9. PMID: 31196499.
28. Chowdhry V, Goldberg S, DeLaney TF, Cote GM, Chebib I, Kim J, Lozano-Calderón SA, De Amorim BK. Myxoid Liposarcoma: treatment outcomes from chemotherapy and radiation therapy. Sarcoma. 2018;2018:8029157. https://doi.org/10.1155/2018/8029157. PMID: 30515050; PMCID: PMC6236966.
29. Roberge D, Skamene T, Nahal A, Turcotte RE, Powell T, Freeman C. Radiological and pathological response following pre-operative radiotherapy for soft-tissue sarcoma. Radiother Oncol. 2010;97(3):404–7. https://doi.org/10.1016/j.radonc.2010.10.007. Epub 2010 Oct 30. PMID: 21040989.
30. Moreau LC, Turcotte R, Ferguson P, Wunder J, Clarkson P, Masri B, Isler M, Dion N, Werier J, Ghert M. Deheshi B; Canadian Orthopaedic oncology society (CANOOS). Myxoid\round cell liposarcoma (MRCLS) revisited: an analysis of 418 primarily managed cases. Ann Surg Oncol. 2012;19(4):1081–8. https://doi.org/10.1245/s10434-011-2127-z. Epub 2011 Nov 4. PMID: 22052112.
31. Chung PW, Deheshi BM, Ferguson PC, Wunder JS, Griffin AM, Catton CN, Bell RS, White LM, Kandel RA, O'Sullivan B. Radiosensitivity translates into excellent local control in extremity myxoid liposarcoma: a comparison with other soft tissue sarcomas. Cancer. 2009;115(14):3254–61. https://doi.org/10.1002/cncr.24375. PMID: 19472403.
32. Lansu J, Bovée JVMG, Braam P, van Boven H, Flucke U, Bonenkamp JJ, Miah AB, Zaidi SH, Thway K, Bruland ØS, Baldini EH, Jebsen NL, Scholten AN, van den Ende PLA, Krol ADG, Ubbels JF, van der Hage JA, van Werkhoven E, Klomp HM, van der Graaf WTA, van Coevorden F, Schrage Y, van Houdt WJ, Haas RL. Dose reduction of preoperative radiotherapy in myxoid liposarcoma: a nonrandomized controlled trial. JAMA Oncol. 2021;7(1):e205865. https://doi.org/10.1001/jamaoncol.2020.5865. Epub 2021 Jan 21. PMID: 33180100; PMCID: PMC7662477.
33. Perera JR, AlFaraidy M, Ibe I, Aoude A, Acem I, van de Sande MAJ, Dessureault M, Turcotte RE, Mottard S, Basile G, Isler M, Saint-Yves H, Eastley N, Stevenson J, Houdek MT, Chung PWM, Griffin AM, Ferguson P, Wunder JS, Tsoi KM. Intermuscular extremity myxoid liposarcoma can be managed by marginal resection following neoadjuvant radiotherapy. Eur J Surg Oncol. 2023;49(2):362–7. https://doi.org/10.1016/j.ejso.2022.09.008. Epub 2022 Sep 27. PMID: 36243649.
34. Gronchi A, Bui BN, Bonvalot S, Pilotti S, Ferrari S, Hohenberger P, Hohl RJ, Demetri GD, Le Cesne A, Lardelli P, Pérez I, Nieto A, Tercero JC, Alfaro V, Tamborini E, Blay JY. Phase II clinical trial of neoadjuvant trabectedin in patients with advanced localized myxoid liposarcoma. Ann Oncol. 2012;23(3):771–6. https://doi.org/10.1093/annonc/mdr265. Epub 2011 Jun 3. PMID: 21642514.
35. Gronchi A, Palmerini E, Quagliuolo V, Martin Broto J, Lopez Pousa A, Grignani G, Brunello A, Blay JY, Tendero O, Diaz Beveridge R, Ferraresi V, Lugowska I, Merlo DF, Fontana V, Marchesi E, Braglia L, Donati DM, Palassini E, Bianchi G, Marrari A, Morosi C, Stacchiotti S, Bagué S, Coindre JM, Dei Tos AP, Picci P, Bruzzi P, Casali PG. Neoadjuvant chemotherapy in high-risk soft tissue sarcomas: final results of a randomized trial from Italian (ISG), Spanish (GEIS), French (FSG), and polish (PSG) sarcoma groups. J Clin Oncol. 2020;38(19):2178–86. https://doi.org/10.1200/JCO.19.03289. Epub 2020 May 18. PMID: 32421444.
36. Sanfilippo R, Hindi N, Cruz Jurado J, Blay JY, Lopez-Pousa A, Italiano A, Alvarez R, Gutierrez A, Rincón-Perez I, Sangalli C, Pérez Aguiar JL, Romero J, Morosi C, Sunyach MP, Fabbroni C, Romagosa C, Ranchere-Vince D, Dei Tos AP, Casali PG, Martin-Broto J, Gronchi A. Effectiveness and safety of Trabectedin and radiotherapy for patients with Myxoid Liposarcoma: a nonrandomized clinical trial. JAMA Oncol. 2023;9(5):656–63. https://doi.org/10.1001/jamaoncol.2023.0056. PMID: 36995731; PMCID: PMC10064283.
37. Huis In't Veld EA, van Coevorden F, Grünhagen DJ, Smith MJ, van Akkooi ACJ, Wouters MWJM, Hayes AJ, Verhoef C, Strauss DC, van Houdt WJ. Outcome after surgical treatment of dermatofibrosarcoma protuberans: is clinical follow-up always indicated? Cancer. 2019;125(5):735–41. https://doi.org/10.1002/cncr.31924. Epub 2019 Jan 15. PMID: 30644528.
38. Rouhani P, Fletcher CD, Devesa SS, Toro JR. Cutaneous soft tissue sarcoma incidence patterns in the U.S.: an analysis of 12,114 cases. Cancer. 2008;113(3):616–27. https://doi.org/10.1002/cncr.23571. PMID: 18618615.

39. Navarrete-Dechent C, Mori S, Barker CA, Dickson MA, Nehal KS. Imatinib treatment for locally advanced or metastatic dermatofibrosarcoma protuberans: a systematic review. JAMA Dermatol. 2019;155(3):361–9. https://doi.org/10.1001/jamadermatol.2018.4940. PMID: 30601909; PMCID: PMC8909640.
40. Rutkowski P, Van Glabbeke M, Rankin CJ, Ruka W, Rubin BP, Debiec-Rychter M, Lazar A, Gelderblom H, Sciot R, Lopez-Terrada D, Hohenberger P, van Oosterom AT, Schuetze SM, European Organisation for Research and Treatment of Cancer Soft Tissue/Bone Sarcoma Group; Southwest Oncology Group. Imatinib mesylate in advanced dermatofibrosarcoma protuberans: pooled analysis of two phase II clinical trials. J Clin Oncol. 2010;28(10):1772–9. https://doi.org/10.1200/JCO.2009.25.7899. Epub 2010 Mar 1. PMID: 20194851; PMCID: PMC3040044.
41. Radaelli S, Pasquali S, Colombo C, Callegaro D, Sanfilippo R, Stacchiotti S, Provenzano S, Sangalli C, Morosi C, Barisella M, Miceli R, Fiore M, Gronchi A. Treatment strategies and outcomes of primary myxofibrosarcomas in a large patients cohort. Eur J Surg Oncol. 2022;48(8):1723–9. https://doi.org/10.1016/j.ejso.2022.01.003. Epub 2022 Jan 21. PMID: 35153104.
42. Fourman MS, Ramsey DC, Kleiner J, Daud A, Newman ET, Schwab JH, Chen YL, DeLaney TF, Mullen JT, Raskin KA, Lozano-Calderón SA. Temporizing wound VAC dressing until final negative margins are achieved reduces myxofibrosarcoma local recurrence. Ann Surg Oncol. 2021;28(13):9171–6. https://doi.org/10.1245/s10434-021-10242-4. Epub 2021 Jun 18. PMID: 34143336.
43. Boughzala-Bennadji R, Stoeckle E, Le Péchoux C, Méeus P, Honoré C, Attal J, Duffaud F, De Pinieux G, Bompas E, Thariat J, Leroux A, Bertucci F, Isambert N, Delcambre C, Blay JY, Sunyach MP, Coindre JM, Sargos P, Penel N, Bonvalot S. Localized myxofibrosarcomas: roles of surgical margins and adjuvant radiation therapy. Int J Radiat Oncol Biol Phys. 2018;102(2):399–406. https://doi.org/10.1016/j.ijrobp.2018.05.055. Epub 2018 Jun 2. PMID: 30191871.
44. Mutter RW, Singer S, Zhang Z, Brennan MF, Alektiar KM. The enigma of myxofibrosarcoma of the extremity. Cancer. 2012;118(2):518–27. https://doi.org/10.1002/cncr.26296. Epub 2011 Jun 29. PMID: 21717447; PMCID: PMC3360945.
45. Tawbi HA, Burgess M, Bolejack V, Van Tine BA, Schuetze SM, Hu J, D'Angelo S, Attia S, Riedel RF, Priebat DA, Movva S, Davis LE, Okuno SH, Reed DR, Crowley J, Butterfield LH, Salazar R, Rodriguez-Canales J, Lazar AJ, Wistuba II, Baker LH, Maki RG, Reinke D, Patel S. Pembrolizumab in advanced soft-tissue sarcoma and bone sarcoma (SARC028): a multicentre, two-cohort, single-arm, open-label, phase 2 trial. Lancet Oncol. 2017;18(11):1493–501. https://doi.org/10.1016/S1470-2045(17)30624-1. Epub 2017 Oct 4. Erratum in: Lancet Oncol. 2017 Dec;18(12):e711. Erratum in: Lancet Oncol. 2018 Jan;19(1):e8. PMID: 28988646; PMCID: PMC7939029.
46. D'Angelo SP, Mahoney MR, Van Tine BA, Atkins J, Milhem MM, Jahagirdar BN, Antonescu CR, Horvath E, Tap WD, Schwartz GK, Streicher H. Nivolumab with or without ipilimumab treatment for metastatic sarcoma (Alliance A091401): two open-label, non-comparative, randomised, phase 2 trials. Lancet Oncol. 2018;19(3):416–26. https://doi.org/10.1016/S1470-2045(18)30006-8. Epub 2018 Jan 19. PMID: 29370992; PMCID: PMC6126546.
47. Keung EZ, Tsai JW, Ali AM, Cormier JN, Bishop AJ, Guadagnolo BA, Torres KE, Somaiah N, Hunt KK, Wargo JA, Lazar AJ, Wang WL, Roland CL. Analysis of the immune infiltrate in undifferentiated pleomorphic sarcoma of the extremity and trunk in response to radiotherapy: rationale for combination neoadjuvant immune checkpoint inhibition and radiotherapy. Onco Targets Ther. 2017;7(2):e1385689. https://doi.org/10.1080/2162402X.2017.1385689. PMID: 29308306; PMCID: PMC5749668.
48. Farid M, Demicco EG, Garcia R, Ahn L, Merola PR, Cioffi A, Maki RG. Malignant peripheral nerve sheath tumors. Oncologist. 2014;19(2):193–201. https://doi.org/10.1634/theoncologist.2013-0328. Epub 2014 Jan 27. PMID: 24470531; PMCID: PMC3926794.
49. Anghileri M, Miceli R, Fiore M, Mariani L, Ferrari A, Mussi C, Lozza L, Collini P, Olmi P, Casali PG, Pilotti S, Gronchi A. Malignant peripheral nerve sheath tumors: prognostic factors and survival in a series of patients treated at a single institution. Cancer. 2006;107(5):1065–74. https://doi.org/10.1002/cncr.22098. PMID: 16881077.
50. Bishop AJ, Zagars GK, Torres KE, Bird JE, Feig BW, Guadagnolo BA. Malignant peripheral nerve sheath tumors: a single institution's experience using combined surgery and radiation therapy. Am J Clin Oncol. 2018;41(5):465–70. https://doi.org/10.1097/COC.0000000000000303. PMID: 27281262; PMCID: PMC5145780.

Soft Tissue Sarcomas: Philosophy of Surgical Approach

19

Peter S. Rose

19.1 Introduction

Soft tissue sarcomas represent a heterogeneous group of rare malignancies of mesenchymal origin. Recent data from the United States suggests that soft tissue sarcomas represent ~0.7% of all new cancer diagnoses [1]. This chapter will focus primarily on the surgical considerations in the evaluation and treatment of patients with truncal and extremity soft tissue sarcomas.

As surgeons evaluate and treat these diseases, they must individualize treatments for unique patient presentations. This will include establishing a philosophy of treatment which balances the goals of cure with the morbidity of treatment options (particularly in light of conflicting evidence of the impact of morbid local control or recurrence on overall survival).

19.2 Diagnosis

Although imaging is frequently suggestive of the underlying diagnosis, histologic confirmation is generally obtained prior to active tumor management. Diagnosis may be via core needle biopsy, excisional surgical biopsy (typically reserved for small lesions), or incisional surgical biopsy depending on local practice patterns and patient presentations. Ideally a biopsy is performed by or with the input of the treating surgeon. A proper biopsy should not traverse unnecessary anatomic compartments, avoid exposure and manipulation of non-involved critical neurovascular structures, and be oriented in line with the planned approach for surgical resection. Poorly planned or executed biopsies may lead to contamination of tissues, compartments, or critical structures that negatively influence surgical options and patient outcomes.

P. S. Rose (✉)
Orthopedic Surgery, Mayo Clinic, Rochester, MN, USA
e-mail: rose.peter@mayo.edu

As soft tissue sarcomas are rare tumors, some centers will necessarily have less experience in their histologic diagnosis. If ambiguity exists, review at a reference center is recommended. A recent study demonstrated a change in diagnosis in 38% of patients with soft tissue sarcomas reviewed at a reference cancer center with 25% of cases having a change in treatment [2]. These results highlight the role of pathologic confirmation in cases with any diagnostic ambiguity.

19.3 Imaging

Once a patient has histologic diagnosis of a soft tissue sarcoma, local and distant imaging is obtained to define disease boundaries and oncologic staging. Magnetic resonance (MR) imaging provides the best anatomic resolution and tissue contrast in defining the local extent of soft tissue sarcomas (see also Chaps. 2 and 3). When impractical, computed tomography (CT) with intravenous contrast is a substitute imaging modality. CT angiography may also be used for closure flap planning or to carefully define vascular anatomy around tumor resections. While ultrasound may be used to confirm the presence of a mass, the lack of axial imaging and tissue discrimination it provides makes it unsuitable for the pre-operative characterization of soft tissue sarcomas.

Classic systemic staging to identify distant metastases is by chest CT. Certain histologies have an increased risk of lymph node metastases (most notability rhabdomyosarcoma, clear cell sarcoma, and epithelioid sarcoma) [3]. In these patients, positron emission tomography (PET) +/− sentinel lymph node biopsy is commonly used to evaluate for regional lymph node metastases. However, this remains a developing and controversial area of sarcoma oncology, and the overall level of evidence supporting lymph node sampling remains low [4]. Additionally, high-grade myxoid liposarcoma (sometimes called round cell liposarcoma) has a known predilection for metastases to the axial bone marrow space. These lesions are not reliably detected by CT or PET imaging. Many centers use spine and pelvic MR or total body MR

H. Özger et al. (eds.), *Diagnosis and Treatment of Soft Tissue Tumors*, https://doi.org/10.1007/978-3-031-77061-6_19

in the staging of these patients (see Chaps. 4 and 5). It is important both practically and philosophically to obtain a complete evaluation of all potential disease in patients at their baseline evaluation.

19.4 Staging

A detailed discussion of staging is found in Chap. 9; the most commonly used current staging system is the American Joint Committee on Cancer (AJCC) Staging Manual; this closely parallels the International Union for Cancer Control T, N, M staging system [5]. The current (8th edition AJCC Staging Manual) provides stage groupings based on size, grade, and presence of lymph node or distant metastases. Stage groups (IA–IV) are generally predictive of patient outcome.

19.5 Treatment

Virtually all patients with soft tissue sarcoma are considered for surgical resection; radiation therapy is strongly considered in most deep and some superficial tumors. The role of chemotherapy remains investigational at this time. Surgeons must carefully balance the extent (and morbidity) of treatment with functional loss and patient outcome.

19.5.1 Radiation Therapy

A detailed discussion of the role of radiation treatment is found in Chaps. 13 and 14; radiation therapy has been proven in randomized trials to improve local control in clinically and statistically significant ways. Rosenberg initially demonstrated that the use of radiation therapy and local excision provided survival equivalent to amputation [6]. Subsequent randomized trials confirmed these results in patients treated with post-operative external beam radiation [7, 8] and brachytherapy [9]. Brachytherapy improved local control in high but not low-grade sarcoma while post-operative external beam radiation improved local control in both low and high-grade histologies. Note that these studies did not demonstrate an improvement in overall survival. The value of radiation likely varies with histology; Callegro demonstrated the largest benefit in myxoid liposarcoma, vascular sarcomas, and myxoid liposarcoma [10].

As radiation therapy became a part of the default treatment protocol for soft tissue sarcoma, local complications of contracture, fibrosis, lymphedema, and fracture were recognized. These complications were logically felt to be the result of radiation dose and treatment volume. A subsequent prospective randomized trial compared pre- versus post-operative radiation therapy [11]. This study demonstrated a significant increase in surgical wound complications but also lower late radiation toxicities; local control was equivalent with either pre- or post-operative treatment [11, 12].

In contemporary practice, radiation is considered for most soft tissue sarcomas to decrease the risk of local recurrence. Surgeons may naturally select pre- or post-operative treatments depending on individual patient presentations and institutional practice patterns. For example, tumors juxtaposed to major neurovascular structures may be better served with pre-operative radiation to minimize the dose and length of irradiated nerves or vessels to decrease late radiation neuropathy or vascular complications. In contrast, situations at high risk or high consequence for wound infection (tumor near a pre-existing arthroplasty, for example) may be better treated with post-operative radiation to decrease infection risk. In approaching individual patients, surgeons should balance the local control benefits of radiation (which may vary by histology) with the morbidity of radiation and lack of overall survival benefit of radiation therapy in prospective, randomized trials.

19.5.2 Chemotherapy

The role of chemotherapy in soft tissue sarcoma is nuanced and covered in detail in Chaps. 11 and 12; a recent meta-analysis demonstrated no clear survival benefit, while a propensity matched study showed a 5% survival benefit at 5- and 10-year timepoints [10, 13]. Given the certain morbidity of chemotherapy treatment and unclear to low overall survival benefit in soft tissue sarcoma patients, its role is generally restricted to high risk presentations or clinical trials. From a philosophical perspective, the use of chemotherapy engenders certain risks to patients with less certain clinical benefits.

19.5.3 Surgical Resection

Surgical resection is the primary curative treatment for soft tissue sarcoma, and incomplete resection is the highest risk factor for local recurrence of tumor [9]. Thus, the execution of the surgical resection defines the primary modifiable risk factor for patient outcome in soft tissue sarcoma. Traditional margin definitions for soft tissue sarcomas defined by Enneking include radical resections (removal of the entire anatomic compartment), wide resections (removal with a cuff of normal tissue surrounding the tumor), marginal resection (dissection through the pseudocapsule or reactive zone surrounding the tumor), or intralesional (dissection which violates the tumor) [14]. Wide resection has generally been advocated as the standard of care for these tumors. However, no standardized definition exists for what cuff of normal tissue defines a "wide margin," either in terms of distance from tumor or tissue quality (e.g., fascia vs. adipose tissue); Chaps. 17 and 18 cover this area in detail.

Local conditions often make a wide margin resection impractical or highly morbid. Soft tissue sarcomas of the posterior thigh (the most common anatomic location for extremity soft tissue sarcomas) often abut the sciatic nerve or femur without involvement or encasement. Clinical experience has shown that the combination of radiation therapy and close margin dissection can preserve function while maintaining oncologic control [15]. Because of the variability in assessing wide margins, many centers have adopted the R classification of margins (residual tumor classification). This system, in common use for retroperitoneal tumors in which anatomic compartmentalization is not present in the same manner as the extremities, defines margins as grossly positive (R2), microscopically positive (R1), or microscopically negative (R0) [16]. Other authors have proposed an "R + 1 mm" margin in which negative margins were defined by at least 1 mm of normal tissue between tumor and the resection plane [17]. This "R + 1 mm" margin does not show clear discriminatory benefit in predicting local recurrence outcome over the traditional R system in patients receiving radiotherapy [18]. These results support the surgical approach of "planned close margin resections" to preserve function and minimize morbidity while not compromising oncologic outcome.

19.5.4 Special Considerations in Management

Several patient populations deserve specific consideration in formulating a treatment approach in patients with soft tissue sarcoma.

- Unplanned excisions remain common in soft tissue sarcoma care (non-oncologic manipulation of a tumor without prior sarcoma diagnosis; see Chap. 19). Even after apparent gross total excision, over one-third of these patients will harbor macroscopic disease at re-excision [19]. Current standard of care for these patients includes radiation therapy and re-excision; studies suggest that patients cared for in this manner can achieve equivalent local recurrence and overall survival rates compared to those patients undergoing primary planned curative resection [20–22]. Patients undergoing unplanned and subsequent salvage excisions do have higher rates of flap coverage and amputations in AJCC Stage III tumors (large, deep, high grade) [22]. This excess morbidity of salvage treatment of unplanned excisions emphasizes the goal of careful disease recognition and treatment planning.
- Up to one-third of soft tissue sarcomas may present in the subcutaneous area [23]. Traditional curative resection of these tumors was provided with wide local resection alone without radiation therapy [24]. However, recent results have suggested a potential role for radiation to decrease local recurrence in subcutaneous sarcomas [25]. As survival is not clearly impacted by subcutaneous local recurrence, surgeons can balance the relative merits of additional treatment with radiation compared to the local morbidity of recurrence and the potential need for re-resection in subcutaneous soft tissue sarcomas.
- Regional lymph node metastases are identified in roughly 5% of patients. While an adverse prognostic factor, isolated lymph node metastases appear to demonstrate a better prognosis that pulmonary metastases, and survival is improved with resection [26, 27].
- Neurologic and vascular structures may be encased and require resection. Neurologic resection, particularly of the femoral nerve, leads to functional morbidity and an increased risk of falls [28, 29]. Formal vascular resection and reconstruction may allow limb salvage in otherwise adverse circumstances. Surgeons should be aware that these procedures entail a high complication profile, particularly for wound dehiscence, thrombosis, and secondary amputation but only slightly lower ultimate functional outcome scores [30].
- Elderly patients may present a challenge in soft tissue sarcoma management due to frailty and medical comorbidities that impact their suitability for aggressive treatments. Elderly patients undergoing R0 surgical resection have an increased 90-day mortality compared to those not undergoing aggressive surgical treatment but improved overall survival [31]. These results highlight the narrow risk benefit ratio and individualization of care necessary in approaching this patient population [32].
- In the case of unclear surgical margins or the need for oncoplastic reconstruction not immediately available or anticipated, a sterile negative pressure wound dressing may be applied after resection. Subsequent definitive closure/reconstruction may be performed when final margins and resources are available [33]. The use of immediate versus staged reconstruction remains center specific based on practice patterns and local resource availability.
- Amputation may be considered for the primary treatment of soft tissue sarcomas or following failed limb salvage. Amputation may be indicated for locally advanced primary presentation of tumor or in the case of recurrent disease (particularly if multifocal). Again, surgeons must carefully consider the unclear impact of local recurrence on overall survival and treatment goals when considering such morbid treatments (see Chap. 24).

19.6 Outcomes

19.6.1 Survival

Survival from soft tissue sarcoma is influenced by histology and presenting stage (see Chap. 10). Nomograms may incorporate histologic and/or anatomic variables in patient presentation [34]. Both traditional static as well as dynamic survival predictors are available [35]. Long-term survival varies from >85% for small, low-grade tumors to ≤50% for large, deep, high-grade sarcomas.

19.6.2 Local Recurrence

Local recurrence is seen in up to 12 + % of patients undergoing limb salvage treatment; tumor size, depth, and histologic grade are most closely associated with risk of recurrence [36]. However, these factors are also associated with increased risk of distant metastases and death from disease, a competing risk factor for local recurrence. The net effect is similar overall local recurrence rates between soft tissue sarcomas as lower risk tumors have greater survival and thus more exposure for local recurrence [36]. The impact of local recurrence on overall survival is controversial with different studies reaching different conclusions [37]; this has obvious implications for the philosophy of how surgeons approach these patients.

19.6.3 Health-Related Quality of Life

Health-related quality of life (HRQOL) is defined separately from traditional oncologic outcomes of disease survival statistics (see Chap. 25). In the context of soft tissue sarcoma treatment, HRQOL refers to the perceived physical and mental health changes over time. The presence and treatment of a malignant musculoskeletal neoplasm obviously has impact on physical health and function; similarly, treatment and prognosis have implications for mental health and outlook. While the overall change in HRQOL in the first year of treatment for soft tissue sarcoma is small, this result masks wide variability in individual patient outcomes [38].

19.6.4 Functional Recovery

Patient functional outcome is heavily influenced by the nature of surgical resection, complications, and the effects of adjuvant treatments. Maximal functional outcome is generally achieved at 12–24 months post-operatively, important information in counseling patients and caregivers during recovery [39–41].

19.6.5 Complications

Complications following soft tissue sarcoma treatment may be divided into early and late phase complications. Wound healing complications and infection dominate early phase complications. Pre-operative radiotherapy and obesity are closely associated with increased risks of early phase complications [11, 42, 43]. However, patients treated with post-operative radiotherapy have greater late radiotherapy effects of fibrosis, stiffness, and edema [11]. Nine percent of patients treated for soft tissue sarcomas develop significant lymphedema, with large and deep tumors defining the high risk cohort [44].

19.7 Follow-Up

Patients require oncologic surveillance post-operatively to detect local and distant tumor recurrence. Individual institutions have different oncologic practice patterns which influence patient follow-up schedules. Traditional follow-up screening is via computed tomography of the chest and MR imaging of the local tumor site every 3–6 months through 5 years post-treatment, with some centers having extended follow-up through 10 years. Routine surveillance MR imaging is demonstrated to improve the detection of local recurrence [45].

However, given the unclear clinical impact of local recurrence on overall survival, the utility of aggressive surveillance strategies to detect asymptomatic local recurrences remains unclear. A prospective randomized trial of intense versus less aggressive post-operative surveillance after soft tissue sarcoma excision is underway to help better define the relative benefits of different surveillance strategies [46]. Pending these results, clinicians can define rationale surveillance strategies based on known risk factors [47].

19.8 Conclusions

Extremity and truncal soft tissue sarcomas represent a group of related diseases which may present with widely variable clinical presentations and outcomes. Surgery remains the mainstay of treatment for these patients, with complete resection of tumor the primary modifiable variable for patient outcome. Treatment and follow-up may be individualized to different clinical presentations.

As surgeons approach these patients, careful consideration must be given to individual patient presentations with attendant oncologic risks and other competing health risks. Morbid treatment for soft tissue sarcoma must be balanced against the unclear influence of local recurrence on overall survival; careful employment of adjuvant treatments often allows function sparing surgery with equivalent survival and improved patient outcomes.

References

1. Siegel RL, Miller KD, Fuchs HE, Jemal A. Cancer statistics, 2022. CA Cancer J Clin. 2022;72:7–33.
2. Rupani A, Hallin M, Jones RL, Fisher C, Thway K. Diagnostic differences in expert second-opinion consultation cases at a tertiary sarcoma center. Sarcoma. 2020;2020:9810170.
3. Liu QK, Yu XJ, Wang YG, et al. Risk factors for lymph node metastasis of soft tissue sarcomas of the head, neck, and extremities, and the clinical significance of negative lymph node dissection. J Orthop Surg Res. 2022;17:167.
4. Woods, R, Cancer Council Australia Sarcoma Guidelines Working Party. Clinical question: what is the role of sentinel lymph node biopsy in patients with BSTT?. In: Clinical practice guidelines for the management of adult onset sarcoma. Sydney: Australia and New Zealand Sarcoma Association (formerly known as the Australian Sarcoma Group). https://wiki.cancer.org.au/australiawiki/index.php?oldid=213635. [Cited 2023 Mar 5]. https://wiki.cancer.org.au/australia/Guidelines:Sarcoma.
5. Amin MB, Edge S, Greene F, Byrd DR, Brookland RK, Washington MK, Gershenwald JE, Compton CC, Hess KR, et al., editors. AJCC cancer staging manual (8th edition). Springer: American Joint Commission on Cancer; 2017.
6. Rosenberg SA, Tepper J, Glatstein L, et al. The treatment of soft-tissue sarcomas of the extremities: prospective randomized evaluations of (1) limb-sparing surgery plus radiation therapy compared with amputation and (2) the role of adjuvant chemotherapy. Ann Surg. 1982;196:305–15.
7. Beane JD, Yang JC, White D, et al. Efficacy of adjuvant radiation therapy in the treatment of soft tissue sarcoma of the extremity : 20-year follow-up of a randomized prospective trial. Ann Surg Oncol. 2014;21:2484–9.
8. Yang JC, Change AE, Baker AE, et al. Randomized prospective study of the benefit of adjuvant radiation therapy in the treatment of soft tissue sarcomas of the extremity. J Clin Oncol. 1998;16(1):197–203.
9. Pisters PW, Harrison LB, Leung DH, et al. Long-term results of a prospective randomized trial of adjuvant brachytherapy in soft tissue sarcoma. J Clin Oncol. 1996;14:859–68.
10. Callegaro D, Miceli R, Bonvalot S, et al. Impact of perioperative chemotherapy and radiotherapy in patients with primary extremity soft tissue sarcoma: retrospective analysis across major histological subtypes and major reference centres. Eur J Cancer. 2018;105:19–27.
11. O'Sullivan B, Davis AM, Turcotte R, et al. Preoperative versus postoperative radiotherapy in soft-tissue sarcoma of the limbs: a randomized trial. Lancet. 2002;359:2235–41.
12. Davis AM, O'Sullivan B, Turcotte R, et al. Late radiation morbidity following randomization to preoperative versus postoperative radiotherapy in extremity soft tissue sarcoma. Radiother Oncol. 2005;75:48–53.
13. Istl AC, Ruck JM, Morris CD. Call for improved design and reporting in soft tissue sarcoma studies: a systematic review and meta-analysis of chemotherapy and survival outcomes in resectable STS. J Surg Oncol. 2019;119:824–35.
14. Enneking WF, Spannier SS, Goodman MA. A system for the surgical staging of musculoskeletal sarcoma. Clin Orthop Relat Res. 1980;153:106–20.
15. Clarkson P, Griffin AN, Catton CM, et al. Epineural dissection is a safe technique that facilitates limb salvage surgery. Clin Orthop Relat Res. 2005;438:92–6.
16. Bearhs OH, Henson DE, Hutter RVP, Myers MH, editors. Manual for staging of cancer. 3rd ed. Philadelphia: American Joint Committee on Cancer/JB Lippincott; 1988.
17. Wittekind C, Compton CC, Greene FL, et al. TNM residual tumor classification revisited. Cancer. 2002;94:2511–6.
18. Gundle KR, Kafchinski L, Gupta S, et al. Analysis of margin classification systems for assessing the risk of local recurrence after soft tissue sarcoma resection. J Clin Oncol. 2018;36:704–9.
19. Noria S, Davis A, Kandel R, et al. Residual disease following unplanned excision of a soft-tissue sarcoma of an extremity. J Bone Joint Surg Am. 1996;78-A:650–5.
20. Funovics PT, Vaselic S, Panotopoulos J, et al. The impact of re-excision of inadequately resected soft tissue sarcomas on surgical therapy, results, and prognosis: a single institution experience with 682 patients. J Surg Oncol. 2010;102:626–33.
21. Manoso MW, Frassica DA, Deune EG, Frassica FJ. Outcomes of re-excision after unplanned excisions of soft tissue sarcomas. J Surg Oncol. 2005;91:153–8.
22. Traub F, Griffin AM, Wunder JS, Ferguson PC. Influence of unplanned excisions on the outcomes of patients with stage III extremity soft tissue sarcoma. Cancer. 2018;124:3868–75.
23. Rydholm A, Gustafson P, Rooser B, Willen H, Berg NO, Subcutaneous sarcoma. A population-based study of 129 patients. J Bone Joint Surg (Br). 1991;73:662–7.
24. Gibbs SP, Peabody TD, Mundt AJ, Montafg AG, Simon MA. Oncologic outcomes of operative treatment of subcutaneous soft-tissue sarcomas of the extremities. J Bone Joint Surg Am. 1997;79:888–97.
25. Fujiwara T, Tsuda Y, Louis-Romee LN, et al. The role of radiotherapy in the treatment of superficial soft-tissue sarcomas. Bone Joint J. 2020;102-B:1088–94.
26. Basile G, Mattei JC, Alshaygy, et al. Curability of lymph node metastases from extremity soft-tissue sarcoma. Cancer. 2020;126:5098–108.
27. Fong Y, Coit DG, Woodruff JM, Brennan MF. Lymph node metastasis from soft tissue sarcoma in adults. Analysis of data from a prospective database of 1772 sarcoma patients. Ann Surg. 1993;217:72–7.
28. Fuchs B, Davis AM, Winder JS. Sciatic nerve resection in the thigh: a functional evaluation. Clin Orthop Relat Res. 2001;382:34–41.
29. Jones KB, Ferguson PC, Deheshi B, et al. Complete femoral nerve resection with soft tissue sarcoma: functional outcomes. Ann Surg Oncol. 2010;17:401–6.
30. Ghert MA, Davis AM, Griffin AM, et al. The surgical and functional outcome of limb-salvage surgery with vascular reconstruction for soft tissue sarcoma of the extremity. Ann Surg Oncol. 2005;12:1102–10.
31. Gingrigh AA, Bateni SB, Monjazeb AM, et al. Extremity soft tissue sarcoma in the elderly: are we overtreating or undertreating this potentially vulnerable patient population? J Surg Oncol. 2019;119:1087–98.
32. Nakamura T, Sudo A. Treatment strategy for elderly patients with soft tissue sarcoma. Curr Oncol Rep. 2022;24:563–71.
33. deVries JA, Abbas A, King DM, et al. Staged reconstruction of soft tissue sarcoma resections using temporizing negative pressure wound therapy is safe and efficacious. Eur J Plastic Surg. 2022;45:799–807.
34. Callegaro D, Miceli R, Mariani L, et al. Soft tissue sarcoma nomograms and their incorporation into practice. Cancer. 2017;123:2802–20.
35. Rueten-Budde AJ, van Praag VM, et al. Dynamic prediction of overall survival for patients with high-grade extremity soft tissue sarcoma. Surg Oncol. 2018;27:695–701.
36. Biau DJ, Ferguson PC, Chung P, et al. Local recurrence of localized soft tissue sarcoma. Cancer. 2012;118:5867–77.
37. Novais EN, Demirapl B, Alderete J, et al. Do surgical margin and local recurrence influence survival in soft tissue sarcomas? Clin Orthop Relat Res. 2010;369:3003–11.

38. Davidson D, Barr RD, Riad S, et al. Health-related quality of life following treatment for extremity soft tissue sarcoma. J Surg Oncol. 2016;114:821–7.
39. Davis AM, O'Sullivan B, Bell R, et al. Function and health status outcomes in a randomized trial comparing preoperative and postoperative radiotherapy in extremity soft tissue sarcoma. J Clin Oncol. 2002;20:4472–7.
40. Oh E, Seo SW, Han KJ. A longitudinal study of functional outcomes in patients with limb salvage surgery for soft tissue sarcoma. Sarcoma. 2018;2018:6846275.
41. Saebye C, Amidi A, Keller J, et al. Changes in functional outcome and quality of life in soft tissue sarcoma patients within the first year after surgery: a prospective observational study. Cancers. 2020;12:463.
42. Houdek MT, Griffin AM, Ferguson PC, Wunder JS. Morbid obesity increase the risk of postoperative wound complications, infection, and repeat surgical procedures following upper extremity limb salvage surgery for soft tissue sarcoma. Hand. 2019;14:114–20.
43. Houdek MT, Hevesi M, Griffin AM, Wunder JS, Ferguson PC. Morbid obesity is associated with an increased risk of wound complications and infection after lower extremity soft-tissue sarcoma resection. J Am Acad Orthop Surg. 2019;27:807–15.
44. Friedmann D, Wunder JS, Ferguson P, et al. Incidence and severity of lymphoedema following limb salvage of extremity soft tissue sarcoma. Sarcoma. 2011;2011:289673.
45. England P, Hong Z, Rhea L, et al. Does advanced imaging have a role in detecting local recurrence of soft-tissue sarcoma? Clin Orthop Relat Res. 2020;478:2812–20.
46. SAFETY Investigators. The surveillance after extremity tumor surgery (SAFETY) trial: protocol for a pilot study to determine the feasibility of a multi-centre randomised controlled trial. BMJ Open. 2019;9:e029054.
47. Wilson DAJ, Gazendam A, Visgauss J, et al. Designing a rationale follow-up schedule for patients with extremity soft tissue sarcoma. Ann Surg Oncol. 2020;27:2033–41.

20 Principles of Upper Extremity Reconstruction Following Soft-Tissue Sarcoma Resection

Matthew T. Houdek, Brooke E. Willborg, Mikaela H. Sullivan, Karim Bakri, and Steven L. Moran

20.1 Introduction

Soft-tissue sarcomas (STS) of the upper extremity are rare, accounting for less than a third of all cases [1, 2]. Often, these tumors are located in the arm and proximal forearm, and less commonly in the hand [3–6]. Due to the association between tumor location and activity limitations [7], treatment for upper extremity STS can have a substantial impact on the patients quality of life.

Limb salvage surgery has become the primary means of treating patients with an upper extremity STS; however, patients with an upper extremity STS are known to have a higher risk of local recurrence; likely due to a high incidence of unplanned excisions and adjacent critical structures [4]. To maximize outcomes following extirpation, a multidisciplinary team is essential for successful reconstruction and subsequent rehabilitation. In order to achieve limb salvage, patients are often treated in part with radiotherapy, which allows for a planned close margin of resection along critical neurovascular and bony structures [8–11]. Due to the higher treatment doses and larger treatment volumes, postoperative radiation can be permanently disabling and associated with joint and soft-tissue fibrosis, lymphedema, and pain [12, 13]. Since preoperative radiotherapy is associated with a high rate of wound-healing complications [14], it is essential for the extirpative and reconstructive surgeons to work closely together to optimize patient outcome through an *oncoplastic* approach with the goals of a negative margin resection and optimization of patient function [15].

The benefits of oncoplastic approach for limb salvage surgery includes the principles and practices of orthopedic oncology to achieve a negative margin of resection and functional reconstruction and wound closure performed by plastic surgery. This combined approach has been shown to reduce the rate of wound-healing complications in the setting of preoperative radiotherapy [6, 16]. The primary goal of any tumor surgery is to obtain negative margin of resection; however, to preserve critical structures, preoperative radiotherapy with a planned close, or planned close and ultimately microscopically margins shows equivalent outcomes [8–11, 17, 18]. In these cases, the reconstructive surgeon must ensure critical structure coverage and reconstruct neurovascular structures when necessary [19]. The purpose of this chapter is to review the concepts of oncoplastic reconstruction following STS extirpation of the upper extremity, and to provide an overview of the various types of flaps available for soft tissue and bone reconstruction and outline options for joint reconstruction.

20.1.1 Surgical Planning and Timing

The team approach to oncoplastic surgery allows both oncologic and reconstructive surgeons to plan the resection and maximize functional reconstruction. In addition, discussion between medical and radiation oncology teams is essential for timing of surgery as delays in surgical care following preoperative radiotherapy have been shown to impact outcome, with the surgery ideally being performed 3–5 weeks following the completion of radiotherapy [20]. It is critical that the surgical margin is never compromised in order to assist with a future reconstruction. As such, ideally the extirpative surgeon *should not be* the reconstructive surgeon, as there is

M. T. Houdek (✉) · M. H. Sullivan
Department of Orthopedic Surgery, Mayo Clinic, Rochester, MN, USA
e-mail: houdek.matthew@mayo.edu; Sullivan.mikaela2@mayo.edu

B. E. Willborg
Division of Plastic and Reconstructive Surgery, Mayo Clinic, Rochester, MN, USA
e-mail: Willborg.brooke@mayo.edu

K. Bakri · S. L. Moran
Department of Orthopedic Surgery, Mayo Clinic, Rochester, MN, USA

Division of Plastic and Reconstructive Surgery, Mayo Clinic, Rochester, MN, USA
e-mail: bakri.karim@mayo.edu; moran.steven@mayo.edu

H. Özger et al. (eds.), *Diagnosis and Treatment of Soft Tissue Tumors*, https://doi.org/10.1007/978-3-031-77061-6_20

always a concern one may under resect to assist with the reconstruction. Preoperative discussion allows the reconstructive surgeon to prepare for the possibility of neurovascular reconstruction, the need for free tissue transfer and bone grafting. At our institution our preference is for immediate reconstruction following confirmation of negative margins on intraoperative frozen pathology performed in the areas where the oncologic surgeon felt the margin of resection would have been closest to residual tumor. We have moved away from intraoperative external beam radiotherapy as studies have shown high rate of complications, without any proven oncologic benefit [21]. If there is a concern for the margin assessment or in the setting of a fungating tumor with an infected wound, temporization of the wound can be performed with a negative pressure dressing until definitive closure is possible [22].

The basis of an oncoplastic approach to limb salvage is based on the algorithm for orthoplastic upper limb reconstruction follows the reconstructive ladder as outlined by Levin [23]. The reconstructive surgeon performs the simplest procedure to cover a wound first (providing it will provide the best functional recovery) and then proceeds up the rungs to more complex procedures to achieve wound closure and coverage (Table 20.1). Free tissue transfer has been found to be safe and reliable, even in the setting of radiotherapy, as such the reconstructive surgeon should feel comfortable performing whichever reconstructive procedure, they feel would provide the best outcome for the patient [24–27]. When a reconstructive procedure will require a flap, a CT angiogram is essential to allow for identification of perforating vessels to determine the possibility and safety of using local, pedicled, or perforator flaps versus free tissue transfer [28].

20.1.2 Soft-Tissue Reconstruction

Following tumor extirpation, the surgical team can be faced with composite soft-tissue defects, including the removal of nerves, vessels, muscles, and tendons. To reconstruct these defects, we generally prefer free tissue transfer for defect reconstruction. At our institution, the major indications for free tissue transfer are coverage of large defects with exposed bone, joint, tendons, or hardware; large resections which received preoperative radiation or a plan for postoperative radiation; composite defects which included multiple tissue types; or in the setting of a failed reconstruction which utilized traditional wound management. When possible, composite flaps can restore function by replacement of missing bone, recreating a gliding tissue plane, obliterate potential space, replacement of tendons, and provide a source of vascularized nerve grafts [29].

Table 20.1 Reconstructive ladder for wound coverage

- Primary closure
- Skin grafting
- Local cutaneous flaps
- Transposition fasciocutaneous flaps
- Island fascial or fasciocutaneous flaps
- Local or distant one-stage muscle or myocutaneous pedicled flaps
- Distant pedicle flaps
- Microvascular free tissue transfer

There are few absolute contraindications to the use of a free flap when needed within the upper extremity. Relative contraindications to free tissue transfer include a hypercoagulable state, infection, recent upper extremity deep venous thrombosis, and inadequate recipient vessels for flap anastomosis.

20.1.2.1 Skin Grafting

Well-vascularized wounds without exposed critical structures and surgical hardware can often be closed with a split thickness skin graft (STSG), even in the setting of preoperative or planned postoperative radiotherapy [30, 31]. In the setting of preoperative radiotherapy, the use of a wound vac can improve the rate of healing for an STSG [32]. Although an STSG is safe to use following oncologic resection, there are draw backs to their use including contracture, scaring, durability and non-pliable nature of the skin. In the distal upper extremity, STSG adherence to underlying muscle and peritenon can complicate tendon gliding and motion across joints, potentially impacting hand function. Full thickness grafts can be used; however, secondary contracture can occur with full thickness grafts as well; as such, STSGs are most appropriate for small defects.

20.2 Flaps for Upper Limb Reconstruction

There are a variety of local pedicled or perforator flaps which can be used for upper limb reconstruction. Familiarity with these flaps can allow the surgeon to cover most tumor defects, permitting the surgeon to choose the flap which will provide the best size match, functional, and aesthetic result.

20.2.1 Fasciocutaneous Flaps

20.2.1.1 Groin Flap

Based on the superficial circumflex iliac artery and the superficial inferior epigastric artery, the groin flap was commonly used for hand and forearm reconstruction prior to the development of microsurgical techniques [33, 34]. The flap is elevated and inset, with the hand and/or forearm sewn-in-place near the pedicle. If the wound is healed at the distal margin, the pedicle can then be divided as early as 3 weeks postoperative. When the hand/forearm is sewn in place against the groin, hand and elbow stiffness can develop. In addition to being utilized as a distant pedicled flap, the flap can be harvested as a free perforator flap based on the superficial circumflex iliac artery (SCIP) which provides thin coverage, minimal donor site morbidity and a rapid return to hand function over the classic sewn-in-place groin flap [35].

20.2.1.2 Radial Forearm Flap

Due to the ease of flap elevation and versatility, the radial forearm flap (RFF) is a workhorse for hand and forearm reconstruction The RFF is a fasciocutaneous flap which can be utilized as a local pedicled flap or free flap. When used as a pedicled flap, the RFF is based on either antegrade or retrograde flow from the radial artery which gives off perforators along its course to the skin of the forearm [36]. Since use of the RFF will sacrifice atrial perfusion to the hand from the radial artery, it is imperative that the surgeon preform the Allen's test to assess the patency of the palmar arch through the ulnar artery. As a local pedicled flap the distal division of the artery allows the RFF to cover defects about the elbow (Fig. 20.1), while proximal division of the artery allows for retrograde flow and the RFF to cover defects on the dorsum and palmar surfaces of the hand. For composite defects, the RFF can be elevated with the palmaris longus, flexor carpi radialis, bone from the radius and portions of the lateral and medial antebrachial cutaneous nerves [37, 38].

Sacrifice of the radial artery and donor site complications/appearance are the main disadvantage to using the radial forearm flap. Following flap elevation, patients can complain of cold intolerance, scarring, and pain at the donor site. Likewise, the donor site often requires STSG for wound closure. Even with these drawbacks, the RFF is one of the most successful flaps for upper extremity reconstruction, in addition can also be elevated as a perforator flap which does not require sacrifice of the radial artery [39–42].

20.2.1.3 Posterior Interosseous Artery Flap

Similar to the RFF, the posterior interosseous artery flap is a fasciocutaneous flap; however, it is based off the posterior interosseous artery which runs in the septum between extensor carpi ulnaris and extensor digiti minimi. Although it is smaller than

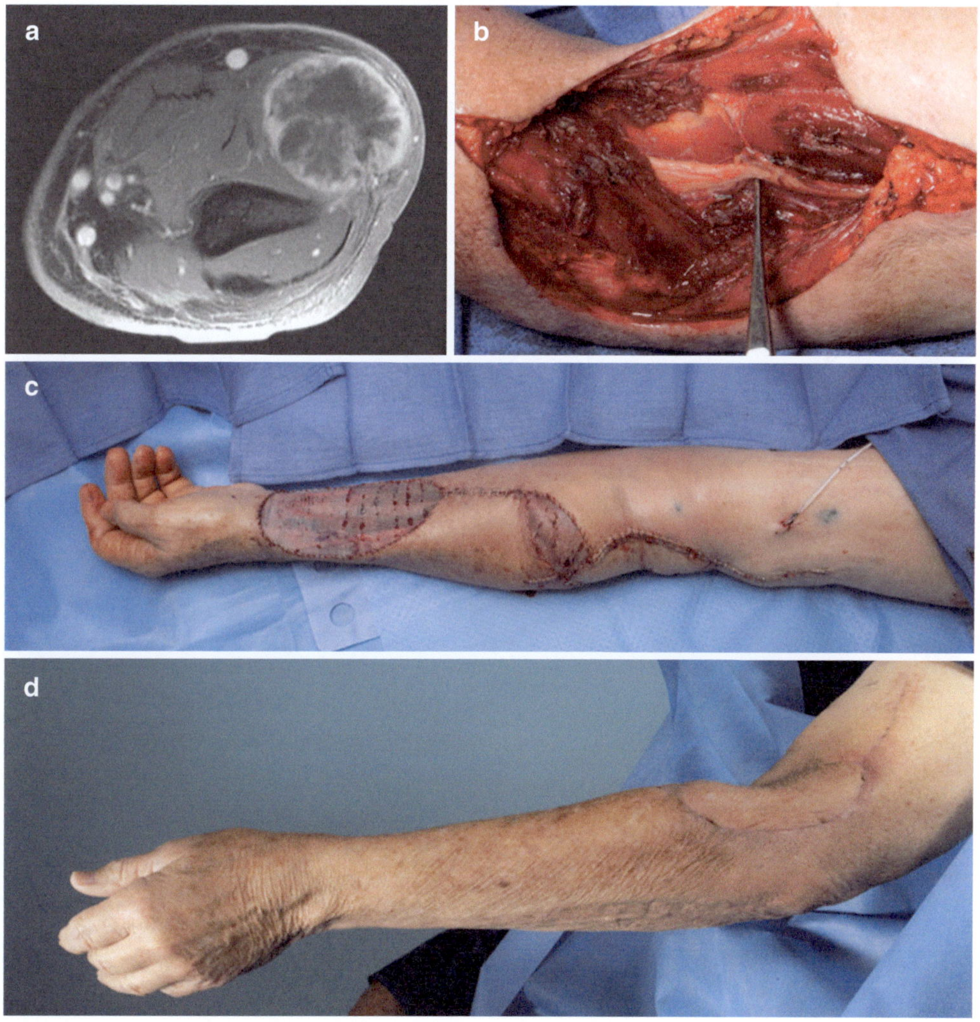

Fig. 20.1 Preoperative axial MRI with contrast showing a heterogeneous mass involving the mobile wad of the forearm and abutting the radial nerve (**a**). The patient was treated with preoperative radiotherapy and a planned close margin of resection was performed on the radial nerve (**b**). The patient was covered with a proximally divided pedicled radial forearm flap. Due to the size of the flap, there was a large donor defect (**c**) that was closed with a split-thickness skin graft. At 3 months postoperative, the flap was healed without functional limitations (**d**)

the RFF, when the radial or ulnar artery are damaged or occluded, negating the use of an RFF, the posterior interosseous artery flap can be used to cover defects of the forearm [43, 44]. In addition although the donor site is more visible, it usually is does not have the cosmetic concerns of an RFF donor site.

20.2.1.4 Lateral Arm and Reverse Lateral Arm Flaps

The lateral arm flap is a fasciocutaneous flap based on the posterior radial collateral artery (Fig. 20.2). It is primarily used as a free flap but may also be considered as a pedicled flap in an antegrade or retrograde fashion. The reverse pedicled lateral arm flap can be used to cover the olecranon and the antecubital fossa, if the radial forearm flap is unavailable. When raised as a free flap, it can include a portion of the humerus to create and osteocutaneous flap and sensory flap [45–47].

20.2.1.5 Anterolateral Thigh Flap

The anterolateral thigh (ALT) flap is considered to be the soft-tissue flap of choice for extremity reconstruction, with a success rate of up to 98% in large series [48–53]. Although the flap harvest can be tedious, it has a very long and reliable pedicle (the descending branch of the lateral femoral circumflex artery) which can be harvested at the suprafascial level allowing for a large thin flap (Fig. 20.3) which can cover defects as large as 40 × 20 cm [54, 55]. When planning for an ALT, it is important to obtain a preoperative CT-angiogram of the thigh to verify perforator location. For composite defects, the flap can be harvested with the rectus femoris or vastus lateralis muscle or with only fascia for coverage of variety of composite defects [56].

20.2.2 Muscle Flaps

For large soft-tissue defects, muscle flaps were traditionally utilized; however, they often required STSG as well. This approach has largely been replaced with fasciocutaneous flaps which are more tolerant to radiotherapy and secondary surgery. Muscle flaps however are still valuable for functional reconstruction as well as in cases of significant soft-tissue contamination.

20.2.2.1 Latissimus Dorsi

Based on the thoracodorsal artery, the latissimus dorsi is a reliable flap which can be raised with a skin paddle, providing a large flap which is one of the most versatile flaps for reconstruction. As a pedicled flap, the latissimus can cover

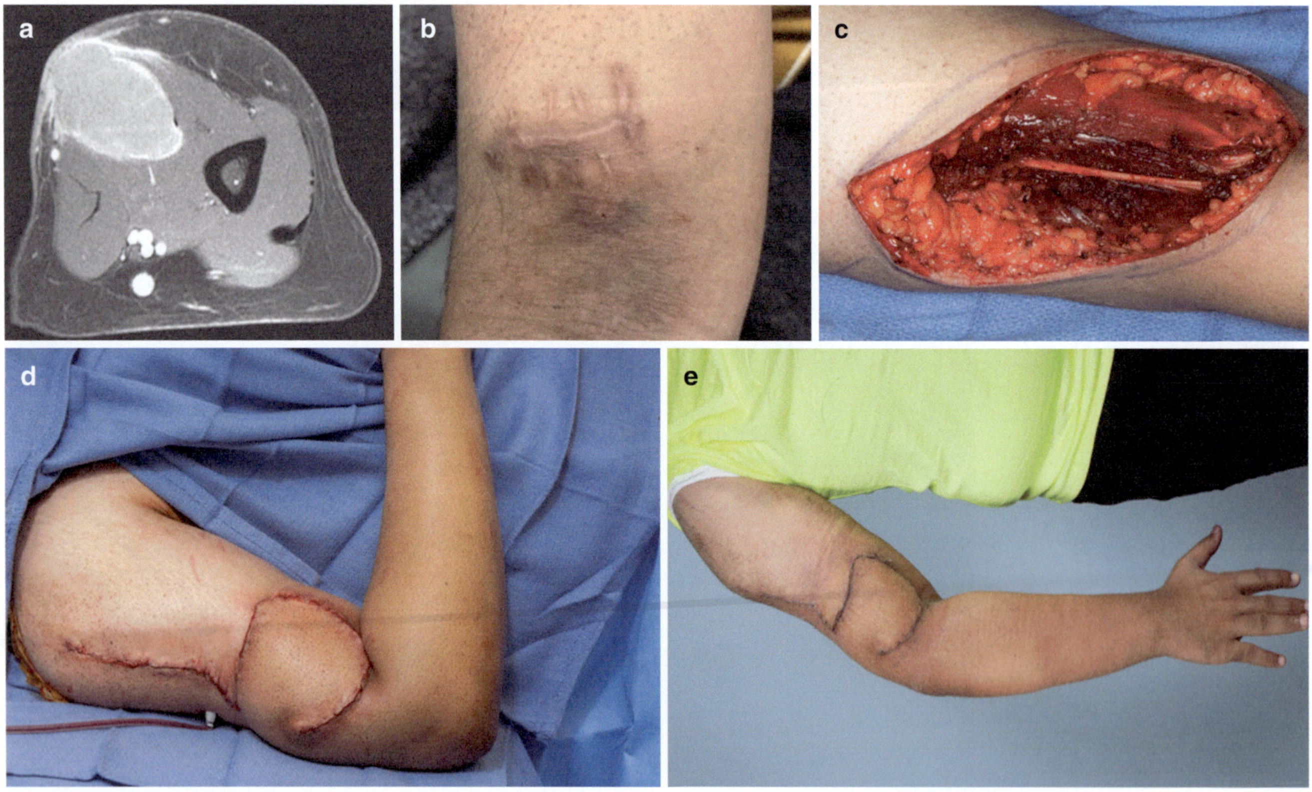

Fig. 20.2 Preoperative axial MRI with contrast showing a soft-tissue sarcoma overlying the radial nerve (**a**). The patient underwent an unplanned biopsy with a poorly performed transverse incision (**b**). A planned close margin of resection over the radial nerve was performed (**c**). The wound was covered with a lateral arm flap (**d**), and at 8 weeks (**e**), the wound was healed and the patient had a fully functional upper extremity

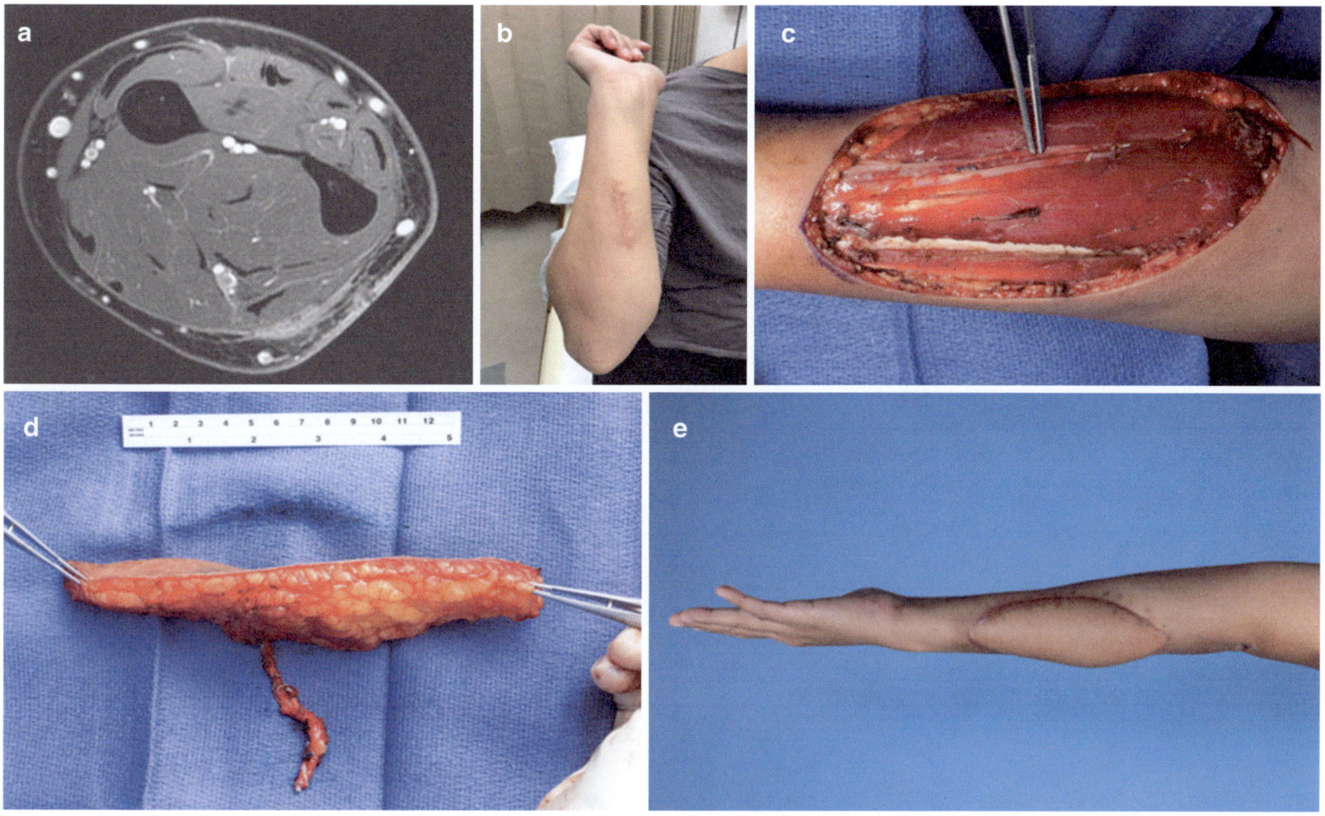

Fig. 20.3 Preoperative axial MRI (**a**) with contrast showing a soft-tissue sarcoma tumor bed overlying the flexor carpi ulnaris (FCU) following an unplanned excision (**b**). Following preoperative radiotherapy the patient underwent a planned close margin resection which included the FCU, exposing the ulnar neurovascular bundle (**c**). The patient was reconstructed with a thin free ALT flap (**d**) allowing for a gliding tissue plan for a reconstruction of the FCU and full elbow range of motion (**e**)

the arm to the level of the elbow. For composite free flap coverage, the latissimus can be harvested with the vascularized rib and/or serratus. Along with soft-tissue coverage, the latissimus can be used as a functioning muscle flap. At our institution it is our preferred flap to restore biceps, triceps, or deltoid function following oncologic resection (Fig. 20.4). The donor site morbidity is minimal, but occasionally patients will some note some loss of shoulder motion and strength.

20.2.2.2 Gracilis

The gracilis can be used as a free functioning muscle to restore flexor tendons of the volar compartment or extensor tendon function in the hand. The gracilis flap is based off the medial femoral circumflex artery, receiving its nerve supply from the obturator nerve. In addition to hand function, it can also be used to restore biceps function at the elbow provided appropriate donor nerves can be isolated [57, 58]; however, for this, we prefer the use of a pedicled latissimus flap.

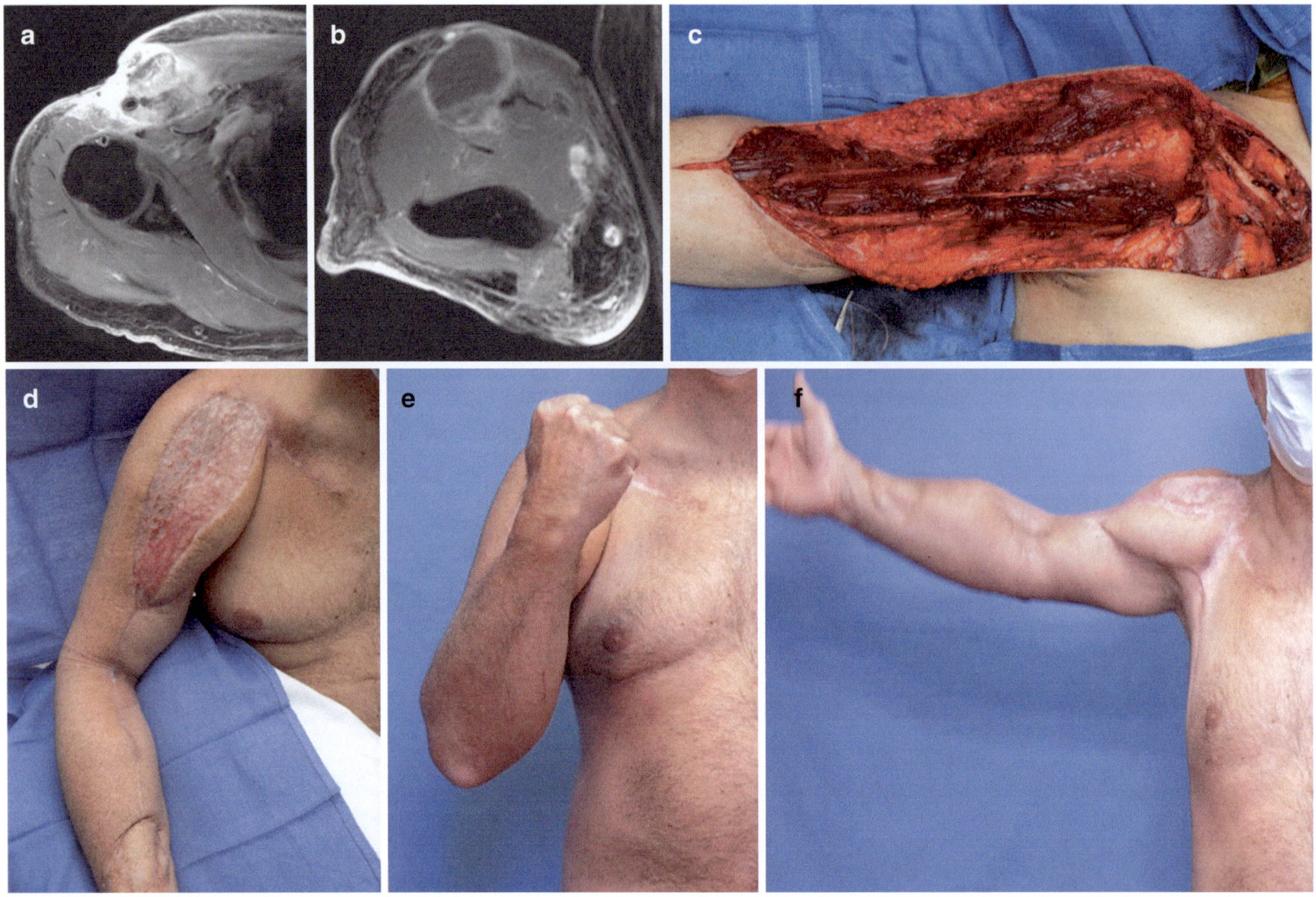

Fig. 20.4 Preoperative axial MRI with contrast showing a multifocal recurrent sarcoma involving the proximal (**a**) and distal (**b**) anterior arm. The patient refused amputation and was treated with preoperative radiotherapy and underwent a planned close margin resection of the entire anterior compartment of the arm (**c**). They were covered with a functional latissimus flap and skin graft that was utilized for both coverage (**d**) and function which allowed for elbow flexion (**e**) and shoulder abduction (**f**)

20.3 Bone and Joint Reconstruction

When a soft-tissue sarcoma is adjacent to the bone, the use of preoperative MRI and physical exam can help the surgeon determine if the bone or joint needs to be sacrificed [59]. On preoperative MRI the presence of cortical erosion or presence of signal change in the bone marrow can signify bony invasion. Intraoperatively this can also be assessed to determine if the STS moves around the bone or remains fixed. The fascia surrounding the tumor is circumferentially mobilized, and if the tumor can be "rolled" over the bone, it is not invading the bone; however, if it remains fixed, the adjacent bone should be resected with the tumor in an en-bloc fashion. If the tumor can be rolled, the periosteum can be stripped with the tumor as the deep margin [59]. In addition to bony invasion, the preoperative MRI can be utilized to evaluate the presence of tumor extending into the joint [60].

If a bony defect is left following tumor excision reconstruction is predicated on the size of the defect and status of the underlying bone. For small bone defects (<5 cm) with surrounding well vascularized bone and soft tissues, bone shortening or non-vascularized cancellous bone grafting can utilized for bony reconstruction. There are multiple options which exist for bone grafting including autologous graft and non-autologous bone substitutes, each with their own pluses and minus, but the choice of bone graft is beyond the scope of this chapter. If cancellous bone graft is to be used, stable bone fixation is imperative for bone consolidation. For defects >5 cm or in the setting of radiated bone, vascularized bone grafting is the preferred option [61–72]. Vascularized bone flaps have been shown to reliably heal in the setting of radiotherapy, reduce the risk of fracture and infection, and remodel under stress allowing for early weight bearing [68–70, 73].

20.3.1 Vascularized Fibula

The free vascularized fibula (FVF) is the workhorse bone flap for intercalary long bone reconstruction following tumor extirpation [65, 67, 68, 70, 74–76]. The fibula has a reliable vascular pedicle from the peroneal artery, and can provide up to 25 cm of straight, cortical bone [74, 77]. In addition to bony reconstruction, the FVF can be harvested with an osseo-cutaneous paddle based on cutaneous perforators which are located in the lower two-thirds of the leg; these skin islands help with flap monitoring and reconstruct of associated soft-tissue defects [78]. Prior to considering an FVF, the surgical team should obtain a CT-angiogram of the leg to evaluate for a peroneal magnus artery, as harvest of the FVF in this situation would lead to devascularization of the foot [79].

For intercalary defects of the forearm, the shape and size of the fibula is similar to the diaphysis of the radius and ulna, allowing for reconstruction with an FVF to provide a stable forearm and wrist, with excellent results [68, 76, 80, 81]. Likewise for intercalary defects of the humerus, when combined with rigid compression plating (Fig. 20.5), the FVF is a reliably option bony reconstruction [82–84] The FVF has also historically been utilized to assist with a glenohumeral arthrodesis when the glenohumeral joint has been sacrificed [82, 83, 85–88]. It was felt that in younger patients the stress placed over a prosthetic component would be too high and lead to early failure [86]. However, new reconstructive options, such as the use of allograft prosthetic composites utilizing a reverse total shoulder, have showed improved functional outcomes, with a low rate of failure [89, 90]. In addition, these reconstructions can be combined with local muscle transfers (deltoid or latissimus dorsi) to improve shoulder function [91].

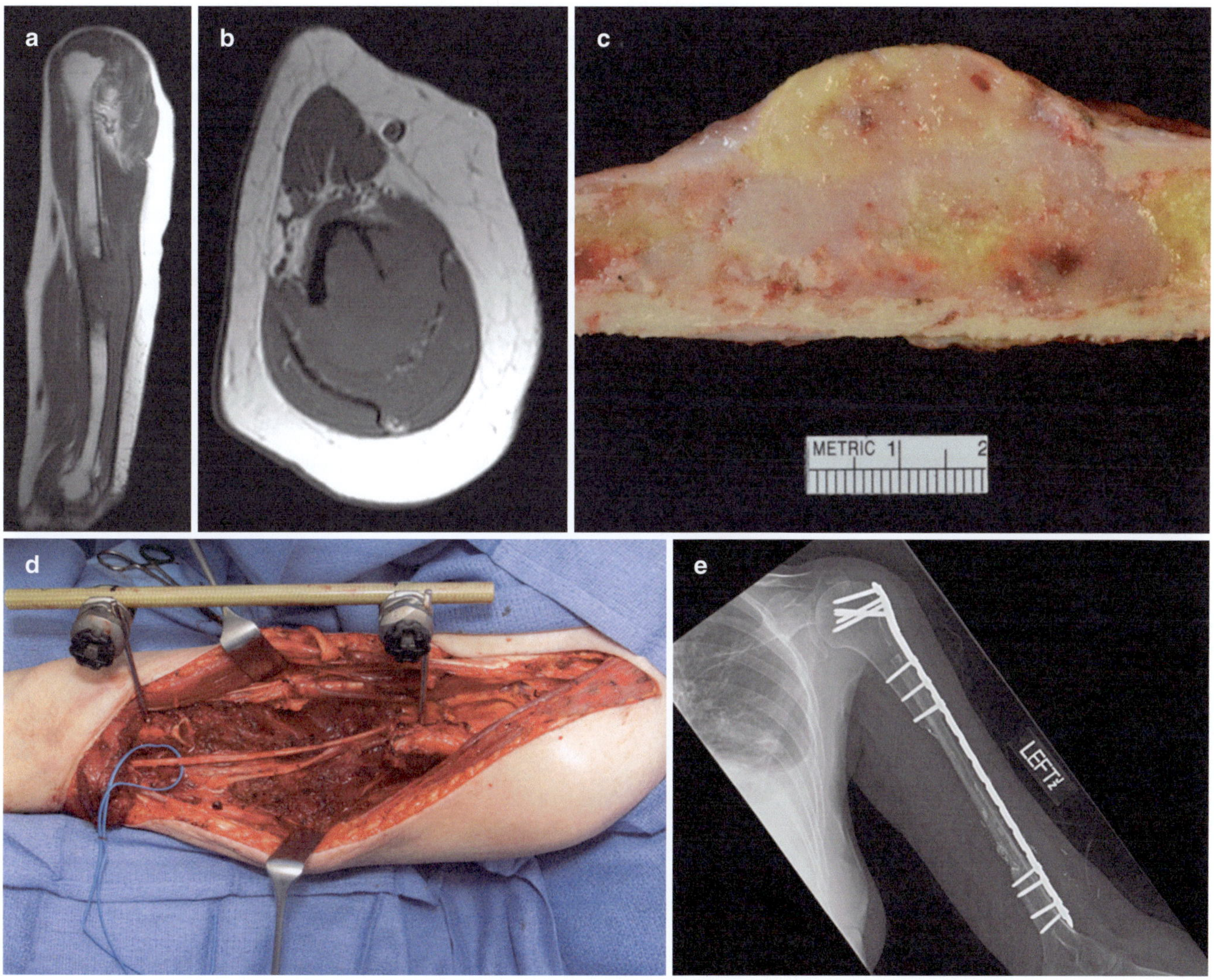

Fig. 20.5 Preoperative sagittal (**a**) and axial (**b**) MRI of the arm showing a leiomyosarcoma which invaded the diaphysis of the humerus. The patient underwent en-bloc resection (**c**) with a planned close margin of resection along the radial nerve following preoperative radiotherapy (**d**). The patient underwent an intercalary reconstruction with a free vascularized fibula flap with fixation provided by a spanning locking plate (**e**)

20.3.2 Vascularized Proximal Fibula Epiphyseal Transfer

In skeletally immature patients, reconstruction of the proximal humerus or wrist is challenging due to the difficulty in preserving physeal growth. In these special cases, the proximal fibula physis can be transferred based on the anterior tibial artery to allow for a "growing" biologic bony reconstruction [92]. In the wrist, the proximal fibula physis has been shown to provide reliable healing, with a growth rate similar to the contralateral radius and the ipsilateral ulna [93–95]. Its use for humeral reconstruction has been associated with a high rate of graft fracture and poor functional outcomes [95, 96]. This is thought to be due to the size mismatch between the fibula and humerus, which can lead to frequent fibular stress fractures. Additionally, the fibular head lacks adequate soft-tissue attachments to reconstruct the rotator cuff following the oncologic resection [95, 96]. One way to potentially mitigate this is to utilize a composite free vascularized proximal fibula epiphysis with a proximal humerus allograft which has the donor rotator cuff [97]. This has been shown to allow for growth of the proximal humerus, while the allograft provides structural support to reduce the risk of fracture and the allograft rotator cuff can be repaired to the host rotator cuff to improve shoulder motion [97].

20.3.3 Vascularized Scapula

In situations where the FVF cannot be utilized, the lateral boarder of the scapula can be harvested to reconstruct bony defects of the forearm as a free flap or the humerus as a pedicled flap [98–106]. The flap is based on the subscapular artery and can be harvested with a large skin paddle to provide an osteocutaneous flap [98–100].

20.3.4 Vascularized Medial Femoral Condyle

The vascularized medial femoral condyle (MFC) is commonly used to reconstruct scaphoid non-unions, the pliable nature of the flap allow it to be wrapped around the tubular bones of the upper extremity to "patch" nonunion sites, with subsequent union rates up to 100% [107–112]. This is especially helpful in the setting of previous radiotherapy, or non-union at allograft native bone junctions [110, 111, 113, 114].

20.3.5 Endoprosthetic Reconstruction

When the joint is sacrificed in the process of tumor extirpation, endoprosthetic reconstructive options for the shoulder, elbow and wrist are limited. In this setting, the reconstruction is utilized either in the form of an allograft prosthetic composite (APC) or endoprosthesis [89, 115–117]. For the shoulder, historically a hemiarthroplasty has been utilized; however, the functional outcomes have been poor [89, 118]. Recent advances in the design of reverse endoprosthesis or reverse APC have improved shoulder function. At our institution for shoulder reconstruction our preference is to utilize an APC (Fig. 20.6) secondary to the improved functional outcomes compared to an endoprosthesis [89]. Unlike the shoulder the options for elbow reconstruction are limited, and associated with a high rate of failure [119–121]. Similar to the shoulder, our institutional preference is to utilize an APC as it allows for selection of any off-shelf elbow implant, and is a reliable option for reconstruction [116, 121].

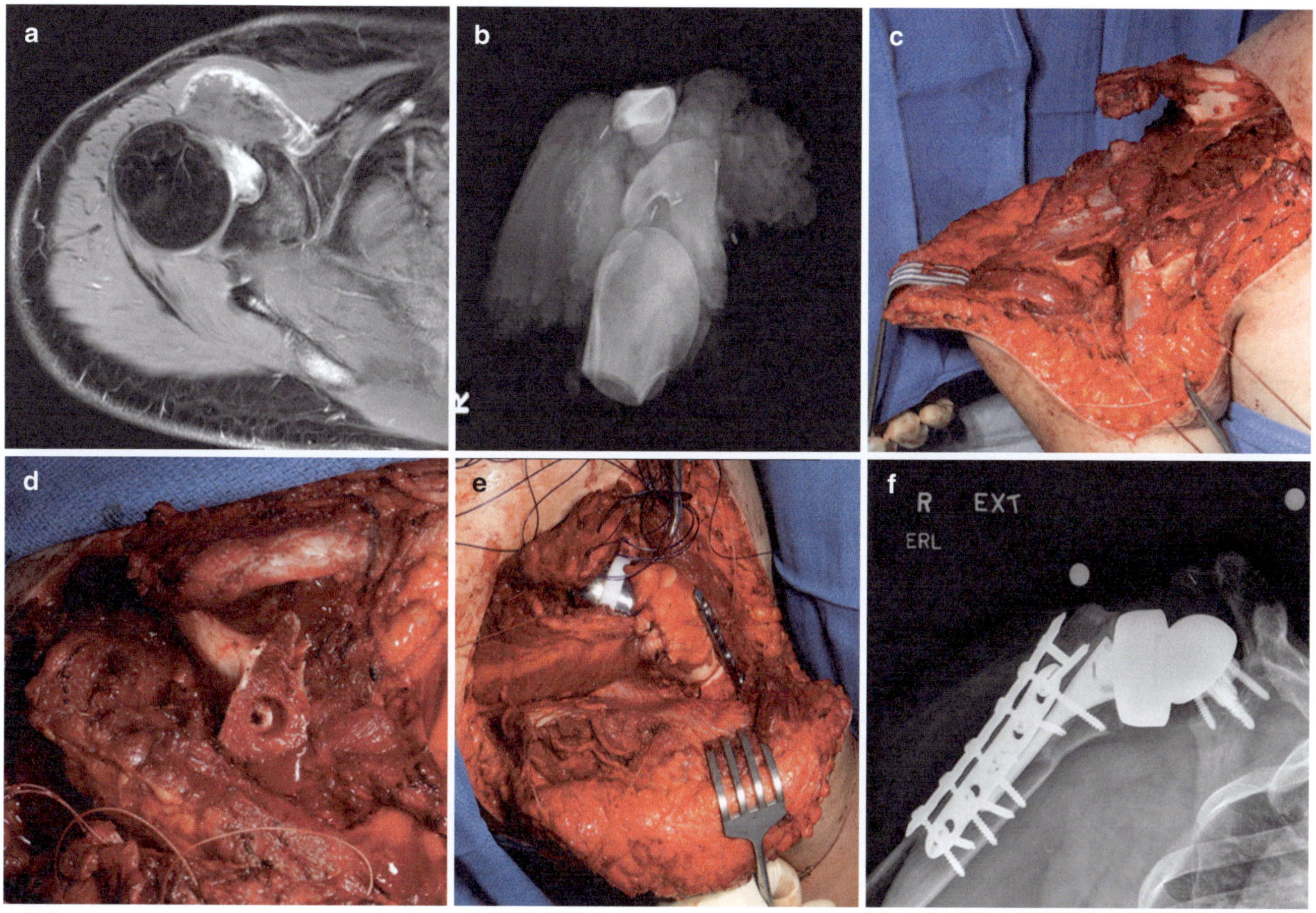

Fig. 20.6 Preoperative axial MRI showing a synovial sarcoma which extended intra-articular into the glenohumeral joint (**a**). The patient underwent an extra-articular resection (**b**) with preservation of the scapular pain (**c**) and the glenoid osteotomy medial to the joint capsule allowing for the placement of a traditional reverse total shoulder glenosphere (**d**). The proximal humerus was reconstructed utilizing an allograft prosthetic composite which allowed for direct repair of the patients' residual rotator cuff (**e**) and 1 year of follow-up the junction had healed (**f**) and the patient had active use of the shoulder

20.4 Neurovascular Reconstruction

Resection of critical neurovascular structures can have a substantial impact on patient function and such resections are associated with a high rate of postoperative complications [11, 122, 123]. Nerve reconstruction is rarely performed for patients following resection of an STS [124]. This is likely due to the fact that resultant motor defects following resection can often be reconstructed with tendon transfers, especially in the upper extremity [125]. For sensory deficits, however, nerve reconstruction is the only hope for return of sensation, which is critical for the ulnar boarder of the hand and the palm. Nerve transfers are theoretically excellent options for reconstruction of proximal nerve defects of the brachial plexus and distally to restore sensation in the hand as shown by data from brachial plexus injuries and traumatic nerve injuries [126]; however, literature nerve reconstruction in sarcoma surgery is limited. For large nerve defects, our preferred reconstructive technique is to utilize cabled sural nerve autografts, which can be vascularized to improve nerve recovery. For smaller diameter nerves, local nerve autograft can also be taken from either the medial or lateral antebrachial cutaneous nerve. For non-critical nerves, reconstruction can be performed with processed decellularized nerve graft and for defects less than 5–8 mm conduits can be utilized [127].

Following resection of an STS, vascular reconstruction may need to be performed [128]. When the vascular structures are circumferentially encased by tumor, resection is necessary in order to provide an oncologic margin. For arterial reconstruction, saphenous vein autograft, in addition to artificial and cryopreserve allografts can restore perfusion and all have been shown to have similar outcomes [129, 130]. The necessity of deep venous reconstruction in these cases is debated, and often not performed due to the high rate of thrombosis [130]. Typically isolated vein resections are not reconstructed if there is appropriate collateral superficial drainage; however, if it is necessary, reconstruction with autogenous vein grafts has been shown to have the lowest rate of failure [130].

20.5 Amputation

Safe limb salvage is achievable in the majority of patients; however, for certain patients, amputations are still necessary [131–133]. Oncoplastic surgery remains important in this patient population, as newer surgical techniques such as targeted muscle reinnervation has minimized post-operative phantom pain and improved patient outcome [134].

20.5.1 Forequarter Amputation

Historically forequarter amputation was the preferred treatment for patients with shoulder girdle sarcoma; however, today, it is rarely performed today [135]. The most common indication for a forequarter amputation is involvement of the brachial vessels and encasement of the brachial plexus [136–140]. Although these procedures are disfiguring, they lead to improvement in the patients' quality of life and reduced narcotic requirements [140]. Unfortunately, the overall 5-year survival rate following this procedure is reported between 20% and 36% [135, 137, 140–142]. Most forequarter amputations can be closed with primary wound closure; however, in situations where a flap is necessary, a fillet flap from the amputated limb is a viable reconstructive option [143].

20.5.2 Transhumeral and Transradial Amputation

Indications for transhumeral and transradial amputation include multifocal tumors, primary or recurrent tumors involving neurovascular bundles which would result in an insensate hand, and for palliative measures [138]. Wound healing of the soft-tissue flaps is often not an issue, even in the setting of radiotherapy due to the robust blood supply to the arm. The muscle bellies should be tensioned over the cut bone through a myodesis to allow for appropriate prosthetic use.

20.5.3 Hand Amputation

Although limb salvage is utilized for a majority of patients with distal STS, partial hand amputations are still necessary for oncologic control; however, partial hand amputations should not be considered to be a failure of limb salvage surgery [144–147]. For larger partial hand amputations, soft-tissue coverage is often needed in the form of either a fillet flap, radial forearm flap, or free flap [147].

20.6 Conclusion

An oncoplastic approach to upper extremity reconstruction leads to the best oncologic and functional outcome for patients with upper extremity soft-tissue sarcomas. A majority of patients can undergo limb salvage surgery, and various bony and soft-tissue flaps are necessary to reconstruct to provide the patient with a functional extremity.

Conflicts of Interest No conflicts of interest are declared by any author on this study.

Funding No disclosures of funding were received for this work from NIH, Wellcome Trust, or HHMI.

References

1. Stiller CA, Trama A, Serraino D, Rossi S, Navarro C, Chirlaque MD, et al. Descriptive epidemiology of sarcomas in Europe: report from the RARECARE project. Eur J Cancer. 2013;49(3):684–95.
2. Lohman RF, Nabawi AS, Reece GP, Pollock RE, Evans GR. Soft tissue sarcoma of the upper extremity: a 5-year experience at two institutions emphasizing the role of soft tissue flap reconstruction. Cancer. 2002;94(8):2256–64.
3. Muller DA, Beltrami G, Scoccianti G, Frenos F, Capanna R. Combining limb-sparing surgery with radiation therapy in high-grade soft tissue sarcoma of extremities—is it effective? Eur J Surg Oncol. 2016;42(7):1057–63.
4. Gerrand CH, Wunder JS, Kandel RA, O'Sullivan B, Catton CN, Bell RS, et al. The influence of anatomic location on functional outcome in lower-extremity soft-tissue sarcoma. Ann Surg Oncol. 2004;11(5):476–82.
5. Baroudi MR, Ferguson PC, Wunder JS, Isler MH, Mottard S, Werier JA, et al. Forearm soft tissue sarcoma: tumors characteristics and oncologic outcomes following limb salvage surgery. J Surg Oncol. 2014;110(6):676–81.
6. Payne CE, Hofer SO, Zhong T, Griffin AC, Ferguson PC, Wunder JS. Functional outcome following upper limb soft tissue sarcoma resection with flap reconstruction. J Plast Reconstr Aesthet Surg. 2013;66(5):601–7.
7. Schreiber D, Bell RS, Wunder JS, O'Sullivan B, Turcotte R, Masri BA, et al. Evaluating function and health related quality of life in patients treated for extremity soft tissue sarcoma. Qual Life Res. 2006;15(9):1439–46.
8. O'Donnell PW, Griffin AM, Eward WC, Sternheim A, Catton CN, Chung PW, et al. The effect of the setting of a positive surgical margin in soft tissue sarcoma. Cancer. 2014;120(18):2866–75.
9. Clarkson PW, Griffin AM, Catton CN, O'Sullivan B, Ferguson PC, Wunder JS, et al. Epineural dissection is a safe technique that facilitates limb salvage surgery. Clin Orthop Relat Res. 2005;438:92–6.
10. Jones KB, Ferguson PC, Deheshi B, Riad S, Griffin A, Bell RS, et al. Complete femoral nerve resection with soft tissue sarcoma: functional outcomes. Ann Surg Oncol. 2010;17(2):401–6.

11. Ghert MA, Davis AM, Griffin AM, Alyami AH, White L, Kandel RA, et al. The surgical and functional outcome of limb-salvage surgery with vascular reconstruction for soft tissue sarcoma of the extremity. Ann Surg Oncol. 2005;12(12):1102–10.
12. Davis AM, O'Sullivan B, Turcotte R, Bell R, Catton C, Chabot P, et al. Late radiation morbidity following randomization to preoperative versus postoperative radiotherapy in extremity soft tissue sarcoma. Radiother Oncol. 2005;75(1):48–53.
13. Davis AM, O'Sullivan B, Bell RS, Turcotte R, Catton CN, Wunder JS, et al. Function and health status outcomes in a randomized trial comparing preoperative and postoperative radiotherapy in extremity soft tissue sarcoma. J Clin Oncol. 2002;20(22):4472–7.
14. O'Sullivan B, Davis AM, Turcotte R, Bell R, Catton C, Chabot P, et al. Preoperative versus postoperative radiotherapy in soft-tissue sarcoma of the limbs: a randomised trial. Lancet. 2002;359(9325):2235–41.
15. Brown A, Spazzoli B, Mah E, May D, Chu J, Spelman T, et al. Planned combined onco-plastic (COP) surgical approach improves oncologic outcomes in soft tissue sarcomas. Eur J Surg Oncol. 2021;47(2):443–9.
16. Chan LWM, Imanishi J, Grinsell DG, Choong P. Preoperative radiotherapy and wide resection for soft tissue sarcomas: achieving a low rate of major wound complications with the use of flaps. Results of a single surgical team. Front Surg. 2017;4:79.
17. Gundle KR, Kafchinski L, Gupta S, Griffin AM, Dickson BC, Chung PW, et al. Analysis of margin classification systems for assessing the risk of local recurrence after soft tissue sarcoma resection. J Clin Oncol. 2018;36(7):704–9.
18. Gundle KR, Gupta S, Kafchinski L, Griffin AM, Kandel RA, Dickson BC, et al. An analysis of tumor- and surgery-related factors that contribute to inadvertent positive margins following soft tissue sarcoma resection. Ann Surg Oncol. 2017;24(8):2137–44.
19. Lerman OZ, Kovach SJ, Levin LS. The respective roles of plastic and orthopedic surgery in limb salvage. Plast Reconstr Surg. 2011;127(Suppl 1):215S–27S.
20. Griffin AM, Dickie CI, Catton CN, Chung PW, Ferguson PC, Wunder JS, et al. The influence of time interval between preoperative radiation and surgical resection on the development of wound healing complications in extremity soft tissue sarcoma. Ann Surg Oncol. 2015;22(9):2824–30.
21. Roeder F, de Paoli A, Saleh-Ebrahimi L, Alldinger I, Bertola G, Boz G, et al. Intraoperative electron radiation therapy combined with external beam radiation therapy after gross total resection in extremity soft tissue sarcoma: a European pooled analysis. Ann Surg Oncol. 2018;25(13):3833–42.
22. Fourman MS, Ramsey DC, Newman ET, Schwab JH, Chen YL, Hung YP, et al. Assessing the safety and utility of wound VAC temporization of the sarcoma or benign aggressive tumor bed until final margins are achieved. Ann Surg Oncol. 2022;29(4):2290–8.
23. Levin LS. The reconstructive ladder. An orthoplastic approach. Orthop Clin North Am. 1993;24(3):393–409.
24. Townley WA, Mah E, O'Neill AC, Wunder JS, Ferguson PC, Zhong T, et al. Reconstruction of sarcoma defects following preoperative radiation: free tissue transfer is safe and reliable. J Plast Reconstr Aesthet Surg. 2013;66(11):1575–9.
25. Gopal S, Majumder S, Batchelor AG, Knight SL, De Boer P, Smith RM. Fix and flap: the radical orthopaedic and plastic treatment of severe open fractures of the tibia. J Bone Joint Surg Br. 2000;82(7):959–66.
26. Fleming ME, O'Daniel A, Bharmal H, Valerio I. Application of the orthoplastic reconstructive ladder to preserve lower extremity amputation length. Ann Plast Surg. 2014;73(2):183–9.
27. Honig RL, Tibbo ME, Mallett KE, Bakri K, Ahmed SK, Petersen IA, et al. Outcome of soft-tissue reconstruction in the setting of combined preoperative and intraoperative radiotherapy for extremity soft-tissue sarcomas. Anticancer Res. 2020;40(12):6941–5.
28. Bogdan MA, Klein MB, Rubin GD, McAdams TR, Chang J. CT angiography in complex upper extremity reconstruction. J Hand Surg Br. 2004;29(5):465–9.
29. Wood MB. Composite free flaps to the hand. Hand Clin. 1997;13(2):231–8.
30. Lal ST, Banipal RP, Bhatti DJ. Tolerance of skin grafts to postoperative radiotherapy. Int J Appl Basic Med Res. 2015;5(3):187–9.
31. Bui DT, Chunilal A, Mehrara BJ, Disa JJ, Alektiar KM, Cordeiro PG. Outcome of split-thickness skin grafts after external beam radiotherapy. Ann Plast Surg. 2004;52(6):551–6; discussion 7.
32. Senchenkov A, Petty PM, Knoetgen J 3rd, Moran SL, Johnson CH, Clay RP. Outcomes of skin graft reconstructions with the use of vacuum assisted closure (VAC(R)) dressing for irradiated extremity sarcoma defects. World J Surg Oncol. 2007;5:138.
33. Smith PJFB, McGregor IA, Jackson IT. The anatomical basis of the groin flap. Plast Reconstr Surg. 1972;49:41–7.
34. Moran SL, Johnson CH. Skin and soft tissue: pedicled flaps. In: Berger RA, Weiss AP, editors. Hand surgery. Philadelphia: Lippincott Williams and Wilkins; 2004. p. 1131–60.
35. Goh TL, Park SW, Cho JY, Choi JW, Hong JP. The search for the ideal thin skin flap: superficial circumflex iliac artery perforator flap—a review of 210 cases. Plast Reconstr Surg. 2015;135(2):592–601.
36. Kaufman MR, Jones NF. The reverse radial forearm flap for soft tissue reconstruction of the wrist and hand. Tech Hand Up Extrem Surg. 2005;9(1):47–51.
37. Foucher G, van Genechten F, Merle N, Michon J. A compound radial artery forearm flap in hand surgery: an original modification of the Chinese forearm flap. Br J Plast Surg. 1984;37(2):139–48.
38. Yajima H, Inada Y, Shono M, Tamai S. Radical forearm flap with vascularized tendons for hand reconstruction. Plast Reconstr Surg. 1996;98(2):328–33.
39. Jones DB Jr, Burger H, Bishop AT, Shin AY. Treatment of scaphoid waist nonunions with an avascular proximal pole and carpal collapse. A comparison of two vascularized bone grafts. J Bone Joint Surg Am. 2008;90(12):2616–25.
40. Zhang J, Zang M, Yu S, Xu L, Liu Y. Reconstruction of forearm soft tissue defects with radial artery perforator-pedicled propeller flaps. J Plast Reconstr Aesthet Surg. 2015;68(1):125–6.
41. Saint-Cyr M, Mujadzic M, Wong C, Hatef D, Lajoie AS, Rohrich RJ. The radial artery pedicle perforator flap: vascular analysis and clinical implications. Plast Reconstr Surg. 2010;125(5):1469–78.
42. Hansen AJ, Duncan SF, Smith AA, Shin AY, Moran SL, Bishop AT. Reverse radial forearm fascial flap with radial artery preservation. Hand (N Y). 2007;2(3):159–63.
43. Angrigiani C, Grilli D, Dominikow D, et al. Posterior interosseous reverse forearm flap: experience with 80 consecutive cases. Plast Reconstr Surg. 1993;92:285–93.
44. Mazzer N, Barbieri CH, Cortez M. The posterior interosseous forearm island flap for skin defects in the hand and elbow. A prospective study of 51 cases. J Hand Surg. 1996;21B:237–43.
45. Ninkovic M, Harpf C, Schwabegger AH, et al. The lateral arm flap. Clin Plast Surg. 2001;28:367–74.
46. Arnez ZM, Kersnic M, Smith RW, et al. Free lateral arm osteocutaneous neurosensory flap for thumb reconstruction. J Hand Surg (Br). 1991;16:395–9.
47. Tung TC, Wang KC, Fang CM, et al. Reverse pedicle lateral arm flap for reconstruction of posterior soft-tissue defects of the elbow. Ann Plast Surg. 1997;38:635–41.
48. Gedebou TM, Wei FC, Lin CH. Clinical experience of 1284 free anterolateral thigh flaps. Handchir Mikrochir Plast Chir. 2002;34(4):239–44.
49. Wang HT, Erdmann D, Fletcher JW, Levin LS. Anterolateral thigh flap technique in hand and upper extremity reconstruction. Tech Hand Up Extrem Surg. 2004;8(4):257–61.

50. Chen HC, Tang YB, Mardini S, Tsai BW. Reconstruction of the hand and upper limb with free flaps based on musculocutaneous perforators. Microsurgery. 2004;24(4):270–80.
51. Bakri K, Moran SL. Initial assessment and management of complex forearm defects. Hand Clin. 2007;23:255–68.
52. Jensen M, Moran SL. Soft tissue coverage of the elbow: a reconstructive algorithm. Orthop Clin North Am. 2008;39:251–64.
53. Wei FC, Jain V, Celik N, Chen HC, Chuang DC, Lin CH. Have we found an ideal soft-tissue flap? An experience with 672 anterolateral thigh flaps. Plast Reconstr Surg. 2002;109(7):2219–26; discussion 27–30.
54. Rajacic N, Gang RK, Krishnan J, Lal Bang R. Thin anterolateral thigh free flap. Ann Plast Surg. 2002;48(3):252–7.
55. Kimura N, Satoh K. Consideration of a thin flap as an entity and clinical applications of the thin anterolateral thigh flap. Plast Reconstr Surg. 1996;97(5):985–92.
56. Fox P, Endress R, Sen S, Chang J. Fascia-only anterolateral thigh flap for extremity reconstruction. Ann Plast Surg. 2014;72(Suppl 1):S9–13.
57. Grinsell D, Di Bella C, Choong PF. Functional reconstruction of sarcoma defects utilising innervated free flaps. Sarcoma. 2012;2012:315190.
58. Chuang DC, Strauch RJ, Wei FC. Technical considerations in two-stage functioning free muscle transplantation reconstruction of both flexor and extensor functions of the forearm. Microsurgery. 1994;15(5):338–43.
59. Ferguson PC, Griffin AM, O'Sullivan B, Catton CN, Davis AM, Murji A, et al. Bone invasion in extremity soft-tissue sarcoma: impact on disease outcomes. Cancer. 2006;106(12):2692–700.
60. Bui-Mansfield LT, O'Brien SD. Magnetic resonance appearance of intra-articular synovial sarcoma: case reports and review of the literature. J Comput Assist Tomogr. 2008;32(4):640–4.
61. Wood MB, Cooney WP 3rd, Irons GB Jr. Skeletal reconstruction by vascularized bone transfer: indications and results. Mayo Clin Proc. 1985;60(11):729–34.
62. Wood MB. Free vascularized bone transfers for nonunions, segmental gaps, and following tumor resection. Orthopedics. 1986;9(6):810–6.
63. de Boer HH, Wood MB. Bone changes in the vascularised fibular graft. J Bone Joint Surg Br. 1989;71(3):374–8.
64. Dell PC, Sheppard JE. Vascularized bone grafts in the treatment of infected forearm nonunions. J Hand Surg Am. 1984;9(5):653–8.
65. Taylor GI, Miller GD, Ham FJ. The free vascularized bone graft. A clinical extension of microvascular techniques. Plast Reconstr Surg. 1975;55(5):533–44.
66. Malizos KN, Zalavras CG, Soucacos PN, Beris AE, Urbaniak JR. Free vascularized fibular grafts for reconstruction of skeletal defects. J Am Acad Orthop Surg. 2004;12(5):360–9.
67. Wood MB. Femoral reconstruction by vascularized bone transfer. Microsurgery. 1990;11(1):74–9.
68. Han CS, Wood MB, Bishop AT, Cooney WP 3rd. Vascularized bone transfer. J Bone Joint Surg Am. 1992;74(10):1441–9.
69. Claxton MR, Shirley MB, Bakri K, Rose PS, Moran SL, Houdek MT. Utility of the free vascularized fibula flap to reconstruct oncologic defects in the upper extremity. Anticancer Res. 2020;40(5):2751–5.
70. Houdek MT, Wagner ER, Bishop AT, Shin AY, Rose PS, Sim FH, et al. Complications and long-term outcomes of free fibula reconstruction following resection of a malignant tumor in the extremities. Plast Reconstr Surg. 2017;139(2):510e–9e.
71. Arata MA, Wood MB, Cooney WP 3rd. Revascularized segmental diaphyseal bone transfers in the canine. An analysis of viability. J Reconstr Microsurg. 1984;1(1):11–9.
72. Berggren A, Weiland AJ, Dorfman H. The effect of prolonged ischemia time on osteocyte and osteoblast survival in composite bone grafts revascularized by microvascular anastomoses. Plast Reconstr Surg. 1982;69(2):290–8.
73. Fujimaki A, Suda H. Experimental study and clinical observations on hypertrophy of vascularized bone grafts. Microsurgery. 1994;15(10):726–32.
74. Lin CH, Wei FC, Chen HC, Chuang DC. Outcome comparison in traumatic lower-extremity reconstruction by using various composite vascularized bone transplantation. Plast Reconstr Surg. 1999;104(4):984–92.
75. Heitmann C, Erdmann D, Levin LS. Treatment of segmental defects of the humerus with an osteoseptocutaneous fibular transplant. J Bone Joint Surg Am. 2002;84-A(12):2216–23.
76. Jupiter JB, Gerhard HJ, Guerrero J, Nunley JA, Levin LS. Treatment of segmental defects of the radius with use of the vascularized osteoseptocutaneous fibular autogenous graft. J Bone Joint Surg Am. 1997;79(4):542–50.
77. Wei FC, Chen HC, Chuang CC, Noordhoff MS. Fibular osteoseptocutaneous flap: anatomic study and clinical application. Plast Reconstr Surg. 1986;78(2):191–200.
78. Stevanovic M, Gutow AP, Sharpe F. The management of bone defects of the forearm after trauma. Hand Clin. 1999;15(2):299–318.
79. Rosson GD, Singh NK. Devascularizing complications of free fibula harvest: peronea arteria magna. J Reconstr Microsurg. 2005;21(8):533–8.
80. Soucacos PN, Korompilias AV, Vekris MD, Zoubos A, Beris AE. The free vascularized fibular graft for bridging large skeletal defects of the upper extremity. Microsurgery. 2011;31(3):190–7.
81. Kremer T, Bickert B, Germann G, Heitmann C, Sauerbier M. Outcome assessment after reconstruction of complex defects of the forearm and hand with osteocutaneous free flaps. Plast Reconstr Surg. 2006;118(2):443–54; discussion 55–6.
82. Rashid M, Hafeez S, Zia ul Islam M, Rizvi ST, ur Rehman S, Tamimy MS, et al. Limb salvage in malignant tumours of the upper limb using vascularised fibula. J Plast Reconstr Aesthet Surg. 2008;61(6):648–61.
83. Rose PS, Shin AY, Bishop AT, Moran SL, Sim FH. Vascularized free fibula transfer for oncologic reconstruction of the humerus. Clin Orthop Relat Res. 2005;438:80–4.
84. Wood MB. Upper extremity reconstruction by vascularized bone transfers: results and complications. J Hand Surg Am. 1987;12(3):422–7.
85. Bilgin SS. Reconstruction of proximal humeral defects with shoulder arthrodesis using free vascularized fibular graft. J Bone Joint Surg Am. 2012;94(13):e94.
86. Fuchs B, O'Connor MI, Padgett DJ, Kaufman KR, Sim FH. Arthrodesis of the shoulder after tumor resection. Clin Orthop Relat Res. 2005;436:202–7.
87. Scalise JJ, Iannotti JP. Glenohumeral arthrodesis after failed prosthetic shoulder arthroplasty. J Bone Joint Surg Am. 2008;90(1):70–7.
88. Viehweger E, Gonzalez JF, Launay F, Legre R, Jouve JL, Bollini G. [Shoulder arthrodesis with vascularized fibular graft after tumor resection of the proximal humerus]. Rev Chir Orthop Reparatrice Appar Mot. 2005;91(6):523–9.
89. Houdek MT, Bukowski BR, Athey AG, Elhassan BT, Barlow JD, Morrey ME, et al. Comparison of reconstructive techniques following oncologic intraarticular resection of proximal humerus. J Surg Oncol. 2021;123(1):133–40.
90. Sanchez-Sotelo J, Wagner ER, Sim FH, Houdek MT. Allograft-prosthetic composite reconstruction for massive proximal humeral bone loss in reverse shoulder arthroplasty. J Bone Joint Surg Am. 2017;99(24):2069–76.
91. Li X, Galvin JW, Zalneraitis BH, Gasbarro G, Parada SA, Eichinger JK, et al. Muscle tendon transfers around the shoulder:

diagnosis, treatment, surgical techniques, and outcomes. J Bone Joint Surg Am. 2022;104(9):833–50.
92. Morsy M, Sur YJ, Akdag O, Sabbagh MD, Suchyta MA, El-Gammal TA, et al. Vascularity of the proximal fibula and its implications in vascularized epiphyseal transfer: an anatomical and high-resolution computed tomographic angiography study. Plast Reconstr Surg. 2019;143(1):172e–83e.
93. Innocenti M, Delcroix L, Manfrini M, Ceruso M, Capanna R. Vascularized proximal fibular epiphyseal transfer for distal radial reconstruction. J Bone Joint Surg Am. 2004;86-A(7):1504–11.
94. Akinbo O, Strauch R. Physeal transfers for skeletal reconstruction. J Hand Surg Am. 2008;33(4):584–90.
95. Medrykowski F, Barbary S, Gibert N, Lascombes P, Dautel G. Vascularized proximal fibular epiphyseal transfer: two cases. Orthop Traumatol Surg Res. 2012;98(6):728–32.
96. Innocenti M, Delcroix L, Romano GF, Capanna R. Vascularized epiphyseal transplant. Orthop Clin North Am. 2007;38(1):95–101. vii
97. Houdek MT, Wellings EP, Saifuddin H, Moran SL. Composite-free vascularized fibular epiphyseal flap and proximal humeral allograft for proximal humerus reconstruction in a pediatric patient. J Am Acad Orthop Surg Glob Res Rev. 2021;5(7).
98. Gilbert A, Teot L. The free scapular flap. Plast Reconstr Surg. 1982;69(4):601–4.
99. Barwick WJ, Goodkind DJ, Serafin D. The free scapular flap. Plast Reconstr Surg. 1982;69(5):779–87.
100. Hamilton SG, Morrison WA. The scapular free flap. Br J Plast Surg. 1982;35(1):2–7.
101. Izadi D, Paget JT, Haj-Basheer M, Khan UM. Fasciocutaneous flaps of the subscapular artery axis to reconstruct large extremity defects. J Plast Reconstr Aesthet Surg. 2012;65(10):1357–62.
102. Sabino J, Franklin B, Patel K, Bonawitz S, Valerio IL. Revisiting the scapular flap: applications in extremity coverage for our U.S. combat casualties. Plast Reconstr Surg. 2013;132(4):577e–85e.
103. Coleman JJ 3rd, Sultan MR. The bipedicled osteocutaneous scapula flap: a new subscapular system free flap. Plast Reconstr Surg. 1991;87(4):682–92.
104. Allen RJ, Dupin CL, Dreschnack PA, Glass CA, Mahon-Deri B. The latissimus dorsi/scapular bone flap (the "latissimus/bone flap"). Plast Reconstr Surg. 1994;94(7):988–96.
105. Guerra AB, Metzinger SE, Lund KM, Cooper MM, Allen RJ, Dupin CL. The thoracodorsal artery perforator flap: clinical experience and anatomic study with emphasis on harvest techniques. Plast Reconstr Surg. 2004;114(1):32–41; discussion 2–3.
106. Datiashvili RO, Yueh JH. Management of complicated wounds of the extremities with scapular fascial free flaps. J Reconstr Microsurg. 2012;28(8):521–8.
107. Sakai K, Doi K, Kawai S. Free vascularized thin corticoperiosteal graft. Plast Reconstr Surg. 1991;87(2):290–8.
108. Friedrich JB, Pederson WC, Bishop AT, Galaviz P, Chang J. New workhorse flaps in hand reconstruction. Hand (N Y). 2012;7(1):45–54.
109. Kakar S, Duymaz A, Steinmann S, Shin AY, Moran SL. Vascularized medial femoral condyle corticoperiosteal flaps for the treatment of recalcitrant humeral nonunions. Microsurgery. 2011;31(2):85–92.
110. Fuchs B, Steinmann SP, Bishop AT. Free vascularized corticoperiosteal bone graft for the treatment of persistent nonunion of the clavicle. J Shoulder Elb Surg. 2005;14(3):264–8.
111. De Smet L. Treatment of non-union of forearm bones with a free vascularised corticoperiosteal flap from the medial femoral condyle. Acta Orthop Belg. 2009;75(5):611–5.
112. Jones DB Jr, Rhee PC, Bishop AT, Shin AY. Free vascularized medial femoral condyle autograft for challenging upper extremity nonunions. Hand Clin. 2012;28(4):493–501.
113. Choudry UH, Bakri K, Moran SL, Karacor Z, Shin AY. The vascularized medial femoral condyle periosteal bone flap for the treatment of recalcitrant bony nonunions. Ann Plast Surg. 2008;60(2):174–80.
114. Del Pinal F, Garcia-Bernal FJ, Regalado J, Ayala H, Cagigal L, Studer A. Vascularised corticoperiosteal grafts from the medial femoral condyle for difficult non-unions of the upper limb. J Hand Surg Eur. 2007;32(2):135–42.
115. Abdeen A, Hoang BH, Athanasian EA, Morris CD, Boland PJ, Healey JH. Allograft-prosthesis composite reconstruction of the proximal part of the humerus: functional outcome and survivorship. J Bone Joint Surg Am. 2009;91(10):2406–15.
116. Morrey ME, Sanchez-Sotelo J, Abdel MP, Morrey BF. Allograft-prosthetic composite reconstruction for massive bone loss including catastrophic failure in total elbow arthroplasty. J Bone Joint Surg Am. 2013;95(12):1117–24.
117. Mayle RE Jr, Paprosky WG. Massive bone loss: allograft-prosthetic composites and beyond. J Bone Joint Surg Br. 2012;94(11 Suppl A):61–4.
118. Arguello AM, Houdek MT, Barlow JD. Management of proximal humeral oncologic lesions. Orthop Clin North Am. 2023;54(1):89–100.
119. Goulding KA, Schwartz A, Hattrup SJ, Randall RL, Lee D, Rispoli DM, et al. Use of compressive osseointegration endoprostheses for massive bone loss from tumor and failed arthroplasty: a viable option in the upper extremity. Clin Orthop Relat Res. 2017;475(6):1702–11.
120. Funovics PT, Schuh R, Adams SB Jr, Sabeti-Aschraf M, Dominkus M, Kotz RI. Modular prosthetic reconstruction of major bone defects of the distal end of the humerus. J Bone Joint Surg Am. 2011;93(11):1064–74.
121. Kruckeberg BM, Lee DR, Barlow JD, Morrey ME, Rose PS, Sanchez-Sotelo J, et al. Total elbow arthroplasty for tumors of the distal humerus and elbow. J Surg Oncol. 2021;124(8):1508–14.
122. Akgul T, Sormaz IC, Aksoy M, Ucar A, Ozger H, Eralp L. Results and functional outcomes of en-bloc resection and vascular reconstruction in extremity musculoskeletal tumors. Acta Orthop Traumatol Turc. 2018;52(6):409–14.
123. Fuchs B, Davis AM, Wunder JS, Bell RS, Masri BA, Isler M, et al. Sciatic nerve resection in the thigh: a functional evaluation. Clin Orthop Relat Res. 2001;382:34–41.
124. Ogura K, Higashi T, Kawai A. Statistics of soft-tissue sarcoma in Japan: report from the Bone and Soft Tissue Tumor Registry in Japan. J Orthop Sci. 2017;22(4):755–64.
125. Martin E, Dullaart MJ, van de Sande MAJ, van Houdt WJ, Schellekens PPA, Coert JH. Resuscitating extremities after soft tissue sarcoma resections: are functional reconstructions an overlooked option in limb salvage? A systematic review. Eur J Surg Oncol. 2019;45(10):1762–9.
126. Forli A, Bouyer M, Aribert M, Curvale C, Delord M, Corcella D, et al. Upper limb nerve transfers: a review. Hand Surg Rehabil. 2017;36(3):151–72.
127. Mauch JT, Bae A, Shubinets V, Lin IC. A systematic review of sensory outcomes of digital nerve gap reconstruction with autograft, allograft, and conduit. Ann Plast Surg. 2019;82(4S Suppl 3):S247–55.
128. Radaelli S, Fiore M, Colombo C, Ford S, Palassini E, Sanfilippo R, et al. Vascular resection en-bloc with tumor removal and graft reconstruction is safe and effective in soft tissue sarcoma (STS) of the extremities and retroperitoneum. Surg Oncol. 2016;25(3):125–31.
129. Park D, Cho S, Han A, Choi C, Ahn S, Min SI, et al. Outcomes after arterial or venous reconstructions in limb salvage surgery for extremity soft tissue sarcoma. J Korean Med Sci. 2018;33(40):e265.

130. Kang J, Choi KW, Han A, Min S, Heo SH, Yang SS, et al. Venous reconstruction in extremity soft tissue sarcoma is not essential. Vasc Endovasc Surg. 2023;57(4):365–72.
131. Bielack SS, Kempf-Bielack B, Delling G, Exner GU, Flege S, Helmke K, et al. Prognostic factors in high-grade osteosarcoma of the extremities or trunk: an analysis of 1,702 patients treated on neoadjuvant cooperative osteosarcoma study group protocols. J Clin Oncol. 2002;20(3):776–90.
132. Goorin AM, Schwartzentruber DJ, Devidas M, Gebhardt MC, Ayala AG, Harris MB, et al. Presurgical chemotherapy compared with immediate surgery and adjuvant chemotherapy for nonmetastatic osteosarcoma: Pediatric Oncology Group Study POG-8651. J Clin Oncol. 2003;21(8):1574–80.
133. Beasley RW. Surgery of hand and finger amputations. Orthop Clin North Am. 1981;12(4):763–803.
134. Alexander JH, Jordan SW, West JM, Compston A, Fugitt J, Bowen JB, et al. Targeted muscle reinnervation in oncologic amputees: early experience of a novel institutional protocol. J Surg Oncol. 2019;120(3):348–58.
135. Sim FH, Pritchard DJ, Ivins JC. Forequarter amputation. Orthop Clin North Am. 1977;8(4):921–31.
136. Qadir R, Sidhu S, Romine L, Meyer MS, Duncan SF. Interscapulothoracic (forequarter) amputation for malignant tumors involving the upper extremity: surgical technique and case series. J Shoulder Elb Surg. 2014;23(6):e127–33.
137. Bhagia SM, Elek EM, Grimer RJ, Carter SR, Tillman RM. Forequarter amputation for high-grade malignant tumours of the shoulder girdle. J Bone Joint Surg Br. 1997;79(6):924–6.
138. Puhaindran ME, Chou J, Forsberg JA, Athanasian EA. Major upper-limb amputations for malignant tumors. J Hand Surg Am. 2012;37(6):1235–41.
139. Williard WC, Collin C, Casper ES, Hajdu SI, Brennan MF. The changing role of amputation for soft tissue sarcoma of the extremity in adults. Surg Gynecol Obstet. 1992;175(5):389–96.
140. Wittig JC, Bickels J, Kollender Y, Kellar-Graney KL, Meller I, Malawer MM. Palliative forequarter amputation for metastatic carcinoma to the shoulder girdle region: indications, preoperative evaluation, surgical technique, and results. J Surg Oncol. 2001;77(2):105–13; discussion 14.
141. Fanous N, Didolkar MS, Holyoke ED, Elias EG. Evaluation of forequarter amputation in malignant diseases. Surg Gynecol Obstet. 1976;142(3):381–4.
142. Rickelt J, Hoekstra H, van Coevorden F, de Vreeze R, Verhoef C, van Geel AN. Forequarter amputation for malignancy. Br J Surg. 2009;96(7):792–8.
143. Kreutz-Rodrigues L, Mohan AT, Moran SL, Carlsen BT, Mardini S, Houdek MT, et al. Extremity free fillet flap for reconstruction of massive oncologic resection-surgical technique and outcomes. J Surg Oncol. 2020;121(3):465–73.
144. Puhaindran ME, Healey JH, Athanasian EA. Single ray amputation for tumors of the hand. Clin Orthop Relat Res. 2010;468(5):1390–5.
145. Kuntscher MV, Erdmann D, Homann HH, Steinau HU, Levin SL, Germann G. The concept of fillet flaps: classification, indications, and analysis of their clinical value. Plast Reconstr Surg. 2001;108(4):885–96.
146. Puhaindran ME, Athanasian EA. Double ray amputation for tumors of the hand. Clin Orthop Relat Res. 2010;468(11):2976–9.
147. Puhaindran ME, Steensma MR, Athanasian EA. Partial hand preservation for large soft tissue sarcomas of the hand. J Hand Surg Am. 2010;35(2):291–5.

Principles of Lower Extremity Reconstruction Following Soft Tissue Sarcoma Resection

21

Gavin L. Mills and Cory G. Couch

21.1 Introduction

The lower extremity is the most common location of soft tissue sarcoma (STS) [1, 2]. Unlike the upper extremity, there is often more local soft tissue available for soft tissue reconstruction after tumor resection. Similarly, due to the advent of modern radiation therapy techniques (see Chap. 13), preoperative radiation allows the surgical team to perform "close margin" resection utilizing fascial margins which often renders neurovascular structures viable [3]. Additionally, radical excision with amputation has not shown to improve overall survival [4]. As such, limb salvage is often attainable following STS excision and has become the primary treatment for extremity STS [5–7].

As previously discussed, prioritizing the quality of the margins of the resection must be the primary goal of the operation. Many authors suggest that the resection phase of the operation should be an independent procedure and separate from the reconstruction phase, going so far as to advocate for using separate surgical teams to avoid preserving tissue to facilitate reconstruction and potentially compromising oncologic margins. Any theorized preservation of function pales in comparison to the detriment of local recurrence. Consequently, there are often significant tissue defects remaining after the resection. Successful soft tissue and bone reconstruction requires a multidisciplinary team and a tailored approach to each patient. Not infrequently, multiple surgical teams work either together or in sequence to optimize surgical outcomes. Similar to the upper extremity, the postradiation complications with regards to wound healing is not insignificant [8–10]. As highlighted in Chap. 21, an *oncoplastics* approach should be utilized for locally advanced lower extremity STS resection and reconstruction whereby negative margin surgery and postoperative function are both prioritized.

In most cases, the treatment philosophy is determined by the treatment team and the patient with either intent to cure or a palliative purpose. Limb salvage and complex lower extremity reconstruction carry a significant complication profile and, in some cases, limited functional outcomes. Especially in cases of large, locally advanced tumors invading critical neurovascular structures, a thorough discussion of limb salvage must include amputation. Depending on the level of proposed amputation, there are significant benefits to limb ablative surgery with regards to decreased rates of local recurrence, improved function, and reoperation rates [11, 12]. The importance of shared decision-making as well as a thorough discussion of the risks and proposed benefits of limb reconstruction with the patient cannot be overstated. The purpose of this chapter is to review the options for soft tissue and bone reconstruction as well as provide an overview of commonly used endoprostheses for joint reconstruction after lower extremity STS excision.

21.2 Surgical Planning and Timing

Utilizing a multidisciplinary team provides the optimal comprehensive care for the patient with soft tissue sarcoma of the lower extremity. The timing of the surgical resection should be discussed among the subspecialists caring for the patient commonly including medical oncology, radiation oncology, and plastic surgery. Optimal surgical timing is typically 3–5 weeks following completion neoadjuvant radiation therapy, when a preoperative radiation protocol is utilized [13]. Working within this window is usually late enough to allow for radiation dermatitis to resolve but prior to extensive tissue fibrosis rending dissection of tissue planes more difficult. Additionally, cytotoxic chemotherapy agents must be held

G. L. Mills (✉)
Department of Orthopaedic Surgery, Brooke Army Medical Center, Fort Sam Houston, TX, USA

Department of Orthopedic Surgery, Mayo Clinic, Rochester, MN, USA
e-mail: mills.gavin@mayo.edu

C. G. Couch
Department of Orthopedic Surgery, Mayo Clinic, Rochester, MN, USA
e-mail: couch.cory@mayo.edu

H. Özger et al. (eds.), *Diagnosis and Treatment of Soft Tissue Tumors*, https://doi.org/10.1007/978-3-031-77061-6_21

preoperatively and not restarted until the wound has appropriately healed.

Postoperative or adjuvant radiation is preferred by some multidisciplinary teams. There are both risks and benefits of adjuvant versus neoadjuvant radiotherapy. An extensive review of these issues is beyond the scope of this chapter, but in brief summation, preoperative/neoadjuvant radiotherapy allows for a smaller field and lower dose of radiation treatment, but a higher wound healing complication rate, whereas postoperative/adjuvant radiation requires a larger field and dosage leading too more extensive fibrosis, but with less wound healing complications.

A standard preoperative workup should be completed to include common blood laboratories. Severely neutropenic patients undergoing cytotoxic chemotherapy may benefit from surgical delay to avoid unnecessarily elevated risk of perioperative infection. In discussion with the plastic surgery team, the likelihood of using skin graft, locoregional, or free tissue transfer should be noted to appropriately position the patient in the operating room. A preoperative CT-angiogram is useful to evaluate vasculature of donor as well as recipient vessels if a free flap is being considered. In most cases, bone and soft tissue reconstruction is performed at the time of tumor excision once negative margins have been confirmed. Immediate reconstruction is associated with less morbidity and a lower risk of wound infection and dehiscence compared with delayed reconstruction [14]. In contrast, some multidisciplinary teams prefer a delayed reconstruction method. The main reason for delayed reconstruction is unknown margin status or potentially infected wound bed from a fungating or hemorrhagic STS. When this scenario arises, which is fortunately uncommon, placement of a negative pressure wound dressing may be applied and a return to the operating room once final margin evaluation has been completed and an appropriate plan has been finalized.

21.3 Soft Tissue Reconstruction

Working closely with a plastic surgery team in the surgical management of lower extremity STS has been shown to decrease rates of failed limb salvage as well as postoperative infections [15]. Even in the setting of preoperative radiation treatment, soft tissue reconstruction can be performed without higher rates of wound complications [16]. In our practice, we use a stepwise algorithm published by Elswick et al., attempting to utilize the simplest reconstructive option possible and elevating to more complex options depending on the wound or expected loss of limb function following tumor extirpation [17]. Familiarity with the commonly used soft tissue flaps and reconstruction techniques used in the lower extremity enables the surgical team to tailor the methods of soft tissue reconstruction to the specific dimensions of the defect.

21.3.1 Skin Grafting

In general, a well-vascularized wound bed can be covered with split thickness skin grafting (STSG) and negative pressure wound therapy. This can be done in radiated tissue as well with predictable wound healing [18]. The advantages of split thickness skin grafting are that it is fairly straightforward to perform, has minimal long-term morbidity, provides a wound bed that can be easily surveilled, and it can be excised in the setting of repeat wound exploration secondary to local recurrency at a later time without concern for violation of a flap pedicle. Because the healing and maturation of a STSG relies on inosculation and neovascularization, it is imperative that the underlying tissue be well-vascularized. Contraindications to STSG are defects containing exposed hardware, tendons, bone, or neurovascular structures.

21.3.2 Lymphatic Resection

Lymphatic resection and reconstructive methods are an often-overlooked portion of lower extremity STS excision. Lymphedema is a common and very disabling long-term complication seen in patients with impaired lymphatic drainage of a limb. In a series by Wu et al., 12% of patients developed lymphedema following STS resection of the lower extremity [19]. Risk factors included resections involving the medial thigh, arterial resection or reconstruction, cardiac disease and radiation therapy [19–22]. Though maintaining a wide margin is critically important, care should be taken to avoid resecting lymphatics unnecessarily, especially in patients at higher risk of developing lymphedema. Further, these higher risk patients should be monitored closely for the development of lymphedema so that treatment can be initiated. Patients can be provided customized compression garments or compression wraps and educated on measures to mitigate symptoms. Additionally, certain centers have utilized lymphovenous anastomosis or lymph node transplant to improve lymphedema in symptomatic patients [23, 24].

21.3.3 Flaps for Lower Limb Reconstruction

The reconstructive flap is chosen based on the location and size of the defect as well as the expected loss of function of the limb [25]. Additionally, ease of access and quality of donor tissue can play a factor in a patient who has been operated on multiple times which may limit tissue available for transfer. Depending on the size of the defect and the quality of remaining tissue, a locoregional flap or free flap may be utilized. In general, if healthy tissue is available, our preference is to use ipsilateral extremity for donor tissue for free flaps to minimize additional morbidity to another extremity.

Familiarity with a number of commonly used tissue flaps will enable surgical teams to modify the reconstructive approach to the location as well as the defect encountered.

21.3.3.1 Proximal and Middle Thigh

Due to the soft tissue redundancy of the proximal and middle thigh, locoregional flaps can frequently be used to cover a defect. Conversely, due to the large anatomic compartments and residual potential space left behind after STS excision, the thigh has the highest rate of postoperative complication [8, 9]. Careful attention should be made to obliterate the residual potential space to help decrease the risk of developing postoperative seroma and wound infection. Additionally, drains are used to help decompress the wound bed and avoid accumulating large fluid collections.

A pedicled rectus abdominus flap with a vertically or transversally oriented skin paddle can be used to cover a proximal thigh defected. Rotational muscle flaps to the region include the gracilis, rectus femoris, vastus lateralis, or sartorius muscles. An anterolateral thigh (ALT) flap is a fasciocutaneous flap that can be used to reliably cover defects on the medial and anterior proximal thigh. Posteriorly, the biceps femoris and gluteus muscles can be used.

Similarly, in the mid-thigh, many of the same muscle flaps can be utilized with the addition of the vastus medialis and adductor longus. This anatomic location is amenable to the use of keystone or perforator-pedicled propeller flaps as well to cover defects (Fig. 21.1). The biceps femoris and semimembranosus are useful to cover posterior soft tissue defects at this level.

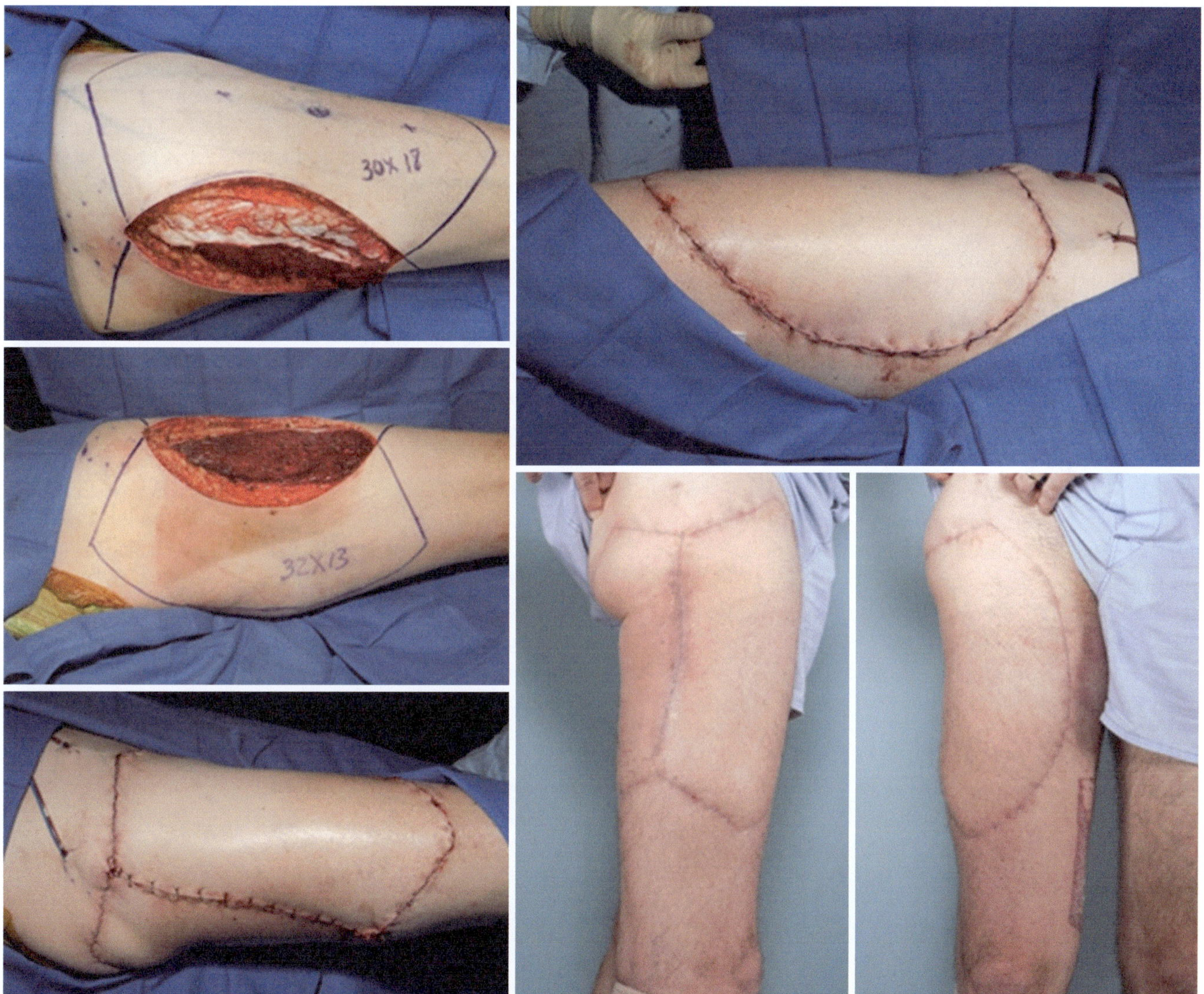

Fig. 21.1 Keystone flap multiperforator advancement

Free flaps to the thigh are used for large defects and those where significant potential space must be filled. The latissimus dorsi and rectus abdominus are frequently used as free flaps to this area and can be taken with a skin paddle. Additionally, the contralateral ALT and parascapular flaps are useful free fasciocutaneous flaps.

21.3.3.2 Distal Thigh and Knee

As the limb narrows in the distal thigh, there are less locoregional flap options to cover defects. The reverse ALT and medial or lateral gastrocnemius flaps are commonly used. When utilizing a reverse ALT flap, the retrograde flow of the lateral femoral circumflex artery and lateral superior geniculate artery must be confirmed [25]. The medial gastrocnemius muscle belly is more frequently used compared to the lateral because of the increased excursed available given the fibula is not blocking the path. Additional length can be gained by dis-originating the muscle from the posterior medial femoral condyle taking care to not over tension the medial sural artery pedicle. The maximum reach of a pedicled medial gastrocnemius flap is typically to the level of the proximal patella, and these flaps commonly require additional skin grafting as skin paddles are not readily transferred with them.

Free tissue flaps to the distal thigh and knee can be difficult to perform due to the limited availability of recipient vessels. Free ALT, rectus abdominis, and latissimus dorsi free flaps are all reasonable options. An arteriovenous loop can be constructed to anastomosis the free flap to if needed allowing the graft to be inset safely without tension and a reliable source of blood flow [25].

Functional muscle transfer or nerve reconstruction must be considered after extensive resections of the anterior thigh. Specifically, resections of the femoral triangle involving motor branches of the femoral nerve can denervate large portions of the intact remaining quadriceps significantly weakening the extensor mechanism of the knee. Cabled sural autografts are used for large defects. For smaller defects less than 5–8 mm, nerve conduits are used [26]. If three or more muscles of the quadriceps muscle complex are resected or devitalized, the strength of knee extension decreases by 55% [27]. In addition to the decreased range of motion, this becomes primarily disabling given the elevated risk of falling due to buckling of the knee. The latissimus dorsi based on the thoracodorsal neurovascular pedicle can be harvested as a free innervated flap with the necessary length as well as strength needed for a function muscle transfer. The contralateral rectus femoris with its innervated femoral nerve branch can be used as well; however, this will likely weaken the contralateral extremity (Fig. 21.2). The muscle flap can be anchored using bone tunnels or suture anchors [28]. The donor nerve is coapted to the remnant femoral nerve branches. This can be done using nerve cabled autograft if excess length is needed. Free functional muscle transfer has been shown to be quite effective; however, reinnervate occurs at a mean of 6 months postoperatively necessitating an prolonged rehabilitation course [29].

21.3.3.3 Lower Leg

As the lower limb further narrows distally, locoregional coverage options become more limited. The proximal third is commonly covered using the gastrocnemius muscle. The soleus is used to cover defects on the middle third of the tibia. Propeller flaps can be fashioned for fasciocutaneous flaps in this area as well. Due to the limited soft tissue of the distal third of the lower leg, a pedicle perforator flap or free flap are frequently required for myocutaneous coverage (Fig. 21.3). If tumor extirpation renders the ankle dorsiflexors incompetent, bracing may be necessary to help the patient overcome the foot drop.

21.3.3.4 Foot and Ankle

Compared to the resection of high-grade tumors of the thigh and lower leg, amputation is required more frequently in the treatment of STS of the foot or ankle due to the close anatomic association with critical neurovascular structures [30]. Additionally, due to the limited soft tissue available, large defects are almost exclusively managed with free tissue flaps. Unfortunately, flaps that replace the plantar glabrous skin have far worse weight bearing characteristics. Furthermore, it can be challenging to fit patients with bulky or edematous flaps with footwear. Amputation is an espe-

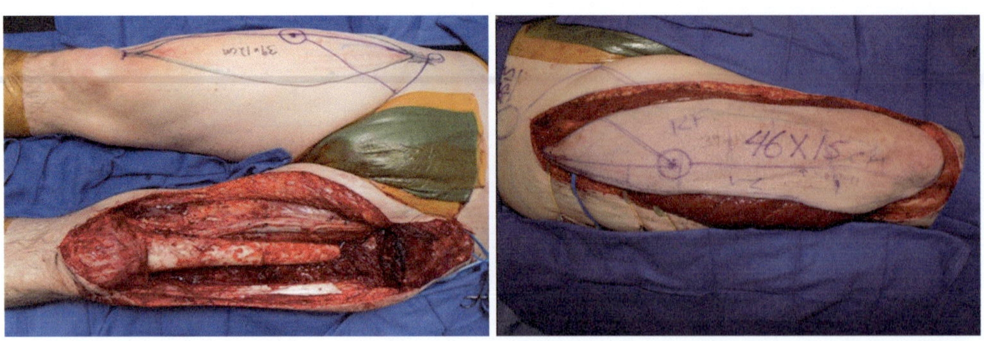

Fig. 21.2 (**a**) Left thigh soft tissue defect after STS resection. (**b**) Quadriceps reconstruction with functional innervated contralateral rectus

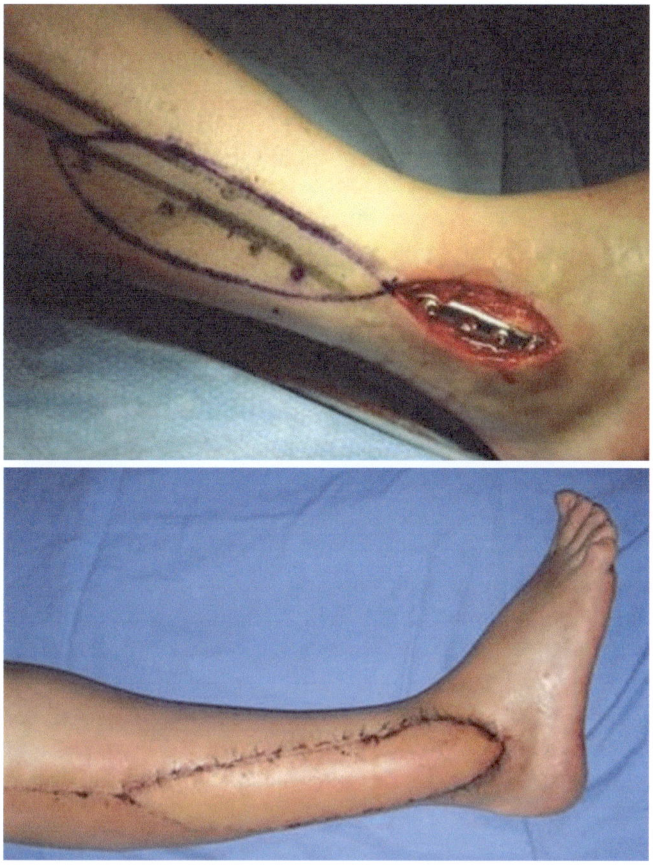

Fig. 21.3 Pedicle perforator flap

cially attractive option for patients left with weight bearing soft tissue defects given the accelerated rehabilitation available to amputees. As discussed later, in otherwise healthy patients, below knee amputees achieve excellent postoperative function. If needed, free flaps such as ALT, latissimus and gracilis can be used to cover both weight bearing and dorsal surface of the foot [31].

A successful outcome can be achieved by utilizing an *oncoplastics* approach coupled with shared decision making with the patient with regards to expected postoperative function and complication profile of the various treatment options for soft tissue reconstruction following STS excision.

21.4 Bone and Joint Reconstruction

Soft tissue sarcoma can arise adjacent to the osseous structures of the lower extremity. A detailed physical examination of the affected limb and axial imaging in the form of a contrast enhanced MRI aid in preoperative decision making of potential bone and joint resection in conjunction with sarcoma resection [32]. Imaging features of bone involvement include bone marrow edema or signal change and cortical erosive changes. MRI can also help practitioners determine the presence of intraarticular invasion by the soft tissue sarcoma [33]. Computed tomography of the concerning area can provide additional fine detail as to cortical involvement. Additional evaluation of osseous involvement occurs intraoperatively, as the limb and tumor are manipulated and mobilized. In the setting of pre- and postoperative radiation therapy, if the bone can be rotated without movement of the tumor, or the tumor rolled independently of the bone, then the tumor is not invading bone, and a periosteal margin can typically be utilized [32]. If the tumor and bone move as one unit, the bone and/or joint should be resected en bloc with the soft tissue component.

Preoperative planning of the extent of bone and joint resection and reconstruction is key to a successful reconstruction when limb salvage is pursued. Bone and joint reconstruction is an extensive topic and varies based on the amount of resection necessary for a negative margin. Summaries of each of the key reconstructive options are discussed in the sections below.

Use of autograft, allograft bone, and bone substitutes can be used in a variety of combinations in instances of bone reconstruction after sarcoma resection. When bone defects have surrounding well vascularized soft tissues and bone, and are relatively small, under 5 cm, cancellous nonvascularized bone grafting or acute limb shortening combined with robust osteosynthesis methods are viable reconstructive options. For biologic reconstruction of larger defects and in previously radiated bone, vascularized autograft is preferred, with the vascularized free fibula as the workhorse bone flap for large intercalary reconstructions [34–41]. Vascularized bone flaps are ideal in biologic reconstruction as they reduce infection risk, fracture risk, allow for bone remodeling under Wolff's law, and can heal in a previously radiated field [42, 43].

21.4.1 Endoprosthetic Reconstruction

Endoprosthetic reconstruction is sought when a joint of the lower extremity is resected due to STS involvement. Fortunately, there are extensive reconstruction options available for the hip, knee and lower leg. The most common reconstruction options utilized currently are an endoprosthesis, and less commonly in 2023 an allograft prosthetic composite (APC).

21.4.2 Periacetabular Reconstruction

After an extraarticular resection of the hip joint, the surgeon is faced with complex acetabular reconstruction if this is to be attempted. When reconstruction is sought, two separate reconstruction methods are frequently utilized by our institution: custom acetabular implants (custom triflange or custom hemi-pelvis) and cup-cage +/− augment reconstruction. Both techniques have been utilized successfully for many patients, each with their own benefits and shortcomings [44]. These techniques can be utilized in conjunction with custom cutting guides manufacture either by in-hospital 3D printing or outsourced to industry partners or, at some centers, with intraoperative navigation (Fig. 21.4). Custom acetabular implant utilization has the added benefit of less intraoperative variability. Once the resection has been performed and the pelvic bone cuts match the implant accurately, the implant can be fastened to the pelvis in an expeditious manner. Additionally, the custom implants often come with preplanned screw lengths and trajectories to assist surgeons in accurate screw length placement. The three main downsides to this approach are significant planning and lead time to manufacture the implants, sometimes up to 3 months or more depending on demand, cost of the implant—which is higher, and lack of intraoperative flexibility. The other preferred surgical reconstructive approach initially designed and extensively utilized at our institution is the use of the cup-cage reconstruction. This technique utilizes readily available off the shelf revision highly porous acetabular components, elliptical cups and highly porous augments depending on the defect shape and size. In addition, an antiprotrusio cage is applied to the concave surface of the acetabular component with a flange spanning to the ilium (half cup-cage) and sometimes to the ischium as well (cup-cage).

21.4.3 Proximal Femur

Proximal femoral replacement (PFR) is utilized when extra-articular resection of the hip is performed, or the resection necessitates the excision of the soft tissue attachments of the proximal femur including the greater trochanter and lesser trochanter. One of the most challenging aspects of the proximal femoral replacement is reconstruction of the hip abductors. Failure to repair the hip abductors results in a Trendelenburg gait, increases the rate of dislocation, and can lead to hip pain [45]. The loss of the gluteus maximus insertion leads to weakness in hip extension and difficulty getting up from seated position. Additionally, the loss of the insertion of the iliopsoas on the lesser trochanter leads to weakness in hip flexion. There are a number of configurations of either suture holes or highly porous ingrowth surfaces to enhance strength and stability of the prosthesis [46]. Some implants offer the ability to fix the greater trochanter directly to the implant. In an effort to preserve acetabular bone stock in younger patients and to decrease the risk of dislocation, bipolar hemiarthroplasty components are used if an acetabular resection is not needed for oncologic margins. This is also used an elderly patient who are not expected to live long enough damage the acetabulum. Stability can be enhanced by utilizing larger head sizes, using a constrained liner or perform trochanteric slide to further tension the abductors. If the capsule is preserved, it can be closed around the femoral neck using a purse string suture [47]. Fortunately, the risk of conversion from bipolar to subsequent total hip arthroplasty is low [48].

21.4.4 Distal Femur

A distal femoral replacement (DFR) is utilized when the distal femur has osseous invasion of the lesions requiring excision rendering the soft tissue attachments nonfunctional. The DFR provides a durable functional knee articulation. Compared to earlier iterations, moderate designs utilize a rotating hinge platform help decrease constraint across the

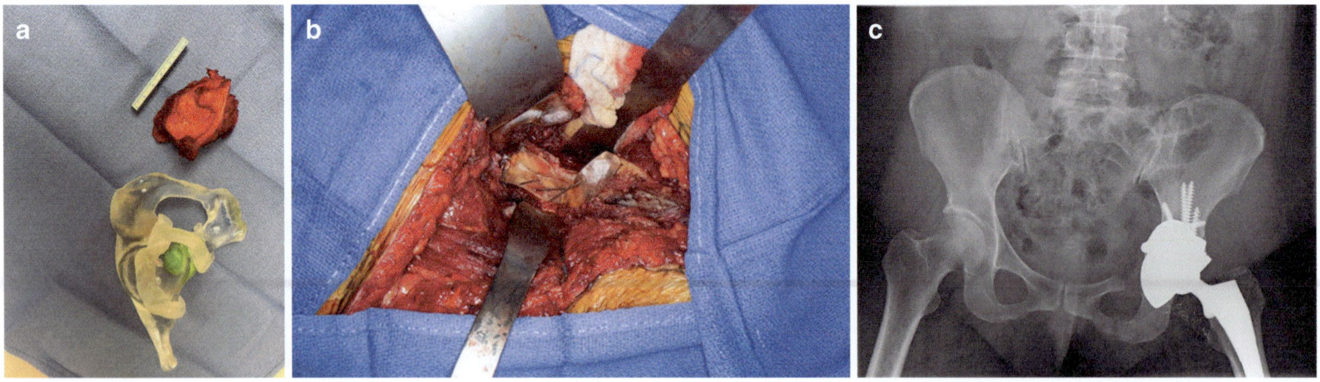

Fig. 21.4 (**a**) 3D-printed custom cutting guide adjacent to 3D model of pelvis and resected specimen. (**b**) 3D-printed custom cutting guide pinned in place for peri-acetabular resection. (**c**) Postoperative radiographs after peri-acetabular resection and reconstruction using total hip arthroplasty with highly porous acetabular cup and augment

mechanical articulation which has improved implant longevity [49]. The length of bone resection and rotation marked prior to making the femoral osteotomy. It can be easy to overstuff the joint given that the collaterals have been resected.

21.4.5 Proximal Tibia

The primary challenge to reconstruction of the proximal tibia with endoprosthesis is securing the extensor mechanism in a reliable manner. Both healing of the extensor mechanism as well as residual extensor lag can be difficult to counter. At our institution, in addition to using suture holes in the prosthesis, the implant is wrapped with nonabsorbable mesh to further augment soft tissue ingrowth. We typically utilize a medial gastrocnemius flap to ensure adequate soft tissue coverage of the implant.

21.4.6 Prophylactic Fixation in Soft Tissue Sarcoma

The periosteum can be used as a deep fascial margin when high-grade tumors are treated with preoperative radiation therapy so long as there is not MRI evidence of intra-osseus extension of the tumor [3]. If a large portion of the periosteum is excised with the tumor, there is concern for postoperative fracture [50]. Risk factors for fracture include female patients over 55 years old who had >60 Gy of radiation, preoperative chemotherapy and extensive periosteal stripping in the anterior compartment of the thigh on the tension side of the femur [50, 51]. These higher risk patients likely benefit from prophylactic fixation commonly in the form of intramedullary nail fixation. This can be done immediately after the primary resection or in a staged fashion to allow for the patient to recover from the initial resection as well as repositioning if needed for efficient placement of intramedullary nail. Some advocate for the use of carbon fiber/polyether ether ketone (PEEK) implants if postoperative radiation is needed (Fig. 21.5). Compared to titanium, there is less radiation dose attenuation as well as decreased artifact on pretreatment template CT scans likely creating more precise radiation delivery. Additionally, if an MRI surveillance protocol is utilized, carbon fiber/PEEK implants significantly decrease artifact on MRI (Fig. 21.5) [52]. Regardless of the type of implant used, it is important to ensure high-risk patients undergo prophylactic fixation to avoid the tremendous morbidity associated with pathologic fracture in previously radiated bone.

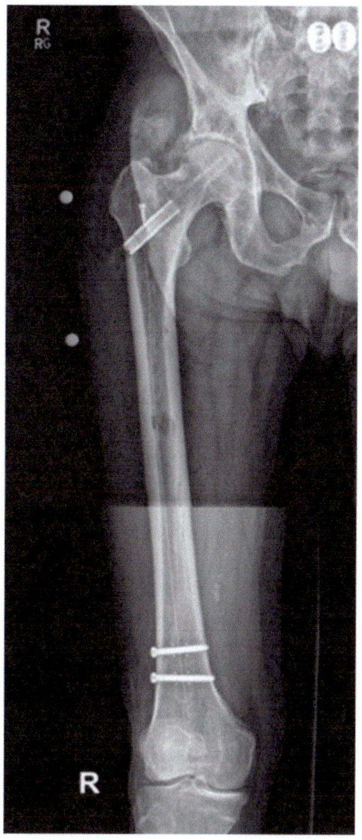

Fig. 21.5 Carbon fiber/PEEK cephalomedullary nail used in this application for prophylactic fixation of impending pathologic fracture in the setting of multiple myeloma

21.5 Amputation

As previously noted, adjuvant radiation therapy and wide local excision utilizing modern limb salvage techniques has replaced amputation as the primary treatment of extremity soft tissue sarcoma. Though local recurrence is decrease with amputation, overall survival is unchanged when compared to limb salvage [5–7]. Unfortunately, there are scenarios where amputation is appropriate and may be preferred by the patient over limb salvage if they are well-informed of the likely outcomes of both courses of treatment. As stated by Barla et al., "Amputation must not be considered as a failure, but a deliberate choice due to the functional impact of complications that occur after limb-salvage" [53]. A balanced approach to even the most sophisticated limb salvage treatment plans must contain an honest appraisal of the patient's reasonable oncologic prognosis and functional goals and identification of the point at which these are best met with limb ablative treatment. A thorough understanding of commonly used lower extremity amputations as well as modern techniques used to optimize their function will enable a more balanced approach to limb salvage.

Targeted muscle reinnervation (TMR) has been used for prophylaxis as well the treatment of painful neuromas and phantom limb pain. Symptomatic neuroma and phantom limb pain significantly impacts the quality of life of amputees [54]. TMR is a surgical technique utilizing the transfer of peripheral nerves to existing motor nerves in target muscles with the intent to restore physiological continuity of residual nerves to decreased neuroma formation. TMR was developed as a method to power myoelectronic prostheses. Serendipitously, patients who underwent TMR were found to have decreased rates of phantom limb pain and neuroma formation [55, 56]. In the setting of curative primary STS resection, we offer most patients TMR either at the time of resection or in a staged manner shortly thereafter.

21.5.1 External Hemipelvectomy and Hindquarter Amputation

Pelvic soft tissue sarcoma is associated with poor overall survival and often requires hemipelvectomy to achieve negative margins [57]. Additionally, treatment of these proximal tumors poses a number of technical challenges given the complex anatomy and proximity to critical neurovascular structures and is associated with significant morbidity and loss of function for the patient. Limb salvage can be pursued utilizing in internal hemipelvectomy. Indications for internal hemipelvectomy include the safe preservation of two of the three following pelvic structures: acetabulum, femoral neurovascular bundle, and sciatic nerve [58]. An external hemipelvectomy is more commonly used in the setting of local recurrence or failed limb salvage when adequate margins are too unpredictable to obtain when preserving critical neurovascular structures [30]. Though challenging, fitting an external hemipelvectomy with a prosthesis is possible to aid in ambulation [59]. Regardless the course of treatment, understanding the complication profile while prioritizing oncologic margins aids in clinic decision making when addressing pelvic soft tissue sarcomas.

21.5.2 Above Knee Amputation

Transfemoral amputation results in a residual limb that is significantly more functional than hip disarticulation or hemipelvectomy given the preservation of the hip joint as well as improvement in prosthetic fitting and sitting balance [60]. Above knee amputation function is improved with longer residual limbs especially if the thigh adductors can be preserved and secured with a myodesis to the residual femur creating a more dynamic muscle balance between adductors and hip abductors/flexors and more efficient ambulation [61]. Additionally, an adductor myodesis can aid in prosthetic fitting as it provides more durable soft tissue envelop over the osteotomy and can help maintain muscle girth by engaging the adductors in the gate cycle. In many countries, there are now transcutaneous osseointegrated (OI) devices available for the use in AKA that shows promise in further improving the function of patient with AKA. It removes the soft tissue-prosthesis interface as well as the frequent pressure injuries that it may cause [62]. OI is particularly advantageous in higher functioning patients with ultra-short residual femurs.

21.5.3 Below Knee Amputation

Amputees in whom the knee articulation is preserved typically achieve a significantly higher level of function relative to AKA. Additionally, due to the more uniform soft tissue envelope, below knee amputations (BKA) are usually easier to fit with a prosthesis. Patients with BKA also use less energy to ambulate when compared to AKA [63]. TMR is quite advantageous in these patients given the high level of function they can achieve with modern prostheses. Pragmatically, most use a length of 10–15 cm distal to the tibial tubercle to perform the osteotomy. This ensures adequate ground clearance with moderate prostheses as well as a long enough lever arm to facilitate prosthetic fitting and the generation of torque through the prosthesis. Additionally, the soft tissue envelope narrows distally about the tibia leading to a less robust soft tissue envelope available to cover the weight bearing portion of the residual limb. Fortunately, most patients achieve a high level of function following BKA so long as the wound heals adequately and they do not develop significant neuroma or phantom limb pain [64].

21.5.4 Foot and Ankle Amputations

Soft tissue sarcoma of the foot and ankle can be challenging to treat given that the anatomic compartments are closely associated with critical neurovascular structures. Achieving a wide margin in high-grade lesions is quite difficult without amputation. STS of the foot and ankle represent only 5% of extremity soft tissue sarcoma which likely leads to misdiagnosis as well as unplanned excision [65]. In contrast to unplanned STS excision in most anatomic locations, when this occurs in the foot and ankle, not only does the rate of amputation and the need for tissue flap increase, so does mortality [66]. More common diagnoses can be confused with high-grade malignancies: osteosarcoma for stress fracture, plantar sarcoma for fibromatosis, and dorsal synovial sarcoma for ganglion [67, 68]. In younger, higher functioning patients, a BKA is often preferred over hindfoot amputations due to the higher level of function achieved in a well-fit BKA prosthesis. However, in older, lower demand individuals, more distal amputations are reasonable when the heel pad or weight bearing plantar skin can be preserved.

Any partial foot amputation should be accompanied by a gastrocnemius recession or Achilles tendon lengthening to ensure the resting position of the ankle is not in equinus, thereby increasing the risk of pressure injury or delayed wound healing. In transmetatarsal amputations in younger, higher-level patients, the residual forefoot should be balance as well utilizing tendon transfers if needed. One option is to use a tenodesis of the extensor digitorum longus into the dorsum of the fourth metatarsal base and tenodesis of the flexor hallucis longus tendon into the base of the first metatarsal [69]. Amputation through the midfoot, or Lisfranc amputation, is prone to equinovarus deformity due to unopposed pull of the tibialis posterior and gastrocnemius-soleus complex. This can be countered by maintaining the insertion of the peroneus brevis as well as an Achilles tendon lengthening. A hindfoot amputation, or a Chopart amputation, is taken through the talonavicular and calcaneocuboid joints. This level of amputation is especially prone to equinus deformity. This can be countered by transfer of the tibialis anterior to the talar neck as well as an Achilles tendon lengthening. Ankle disarticulation, or Syme amputation, requires a viable, stable heel pad to be a durable weight-bearing surface for the patient. This level of amputation has the added advantage of avoiding hindfoot deformity and the subsequent pressure injuries that may develop. Additionally, in elderly patients, this obviates the need for an end bearing prosthesis in most cases and provides the proprioception inherent to native weight-bearing tissue. In contrast, the significant disadvantage of amputations distal to a BKA for higher functioning patients is the inability to utilize modern dynamic prostheses inhibiting the patient's ability to dissipate force when attempting to run [70]. Additionally, energy consumption is usually higher for partial foot amputations when compared to below-knee amputation [63].

Ultimately, educating the patient on the expected functional outcomes and postoperative wound complications is important in shared decision-making when determining the level of amputation in the lower leg. There are several durable options for foot and ankle amputations as long as care is taken avoid postoperative deformity. Fortunately, with regards to high-grade malignancy of the foot and ankle, a BKA has the added benefit of providing a truly radical margin avoiding the tendency to compromise margin status in an effort to preserve critical structures.

21.6 Conclusion

There are a number of durable, long-term reconstructive options for patients with lower extremity soft tissue sarcoma even when relying on limb ablative surgery to ensure the quality of oncologic margins. A multidisciplinary approach to soft tissue and bony reconstruction of the lower extremity will optimize both oncologic and functional outcomes for patients with lower extremity soft tissue sarcoma.

Conflicts of Interest No conflicts of interest are declared by any author on this study.

Funding No disclosures of funding were received for this work from NIH, Wellcome Trust, or HHMI.

References

1. Baldini EH, Lapidus MR, Wang Q, Manola J, Orgill DP, Pomahac B, et al. Predictors for major wound complications following preoperative radiotherapy and surgery for soft-tissue sarcoma of the extremities and trunk: importance of tumor proximity to skin surface. Ann Surg Oncol. 2013;20(5):1494–9.
2. Lahat G, Lazar A, Lev D. Sarcoma epidemiology and etiology: potential environmental and genetic factors. Surg Clin North Am. 2008;88(3):451–81. v
3. Dagan R, Indelicato DJ, McGee L, Morris CG, Kirwan JM, Knapik J, et al. The significance of a marginal excision after preoperative radiation therapy for soft tissue sarcoma of the extremity. Cancer. 2012;118(12):3199–207.
4. Shiu MH, Castro EB, Hajdu SI, Fortner JG. Surgical treatment of 297 soft tissue sarcomas of the lower extremity. Ann Surg. 1975;182(5):597–602.
5. Ferrone ML, Raut CP. Modern surgical therapy: limb salvage and the role of amputation for extremity soft-tissue sarcomas. Surg Oncol Clin N Am. 2012;21(2):201–13.
6. Rosenberg SA, Tepper J, Glatstein E, Costa J, Baker A, Brennan M, et al. The treatment of soft-tissue sarcomas of the extremities: prospective randomized evaluations of (1) limb-sparing surgery plus radiation therapy compared with amputation and (2) the role of adjuvant chemotherapy. Ann Surg. 1982;196(3):305–15.
7. Yang JC, Chang AE, Baker AR, Sindelar WF, Danforth DN, Topalian SL, et al. Randomized prospective study of the benefit of adjuvant radiation therapy in the treatment of soft tissue sarcomas of the extremity. J Clin Oncol. 1998;16(1):197–203.
8. Gerrand CH, Wunder JS, Kandel RA, O'Sullivan B, Catton CN, Bell RS, et al. The influence of anatomic location on functional outcome in lower-extremity soft-tissue sarcoma. Ann Surg Oncol. 2004;11(5):476–82.
9. Tseng JF, Ballo MT, Langstein HN, Wayne JD, Cormier JN, Hunt KK, et al. The effect of preoperative radiotherapy and reconstructive surgery on wound complications after resection of extremity soft-tissue sarcomas. Ann Surg Oncol. 2006;13(9):1209–15.

10. O'Sullivan B, Davis AM, Turcotte R, Bell R, Catton C, Chabot P, et al. Preoperative versus postoperative radiotherapy in soft-tissue sarcoma of the limbs: a randomised trial. Lancet. 2002;359(9325):2235–41.
11. Allami M, Yavari A, Karimi A, Masoumi M, Soroush M, Faraji E. Health-related quality of life and the ability to perform activities of daily living: a cross-sectional study on 1079 war veterans with ankle-foot disorders. Mil Med Res. 2017;4(1):37.
12. Jauregui JJ, Nadarajah V, Munn J, Pivec R, Kapadia BH, Lerman DM, et al. Limb salvage versus amputation in conventional appendicular osteosarcoma: a systematic review. Indian J Surg Oncol. 2018;9(2):232–40.
13. Griffin AM, Dickie CI, Catton CN, Chung PW, Ferguson PC, Wunder JS, et al. The influence of time interval between preoperative radiation and surgical resection on the development of wound healing complications in extremity soft tissue sarcoma. Ann Surg Oncol. 2015;22(9):2824–30.
14. Sanniec KJ, Velazco CS, Bryant LA, Zhang N, Casey WJ III, Mahabir RC, et al. Immediate versus delayed sarcoma reconstruction: impact on outcomes. Sarcoma. 2016;2016:7972318.
15. Agrawal N, Wan D, Bryan Z, Boehmler J, Miller M, Tiwari P. Outcomes analysis of the role of plastic surgery in extremity sarcoma treatment. J Reconstr Microsurg. 2013;29(2):107–11.
16. Chao AH, Chang DW, Shuaib SW, Hanasono MM. The effect of neoadjuvant versus adjuvant irradiation on microvascular free flap reconstruction in sarcoma patients. Plast Reconstr Surg. 2012;129(3):675–82.
17. Elswick SM, Wu P, Arkhavan AA, Molinar VE, Mohan AT, Sim FH, et al. A reconstructive algorithm after thigh soft tissue sarcoma resection including predictors of free flap reconstruction(☆). J Plast Reconstr Aesthet Surg. 2019;72(8):1304–15.
18. Senchenkov A, Petty PM, Knoetgen J 3rd, Moran SL, Johnson CH, Clay RP. Outcomes of skin graft reconstructions with the use of vacuum assisted closure (VAC(R)) dressing for irradiated extremity sarcoma defects. World J Surg Oncol. 2007;5:138.
19. Wu P, Elswick SM, Arkhavan A, Molinar VE, Mohan AT, Curiel D, et al. Risk factors for lymphedema after thigh sarcoma resection and reconstruction. Plast Reconstr Surg Glob Open. 2020;8(7):e2912.
20. Cheville AL, McGarvey CL, Petrek JA, Russo SA, Thiadens SR, Taylor ME. The grading of lymphedema in oncology clinical trials. Semin Radiat Oncol. 2003;13(3):214–25.
21. Bedi M, King DM, Whitfield R, Hackbarth DA, Neilson JC, Charlson JA, et al. The effect of smoking and major vein resection on post-therapy lymphedema in soft tissue sarcomas treated with neoadjuvant radiation and limb-salvage surgery. Am J Clin Oncol. 2015;38(2):184–8.
22. Rimner A, Brennan MF, Zhang Z, Singer S, Alektiar KM. Influence of compartmental involvement on the patterns of morbidity in soft tissue sarcoma of the thigh. Cancer. 2009;115(1):149–57.
23. Verhey EM, Kandi LA, Lee YS, Morris BE, Casey WJ, Rebecca AM, et al. Outcomes of lymphovenous anastomosis for lower extremity lymphedema: a systematic review. Plast Reconstr Surg Glob Open. 2022;10(10):e4529.
24. Gould DJ, Mehrara BJ, Neligan P, Cheng MH, Patel KM. Lymph node transplantation for the treatment of lymphedema. J Surg Oncol. 2018;118(5):736–42.
25. Parikh RP, Sacks JM. Lower extremity reconstruction after soft tissue sarcoma resection. Clin Plast Surg. 2021;48(2):307–19.
26. Mauch JT, Bae A, Shubinets V, Lin IC. A systematic review of sensory outcomes of digital nerve gap reconstruction with autograft, allograft, and conduit. Ann Plast Surg. 2019;82(4S Suppl 3):S247–55.
27. Markhede G, Stener B. Function after removal of various hip and thigh muscles for extirpation of tumors. Acta Orthop Scand. 1981;52(4):373–95.
28. Garcia RM, Ruch DS. Free flap functional muscle transfers. Hand Clin. 2016;32(3):397–405.
29. Ihara K, Shigetomi M, Kawai S, Doi K, Yamamoto M. Functioning muscle transplantation after wide excision of sarcomas in the extremity. Clin Orthop Relat Res. 1999;(358):140–8.
30. Erstad DJ, Ready J, Abraham J, Ferrone ML, Bertagnolli MM, Baldini EH, et al. Amputation for extremity sarcoma: contemporary indications and outcomes. Ann Surg Oncol. 2018;25(2):394–403.
31. Franco MJ, Nicoson MC, Parikh RP, Tung TH. Lower extremity reconstruction with free gracilis flaps. J Reconstr Microsurg. 2017;33(3):218–24.
32. Ferguson PC, Griffin AM, O'Sullivan B, Catton CN, Davis AM, Murji A, et al. Bone invasion in extremity soft-tissue sarcoma: impact on disease outcomes. Cancer. 2006;106(12):2692–700.
33. Bui-Mansfield LT, O'Brien SD. Magnetic resonance appearance of intra-articular synovial sarcoma: case reports and review of the literature. J Comput Assist Tomogr. 2008;32(4):640–4.
34. Han CS, Wood MB, Bishop AT, Cooney WP 3rd. Vascularized bone transfer. J Bone Joint Surg Am. 1992;74(10):1441–9.
35. Wood MB. Free vascularized bone transfers for nonunions, segmental gaps, and following tumor resection. Orthopedics. 1986;9(6):810–6.
36. de Boer HH, Wood MB. Bone changes in the vascularised fibular graft. J Bone Joint Surg. 1989;71(3):374–8.
37. Taylor GI, Ham FJ. The free vascularized nerve graft. A further experimental and clinical application of microvascular techniques. Plast Reconstr Surg. 1976;57(4):413–26.
38. Malizos KN, Zalavras CG, Soucacos PN, Beris AE, Urbaniak JR. Free vascularized fibular grafts for reconstruction of skeletal defects. J Am Acad Orthop Surg. 2004;12(5):360–9.
39. Wood MB. Femoral reconstruction by vascularized bone transfer. Microsurgery. 1990;11(1):74–9.
40. Houdek MT, Wagner ER, Stans AA, Shin AY, Bishop AT, Sim FH, et al. What is the outcome of allograft and intramedullary free fibula (Capanna technique) in pediatric and adolescent patients with bone tumors? Clin Orthop Relat Res. 2016;474(3):660–8.
41. Arata MA, Wood MB, Cooney WP 3rd. Revascularized segmental diaphyseal bone transfers in the canine. An analysis of viability. J Reconstr Microsurg. 1984;1(1):11–9.
42. Houdek MT, Wagner ER, Bishop AT, Shin AY, Rose PS, Sim FH, et al. Complications and long-term outcomes of free fibula reconstruction following resection of a malignant tumor in the extremities. Plast Reconstr Surg. 2017;139(2):510e–9e.
43. Fujimaki A, Suda H. Experimental study and clinical observations on hypertrophy of vascularized bone grafts. Microsurgery. 1994;15(10):726–32.
44. Houdek MT, Abdel MP, Perry KI, Salduz A, Rose PS, Sim FH, et al. Outcome of patients treated with porous tantalum acetabular implants for neoplastic periacetabular lesions. J Am Acad Orthop Surg. 2020;28(6):256–62.
45. Lozano Calderon SA, Kuechle J, Raskin KA, Hornicek FJ. Lower extremity megaprostheses in orthopaedic oncology. J Am Acad Orthop Surg. 2018;26(12):e249–57.
46. Henderson ER, Marulanda GA, Cheong D, Temple HT, Letson GD. Hip abductor moment arm—a mathematical analysis for proximal femoral replacement. J Orthop Surg Res. 2011;6:6.
47. Jawad MU, Brien EW. Proximal femoral reconstruction with a constrained acetabulum in oncologic patients. Orthopedics. 2014;37(2):e187–93.
48. Houdek MT, Wyles CC, Labott JR, Rose PS, Taunton MJ, Sim FH. Durability of hemiarthroplasty for pathologic proximal femur fractures. J Arthroplast. 2017;32(12):3607–10.
49. Ogura K, Yakoub MA, Boland PJ, Healey JH. Finn/orthopaedic salvage system distal femoral rotating-hinge megaprostheses in oncologic patients: long-term complications, reoperations, and amputations. J Bone Joint Surg Am. 2021;103(8):705–14.

50. Lin PP, Schupak KD, Boland PJ, Brennan MF, Healey JH. Pathologic femoral fracture after periosteal excision and radiation for the treatment of soft tissue sarcoma. Cancer. 1998;82(12):2356–65.
51. Holt GE, Griffin AM, Pintilie M, Wunder JS, Catton C, O'Sullivan B, et al. Fractures following radiotherapy and limb-salvage surgery for lower extremity soft-tissue sarcomas. A comparison of high-dose and low-dose radiotherapy. J Bone Joint Surg Am. 2005;87(2):315–9.
52. Laux CJ, Villefort C, Ehrbar S, Wilke L, Guckenberger M, Muller DA. Carbon fiber/polyether ether ketone (CF/PEEK) implants allow for more effective radiation in long bones. Materials. 2020;13(7):1754.
53. Barla M, Gavanier B, Mangin M, Parot J, Bauer C, Mainard D. Is amputation a viable treatment option in lower extremity trauma? Orthop Traumatol Surg Res. 2017;103(6):971–5.
54. Bowen JB, Wee CE, Kalik J, Valerio IL. Targeted muscle reinnervation to improve pain, prosthetic tolerance, and bioprosthetic outcomes in the amputee. Adv Wound Care. 2017;6(8):261–7.
55. Souza JM, Cheesborough JE, Ko JH, Cho MS, Kuiken TA, Dumanian GA. Targeted muscle reinnervation: a novel approach to postamputation neuroma pain. Clin Orthop Relat Res. 2014;472(10):2984–90.
56. Daugherty THF, Parikh R, Mailey BA, Felder JM, Bueno RA Jr. Surgical technique for below-knee amputation with concurrent targeted muscle reinnervation. Plast Reconstr Surg Glob Open. 2020;8(7):e2990.
57. Apffelstaedt JP, Zhang PJ, Driscoll DL, Karakousis CP. Various types of hemipelvectomy for soft tissue sarcomas: complications, survival and prognostic factors. Surg Oncol. 1995;4(4):217–22.
58. Sherman CE, O'Connor MI, Sim FH. Survival, local recurrence, and function after pelvic limb salvage at 23 to 38 years of followup. Clin Orthop Relat Res. 2012;470(3):712–27.
59. Houdek MT, Kralovec ME, Andrews KL. Hemipelvectomy: high-level amputation surgery and prosthetic rehabilitation. Am J Phys Med Rehabil. 2014;93(7):600–8.
60. Hendershot BD, Nussbaum MA. Persons with lower-limb amputation have impaired trunk postural control while maintaining seated balance. Gait Posture. 2013;38(3):438–42.
61. Jeans KA, Browne RH, Karol LA. Effect of amputation level on energy expenditure during overground walking by children with an amputation. J Bone Joint Surg Am. 2011;93(1):49–56.
62. Branemark R, Branemark PI, Rydevik B, Myers RR. Osseointegration in skeletal reconstruction and rehabilitation: a review. J Rehabil Res Dev. 2001;38(2):175–81.
63. Goktepe AS, Cakir B, Yilmaz B, Yazicioglu K. Energy expenditure of walking with prostheses: comparison of three amputation levels. Prosthetics Orthot Int. 2010;34(1):31–6.
64. Jarvis HL, Bennett AN, Twiste M, Phillip RD, Etherington J, Baker R. Temporal spatial and metabolic measures of walking in highly functional individuals with lower limb amputations. Arch Phys Med Rehabil. 2017;98(7):1389–99.
65. Kennedy JG, Ross KA, Smyth NA, Hogan MV, Murawski CD. Primary tumors of the foot and ankle. Foot Ankle Spec. 2016;9(1):58–68.
66. Karaca MO, Basarir K, Merter A, Acar E, Ozbek EA, Ozyildiran M, et al. Malignant tumors of the foot and ankle. Foot Ankle Int. 2022;43(9):1232–41.
67. Azevedo CP, Casanova JM, Guerra MG, Santos AL, Portela MI, Tavares PF. Tumors of the foot and ankle: a single-institution experience. J Foot Ankle Surg. 2013;52(2):147–52.
68. Bos GD, Esther RJ, Woll TS. Foot tumors: diagnosis and treatment. J Am Acad Orthop Surg. 2002;10(4):259–70.
69. Roukis TS. Flexor hallucis longus and extensor digitorum longus tendon transfers for balancing the foot following transmetatarsal amputation. J Foot Ankle Surg. 2009;48(3):398–401.
70. Philbin TM, Leyes M, Sferra JJ, Donley BG. Orthotic and prosthetic devices in partial foot amputations. Foot Ankle Clin. 2001;6(2):215–28. v

Extremity Soft Tissue Sarcoma: Assessing Treatment-Related Morbidity

22

Patrick Qi Wang, Nicholas C. Eastley, Meshal Alfaraidy, Anthony M. Griffin, Kim M. Tsoi, Peter C. Ferguson, and Jay S. Wunder

22.1 Introduction

Soft tissue sarcomas (STS) are rare extra-skeletal tumours arising from mesenchymal cells that occur most commonly in the extremities and trunk [1, 2]. The advent of radiation therapy has shifted the treatment paradigm from primary amputation to limb-salvage surgery without negatively impacting local recurrence, distant metastatic disease, and overall survival [1, 3, 4]. This has allowed for improved functional outcomes while decreasing the morbidity related to amputations. However, treatment-related morbidity and high complication rates following limb-salvage surgery continue to affect patient outcomes and quality of life [3, 5–7]. Thus, minimizing surgical complications and patient morbidity is a critical element in optimizing patient outcomes related to STS management.

22.2 Wound Complications

Wound complications remain the most common issue following resection of extremity STS. Various studies have reported wound healing complications in upwards of 56% of patients following resection of extremity STS, with the highest rates occurring when radiation therapy is utilized as part of multimodality treatment [5, 6]. Wound complications are often classified as *major* or *minor* with a major wound complication involving the need for a re-operation, invasive wound care procedure, or specialized wound care [4, 8]. They can also be categorized between superficial and deep wound complications which range from cellulitis, wound dehiscence, and skin necrosis to seroma, hematoma, abscess formation, persistent wound drainage, and full thickness tissue necrosis [5, 9]. Reported risk factors include radiation therapy, tumour location, large tumour size/volume, thin skin flaps, residual dead space following closure, prolonged surgical duration, intraoperative blood loss, increasing age, smoking, diabetes, and obesity [5, 8, 10]. A systematic review and meta-analysis of 21 pooled studies by Slump et al. (2019) demonstrated that lower extremity STS, radiation, diabetes, obesity, and smoking were independent predictors of major wound complications following resection of extremity STS [11].

22.2.1 Radiation Therapy

High wound complication rates related to the combination of radiation therapy and surgical resection for extremity STS have been well documented in the literature. Multiple reviews have reported no differences in distant metastasis and overall survival between the use of adjuvant or neoadjuvant radiation, although there are some reports suggesting that preoperative radiation may have a slight advantage in terms of lower rates of local recurrence [12–15]. The addition of radiation therapy to surgical resection in the management of extremity STS is a significant predictor of postoperative wound healing complications compared to patients treated by surgery alone. However, patients undergoing perioperative radiation often have large, deep, and high-grade tumours [16–18]. In the early 2000s, the Canadian SR-2 randomized controlled trial reported by

P. Q. Wang (✉) · N. C. Eastley · M. Alfaraidy · A. M. Griffin
The University of Toronto Musculoskeletal Oncology Unit, Mount Sinai Hospital, Toronto, ON, Canada

Department of Surgery, University of Toronto, Toronto, ON, Canada
e-mail: patrick-qi.wang.med@ssss.gouv.qc.ca; Neastley@doctors.org.uk; MKAlFaraidy@moh.gov.sa; Anthony.Griffin@sinaihealth.ca

K. M. Tsoi · P. C. Ferguson · J. S. Wunder
The University of Toronto Musculoskeletal Oncology Unit, Mount Sinai Hospital, Toronto, ON, Canada

Department of Surgery, University of Toronto, Toronto, ON, Canada

Department of Surgical Oncology, Princess Margaret Cancer Centre, Toronto, ON, Canada
e-mail: Kim.Tsoi@sinaihealth.ca; Peter.Ferguson@sinaihealth.ca; Jay.Wunder@sinaihealth.ca

H. Özger et al. (eds.), *Diagnosis and Treatment of Soft Tissue Tumors*, https://doi.org/10.1007/978-3-031-77061-6_22

O'Sullivan et al. (2002) demonstrated double the rate of wound healing complications in patients treated with preoperative compared to postoperative radiation in addition to surgical resection of extremity STS (35% vs. 17%, respectively) [4]. Multiple studies have reported consistent rates of wound healing problems [2, 5, 8, 9, 19]. Furthermore, there is a tendency to favour the use of neoadjuvant radiation therapy for management of younger patients, large tumours (>5 cm), when vascularized tissue transfers and/or skin grafts are required, and when tumours are near vital organs (e.g. lung, liver) and critical structures (e.g. major nerves, vessels, and bone) [2, 4, 13, 20, 21].

22.2.2 Tumour Location and Size

Important treatment considerations are made based on tumour location and size. Extremity STS account for nearly 60% of all STS [6, 10, 22], with lower extremity tumours being two to four times more common than upper extremity STS [2, 5, 8, 10]. However, wound healing complications occur significantly more often following treatment of lower extremity STS. Tseng et al. (2006) reported 36% vs. 17% complication rates following resection of lower extremity tumours compared to the upper extremity [23], while Korah et al. (2012) found a much larger difference between lower and upper extremity sites of 29% and 4%, respectively [10]. In the Canadian SR-2 randomized trial, there was only one wound complication in the 37 patients (2.7%) with upper extremity STS compared to 46 of 145 (31.7%) in those with lower extremity tumours [4]. In a study of 798 STS patients treated with preoperative radiation and resection, Griffin et al. (2015) reported complication rates of 36.4% (206/565) in the lower extremity and 15.5% (36/233) for upper extremity tumours [24]. It is important to note that lower extremity STS are on average 1.5 to two times larger than upper extremity tumours [10, 25].

Tumours greater than 8–10 cm in diameter are an independent risk factor for increased wound complications, although other studies also reported higher wound complication rates following treatment of tumours greater than 5 cm. Larger tumours are most commonly found in the thigh compared to distal lower extremity and upper extremity locations. Recognizing the risk presented by large tumours, the Canadian SR-2 randomized trial first stratified STS patients by tumour size using a cut-off of 10 cm prior to randomization to pre-operative vs. post-operative radiation [4, 8, 10, 26, 27]. In contrast, Ziegele et al. (2016) argued that tumour volume is a more accurate predictor of wound complications compared to the more commonly utilized variable tumour diameter. They demonstrated a strong correlation between tumour volume, but not tumour diameter, and the rate of wound complications, which they suggested is, at least, partially related to the increased residual dead space following resection of larger tumours [28, 29]. Additionally, Geller et al. (2007) demonstrated that patients with major wound complications had, on average, twice the volume of tissue resected compared to those without wound healing issues (919 cm^3 vs. 456 cm^3, respectively) [6].

Of all anatomic locations, the proximal thigh is associated with the highest risk of wound complication as thigh STS are more likely to be greater in size compared to other sites [5, 30]. Cannon et al. (2006) found a four-fold increase in chronic wound complications (greater than 3 months) in the groin and thigh regions compared to more distal lower extremity STS [9]. In a study by Korah et al. (2012), 84% of all re-operations for wound complications occurred following management of thigh STS [10]. Additionally, it is believed that disruption of the lymphatic drainage as well as the vascular system due to extensive dissections during resection of thigh STS also increases the risk of fluid collections and seroma, thereby contributing to increased rates of infection and other wound complications [5, 9, 10, 26, 28].

Baldini et al. (2013) reported increased wound complications when the tumour was within 3 mm of the skin surface, as the skin could not be spared and received a full dose of radiation [8]. In a Phase 2 study of pre-operative intensity-modulated radiation therapy (IMRT) for lower extremity STS, O'Sullivan et al. (2013) also found higher radiation doses to the skin overlying the tumour in patients suffering wound complications, and this predominantly occurred when the tumour was closer to the skin surface [31]. However, controversy remains as to whether tumour proximity to the skin affects the rate of wound complications as these findings were not reproduced in subsequent studies [5, 28].

22.2.3 Host Factors

Host factors must also be considered in the management of extremity STS. However, given the time-sensitive nature of the disease, most host-related risk factors are not modifiable. Independent host risk factors identified include increasing age, diabetes, tobacco use, and elevated body mass index (BMI) ≥30 [2, 5, 8, 32, 33]. However, these variables are not consistently included in sarcoma outcome studies [11, 32]. Peripheral vascular disease has not been shown to correlate with major wound complications following management of extremity sarcoma [8], but likely does play a role as well.

22.2.4 Surgical Risk Factors

Several other risk factors have been proposed to increase the rate of major wound complications following resection of STS. Increased intraoperative blood loss [5, 26], increasing surgical duration [34], as well as major vascular resection and reconstruction [35] have all been associated with increased postoperative wound complications. Meanwhile, tumour grade, periosteal stripping, and chemotherapy have not been found to increase wound complication rates [2, 5, 9, 23, 28].

22.2.5 Surgical Timing

There is scarce data regarding surgical timing following preoperative radiation in relation to wound complication risk in extremity STS. In general, surgical resection is performed 4–6 weeks following radiation [4, 8]. Griffin et al. (2015) identified a trend towards increasing wound complications when surgery was performed within 3 weeks or greater than 6 weeks following completion of radiation, although these findings did not reach statistical significance [24]. Louie et al. (2020) found an increased rate of perioperative complication (38%) in sarcomas resected more than 6 weeks after radiation in their review of 269 patients compared to those who underwent surgery within 6 weeks (15%) of preoperative treatment. However, their data is derived from patients with a combination of head and neck, chest, retroperitoneal, and extremity STS [36]. Meanwhile, postoperative radiation is typically given within 6 weeks of surgery provided that the wound has healed and there are no other active perioperative complications [10, 37].

22.2.6 Predictive Model

Bedi et al. (2020) developed a nomogram predicting postoperative wound complications in a study of 1669 patients who underwent limb-salvage resection for localized extremity STS. Following univariate and multiple logistic regression analysis, they concluded that increasing age and BMI, lower extremity location, and neoadjuvant radiation were significantly associated with increased wound complications and were included in their predictive model. However, this model is limited by its retrospective design and data collection. Further studies could help by evaluating other contributing variables which may strengthen the model [32]. At present, this is the only published predictive model for major wound complications in extremity STS.

22.2.7 Quality of Life and Function with Wound Complications

Wound complications have a profound effect on patients' quality of life and function. Davis et al. (2000) demonstrated significant disability in both univariate and multivariate analysis based on Musculoskeletal Tumour Society (MSTS) 1993 and MSTS 1987 scores when patients sustained treatment-related complications. Of the 172 patients who underwent combined surgery and radiation for lower-extremity STS, 48 suffered major wound complications or infection [38]. A subsequent analysis demonstrated that wound complications significantly impacted MSTS scores for up to 2 years after surgery (which was the end point of the study). The Toronto Extremity Salvage Score (TESS) was negatively affected within the first 6 months postoperatively but improved by 12 months. Pain management issues were common at 6 weeks and 6 months but not beyond [39]. Whereas the TESS score assesses daily functional outcomes and activity level, MSTS scores assess objective and subjective metrics such as range of motion, strength, deformity, and pain. Wound complications are associated with increased impairments, activity limitations, and decreased health-related quality of life (HRQOL) scores [39, 40].

22.2.8 Treatment and Prevention of Wound Complications

Most major wound complications are usually successfully treated using various combinations of percutaneous drainage, irrigation and debridement, vacuum-assisted closure (VAC), antibiotic treatment, and soft tissue reconstruction surgery [6, 8]. Depending on the severity, complete wound healing may take anywhere between 1 month to upwards of 2 years. Therefore, it is imperative to counsel the patient about this risk ahead of combined surgery and radiation treatment for extremity STS and again if a major wound complication develops [8].

During surgical planning for STS resection, important decisions must be made regarding the optimal method for wound closure. There are currently no standardized guidelines for primary closure versus soft tissue reconstructive surgery. Instead, decisions are generally made as part of a multidisciplinary approach and typically involve Plastic Surgery for high-risk situations or when large defects are anticipated that will not be amenable to primary wound closure. The goal in limb-salvage resections is to obtain a tension-free, stable, and viable tissue closure while ensuring adequate soft tissue coverage of critical structures such as nerves, vessels, bone, and joints [6, 8, 23]. Closure options include primary closure with or without incisional VAC, split-thickness skin graft, pedicled flap, and free flap. In the Phase 2 study utilizing preoperative IMRT for patients with lower extremity STS, O'Sullivan et al. (2013) reported that primary wound closure was frequently possible (55/59, 93.2%) with minimal need for flaps [31]. Bedi et al. (2019) recently demonstrated the benefits of vacuum-assisted wound closure in decreasing wound complications following resection of STS, especially in the proximal lower extremity [41].

In general, the rate of major wound complications is similar between primary closure and soft tissue reconstruction. In the systematic review and meta-analysis of 11 studies by Slump et al. (2019), there were no significant differences in wound complications between the primary closure and flap reconstruction groups [11]. On the other hand, Ziegele et al. (2016) found a 19% higher wound complication rate following use of vascularized flaps compared to primary closure in an 81-patient cohort [28]; however, this result may be largely influenced by selection bias. Independent risk factors for flap reconstruction failures include high grade tumours, cerebrovascular event, cardiac disease, obesity (BMI ≥30), and previous re-operations. Barwick et al. (1992) had previously demonstrated significant reduction in wound complications (19% vs. 51%), re-operation rate (10% vs. 35%), and average hospitalization (15 vs. 48 days) in an 82-patient study comparing prophylactic flap coverage and primary wound closure, respectively, in patients treated with preoperative radiation [42]. These results were also reflected in a subsequent study with an 11% wound complication rate in the vascularized tissue transfer group compared to 30% in the primary closure group [16]. O'Sullivan et al. (2002) did not find differences in wound complications in patients treated with preoperative radiation comparing primary closure and vascularized soft tissue transfer or split-thickness skin graft [4].

In a meta-analysis, Tasch et al. (2022) reported a significantly elevated risk of total and partial flap failures in the preoperative radiation group vs. the non-radiated group. However, this data is mostly derived from head and neck as well as breast reconstruction surgery [43]. In sarcoma-specific studies, Townley et al. (2013) compared 46 patients who underwent free flap reconstruction with neoadjuvant radiation or without radiation. They demonstrated no significant difference in microvascular flap-related complications but increased wound healing issues in the neoadjuvant radiation group [44]. In a 119-patient cohort study, Chao et al. (2012) found that none of the 73 patients in the neoadjuvant therapy group suffered a total flap failure and only 6.8% suffered late wound complications compared to 8.7% total free flap loss and 26.1% late wound complications among the 46 patients in the adjuvant radiation group. That study included patients with STS located in both the head and neck and extremities [45]. A more recent study of 57 patients who underwent vascularized tissue reconstruction following STS resection showed no difference in microvascular or wound complications in the radiated vs. non-radiated group [46]. Vascularized soft tissue reconstruction has shown great benefit following STS resection allowing for closure of large defects and facilitating high-risk primary closures, with, at least, comparable results to 'lower risk' wounds closed primarily. Flap reconstruction failures are more likely a reflection of large tumour size, anatomic location, and medical host factors [3, 8, 23].

VAC devices were introduced to help improve healing speed in open wounds and decrease time to primary skin closure using negative pressure wound therapy. Its effects in non-oncologic wound healing have been previously well documented, while its use in the oncology setting has been steadily increasing. Previous reluctance to using incisional VAC dressing was due to the fear of promoting malignancy when subatmospheric pressures were applied. However, no reports have confirmed the theory [6, 41, 47]. Several retrospective studies demonstrated decreased rates of wound healing complications in STS treated with neoadjuvant radiation and VAC dressings. However, selection bias remains as wound risk profiles and incisional VAC dressing candidates are often determined preoperatively as well as intraoperatively. Furthermore, depending on surgeon experience or institutional preference, soft tissue flap coverage may be favoured in higher risk wound closures over the use of an incisional VAC [41, 47–49]. Incisional VAC dressings (including VAC overlying STSG) have also demonstrated its usefulness in treating wound complications with reports of decreased hospital stay, length of treatment, number of re-operations, and need for soft tissue reconstruction [50]. At present, a pressure of 125 mmHg in continuous mode is the most commonly reported setting. However, heterogeneity remains regarding the actual type of VAC dressing and protocols [51]. Two systematic reviews and meta-analyses which include studies of all cancers including soft tissue sarcomas, demonstrated favourable outcomes when negative pressure wound therapy was applied over standard surgical dressings [51, 52].

22.3 Radiation Therapy Morbidity

Radiation therapy combined with surgical resection significantly improves local control following limb salvage resection of extremity STS and has become a standard (neo) adjuvant treatment paradigm [4, 53, 54]. This is critical, especially in large (>5 cm), deep (to fascia), and intermediate-to-high-grade tumours, as well as STS near critical structures such as major nerves, vessels, and bone. Meanwhile, small, superficial, low-grade tumours that are away from critical structures can be treated with or without radiation at the discretion of the clinical team. Current guidelines suggest a radiation dose of 50 Gray (Gy) in 25 fractions once daily for preoperative radiation, while postoperative radiation dose is approximately 66 Gy based on radiobiologic principles including presumed hypoxia in the surgical wound, although institutional protocols may vary. At present, various treatment guidelines detail when radiation is required as part of limb-salvage surgery for extremity STS. Ultimately, its usage should be predominantly based on the adequacy of the surgical resection margins [4, 7, 9, 37, 55].

The utilization of radiation treatment increases patient morbidity and disability. Preoperative radiation increases the rate of early major wound complications, nearly doubled compared to the use of postoperative treatment. Meanwhile, the disadvantage of postoperative radiation is the increased rates of late sequalae including soft tissue fibrosis, reduced joint range of motion, pain, lymphedema, and pathologic fractures, all of which also contribute to worse functional outcomes [2, 4, 7, 37]. While most early wound complications can be successfully treated, late radiation-associated toxicities are generally irreversible and can also be progressive. As such, there is a tendency to favour the use of preoperative radiation therapy, whenever feasible. Morbidity specifically related to radiation therapy will be discussed in this section. Major wound complications secondary to radiation were discussed above in Sect. 22.2.

22.3.1 Late Radiation Complications

Late radiation toxicity including soft tissue fibrosis, joint stiffness, and lymphedema can lead to significant functional impairments and disability. These sequalae are especially associated with the utilization of postoperative radiation, based on the combination of its higher dosage and larger field size [7]. A randomized controlled trial evaluating late radiation morbidity included 73 and 56 patients in the preoperative and postoperative arms, respectively. The Canadian Sarcoma Group demonstrated a significantly higher proportion of grade ≥2 fibrosis in the postoperative radiation group (on a scale of 0–3 as per the European Organization for Research and Treatment of Cancer/Radiation Therapy Oncology). Meanwhile, joint stiffness and oedema were also more common in the postoperative group, but this did not reach significance. Patients with grade ≥2 fibrosis, joint stiffness, and oedema reported significantly greater physical disability and functional impairment based on their TESS and MSTS scores [7, 56]. In a retrospective review of 517 patients by Zagars et al. (2003), late radiation-related complications were reported in 33 patients including soft tissue necrosis, fibrosis, oedema, osteonecrosis, fracture, and brain necrosis. In their multivariate analysis, only treatment sequence (preoperative vs. postoperative radiation) was statistically significant, with postoperative radiation leading to increased late complications [13]. In another retrospective review of 214 patients who underwent external beam radiation therapy (EBRT) combined with brachytherapy or EBRT alone postoperatively, three patients sustained peripheral nerve injuries and five had severe limb dysfunction from fibrosis. These complications occurred when brachytherapy was added but not with EBRT alone [57]. In a review of 220 patients, among the 81 patients who received postoperative radiation, 38.3% suffered from grade ≥2 acute radiation dermatitis. Meanwhile, late complications including joint stiffness, oedema, and radiation-induced peripheral nerve damage were observed in eight (9.9%), ten (12.3%), and one (1.2%) patient(s), respectively [58]. In a review of 54 patients, of the 41 who had undergone radiation therapy with surgery (sequence not delineated), 32 patients had moderate to severe joint stiffness, 30 patients had reduced muscle power, and 15 patients suffered from lymphedema. The use of radiation was determined to be a significant factor associated with functional limitations [27]. Yang et al. (1998) observed increased joint stiffness and oedema, as well as decreased muscle power in patients receiving postoperative radiation compared to patients who underwent surgery alone. However, their global quality-of-life scale and activities of daily living scores remain similar in both groups [54]. Significant risk factors for chronic radiation-induced complications include the proximal thigh and groin location, higher doses of radiation, and previous acute wound complications [9].

Although major acute wound healing complications are predominantly associated with the use of preoperative radiation, acute dermatitis/skin toxic side effects occur more commonly in the postoperative treatment group. Acute skin toxic side effects have been reported in up to 40% of patients undergoing radiation, with nearly twice as many cases in postoperatively treated patients, likely related to the larger treatment field and higher dose [7, 58]. However, these complications are generally self-limiting compared to major wound complications [4].

Patients presenting with debilitating pain and functional limitations, fungating masses, active tumour bleeding often require urgent surgery followed by postoperative radiation. Nonetheless, even for patients who present with fungating tumours, an attempt to administer preoperative radiation can be considered in conjunction with formalized wound care due to the potential long-term functional benefits associated with this approach [3, 7, 23, 37]. Otherwise, the high risk of morbidity and mortality related to the need for additional treatments including surgery to manage early wound complications may outweigh the long-term functional deficits associated with postoperative radiation therapy. For example, elderly patients, especially those with multiple co-morbidities including diabetes and cardiovascular disease should be considered for postoperative radiation therapy to minimize the negative impacts associated with the high rate of early wound complications [59]. Therefore, careful consideration and multidisciplinary team discussion should be undertaken on an individual basis [37, 60].

22.3.2 Booster Dose of Radiation

Controversy exists regarding the need for a secondary post-operative radiation boost following preoperative radiation and a positive resection margin. When possible, re-resection of a positive margin to obtain a negative final margin is preferable if the risks and morbidity are within acceptable range. This is more likely to be feasible following resection of superficial STS. Some reports documented improved local control with a postoperative radiation boost and final total dose >64 Gy [37, 61], while two other large studies did not demonstrate any improvement in local control with this approach [62, 63]. Further studies may shed additional insight into this controversy, but in the meantime, the treating team must individualize treatment when managing this scenario and consider the potential negative impact of additional radiation.

22.3.3 Delivery of Radiation and Alternative Protocols

Several different techniques and protocols of delivering radiation have been proposed. Traditional high dose conventional EBRT led to increased late complications including radiation-induced fractures due to the large non-conformal treatment fields. The evolution of conformal IMRT has allowed for more targeted radiation treatment resulting in decreased morbidity [31, 64, 65].

Brachytherapy was introduced to deliver radiation interstitially via brachytherapy catheters, usually implanted during surgery to provide intraoperative and/or postoperative treatment. The advantage of this modality is to provide more targeted radiation, preserve normal tissue, and especially shorten the duration of treatment. However, brachytherapy is limited by lower volume targets, making it less suitable for very large, high-grade STS when administered alone. As a result, brachytherapy has often been used in combination with EBRT. Yet, this approach has not demonstrated consistent benefits in local control, systemic recurrence, and overall survival rate while radiation-related morbidity remains similar [66–71].

More recently, hypofractionated radiotherapy protocols have been reported. This involves using larger doses per fraction over a shorter time period and is utilized preoperatively. Image-guided intensity-modulated radiation therapy is often utilized in these protocols to allow for better precision. Current protocols include receiving between 25 and 35 Gy of radiation in as few as five fractions preoperatively. The timing of surgical resection varies depending on the protocol and may be performed as early as 3–7 days or up to 6 weeks from completion of radiation. The goal is to safely reduce treatment time, healthcare costs, patient anxiety with a shorter treatment course, and allowing quicker resumption of systemic treatment in patients with metastatic disease. Several hypofractionated radiotherapy studies reported major wound complications between 7% and 41%, and late radiation-related complications in nearly 10% of patients. While early data on local recurrence and overall survival are encouraging, long-term oncologic and toxicity profile outcomes are mandatory [72–76].

22.4 Pain

Long-term pain following soft tissue sarcoma treatment leads to significant disability for patients. Narcotic requirements beyond 1 year are observed in 7–11% of patients with extremity STS, although more than half of STS patients may suffer from some degree of chronic pain. The ongoing need for a long-term gait aid is seen in up to 16% of patients [27, 77]. Pain is often described as either musculoskeletal from altered biomechanics, neuropathic from nerve injury/resection, and phantom limb pain following amputation [78]. Independent risk factors for chronic pain include lower extremity tumour resection and high dose radiation (>63 Gy). When compared with postoperative radiation, preoperative radiation led to significantly higher pain scores in the first 6 weeks only, with no significant differences beyond 6 weeks [7, 39, 77]. There is currently a paucity of research assessing pain outcomes following STS treatment. Most reported pain outcomes are derived from functional outcome scores and HRQOL assessments in which pain is only a minor component. Further pain-specific studies would be beneficial.

22.5 Lymphedema

Lymphedema is identified in up to 30% of patients following extremity STS treatment. It is often unavoidable as it results from either the surgical resection disrupting the lymphatic system and major blood vessels or as a consequence of chronic fibrosis related to the use of radiation. Lymphedema is associated with an increased risk of infection and wound complication, as well as abnormal skin changes including hyperkeratosis and papillomatosis [7, 79, 80]. Multiple risk factors for lymphedema identified in several studies include tumours in the medial thigh compartment, tumour size >5 cm, location deep to fascia, lower extremity tumours compared to the upper extremity sites, radiation field length >35 cm, high radiation dose, female sex, smoking, arterial and venous resections with or without reconstruction, as well as a history of cardiac disease [5, 35, 64, 77, 79–81].

The effect of lymphedema on functional outcomes remains largely unknown. In the study by Friedman et al. (2011), of the 289 patients who underwent STS resection with or without adjuvant radiation, the rate of lymphedema was 28.8% and 9%, respectively. Higher radiation doses led to significantly lower TESS scores but not MSTS scores. Meanwhile higher radiation dose was also found to be correlated with lymphedema on univariate analysis, but was not found to be an independent predictor [79]. A previous study in patients receiving conservative treatment for extremity lymphedema found significant improvement in the Nottingham Health Profile Part-1 (NHP-1) assessment as a surrogate for HRQOL, specifically in the *physical* domain but not the psychological or emotional domains [82]. Lower functional outcomes following treatment that included radiation are a consequence of a combination of fibrosis, joint stiffness, and lymphedema. However, whether lymphedema is an independent predictor for worse functional scores and higher rates of wound complication is yet to be determined.

22.6 Pathologic Fracture

Radiation-associated pathologic fractures are devastating complications following combined management of extremity STS with radiation. Fortunately, the incidence of pathologic fracture remains low. The incidence varies between 1.2% and 8.6% [9, 57, 83]. Risk factors, although inconsistently reported, include surgery adjacent to a weight-bearing bone, periosteal stripping, thigh location especially anterior compartment involvement, positive tumour resection margins, high dose of postoperative radiation, radiation involving the entire circumference of the bone, chemotherapy, female gender, and increasing age >55 years old [9, 57, 83–87].

Considering the heterogeneous data, predictive models for radiation-induced pathologic fractures of the femur have been developed to help guide clinical decision-making. Gortzak et al. (2010) performed a retrospective study using prospectively collected data from 101 patients treated surgically for STS of the thigh combined with radiation. Univariate analysis revealed a significant relationship between radiation-related pathologic fracture with age, tumour size, length of periosteal stripping, and thigh muscle involved. Gender and radiation dose were not found to be significant predictors. In the multiple logistic regression analysis, only age and tumour size were identified as significant risk factors for pathologic fracture. From this data, a predictive nomogram model was produced incorporating the six variables even if they did not necessarily reach significance on univariate and/or multivariate analysis given that they are commonly reported as independent predictors in the literature [88]. Dickie et al. (2009) reviewed 691 patients treated with resection of lower extremity STS and radiation therapy, of which 31 sustained a radiation-induced pathologic fracture. Their analysis demonstrated that the risk of radiation-induced pathologic fracture was reduced when (1) the proportional volume of radiated bone ≥40 Gy (V40) was <64%, (2) the mean dose to bone was less than 37 Gy, and (3) the maximum dose along the bone was less than 59 Gy. There was a trend indicating a lower risk of fracture with lower radiation field sizes, but this did not reach significance for risk reduction [85]. The results of these studies can be used to help identify patients at high risk for radiation-related fractures in the lower extremity who might benefit from prophylactic surgical stabilization or potential modification of the radiation therapy treatment plan.

The management of radiation-related pathologic fractures is problematic. Lin et al. (1998) reported four non-unions and three delayed unions out of nine patients. Subsequent management options included secondary bone grafting, endoprosthetic replacement, and amputation [86]. Sternheim et al. (2013) reported complications in 86% of STS patients with radiation-induced femur fractures. Among the 19 patients analysed, 18 demonstrated radiographic non-union at 1 year, 13 underwent revision surgery, and six underwent multiple re-operations. Surgeries included revision intramedullary nail, open reduction and internal fixation of a second fracture, endoprostheses, and amputation [89]. Multiple surgeries to address pathologic fractures also increase the risk of deep infection. Prophylactic intramedullary nailing in high-risk patients has been proposed but has not been routinely implemented. However, fracture risk in this setting has been further decreased with the implementation of preoperative IMRT. Consequently, the decision to proceed with prophylactic fixation should be made on an individual basis with a multidisciplinary input [31, 85, 88, 89].

22.7 Radiation-Induced Sarcoma

Radiation-induced sarcoma (RIS), although rare, is a known late-occurring complication following radiation therapy. The risk of developing RIS is estimated at one in 10,000 following radiation treatment. Nonetheless, 40% of radiation-induced sarcomas affect the extremities or trunk and account for between 0.5% and 5% of all STS. The median latent period from radiation to onset of disease ranges between 10 and 17 years. The diagnostic criteria include: (1) sarcoma arising within a previously radiated field or adjacent to it, (2) at least 2 years separating radiation therapy and onset of a new malignant tumour, (3) the histology confirms a high-grade sarcoma which is distinct from the initial malignancy [90–92]. RIS are associated with a poor prognosis with 5-year overall survival between 10% and 52.9% and 10-year overall survival of 41% [93–96]. The rate of local recurrence and metastatic disease following treatment has been reported to be as high as 68% and 50%, respectively [91, 95]. Controversy exists as to whether there is a role for chemotherapy and/or radiation in the management of patients with RIS. Several studies showed no therapeutic effects of chemotherapy on the treatment of localized radiation-induced STS although it is commonly used in the palliative setting or in the presence of metastatic disease [92–94]. Conversely, repeat radiation has been shown to decrease local recurrence below the very high rates listed above, although still greater than following management of primary STS. However, the functional outcomes, complication rates, and toxicity profile appear to be similar to the treatment of de novo STS, although using a modified twice-a-day treatment protocol [95].

22.8 Chemotherapy

The use of perioperative chemotherapy remains controversial in the curative treatment of extremity STS. While neoadjuvant or adjuvant chemotherapy alone has failed to demonstrate consistent survival benefits, sequential neoadjuvant chemotherapy and radiation (referred as chemoradiation) has shown some promising results with local control, metastatic rate, and overall survival benefits, especially with certain sarcoma subtypes, including synovial sarcoma, high-grade myxoid liposarcoma, undifferentiated pleomorphic sarcoma, malignant peripheral nerve sheath tumour, and vascular sarcomas. Current indications for chemotherapy as part of multimodal management for patients with extremity STS include younger age, high-grade STS, borderline resectability and/or presence of metastatic disease. However, chemoradiation does not demonstrate superior outcomes compared to radiation and surgical resection alone, while having potentially severe side effects. Thus, the use of chemoradiation is not widespread [97–100]. Additionally, effective histologic-specific chemotherapy regimens are still lacking.

Chemotherapy toxicity also needs to be considered, especially since most patients are older and cannot tolerate the high-dose regimens used for STS. The most common side effects include nausea, vomiting, and alopecia, which are mostly self-limited; however, acute hematologic toxicity (anaemia, leukopenia, thrombocytopenia) requiring treatment affects more than 80% of patients. Febrile neutropenia requiring hospital admission and antibiotic treatment also occurs frequently (25–40%). Although less common, neurologic toxicities, amputation due to sepsis at the biopsy or surgical site, pulmonary embolism, death from septic shock, or late complications of acute myelogenous leukaemia, and fatal myelodysplasia have also been reported. Cardiotoxicity is another longer-term complication associated with the use of high-dose Doxorubicin. Surgery-related complication rates are similar with or without the use of chemotherapy [97, 101–104].

Perioperative radiation and surgical resection for large, deep, and intermediate-to-high-grade tumours remain the standard of care in STS treatment. Despite promising results, there is still a lack of universally accepted data favouring the use of chemotherapy alone or chemoradiation as part of the management of localized curable extremity STS. Specifically, there is a paucity of data supporting histology-specific chemotherapy regimens [105, 106]. Meanwhile, the use of chemoradiation needs to be balanced against the toxicity profile, which in many instances, remains unacceptable [107].

22.9 Anatomic Considerations

22.9.1 Bone Involvement

Direct invasion of bone by extremity STS has been reported in 5.5% of cases and usually requires *en bloc* resection of the involved bone together with a form of osseous/joint reconstruction. This is distinct from tumours that directly abut a bone in which case subperiosteal resection is favoured in conjunction with radiation therapy to allow for bone-preservation, in order to avoid the need for endoprosthetic or structural bone graft reconstruction, which is often associated with high rates of complications and re-operations [108–110].

22.9.2 Nerve Involvement

Major and minor nerves usually require resection together with the tumour when they are encased within the STS. While this contributes to worse functional outcomes, the need for major nerve sacrifice alone is not an indication for amputation [111]. Additionally, planned close but ultimately positive resection margins as a result of epineural and adventitial dissection to salvage major nerves and blood vessels, respectively, located directly adjacent to extremity STS provides similar local recurrence rates compared with negative margins when combined with radiation therapy [20, 21]. Clarkson et al. (2005) studied the outcomes of epineural dissection, specifically of the sciatic nerve. When they compared STS located directly adjacent but not encasing the sciatic nerve with tumours clearly separate from major nerves with otherwise similar characteristics, they found no difference in the local or systemic recurrence rates [112].

Involvement and injury to the sciatic nerve during surgical resection of STS is more common than for other nerves in the thigh [10, 64]. Nonetheless, even sciatic nerve resection is not an indication for amputation. Several studies have shown that functional outcomes are moderate to good based on patient-rated assessments indicating only mild to moderate disability. Ambulation without gait aids is achieved in more than 50% of patients, and ankle braces/splints are often the only other adjunct required to facilitate independent ambulation [111, 113, 114]. As another example, following complete femoral nerve resection most patients either develop compensatory hyperextension and a back-knee gait or utilize braces and/or other gait aids. However, sacrificing the femoral nerve is often associated with falls leading to lower extremity fractures and is predictive of lower functional scores [22, 30, 38, 39, 115].

In the upper extremity, nerve transfers as well as tendon transfers can facilitate satisfactory outcomes in some instances following the need for major motor nerve resection. However, restoration of motor function and sensation through primary nerve reconstruction is rarely effective, especially in adults when radiation is used as part of STS management. Reconstruction techniques are usually more successful in upper compared to lower extremity sites. A thorough discussion with a peripheral nerve and/or Plastic surgeon is highly recommended preoperatively when major nerve sacrifice is anticipated [116, 117].

22.9.3 Vascular Reconstruction

Vascular reconstructions allow for limb-sparing procedures when STS resection includes major arteries, usually due to vessel encasement or invasion. Limb-salvage is possible in over 90% of cases following vascular resection/reconstruction but is associated with post-surgical complication rates greater than 50% including infection, hematoma, thrombosis, thromboembolism, significant limb oedema, reconstruction failure, and ischaemic injury leading to compartment syndrome, though rarely amputation. Reported functional outcomes tend to be similar compared to STS patients not requiring vascular reconstructions [111, 118–121].

22.10 Amputation

The evolution of surgical techniques and multidisciplinary management of STS has led to the ability of obtaining equivalent local control, metastasis-free survival, and overall survival with limb-salvage surgery compared to amputations. Current rates of primary amputations for STS treatment in tertiary sarcoma centres are less than 10%. Contemporary indications for primary amputation include limb-sparing STS resection which would otherwise result in unacceptable functional outcomes, major nerve and vessel resections which would otherwise result in unacceptable functional outcomes (although sacrificing a major nerve or vessel in itself is not a contraindication to limb-salvage surgery as mentioned above), tumour multifocality, prior unplanned excision or local recurrence with extensively contaminated tissues including critical anatomical structures, major medical co-morbidities precluding complex and extensive surgery especially in the elderly, multiple re-operations for infection, and sepsis [1, 111, 122, 123].

Following lower extremity amputations for STS, performance scores are generally lower than limb-salvage surgery. Additionally, more proximal amputations have significantly lower scores than distal amputations. Nonetheless, with prosthetic fitting, most patients report similar quality of life long-term compared to limb-salvage. Furthermore, sarcoma-related amputees are generally healthier and have less co-morbidities compared to amputees due to underlying diabetes and vascular disorders. Most patients with lower extremity amputations for sarcoma, especially transtibial and trans-femoral are community ambulators by 6 months following surgery. Younger patients with lower extremity amputations are often able to return to high level sports [1, 123–126].

Hindquarter amputations are one of the most morbid interventions in surgical oncology. They are life-altering, negatively affect quality of life and mobility, and can be extremely disfiguring. Postoperative complications can be observed in up to 70% of patients with major wound complications, infections, and flap necrosis, with a perioperative mortality between 1.3% and 8.8%. Other complications include gastro-intestinal and genitourinary injuries, arterial bleeding following closure, aspiration, deep vein thrombosis, cardiac events, and stroke [1, 122, 127]. Anxiety, depression, and impaired sexual function following hindquarter amputation are common. Psychosocial interventions are often required to help patients adapt and cope [1, 128]. One study assessing functional outcomes for patients who survived more than 1 year showed that most patients regained a social life and many were able to perform some types of work. In general, younger patients <45 years of age reached a better ambulatory status; however, older patients had better pain scores, which may reflect their functional status and level of activity. A multidisciplinary approach to rehabilitation is highly recommended to optimize outcomes for these patients [122, 123].

In general, limb-salvage surgery of the upper extremity is more critical than for patients with lower extremity sarcomas since arm prosthetics generally yield poor function, and in some cases, are purely cosmetic. Current upper extremity prostheses have yet to incorporate the multiple tactile functions and fine motor skills required for arm and hand function [1, 129, 130].

Although life-altering, forequarter amputation is associated with low rates of complications. Given the lack of prosthetics, most patients either prefer simply padding the shoulder to allow for a more symmetric appearance of the torso or a prosthetic fitting for cosmetic reasons. Most patients usually adapt well following forequarter amputations and can perform their activities of daily living [1, 131].

22.11 Conclusion

Complications following management of STS are frequent and can be quite challenging to manage. Tumour characteristics, anatomic considerations, surgical factors, patient factors, and adjuvant therapies all contribute to the various treatment complications. A multidisciplinary approach is useful in optimizing outcomes and decreasing long-term morbidity.

References

1. Clark MA, Thomas JM. Amputation for soft-tissue sarcoma. Lancet Oncol. 2003;4(6):335–42.
2. Potkrajcic V, Kolbenschlag J, Sachsenmaier S, Daigeler A, Ladurner R, Golf A, et al. Postoperative complications and oncologic outcomes after multimodal therapy of localized high risk soft tissue sarcoma. Radiat Oncol. 2022;17(1):210.
3. Stevenson MG, Ubbels JF, Slump J, Huijing MA, Bastiaannet E, Pras E, et al. Identification of predictors for wound complications following preoperative or postoperative radiotherapy in extremity soft tissue sarcoma. Eur J Surg Oncol. 2018;44(6):816–22.
4. O'Sullivan B, Davis AM, Turcotte R, Bell R, Catton C, Chabot P, et al. Preoperative versus postoperative radiotherapy in soft-tissue sarcoma of the limbs: a randomised trial. Lancet. 2002;359(9325):2235–41.
5. Moore J, Isler M, Barry J, Mottard S. Major wound complication risk factors following soft tissue sarcoma resection. Eur J Surg Oncol EJSO. 2014;40(12):1671–6.
6. Geller DS, Hornicek FJ, Mankin HJ, Raskin KA. Soft tissue sarcoma resection volume associated with wound-healing complications. Clin Orthop. 2007;459:182–5.
7. Davis A, Osullivan B, Turcotte R, Bell R, Catton C, Chabot P, et al. Late radiation morbidity following randomization to preoperative versus postoperative radiotherapy in extremity soft tissue sarcoma. Radiother Oncol. 2005;75(1):48–53.
8. Baldini EH, Lapidus MR, Wang Q, Manola J, Orgill DP, Pomahac B, et al. Predictors for major wound complications following preoperative radiotherapy and surgery for soft-tissue sarcoma of the extremities and trunk: importance of tumor proximity to skin surface. Ann Surg Oncol. 2013;20(5):1494–9.
9. Cannon CP, Ballo MT, Zagars GK, Mirza AN, Lin PP, Lewis VO, et al. Complications of combined modality treatment of primary lower extremity soft-tissue sarcomas. Cancer. 2006;107(10):2455–61.
10. Korah MP, Deyrup AT, Monson DK, Oskouei SV, Weiss SW, Landry J, et al. Anatomic tumor location influences the success of contemporary limb-sparing surgery and radiation among adults with soft tissue sarcomas of the extremities. Int J Radiat Oncol. 2012;82(2):933–9.
11. Slump J, Bastiaannet E, Halka A, Hoekstra HJ, Ferguson PC, Wunder JS, et al. Risk factors for postoperative wound complications after extremity soft tissue sarcoma resection: a systematic review and meta-analyses. J Plast Reconstr Aesthet Surg. 2019;72(9):1449–64.
12. Yang X, Zhang L, Yang X, Yu W, Fu J. Oncologic outcomes of pre- versus post-operative radiation in resectable soft tissue sarcoma: a systematic review and meta-analysis. Radiat Oncol. 2020;15(1):158.
13. Zagars GK, Ballo MT, Pisters PWT, Pollock RE, Patel SR, Benjamin RS. Preoperative vs. postoperative radiation therapy for soft tissue sarcoma: a retrospective comparative evaluation of disease outcome. Int J Radiat Oncol. 2003;56(2):482–8.
14. Al-Absi E, Farrokhyar F, Sharma R, Whelan K, Corbett T, Patel M, et al. A systematic review and meta-analysis of oncologic outcomes of pre- versus postoperative radiation in localized resectable soft-tissue sarcoma. Ann Surg Oncol. 2010;17(5):1367–74.
15. Albertsmeier M, Rauch A, Roeder F, Hasenhütl S, Pratschke S, Kirschneck M, et al. External beam radiation therapy for resectable soft tissue sarcoma: a systematic review and meta-analysis. Ann Surg Oncol. 2018;25(3):754–67.
16. Peat BG, Bell RS, Davis A, O'Sullivan B, Mahoney J, Manktelow RT, et al. Wound-healing complications after soft-tissue sarcoma surgery. Plast Reconstr Surg. 1994;93:980–7.
17. Karthik N, Ward MC, Juloori A, Scott J, Mesko N, Shah C. Factors associated with acute and chronic wound complications in patients with soft tissue sarcoma with long-term follow-up. Am J Clin Oncol. 2018;41(10):1019–23.
18. Davidge KM, Wunder J, Tomlinson G, Wong R, Lipa J, Davis AM. Function and health status outcomes following soft tissue reconstruction for limb preservation in extremity soft tissue sarcoma. Ann Surg Oncol. 2010;17(4):1052–62.
19. Cheng EY, Dusenbery KE, Winters MR, Thompson RC. Soft tissue sarcomas: preoperative versus postoperative radiotherapy. J Surg Oncol. 1996;61(2):90–9.
20. O'Donnell PW, Griffin AM, Eward WC, Sternheim A, Catton CN, Chung PW, et al. The effect of the setting of a positive surgical margin in soft tissue sarcoma: positive margins in soft tissue sarcoma. Cancer. 2014;120(18):2866–75.
21. Gundle KR, Kafchinski L, Gupta S, Griffin AM, Dickson BC, Chung PW, et al. Analysis of margin classification systems for assessing the risk of local recurrence after soft tissue sarcoma resection. J Clin Oncol. 2018;36(7):704–9.
22. Ramu EM, Houdek MT, Isaac CE, Dickie CI, Ferguson PC, Wunder JS. Management of soft-tissue sarcomas; treatment strategies, staging, and outcomes. SICOT-J. 2017;3:20.
23. Tseng JF, Ballo MT, Langstein HN, Wayne JD, Cormier JN, Hunt KK, et al. The effect of preoperative radiotherapy and reconstructive surgery on wound complications after resection of extremity soft-tissue sarcomas. Ann Surg Oncol. 2006;13(9):1209–15.
24. Griffin AM, Dickie CI, Catton CN, Chung PWM, Ferguson PC, Wunder JS, et al. The influence of time interval between preoperative radiation and surgical resection on the development of wound healing complications in extremity soft tissue sarcoma. Ann Surg Oncol. 2015;22(9):2824–30.
25. Gerrand CH, Wunder JS, Kandel RA, O'Sullivan B, Catton CN, Bell RS, et al. The influence of anatomic location on functional outcome in lower-extremity soft-tissue sarcoma. Ann Surg Oncol. 2004;11(5):476–82.
26. Nakamura T, Nakamura K, Hagi T, Asanuma K, Sudo A. Soft tissue sarcoma at the adductor compartment of the thigh may have a greater risk of tumor-associated events and wound complications. J Orthop Surg. 2019;27(2):230949901984081.
27. Robinson MH, Spruce L, Eeles R, Fryatt I, Harmer CL, Thomas JM, et al. Limb function following conservation treatment of adult soft tissue sarcoma. Eur J Cancer Clin Oncol. 1991;27(12):1567–74.
28. Ziegele M, King DM, Bedi M. Tumor volume is a better predictor of post-operative wound complications compared to tumor size in soft tissue sarcomas of the proximal lower extremity. Clin Sarcoma Res. 2016;6(1):1.
29. Novak R, Nevin JL, Rowell PD, Griffin A, Mazin S, Hofer SOP, et al. A size-based criteria for flap reconstruction after thigh-adductor, soft-tissue sarcoma resection. Ann Surg Oncol. 2023;30(6):3701–11.
30. Bell RS, O'Sullivan B, Davis A, Langer F, Cummings B, Fornasier VL. Functional outcome in patients treated with surgery and irradiation for soft tissue tumours. J Surg Oncol. 1991;48(4):224–31.
31. O'Sullivan B, Griffin AM, Dickie CI, Sharpe MB, Chung PWM, Catton CN, et al. Phase 2 study of preoperative image-guided intensity-modulated radiation therapy to reduce wound and combined modality morbidities in lower extremity soft tissue sarcoma: phase 2 IMRT sarcoma study. Cancer. 2013;119(10):1878–84.
32. Bedi M, Ethun CG, Charlson J, Tran TB, Poultsides G, Grignol V, et al. Is a nomogram able to predict postoperative wound com-

plications in localized soft-tissue sarcomas of the extremity? Clin Orthop. 2020;478(3):550–9.
33. Houdek MT, Griffin AM, Ferguson PC, Wunder JS. Morbid obesity increases the risk of postoperative wound complications, infection, and repeat surgical procedures following upper extremity limb salvage surgery for soft tissue sarcoma. Hand. 2019;14(1):114–20.
34. Nakamura T, Matsumine A, Matsubara T, Asanuma K, Uchida A, Sudo A. Clinical characteristics of patients with large and deep soft tissue sarcomas. Oncol Lett. 2015;10(2):841–4.
35. Ghert MA, Davis AM, Griffin AM, Alyami AH, White L, Kandel RA, et al. The surgical and functional outcome of limb-salvage surgery with vascular reconstruction for soft tissue sarcoma of the extremity. Ann Surg Oncol. 2005;12(12):1102–10.
36. Louie RJ, Wang K, Royce TJ, Beaty BT, Esther RJ, Tepper JE, et al. Does timing matter? Surgical outcomes in high-grade sarcomas after neoadjuvant radiation therapy. J Surg Res. 2020;254:118–24.
37. Salerno KE, Alektiar KM, Baldini EH, Bedi M, Bishop AJ, Bradfield L, et al. Radiation therapy for treatment of soft tissue sarcoma in adults: executive summary of an ASTRO clinical practice guideline. Pract Radiat Oncol. 2021;11(5):339–51.
38. Davis AM, Sennik S, Griffin AM, Wunder JS, O'Sullivan B, Catton CN, et al. Predictors of functional outcomes following limb salvage surgery for lower-extremity soft tissue sarcoma. J Surg Oncol. 2000;73(4):206–11.
39. Davis AM, O'Sullivan B, Bell RS, Turcotte R, Catton CN, Wunder JS, et al. Function and health status outcomes in a randomized trial comparing preoperative and postoperative radiotherapy in extremity soft tissue sarcoma. J Clin Oncol. 2002;20(22):4472–7.
40. Schreiber D, Bell RS, Wunder JS, O'Sullivan B, Turcotte R, Masri BA, et al. Evaluating function and health related quality of life in patients treated for extremity soft tissue sarcoma. Qual Life Res. 2006;15(9):1439–46.
41. Bedi M, King DM, DeVries J, Hackbarth DA, Neilson JC. Does vacuum-assisted closure reduce the risk of wound complications in patients with lower extremity sarcomas treated with preoperative radiation? Clin Orthop. 2019;477(4):768–74.
42. Barwick WJ, Goldberg JA, Scully SP, Harrelson JM. Vascularized tissue transfer for closure of irradiated wounds after soft tissue sarcoma resection. Ann Surg. 1992;216(5):591–5.
43. Tasch C, Pattiss A, Maier S, Lanthaler M, Pierer G. Free flap outcome in irradiated recipient sites: a systematic review and meta-analysis. Plast Reconstr Surg Glob Open. 2022;10(3):e4216.
44. Townley WA, Mah E, O'Neill AC, Wunder JS, Ferguson PC, Zhong T, et al. Reconstruction of sarcoma defects following pre-operative radiation: free tissue transfer is safe and reliable. J Plast Reconstr Aesthet Surg. 2013;66(11):1575–9.
45. Chao AH, Chang DW, Shuaib SW, Hanasono MM. The effect of neoadjuvant versus adjuvant irradiation on microvascular free flap reconstruction in sarcoma patients. Plast Reconstr Surg. 2012;129(3):675–82.
46. Azzi AJ, Zhou S, Safran T, Xu L, Alnaif N, Zadeh T. Vascularized tissue reconstruction in previously irradiated sarcoma defects. Ann Plast Surg. 2019;82(1):89–92.
47. Delman KA, Johnstone PAS. Vacuum-assisted closure for surgical wounds in sarcoma. J Surg Oncol. 2007;96(7):545–6.
48. Bickels J, Kollender Y, Wittig JC, Cohen N, Meller I, Malawer MM. Vacuum-assisted wound closure after resection of musculoskeletal tumors. Clin Orthop. 2005;441:346–50.
49. Sakellariou VI, Mavrogenis AF, Papagelopoulos PJ. Negative-pressure wound therapy for musculoskeletal tumor surgery. Adv Skin Wound Care. 2011;24(1):25–30.
50. Siegel HJ, Long JL, Watson KM, Fiveash JB. Vacuum-assisted closure for radiation-associated wound complications. J Surg Oncol. 2007;96(7):575–82.
51. Hays TR, Singh G, Saragossi J, Park J, Shekar S, Marquez JE, et al. Negative-pressure wound therapy versus standard surgical dressings after malignant tumor resection: a systematic review and meta-analysis. Plast Reconstr Surg. 2022;150(3):655e–70e.
52. Wang Y, Yao X, Lin Y, Wang J, Chang C. Oncologic feasibility for negative pressure wound therapy application in surgical wounds: a meta-analysis. Int Wound J. 2022;19(3):573–82.
53. Pisters PW, Harrison LB, Leung DH, Woodruff JM, Casper ES, Brennan MF. Long-term results of a prospective randomized trial of adjuvant brachytherapy in soft tissue sarcoma. J Clin Oncol. 1996;14(3):859–68.
54. Yang JC, Chang AE, Baker AR, Sindelar WF, Danforth DN, Topalian SL, et al. Randomized prospective study of the benefit of adjuvant radiation therapy in the treatment of soft tissue sarcomas of the extremity. J Clin Oncol. 1998;16(1):197–203.
55. Biau DJ, Ferguson PC, Chung P, Griffin AM, Catton CN, O'Sullivan B, et al. Local recurrence of localized soft tissue sarcoma: a new look at old predictors. Cancer. 2012;118(23):5867–77.
56. Cox JD, Stetz J, Pajak TF. Toxicity criteria of the radiation therapy oncology group (RTOG) and the European organization for research and treatment of cancer (EORTC). Int J Radiat Oncol. 1995;31(5):1341–6.
57. Livi L, Santoni R, Paiar F, Bastiani P, Beltrami G, Caldora P, et al. Late treatment–related complications in 214 patients with extremity soft-tissue sarcoma treated by surgery and postoperative radiation therapy. Am J Surg. 2006;191(2):230–4.
58. Zhao RP, Yu XL, Zhang Z, Jia LJ, Feng Y, Yang ZZ, et al. The efficacy of postoperative radiotherapy in localized primary soft tissue sarcoma treated with conservative surgery. Radiat Oncol. 2016;11(1):25.
59. Andrä C, Klein A, Dürr HR, Rauch J, Lindner LH, Knoesel T, et al. External-beam radiation therapy combined with limb-sparing surgery in elderly patients (>70 years) with primary soft tissue sarcomas of the extremities: a retrospective analysis. Strahlenther Onkol. 2017;193(8):604–11.
60. Larrier NA, Czito BG, Kirsch DG. Radiation therapy for soft tissue sarcoma. Surg Oncol Clin N Am. 2016;25(4):841–60.
61. DeLaney TF, Kepka L, Goldberg SI, Hornicek FJ, Gebhardt MC, Yoon SS, et al. Radiation therapy for control of soft-tissue sarcomas resected with positive margins. Int J Radiat Oncol. 2007;67(5):1460–9.
62. Al Yami A, Griffin AM, Ferguson PC, Catton CN, Chung PWM, Bell RS, et al. Positive surgical margins in soft tissue sarcoma treated with preoperative radiation: is a postoperative boost necessary? Int J Radiat Oncol Biol Phys. 2010;77(4):1191–7.
63. Pan E, Goldberg SI, Chen YL, Giraud C, Hornick JL, Nielsen GP, et al. Role of post-operative radiation boost for soft tissue sarcomas with positive margins following pre-operative radiation and surgery: RT boost for positive margin sarcomas. J Surg Oncol. 2014;110(7):817–22.
64. Rimner A, Brennan MF, Zhang Z, Singer S, Alektiar KM. Influence of compartmental involvement on the patterns of morbidity in soft tissue sarcoma of the thigh: sarcoma morbidity by thigh compartments. Cancer. 2009;115(1):149–57.
65. Le Péchoux C, Llacer C, Sargos P, Moureau-Zabotto L, Ducassou A, Sunyach MP, et al. Conformal radiotherapy in management of soft tissue sarcoma in adults. Cancer Radiothér. 2022;26(1–2):377–87.
66. Naghavi AO, Fernandez DC, Mesko N, Juloori A, Martinez A, Scott JG, et al. American brachytherapy society consensus statement for soft tissue sarcoma brachytherapy. Brachytherapy. 2017;16(3):466–89.
67. Emory CL, Montgomery CO, Potter BK, Keisch ME, Conway SA. Early complications of high-dose-rate brachytherapy in soft tissue sarcoma: a comparison with traditional external-beam radiotherapy. Clin Orthop. 2012;470(3):751–8.

68. Alektiar KM, McKee AB, Jacobs JM, McKee BJ, Healey JH, Brennan MF. Outcome of primary soft tissue sarcoma of the knee and elbow. Int J Radiat Oncol. 2002;54(1):163–9.
69. Klein J, Ghasem A, Huntley S, Donaldson N, Keisch M, Conway S. Does an algorithmic approach to using brachytherapy and external beam radiation result in good function, local control rates, and low morbidity in patients with extremity soft tissue sarcoma? Clin Orthop. 2018;476(3):634–44.
70. Holloway CL, Delaney TF, Alektiar KM, Devlin PM, O'Farrell DA, Demanes DJ. American brachytherapy society (abs) consensus statement for sarcoma brachytherapy. Brachytherapy. 2013;12(3):179–90.
71. Lloyd S, Alektiar KM, Nag S, Huang YJ, Deufel CL, Mourtada F, et al. Intraoperative high-dose-rate brachytherapy: an American brachytherapy society consensus report. Brachytherapy. 2017;16(3):446–65.
72. Bedi M, Singh R, Charlson JA, Kelly T, Johnstone C, Wooldridge A, et al. Is 5 the new 25? Long-term oncologic outcomes from a phase ii, prospective, 5-fraction preoperative radiation therapy trial in patients with localized soft tissue sarcoma. Adv Radiat Oncol. 2022;7(3):100850.
73. Parsai S, Lawrenz J, Kilpatrick S, Rubin B, Hymes C, Gray M, et al. Early outcomes of preoperative 5-fraction radiation therapy for soft tissue sarcoma followed by immediate surgical resection. Adv Radiat Oncol. 2020;5(6):1274–9.
74. Mayo ZS, Parsai S, Asha W, Dinh M, Mesko N, Nystrom L, et al. Early outcomes of ultra-hypofractionated preoperative radiation therapy for soft tissue sarcoma followed by immediate surgical resection. Radiother Oncol. 2023 Mar;180:109439.
75. Koseła-Paterczyk H, Szacht M, Morysiński T, Ługowska I, Dziewirski W, Falkowski S, et al. Preoperative hypofractionated radiotherapy in the treatment of localized soft tissue sarcomas. Eur J Surg Oncol EJSO. 2014;40(12):1641–7.
76. Guadagnolo BA, Bassett RL, Mitra D, Farooqi A, Hempel C, Dorber C, et al. Hypofractionated, 3-week, preoperative radiotherapy for patients with soft tissue sarcomas (HYPORT-STS): a single-centre, open-label, single-arm, phase 2 trial. Lancet Oncol. 2022;23(12):1547–57.
77. Stinson SF, Delaney TF, Greenberg J, Yang JC, Lampert MH, Hicks JE, et al. Acute and long-term effects on limb function of combined modality limb sparing therapy for extremity soft tissue sarcoma. Int J Radiat Oncol Biol Phys. 1991;21(6):1493–9.
78. Andrews CC, Siegel G, Smith S. Rehabilitation to improve the function and quality of life of soft tissue and bony sarcoma patients. Patient Relat Outcome Meas. 2020;10:417–25.
79. Friedmann D, Wunder JS, Ferguson P, O'Sullivan B, Roberge D, Catton C, et al. Incidence and severity of lymphoedema following limb salvage of extremity soft tissue sarcoma. Sarcoma. 2011;2011:1–6.
80. Wu P, Elswick SM, Akhavan A, Molinar VE, Mohan AT, Curiel D, et al. Risk factors for lymphedema after thigh sarcoma resection and reconstruction. Plast Reconstr Surg Glob Open. 2020;8(7):e2912.
81. Bedi M, King DM, Whitfield R, Hackbarth DA, Neilson JC, Charlson JA, et al. The effect of smoking and major vein resection on post-therapy lymphedema in soft tissue sarcomas treated with neoadjuvant radiation and limb-salvage surgery. Am J Clin Oncol. 2015;38(2):184–8.
82. Sitzia J, Sobrido L. Measurement of health-related quality of life of patients receiving conservative treatment for limb lymphoedema using the Nottingham Health Profile. Qual Life Res. 1997;6(5):373–84.
83. Prendergast B, Fiveash JB, Gibbs CP, Scarborough MT, Indelicato DJ. Radiotherapy for soft tissue sarcoma of the proximal lower extremity. Sarcoma. 2010;2010:1–10.
84. Helmstedter CS, Goebel M, Zlotecki R, Scarborough MT. Pathologic fractures after surgery and radiation for soft tissue tumors. Clin Orthop. 2001;389:165–72.
85. Dickie CI, Parent AL, Griffin AM, Fung S, Chung PWM, Catton CN, et al. Bone fractures following external beam radiotherapy and limb-preservation surgery for lower extremity soft tissue sarcoma: relationship to irradiated bone length, volume, tumor location and dose. Int J Radiat Oncol Biol Phys. 2009;75(4):1119–24.
86. Lin PP, Schupak KD, Boland PJ, Brennan MF, Healey JH. Pathologic femoral fracture after periosteal excision and radiation for the treatment of soft tissue sarcoma. Cancer. 1998;82(12):2356–65.
87. Holt GE, Griffin AM, Pintilie M, Wunder JS, Catton C, O'Sullivan B, et al. Fractures following radiotherapy and limb-salvage surgery for lower extremity soft-tissue sarcomas. A comparison of high-dose and low-dose radiotherapy. J Bone Joint Surg Am. 2005;87(2):315–9.
88. Gortzak Y, Lockwood GA, Mahendra A, Wang Y, Chung PWM, Catton CN, et al. Prediction of pathologic fracture risk of the femur after combined modality treatment of soft tissue sarcoma of the thigh. Cancer. 2010;116(6):1553–9.
89. Sternheim A, Saidi K, Lochab J, O'Donnell PW, Eward WC, Griffin A, et al. Internal fixation of radiation-induced pathological fractures of the femur has a high rate of failure. Bone Jt J. 2013;95-B(8):1144–8.
90. Renn A, Adejolu M, Messiou C, Bhaludin B, Strauss DC, Thway K, et al. Overview of malignant soft-tissue sarcomas of the limbs. Clin Radiol. 2021;76(12):940.e1–16.
91. Mavrogenis A, Angelini A, Pala E, Calabro T, Bianchi G, Casadei R, et al. Radiation-induced sarcomas. J Long-Term Eff Med Implants. 2011;21(3):233–40.
92. Callesen LB, Safwat A, Rose HK, Sørensen FB, Baad-Hansen T, Aggerholm-Pedersen N. Radiation-induced sarcoma: a retrospective population-based study over 34 years in a single institution. Clin Oncol. 2021;33(5):e232–8.
93. Patel SR. Radiation-induced sarcoma. Curr Treat Options in Oncol. 2000;1(3):258–61.
94. Italiano A, Bringer S, Blay JY, Bonvalot S, Le Cesne A, Le Loarer F, et al. Patterns of care and outcome radiation-induced soft tissue sarcomas. Int J Radiat Oncol Biol Phys. 2019;103(2):449–52.
95. Riad S, Biau D, Holt GE, Werier J, Turcotte RE, Ferguson PC, et al. The clinical and functional outcome for patients with radiation-induced soft tissue sarcoma: radiation-induced soft tissue sarcoma. Cancer. 2012;118(10):2682–92.
96. Gladdy RA, Qin LX, Moraco N, Edgar MA, Antonescu CR, Alektiar KM, et al. Do radiation-associated soft tissue sarcomas have the same prognosis as sporadic soft tissue sarcomas? J Clin Oncol. 2010;28(12):2064–9.
97. Pasquali S, Gronchi A. Neoadjuvant chemotherapy in soft tissue sarcomas: latest evidence and clinical implications. Ther Adv Med Oncol. 2017;9(6):415–29.
98. Bedi M, King DM, Shivakoti M, Wang T, Zambrano EV, Charlson J, et al. Prognostic variables in patients with primary soft tissue sarcoma of the extremity and trunk treated with neoadjuvant radiotherapy or neoadjuvant sequential chemoradiotherapy. Radiat Oncol. 2013;8(1):60.
99. Curtis KK, Ashman JB, Beauchamp CP, Schwartz AJ, Callister MD, Dueck AC, et al. Neoadjuvant chemoradiation compared to neoadjuvant radiation alone and surgery alone for stage II and III soft tissue sarcoma of the extremities. Radiat Oncol. 2011;6(1):91.
100. Hong NJL, Hornicek FJ, Harmon DC, Choy E, Chen YL, Yoon SS, et al. Neoadjuvant chemoradiotherapy for patients with high-risk extremity and truncal sarcomas: a 10-year single institution retrospective study. Eur J Cancer. 2013;49(4):875–83.
101. Gortzak E, Azzarelli A, Buesa J, Bramwell VHC, van Coevorden F, van Geel AN, et al. A randomised phase ii study on neo-

adjuvant chemotherapy for 'high-risk' adult soft-tissue sarcoma. Eur J Cancer. 2001;37(9):1096–103.

102. DeLaney TF, Spiro IJ, Suit HD, Gebhardt MC, Hornicek FJ, Mankin HJ, et al. Neoadjuvant chemotherapy and radiotherapy for large extremity soft-tissue sarcomas. Int J Radiat Oncol Biol Phys. 2003;56(4):1117–27.
103. Kobus M, Roohani S, Ehret F, Flörcken A, Striefler JK, Brandes F, et al. The role of neoadjuvant radiochemotherapy in the management of localized high-grade soft tissue sarcoma. Radiat Oncol. 2022;17(1):139.
104. Sarcoma Meta-analysis Collaboration (SMAC)—see acknowledgement section for list of authors. Adjuvant chemotherapy for localised resectable soft tissue sarcoma in adults. Cochrane Gynaecological, Neuro-oncology and Orphan Cancer Group, editor. Cochrane Database Syst Rev. 2000. [cited 2023 Mar 6]. https://doi.wiley.com/10.1002/14651858.CD001419.
105. Gronchi A, Ferrari S, Quagliuolo V, Broto JM, Pousa AL, Grignani G, et al. Histotype-tailored neoadjuvant chemotherapy versus standard chemotherapy in patients with high-risk soft-tissue sarcomas (ISG-STS 1001): an international, open-label, randomised, controlled, phase 3, multicentre trial. Lancet Oncol. 2017;18(6):812–22.
106. Gronchi A, Palmerini E, Quagliuolo V, Martin Broto J, Lopez Pousa A, Grignani G, et al. Neoadjuvant chemotherapy in high-risk soft tissue sarcomas: final results of a randomized trial from Italian (ISG), Spanish (GEIS), French (FSQ), and Polish (PSG) sarcoma groups. J Clin Oncol. 2020;38(19):2178–86.
107. Baldini EH, Le Cesne A, Trent JC. Neoadjuvant chemotherapy, concurrent chemoradiation, and adjuvant chemotherapy for high-risk extremity soft tissue sarcoma. Am Soc Clin Oncol Educ Book. 2018;38:910–5.
108. Ferguson PC, Griffin AM, O'Sullivan B, Catton CN, Davis AM, Murji A, et al. Bone invasion in extremity soft-tissue sarcoma: impact on disease outcomes. Cancer. 2006;106(12):2692–700.
109. Yan TQ, Zhou WH, Guo W, Yang RL, Dong S, Liang WM, et al. Endoprosthetic reconstruction for large extremity soft-tissue sarcoma with juxta-articular bone involvement: functional and survival outcome. J Surg Res. 2014;187(1):142–9.
110. Özger H, Sim FH, Puri A, Eralp L, editors. Orthopedic surgical oncology for bone tumors: a case study atlas. Cham: Springer; 2022. [cited 2023 Mar 6]. https://link.springer.com/10.1007/978-3-030-73327-8.
111. Ghert MA, Abudu A, Driver N, Davis AM, Griffin AM, Pearce D, et al. The indications for and the prognostic significance of amputation as the primary surgical procedure for localized soft tissue sarcoma of the extremity. Ann Surg Oncol. 2005;12(1):10–7.
112. Clarkson PW, Griffin AM, Catton CN, O'Sullivan B, Ferguson PC, Wunder JS, et al. Epineural dissection is a safe technique that facilitates limb salvage surgery. Clin Orthop. 2005;438:92–6.
113. Brooks AD, Gold JS, Graham D, Boland P, Lewis JJ, Brennan MF, et al. Resection of the sciatic, peroneal, or tibial nerves: assessment of functional status. Ann Surg Oncol. 2002;9(1):41–7.
114. Fuchs B, Davis AM, Wunder JS, Bell RS, Masri BA, Isler M, et al. Sciatic nerve resection in the thigh: a functional evaluation. Clin Orthop. 2001;382:34–41.
115. Jones KB, Ferguson PC, Deheshi B, Riad S, Griffin A, Bell RS, et al. Complete femoral nerve resection with soft tissue sarcoma: functional outcomes. Ann Surg Oncol. 2010;17(2):401–6.
116. Martin E, Dullaart MJ, Verhoef C, Coert JH. A systematic review of functional outcomes after nerve reconstruction in extremity soft tissue sarcomas: a need for general implementation in the armamentarium. J Plast Reconstr Aesthet Surg. 2020;73(4):621–32.
117. Karakawa R, Yoshimatsu H, Fuse Y, Tanakura K, Imai T, Sawaizumi M, et al. Immediate tendon transfer for functional reconstruction of a dorsal forearm defect after sarcoma resection. J Plast Surg Hand Surg. 2023;57(1–6):157–62.
118. Shah A, Ramanujan V, Muralidharan K, AnRaja A. Outcomes of vascular resection and reconstruction in extremity soft tissue sarcoma and bone tumors. Vasc Spec Int. 2021;37(1):22–8.
119. Angelini A, Piazza M, Pagliarini E, Trovarelli G, Spertino A, Ruggieri P. The orthopedic-vascular multidisciplinary approach improves patient safety in surgery for musculoskeletal tumors: a large-volume center experience. J Pers Med. 2021;11(6):462.
120. Schwarzbach MHM, Hormann Y, Hinz U, Bernd L, Willeke F, Mechtersheimer G, et al. Results of limb-sparing surgery with vascular replacement for soft tissue sarcoma in the lower extremity. J Vasc Surg. 2005;42(1):88–97.
121. Muramatsu K, Ihara K, Miyoshi T, Yoshida K, Taguchi T. Clinical outcome of limb-salvage surgery after wide resection of sarcoma and femoral vessel reconstruction. Ann Vasc Surg. 2011;25(8):1070–7.
122. van Houdt WJ, Griffin AM, Wunder JS, Ferguson PC. Oncologic outcome and quality of life after hindquarter amputation for sarcoma: is it worth it? Ann Surg Oncol. 2018;25(2):378–86.
123. Smith SR. Rehabilitation strategies and outcomes of the sarcoma patient. Phys Med Rehabil Clin N Am. 2017;28(1):171–80.
124. Bekkering WP, Vliet Vlieland TPM, Koopman HM, Schaap GR, Bart Schreuder HW, Beishuizen A, et al. Functional ability and physical activity in children and young adults after limb-salvage or ablative surgery for lower extremity bone tumors: functioning after bone tumor surgery. J Surg Oncol. 2011;103(3):276–82.
125. Davis AM, Devlin M, Griffin AM, Wunder JS, Bell RS. Functional outcome in amputation versus limb sparing of patients with lower extremity sarcoma: a matched case-control study. Arch Phys Med Rehabil. 1999;80(6):615–8.
126. Hoftiezer YAJ, Lans J, Heijden BEPA, Chen NC, Eberlin KR, Lozano-Calderón SA. Long-term patient-reported outcome measures following limb salvage with complex reconstruction or amputation in the treatment of upper extremity sarcoma. J Surg Oncol. 2021;123(5):1328–35.
127. Grimer RJ, Chandrasekar CR, Carter SR, Abudu A, Tillman RM, Jeys L. Hindquarter amputation: is it still needed and what are the outcomes? Bone Jt J. 2013;95-B(1):127–31.
128. Yari P, Dijkstra PU, Geertzen JH. Functional outcome of hip disarticulation and hemipelvectomy: a cross-sectional national descriptive study in The Netherlands. Clin Rehabil. 2008;22(12):1127–33.
129. Stevenson MG, Musters AH, Geertzen JHB, van Leeuwen BL, Hoekstra HJ, Been LB. Amputations for extremity soft tissue sarcoma in an era of limb salvage treatment: local control and survival. J Surg Oncol. 2018;117(3):434–42.
130. Jubbal KT, D'Souza G, Abrams RA, Kulidjian AA. Management of soft tissue tumors of the upper extremity: a review. SICOT-J. 2017;3:47.
131. Dimas V, Kargel J, Bauer J, Chang P. Forequarter amputation for malignant tumours of the upper extremity: case report, techniques and indications. Can J Plast Surg. 2007;15(2):83–5.

Assessing Functional Outcomes

23

Thomas Baad-Hansen and Sarah Stammose Freund

23.1 Introduction

Evaluating functional outcome after sarcoma surgery is essential for numerous reasons. First, functional outcome measures can provide insight into how well a patient is able to perform activities of daily living and other tasks that are important after surgery. This can help healthcare providers and patients understand the impact of surgery on the patient's overall quality of life. Second, functional outcome measures can be used to assess the effectiveness of surgery in achieving its intended goals. Third, functional outcome measures can be used to identify any potential areas of difficulty or limitations that a person may have after surgery, which can help guide the development of a rehabilitation plan or other interventions to support the patient's recovery. Finally, functional outcome measures can be useful in comparing the outcomes of different treatment approaches or surgical techniques, which can help inform future treatment decisions and improve the overall care of patients with sarcoma.

23.2 What Makes a Good Clinical Score?

When investigating functional outcomes in patient populations, it is important to have a clear understanding of how function is defined. Physical function has by the World Health Organization been classified as a functional impairment defined by Classification of Impairments, Disabilities and Handicap as 'any loss or abnormality of psychological, physiological or anatomical structure or function' [1]. At the same time, functional disability can be understood as 'any restriction or lack of ability to perform an activity in the manner or within the range considered normal for a human being' [1].

T. Baad-Hansen (✉) · S. S. Freund
Sarcoma Division, Department of Orthopaedic Oncology, Aarhus University Hospital, Aarhus, Denmark
e-mail: thombaad@rm.dk; Sarah.freund@auh.rm.dk

Having that in mind, a good clinical test is one that is validated, reliable, and accurate. It should also be based on easily recordable variables, be applied to all groups of patients, be applicable to all geographical locations, ethical, and cost-effective.

23.2.1 Validation

It is important to test the measurement properties of an instrument to ensure that the score measures correctly and is reliable. Measurement properties are also known as psychometric properties. Mokkink et al. [2] found an international consensus on the taxonomy used in studies with respect to the report of psychometric properties. The COSMIN study reached agreement among several international experts on taxonomy, terminology, and definitions of psychometric properties, such as validity and reliability [2]. The COSMIN study is intended for newly developed instruments. The concept of the COSMIN study is however still valid when testing a culturally and linguistically adapted questionnaire.

Validity and reliability are two main domains in the COSMIN taxonomy, in which validity can be subdivided into construct validity, criterion validity, and content validity. Reliability can be subdivided into reliability, internal consistency, and measurement of error.

23.2.2 Validity

The validity of the construct is a measurement of the amount to which the instrument score can measure the concept for which it has been developed, for example, the functional outcome or the quality of life. This is usually tested by hypotheses or comparisons with another instrument developed for that specific outcome [2, 3].

H. Özger et al. (eds.), *Diagnosis and Treatment of Soft Tissue Tumors*, https://doi.org/10.1007/978-3-031-77061-6_23

23.2.3 Reliability

The internal consistency is a measure according to which each item in an instrument measure the same aspect. This is an important measurement property for a questionnaire which intends to measure one concept through several items [2, 3].

Reliability as a subdomain is also known as the reproducibility of an instrument. However, in the COSMIN study, a consensus was established to refer to it as reliability [2]. The reliability sub-domain is the measurement property according to which the instrument can distinguish the patients from each other when measurement error is considered. However, this can be evaluated between patients and within patients (test–retest, over time). One method to assess reliability is to use the intraclass correlation coefficient (ICC) [3, 4].

The measurement error is also a subdomain of reliability. It is defined as the systematic and random error of the score of a patient that is not caused by real changes in the concept to be measured [2]. Measurement error can be investigated between subjects over time or between different raters. A Bland–Altman plot with limits of agreement is an easy and reliable way to identify the systematic and random error [5].

The ceiling and floor effect refers to the situation where a measure or score is unable to detect or capture changes in the highest range of the scale and are defined as the number of patients who achieve the lowest or highest possible scores on a measurement instrument. For example, if a measure has a ceiling of 100, it will be unable to detect changes in scores above 100. If more than 15% of the patients receive the lowest or highest score, an effect of the floor or ceiling is considered present [3]. These effects are important parameters to look for, as their presence can result in reduced reliability due to the difficulties of distinguishing between those patients who have the lowest or highest score, respectively [3].

Ethics refers to the ethical considerations involved in administering the test. The test should be administered in a way that respects the rights and dignity of the individuals being tested.

Cost-effectiveness refers to the balance between the benefits and costs of the test. A good clinical test should provide sufficient benefits to justify the costs involved in administering it. Ease of use refers to the simplicity and practicality of administering the score. A score that is easy to use will be quick to administer and require minimal training.

23.3 Clinical Score Systems and Methods Evaluating Function Outcome

An extensive number of methods are used to assess functional outcome after sarcoma surgery.

After a simple search on Medline with the following search strings: Sarcoma and 'functional outcome', Sarcoma and 'Recovery of Function', and Sarcoma and 'Motor Activity', a total of 661 published articles were identified in the period from 1 January 2004 to 30 November 2022. Of these, 421 of the abstracts explained which methods (one or more) were used to report functional outcome.

As shown in Table 23.1, the Musculoskeletal Tumour Society Score (MSTS) is by far the most used method for reporting functional outcome in sarcoma patients. The MSTS is a physician completed questionnaire [6], whereas the Toronto Extremity Salvage Score (TESS) is a patient completed questionnaire [7].

The MSTS and the TESS should however be considered as more subjective measurements since they are possibly influenced by the physician/patient completing it. New specific tools have been introduced in recent years to assess physical activity levels in long-term survivors of sarcoma, e.g. the UCLA score system that evaluates sport activity levels after treatment [8], but also objective measurements of physical function, such as the TUG and range of motion, are less likely to be subjectively influenced; however, they are rarely used in sarcoma research [9, 10], as reported in Table 23.1.

23.3.1 Clinical Score Systems

23.3.1.1 The Musculoskeletal Tumour Society Score (MSTS)

MSTS was developed in 1987 as a disease-specific measurement of function in patients who had undergone surgery for neoplasms in the extremities.

Table 23.1 Methods used to measure physical function in patients with sarcomas

	No. (% of studies)
Musculoskeletal Tumour Society Score (MSTS)	292 (69%)
Toronto Extremity Salvage Score (TESS)	82 (19%)
Range of Motion (ROM)	14 (3%)
Patient-Reported Outcomes Measurement Information System (PROMIS)	12 (3%)
SF-36	8 (2%)
Reintegration to normal	7 (2%)
Disabilities of the Arm, Shoulder, and Hand (DASH)	7 (2%)
Isokinetic test	5 (1%)
Timed Up & Go (TUG)	5 (1%)
Timed Up & Down Stairs	4 (1%)
UCLA Score	3 (1%)
Functional Mobility Assessment	3 (1%)
9-Minute Walk	2 (less than 1%)
American Orthopaedic Foot and Ankle Score	2 (less than 1%)

The initial MSTS consisted of seven elements: pain, range of motion, emotional acceptance, strength, general function, joint stability, and joint deformity. Each of these items was rated by the physician and a total score (ranging from 0 to 35) was calculated [6]. However, to improve the evaluation of the entire extremity and patients with sarcoma as a whole, the MSTS was revised by Enneking et al. [11] in 1993 so the MSTS questionnaire now consists of six items, where three items (pain, functional activities, and emotional acceptance) are generic and three items are specific for either the upper extremity (dexterity, lifting ability and positioning of the hand) or the lower extremity (use of external supports, walking ability, and gait). Each item is scored on a scale from 0 to 5, where the total score is calculated as a percentage, thus ranging from 0 to 100 (Tables 23.2 and 23.3). The original English MSTS has never been properly validated in terms of its psychometric properties, except for the interrater reliability, which was found to be good [11]. The MSTS has been translated according to international guidelines into Brazilian Portuguese, Danish, Japanese, and Chinese [12–15].

23.3.1.2 The Toronto Extremity Salvage Score (TESS)

TESS was developed in the mid-1990s by Davis et al. [7] and is intended as a disease-specific functional status instrument that measures disability as perceived by patients, where disability is based on the classification from the ICIDH. It is divided into an upper and lower extremity version consisting of 29 and 30 items respectively, which concerns daily activities. The questionnaire is solely completed by the patient, Patient-Reported Outcome Measure (PROM). Each item is scored from 1 to 5. A total score of the elements is calculated, ranging from 0 to 100. During the development of the questionnaire, psychometric properties were tested and found to be good. The TESS has been translated according to international guidelines into Brazilian Portuguese (lower extremity version only) [16], Korean, Japanese, Chinese, and Dutch [17–20]. The English TESS has also been tested for sensitivity to age, gender and cultural background in a normal population, where age is found to be the only significant factor influencing the TESS score [21]. Furthermore, the TESS has been validated for online use [22].

23.3.1.3 Disabilities of the Arm, Shoulder, and Hand (DASH)

The DASH is a questionnaire designed to describe the disability experienced by patients with upper extremity disorders. It is a 30-item self-report questionnaire and has been applied in several articles on upper limb sarcomas [23, 24] and a strong correlation with the TESS score [25] has been reported.

23.3.1.4 Patient-Reported Outcomes Measurement Information System (PROMIS)

In 2004, the National Institute of Health (NIH) initiated PROMIS with the intention of providing more accurate, reliable, and generalizable measures of outcomes that are relevant to the patients [25]. PROMIS are non-disease-specific measures that evaluate physical, mental, and social health. PROMIS is constructed with Item Response Theory (IRT), where an IRT-calibrated item bank consists of items (questions), each denoting a level of symptom (e.g. pain) or function (e.g. physical function). Items can be scored and compared to all other measures derived from the same item bank.

PROMIS has the advantage of using Computer Adaptive Tests (CATs), where the items are tailored to the respondent. An item in the middle of the range of function is administered and an estimated score is calculated on the patient's

Table 23.2 Revised MSTS score lower limb

	Pain	Function	Emotional acceptance	Supports	Walking	Gait
5	None	No restrictions	Enthused	None	Unlimited	Normal
4	Intermediate					
3	Modest	Recreational restrictions	Satisfied	Brace	Limited	Minor cosmetic
2	Intermediate					
1	Moderate	Partial disability	Accepts	One cane/crutch	Inside only	Major cosmetic
0	Severe	Total disability	Dislikes	Two canes/crutches	Unable unaided	Major handicap

Table 23.3 Revised MSTS score upper limb

	Pain	Function	Emotional acceptance	Hand positioning	Dexterity	Lifting ability
5	None	No restrictions	Enthused	Unlimited	Normal	Normal
4	Intermediate					
3	Modest	Recreational restrictions	Satisfied	Not above shoulder or no pro/sup	Loss of fine movements	Limited
2	Intermediate					
1	Moderate	Partial disability	Accepts	Not above waist	Cannot pinch	Helping only
0	Severe	Total disability	Dislikes	Flail	Cannot grasp	Cannot

response. The most suited item for refining the patients score is then selected by the CAT algorithm. The CAT will continue until either the standard error drops below a specified level, or the participant has answered the maximum number of items (e.g. 12). Each item usually has five response options on a Likert scale. The final score for PROMIS measures is represented by the T-score, a standardized score with a mean of 50 (United States general population) and a standard deviation of 10 [26–28]. In addition to being psychometrically sound, PROMIS-CAT has been validated in Orthopaedic oncology populations with reduced floor and ceiling effect along with reduced question burden [29–32].

According to NIH, approximately 70 PROMIS domains have been developed and translated according to international guidelines into more than 40 languages [33].

23.3.2 Objective Measurement Tests

23.3.2.1 Range of Motion

Joint specific range of motions are often stated in combination with a clinical score systems [34] and are typically reported in degrees based on instruments such as goniometers or inclinometers. Range of motion can both be expressed as active or passive range of motion, depending on assistance by the examiner.

23.3.2.2 The Timed Up & Go (TUG)

The TUG originates from the 'Get-up and go test' developed by Mathias et al. [35]. The get-up and go test consists of a patient sitting in a chair who on the command 'go' rises, walks 3 m at a safe and comfortable speed, turns, walks back to the chair, and sits down. Afterwards an observer scores the patient between 1 and 5 based on the observer's assessment of the patient's risk of falling during the test. Podsiadlo et al. [36] have since suggested using the time between the command 'go' and until the patient sat down in the chair again. After this amendment in the scoring approach, the test has been known as the 'Timed Up & Go' test. The TUG has been found to have good validity and reliability [37, 38] and are used to measure a combined aspect of patients' gait and balance, in a variety of populations, including the sarcoma population [9, 10].

23.3.2.3 The 10-Metre Walk Test (10-MWT)

The 10-MWT is a standardized test in which patients are instructed to walk at their normal comfortable speed or at their maximum speed of 10 m. The middle six meters are timed, allowing patients to have an acceleration/deceleration of 2 m [39]. Normative data exist for adults aged 20–79 years [39, 40]. The 10-MWT has shown excellent test–retest reliability in cancer patients [41].

23.3.3 The 6-Minute Walking Test (6-MWT)

The 6-MWT has since been used in many different patient populations, including cancer patients [42]. 6-MWT is a simple and easy test to assess exercise capacity, and specific guidelines have been established for carrying out the test [43]. To perform the test, a 20- to 30-m hallway is required, patients are instructed to walk at their fastest pace covering as much distance as possible in 6 min, during which the test supervisor gives standardized encouragements every minute. Psychometric properties tests have shown that 6-MWT has good validity and reliability in various populations, including cancer patients [42, 44].

23.3.4 Isokinetic Tests

The Biodex System 3 PRO® dynamometer is a method to objectively measure the strength of a joint in the upper and lower extremities. Biodex can be used as an isokinetic dynamometer, which means that the dynamometer provides a constant velocity with accommodating resistance throughout the range of motion of the joint. The Biodex dynamometer has been proven to be reliable and valid for measuring muscle strength in patients [45]. Only a few studies have previously measured strength in patients with sarcoma using a dynamometer [46–48].

23.3.5 Nine-Hole Peg Test (9-HPT)

The 9-HPT is one of the most widely used methods for measuring dexterity in the hand. It was introduced for the first time in 1971, although reintroduced in 1985 when Mathiowetz et al. created a guideline for its use and tested the reliability and normative data [49]. The 9-HPT consists of a plastic console consisting of a shallow round dish for the pegs, and the nine holes on the other side of the console. The patient is asked to centre the console in front of him so that the shallow dish is on the dominant side of the patient. Reliability has been tested, and normative data are available for 9-HPT [49, 50]; however, 9-HPT has not been used in sarcoma clinical research, although it has been used in other cancer patients [51].

References

1. WHO. WHO classification of impairments, disabilities and handicaps. 1993.
2. Mokkink LB, Terwee CB, Patrick DL, Alonso J, Stratford PW, Knol DL, et al. The COSMIN study reached international consensus on taxonomy, terminology, and definitions of measurement properties

for health-related patient-reported outcomes. J Clin Epidemiol. 2010;63(7):737–45.
3. Terwee CB, Bot SD, de Boer MR, van der Windt DA, Knol DL, Dekker J, et al. Quality criteria were proposed for measurement properties of health status questionnaires. J Clin Epidemiol. 2007;60(1):34–42.
4. de Vet HC, Terwee CB, Knol DL, Bouter LM. When to use agreement versus reliability measures. J Clin Epidemiol. 2006;59(10):1033–9.
5. Bland JM, Altman DG. Statistical methods for assessing agreement between two methods of clinical measurement. Lancet. 1986;1(8476):307–10.
6. Enneking WF. [The training of future orthopedic specialists]. Chir Organi Mov. 1987;72(4):309–11.
7. Davis AM, Wright JG, Williams JI, Bombardier C, Griffin A, Bell RS. Development of a measure of physical function for patients with bone and soft tissue sarcoma. Qual Life Res. 1996;5(5):508–16.
8. Lang NW, Hobusch GM, Funovics PT, Windhager R, Hofstaetter JG. What sports activity levels are achieved in patients with modular tumor endoprostheses of osteosarcoma about the knee? Clin Orthop Relat Res. 2015;473(3):847–54.
9. Marchese VG, Ogle S, Womer RB, Dormans J, Ginsberg JP. An examination of outcome measures to assess functional mobility in childhood survivors of osteosarcoma. Pediatr Blood Cancer. 2004;42(1):41–5.
10. Marchese VG, Spearing E, Callaway L, Rai SN, Zhang L, Hinds PS, et al. Relationships among range of motion, functional mobility, and quality of life in children and adolescents after limb-sparing surgery for lower-extremity sarcoma. Pediatr Phys Ther. 2006;18(4):238–44.
11. Enneking WF, Dunham W, Gebhardt MC, Malawar M, Pritchard DJ. A system for the functional evaluation of reconstructive procedures after surgical treatment of tumors of the musculoskeletal system. Clin Orthop Relat Res. 1993;286:241–6.
12. Iwata S, Uehara K, Ogura K, Akiyama T, Shinoda Y, Yonemoto T, et al. Reliability and validity of a Japanese-language and culturally adapted version of the Musculoskeletal Tumor Society scoring system for the lower extremity. Clin Orthop Relat Res. 2016;474(9):2044–52.
13. Rebolledo DC, Vissoci JR, Pietrobon R, de Camargo OP, Baptista AM. Validation of the Brazilian version of the Musculoskeletal Tumor Society rating scale for lower extremity bone sarcoma. Clin Orthop Relat Res. 2013;471(12):4020–6.
14. Saebye CKP, Keller J, Baad-Hansen T. Validation of the Danish version of the Musculoskeletal Tumour Society score questionnaire. World J Orthop. 2019;10(1):23–32.
15. Xu L, Li X, Wang Z, Xiong J, Wang S. Functional evaluation for patients with lower extremity sarcoma: application of the Chinese version of Musculoskeletal Tumor Society scoring system. Health Qual Life Outcomes. 2017;15(1):107.
16. Saraiva D, de Camargo B, Davis AM. Cultural adaptation, translation and validation of a functional outcome questionnaire (TESS) to Portuguese with application to patients with lower extremity osteosarcoma. Pediatr Blood Cancer. 2008;50(5):1039–42.
17. Akiyama T, Uehara K, Ogura K, Shinoda Y, Iwata S, Saita K, et al. Cross-cultural adaptation and validation of the Japanese version of the Toronto Extremity Salvage Score (TESS) for patients with malignant musculoskeletal tumors in the upper extremities. J Orthop Sci. 2017;22(1):127–32.
18. Kim HS, Yun J, Kang S, Han I. Cross-cultural adaptation and validation of the Korean Toronto Extremity Salvage Score for extremity sarcoma. J Surg Oncol. 2015;112(1):93–7.
19. Willeumier JJ, van der Wal C, van der Wal RJP, Dijkstra PDS, Vliet Vlieland TPM, van de Sande MAJ. Cross-cultural adaptation, translation, and validation of the Toronto Extremity Salvage Score for extremity bone and soft tissue tumor patients in Netherlands. Sarcoma. 2017;2017:6197525.
20. Xu L, Sun M, Sun W, Qin X, Zhu Z, Wang S. Cross-cultural adaptation and validation of the Chinese version of Toronto Extremity Salvage Score for patients with extremity sarcoma. Springerplus. 2016;5(1):1118.
21. Clayer M, Doyle S, Sangha N, Grimer R. The Toronto Extremity Salvage Score in unoperated controls: an age, gender, and country comparison. Sarcoma. 2012;2012:717213.
22. Clayer M, Davis A. Can the Toronto Extremity Salvage Score produce reliable results when used online? Clin Orthop Relat Res. 2011;469(6):1750–6.
23. Barret H, Bozon O, Fassot G, Chammas M, Coulet B, Lazerges C. What is the patient acceptance when only scapulectomy is possible in case of malignant tumor? A case series. JSES Int. 2022;6(6):1034–41.
24. Yamada Y, Nishida Y, Nakashima H, Sugiura H, Tsukushi S, Kamei Y, et al. Oncologic and functional outcomes of soft tissue sarcomas of the distal upper extremity: comparison with those of the proximal upper extremity. Int Surg. 2010;95(1):33–9.
25. Cella D, Riley W, Stone A, Rothrock N, Reeve B, Yount S, et al. The Patient-Reported Outcomes Measurement Information System (PROMIS) developed and tested its first wave of adult self-reported health outcome item banks: 2005-2008. J Clin Epidemiol. 2010;63(11):1179–94.
26. Cella D, Gershon R, Lai JS, Choi S. The future of outcomes measurement: item banking, tailored short-forms, and computerized adaptive assessment. Qual Life Res. 2007;16(Suppl 1):133–41.
27. Garcia SF, Cella D, Clauser SB, Flynn KE, Lad T, Lai J-S, et al. Standardizing patient-reported outcomes assessment in cancer clinical trials: a patient-reported outcomes measurement information system initiative. J Clin Oncol. 2007;25(32):5106–12.
28. Rose M, Bjorner JB, Becker J, Fries JF, Ware JE. Evaluation of a preliminary physical function item bank supported the expected advantages of the Patient-Reported Outcomes Measurement Information System (PROMIS). J Clin Epidemiol. 2008;61(1):17–33.
29. Reeve BB, Hays RD, Bjorner JB, Cook KF, Crane PK, Teresi JA, et al. Psychometric evaluation and calibration of health-related quality of life item banks: plans for the Patient-Reported Outcomes Measurement Information System (PROMIS). Med Care. 2007;45(5 Suppl 1):S22–31.
30. Jensen RE, Potosky AL, Reeve BB, Hahn E, Cella D, Fries J, et al. Validation of the PROMIS physical function measures in a diverse US population-based cohort of cancer patients. Qual Life Res. 2015;24(10):2333–44.
31. Janssen SJ, Paulino Pereira NR, Raskin KA, Ferrone ML, Hornicek FJ, van Dijk CN, et al. A comparison of questionnaires for assessing physical function in patients with lower extremity bone metastases. J Surg Oncol. 2016;114(6):691–6.
32. Ploetze KL, Dalton JF, Calfee RP, McDonald DJ, O'Keefe RJ, Cipriano CA. Patient-Reported Outcomes Measurement Information System physical function correlates with Toronto Extremity Salvage Score in an orthopaedic oncology population. J Orthop Translat. 2019;19:143–50.
33. Patient-Reported Outcomes Measurement Information System (PROMIS): National Institute of Health; 2019. https://commonfund.nih.gov/promis.
34. Houdek MT, Wellings EP, Mallett KE, Honig RL, Rose PS, Moran SL. Free functional latissimus dorsi reconstruction of the quadriceps and hamstrings following oncologic resection of soft tissue sarcomas of the thigh. Sarcoma. 2021;2021:8480737.
35. Mathias S, Nayak US, Isaacs B. Balance in elderly patients: the "get-up and go" test. Arch Phys Med Rehabil. 1986;67(6):387–9.
36. Podsiadlo D, Richardson S. The timed "up & go": a test of basic functional mobility for frail elderly persons. J Am Geriatr Soc. 1991;39(2):142–8.

37. Lin MR, Hwang HF, Hu MH, Wu HD, Wang YW, Huang FC. Psychometric comparisons of the timed up and go, one-leg stand, functional reach, and Tinetti balance measures in community-dwelling older people. J Am Geriatr Soc. 2004;52(8):1343–8.
38. Schoppen T, Boonstra A, Groothoff JW, de Vries J, Goeken LN, Eisma WH. The timed "up and go" test: reliability and validity in persons with unilateral lower limb amputation. Arch Phys Med Rehabil. 1999;80(7):825–8.
39. Bohannon RW, Andrews AW, Thomas MW. Walking speed: reference values and correlates for older adults. J Orthop Sports Phys Ther. 1996;24(2):86–90.
40. Bohannon RW. Comfortable and maximum walking speed of adults aged 20-79 years: reference values and determinants. Age Ageing. 1997;26(1):15–9.
41. Eden MM, Tompkins J, Verheijde JL. Reliability and a correlational analysis of the 6MWT, ten-meter walk test, thirty second sit to stand, and the linear analog scale of function in patients with head and neck cancer. Physiother Theory Pract. 2018;34(3):202–11.
42. Schmidt K, Vogt L, Thiel C, Jager E, Banzer W. Validity of the six-minute walk test in cancer patients. Int J Sports Med. 2013;34(7):631–6.
43. Enright PL. The six-minute walk test. Respir Care. 2003;48(8):783–5.
44. Gibbons WJ, Fruchter N, Sloan S, Levy RD. Reference values for a multiple repetition 6-minute walk test in healthy adults older than 20 years. J Cardpulm Rehabil. 2001;21(2):87–93.
45. Nordez A, Casari P, Cornu C. Accuracy of Biodex system 3 pro computerized dynamometer in passive mode. Med Eng Phys. 2008;30(7):880–7.
46. Tanaka A, Yoshimura Y, Aoki K, Okamoto M, Kito M, Suzuki S, et al. Prediction of muscle strength and postoperative function after knee flexor muscle resection for soft tissue sarcoma of the lower limbs. Orthop Traumatol Surg Res. 2017;103(7):1081–5.
47. Fernandez-Pineda I, Hudson MM, Pappo AS, Bishop MW, Klosky JL, Brinkman TM, et al. Long-term functional outcomes and quality of life in adult survivors of childhood extremity sarcomas: a report from the St. Jude Lifetime Cohort Study. J Cancer Surviv. 2017;11(1):1–12.
48. Saebye C, Amidi A, Keller J, Andersen H, Baad-Hansen T. Changes in functional outcome and quality of life in soft tissue sarcoma patients within the first year after surgery: a prospective observational study. Cancers (Basel). 2020;12(2):463.
49. Mathiowetz V, Volland G, Kashman N, Weber K. Adult norms for the Box and Block Test of manual dexterity. Am J Occup Ther. 1985;39(6):386–91.
50. Oxford Grice K, Vogel KA, Le V, Mitchell A, Muniz S, Vollmer MA. Adult norms for a commercially available Nine Hole Peg Test for finger dexterity. Am J Occup Ther. 2003;57(5):570–3.
51. Gorter RR, Vos CG, Halmans J, Hartemink KJ, Paul MA, Oosterhuis JW. Evaluation of arm function and quality of life after trimodality treatment for superior sulcus tumours. Interact Cardiovasc Thorac Surg. 2013;16(1):44–8.

Prevention and Treatment of Complications

24

Levent Eralp, Buğra Alpan, Melih Civan, and Harzem Özger

In the constantly evolving field of medical science, the past three decades have seen tremendous advancements that have significantly transformed patient care approaches, especially in the realm of oncology. Major developments in imagining, pathology, surgery and radiotherapy techniques have heralded a new are in the treatment of soft tissue sarcomas. These advancements have made limb-sparing surgery (LSS) a viable option for approximately 90% of patients diagnosed with this condition.

As is the case with any medical progression, the new techniques bring a set of challenges alongside the benefits. The acceptance of more complex tumors as surgically removable has, for instance, led to an increase in complications rates. It is imperative that these potential complications are mitigated effectively to ensure the best possible patient outcomes. Surgeons can evaluate and improve their abilities in order to enhance patient outcomes and avoid complications through various means.

First and foremost, complication reporting and analysis is a crucial step. This involves documenting and deviations from the expected course during or after surgery and performing thorough investigation of each case [1]. These deviations may range from minor postoperative to severe unexpected outcomes. By analyzing these incidents, surgeons can glean valuable insights into the factors that led to the complications, and subsequently develop strategies to avoid such events in the future.

L. Eralp · H. Özger
Department of Orthopedics and Traumatology, Istanbul University, Istanbul Medical Faculty, Istanbul, Türkiye
e-mail: drleventeralp@gmail.com; harzemo@yahoo.com

B. Alpan
Department of Orthopedics and Traumatology, Acıbadem Mehmet Ali Aydınlar University, School of Medicine, Istanbul, Türkiye
e-mail: bugra.alpan@acibadem.edu.tr

M. Civan (✉)
Department of Orthopedics and Traumatology, Başakşehir Çam ve Sakura City Hospital, Istanbul, Türkiye
e-mail: melihcivan@gmail.com

When it comes to the specifics of soft tissue sarcomas, complications can be evaluated in terms of chronology, treatment stage-related and their severity. While the first two assessments are grounded in our accumulated knowledge, the latter will unveil the current scoring systems, accompanying statistical analyses, and most importantly, the risk factors these analyses predict. Knowing or expecting risk factors will guide us in incorporating medical or surgical measures to prevent them into our game plan.

To elaborate:

1. Chronological evaluation: This involves stages of diagnosis (examination, imaging, biopsy), determination of the treatment strategy, preoperative/intraoperative/postoperative course, and follow-up processes.
2. The stages of treatment-related complications, specifically; consist of biopsy, preoperative oncological treatment choice, intraoperative period, and early postoperative periods.
3. For determining severity; nonspecific classifications like problems/complications/sequelae or numerical classifications such as the Clavien–Dindo scoring system can be used.

This systematic approach helps in the comprehensive understanding of the potential risks and effective planning to mitigate these risks, thereby improving the overall patient outcomes.

During the diagnostic stage, three fundamental problems can arise: inadequate imaging, insufficient evaluation of the imaging, and incorrect biopsy procedures. In case of soft tissue sarcomas, the gold-standard imagining method for initial diagnosis, preparing for surgery after neoadjuvant treatments, and postoperative follow-ups is MRI with intravenous contrast. Basic mistakes in MRI interpretation may not include imaging the entire compartment, inability to perceive the border characteristics of the inflammatory area around the tumor, overlooking possible periosteal and bone cortex invasion, missing the potential gelatinous content of the

H. Özger et al. (eds.), *Diagnosis and Treatment of Soft Tissue Tumors*, https://doi.org/10.1007/978-3-031-77061-6_24

tumor, overlooking the tail sign in surgical planning, and confusing postoperative changes and recurrent tumors in follow-up MRIs.

To prevent complications in radiological evaluation, the understanding philosophy could be described as "not missing the unseen behind the visible." That is to say, while the imaging may provide a substantial amount of information, it's crucial to interpret these findings correctly and to look beyond the obvious, recognizing subtle clues and signs that may indicate potential complications or specific characteristics of the tumor.

In addition to radiological diagnosis, biopsy procedure and its correct implementation also plays a vital role in the diagnostic process. Mistakes in biopsy procedure can lead to inaccurate diagnosis and staging, inappropriate treatment strategy, and even inadvertent tumor spread. Therefore, conducting the biopsy in a systematic and precise manner, ideally by a surgeon experienced in managing soft tissue sarcomas, is vital to ensure accurate diagnosis and appropriate treatment planning. This procedure should follow an incision line that could be used for potential surgery, employing a technique that controls the hematoma formation. Considering that the biopsy pathway will be removed with the tumor during surgery, the needle entry point should be marked with a 2 mm cross incision line using a number 11 scalpel. The primary resection incision and the biopsy incision, if performed openly, should not intersect at a right angle.

Most avoidable or treatable complications are primarily associated with surgical technique and radiotherapy. Thus, the remainder of this discussion will focus on these particular events. In contemporary practice, the treatment of soft tissue sarcomas with safe margin resection combined with radiotherapy has yielded local control rates expressed in the 90th percentile [2–5]. However, various studies have examined the influence of the timing of radiotherapy (preoperative vs. postoperative) on local and systemic survival rates and have produced different findings [6–10]. The authors of this section, following the approach proposed by O'Sullivan et al., generally prefer preoperative radiotherapy [11]. Postoperative radiotherapy's main disadvantages include a larger radiation field, the requirement for a higher dose and increased risk of long-term fibrosis and functional loss [4]. On the other hand, preoperative radiotherapy is favored for two main reasons: it involves a smaller radiation field and a lower dose, therefore resulting in better functional outcomes. However, this approach's primary drawback is an increased risk of postoperative wound complications [6, 10, 12].

At this stage, immediate flap surgery or VAC (vacuum-assisted closure) applications, which we will detail below, are utilized to minimize the mentioned risks [7, 13]. To assist in planning, studies or nomograms predicting wound healing problems can provide data-driven support for decision-making. In this context, risk factors have been identified as diabetes, age, smoking, body mass index, tumor localization and proximity to the skin of less than 3 mm, timing of radiotherapy, applications of local pedicled flaps, and neurovascular involvement. Studies have also shown that preoperative laboratory findings, such as a poor ratio of C-reactive protein (CRP) to albumin and a high neutrophil-to-platelet score (NPS), significantly increase the risk of major wound complications [6]. These patients should be followed with VAC for a period, even if the incision can be easily closed. If the orthopedic oncology team recognizes these risk factors in advance, they can take significant steps to prevent wound healing problems with proactive interventions before or during surgery.

Improving the patient's nutritional parameters before surgery, controlling weight, utilizing different radiotherapy techniques if necessary (like IMRT, brachytherapy, etc.) or choosing the appropriate flap are impactful parameters of the outcome. Although not yet in routine use, it is possible to identify hypovascular areas in the skin by performing indocyanine green fluorescence angiography before the surgery concludes. Subsequently, these areas can be covered with healthier tissues through resections [9].

Another group that may experience soft tissue complications consists of those where a previous incorrect resection (known as a "whoops procedure") cannot be completely removed with the new extensive resection incision. In these situations, the contaminated area should be removed through the "tunnel technique" employing broad margins from the opposite side. If the previous incision can be entirely removed with a single cut, even when it results in a significant loss of skin tissue, reconstructive techniques should not be avoided. Methods such as delayed primary closure with vacuum-assisted closure (VAC), rotational flaps, and even free flap procedures can be effectively used in these situations (Fig. 24.1a–m).

In patients treated with surgery and radio/chemotherapy due to soft tissue sarcoma, surgeries aiming to preserve the limb and its function can be complicated by wound healing issues. In these unwanted situations, plastic surgical reconstructions become necessary. The preferred approach is for these interventions to occur in the same session as the primary resection, thus taking on a preventative rather than remedial role [14].

Wound healing occurs in three phases: inflammation, repair, and remodeling. All of these stages can be adversely affected by radiotherapy and even chemotherapy. Particularly in irradiated anatomical areas, factors like hypovascularity, slowed cell division, and the fibrosis process can hinder wound healing. Theoretically, regular wound care, vacuum-assisted closure (VAC), improving the patient's nutritional parameters, and even hyperbaric oxygen therapy (HBOT) can be used to manage the adverse conditions of the wound

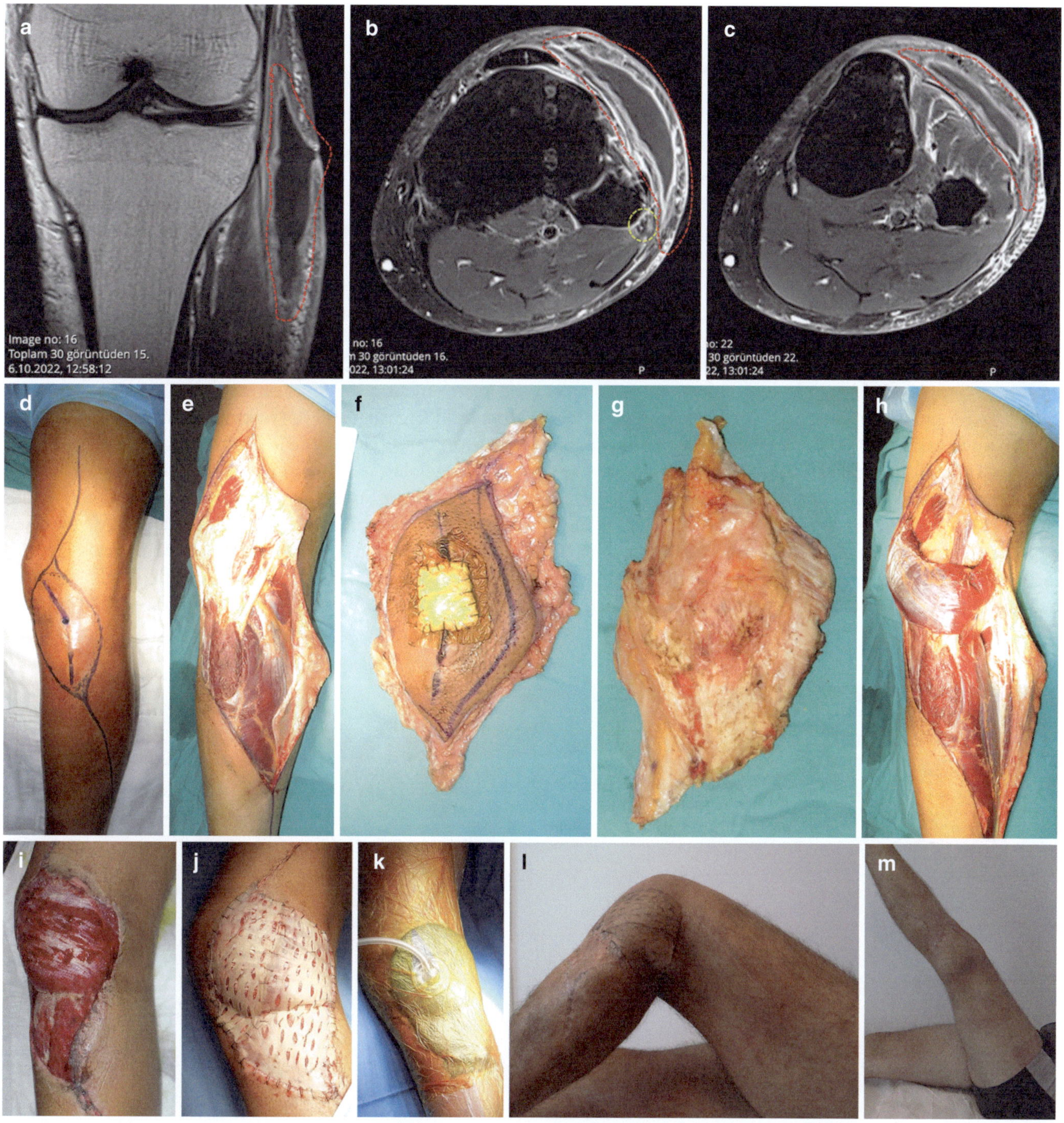

Fig. 24.1 (**a**–**m**) 43-year-old male patient presented to us following a "whoops procedure" performed elsewhere on the lateral aspect of his left knee. His history revealed that a soft tissue mass was excised piecemeal with a presumed diagnosis of subcutaneous hematoma and without preoperative imaging. However, the postoperative pathology report confirmed a diagnosis of low-grade myxoid fibrosarcoma. An infected seroma with a fistula had formed at the site of the operation. Coronal and axial contrast-enhanced MRI sections demonstrate the extent of fluid collection and the tumor-contaminated area (red-dashed line) at presentation (**a**–**c**). Close proximity of the fibular nerve (yellow-dashed circle) to the unplanned resection site is also observed (**b**). Images show tumor bed resection following neoadjuvant radiotherapy. The cavity was injected with methylene blue through the fistula green-dashed circle (**d**), and macroscopic examination of the resected specimen (**f** and **g**) confirmed wide resection of the cavitary lesion. Intraoperative images show soft tissue reconstruction with lateral gastrocnemius rotational flap, which was aimed at covering the lateral aspect of the knee joint as well as obliterating dead space (**h**). After an initial episode of negative-pressure wound treatment, sufficient granulation was observed on the muscle flap (**i**), and split-thickness skin grafting (**j**) was performed with the aid of further negative-pressure wound treatment (**k**). Clinical images at postoperative 7 months show excellent soft tissue healing and function (**l** and **m**). The case illustrates both complication management and complication prevention in soft tissue sarcomas

healing environment. However, plastic surgical reconstructions play a decisive role [4, 12, 14, 15].

Although we consider VAC a supportive method, we believe its preventative role in wound complications is increasingly being recognized. We will devote a separate paragraph to this method.

The primary aim of plastic surgical methods is to close the fascia, subcutaneous tissues, and skin left behind following resection using loose stiches. If this cannot be achieved with primary sutures, the use of local or free flaps will be necessary. If the local flap planned to be used remains within the preoperative radiotherapy area, it should be kept in mind that this tissue may also experience issues due to problems with vascularity and elasticity.

While "propeller" flaps, which are based on perforators and allow for up to 180° rotation, can be easily applied, they are known to carry a 10–25% complication risk even in non-irradiated limbs. Therefore, free (myocutaneous) flaps, which have a lower complication rate, may be the preferred choice [14].

As a general approach, reconstruction of defects on the torso should be performed with perforator flaps, while defects on the extremities should be reconstructed using free flaps. The need for a free flap increases as one moves distally in the lower extremity (Fig. 24.2a–f).

Particularly following Limb-Sparing Surgery (LSS) applied to patients involving neurovascular structures, defect repair with free flaps significantly reduces major wound healing problems, regardless of the timing of radiotherapy [2, 5].

Vacuum-assisted closure (VAC), also known as negative pressure wound therapy, affects wound healing through direct and indirect mechanisms. The direct mechanism involves the approximation of wound edges through suction and negative pressure. Indirect mechanisms include enhancing local blood flow, reducing bacterial load through exudate absorption, facilitating the migration of fibroblastic growth factors to the healing area, directing collagen fiber orientation, and increasing VEGF (vascular endothelial growth factor) expression. The theoretical concern with VAC treatment is the possible promotion of malignant cell growth due to sub-atmospheric pressure. However, randomized studies examining this issue suggest that the use of VAC does not increase local recurrence rates. One detail that may contribute to the safety of the method is determining boundary characteristics intraoperatively with a "frozen section" [7, 10].

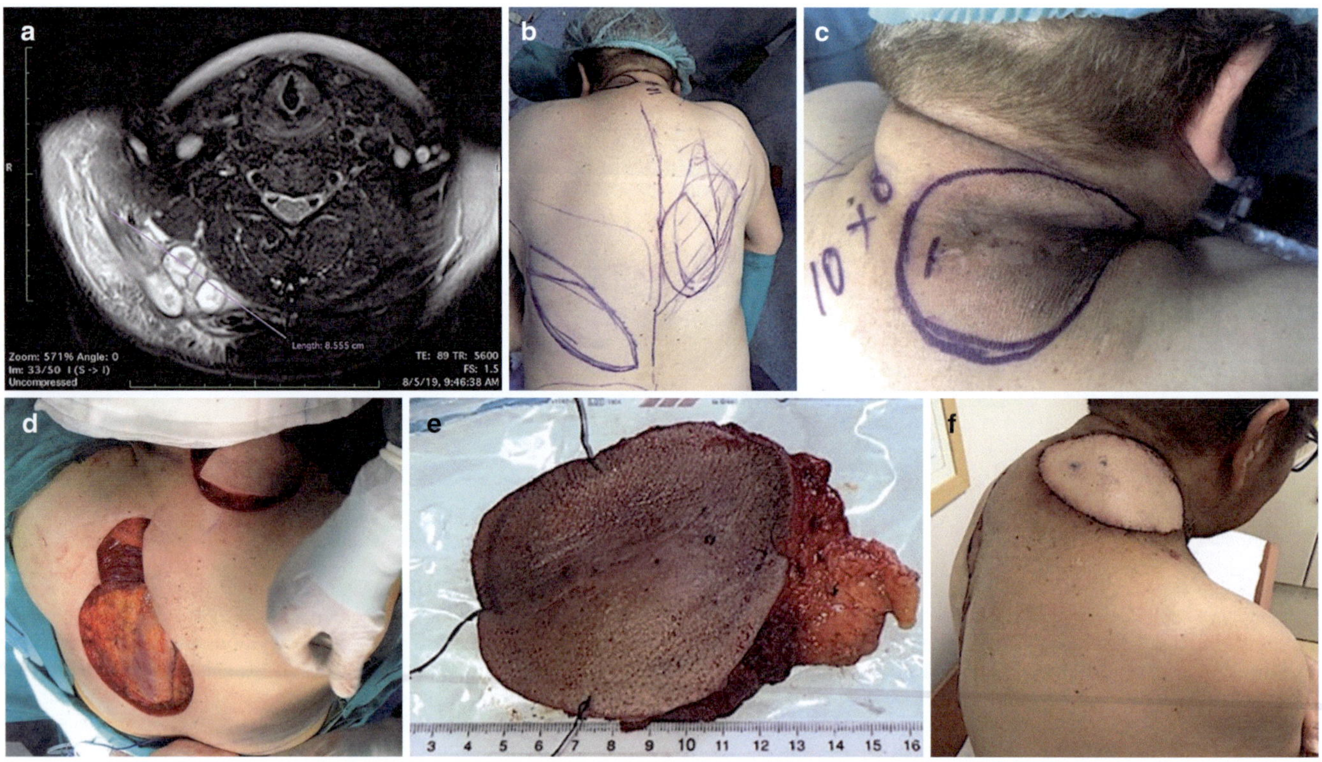

Fig. 24.2 (**a**–**f**) In a 56-year-old male patient who underwent a mass excision due to swelling that occurred in the posterior vicinity of the right cervicothoracic region 3 months ago without consulting the senior author (LE), a recurrent tumor was detected in the control MRIs (**a**). Before surgery, it was planned to close the planned skin and soft tissue defect with a latissimus dorsi flap (**b**, **c**). During the operation of the patient, clinical photographs during the flap stage (**d**) and the excised material removed with wide boundaries (**e**) are seen with marker sutures. Healthy tissue healing is observed in the reconstructed defect area in the first month postoperative control of the patient (**f**)

Particularly in patients where wound closure has been achieved with increased tension, or in areas with high contamination risk such as the groin, the use of VAC has been shown to significantly reduce early postoperative infection and wound dehiscence [7]. Generally, VAC can be discontinued 5–7 days after the application, or when the surgeon is confident that the incision has been securely "sealed."

We previously discussed the advantages and disadvantages of administering radiotherapy before or after surgery. A significant area of research for preoperative radiotherapy application, preferred by the authors of this section, is whether it alters local and systemic survival rates. Current literature knowledge is based on univariate analysis (UVA) and multivariate analysis (MVA) data. Neoadjuvant radiotherapy application has been shown via UVA to provide superior local survival. MVA data also indicate a trend in this direction. Similarly, UVA data demonstrate a significant increase in overall survival in patients who have received neoadjuvant radiotherapy, although this finding is not supported by MVA data. However, a decrease in the rate of distant metastasis has been proven with UVA and shown to be a trend with MVA. Therefore, it is understood that the use of neoadjuvant radiotherapy carries a positive predictive value on local control and the development rate of distant metastasis. However, radiotherapy toxicity also significantly increased in neoadjuvant applications. Thus, our current perspective is that, considering morbidity factors, local anatomical characteristics of the tumor, and the properties of the resultant dead space, the goal should be to administer radiotherapy before surgery and benefit from the oncological superiority of this timing. This should be achieved through the use of medical treatments that control adverse factors but, more importantly, early reconstructive interventions, while also preventing the patient from experiencing complications [12, 15, 16].

24.1 Conclusion

Resection with negative (safe) margins is the primary goal in the treatment of soft tissue sarcomas. Naturally, these types of surgeries often leave defects of various sizes and containing various tissue groups, where primary wound closure is often impossible. The use of radiotherapy, regardless of its timing, and patient-related comorbid factors, as well as characteristics related to the tumor size and location, all increase the complication rate.

Today, the treatment options and outcomes for soft tissue sarcomas are steadily improving. Nevertheless, postoperative complication rates, particularly the rate of wound healing problems, remain high. The early recognition of risk factors that lead to these adverse outcomes, particularly those that can be modified, is crucial in reducing postoperative morbidity, thereby determining the treatment outcome and preserving the quality of life.

For the prevention of major wound problems, especially in patients undergoing preoperative radiotherapy, the application of a free flap during resection ensures equal or fewer complications compared to patients undergoing postoperative radiotherapy [2]. Compared to local flaps, the use of free flaps, especially those unaffected by the radiotherapy field, helps ensure smooth healing of the resection area with well-vascularized tissue. Even in patients whose wounds can easily be closed primarily, VAC applications controlling exudation in the surgical field increase the rates of successful wound healing.

In conclusion, the adoption of a comprehensive approach involving effective surgical techniques, careful radiotherapy planning, and utilization of advanced wound care strategies, including VAC and free flap application, plays an integral role in improving treatment outcomes and quality of life in patients with soft tissue sarcomas.

References

1. Bolliger M, et al. Experiences with the standardized classification of surgical complications (Clavien-Dindo) in general surgery patients. Eur Surg. 2018;50(6):256–61.
2. Moore J, et al. Major wound complication risk factors following soft tissue sarcoma resection. Eur J Surg Oncol. 2014;40(12):1671–6.
3. Baldini EH, et al. Predictors for major wound complications following preoperative radiotherapy and surgery for soft-tissue sarcoma of the extremities and trunk: importance of tumor proximity to skin surface. Ann Surg Oncol. 2013;20(5):1494–9.
4. Ouyang Z, et al. Nomogram predicting the risk of postoperative major wound complication in soft tissue sarcoma of the trunk and extremities after preoperative radiotherapy. Cancers (Basel). 2022;14(17):4096.
5. Schwartz A, et al. Risk factors for significant wound complications following wide resection of extremity soft tissue sarcomas. Clin Orthop Relat Res. 2013;471(11):3612–7.
6. Farhan-Alanie OM, et al. Inflammatory prognostic scoring systems are risk factors for surgical site infection following wide local excision of soft tissue sarcoma. Eur J Orthop Surg Traumatol. 2022;32(8):1591–9.
7. Bedi M, et al. Does vacuum-assisted closure reduce the risk of wound complications in patients with lower extremity sarcomas treated with preoperative radiation? Clin Orthop Relat Res. 2019;477(4):768–74.
8. Bridgham KM, et al. Reconstructive limb-salvage surgery after lower extremity soft tissue sarcoma resection: a 20-year experience. J Surg Oncol. 2019;119(6):708–16.
9. Wilke BK, et al. A prospective evaluation of intraoperative indocyanine green fluorescence angiography for soft tissue sarcomas. J Am Acad Orthop Surg Glob Res Rev. 2021;5(8):e21.00187-6.
10. Yilmaz M, et al. Effect of negative pressure wound therapy after surgical removal of deep-seated high-malignant soft tissue sarcomas of the extremities and trunk wall-study protocol for a randomized controlled trial. Trials. 2022;23(1):507.
11. O'Sullivan B, et al. Preoperative versus postoperative radiotherapy in soft-tissue sarcoma of the limbs: a randomised trial. Lancet. 2002;359(9325):2235–41.

12. Abouarab MH, et al. Therapeutic options and postoperative wound complications after extremity soft tissue sarcoma resection and postoperative external beam radiotherapy. Int Wound J. 2018;15(1):148–58.
13. Siegel HJ, et al. Vacuum-assisted closure for radiation-associated wound complications. J Surg Oncol. 2007;96(7):575–82.
14. Lafaye G, et al. Clinical reliability of pedicled perforator flaps in the management of adult limb and trunk soft tissue sarcomas: experience of two French expert centres. J Plast Reconstr Aesthet Surg. 2022;75(12):4361–70.
15. Lansu J, et al. Time dependent dynamics of wound complications after preoperative radiotherapy in extremity soft tissue sarcomas. Eur J Surg Oncol. 2019;45(4):684–90.
16. Kobus M, et al. The role of neoadjuvant radiochemotherapy in the management of localized high-grade soft tissue sarcoma. Radiat Oncol. 2022;17(1):139.

25 Management Algorithm for Extremity Soft Tissue Sarcomas

Harzem Özger, Franklin H. Sim, Ajay Puri, Levent Eralp, and Buğra Alpan

25.1 Introduction

The authors want to clarify repeated terminology and concepts in the following algorithms.

The "feasibility of excision" denotes oncologically safe margins with no or acceptable morbidity in terms of limb salvage. Excision is classified as unfeasible if oncologically safe margins are questionable or impossible. Excision is also classified as unfeasible if safe margins can be achieved; however, the required reconstruction for limb salvage is too complex and has a prolonged recovery time, in which case a crucial systemic treatment will be delayed.

A "superficial" extremity lesion describes one that is above the fascia and involves the subcutaneous tissue. For anatomical parts lacking fascia, such as inguinal, popliteal, or antecubital fossae, superficiality still denotes subcutaneous localization, superficial to the major neurovascular structures. A "deep" extremity lesion describes one that involves the fascia or is seated below the fascia. Involvement of or being seated below major neurovascular structures in the flexor fossae also denotes "deep" localization. A "critically located" lesion can be described as one that is juxta-articular or in contact with or adherent to the adventitia, epineurium, or periosteum, regardless of the depth of the lesion.

H. Özger (✉) · L. Eralp
Department of Orthopedics and Traumatology, Istanbul University, Istanbul Medical Faculty, Istanbul, Türkiye
e-mail: harzemo@yahoo.com

F. H. Sim
Department of Orthopaedic Surgery, Mayo Clinic, Rochester, MN, USA

A. Puri
Department of Surgical Oncology, Tata Memorial Hospital, Mumbai, Maharashtra, India

B. Alpan
Department of Orthopedics and Traumatology, Acıbadem Mehmet Ali Aydınlar University, School of Medicine, Istanbul, Türkiye
e-mail: bugra.alpan@acibadem.edu.tr

Tumor size (the largest diameter or approximate volume) is an important prognostic factor and a crucial component of staging systems such as the American Joint Committee on Cancer (AJCC). However, for simplicity, it has not been utilized in this algorithm. Instead, it has been practically incorporated into the "feasibility of excision."

R0 margins are oncologically acceptable and microscopically negative margins. R1 margins denote microscopically positive margins or margins less than 1 mm from the tumor. R2 margins are used for macroscopically positive margins.

Routine follow-up, while it may differ slightly among institutions and according to patient and tumor characteristics, involves a local MRI and thorax CT scan at each visit every 3 months for the first two postoperative years, every 6 months for the third, fourth, and fifth years, and annually from the sixth to tenth postoperative year. Annual whole-body screening (preferably whole-body MRI, alternatively PET-CT scan) might be requested to monitor possible non-pulmonary distant metastases.

25.2 Primary Cases

Primary cases are those that present to or are referred to the orthopedic oncologist without any prior planned or inadvertent intervention, which would increase the possibility of iatrogenic tumor contamination. These cases are theoretically the best candidates for ideal management (Fig. 25.1).

25.2.1 Superficial Low-Grade Primary Lesion

Wide local excision is the treatment of choice [1–3].

- If R0 margins are present, routine follow-up is adequate [3].
- If R1 margins are present, re-excision with wide margins is required, provided that re-excision is feasible. If re-excision is not feasible, then the patient can be closely

H. Özger et al. (eds.), *Diagnosis and Treatment of Soft Tissue Tumors*, https://doi.org/10.1007/978-3-031-77061-6_25

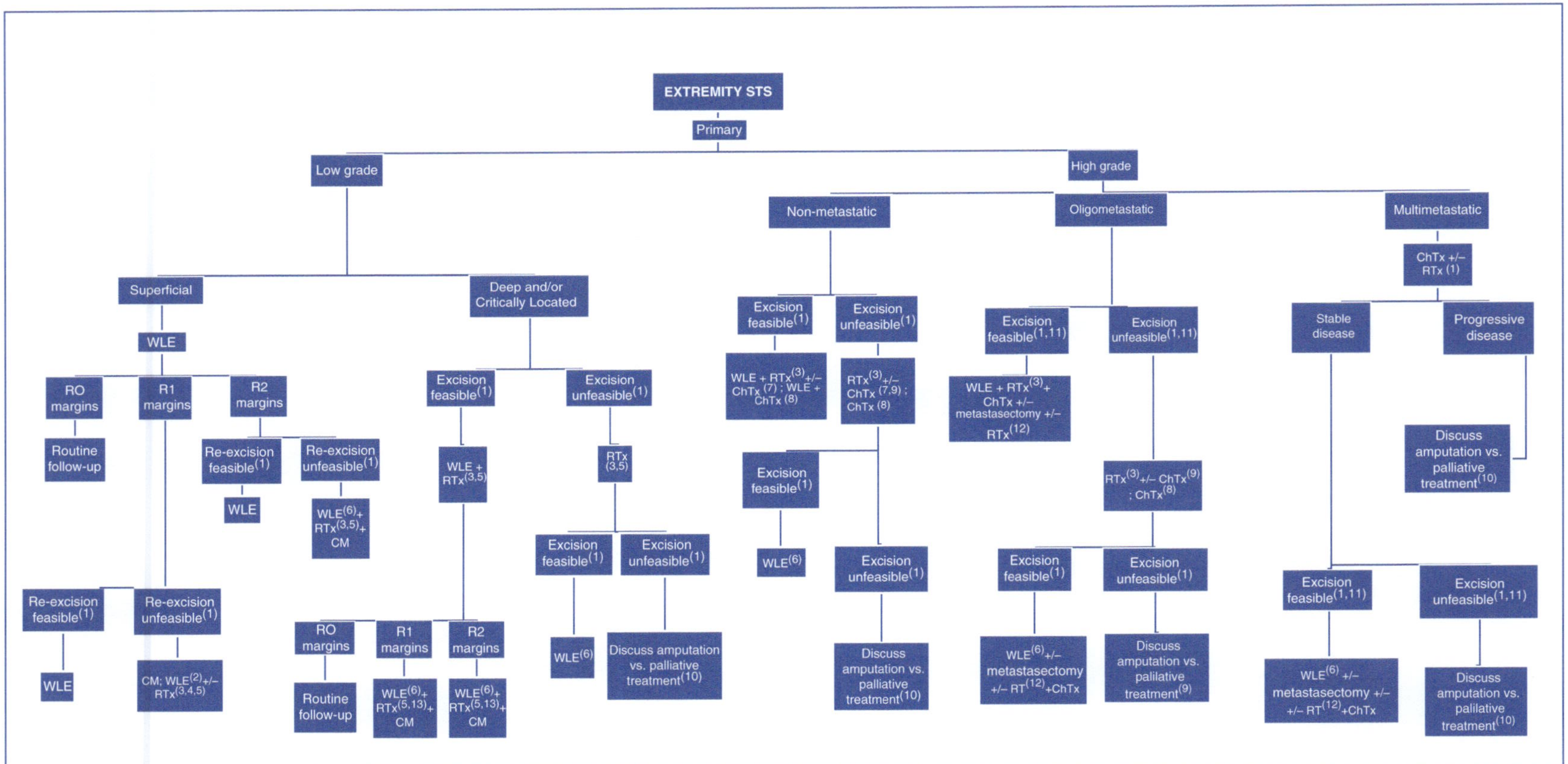

1. Feasibility denotes oncologically safe margins with no or acceptable morbidity. If oncologically safe margins are questionable or impossible, the excision is classified as unfeasible. Excision is also classified as unfeasible if the required reconstruction is too complex with a prolonged recovery time, in which case a crucial systemic treatment will be delayed.
2. Wide local excision can be performed with more predictable margins, if and when, local recurrence(LR) is observed.
3. Pre- or postoperative application of radiotherapy depends on surgeon preference and/or institutional policy. If resectability is in question, preoperative application can help provide tumor regression and/or create a marginal safety zone with a pseudocapsule.
4. If close monitoring is planned for LR of low-grade tumors, withholding radiotherapy until, if and when, LR is observed might be discused by the multidisciplinary team
5. Benefit from radiotherapy is not clear in low-grade tumors.
6. Consider advanced reconstruction following an uncompromising resection.
7. The use and the timing of chemotherapy (neoadjuvant, adjuvant, both) is to be decided by the multidisciplinary team, depending on patient characteristics and the specific tumor histology.
8. Neoadjuvant chemotherapy is proven beneficial in certain soft tissue sarcomas as it considerably improves resectability.
9. Radiotherapy and chemotherapy can be used concurrently in the neoadjuvant setting to facilitate resection with safe margins in extreme limb salvage cases.
10. Amputation can be used both as a curative or a life-saving palliative measure. Palliative treatment methods include various modalities, which aim to improve survival or quality-of-life.
11. Excision refers to "the primary lesion" and not all lesions in metastatic patients.
12. Definitive radiotherapy can be administered to unresectable metastases.
13. Feasibility of radiotherapy depends on whether the same site was irradiated and at what dosage previously. Advanced radiotherapy modalities (carbon ion, proton, intraoperative, brachytherapy) can be considered to limit local adverse effects.

WLE: wide local excision; RTx: radiotherapy; ChTx: chemotherapy; CM: closely monitor; RO: clear surgical margins; R1: microscopic residual disease; R2: macroscopic residual disease.

Fig. 25.1 Management algorithm for primary soft tissue sarcoma of the extremities monitored for LR and wide local excision can be performed with more predictable margins if and when local recurrence is observed. While the benefit of radiotherapy is not clear in low-grade tumors, its use can be discussed by the multidisciplinary team to improve local control when margins are microscopically positive. The multidisciplinary team might also discuss withholding radiotherapy until if and when local recurrence develops so that the option of radiotherapy is still available when needed. The timing of radiotherapy (pre-/postoperative) in relation to local recurrence will depend on surgeon preference and institutional policy [1–4].

- If R2 margins are present, re-excision with wide margins is required, provided that re-excision is feasible. If a straightforward re-excision is not feasible, then a wide re-excision, which might commonly involve local/free flap reconstruction and split-thickness skin grafting and occasionally involve neurovascular reconstruction, is required. While the benefit of radiotherapy is not clear in low-grade tumors, its use can be discussed by the multidisciplinary team to improve local control. The timing of radiotherapy (pre-/postoperative) in relation to local recurrence will depend on surgeon preference and institutional policy. Subsequent close monitoring for local recurrence is imperative [1–4].

25.2.2 Deep and/or Critically Located Primary Lesion

- If wide local excision is feasible, then excision must be performed. While the benefit of radiotherapy is not clear in low-grade tumors, its use is encouraged in deep and/or critically located lesions to improve local control. The timing of radiotherapy (pre-/postoperative) will depend on surgeon preference and institutional policy [1–4].
  - If R0 margins are present, routine follow-up is adequate [3].
  - If R1 or R2 margins are present, then a re-excision with wide margins is required. If a straightforward re-excision is not feasible, then options for advanced reconstruction (osteoarticular, neurovascular, local/free flap) must be considered. If conventional radiotherapy modalities were used previously, advanced modalities such as intraoperative radiotherapy or brachytherapy might be considered to improve local control and limit adverse effects. Subsequent close monitoring for local recurrence is imperative [1–3].
- If a straightforward wide local excision is not feasible, preoperative radiotherapy can occasionally improve resectability in low-grade tumors [1–4].
  - If wide local excision becomes feasible following radiotherapy, then excision must be performed. Following resection, advanced reconstruction might be required [1–4].
  - If resection with safe margins is still unlikely or incompatible with limb salvage (even with advanced reconstruction), then amputation must be discussed with the patient/family as a curative option. In cases where amputation is refused due to psychological and socio-religious factors, then palliative treatment options, such as surgical interventions (emergency amputation for intractable pain, hemorrhage, gangrene, sepsis; non-functional limb salvage; pathologic fracture fixation), radiotherapy, conventional chemotherapy, targeted therapies and immunotherapy, interventional radiology procedures, which are not curative but aim to improve survival and quality of life, should be discussed. Next-generation sequencing (NGS) of biopsy and resection specimens might help guide medical palliative treatment [1–5].

25.2.3 Non-metastatic Patient with High-Grade Lesion

- If wide local excision is feasible, then excision must be performed. Radiotherapy is particularly beneficial for local control in high-grade tumors. The timing of radiotherapy (pre-/postoperative) will depend on surgeon preference and institutional policy. While high-grade tumors might also benefit from chemotherapy, the use, and the timing of chemotherapy (neoadjuvant, adjuvant, both) are to be decided by the multidisciplinary team, depending on patient characteristics and the specific tumor histology. Contrary to most soft tissue sarcomas, neoadjuvant chemotherapy is proven beneficial in specific pathologies such as non-pleomorphic rhabdomyosarcoma and infantile fibrosarcoma since it can downstage the tumor and considerably improve resectability [1–6].
- If a straightforward wide local excision is not feasible, resectability must be re-evaluated following radiotherapy. Radiotherapy and chemotherapy can be used concurrently in the neoadjuvant setting to facilitate resection with safe margins in extreme limb salvage cases such as large, exophytic, and hemorrhagic tumors, which are otherwise candidates for immediate amputation at first impression. For certain pathologies, such as non-pleomorphic rhabdomyosarcoma and infantile fibrosarcoma, resectability must be re-evaluated following neoadjuvant chemotherapy [1–3].
  - If wide local excision becomes feasible following neoadjuvant treatment, then excision must be performed. Advanced reconstruction might be required following resection [1–3].

- If resection with safe margins is still unlikely or incompatible with limb salvage (even with advanced reconstruction), then amputation must be discussed with the patient/family as a curative option. In cases where amputation is refused due to psychological and socio-religious factors, palliative treatment options, such as surgical interventions (emergency amputation for intractable pain, hemorrhage, gangrene, sepsis, non-functional limb salvage, pathologic fracture fixation), radiotherapy, conventional chemotherapy, targeted therapies, and immunotherapy, and interventional radiology procedures, which are not curative but aim to improve survival and quality of life, should be discussed. Next-generation sequencing (NGS) of biopsy and resection specimens might help guide medical palliative treatment [1–6].

25.2.4 Oligometastatic Patient with High-Grade Lesion

- If wide local excision is feasible, then excision must be performed. Radiotherapy is particularly beneficial for local control in high-grade tumors. The timing of radiotherapy (pre-/postoperative) will depend on surgeon preference and institutional policy. Administration of neoadjuvant chemotherapy should be discussed by the multidisciplinary team for both facilitating the resection and for systemic control as the patient is already metastatic. Metastasectomy for resectable lesions should also be considered subsequently. Definitive radiotherapy can be administered to unresectable metastases. The multidisciplinary team will discuss the course of adjuvant chemotherapy, which might range from conventional agents like doxorubicin and ifosfamide to biological therapies (targeted therapies, immunotherapy) depending on staging following initial management. Next-generation sequencing (NGS) of biopsy and resection specimens might help guide advanced medical treatment [1–10].
- If a straightforward wide local excision is not feasible, resectability must be re-evaluated following radiotherapy. Radiotherapy and chemotherapy can be used concurrently in the neoadjuvant setting to facilitate resection with safe margins in extreme limb salvage cases such as large, exophytic, and hemorrhagic tumors, which are otherwise candidates for immediate amputation at first impression. For certain pathologies, such as non-pleomorphic rhabdomyosarcoma and infantile fibrosarcoma, resectability must be re-evaluated following neoadjuvant chemotherapy [1–6].
  - If wide local excision becomes feasible following neoadjuvant treatment, then excision must be performed. Advanced reconstruction might be required following resection. Metastasectomy for resectable lesions should also be considered subsequently. Definitive radiotherapy can be administered to unresectable metastases. The multidisciplinary team will discuss the course of adjuvant chemotherapy, which might range from conventional agents like doxorubicin and ifosfamide to biological therapies (targeted therapies, immunotherapy) depending on staging following initial management. Next-generation sequencing (NGS) of biopsy and resection specimens might help guide advanced medical treatment [1–10].
  - If resection with safe margins is still unlikely or incompatible with limb salvage (even with advanced reconstruction), then amputation must be discussed with the patient/family if it is going to improve survival or quality of life. Amputation should be avoided in metastatic patients if it is not going to provide an advantage in terms of survival or quality of life. In cases where amputation is indicated but refused due to psychological and socioreligious factors, palliative treatment options, such as surgical interventions (emergency amputation for intractable pain, hemorrhage, gangrene, sepsis; non-functional limb salvage; pathologic fracture fixation), radiotherapy, conventional chemotherapy, biological therapies (targeted therapies, immunotherapy), interventional radiology procedures, which are not curative but aim to improve survival and quality of life, should be discussed. Next-generation sequencing (NGS) of biopsy and resection specimens might help guide medical palliative treatment [1–10].

25.2.5 Multimetastatic Patient with High-Grade Lesion

- Chemotherapy should be the mainstay of initial management. Radiotherapy might be applied to the primary lesion and to the metastases, which are either symptomatic or likely to cause imminent morbidity. Subsequently, the patient must be re-evaluated comprehensively.
  - If the disease is stable following initial management and the excision of the primary lesion is feasible, then excision must be performed. Advanced reconstruction might be required following resection. Metastasectomy for resectable lesions should also be considered subsequently. Definitive radiotherapy and adjuvant chemotherapy can be administered to unresectable metastases. The multidisciplinary team will discuss the course of adjuvant chemotherapy, which might range from conventional agents like doxorubicin and ifosfamide to biological therapies (targeted therapies, immunotherapy) depending on staging following initial management. Next-generation sequencing (NGS) of biopsy

and resection specimens might help guide advanced medical treatment [1–10].

- If the disease is stable following initial management, however, the excision of the primary lesion is not feasible, then amputation must be discussed with the patient/family if it is going to improve survival or quality of life. Amputation should be avoided in metastatic patients if it is not going to provide an advantage in terms of survival or quality of life. In cases where amputation is indicated but refused due to psychological and socioreligious factors, palliative treatment options, such as surgical interventions (emergency amputation for intractable pain, hemorrhage, gangrene, sepsis; non-functional limb salvage; pathologic fracture fixation), radiotherapy, conventional chemotherapy, biological therapies (targeted therapies, immunotherapy), interventional radiology procedures, which are not curative but aim to improve survival and quality of life, should be discussed. Next-generation sequencing (NGS) of biopsy and resection specimens might help guide medical palliative treatment [1–10].
- If the disease is progressive following initial management, then amputation must be discussed with the patient/family if it is going to improve quality of life. Amputation should be avoided in metastatic patients if it is not going to provide an advantage in terms of survival or quality of life. In cases where amputation is indicated but refused due to psychological and socioreligious factors, palliative treatment options, such as surgical interventions (emergency amputation for intractable pain, hemorrhage, gangrene, sepsis; non-functional limb salvage; pathologic fracture fixation), radiotherapy, conventional chemotherapy, biological therapies (targeted therapies, immunotherapy), interventional radiology procedures, which are not curative but aim to improve survival and quality of life, should be discussed. Next-generation sequencing (NGS) of biopsy and resection specimens might help guide medical palliative treatment [1–10].

25.3 Relapse Cases

A biopsy of the recurring lesion and re-staging are required. Management is similar to primary lesions (Fig. 25.2). However, previous treatments might affect or limit adjuvant treatment options.

25.3.1 Superficial Low-Grade Relapse Lesion

Wide local excision is the treatment of choice. Following resection, advanced reconstruction might be required [1–3].

25.3.2 Deep or Critically Located Low-Grade Relapse Lesion

- If wide local excision is feasible, then excision must be performed. Advanced reconstruction might be required following resection. While the benefit of radiotherapy is not clear in low-grade tumors, its use is encouraged in deep and/or critically located and recurring lesions to improve local control. The timing of radiotherapy (pre-/postoperative) will depend on surgeon preference and institutional policy. The feasibility of radiotherapy depends on whether the same site was irradiated and at what dosage previously. Advanced radiotherapy modalities (carbon ion, proton, intraoperative, brachytherapy) can limit local adverse effects [1–4].
- If a straightforward wide local excision is not feasible, preoperative radiotherapy can be administered to improve resectability [1–4].
  - If wide local excision becomes feasible following radiotherapy, then excision must be performed. Advanced reconstruction might be required following resection.
  - If resection with safe margins is still unlikely or incompatible with limb salvage (even with advanced reconstruction), then amputation must be discussed with the patient/family as a curative option. In cases where amputation is refused due to psychological and socioreligious factors, then palliative treatment options, such as surgical interventions (emergency amputation for intractable pain, hemorrhage, gangrene, sepsis; non-functional limb salvage; pathologic fracture fixation), radiotherapy, conventional chemotherapy, targeted therapies and immunotherapy, interventional radiology procedures, which are not curative but aim to improve survival and quality of life, should be discussed. Next-generation sequencing (NGS) of biopsy and resection specimens might help guide medical palliative treatment [1–10].

25.3.3 High-Grade Relapse Lesion

- If wide local excision is feasible, then excision must be performed. The timing of radiotherapy (pre-/postoperative) will depend on surgeon preference and institutional policy. The feasibility of radiotherapy depends on whether the same site was irradiated and at what dosage previously. Advanced radiotherapy modalities (carbon ion, proton, intraoperative, brachytherapy) can be considered to limit local adverse effects. While high-grade tumors might also benefit from chemotherapy, the use and the timing of chemotherapy (neoadjuvant, adjuvant, both) are to be decided by the multidisciplinary team, depending on

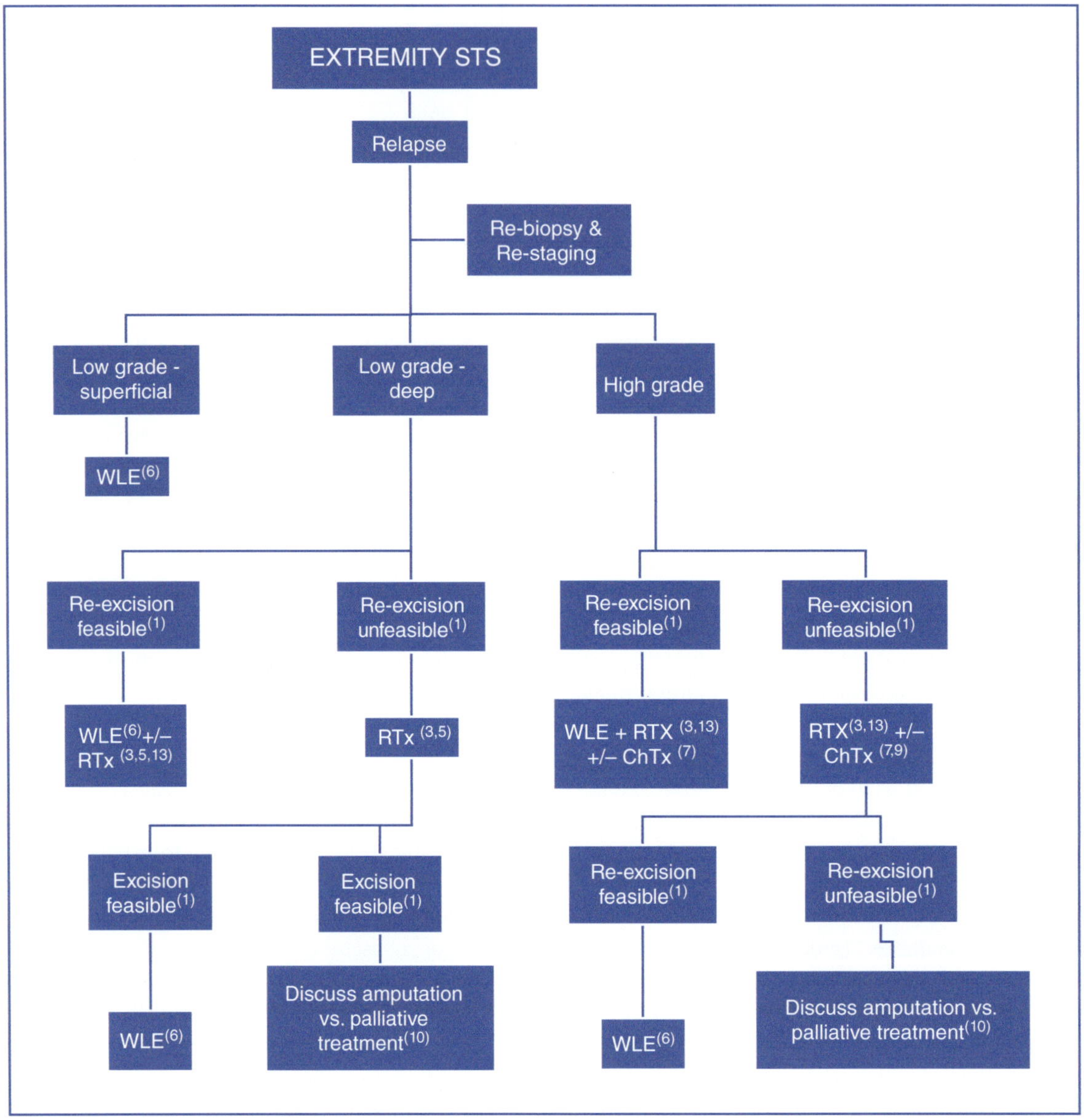

1. Feasibility denotes oncologically safe margins with no or acceptable morbidity. If oncologically safe margins are questionable or impossible, the excision is classified as unfeasible. Excision is also classified as unfeasible if the required reconstruction is too complex with a prolonged recovery time, in which case a crucial systemic treatment will be delayed.
2. Wide local excision can be performed with more predictable margins, if and when, local recurrence(LR) is observed.
3. Pre- or postoperative application of radiotherapy depends on surgeon preference and/or institutional policy. If resectability is in question, preoperative application can help provide tumor regression and/or create a marginal safety zone with a pseudocapsule.
4. If close monitoring is planned for LR of low-grade tumors, withholding radiotherapy until, if and when, LR is observed might be discussed by the multidisciplinary team.
5. Benefit from radiotherapy is not clear in low-grade tumors.
6. Consider advanced reconstruction following an uncompromising resection.
7. The use and the timing of chemotherapy (neoadjuvant, adjuvant, both) is to be decided by the multidisciplinary team, depending on patient characteristics and the specific tumor histology.
8. Neoadjuvant chemotherapy is proven beneficial in certain soft tissue sarcomas as it considerably improves resectability.
9. Radiotherapy and chemotherapy can be used concurrently in the neoadjuvant setting to facilitate resection with safe margins in extreme limb salvage cases.
10. Amputation can be used both as a curative or a life-saving palliative measure. Palliative treatment methods include various modalities, which aim to improve survival or quality-of-life.
11. Excision refers to "the primary lesion" and not all lesions in metastatic patients.
12. Definitive radiotherapy can be administered to unresectable metastases.
13. Feasibility of radiotherapy depends on whether the same site was irradiated and at what dosage previously. Advanced radiotherapy modalities (carbon ion, proton, intraoperative, brachytherapy) can be considered to limit local adverse effects.

WLE: wide local excision; RTx: radiotherapy; ChTx: chemotherapy; CM: closely monitor; RO: clear surgical margins; R1: microscopic residual disease; R2: macroscopic residual disease.

Fig. 25.2 Management algorithm for relapse soft tissue sarcoma of the extremities patient characteristics and the specific tumor histology [1–3].

- If a straightforward wide local excision is not feasible, resectability must be re-evaluated following radiotherapy. The feasibility of radiotherapy depends on whether the same site was irradiated and at what dosage previously. Advanced radiotherapy modalities (carbon ion, proton, intraoperative, brachytherapy) can be considered to limit local adverse effects. Radiotherapy and chemotherapy can be used concurrently in the neoadjuvant setting to facilitate resection with safe margins in extreme limb salvage cases such as large, exophytic, and hemorrhagic tumors, which are otherwise candidates for immediate amputation at first impression [1–4].
  - If wide local excision becomes feasible following neoadjuvant treatment, then excision must be performed. Following resection, advanced reconstruction might be required.
  - If resection with safe margins is still unlikely or incompatible with limb salvage (even with advanced reconstruction), then amputation must be discussed with the patient/family as a curative option. In cases where amputation is refused due to psychological and socioreligious factors, palliative treatment options, such as surgical interventions (emergency amputation for intractable pain, hemorrhage, gangrene, sepsis; non-functional limb salvage; pathologic fracture fixation), radiotherapy, conventional chemotherapy, targeted therapies and immunotherapy, interventional radiology procedures, which are not curative but aim to improve survival and quality of life, should be discussed. Next-generation sequencing (NGS) of biopsy and resection specimens might help guide medical palliative treatment [1–10].

25.4 Whoops Cases

Whoops procedure can be described as any intervention aiming at the excision of a soft tissue mass without the knowledge of diagnosis and concern or consideration for an adverse outcome (e.g., malignancy). The procedure is typically performed by a surgeon who is not an orthopedic oncologist and is unaware of the principles of orthopedic oncology. Unfortunately, a convenient pathology outcome of "R0" margins is inadequate to guarantee a favorable outcome since the procedure might involve other technical errors like a transverse incision or neglecting to place a drain. Furthermore, the pathology is very commonly reported in a non-specialized center by a pathologist who is experienced in musculoskeletal tumors. The evaluation must start with consulting the pathology with the pathologist of the multidisciplinary team to confirm or correct the diagnosis in the "whoops" case (Fig. 25.3). Local and systemic imaging must be performed immediately to evaluate the contaminated volume in the operation site and to complete staging. The radiology before the "whoops procedure" must be obtained if available.

25.4.1 Low-Grade Whoops Lesion with R0 Margins

Close monitoring for local recurrence is essential despite R0 margins since the index procedure was probably performed elsewhere without the intent to perform wide local excision. Preoperative radiology and intraoperative documentation are often missing in these cases. Wide local excision can be performed with more predictable margins if and when local recurrence is observed.

25.4.2 High-Grade Whoops Lesion with R0 Margins

Adjuvant radiotherapy might be administered to complete the inadvertent procedure with an acceptable outcome. While high-grade tumors might also benefit from chemotherapy, the multidisciplinary team will decide whether to use chemotherapy in this setting, depending on patient characteristics and the specific tumor histology. Subsequent close monitoring for local recurrence and regional / and/or distant metastasis is imperative.

25.4.3 Low-Grade Whoops Lesion with R1 Margins

- If re-excision is feasible, wide local excision is the treatment of choice [1–3, 11].
- If re-excision is not feasible, then the patient can be closely monitored for LR and wide local excision can be performed with more predictable margins if and when local recurrence is observed. Advanced reconstruction might be considered. While the benefit of radiotherapy is not clear in low-grade tumors, its use can be discussed by the multidisciplinary team to improve local control when margins are microscopically positive. The multidisciplinary team might also discuss withholding radiotherapy until if and when local recurrence develops so that the option of radiotherapy is still available when needed. The timing of radiotherapy (pre-/postoperative) in relation to local recurrence will depend on surgeon preference and institutional policy. Advanced radiotherapy modalities such as intraoperative radiotherapy or brachytherapy might improve local control and limit adverse effects if the re-excision margins are known or predicted to be positive [1–3, 11, 12].

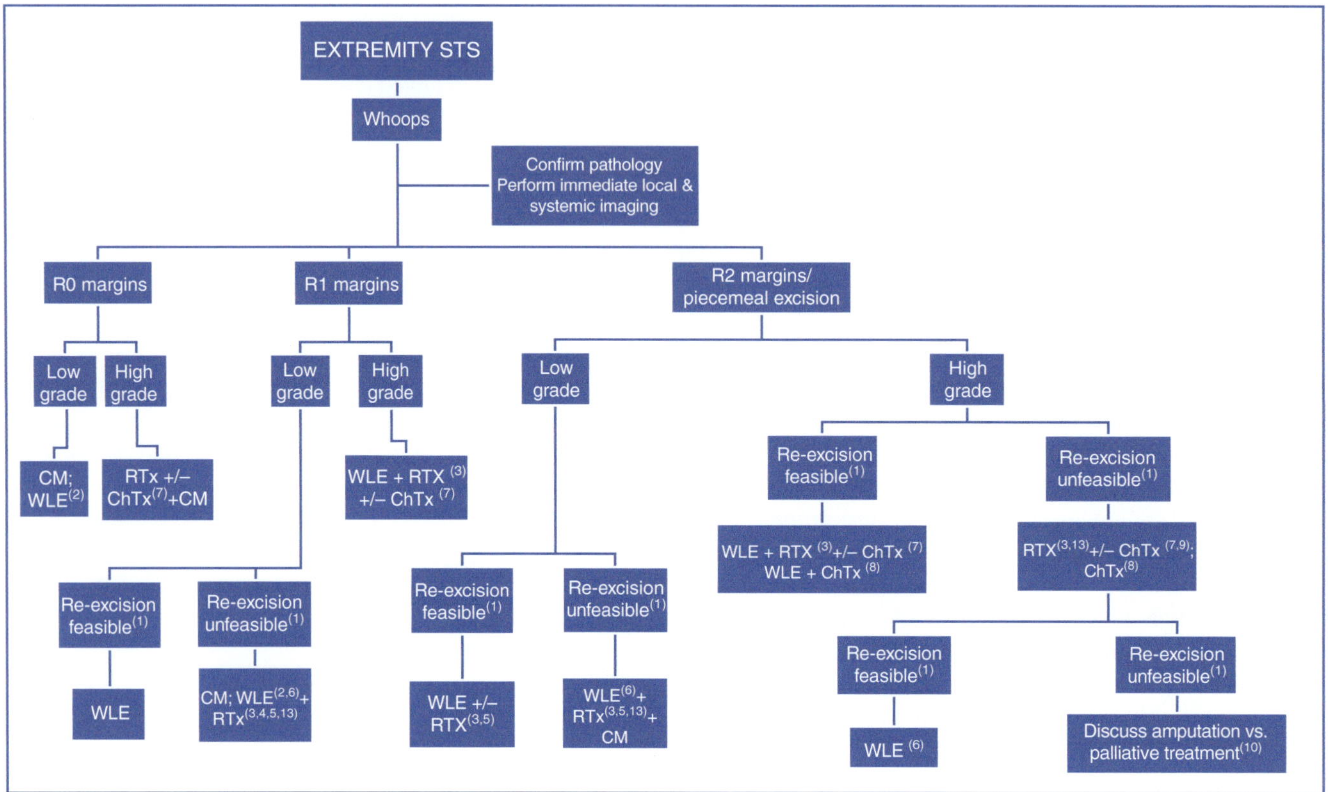

1. Feasibility denotes oncologically safe margins with no or acceptable morbidity. If oncologically safe margins are questionable or impossible, the excision is classified as unfeasible. Excision is alsoclassified as unfeasible if the required reconstruction is too complex with a prolonged recovery time, in which case a crucial systemic treatment will be delayed.
2. Wide local excision can be performed with more predictable margins, if and when, local recurrence(LR) is observed.
3. Pre- or postoperative application of radiotherapy depends on surgeon preference and/or institutional policy. If resectability is in question, preoperative application can help provide tumor regression and/or create a marginal safety zone with a pseudocapsule.
4. If close monitoring is planned for LR of low-grade tumors, withholding radiotherapy until, if and when, LR is observed might be discussed by the multidisciplinary team.
5. Benefit from radiotherapy is not clear in low-grade tumors.
6. Consider advanced reconstruction following an uncompromising resection.
7. The use and the timing of chemotherapy (neoadjuvant, adjuvant, both) is to be decided by the multidisciplinary team, depending on patient characteristics and the specific tumor histology.
8. Neoadjuvant chemotherapy is proven beneficial in certain soft tissue sarcomas as it considerably improves resectability.
9. Radiotherapy and chemotherapy can be used concurrently in the neoadjuvant setting to facilitate resection with safe margins in extreme limb salvage cases.
10. Amputation can be used both as a curative or a life-saving palliative measure. Palliative treatment methods include various modalities, which aim to improve survival or quality-of-life.
11. Excision refers to "the primary lesion" and not all lesions in metastatic patients.
12. Definitive radiotherapy can be administered to unresectable metastases.
13. Feasibility of radiotherapy depends on whether the same site was irradiated and at what dosage previously. Advanced radiotherapy modalities (carbon ion, proton, intraoperative, brachytherapy) can be considered to limit local adverse effects.

WLE: wide local excision; RTx: radiotherapy; ChTx: chemotherapy; CM: closely monitor; RO: clear surgical margins; R1: microscopic residual disease; R2: macroscopic residual disease.

Fig. 25.3 Management algorithm for Whoops procedures resulting in soft tissue sarcoma of the extremities

25.4.4 High-Grade Whoops Lesion with R1 Margins

Re-excision with wide margins must be performed. While radiotherapy is essential in this setting, the timing (pre-/postoperative) will depend on surgeon preference and institutional policy. High-grade tumors might also benefit from chemotherapy. However, the multidisciplinary team will decide the use and timing of chemotherapy (neoadjuvant, adjuvant, both), depending on patient characteristics and the specific tumor histology [1–3, 11, 12].

25.4.5 Low-Grade Whoops Lesion with R2 Margins or Following Piecemeal Excision

- If re-excision is feasible, then re-excision with wide margins is indicated. While the benefit of radiotherapy is not clear in low-grade tumors, the multidisciplinary team can discuss its use to improve local control. The timing of radiotherapy (pre-/postoperative) in relation to re-excision will depend on surgeon preference and/or institutional policy [1–3, 11, 12].

- If a straightforward re-excision is not feasible, then options for advanced reconstruction (osteoarticular, neurovascular, local/free flap) must be considered. While the benefit of radiotherapy is not clear in low-grade tumors, its use can be discussed by the multidisciplinary team to improve local control. The timing of radiotherapy (pre-/postoperative) in relation to re-excision will depend on surgeon preference and institutional policy. Advanced modalities such as intraoperative radiotherapy or brachytherapy might improve local control and limit adverse effects if the re-excision margins are known or predicted to be positive. Subsequent close monitoring for local recurrence is imperative [1–3, 11, 12].

25.4.6 High-Grade Whoops Lesion with R2 Margins or Following Piecemeal Excision

- If wide local excision is feasible, then excision must be performed. While radiotherapy is essential in this setting, the timing (pre-/postoperative) will depend on surgeon preference and/or institutional policy. While high-grade tumors might also benefit from chemotherapy, the use and the timing of chemotherapy (neoadjuvant, adjuvant, both) are to be decided by the multidisciplinary team, depending on patient characteristics and the specific tumor histology. Contrary to most soft tissue sarcomas, neoadjuvant chemotherapy is proven beneficial in specific pathologies such as non-pleomorphic rhabdomyosarcoma and infantile fibrosarcoma since it can downstage the tumor and considerably improve resectability [1–5, 11, 12].
- If a straightforward wide local excision is not feasible, resectability must be re-evaluated following radiotherapy. Radiotherapy and chemotherapy can be used concurrently in the neoadjuvant setting to facilitate resection with safe margins in extreme limb salvage cases such as large, exophytic, and hemorrhagic tumors, which are otherwise candidates for immediate amputation at first impression. For certain pathologies such as non-pleomorphic rhabdomyosarcoma and infantile fibrosarcoma, resectability must be re-evaluated following neoadjuvant chemotherapy [1–5, 11, 12].
  - If wide local excision becomes feasible following neoadjuvant treatment, then excision must be performed. Advanced reconstruction might be required following resection [1–3].
  - If resection with safe margins is still unlikely or incompatible with limb salvage (even with advanced reconstruction), then amputation must be discussed with the patient/family as a curative option. In cases where amputation is refused due to psychological and socio-religious factors, palliative treatment options, such as surgical interventions (emergency amputation for intractable pain, hemorrhage, gangrene, sepsis; non-functional limb salvage; pathologic fracture fixation), radiotherapy, conventional chemotherapy, targeted therapies and immunotherapy, interventional radiology procedures, which are not curative but aim to improve survival and quality of life, should be discussed. Next-generation sequencing (NGS) of biopsy and resection specimens might help guide medical palliative treatment [1–10].

References

1. Gronchi A, Colombo C, Raut CP. Surgical management of localized soft tissue tumors. Cancer. 2014;120:2638–48. Wiley.
2. Gamboa AC, Gronchi A, Cardona K. Soft-tissue sarcoma in adults: an update on the current state of histiotype-specific management in an era of personalized medicine. CA Cancer J Clin. 2020;70(3):200–29.
3. NCCN clinical practice guidelines in oncology (NCCN guidelines®) soft tissue sarcoma version 2.2021—April 28, 2021. [cited 2023 May 11]. http://nccn.ir/Guidelines/Summary/sarcoma.html#pf23.
4. Allignet B, Meurgey A, Bouhamama A, Karanian M, Meeus P, Vaz G, et al. Impact of histological subtype on radiological and pathological response after neoadjuvant radiotherapy in soft tissue sarcoma. Eur J Surg Oncol. 2021;47(12):2995–3003.
5. Stevenson MG, Musters AH, Geertzen JHB, van Leeuwen BL, Hoekstra HJ, Been LB. Amputations for extremity soft tissue sarcoma in an era of limb salvage treatment: local control and survival. J Surg Oncol. 2018;117(3):434–42.
6. Thacker MM. Malignant soft tissue tumors in children. Orthop Clin North Am. 2013;44:657–67.
7. Singhi EK, Moore DC, Muslimani A. Metastatic soft tissue sarcomas: a review of treatment and new pharmacotherapies. P T. 2018;43(7):410–29.
8. Gutkin PM, von Eyben R, Chin A, Donaldson SS, Oh J, Jiang A, et al. Local control outcomes using stereotactic body radiation therapy or surgical resection for metastatic sarcoma. Int J Radiat Oncol Biol Phys. 2022;114(4):771–9.
9. Smolle MA, van Praag VM, Posch F, Bergovec M, Leitner L, Friesenbichler J, et al. Surgery for metachronous metastasis of soft tissue sarcoma—a magnitude of benefit analysis using propensity score methods. Eur J Surg Oncol. 2019;45(2):242–8.
10. Krishnan CK, Kim HS, Park JW, Han I. Outcome after surgery for extremity soft tissue sarcoma in patients presenting with metastasis at diagnosis. Am J Clin Oncol. 2018;41(7):681–6.
11. Grimer R, Parry M, James S. Inadvertent excision of malignant soft tissue tumors. EFORT Open Rev. 2019;4(6):321–9.
12. Jones DA, Shideman C, Yuan J, Dusenbery K, Carlos Manivel J, Ogilvie C, et al. Management of unplanned excision for soft-tissue sarcoma with preoperative radiotherapy followed by definitive resection. Am J Clin Oncol. 2016;39(6):586–92.

Part II

Case Studies

Soft-Tissue Sarcoma of the Thigh with Extensive Osseous Involvement

26

Ajay Puri

26.1 Introduction

Soft-tissue sarcomas account for about 1% of all malignancies, and the extremities are the commonest site with about 60% of soft-tissue sarcomas arising in the extremities.

Before planning any intervention, appropriate imaging and a biopsy are essential investigations. The principles of biopsy should always be respected with all local imaging being completed prior to biopsy (contrast-enhanced MRI is the preferred method for limb lesions). The entire biopsy tract needs to be excised at definitive surgery; hence, the position of biopsy incision is critical and must always be in the line of planned definitive surgery. If a core needle biopsy is preferred, the biopsy site must be clearly documented to enable easy identification for excision at definitive surgery.

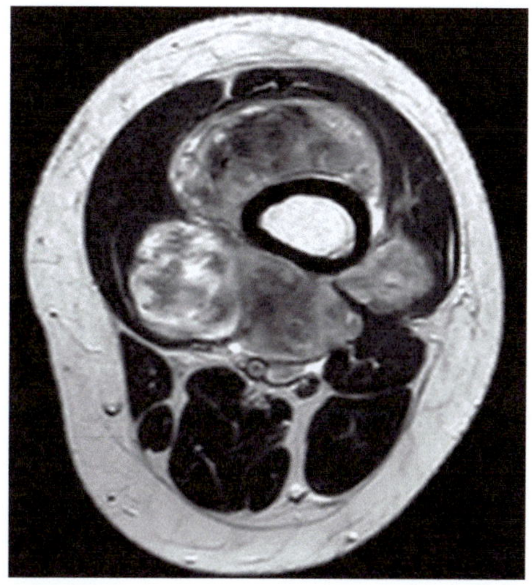

Fig. 26.1 MRI demonstrating a soft-tissue lesion in the thigh, circumferentially surrounding the femur in the middle and lower third part of the thigh

26.2 Brief Clinical History

A 42-year-old female, presented with swelling and pain in the mid-thigh of 3–4 months duration. MRI demonstrated a soft-tissue lesion in the thigh. The lesion circumferentially surrounded the femur in the middle and lower third part of the thigh, Fig. 26.1. There was encasement of the vessel (Fig. 26.2—yellow arrow) with the presence of marrow lesions/metastases in the upper third of the femur (Fig. 26.3—yellow arrow). The lady had no distal neurovascular deficit, and there was no distal limb edema.

A needle biopsy diagnosed it as a high-grade soft-tissue sarcoma. Staging investigations were negative for distant spread (apart from the marrow lesions).

A. Puri (✉)
Department of Surgical Oncology, Tata Memorial Hospital, Mumbai, Maharashtra, India
e-mail: docpuri@gmail.com

H. Özger et al. (eds.), *Diagnosis and Treatment of Soft Tissue Tumors*, https://doi.org/10.1007/978-3-031-77061-6_26

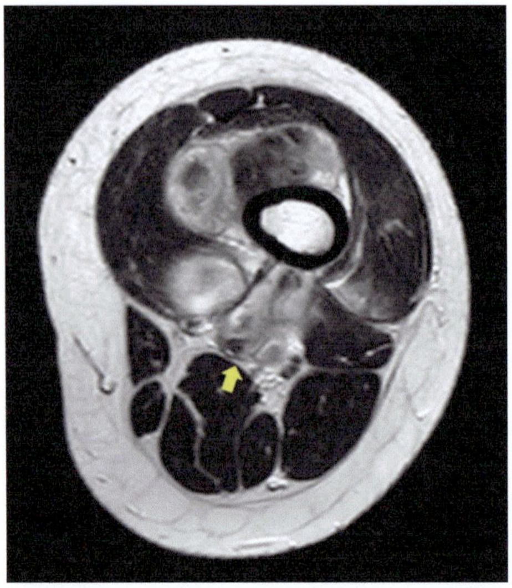

Fig. 26.2 MRI demonstrating encasement of the vessel (yellow arrow)

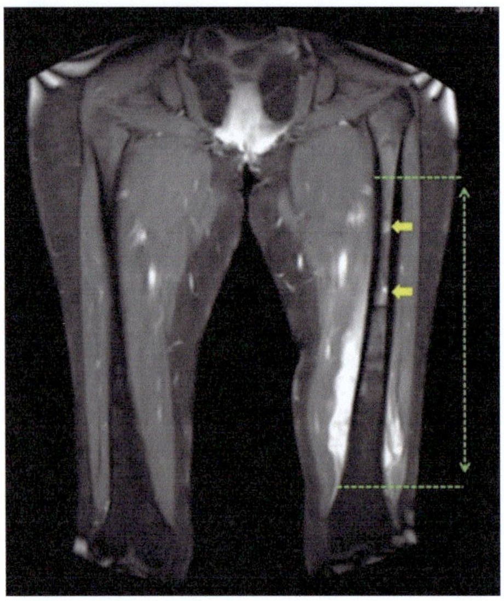

Fig. 26.3 MRI demonstrating the presence of marrow lesions/metastases in the upper third of the femur (yellow arrow) and segment of intercalary femur resection necessary with very short residual bony remnants at the proximal and distal end of femur (green dotted line)

26.3 Preoperative Local Imaging

Contrast-enhanced magnetic resonance imaging as detailed in the paragraph above, Figs. 26.1, 26.2, and 26.3.

Dynamic contrast-enhanced MRI demonstrating the circumferential extent of the soft-tissue lesion, Fig. 26.4

A plain radiograph of the femur was noncontributory except for some soft-tissue calcification seen at the middle third–lower third junction of the thigh, Fig. 26.5.

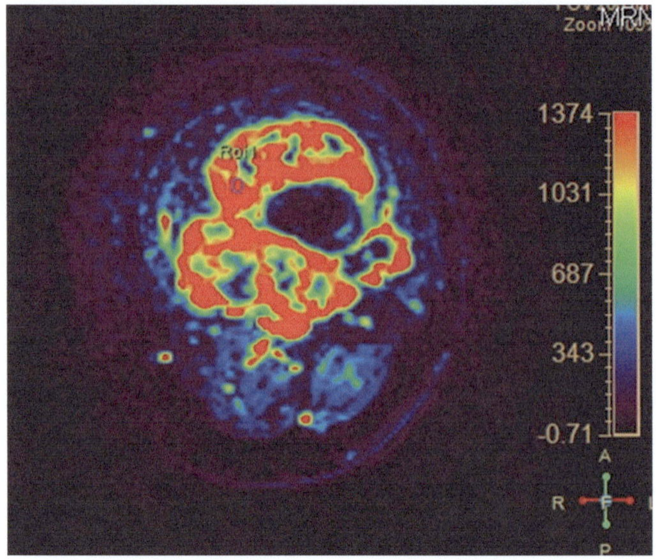

Fig. 26.4 Dynamic contrast-enhanced MRI demonstrating the circumferential extent of the soft tissue

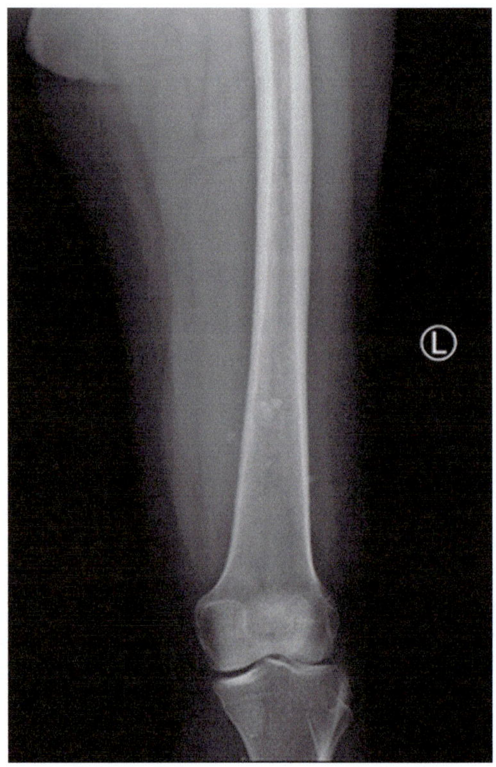

Fig. 26.5 Radiograph of the femur demonstrating some soft-tissue calcification seen at the middle third–lower third junction of the thigh

26.4 Preoperative Problem List

(a) A soft-tissue sarcoma of the thigh circumferentially surrounding the femur necessitating bony resection.
(b) Presence of marrow lesions/metastases in the upper third of the femur resulting in a long segment of intercalary femur resection with very short residual bony remnants at the proximal and distal ends of femur (Fig. 26.3—*green dotted line*).
(c) Need to reconstruct the bony defect to restore structural and skeletal stability.
(d) Associated vascular involvement necessitating vascular resection and reconstruction.

26.5 Treatment Strategy

(a) Multidisciplinary treatment including surgical resection (mandatory) + radiation (mandatory) + discussion regarding chemotherapy [1].
(b) Chemotherapy—with limited evidence for the benefit of neoadjuvant chemotherapy, it was decided to proceed with local therapy and reevaluate the option of subsequent adjuvant chemotherapy after surgery [2].
(c) Radiation—our institute policy favors postoperative radiation and hence the patient was planned for radiation after surgical excision.
(d) Surgical resection—oncologically adequate excision of the soft-tissue sarcoma of the thigh with intercalary femur resection and vascular resection.
(e) Reconstruction of the bony defect. Various options were considered for reconstruction of the resultant post excision bony defect
   - in view of intercalary femur resection with very short residual bony remnants at the proximal and distal end of femur, an intercalary prosthesis would have been very challenging because of the short segments for stem anchorage
   - reconstruction with a total femur prosthesis would result in sacrifice of the proximal and distal articular segments which was avoidable
   - reconstruction with a biological alternative (allograft or reimplanted sterilized tumor bone) had a high risk of nonunion as the patient would receive postoperative radiation. The segmental vascular resection would also reduce vasculature of the surrounding muscles and soft-tissue increasing the chance of infection
   - hence it was decided to reconstruct the defect with an antibiotic impregnated cement spacer with stable internal fixation [3]. This would restore skeletal stability, permit immediate weight-bearing ambulation, possibly reduce the incidence of postoperative infection and permit postoperative radiation without fearing the deleterious effects of radiation on a biological reconstruction

26.6 Basic Principles

(a) Preoperative planning is vital. Adequate oncological resection with appropriate margins needs to be ensured with imaging studies that include an MRI. MRI helps to evaluate the extent of the lesion, the relation to the neurovascular bundle, and plan the planes of dissection when resecting the tumor. Occasionally, a CT scan may better delineate cortical erosion or a reactive periosteal reaction in lesions that closely abut the bone.
(b) Sarcomas respect anatomical borders, and local anatomy influences tumor growth by setting natural boundaries to spread. While it may not always be possible to get a "quantitative" wide margin in soft-tissue sarcomas, negative margin excision ensures a layer of healthy tissue (intact anatomical barrier) around the tumor [4]. The excision should also include the biopsy tract en bloc.
(c) The incision (which includes the biopsy scar) is sited on the medial aspect of the thigh as this enables adequate vascular dissection (and resection/reconstruction) while permitting safe oncologic resection.
(d) Proximal and distal dissection in the sub sartorial canal is accomplished to secure proximal and distal vascular access and obtain control of the tumor-free sections of the femoral arterio-venous bundle.
(e) Ensuring that a layer of healthy tissue is maintained around the tumor, dissection is done to circumferentially isolate the tumor as much as possible.
(f) As in this case bony resection is also required, the site of distal osteotomy based on preoperative planning is identified. Completing this distal osteotomy (while ensuring that the femoral arterio-venous bundle is safeguarded) enables multiplanar mobility of the femur thus facilitating further circumferential dissection of the tumor.
(g) Similarly, the site of proximal osteotomy is identified and the osteotomy completed.
(h) Further dissection around the tumor facilitated by the multiplanar mobility after bony osteotomies results in the tumor (with intercalary resected femur) being attached to the host only by the earlier identified and secured proximal and distal tumor free segments of the femoral arterio-venous bundle.
(i) Dissection is continued proximally and distally along the femoral arterio-venous bundle till the area of vascular involvement.
(j) Appropriate anti coagulation (5000 IU intravenous heparin as a bolus) is administered just prior to vessel

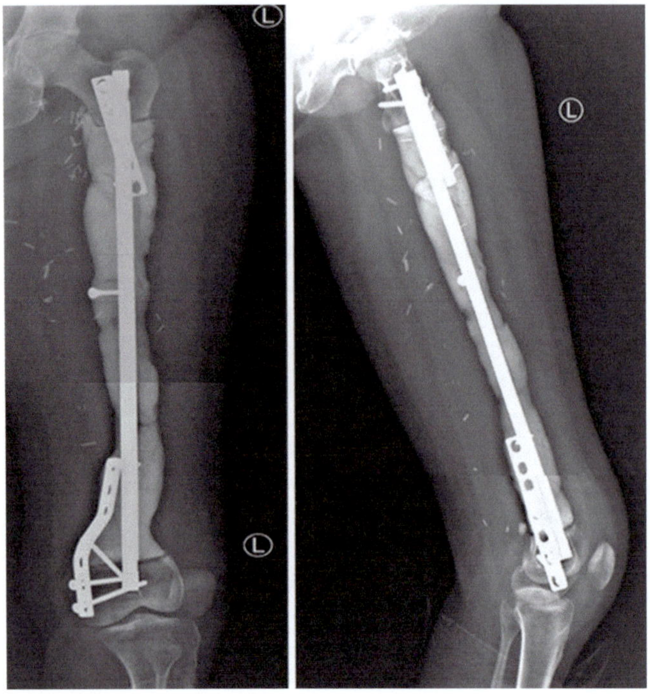

Fig. 26.6 Radiograph of "nail–plate–cement" construct

resection, the vessels are clamped proximally and distally and transected.

(k) A note is made of time of vessel transection—"ischemia time" till reestablishment of vascular continuity is documented.

(l) The specimen is now delivered, and the length of transected intercalary bone segment is measured.

(m) Adequate hemostasis is accomplished.

(n) Reconstruction of skeletal stability—the aim is to obtain and ensure correct length and longitudinal and rotational alignment of the limb. An intramedullary Kuntscher nail is anchored in the intramedullary canal on either side of the residual femur segments. Rotational stability is provided with plates fixed in both bony fragments and appropriately contoured to lie in close proximity to the intramedullary nail proximally and distally in the region of the bony defect, Figs. 26.6 and 26.7. Antibiotic impregnated cement is then molded around the implants to form a construct that bridges the defect. The combined "nail–plate–cement" construct provides adequate skeletal and rotational stability, Fig. 26.6.

(o) Vascular reconstruction is then completed—for reestablishing arterial continuity, we use an autologous reversed saphenous vein interposition graft (Fig. 26.7—*white arrow*), while venous continuity is established using a PTFE vascular graft (Fig. 26.7—*blue arrow*) [5].

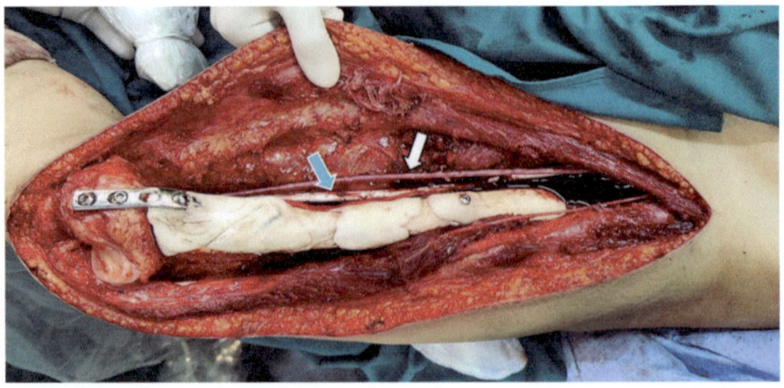

Fig. 26.7 Intraoperative picture of the combined "nail–plate–cement" construct and vascular reconstruction using an autologous reversed saphenous vein interposition graft (white arrow) for the artery and a PTFE vascular graft (blue arrow) for the vein

(p) Distal pulsations and vascularity are checked, and adequate hemostasis is reconfirmed.

(q) The wound is closed in layers over negative suction drains.

(r) Limb elevation in the postoperative period promotes wound healing and decreases postoperative edema.

(s) The patient is allowed to mobilize immediately after surgery. Unrestricted postoperative range of motion of the adjacent joints is permitted.

26.7 Intraoperative Image (Fig. 26.7)

The combined "nail–plate–cement" construct and vascular reconstruction using an autologous reversed saphenous vein interposition graft (Fig. 26.7—*white arrow*) for the artery and a PTFE vascular graft (Fig. 26.7—*blue arrow*) for the vein.

26.8 Technical Pearls

(a) In a soft-tissue sarcoma that requires multimodality reconstruction (bony + vascular) with radiation, it is best to choose a mode of skeletal reconstruction that has a low incidence of early postoperative complications so that adjuvant treatment modalities are not delayed; hence we chose an antibiotic cement spacer construct over a biological option. It has been suggested that massive amounts of methyl methacrylate in such a spacer could be responsible for inhibition of inflammatory cell activity thus helping to reduce the rate of infection [6].

(b) Completing the distal bony osteotomy at an early stage in the surgery enables multiplanar mobility of the femur, facilitating safe oncologic circumferential dissection of the tumor.

(c) After tumor resection it is important to ensure that excessive traction of the distal limb does not occur, as this can result in subsequent neurological deficit. This may occasionally happen because the absence of intact vessels (after vascular resection) removes a "visual guide" that safeguards against excessive traction.
(d) To maintain correct rotational alignment of the limb after reconstruction, longitudinal markings should be made using a cautery/ink on the remaining bony fragments prior to osteotomy to serve as reference points that should be in correct alignment after reconstruction.
(e) Even though it results in a relative increase of "ischemia time," vascular reconstruction should be accomplished after reconstituting bony stability. If vascular reconstruction precedes bony reconstruction there is a danger of disrupting the anastomosis during manipulation/traction while completing the bony reconstruction. Additionally, completion of the bony reconstruction before vascular reconstruction enables the correct estimation of reconstituted vessel length, preventing kinks/folds due to excessive length which can result in postoperative vascular complications.

26.9 Outcome Radiographs and Images

Figure 26.6—Radiograph—"nail–plate–cement" construct provides adequate skeletal and rotational stability.

Figures 26.8 and 26.9—Scar of surgery and post operative knee flexion/extension.

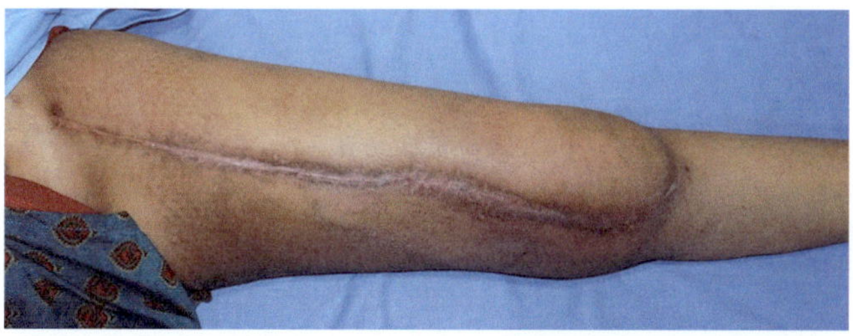

Fig. 26.8 Scar of surgery

26.10 Avoiding and Managing Problems

(a) Seroma formation and infection are not uncommon after large resections of soft-tissue sarcoma in the thigh [7]. Closed system suction drains may need to be retained for a longer duration. Regular clinical examination for detection of seroma formation in the early post operative period is recommended. If a large seroma is detected, an ultrasound-guided aspiration under strict aseptic conditions may be considered.
(b) Postoperative limb elevation and early ambulation are recommended to help reduce limb edema after vascular reconstruction.
(c) Appropriate antithrombotic medication is administered in the postoperative period after vascular reconstruction. While parenteral administration is used in the immediate postoperative period, long-term oral antithrombotics and anti-platelet therapy is continued for varying durations depending on the type of graft used (autologous/PTFE).
(d) Vacuum-assisted closure (VAC) may potentially lower the risk of postoperative wound complications in proximal lower extremity soft-tissue sarcomas without compromising local control or the risk of distant metastasis. [8]
(e) The cement spacer as a reconstruction modality has the advantage of a low incidence of early postoperative complications. However, if the patient is a long-term survivor, a more durable reconstruction option may be needed if failure of the cement spacer construct occurs. It is possible to revise the cement spacer to a prosthesis or biological reconstruction when needed [6, 9]. Reconstruction options that had limitations during index surgery offer multiple alternatives. A custom designed prosthesis (that has a lead time to manufacture that may have delayed index surgery) with innovative short stem anchorage options can be utilized [10]. A vascularized fibula autograft (which was challenging because of paucity of local vessels for anastomosis due to concomitant vascular resection at index surgery) can be an option either as a stand-alone graft [11] or in combination with an allograft (Capanna technique) [12].
[Representative examples are shown: Fig. 26.10—radiographs of an intercalary cement spacer in the tibia that was revised with a vascular fibula graft after failure; Fig. 26.11—radiographs of an intercalary cement spacer in the humerus that was revised with a vascular fibula graft after failure].

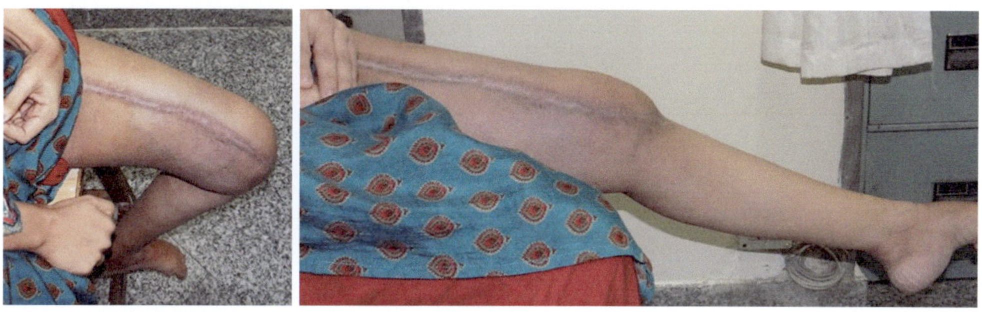

Fig. 26.9 Postoperative knee flexion/extension

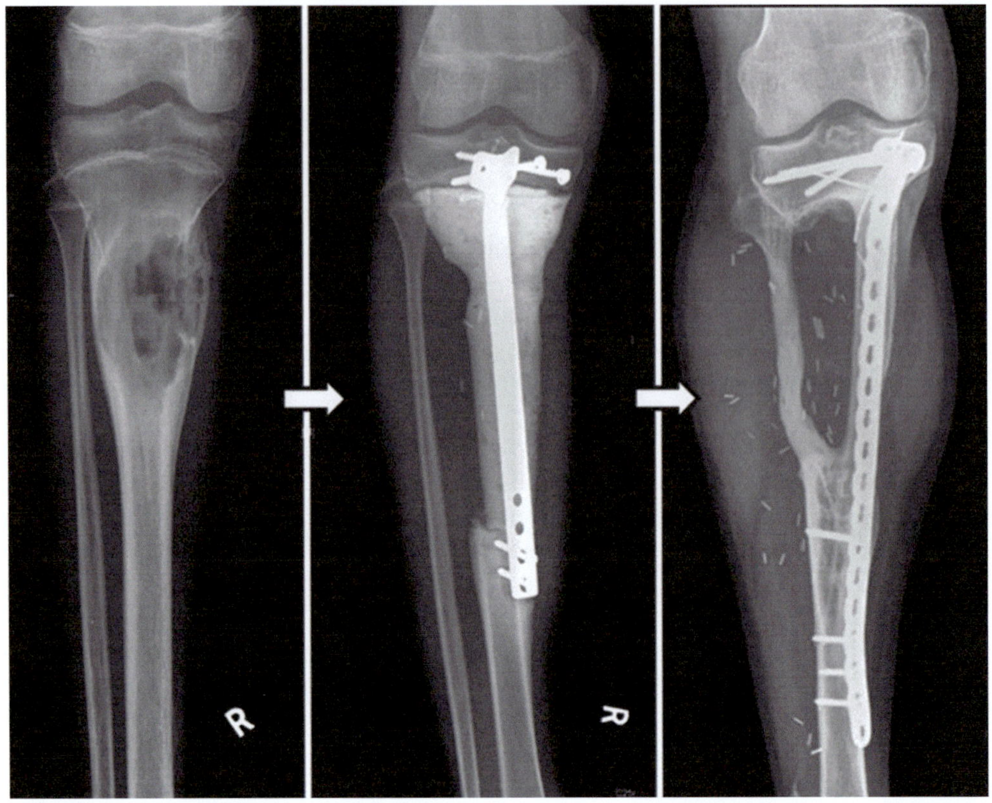

Fig. 26.10 Radiographs of an intercalary cement spacer in the tibia that was revised with a vascular fibula graft after failure

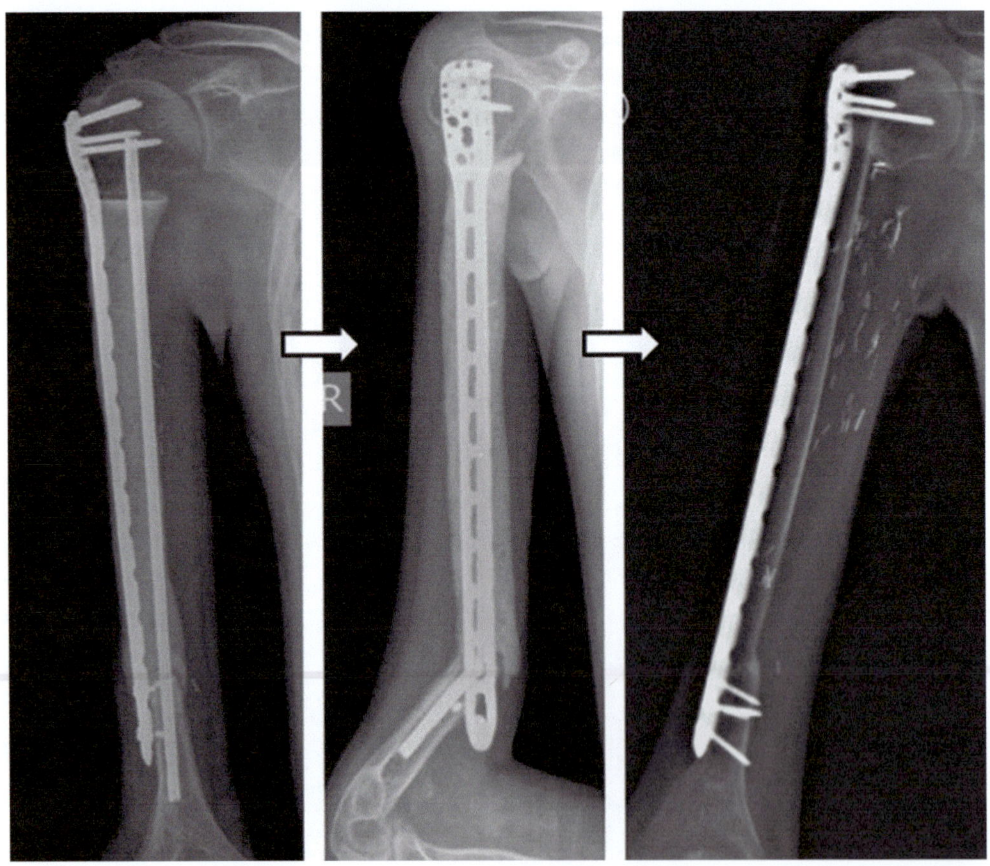

Fig. 26.11 Radiographs of an intercalary cement spacer in the humerus that was revised with a vascular fibula graft after failure

References

1. Roland CL, van Houdt W, Gronchi A. The landmark series: multimodality treatment of extremity sarcoma. Ann Surg Oncol. 2020;27(10):3672–82.
2. George S, Wagner AJ. Low levels of evidence for neoadjuvant chemotherapy to treat soft-tissue sarcoma. JAMA Oncol. 2018;4(9):1169–70.
3. Puri A, Gulia A, Pruthi M, Koushik S. Primary cement spacers: a cost-effective, durable limb salvage option for knee tumors. Knee. 2012;19(4):320–3.
4. Kawaguchi N, Ahmed AR, Matsumoto S, Manabe J, Matsushita Y. The concept of curative margin in surgery for bone and soft tissue sarcoma. Clin Orthop Relat Res. 2004;419:165–72.
5. Mahendra A, Gortzak Y, Ferguson PC, Deheshi BM, Lindsay TF, Wunder JS. Management of vascular involvement in extremity soft tissue sarcoma. Recent Results Cancer Res. 2009;179:285–99.
6. Capanna R, Biagini R, Ruggieri P, Bettelli G, Casadei R, Campanacci M. Temporary resection-arthrodesis of the knee using an intramedullary rod and bone cement. Int Orthop. 1989;13(4):253–8.
7. Elswick SM, Curiel DA, Wu P, Akhavan A, Molinar VE, Mohan AT, et al. Complications after thigh sarcoma resection. J Surg Oncol. 2020;121(6):945–51.
8. Bedi M, King DM, DeVries J, Hackbarth DA, Neilson JC. Does vacuum-assisted closure reduce the risk of wound complications in patients with lower extremity sarcomas treated with preoperative radiation? Clin Orthop Relat Res. 2019;477(4):768–74.
9. Ruggieri P, Kasimatis G, Errani C, Bosco G, Mercuri M. Desarthrodesis and prosthetic reconstruction of the knee after resection of bone tumors. J Surg Oncol. 2010;102(7):832–7.
10. Wang J, An J, Lu M, Zhang Y, Lin J, Luo Y, et al. Is three-dimensional-printed custom-made ultra-short stem with a porous structure an acceptable reconstructive alternative in peri-knee metaphysis for the tumorous bone defect? World J Surg Oncol. 2021;19(1):235.
11. Ozger H, Akgul T, Yildiz F, Topalan M. Biological reconstruction of the femur using double free vascularized fibular autografts in a vertical array because of a large defect following wide resection of an osteosarcoma: a case report with 7 years of follow-up. J Pediatr Orthop B. 2013;22(1):52–8.
12. Li M, Xiao X, Fan J, Lu Y, Chen G, Huang M, et al. Is the capanna technique a reliable method for revision surgery after failure of previous limb-salvage surgery? Ann Surg Oncol. 2022;29(2):1122–9.

Liposarcoma of the Thigh: Multimodal Treatment and Long-Term Concerns

27

Maria Anna Smolle, Iva Brcic, Marko Bergovec, Jasminka Igrec, Bernadette Liegl-Atzwanger, and Andreas Leithner

27.1 Basic Clinical History

A 43-year-old female patient presented to the outpatient clinic with a swelling of her left thigh she had noticed 1 week ago. Magnetic resonance imaging (MRI) examination revealed a contrast-enhancing soft tissue tumour sized 12 × 7 × 7.5 cm encompassing more than half of the distal femoral bone and displacing the vastus intermedius and medialis. Following incisional biopsy via a lateral incision to the lesion, histopathological analysis revealed a myxoid liposarcoma G1. FISH analysis with CHOP probes showed break apart signal within tumour cells confirming the diagnosis. Initial staging with CT-scan of the thorax, abdomen, and pelvis ruled the presence of distant metastases.

27.1.1 Treatment and Clinical Course

Limb salvage surgery with wide resection and prophylactic osteosynthesis of the distal femur following periosteal stripping was carried out. Definite histological work-up revealed myxoid liposarcoma G2 with focal close margins (1 mm). Postoperative radiotherapy (66 Gray [Gy] at gross tumour volume, 55 Gy at safety margin) was carried out uneventful. Two years after surgery, the patient fractured her left patella during a fall and underwent tension band wiring. The osteosynthesis was removed 1 year thereafter. Oncological follow-up was carried out in 3-month intervals for the first 3 years, every 6 months until the end of the fifth postoperative year and yearly thereafter using local MRI and radiography, abdominal ultrasonography, as well as alternating thoracic radiography or CT-scan.

27.1.2 Long-Term Follow-Up and Subsequent Clinical Course

Follow-up was uneventful until 83 months after definite surgery the patient visited our outpatient clinic unscheduled, as having recently felt "strange" around the operating field. On the promptly performed imaging, including radiography and MRI, a novel intramedullary, contrast-enhancing lesion with cortical penetration and extraosseous component was found. CT-guided biopsy (carried out inadequately directly through the remaining knee extensors) revealed inconclusive results. Subsequent open biopsy through lateral approach led to the diagnosis of a secondary, radiation-induced osteosarcoma G3. Staging (CT-scan of thorax/abdomen/pelvis) at that time point ruled out secondary metastases. Within the multidisciplinary sarcoma meeting, decision against neoadjuvant chemotherapy was reached. After careful patient counselling towards risks and benefits of limb-salvage surgery, due to the now also contaminated anterior aspect of the left distal femur, a wide resection with distal femoral endoprosthetic replacement through an extended lateral approach was carried out. The patient underwent adjuvant chemotherapy according to the EURO BOSS protocol with Cisplatin, Adriamycin, and Ifosfamide. She is currently (7.8 years after surgery) receiving her eighth cycle. The limb function is limited with active flexion up to 60°, and passive extension to 0°, whilst active extension is impossible.

M. A. Smolle · M. Bergovec · A. Leithner (✉)
Department of Orthopaedics and Trauma, Medical University of Graz, Graz, Austria
e-mail: maria.smolle@medunigraz.at; marko.bergovec@medunigraz.at; andreas.leithner@medunigraz.at

I. Brcic · B. Liegl-Atzwanger
Institute of Pathology, Medical University of Graz, Graz, Austria
e-mail: iva.brcic@medunigraz.at; Bernadette.liegl-atzwanger@medunigraz.at

J. Igrec
Department of Radiology, Medical University of Graz, Graz, Austria
e-mail: Jasminka.igrec@medunigraz.at

H. Özger et al. (eds.), *Diagnosis and Treatment of Soft Tissue Tumors*, https://doi.org/10.1007/978-3-031-77061-6_27

27.2 Preoperative/Pretreatment Clinical and Radiological Images

Preoperative radiographs of the left knee show displacement of the fatty plains in the suprapatellar region due to soft tissue mass extending along the distal femur. Note intact underlying cortex and no intralesional calcifications (Fig. 27.1).

Preoperative MRI images show the large lesion within the quadriceps femoris muscle, encompassing more than half of the femoral circumference. Strong and inhomogeneous contrast enhancement is visible, corresponding to myxoid tissue (Fig. 27.2).

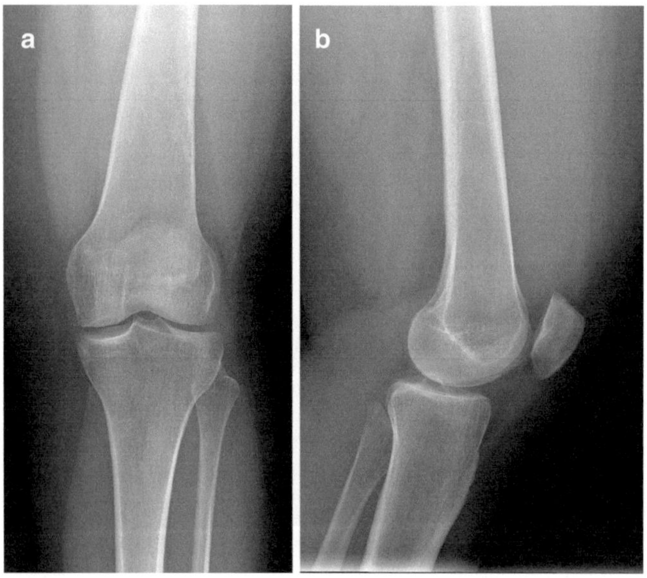

Fig. 27.1 Preoperative a.p. (**a**) and lateral (**b**) radiographs of left knee joint

27.3 Problem List

(a) Low-grade soft-tissue sarcoma encompassing more than half of femoral bone at the distal diaphysis.
(b) Consequences of extensive periosteal stripping following partial bone resection in order to achieve clear margins.
(c) Neoadjuvant versus adjuvant therapy (RTX), taking into consideration long-term toxicities and potential secondary malignancies.
(d) Neoadjuvant RTX dose-reduction in myxoid liposarcoma (36 Gy) versus other soft tissue sarcomas (50 Gy) based on findings of the Dose Reduction of Preoperative Radiotherapy in Myxoid Liposarcoma (DOREMY) trial [1].
(e) Modality and timing of follow-up.
(f) Dealing with post-treatment complications (movement restriction, insufficiency fractures).
(g) Diagnostic work-up of suspected local recurrences, including planning of biopsy tract.

For subsequent complication

(h) Management of secondary, radiation-induced osteosarcoma.

27.4 Treatment Strategy

(a) Wide resection of soft tissue sarcoma, with clear soft tissue and bony margins.
(b) Support of femoral bone with osteosynthesis to prevent insufficiency fracture after periosteal stripping and postoperative radiotherapy.
(c) Postoperative radiotherapy administered due to focal close margins.

Fig. 27.2 Preoperative MRI examination of left distal femur showing the large soft tissue mass encasing more than half of the femoral circumference and extending up to the suprapatellar recess (**a**—axial T1-weighted turbo spin echo [T1w TSE]; **b**—axial T2wfat-saturated TSE; **c**—sagittal proton density TSE; **d**—coronal T1w TSE after gadolinium application)

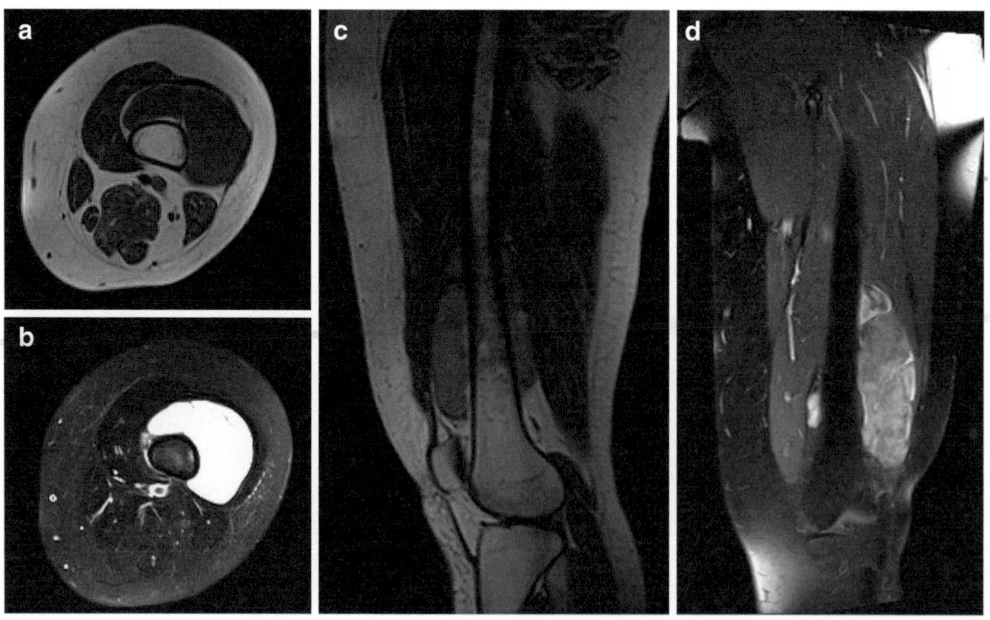

(d) Knee flexion restriction during early postoperative period to allow for adequate healing and scar formation.
(e) Consider reconstruction of knee extensor apparatus (quadriceps muscle, patella tendon) or tendon transfer to allow for active knee extension.
(f) Close oncological follow-up, including local (MRI with contrast agent, radiography) and systemic (chest CT scans) surveillance. Furthermore, consider whole-body MRI in patients with myxoid liposarcoma to eventually detect metastases at atypical locations (e.g., bone, abdomen).

For subsequent complication

(g) Biopsy for suspected recurrence, taking into consideration potential further surgeries.

Consider open re-biopsy after inconclusive CT-guided biopsy.

(h) Distal femoral replacement for secondary osteosarcoma, followed by systemic chemotherapy according to EURO BOSS protocol.

27.5 Basic Principles

(a) Myxoid liposarcomas, particularly high-grade ones, respond well to preoperative radiotherapy [2–4]. However, the size-reducing effect of neoadjuvant radiotherapy is rather minor in low-grade tumours. Moreover, the negative impact of (anticipated) close margins upon definite surgery is reduced to a greater amount by neoadjuvant than adjuvant radiotherapy (RTX) [5]. As in the present case histopathological work-up of the biopsy revealed G1 myxoid liposarcoma and wide margins upon definite surgery appeared technically possible, preoperative irradiation was omitted. In case of close or contaminated margins, postoperative radiotherapy may be considered [6]. Yet, the larger irradiation field, long-term toxicities occurring in irradiated tissues have to be taken into consideration [7–9]. As histopathology of the surgical specimen led to the diagnosis of G2 myxoid liposarcoma with focal close margins, postoperative RTX was recommended.
(b) Periosteal stripping can be performed to achieve clear margins in case a soft-tissue sarcoma is encompassing, but not infiltrating, the bone. Preoperative radiography and CT help to visualise the integrity of the cortical bone [10]. However, periosteal stripping reduces blood supply, eventually leading to subsequent fracture [11, 12]. In weight-bearing bones, prophylactic osteosynthesis to prevent fracture should thus be performed [13]. This seems to particularly apply to tumours involving the anterior thigh [13]. Furthermore, the more extensive the periosteal stripping, the more likely a radiation-induced pathological fracture may occur, strengthening the indication for prophylactic stabilisation [11, 13].
(c) The resected knee extensor apparatus may in part be reconstructed by re-attaching remaining muscles to the patella [14]. In the current case, the patient was counselled beforehand that active knee extension will most likely be impossible, and that a knee orthosis may then become necessary.

For subsequent complication

(d) In case of suspected local recurrence or distant metastasis, interdisciplinary discussion, followed by diagnostic work-up (biopsy) is needed. With a high accuracy rate and low complication rate, CT-guided biopsy constitutes an ideal diagnostic tool [15].
(e) The planned biopsy tract has to be discussed with the sarcoma surgeon in charge, in light of potential later surgical approaches in order to allow for safe removal of the tract upon definite surgery [5]. In particular, it must not contaminate any structures necessary for sufficient limb and/or joint function, e.g., in the present case the quadriceps femoris muscle to maintain active knee extension.
(f) Upon endoprosthetic replacement, sufficient soft tissue coverage of the implant has to be obtained in order to reduce the risk of periprosthetic joint infection.
(g) Radiation-induced secondary malignancies may occur 8–14 years after radiotherapy [16–19], with a 10-year cumulative risk between 0.03% and 0.8% [18, 20]. Undifferentiated pleomorphic sarcomas and osteosarcomas are the most common histological subtypes diagnosed [16–19]. Patients with tumour-predisposition syndromes such as Li–Fraumeni syndrome [21], retinoblastoma syndrome [22] and Nijmegen breakage syndrome [23] may be at higher risk to develop radiation-induced sarcomas [24].
(h) Radiation-induced high-grade osteosarcomas require systemic chemotherapy. In adult patients, treatment doses may have to be reduced owing to occurrence of adverse events [25].

27.6 Photos and Imaging During Treatment

Histopathological image of myxoid liposarcoma biopsy (Fig. 27.3a) and definite surgery specimen (Fig. 27.3b).

Postoperative radiography of the left femur with a LISS plate in place to prevent later insufficiency fracture due to extensive periosteal stripping (Fig. 27.4a, b).

Radiographs of the left distal femur and knee 1.2 years (a, b) and 3.3 years (c, d), respectively, after surgery. Note the posttraumatic/postoperative changes of the patella, with a suture anchor still in place following patella fracture, osteosynthesis and hardware removal (Fig. 27.5c, d).

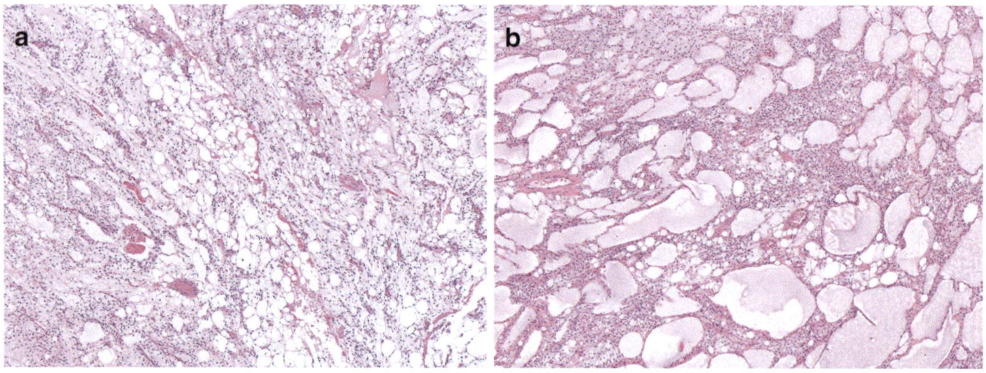

Fig. 27.3 Histopathological image (hematoxylin-eosin staining) of myxoid liposarcoma biopsy (**a**) and resection specimen (**b**). The tumour is composed of monotonous small ovoid cells embedded in a myxoid to hyalinised matrix with prominent plexiform capillary network and uni- and bivacuolated lipoblasts (**a/b**). Pools of mucin ("pulmonary oedema-like" pattern) can be seen (**b**), as well as even more cellular areas

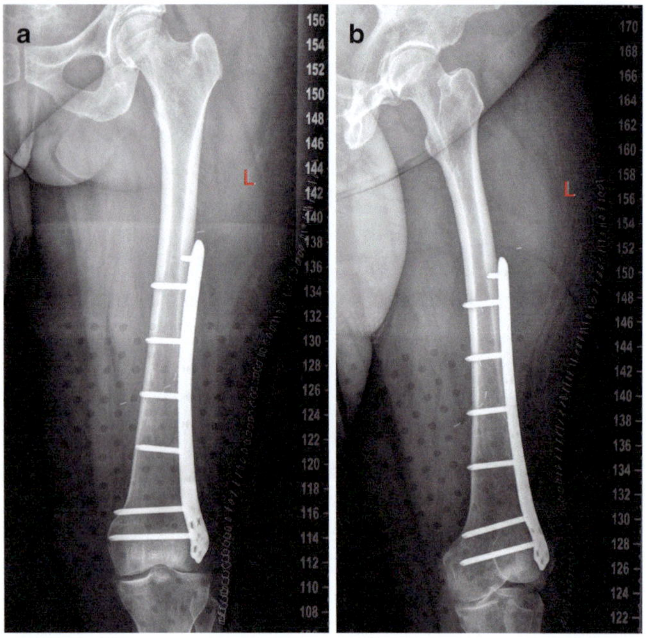

Fig. 27.4 Postoperative a.p. (**a**) and oblique lateral (**b**) radiographs of the left femur

Radiographs of the left femur 7.3 years after primary surgery, depicting a newly developed intramedullary mass at the distal femur with immature cloudlike bone formation and extraosseous component (Fig. 27.6).

Bone scintigraphy with images taken 5 min (a, b) and 3 h after injection (c, d), both showing the increased activity at the tumour site (Fig. 27.7).

High-resolution axial CT-images in bone window during image-guided biopsy, with the biopsy tract inadequately passing directly through the rectus femoris muscle (Fig. 27.8).

Histopathological image of open biopsy (Fig. 27.9a) and definite surgery specimen (Fig. 27.9b–d) showing secondary osteosarcoma.

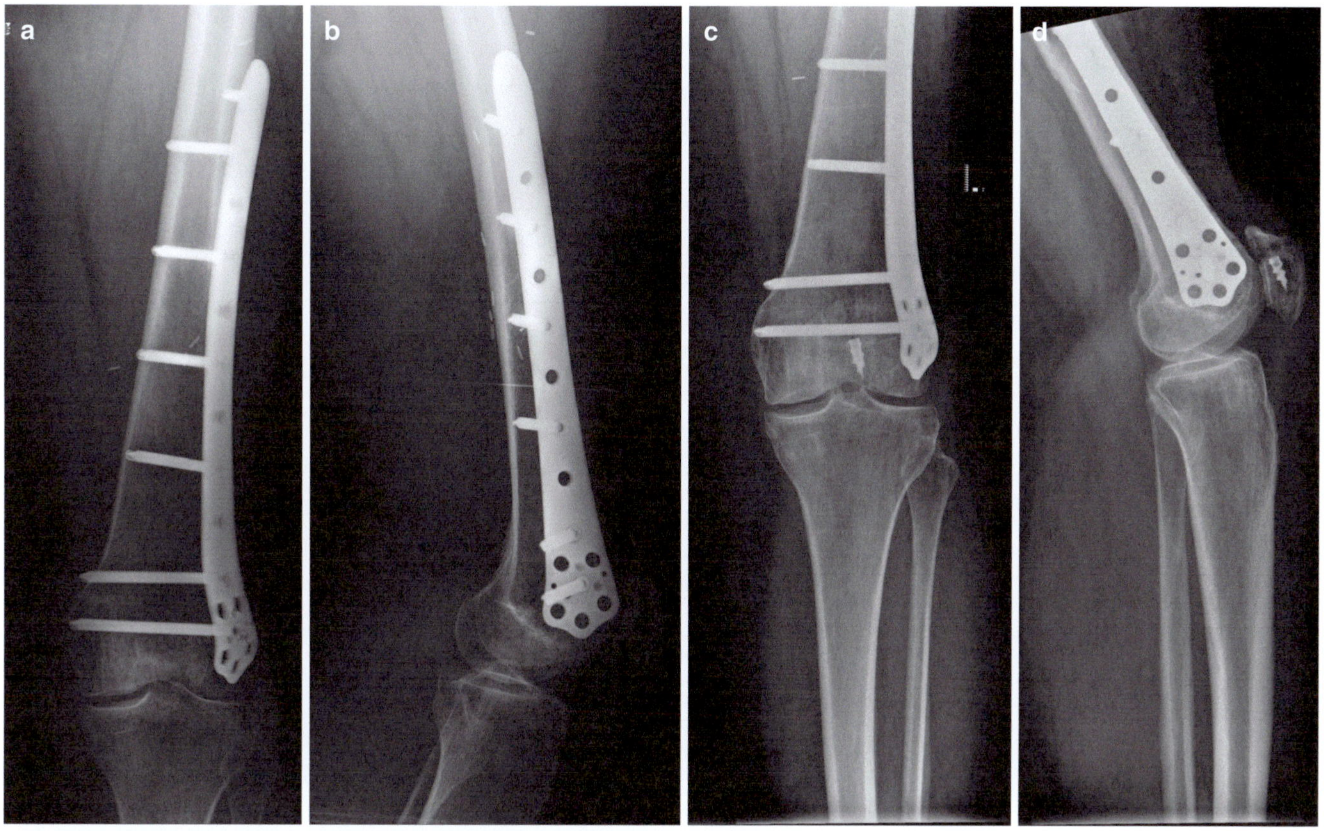

Fig. 27.5 A.p. (**a**, **c**) and lateral (**b**, **d**) radiographs of the left knee 1.2 years (**a**, **b**) and 3.3 years (**c**, **d**) after surgery

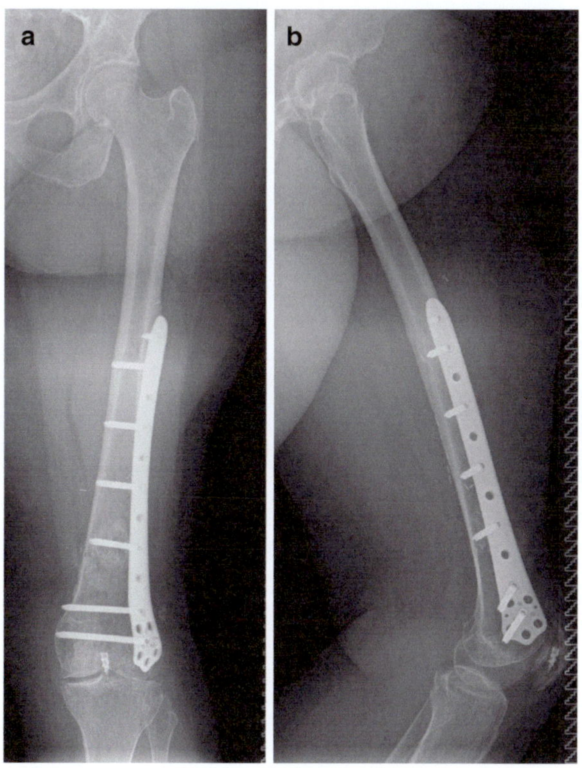

Fig. 27.6 A.p. (**a**) and lateral (**b**) radiographs depict a newly developed sclerotic lesion of the left distal femur 83 months following initial surgery

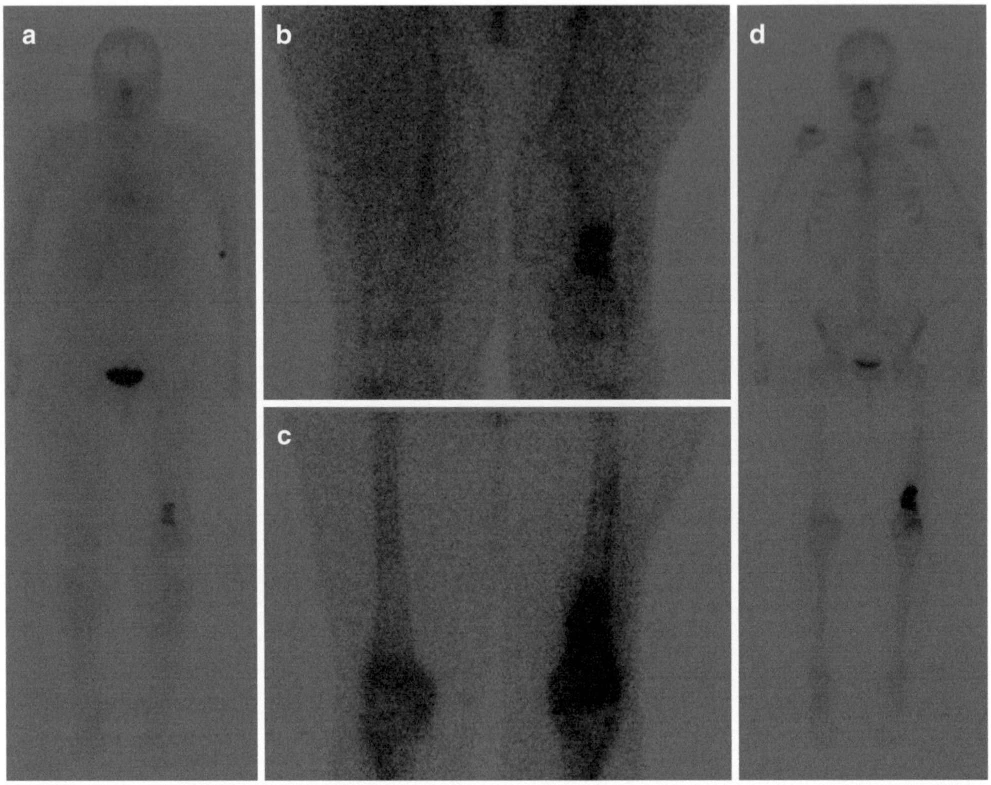

Fig. 27.7 Early (**a**, **b**) and late-phase bone scintigraphy (**c**, **d**) showing increased activity at the left distal femur

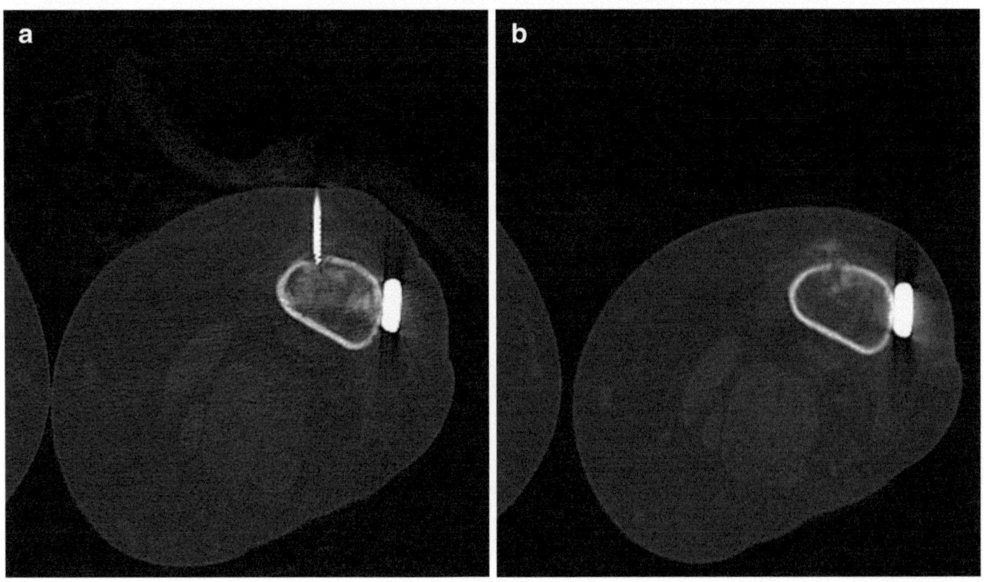

Fig. 27.8 High-resolution CT-images in bone window during image-guided biopsy (**a**, **b**) showing biopsy tract going inappropriately directly through knee extensor mechanism

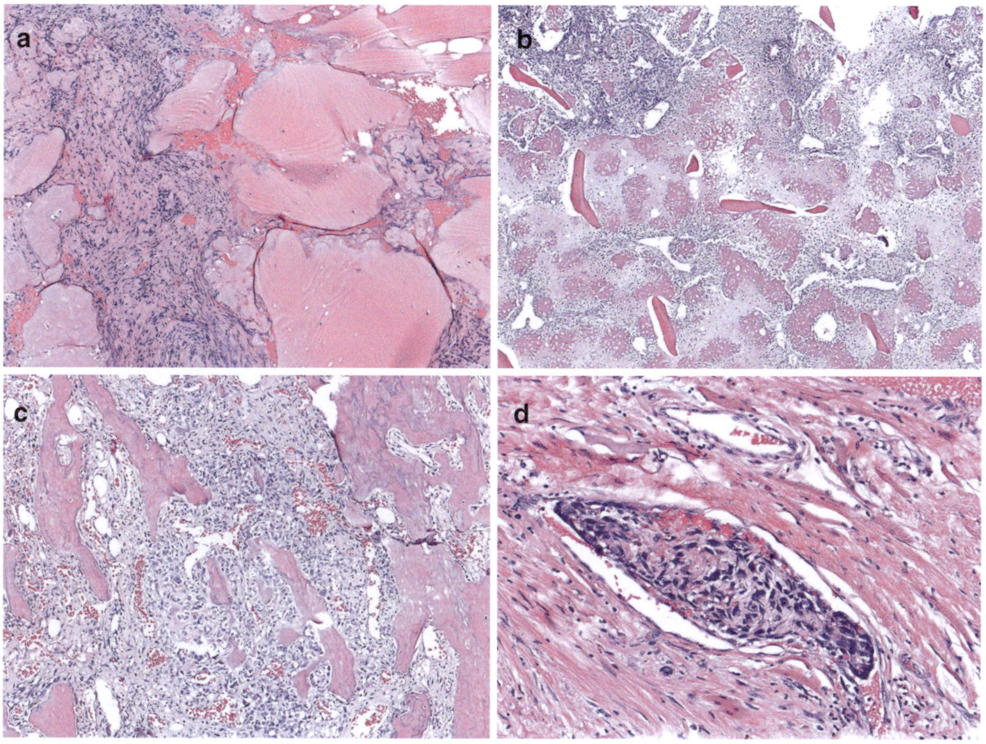

Fig. 27.9 Histopathological image (hematoxylin-eosin staining) of secondary osteosarcoma G3 open biopsy (**a**) and definite surgery specimen (**b–d**). Bone fragment is infiltrated by an atypical spindle cell proliferation with focal osteoid production (**a**). The resection specimen shows tumour comprised of atypical cell proliferation with abundant irregular interconnecting purple trabeculae of neoplastic woven bone replacing the marrow and encasing the preexisting cancellous bone (**b**; 10× magnification). Atypical spindle- to epithelioid cells with focal osteoid production are visible (**c**; 20× magnification). Neoplastic cells are seen within blood vessels (vascular invasion; **d**; 40× magnification)

27.7 Technical Pearls

(a) Upon definite surgery, wide resection via a lateral incision to the femur, encompassing the biopsy tract, is performed. In the herein presented case, this requires removal of the entire vastus intermedius, as well as partial resection of the vastus lateralis and medialis. In order to achieve clear margins at the femur and suprapatellar recess, subperiosteal stripping and resection of the recess, respectively, are carried out.

(b) Due to periosteal stripping of more than half of the femur's circumference and the prospect of additional radiotherapy, prophylactic osteosynthesis with a LISS plate is performed.

(c) Wound is closed meticulously by re-adapting the remaining muscle bellies to achieve sufficient soft tissue coverage of the bone. Suction drainage is inserted in the deep to reduce haematoma—and later on—seroma formation.

(d) Patient's knee flexion is limited to free extension but 15° flexion for 6 weeks. Thereafter, allowed flexion is increased by 30° every 2 weeks. An extension-locking orthosis is prescribed to compensate for (partial) loss of the knee extensor apparatus.

(e) Adjuvant radiotherapy is started after definite wound healing with daily doses of 2 Gray (Gy), reaching 66 Gy at the original tumour bed (reconstructed from preoperative images as the "resected" gross tumour volume [GTV]), and 50 Gy at the surrounding safety margin (i.e., elective clinical target volume [CTV]) [26].

(f) Regular postoperative check-ups every 3 months for the first 3 years, with contrast-enhanced MRI scans and radiographs of the left distal femur, thoracic CT-scans alternated with chest radiographs and ultrasonography of the abdomen, are carried out. In postoperative years 4 and 5, follow-up appointments are extended to 6 monthly intervals. Thereafter, yearly check-ups are recommended [5]. However, patients may counsel their doctors regardless of the intervals in case they notice a novel growing mass, pain, or discomfort. According to the study by *Puri* et al., especially local recurrences seem to be identified by patients themselves in the majority of cases [27]. Furthermore, long-time follow-up with frequently performed radiographs and CT-scans leads to considerable cumulative radiation exposure, wherefore more individualised follow-up approaches, taking into consideration patient-specific risks, have been proposed

[27–29]. Related to this, the ongoing multicentre *Surveillance After Extremity Tumor Surgery* (SAFETY) trial currently evaluates different intervals between appointments (3 vs. 6 months), as well as imaging modalities (thoracic CT-scan vs. radiography) [28]. A relatively innovative approach to monitoring tumour patients during follow-up is through liquid biopsy, a non-invasive method based on the detection of tumour cell fragments in the bloodstream. In patients with sarcomas exhibiting specific mutations (e.g., Ewing sarcoma, rhabdomyosarcoma, myxoid liposarcoma), these genetic alterations can be found in the bloodstream and thus be used to monitor disease activity [30].

(g) Upon biopsy, several issues have to be considered: Plan biopsy together with sarcoma surgeon, contaminate one compartment only, use direct approach to tumour, stay away from neurovascular structures, obtain a sufficient amount of material, and reduce haematoma formation by inserting suction drainages [31].

(h) In case of inconclusive first biopsy but radiological suspicion of malignancy, repeat biopsy with extensive tissue sampling [32].

(i) Adequate soft tissue coverage upon megaprosthetic replacement can be achieved via careful myodesis of remaining muscles, local flaps (e.g., gastrocnemius for the proximal tibia) or free muscular flaps [14].

(j) According to the DOREMY trial, administration of neoadjuvant RTX in myxoid liposarcoma with 36 Gy (rather than usually 50 Gy) in 2 Gy fractions daily results in local control rates comparable to those achieved upon standard RTX dosage [1]. On the other hand, local complications occur at lower levels [1]. In light of this recently gained knowledge, preoperative radiation therapy at lower doses may have reduced the likelihood for secondary insufficiency fracture of the patella, as well as development of radiation-induced osteosarcoma in the present case.

27.8 Outcome Clinical and Radiological Images

Radiographs of the left femur at latest follow-up, 3 months following distal femoral replacement, and 7.8 years after primary tumour diagnosis (Fig. 27.10a, b).

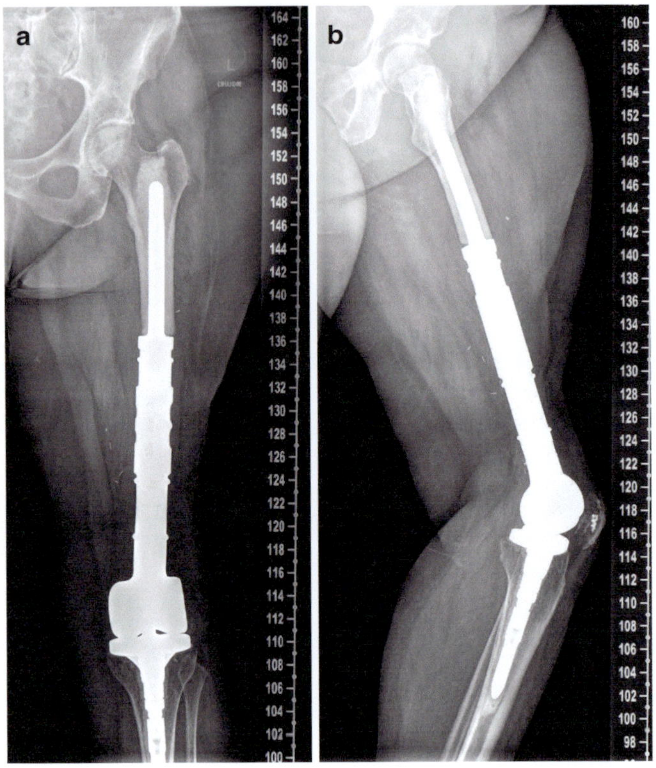

Fig. 27.10 A.p. (**a**) and lateral (**b**) radiographs of distal femur with distal femoral endoprosthesis in place. Images taken 3 months after last surgery (7.8 years after primary tumour diagnosis)

27.9 Avoiding and Managing Complications

(a) Seroma formation can be minimised by meticulous haemostasis and the use of suction drainages. Postoperative seromas may yet occur but often spontaneously regress during follow-up. Vaccum-assisted closure (VAC) may be used to reduce wound complication risk, especially in patients with proximal lower limb soft tissue sarcomas following preoperative radiotherapy [33]. Notably, this surgical strategy does not seem to negatively influence local control rate [33].

(b) Joint stiffness is a common complication following prolonged movement restriction, as well as radiotherapy. Early rehabilitation with standardised physiotherapy protocols may help to reduce the extent of joint stiffness [34, 35].

(c) Insufficiency fractures can occur after radiotherapy [11]. Therefore, prophylactic osteosynthesis or intramedullary nailing of the distal femur can be performed, as periosteal stripping itself already weakens bony blood supply [36]. Notably, in the current case, the patient fractured her left patella 24 months after the initial surgery that was subsequently fixed with tension band wiring at an external hospital. Osteosynthesis was removed 1 year postoperatively.
(d) Inappropriate biopsy tracts eventually require surgeries via suboptimal approaches and, even more significant, the resection of vital structures. Although the CT-guided biopsy had been performed directly through the remaining knee extensor apparatus, the open biopsy was carried out from lateral via the original scar and thus planned later surgical approach.
(e) Necessary resection of parts of the extensor apparatus during distal femoral replacement further increases the risk for periprosthetic joint infection, as soft tissue coverage around the implant is poor.

References

1. Lansu J, Bovée J, Braam P, van Boven H, Flucke U, Bonenkamp JJ, et al. Dose reduction of preoperative radiotherapy in myxoid liposarcoma: a nonrandomized controlled trial. JAMA Oncol. 2021;7(1):e205865. https://doi.org/10.1001/jamaoncol.2020.5865.
2. Chung PW, Deheshi BM, Ferguson PC, Wunder JS, Griffin AM, Catton CN, et al. Radiosensitivity translates into excellent local control in extremity myxoid liposarcoma: a comparison with other soft tissue sarcomas. Cancer. 2009;115(14):3254–61. https://doi.org/10.1002/cncr.24375.
3. Pitson G, Robinson P, Wilke D, Kandel RA, White L, Griffin AM, et al. Radiation response: an additional unique signature of myxoid liposarcoma. Int J Radiat Oncol Biol Phys. 2004;60(2):522–6. https://doi.org/10.1016/j.ijrobp.2004.03.009.
4. Engström K, Bergh P, Cederlund CG, Hultborn R, Willen H, Aman P, et al. Irradiation of myxoid/round cell liposarcoma induces volume reduction and lipoma-like morphology. Acta Oncol. 2007;46(6):838–45. https://doi.org/10.1080/02841860601080415.
5. Gronchi A, Miah AB, Dei Tos AP, Abecassis N, Bajpai J, Bauer S, et al. Soft tissue and visceral sarcomas: ESMO-EURACAN-GENTURIS clinical practice guidelines for diagnosis, treatment and follow-up(☆). Ann Oncol. 2021;32(11):1348–65. https://doi.org/10.1016/j.annonc.2021.07.006.
6. Hatano H, Ogose A, Hotta T, Kawashima H, Sugita T, Sasamoto R, et al. Treatment of myxoid liposarcoma by marginal or intralesional resection combined with radiotherapy. Anticancer Res. 2003;23(3c):3045–9.
7. le Grange F, Cassoni AM, Seddon BM. Tumour volume changes following pre-operative radiotherapy in borderline resectable limb and trunk soft tissue sarcoma. Eur J Surg Oncol. 2014;40(4):394–401. https://doi.org/10.1016/j.ejso.2014.01.011.
8. Davis AM, O'Sullivan B, Turcotte R, Bell R, Catton C, Chabot P, et al. Late radiation morbidity following randomization to preoperative versus postoperative radiotherapy in extremity soft tissue sarcoma. Radiother Oncol. 2005;75(1):48–53. https://doi.org/10.1016/j.radonc.2004.12.020.
9. Tfayli Y, Baydoun A, Naja AS, Saghieh S. Management of myxoid liposarcoma of the extremity. Oncol Lett. 2021;22(2):596. https://doi.org/10.3892/ol.2021.12857.
10. Caracciolo JT, Letson GD. Radiologic approach to bone and soft tissue sarcomas. Surg Clin North Am. 2016;96(5):963–76. https://doi.org/10.1016/j.suc.2016.05.007.
11. Lin PP, Schupak KD, Boland PJ, Brennan MF, Healey JH. Pathologic femoral fracture after periosteal excision and radiation for the treatment of soft tissue sarcoma. Cancer. 1998;82(12):2356–65.
12. Folkert MR, Casey DL, Berry SL, Crago A, Fabbri N, Singer S, et al. Femoral fracture in primary soft-tissue sarcoma of the thigh and groin treated with intensity-modulated radiation therapy: observed versus expected risk. Ann Surg Oncol. 2019;26(5):1326–31. https://doi.org/10.1245/s10434-019-07182-5.
13. Helmstedter CS, Goebel M, Zlotecki R, Scarborough MT. Pathologic fractures after surgery and radiation for soft tissue tumors. Clin Orthop Relat Res. 2001;389:165–72. https://doi.org/10.1097/00003086-200108000-00023.
14. Ek EW, Rozen WM, Ek ET, Rudiger HA. Surgical options for reconstruction of the extensor mechanism of the knee after limb-sparing sarcoma surgery: an evidence-based review. Arch Orthop Trauma Surg. 2011;131(4):487–95. https://doi.org/10.1007/s00402-010-1158-4.
15. Trieu J, Schlicht SM, Choong PF. Diagnosing musculoskeletal tumours: how accurate is CT-guided core needle biopsy? Eur J Surg Oncol. 2016;42(7):1049–56. https://doi.org/10.1016/j.ejso.2016.02.242.
16. Thijssens KM, van Ginkel RJ, Suurmeijer AJ, Pras E, van der Graaf WT, Hollander M, et al. Radiation-induced sarcoma: a challenge for the surgeon. Ann Surg Oncol. 2005;12(3):237–45. https://doi.org/10.1245/aso.2005.03.041.
17. Wiklund TA, Blomqvist CP, Räty J, Elomaa I, Rissanen P, Miettinen M. Postirradiation sarcoma. Analysis of a nationwide cancer registry material. Cancer. 1991;68(3):524–31. https://doi.org/10.1002/1097-0142(19910801)68:3<524::aid-cncr2820680313>3.0.co;2-e.
18. Callesen LB, Safwat A, Rose HK, Sørensen FB, Baad-Hansen T, Aggerholm-Pedersen N. Radiation-induced sarcoma: a retrospective population-based study over 34 years in a single institution. Clin Oncol (R Coll Radiol). 2021;33(5):e232–8. https://doi.org/10.1016/j.clon.2020.12.009.
19. Bjerkehagen B, Småstuen MC, Hall KS, Skjeldal S, Smeland S, Fosså SD. Why do patients with radiation-induced sarcomas have a poor sarcoma-related survival? Br J Cancer. 2012;106(2):297–306. https://doi.org/10.1038/bjc.2011.559.
20. Mark RJ, Poen J, Tran LM, Fu YS, Selch MT, Parker RG. Postirradiation sarcomas. A single-institution study and review of the literature. Cancer. 1994;73(10):2653–62. https://doi.org/10.1002/1097-0142(19940515)73:10<2653::aid-cncr2820731030>3.0.co;2-g.
21. Hisada M, Garber JE, Fung CY, Fraumeni JF Jr, Li FP. Multiple primary cancers in families with Li-Fraumeni syndrome. J Natl Cancer Inst. 1998;90(8):606–11. https://doi.org/10.1093/jnci/90.8.606.
22. Yu CL, Tucker MA, Abramson DH, Furukawa K, Seddon JM, Stovall M, et al. Cause-specific mortality in long-term survivors of retinoblastoma. J Natl Cancer Inst. 2009;101(8):581–91. https://doi.org/10.1093/jnci/djp046.
23. Taalman RD, Jaspers NG, Scheres JM, de Wit J, Hustinx TW. Hypersensitivity to ionizing radiation, in vitro, in a new chromosomal breakage disorder, the Nijmegen Breakage Syndrome. Mutat Res. 1983;112(1):23–32. https://doi.org/10.1016/0167-8817(83)90021-4.
24. Berrington de Gonzalez A, Kutsenko A, Rajaraman P. Sarcoma risk after radiation exposure. Clin Sarcoma Res. 2012;2(1):18. https://doi.org/10.1186/2045-3329-2-18.

25. Ferrari S, Bielack SS, Smeland S, Longhi A, Egerer G, Sundby Hall K, et al. EURO-B.O.S.S.: a European study on chemotherapy in bone-sarcoma patients aged over 40: outcome in primary high-grade osteosarcoma. Tumori. 2018;104(1):30–6. https://doi.org/10.5301/tj.5000696.
26. Haas RL, Delaney TF, O'Sullivan B, Keus RB, Le Pechoux C, Olmi P, et al. Radiotherapy for management of extremity soft tissue sarcomas: why, when, and where? Int J Radiat Oncol Biol Phys. 2012;84(3):572–80. https://doi.org/10.1016/j.ijrobp.2012.01.062.
27. Puri A, Ranganathan P, Gulia A, Crasto S, Hawaldar R, Badwe RA. Does a less intensive surveillance protocol affect the survival of patients after treatment of a sarcoma of the limb? Updated results of the randomized TOSS study. Bone Joint J. 2018;100-B(2):262–8. https://doi.org/10.1302/0301-620X.100B2.BJJ-2017-0789.R1.
28. The Surveillance After Extremity Tumor Surgery (SAFETY) trial: protocol for a pilot study to determine the feasibility of a multicentre randomised controlled trial. BMJ Open. 2019;9(9):e029054. https://doi.org/10.1136/bmjopen-2019-029054.
29. Smolle MA, Sande MV, Callegaro D, Wunder J, Hayes A, Leitner L, et al. Individualizing follow-up strategies in high-grade soft tissue sarcoma with flexible parametric competing risk regression models. Cancers (Basel). 2019;12(1):47. https://doi.org/10.3390/cancers12010047.
30. Seidel MG, Kashofer K, Moser T, Thueringer A, Liegl-Atzwanger B, Leithner A, et al. Clinical implementation of plasma cell-free circulating tumor DNA quantification by digital droplet PCR for the monitoring of Ewing sarcoma in children and adolescents. Front Pediatr. 2022;10:926405. https://doi.org/10.3389/fped.2022.926405.
31. Leithner A, Maurer-Ertl W, Windhager R. Biopsy of bone and soft tissue tumours: hints and hazards. Recent Results Cancer Res. 2009;179:3–10. https://doi.org/10.1007/978-3-540-77960-5_1.
32. Pohlig F, Kirchhoff C, Lenze U, Schauwecker J, Burgkart R, Rechl H, et al. Percutaneous core needle biopsy versus open biopsy in diagnostics of bone and soft tissue sarcoma: a retrospective study. Eur J Med Res. 2012;17(1):29. https://doi.org/10.1186/2047-783x-17-29.
33. Bedi M, King DM, DeVries J, Hackbarth DA, Neilson JC. Does vacuum-assisted closure reduce the risk of wound complications in patients with lower extremity sarcomas treated with preoperative radiation? Clin Orthop Relat Res. 2019;477(4):768–74. https://doi.org/10.1097/corr.0000000000000371.
34. Shehadeh A, El Dahleh M, Salem A, Sarhan Y, Sultan I, Henshaw RM, et al. Standardization of rehabilitation after limb salvage surgery for sarcomas improves patients' outcome. Hematol Oncol Stem Cell Ther. 2013;6(3–4):105–11. https://doi.org/10.1016/j.hemonc.2013.09.001.
35. Tobias K, Gillis T. Rehabilitation of the sarcoma patient-enhancing the recovery and functioning of patients undergoing management for extremity soft tissue sarcomas. J Surg Oncol. 2015;111(5):615–21. https://doi.org/10.1002/jso.23830.
36. Sambri A, Gardini L, Dalla Rosa M, Zavatta G, Keskinbora M, Ferrari C, et al. Femoral fracture in primary soft-tissue sarcoma of the thigh treated with radiation therapy: indications for prophylactic intramedullary nail. Arch Orthop Trauma Surg. 2021;141(8):1277–82. https://doi.org/10.1007/s00402-020-03544-x.

28 Malignant Tenosynovial Giant Cell Tumor of the Foot

Chandhanarat Chandhanayingyong

28.1 Introduction

Malignant tenosynovial giant cell tumors (T-GCT) or malignant pigmented villonodular synovitis (PVNS) is extremely rare, accounting for less than 50 reported cases worldwide [1–3]. Enzinger et al. first described malignant TGCT as uncontrolled growth within a benign lesion or as the recurrence of a previously benign lesion [4]. The feature characteristics that suggest malignancy are nodular and/or solid infiltrative growth pattern, large round or oval cells, cells with large nuclei and nucleoli, areas of necrosis, and atypical mitoses [3, 5]. Histology diagnostic criteria for malignant TGCT by the Armed Forces Institute of Pathology (AFIP), including five out of eight characteristics, are (1) diffuse pleomorphism, (2) prominent nucleoli, (3) high cytoplasmic to nuclear ratios, (4) mitotic ratio greater than 10 per 10 HPFs, (5) necrosis, (6) discohesion of tumor cells, (7) paucity of giant cells, and (8) diffuse growth pattern [6]. Molecular characteristics of malignant T-GCT involve deregulated CFS1 overexpression, aberrations of cyclin A, P53, and chromosome arm 15q [7]. Malignant T-GCT is a highly aggressive tumor with potential for local destruction, distant metastases to the regional lymph nodes and lung, and death from disease. Despite aggressive management, including surgical resection, chemotherapy, and radiation, studies showed a median survival of 22.5 months after diagnosis [2, 3]. A limited number of limb-salvage procedures have been reported for malignant T-GCT following wide resection.

28.2 Brief Clinical History

A previously healthy, 47-year-old female presented with a year's history of right mid-foot progressive swelling, but walked well with a normal gait (Fig. 28.1a). The patient seeks for treatment because she cannot wear shoes to work. Open biopsy established a diagnosis of a malignant tenosynovial giant cell tumor (malignant TGCT) or malignant pigmented villonodular synovitis (malignant PVNS). No distant metastasis was detected. She did not take medication regularly and denied a family history of genetic disorders. The patient understood her health condition but denied below-knee amputation. She agreed to undergo wide resection and reconstruction after a critical discussion of methods of treatment.

C. Chandhanayingyong (✉)
Faculty of Medicine Siriraj Hospital, Mahidol University, Bangkok, Thailand
e-mail: chandhanarat.cha@mahidol.ac.th

H. Özger et al. (eds.), *Diagnosis and Treatment of Soft Tissue Tumors*, https://doi.org/10.1007/978-3-031-77061-6_28

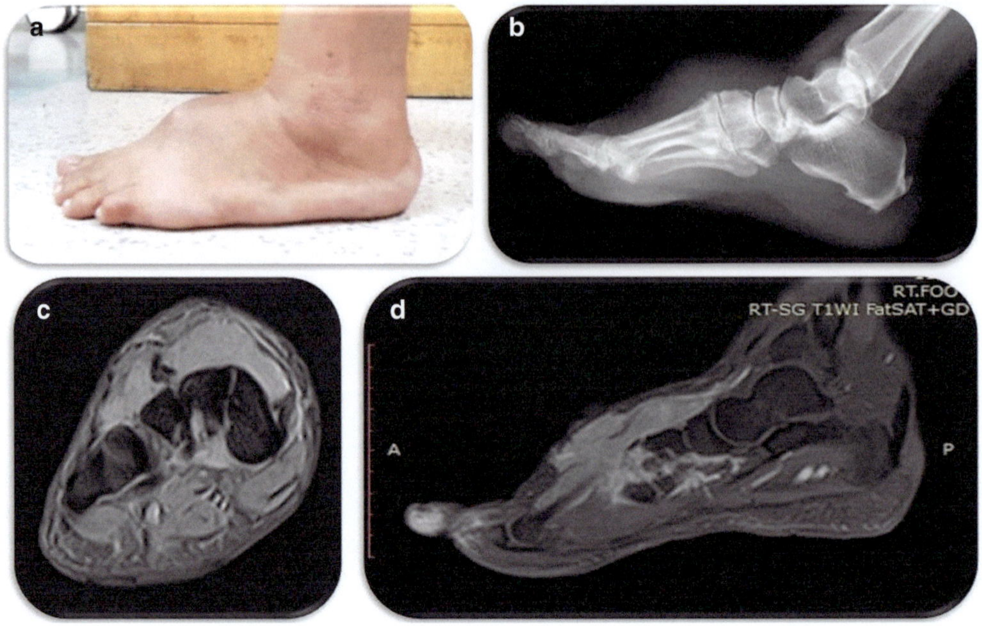

Fig. 28.1 (**a**) Physical examination reveals soft tissue mass at the mid-foot observes from the lateral side. (**b**) show a soft tissue mass at the dorsum of mid-foot without osteolytic lesions. MRI T1W1 fat sat with gadolinium axial and sagittal view (**c**, **d**) show infiltrative soft tissue tumor with the destruction of the cortex and intra-articular invasion

28.3 Preoperative Local Imaging

Radiographs revealed soft tissue mass around the mid-foot area without osteolytic lesions of the underlying base of first to fifth metatarsi, navicular, cuboid, and cuneiforms (Fig. 28.1b). Magnetic resonance imaging showed infiltrative soft tissue mass with heterogeneous signal intensity on T2W and enhanced with gadolinium, axial, and sagittal view (Fig. 28.1c, d) showing infiltrative soft tissue tumor with the destruction of the cortex and intra-articular invasion.

28.4 Preoperative Problem List

1. Tenosynovial soft tissue sarcoma of the forefoot, mid-foot, and proximal part of the hindfoot involving at least five toes.
2. Sarcoma extended superiorly to the skin and inferiorly to the intrinsic muscle, but did not invade neurovascular structures.
3. Need to reconstruct the bone defect to restore structural and skeletal stability.
4. Skin and soft tissue involvement necessitating skin graft or flap coverage.

28.5 Treatment Strategies

- Multidisciplinary including surgical resection (mandatory) + radiation + discussion regarding chemotherapy.
- Chemotherapy—with limited evidence for the benefit of neoadjuvant chemotherapy, it was decided to proceed with local therapy and re-evaluate the option of subsequent adjuvant chemotherapy after surgery.
- Surgical resection—the patient was planned for re-evaluation after receiving free pathological margins and postoperative radiation.
- Reconstruction of the bony defect. Various options were considered for the reconstruction of the remaining bone defect.
  - For nonreconstruction: the defect could be left and wait for scar healing, later covered with a skin graft. However, this method could be achieved with prolonged hospitalization on vacuum dressing and may result in rocker button foot deformity and weakened arc of the foot structure.
  - For biological reconstruction: bone grafting including iliac crest bone graft, or fibular autograft, and fixation with miniplate or screws. The problem with this method is there were 5 toes to reconstruct which may result in delay and nonunion, especially after radiation. Flap coverage with bone reconstruction including vascularized fibular graft with skin indicator or reverse sural flap is the reasonable option for this situation.
  - For nonbiological reconstruction: There is no conventional prosthesis for midfoot and forefoot reconstruction. For 3D-printed prosthesis, customized for the defect could be an option for this patient.

28.6 Surgical Procedure

- Surgery was performed by an orthopedic oncologist, using a longitudinal incision via a dorsal approach (Fig. 28.2a). The skin was retracted medially, and laterally, enabling access to the entire tumor that involved metatarsal bone of first to fourth digit, navicular, all cuneiform, and parts of the cuboid.

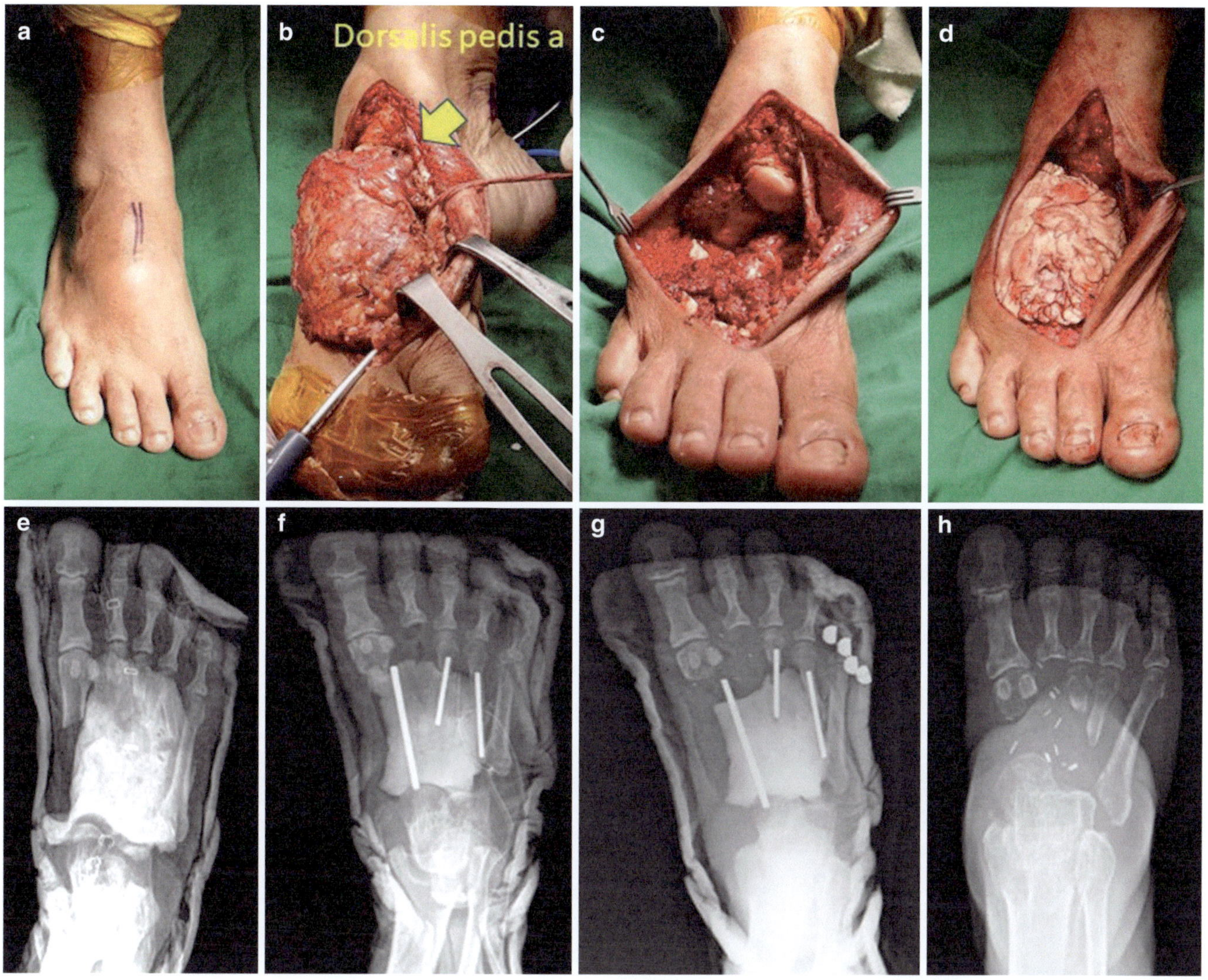

Fig. 28.2 Intraoperative procedures. Wide resection of the malignant tenosynovial giant cell tumor of the mid-foot, with the sacrifice of the extensor tendon (**a–c**). A cement spacer was applied (**d**). Postoperative anteroposterior view radiographs after first wide resection (**e**), second resection (**f**), and third resection (**g**), and the final X-Ray (**h**) represented free surgical margins

- The dorsalis pedis vessels, the deep peroneal nerve, and the extensor tendon were sacrificed (Fig. 28.2b). However, the plantar arch, digital arteries of all digits, and plantar interossei muscles remained intact.
- Removal of the entire tumor mass was done with no local adjuvant therapy at the first surgery (Fig. 28.2c). Antibiotic cement spacer was inserted (Fig. 28.2d).
- The skin was closed successfully.

Pathological report was in accordance with the previous biopsy. Gross pathology, axial cut showed tumor involved all extender tendons, cuneiform and navicular bone (Fig. 28.3a). Hematoxylin and eosin staining revealed infiltrative nodular growing pattern, proliferation of mononuclear cells with minimal pleomorphism and indistinct cellular borders, abundant pink-stained cytoplasm, enlarged nuclei with prominent nucleoli, lack of zoning and few giant cells and rare xanthomatous cells. Mitotic activity is low (2/10 HPF) (Fig. 28.3b). Section showed soft tissue and bone invasion (Fig. 28.3c, d). Immunohistochemistry was positive for CD68, CD163, vimentin, CK33 and INI1, but negative for AE1AE3, CD34, CD30, desmin, SMA, myogenin, CD45, S100, SatB2, CD3, CD20, CK1a, CK13, CK14, CK15, CK21, and CK25.

- After a thorough pathological examination, the margins were not free. Second (Fig. 28.2f) and third (Fig. 28.2g) wide excision surgery was done to remove the whole second metatarsal bone and the surrounding soft tissue. Then, the margins were called free <1 mm.
- The patient was treated by brachytherapy with four retained radio-passing tubes for 2 weeks (Fig. 28.4b, c). The dorsal skin was necrosis during multiple tumor re-

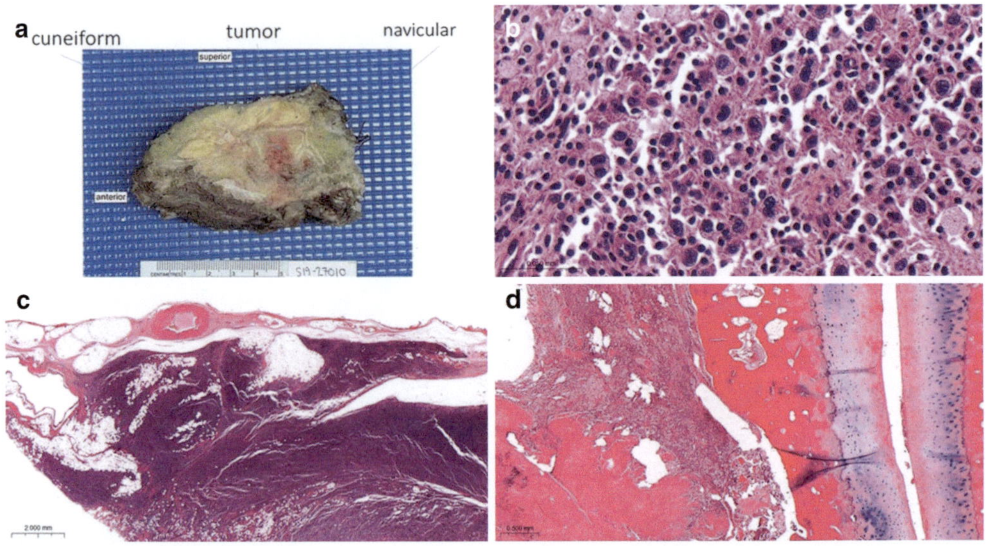

Fig. 28.3 Gross pathology, axial cut showed tumor involving all extender tendons, cuneiform, and navicular bone (**a**). Hematoxylin and eosin stains show histiocytoid cells with prominent nucleoli (**b**), soft tissue and bone invasion (**c**, **d**)

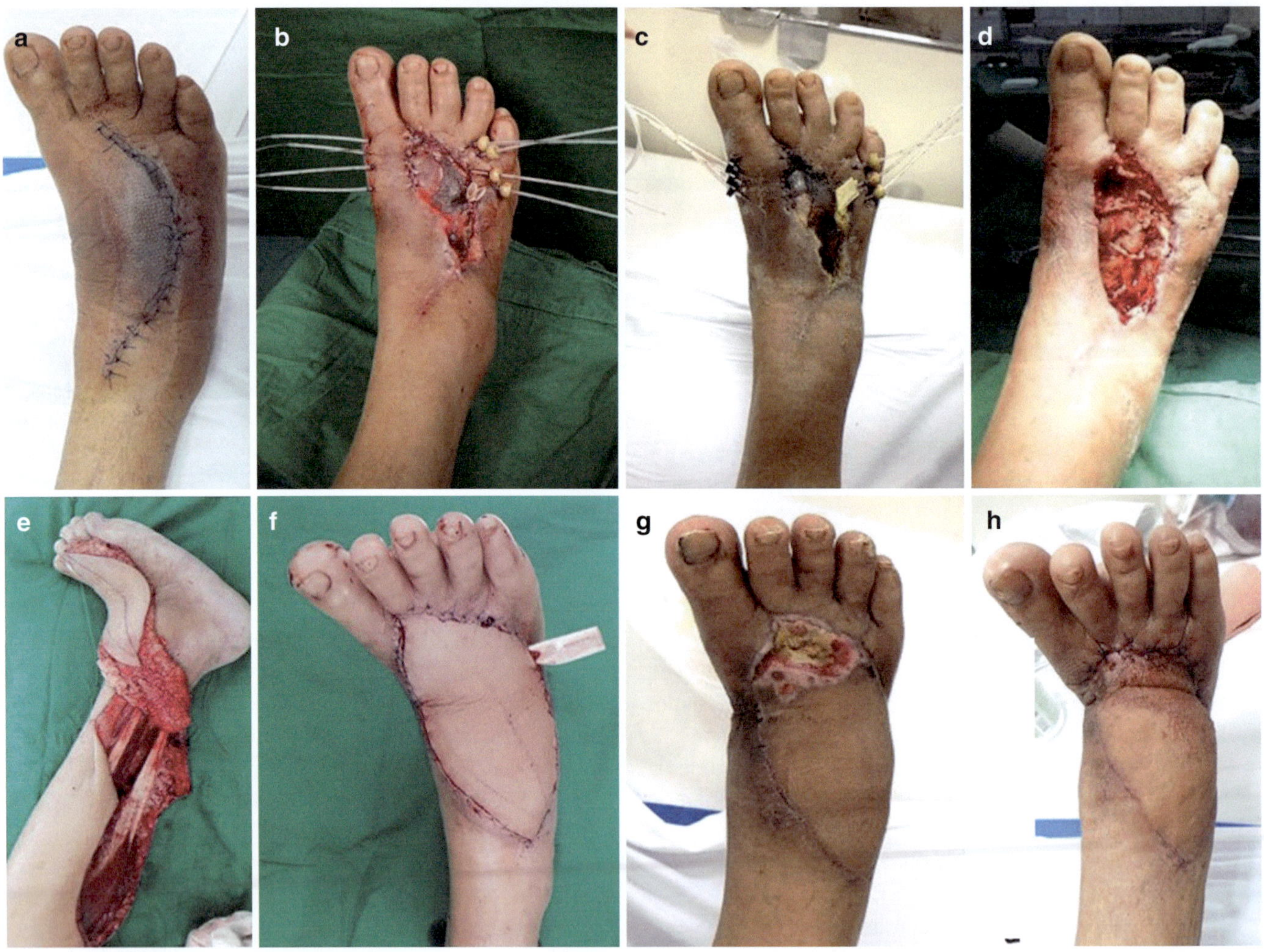

Fig. 28.4 Two weeks after the tumor section and cement spacer application, dorsal skin necrosis occurred after primary closure after the second and third resections (**a**). Brachytherapy was performed postoperatively (**b**, **c**). The skin was removed, and serial debridement was performed because of subcutaneous infection (**d**). When the infection was cleared, a reverse sural flap was performed to close the defect (**e**, **f**). Distal part of the flap was necrosis and removed (**g**, **h**)

resections, before the brachytherapy and progressed during brachytherapy. The necrosis skin was removed (Fig. 28.4d).
- Vacuum dressing of 75 mmHg was applied for 3 weeks.
- The mid-foot 3D-printed prosthesis was designed and manufactured aiming to fill the defect. However, because of fungal and bacterial infection of the wound, we treated it with multiple debridements and subsequently closed it with a reverse sural flap (Fig. 28.4e, f).
- The distal edge of the flap was necrosis (Fig. 28.4g) and was debrided and sutured (Fig. 28.4h).

28.7 Postoperative Care

A short-leg posterior slab with a toe plate was applied for 3 weeks after surgery. Weight-bearing was then permitted gradually to have full weight-bearing over 3 months. During the first 4–5 months, the postoperative course was uneventful.

28.8 Outcome

- The patient walked well on bare feet without support. No pain medication was taken. She has no limitation of daily activities, but limitation of recreational activities. The maximum walking distance was 4–6 blocks. She is wearing sandals without inserts.
- However, scar contraction (Fig. 28.5a) and rocker bottom foot (Fig. 28.5b, c) were evident. Although this was managed with massage, the method did not soften the scar or reduce hyperextension.
- The American Orthopedic Foot and Ankle Society (AOFAS) [8] mid-foot score for this patient was 85 (pain, 40/40; function, 37/50; alignment, 8/10).
- The Musculoskeletal Tumor Society scoring was 25 (83%: no pain, 5; minimal restriction of function, 4; emotional acceptance, 3; no gait support, 5; an intermediate range of walking, 4; normal gait, 4).
- Serial radiographs showed fair alignment, plantigrade foot with some mid-foot malalignment, and shortening of the foot length. MRI showed no tumor recurrence at the time of the last follow-up of 42 months. No lymph node or pulmonary metastasis was observed by PET CT.

28.9 Discussion

Our patient has six out of eight diagnostic criteria for malignant TGCT by the Armed Forces Institute of Pathology (AFIP) [6], specifically 1) diffuse pleomorphism, 2) prominent nucleoli, 3) high cytoplasmic to nuclear ratios, 6) discohesion of tumor cells, 7) paucity of giant cells, and 8) diffuse growth pattern, but lacks 4) mitotic ratio greater than 10 per 10 HPFs and 5) necrosis.

Soft tissue sarcoma of the forefoot and midfoot often presents as small, but infiltrative due to its complex structure that involves the deep arch and intrinsic muscle that requires extensive en bloc resection [9–11]. Reconstruction of this area is challenging and often results in Chopart or below-knee amputation [12, 13]. Recently, limb-sparing technique in foot sarcoma with safe margins and/or adjuvant therapy has proven to equal survival rate compared with amputation, but improved functional outcome [14–17]. Reconstruction methods often involve

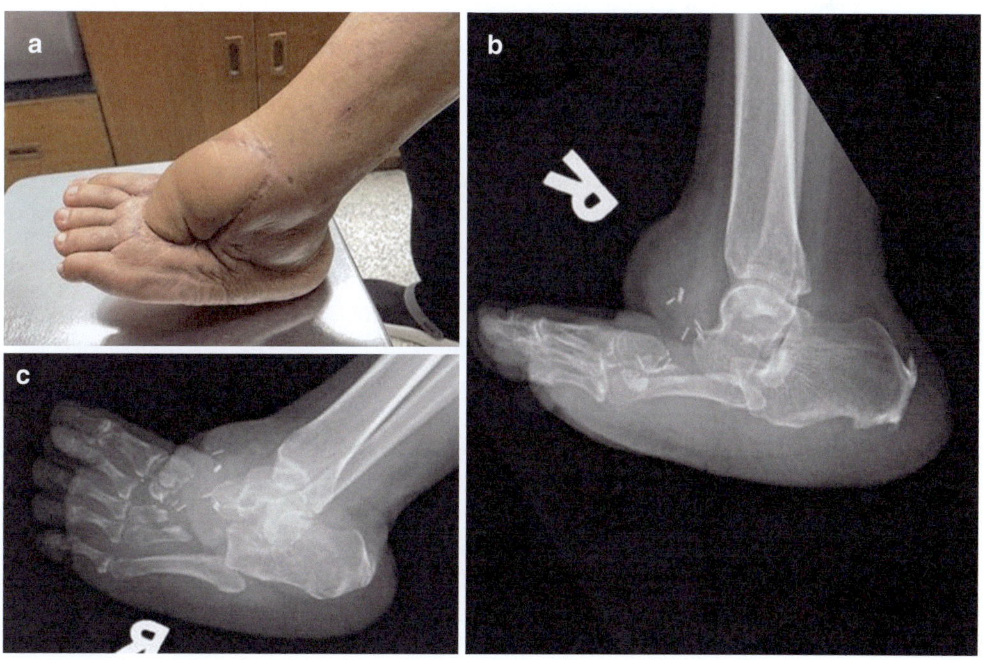

Fig. 28.5 After 5 years, a fibrotic scar formed and retracted the mid-foot area to hyperextend with a rocker-bottom foot (**a**–**c**). However, the patient walks without pain and support in near normal gait. And, she is free of the disease

local or free flap such as medial plantar flap, reverse sural flap, fasciocutaneous free flap, anterolateral thigh flap, vascularized fibular graft, or serratus anterior rib free flap [18–21].

In the present study, we described a technique of wide resection, followed by brachytherapy and reconstruction utilizing a reverse sural flap.

Wide resection: This patient presented with an unusual location of the soft tissue sarcoma of the foot. It is the tenosynovial sarcoma of the extensor tendon and the bone of the forefoot at the dorsum, which did not involve the deep plantar arch or the plantar muscle, including quadratus plantae or plantar interossei. This makes wide resection possible without resection of the blood vessels or digital nerve to the toes. After resection, the distal neurovascular structures are intact with no toe gangrene or loss of foot sensation. The patient achieved satisfactory clinical outcomes with near-normal weight-bearing. There were no symptoms of irritation. However, because of the distal flap necrosis, the patient showed dorsiflexion contracture of the forefoot and eventually developed a full-fixed, rocker bottom deformity at 12 months (Fig. 28.5). Early recognition and prompt treatment by massaging was started; however, it did not change the degree of foot deformity. Finally, the push-off power was decreased and the longitudinal axis of the foot was shortened; however, the patient can walk without gait aid and no pain.

Adjuvant therapy: This case primarily did not achieve clear surgical margins (R0) of over 1 mm pathological margin free. The radiotherapy locally controlled the tumor in the complex mid-foot area. Neoadjuvant radiotherapy might be beneficial in the foot setting, where critical structures are cramped in a very small volume, and it is very difficult to achieve adequate margins compatible with limb salvage by surgery alone. While wound complications might commonly be expected with preop radiotherapy, it might reduce the need for re-resections. However, due to a low-grade tumor found in the biopsy specimen (mitotic of 2/10 HPF), accompanied by the preference of the reconstructive surgeon, this patient was treated by brachytherapy after resection, and before reconstruction with reverse sural flap. The choice between neoadjuvant radiotherapy and adjuvant brachytherapy depends on several factors, including the type of cancer, the location of the tumor, and the patient's plan of reconstruction. It is important to discuss the potential benefits and risks of these treatment approaches to make an informed decision about the best course of action for each specific situation.

Longer follow-up is needed to ascertain if the patient is still disease-free and whether soft-tissue stiffness affects the foot function. However, we can report that this method is an effective alternative for foot reconstruction rather than Chopart or below-knee amputation. Further study of reconstruction procedures, especially in rare areas, is needed to facilitate limb-sparing surgery and reduce complications.

28.10 Conclusions

We reported successful limb-sparing surgery of malignant T-GCT tumor of the mid-foot by wide excision, adjuvant brachytherapy, and reconstruction with reverse sural flap. And, the patient still survived without disease progression after 5 years. The short-term clinical and oncologic outcomes were satisfactory, with early rehabilitation. The patient walks without pain or gait aid, even though, scar contracture led to a rocker-bottom foot postoperatively. Although multiple resection with brachytherapy for limb sparing procedures can be considered as an option to treat extremity malignant T-GCT, longer follow-ups and other treatment modalities should be studied to improve treatment quality.

References

1. Nakayama R, Jagannathan JP, Ramaiya N, Ferrone ML, Raut CP, Ready JE, et al. Clinical characteristics and treatment outcomes in six cases of malignant tenosynovial giant cell tumor: initial experience of molecularly targeted therapy. BMC Cancer. 2018;18(1):1296. https://doi.org/10.1186/s12885-018-5188-6.
2. Yoon HJ, Cho YA, Lee JI, Hong SP, Hong SD. Malignant pigmented villonodular synovitis of the temporomandibular joint with lung metastasis: a case report and review of the literature. Oral Surg Oral Med Oral Pathol Oral Radiol Endod. 2011;111(5):e30–6. https://doi.org/10.1016/j.tripleo.2010.11.031.
3. Li CF, Wang JW, Huang WW, Hou CC, Chou SC, Eng HL, et al. Malignant diffuse-type tenosynovial giant cell tumors: a series of 7 cases comparing with 24 benign lesions with review of the literature. Am J Surg Pathol. 2008;32(4):587–99. https://doi.org/10.1097/PAS.0b013e318158428f.
4. Weiss SWGJ. Enzinger and Weiss's soft tissue tumors. St. Louis: CV Mosby; 2008.
5. Bertoni F, Unni KK, Beabout JW, Sim FH. Malignant giant cell tumor of the tendon sheaths and joints (malignant pigmented villonodular synovitis). Am J Surg Pathol. 1997;21(2):153–63. https://doi.org/10.1097/00000478-199702000-00004.
6. Bhadra AK, Pollock R, Tirabosco RP, Skinner JA, Cannon SR, Briggs TW, et al. Primary tumours of the synovium. A report of four cases of malignant tumour. J Bone Joint Surg Br. 2007;89(11):1504–8. https://doi.org/10.1302/0301-620X.89B11.18963.
7. Huang HY, West RB, Tzeng CC, van de Rijn M, Wang JW, Chou SC, et al. Immunohistochemical and biogenetic features of diffuse-type tenosynovial giant cell tumors: the potential roles of cyclin A, P53, and deletion of 15q in sarcomatous transformation. Clin Cancer Res. 2008;14(19):6023–32. https://doi.org/10.1158/1078-0432.CCR-08-0252.
8. Kitaoka HB, Alexander IJ, Adelaar RS, Nunley JA, Myerson MS, Sanders M. Clinical rating systems for the ankle-hindfoot, midfoot, hallux, and lesser toes. Foot Ankle Int. 1994;15(7):349–53. https://doi.org/10.1177/107110079401500701.
9. Mascard E, Gaspar N, Brugieres L, Glorion C, Pannier S, Gomez-Brouchet A. Malignant tumours of the foot and ankle. EFORT Open Rev. 2017;2(5):261–71. https://doi.org/10.1302/2058-5241.2.160078.

10. Kozawa E, Nishida Y, Nakashima H, Tsukushi S, Toriyama K, Kamei Y, et al. Foot sarcomas: factors affecting oncological and functional outcomes. Oncol Lett. 2012;3(1):82–8. https://doi.org/10.3892/ol.2011.427.
11. Latt LD, Turcotte RE, Isler MH, Wong C, Case series. Soft-tissue sarcoma of the foot. Can J Surg. 2010;53(6):424–31.
12. van der Wal GE, Dijkstra PU, Geertzen JHB. Lisfranc and Chopart amputation: a systematic review. Medicine (Baltimore). 2023;102(10):e33188. https://doi.org/10.1097/MD.0000000000033188.
13. Sage RA. Tumor as an indication for amputation in the foot. Clin Podiatr Med Surg. 1997;14(4):613–20.
14. Tsuda Y, Fujiwara T, Stevenson JD, Abudu A. Surgical outcomes of bone sarcoma of the foot. Jpn J Clin Oncol. 2021;51(10):1541–6. https://doi.org/10.1093/jjco/hyab118.
15. Patel RR, Lupo PJ, Bishop AJ, Lin PP, Delclos GL, Lazar AJ, et al. Synovial sarcoma of the hand and foot: an institutional review. Am J Clin Oncol. 2021;44(7):361–8. https://doi.org/10.1097/COC.0000000000000822.
16. Ozger H, Alpan B, Aycan OE, Valiyev N, Kir MC, Agaoglu F. Management of primary malignant bone and soft tissue tumors of foot and ankle: is it worth salvaging? J Surg Oncol. 2018;117(2):307–20. https://doi.org/10.1002/jso.24817.
17. Ahmed SK, Kaggal S, Harmsen WS, Sawyer JW, Houdek MT, Rose PS, et al. Patient-reported functional outcomes in a cohort of hand and foot sarcoma survivors treated with limb sparing surgery and radiation therapy. J Surg Oncol. 2021;123(1):110–6. https://doi.org/10.1002/jso.26258.
18. Li P, Zhang H, Zhu J, Qiu H, Ni X, Yu F, et al. Foot and ankle reconstruction using the lateral supramalleolar flap versus the anterolateral thigh flap in the elderly: a comparative study. Int Wound J. 2022;19(6):1518–27. https://doi.org/10.1111/iwj.13751.
19. Mallett KE, Houdek MT, Honig RL, Bakri K, Rose PS, Moran SL. Comparison of flap reconstruction for soft tissue sarcomas of the foot and ankle. J Surg Oncol. 2021;124(7):995–1001. https://doi.org/10.1002/jso.26605.
20. Ozger H, Akgul T, Eren I, Topalan M. Midfoot reconstruction with free vascularized fibular graft after wide resection: a case report. Acta Orthop Belg. 2011;77(5):702–6.
21. Tapan M, Ozkan O, Ozkan O. Versatility of the peroneal perforator propeller sural flap for various types of injuries in the ankle and foot regions. Ann Plast Surg. 2021;87(6):e121–8. https://doi.org/10.1097/SAP.0000000000002969.

Synovial Sarcoma of the Forearm: Diagnostic Pitfalls and Biological Reconstruction

29

Harzem Özger, Cihangir Tetik, and Buğra Alpan

29.1 Introduction

Synovial sarcoma (SS) is a well-defined soft tissue neoplasm often seated in a deep extra-articular extremity location and is most prevalent between ages 15 and 40. An important clinical feature is a slow-growing, well-bordered, tender soft tissue tumor, which is sometimes accompanied by significant long-standing local pain. Most lesions are firmly attached to adjacent structures. The indolent behavior and well-circumscribed appearance are commonly misleading toward a benign clinical diagnosis. In most cases, the preoperative duration of symptoms ranges from 2 to 4 years. Adequate surgical excision is the primary treatment modality, while radiotherapy is an essential adjunct for improved local control. Excision of regional lymph nodes might be indicated. Local recurrence commonly develops within the first 2 years. Five-year overall survival rates range from 56% to 76%. Late metastases and long periods of survival after metastasis are not infrequent. Young age, tumor size smaller than 5 cm, distal extremity location, and low tumor grade (absence of poorly differentiated areas) are good prognostic factors. The significance of the histologic subtype (biphasic/monophasic) is unclear. While routine use of chemotherapy in uncomplicated localized disease is not supported by evidence, SS is a chemosensitive tumor, and chemotherapy can offer significant survival benefits in selected cases such as with locally advanced disease [1–4].

Only about 15% of soft tissue sarcomas (STS) are localized to the upper extremity, and synovial sarcomas comprise approximately 10% of all extremity STS, thus making a forearm SS a rare entity [3, 5, 6]. Most cases of upper extremity SS present after an unplanned excision elsewhere. Although re-excision following unplanned resection in forearm STS is usually associated with increased morbidity, it is not clear if these unplanned interventions eventually lead to adverse oncological outcomes. The compact and unique anatomy of the forearm is challenging regarding adequate resection, functional outcomes, and morbidity of local therapies. Some authors suggest that tumor depth and whether the tumor is intra- or extra-compartmental are independent risk factors for oncological outcomes in forearm STS [5, 6].

The histopathology of the tumor, in terms of radio- and chemosensitivity, is equally important as the tumor's location and directly impacts the treatment strategy. Neoadjuvant radiotherapy is essential to facilitate safe resection in primary high-grade soft tissue sarcomas where straightforward wide local excision is not feasible. On the other hand, concurrent neoadjuvant chemoradiotherapy might also be utilized if the predicted benefit from radiotherapy alone is deemed inadequate in terms of resectability or the patient is already metastatic or under significant risk of metastasis at the time of presentation and, therefore, systemic treatment is also urgently indicated.

Preserving the hand function is the primary objective in upper extremity reconstructions. It can be argued that limb salvage in the setting of upper extremity tumors has higher priority due to the more sophisticated functional capacity associated with the distal upper extremity, in comparison to the distal lower extremity, which is relatively more expendable in exchange for acceptable functional outcome even with external prosthetics. Resection with safe margins is the prerequisite for limb salvage, as in tumors of all other anatomic locations, regardless of the reconstruction method. The plausibility of an intercalary resection should be thoroughly evaluated in tumors of the radius and ulna, as in all long bones, to salvage the adjacent joints and to facilitate

H. Özger (✉)
Department of Orthopedics and Traumatology, Istanbul University, Istanbul Medical Faculty, Istanbul, Türkiye
e-mail: harzemo@yahoo.com

C. Tetik
Department of Orthopedics and Traumatology, Acıbadem Maslak Hospital, Istanbul, Türkiye

B. Alpan
Department of Orthopedics and Traumatology, Acıbadem Mehmet Ali Aydınlar University, School of Medicine, Istanbul, Türkiye
e-mail: bugra.alpan@acibadem.edu.tr

H. Özger et al. (eds.), *Diagnosis and Treatment of Soft Tissue Tumors*, https://doi.org/10.1007/978-3-031-77061-6_29

biological reconstruction. Restoring the original two-bone anatomy is the ideal reconstruction for forearm intercalary (diaphyseal) defects. Biological reconstruction is the treatment of choice. Conventionally, defects shorter than 6 cm can be reconstructed with nonvascular fibula or tricortical iliac autografts, while defects measuring 6 cm or more require a vascularized graft. The free vascular fibula is the gold standard for the biological reconstruction of large bone defects in the upper extremities of children and adolescents. It is particularly suitable for intercalary forearm bone defect reconstruction due to its excellent anatomical fit [7–9].

29.2 Brief Clinical History

A 13-year-old male patient presented to our clinic with swelling in his left forearm. A slightly painful swelling had first been noticed 7 years ago, and the patient's family had sought medical attention, upon which an orthopedic surgeon had requested an MRI. A nodular 1.0 × 1.5 cm soft tissue lesion had been detected adjacent to the anteromedial aspect of the proximal ulnar diaphysis. The family had been reassured that the radiologic characteristics were consistent with hemangioma and had been informed that clinical and radiological follow-up would be adequate. The patient's complaints of swelling and mild-to-sometimes-moderate localized pain had remained steady over the following years. Follow-up MRI examinations, respectively, 2 and 5 years after the first detection in the elsewhere institution, had revealed slight progression in size with hypointense foci inside the lesion. These were interpreted as phleboliths, and the decision of radiologic follow-up had been upheld. However, during the seventh year of follow-up, the patient had noticed that the lesion had started to grow rapidly and become much more painful, upon which an MRI examination had demonstrated significant progression of the soft tissue lesion, with a contrast-enhancing solid component and 180° engulfment of the proximal ulna. The patient had then been informed that this could be a malignant lesion. Subsequently, the patient presented to our clinic, and a CT scan was performed to reveal marked calcifications inside the tumor. A trucut biopsy was performed immediately to reveal synovial sarcoma. The diagnosis was confirmed with spindle-cell morphology, Epithelial membrane antigen (EMA) positivity in immunohistochemistry, and SS18 gene rearrangement in Fluorescence in situ hybridization (FISH) analysis. Retrospective consideration of the clinical findings, including the long history of subtle symptoms and very slow tumor growth, and the radiologic findings, including the typical soft tissue calcifications, were consistent with the pathology report. The initial staging did not reveal any regional or systemic evidence. The family was informed about the behavior and natural history of the disease, and limb salvage surgery following neoadjuvant treatment was planned. The patient received two cycles of Ifosfamide and Etoposide chemotherapy concurrent with a total dose of 4500 cGy radiotherapy in 25 fractions. The patient then received a third cycle of neoadjuvant chemotherapy. Wide local excision and vascular fibula reconstruction of the proximal ulnar diaphysis were performed. Tumor necrosis was reported as 50%, while the surgical margins were negative. He also received three cycles of adjuvant chemotherapy and completed his treatment without any incident to continue with his rehabilitation.

29.3 Preoperative Local Imaging

See Figs. 29.1, 29.2, 29.3, and 29.4.

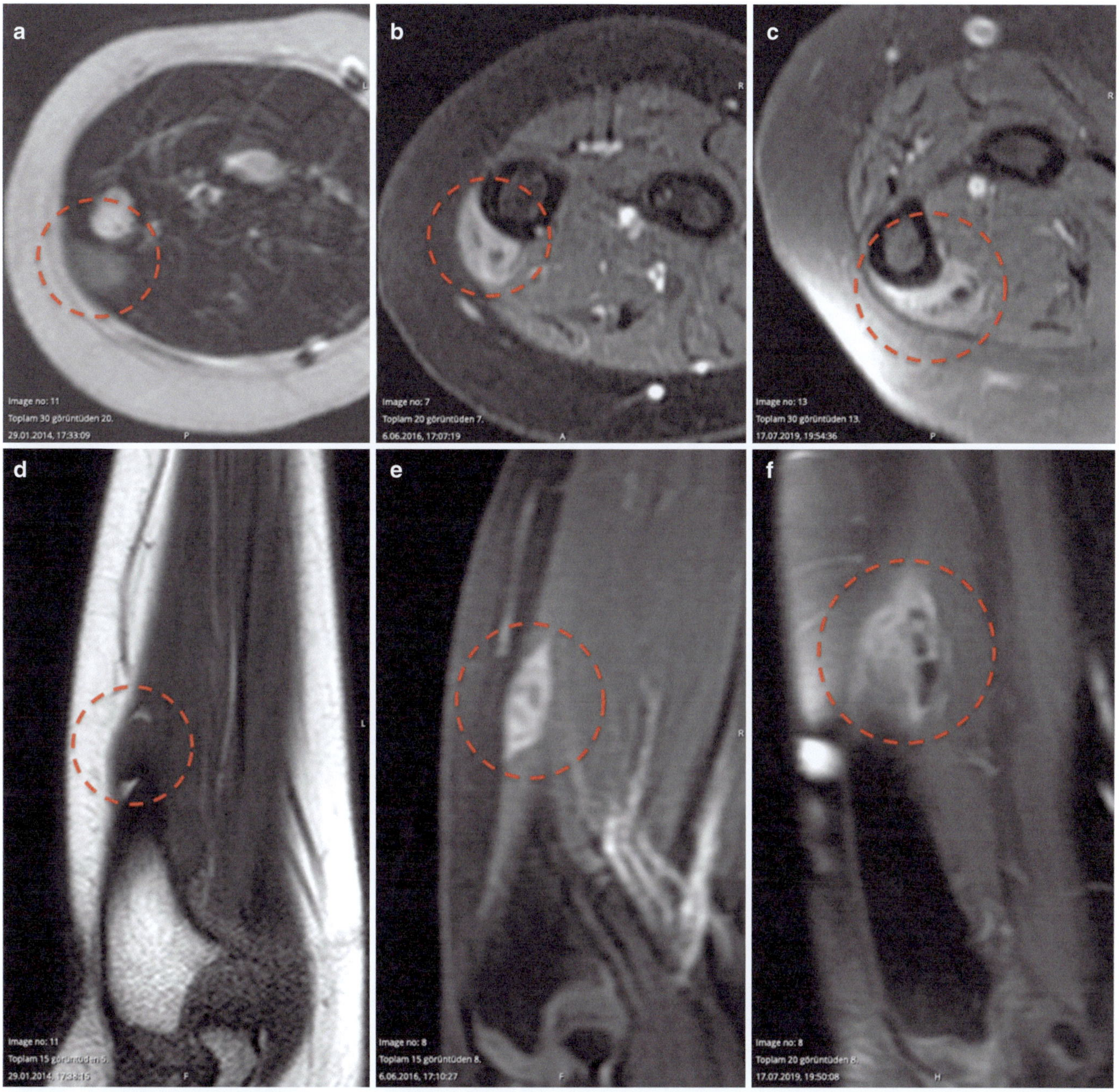

Fig. 29.1 Serial MR images demonstrate the slight changes in the lesion (marked with red-dotted circles) over 5 years of surveillance in another institution with the presumed diagnosis of hemangioma. The lesion is located adjacent to the anteromedial aspect of the proximal ulnar diaphysis. The transverse T2W MR section in (**a**) was obtained at first detection, while T1W fat-saturated contrast-enhanced images in (**b** and **c**) were obtained after 2 and 5 years, respectively. The sagittal T1W MR image in (**d**) shows the lesion at first detection, while T1W fat-saturated contrast-enhanced images in (**e** and **f**) were obtained after 2 and 5 years, respectively. The increase in tumor size is not striking in this period. However, the close relationship with the ulnar cortex, albeit without destruction, is apparent in axial images. The hypointense foci within the lesion are consistent with soft tissue calcifications

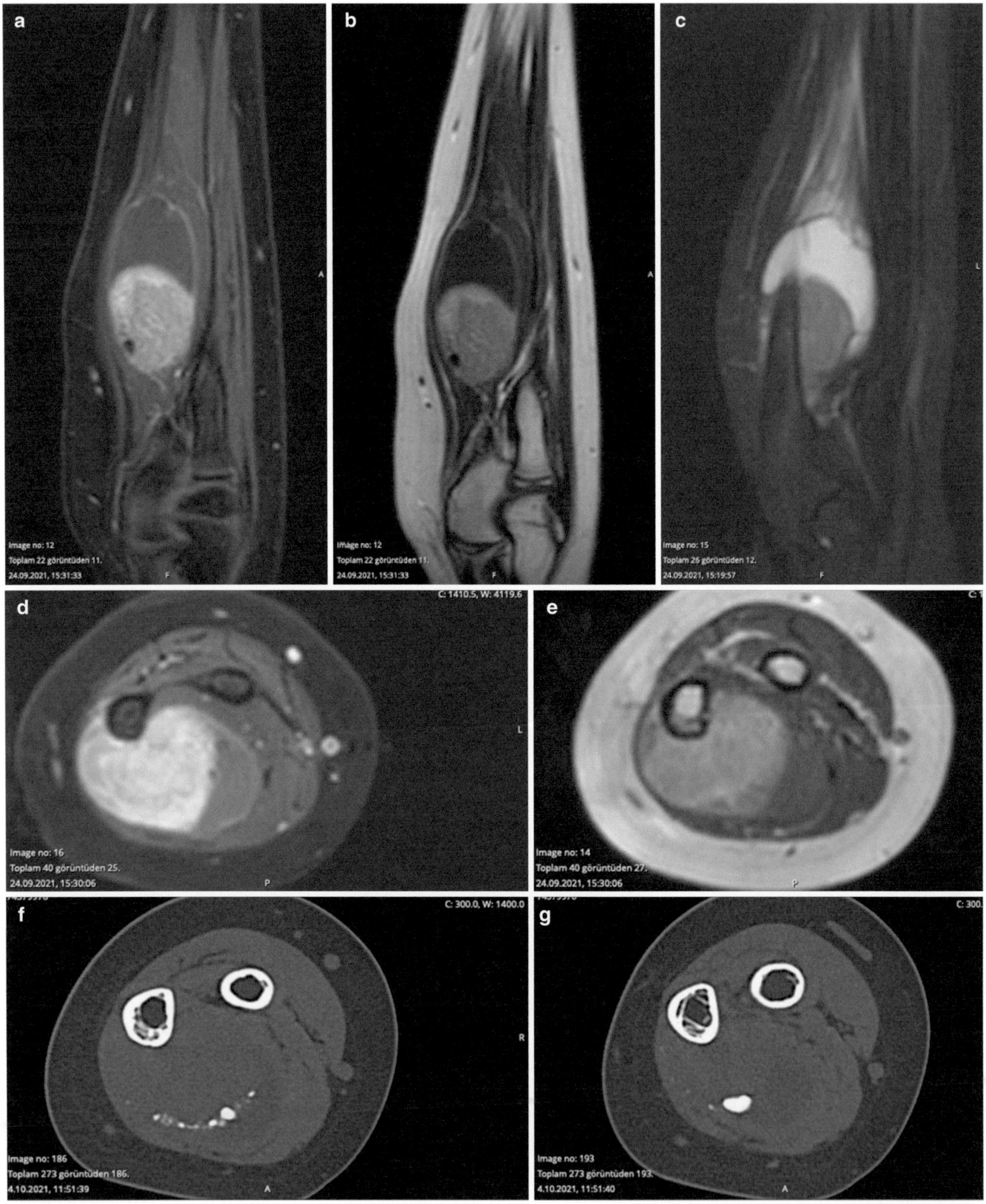

Fig. 29.2 The marked progression in size and the bone-engulfing behavior can be seen in the MR images at presentation to our institution 7 years after the first detection of the lesion. (**a**) Shows a T1W fat-saturated contrast-enhanced sagittal image, while the sagittal sections in (**b** and **c**) demonstrate T1W and T2W sequences, respectively. (**d** and **e**) Show T1W fat-saturated contrast-enhanced and T1W transverse MR images, respectively. Transverse CT sections in (**f** and **g**) reveal the calcifications within the lesion. The tumor has a solid and a cystic component, and its borders are well demarcated in all sections despite the edematous appearance of the muscle compartment in the distal aspect of the tumor (**c**)

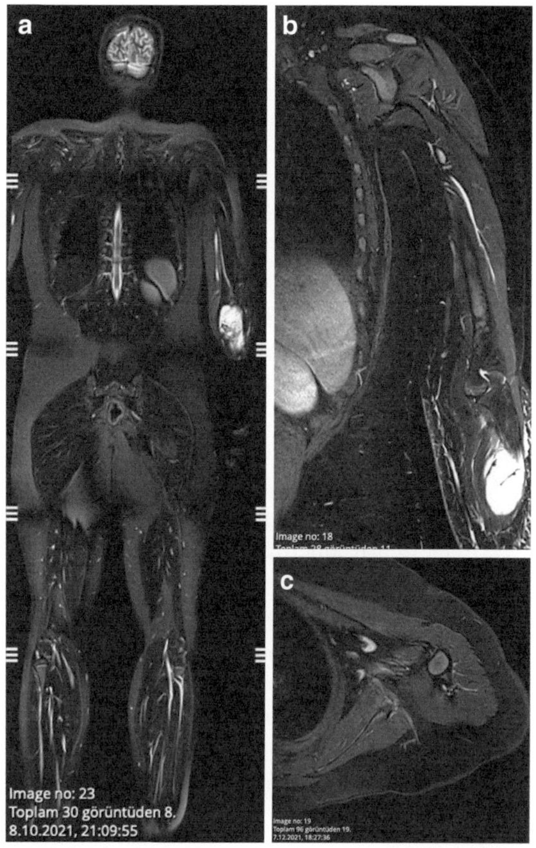

Fig. 29.3 Following the diagnosis of synovial sarcoma upon trucut biopsy, systemic screening was performed with whole-body MRI (wbMRI) to complete staging. A Thorax CT scan was also done, although not shown here. (**a**) Shows the whole-body coronal STIR image. No distant metastasis was observed. In the same session with wbMRI, dedicated imaging of the left upper extremity and the left axilla (**b** and **c**) was also performed to specifically search for any pathologic lymph nodes as synovial sarcoma tends to metastasize via the lymphatic route besides the hematogenous route

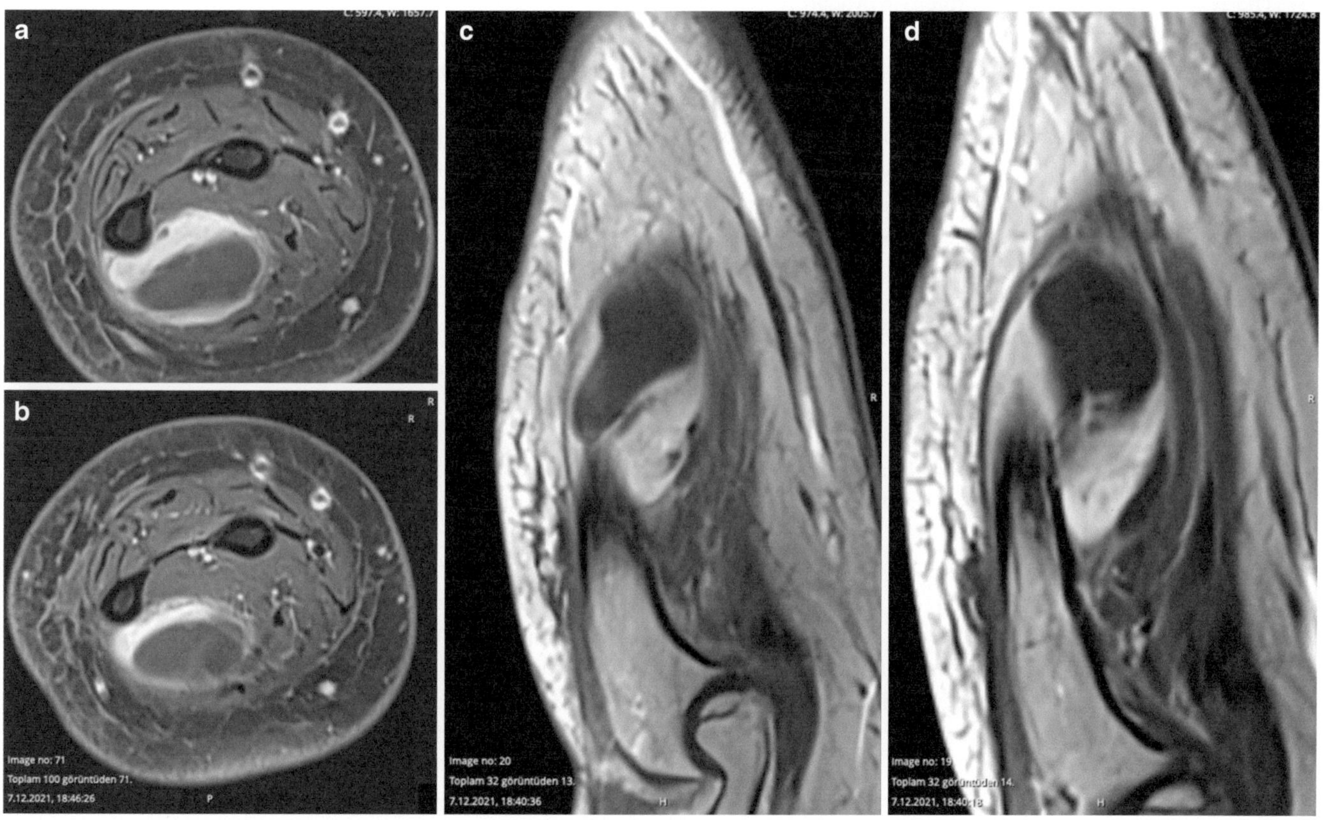

Fig. 29.4 T1W fat-saturated contrast-enhanced transverse MR images in (**a** and **b**) and sagittal T1W images in (**c** and **d**) demonstrate significant tumor regression following concurrent neoadjuvant chemoradiotherapy. While the solid component of the tumor has markedly shrunk, the cystic component has also shown some shrinkage. The contact area between the ulna and the tumor has decreased. Compression of the neurovascular structures in the volar compartment of the forearm has also been reduced, facilitating safe dissection

29.4 Preoperative Problem List

(a) Since the patient is a pediatric patient, the functional expectation is high for any proposed limb salvage procedure.
(b) The diagnosis has been delayed due to the presumption of a benign soft tissue tumor, hemangioma in this case.
  1. While the same MRI features could be attributed to hemangioma at first detection, wide local excision rather than radiologic follow-up could be a better management strategy since the lesion was small, surgical excision with safe margins and without morbidity was feasible, and the patient was already symptomatic.
  2. The significant delay in diagnosis could have already facilitated microscopic metastases.
(c) The radial and ulnar vessels, as well as the median nerve, are compressed by the tumor in the proximal flexor compartment of the forearm. These neurovascular structures are specifically at risk of injury during dissection. Furthermore, marginal safety might be compromised while trying to dissect these structures.
(d) The osseous involvement of the tumor necessitates osseous resection, even if the tumor originates in the soft tissues.
(e) The resection of the ulnar segment will lead to transection of muscles originating from the proximal ulna (extensor carpi ulnaris, flexor pollicis longus, extensor carpi ulnaris, abductor pollicis longus, and extensor pollicis longus) and might lead to weakness associated with these muscles.
(f) The planned length of the ulnar segment to be resected is longer than 6 cm (approximately 10–11 cm, depending on imaging after neoadjuvant treatment). This ideally necessitates reconstruction with a graft, which has biological potential. A vascular fibula will be the best option for such an intercalary reconstruction, and therefore, microsurgery will be needed.
(g) Preoperative radiotherapy might be a predisposing factor specifically for complications like wound problems, deep infection, and bone healing problems.

29.5 Treatment Strategy

(a) The patient's and the family's expectations must be well understood, and they must be well informed about the advantages and disadvantages of various treatment strategies.
(b) Limb salvage surgery is the main treatment objective, and resection with safe margins is the most crucial aspect of LSS.
(c) The preferred method of limb salvage is intercalary resection of the involved osseous segment and restoration of the two-bone forearm anatomy with biological reconstruction.
(d) A multidisciplinary approach is essential for the best functional and oncological outcome. The multidisciplinary board should discuss thoroughly whether adjuvant treatment modalities are indicated and the timing of these possible interventions to facilitate safe resection, improve systemic disease control, and minimize complications [10].
(e) Meticulous postoperative rehabilitation, not compromising the biological reconstruction, is critical for the best functional outcome.

29.6 Basic Principles

(a) Tumor resection with adequately wide margins must be the primary goal. Shrinkage of the tumor with the most appropriate neoadjuvant treatment modalities should be provided for resection with safe margins and preservation of critical anatomical structures in a constrained anatomical compartment. Even if tumor shrinkage cannot be achieved, the neoadjuvant treatment must create a pseudocapsule and neutralize the reactive zone for marginal safety.
(b) Elaborate preoperative planning must be done based on high-quality and detailed local MR imaging obtained at presentation and after the completion of neoadjuvant chemotherapy to decide on surgical margins. The anatomical boundaries of the tumor in the soft tissue compartment (especially the presence of any tail sign along fascial planes), along the periosteum, and whether cortical destruction and intramedullary extension are present must be assessed very carefully. Preoperative imaging must include the upper arm and the axilla to detect lymph node metastasis, which is common for synovial sarcoma.
(c) Necessary technical preparations (surgical equipment, instruments, and implants) must be done for fine dissection of the soft tissue margins and neurovascular structures, precise resection of the involved osseous segment, stable osteosynthesis of the reconstructed segment, and microsurgical anastomosis.
(d) Close postoperative care and monitoring are necessary for the timely management of possible complications (e.g., hematoma, wound dehiscence, compartment syndrome) since the patient must continue with adjuvant chemotherapy.
(e) If adjuvant treatment is indicated, the patient should be referred to the pediatric oncologist as soon as early postoperative complications have been ruled out.

(f) The patient should be scheduled for long-term orthopedic oncology follow-up, including monitoring bone healing and extremity functions, especially in the first 2 postoperative years, and surveillance of any local, regional, or systemic oncological events for at least 10 years postoperatively.

29.7 Intraoperative Images

See Fig. 29.5.

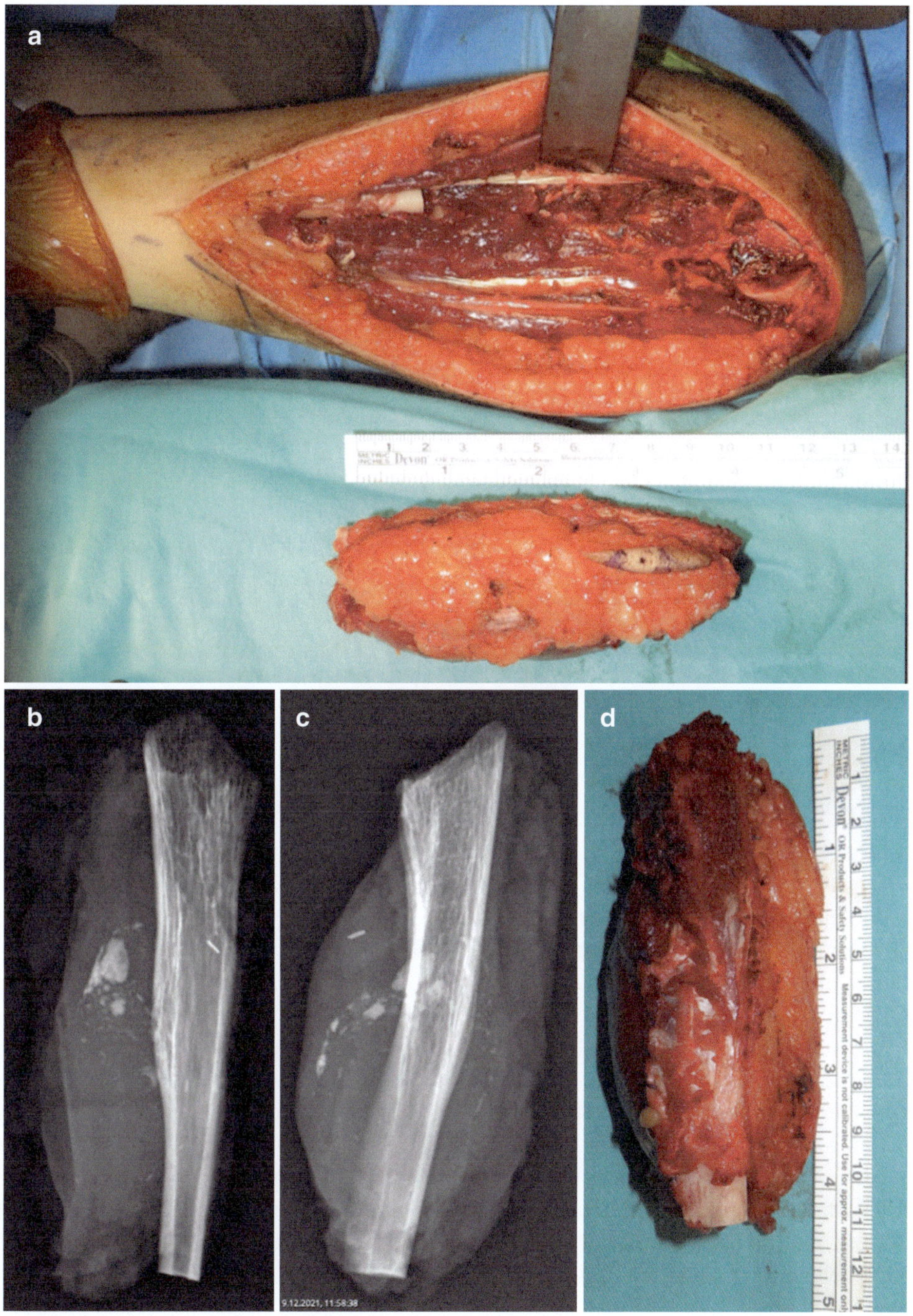

Fig. 29.5 The intraoperative photo in (**a**) shows the resection site following wide local excision and the resected specimen, including the biopsy tract. Radiographs of the resected specimen in (**b** and **c**) show the impression caused by the long-standing soft tissue tumor on the bone and the soft tissue calcifications. The resection length was 11.5 cm (**d**), while the harvested vascular fibula was approximately 15 cm, as shown in (**e**). Harvesting the fibula at least 1 cm longer than planned is advisable to provide flexibility when positioning the bone, and it can be shortened from one or both ends according to pedicle orientation and length. The intraoperative photo (**f**) shows the segmental reconstruction with the vascular fibula and locking plate. The diagnosis of monophasic synovial sarcoma was confirmed after the histopathological examination of the resected specimen. Tumor necrosis was reported as 50%, while the surgical margins were negative

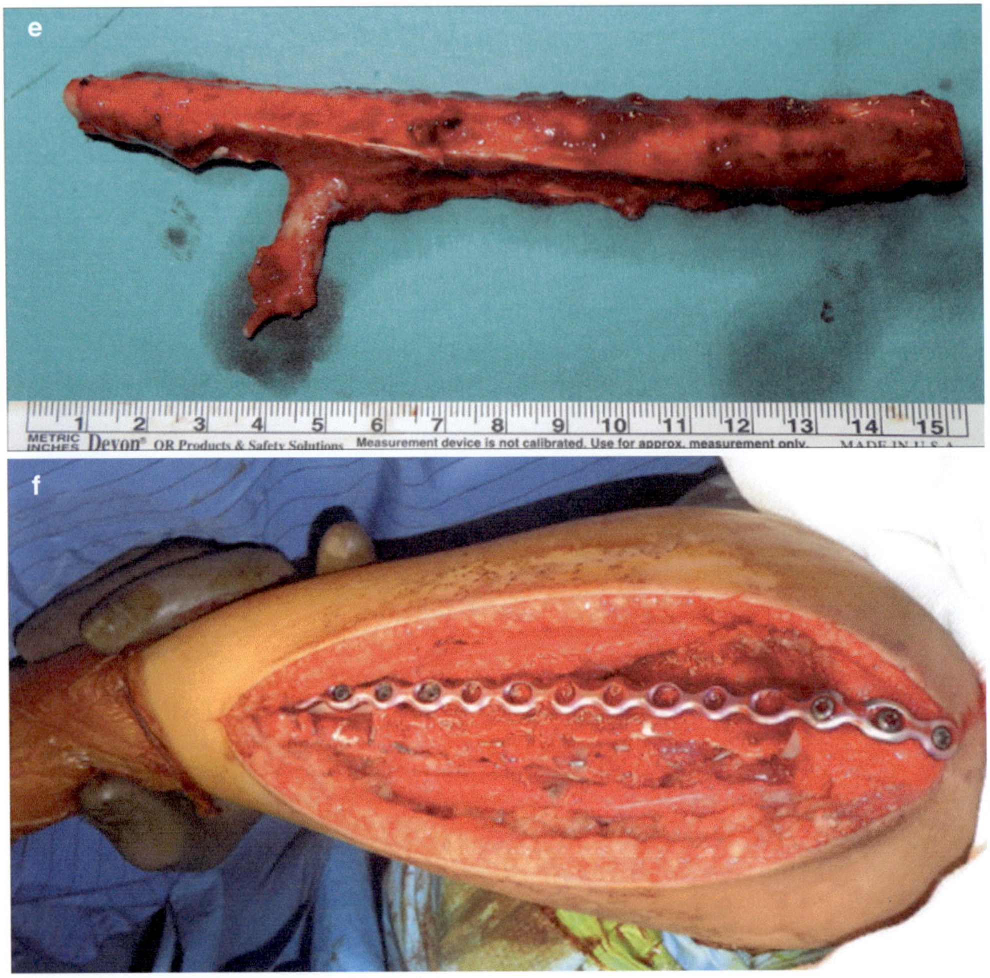

Fig. 29.5 (continued)

29.8 Technical Pearls

(a) A CT or MR angiography of the fibula donor site must be performed preoperatively to reveal the vascular anatomy at the level of popliteal trifurcation and rule out any vascular variation that might interfere with free vascular fibula graft (FVFG) harvesting.
(b) The patient should be supine, and the upper extremity must be stretched onto a radiolucent hand table mounted on the main operating table.
(c) The use of a tourniquet wrapped around the upper arm will dramatically improve the quality of dissection and, thus, marginal safety. The extremity must not be exsanguinated but only elevated before the tourniquet is inflated.
(d) The biopsy tract must be excised with the tumor.
(e) Critical anatomical structures are cramped in a small volume in the forearm, so circumferential dissection is rather challenging. While pronating and supinating the forearm greatly facilitates dissection around the ulna, the soft tissue dissection might alternatively be completed after the proximal and distal osteotomies are performed, and the tumor-bearing segment can be freely rotated.
(f) As soon as the resection is complete, the recipient vessels for the vascular fibula should be explored and marked by the microsurgeon. Then, the tourniquet should be deflated, and meticulous hemostasis should be performed at the resection site, taking care not to injure the recipient vessels.
(g) Subsequently, the FVFG will be prepared for harvest by the microsurgeon. The length of the FVFG will be determined according to the actual length of the resected specimen. A gel positioner might be placed under the ipsilateral buttock for easier access to the lateral aspect of the calf, and a tourniquet must be placed around the ipsilateral thigh for use during FVFG harvest. Harvesting the ipsilateral FVFG allows using a single crutch on the contralateral side.
(h) The FVFG will then be transferred to the proximal ulnar defect, and osteosynthesis will be performed to achieve absolute stability and proper alignment. A locking

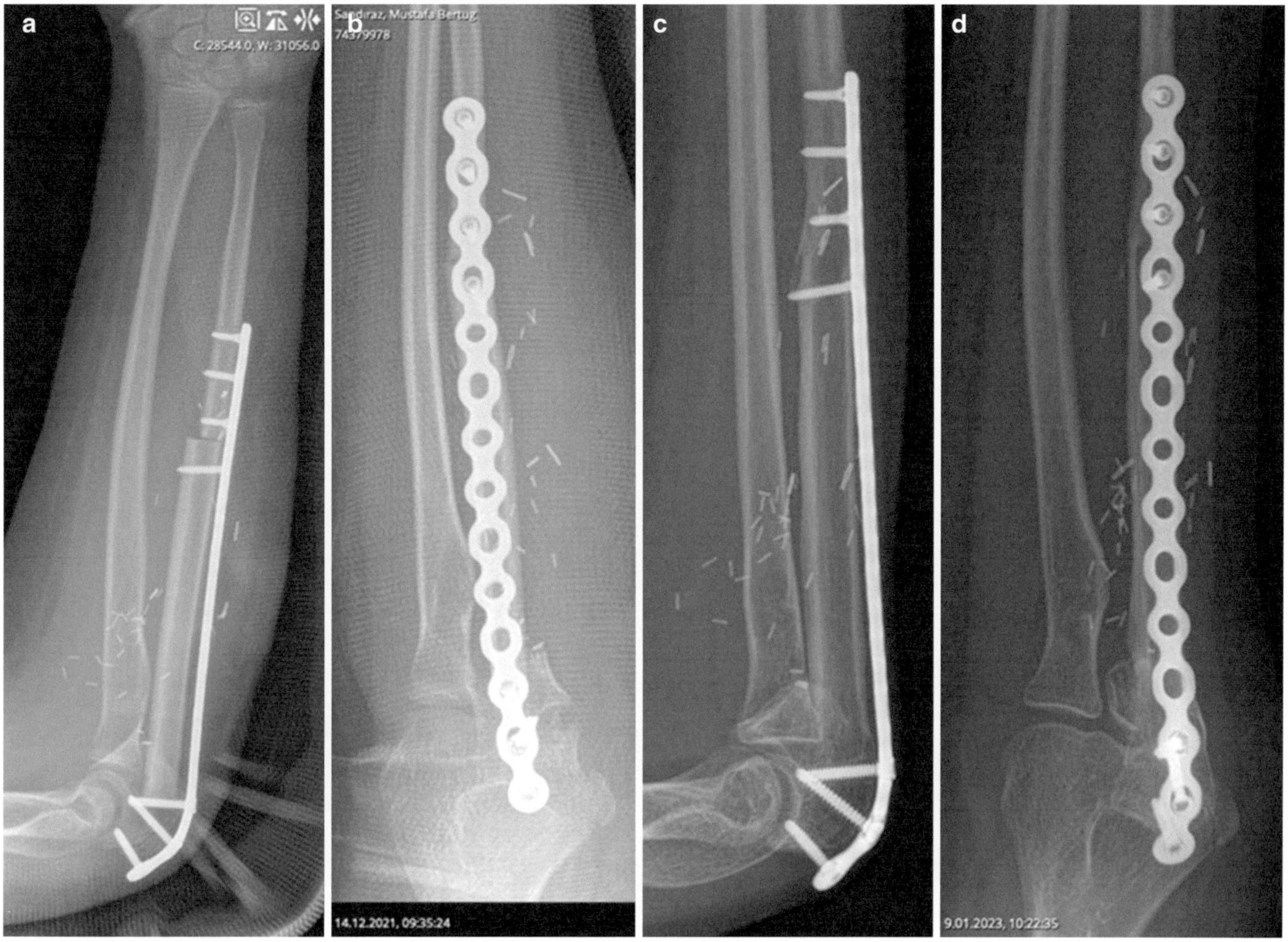

Fig. 29.6 (**a** and **b**) Demonstrate the AP and lateral early postoperative radiographs, while follow-up radiographs at postoperative 13 months in (**c** and **d**) show excellent bone healing. The proximal end of the vascular fibula was partially inserted into the proximal ulna metaphysis. In contrast, the distal end of the vascular fibula was fixed in apposition with the ulnar diaphysis

3.5 mm anatomical olecranon plate or reconstruction plate can be used for this purpose.

(i) Pedicle anastomosis of the FVFG will conclude the reconstruction. If an end-to-end anastomosis is planned between the pedicle artery and either one of the radial or ulnar arteries, then the Allen test must be performed to guarantee the distal circulation at the level of the hand. Two-vein anastomosis is preferable to one-vein anastomosis.

(j) During wound closure, drains must be placed both in the reconstruction and donor sites.

(k) A long-arm splint will be placed in the immediate postoperative period. As soon as soft tissue edema and pain start to subside, elbow flexion and extension will be allowed with a short-arm splint and simple arm sling. Active pronation and supination will be allowed after 1 month, and the patient will continue using an arm sling until radiographic signs of bone healing are visible.

(l) A short-leg splint will be applied to the fibula donor site. It can be removed after 5–7 days when the donor site pain starts to subside.

29.9 Outcome Radiographs and Images

See Figs. 29.6, 29.7, and 29.8.

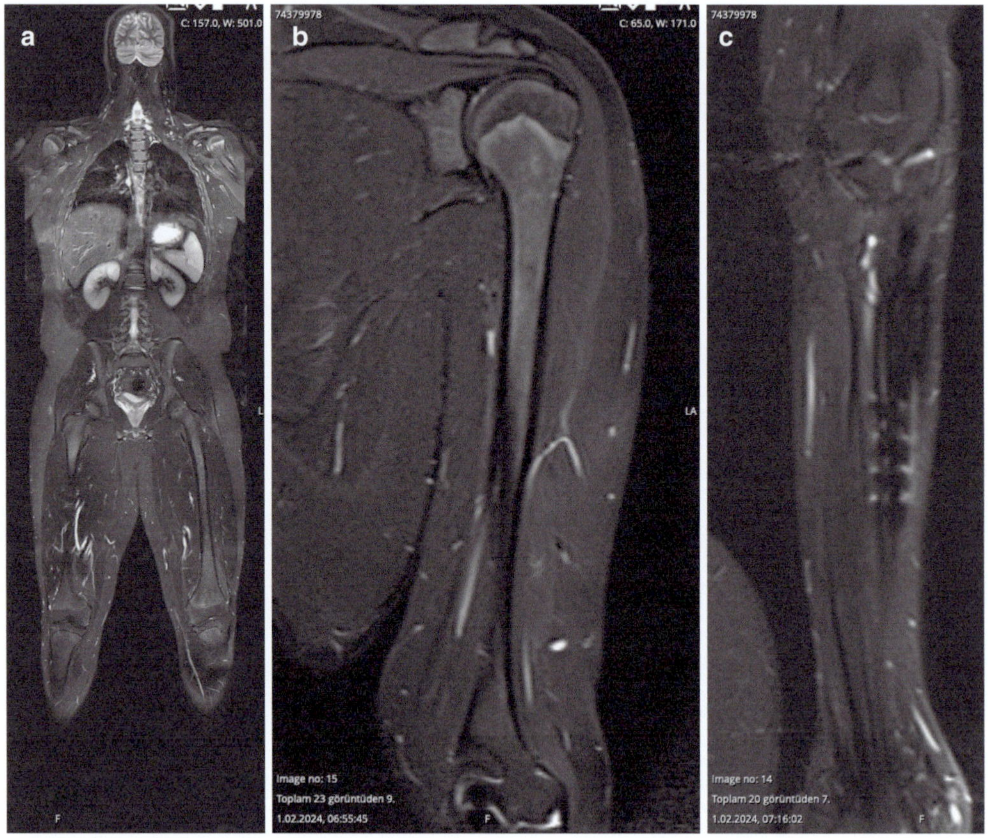

Fig. 29.7 Follow-up imaging at postoperative 26 months shows no evidence of disease. Our institutional policy is to perform an annual whole-body MRI (**a**) routinely for surveillance of distant metastasis for 10 years. Lung metastases are screened with serial CT scans of the chest but sticking to a tighter schedule, especially in the first 5 postoperative years. Upper extremity coronal MR images in (**b** and **c**) show no axillary lymph node involvement, regional metastasis, or local recurrence

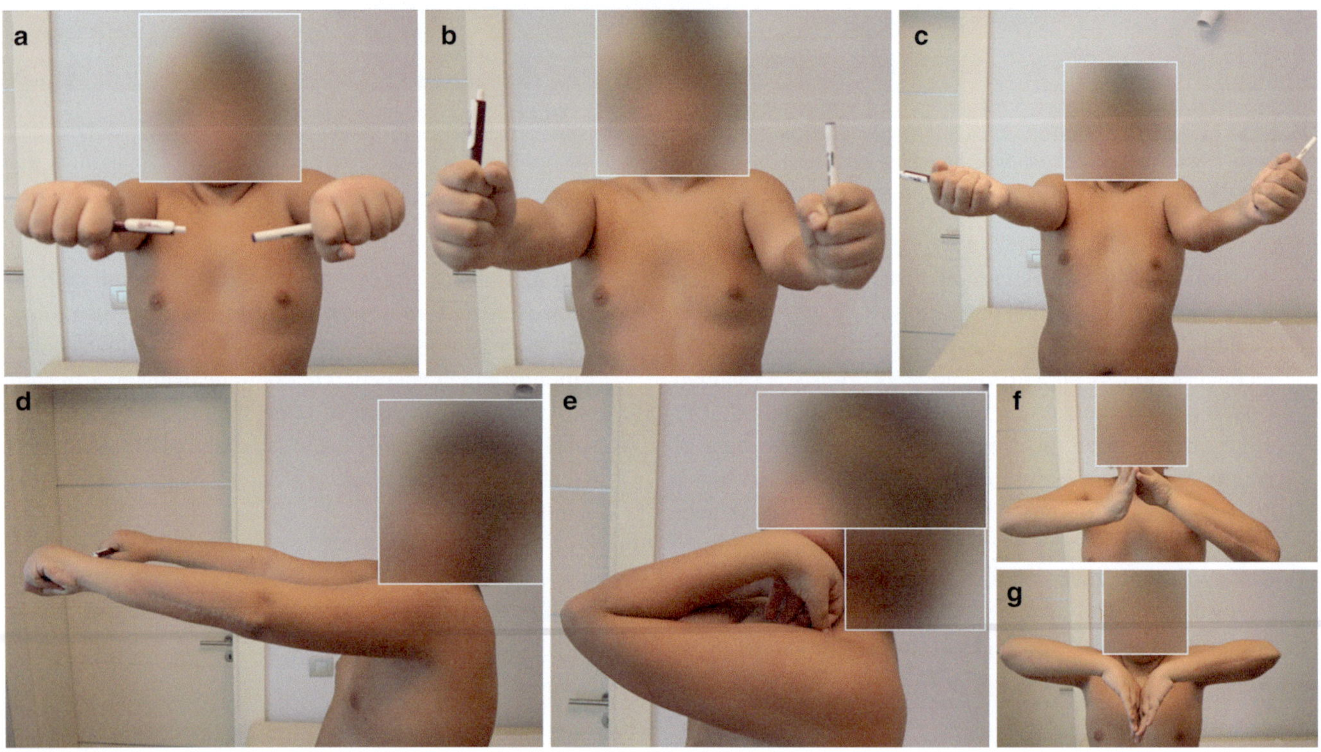

Fig. 29.8 Clinical images at postoperative 13 months show excellent function. Neurovascular examination and grip strength were unremarkable. (**a**) Shows full pronation, while 15° of residual flexion contracture and 45° of supination deficit can be observed in (**b** and **c**). (**d**) Shows the incision scar extending from the olecranon distally along the ulna in full extension and pronation, while (**e**) shows full elbow flexion. Although (**f**) shows limitation in wrist extension, his wrist flexion (**g**) was near normal and he had no complaints about hand dexterity

29.10 Avoiding and Managing Problems

(a) The orthopedic team should regularly check the patient during the neoadjuvant treatment period to detect complications like tumor progression under treatment, severe radiation dermatitis, skin breakdown, and/or tumor-necrosis-related abscess formation. The timely detection of such complications might impact the planning of limb salvage surgery.

(b) Concurrent neoadjuvant chemoradiotherapy is a very effective but demanding treatment protocol. It can only be applied in a specialized center by an experienced multidisciplinary team to achieve the best local control and provide systemic protection until limb salvage surgery.

(c) To prevent tumor contamination of the donor site, different surgical trays and sets of instruments must be used for tumor resection and graft harvest.

(d) Extreme care must be taken not to damage the periosteum and the pedicle of the FVFG during osteosynthesis.

(e) Drain(s) must not be placed in contact with the microvascular anastomosis.

(f) The microsurgeon decides whether to use an anticoagulant or antiaggregant to ensure the patency of the anastomosis. However, both types of medications carry the risk of hematoma formation and, thus, compression of the pedicle. Alternatively, intravenous Dextran infusion can be administered for the first 5 postoperative days to prevent thrombosis in the FVFG pedicle.

(g) If primary wound closure is not possible or is too tight in the setting of preoperative radiotherapy, it must be avoided, and negative pressure wound treatment must be applied. Delayed primary wound closure, split-thickness skin grafting, or flap reconstruction might be indicated depending on the resolution of soft tissue edema in the early postoperative period.

(h) A hospital stay of 5–7 days is recommended for close monitoring, particularly of hematoma formation and wound problems. The microsurgeon and microsurgical equipment should be available in case of hematoma evacuation or debridement.

(i) In the long term, possible complications such as graft fractures, nonunion, or implant failures can often be treated similarly to trauma patients if the FVFG maintains its vascularity and, thus, vitality.

(j) Due to the increased risk of joint contracture, starting physiotherapy as soon as adequate soft tissue healing is observed is especially critical in a joint-sparing resection preceded by radiotherapy and flap reconstruction.

(k) Adjuvant chemotherapy should be strongly considered in a locally advanced soft tissue sarcoma, which is chemosensitive.

(l) The patient must be monitored for donor-site morbidities such as ankle valgus in the long term.

References

1. Gambarotti M. Synovial sarcoma. In: Picci P, Manfrini M, Fabbri N, Gambarotti M, Vanel D, editors. Atlas of musculoskeletal tumors and tumorlike lesions. Cham: Springer; 2014. p. 359–64. https://doi.org/10.1007/978-3-319-01748-8.
2. Goldblum JR, Folpe AL, Weiss SW. Other malignant soft tissue tumors, including those of uncertain type. In: Goldblum JR, Folpe AL, Weiss SW, editors. Enzinger and Weiss's soft tissue tumors. 7th ed. Elsevier; 2020. p. 1175–268.
3. Puri A, Gulia A. Management of extremity soft tissue sarcomas. Indian J Orthop. 2011;45(4):301–6. https://doi.org/10.4103/0019-5413.82332.
4. Suurmeijer AJH, Ladanyi M, Nielsen TO. Synovial sarcoma. In: WHO Classification of Tumours Editorial Board, editor. WHO classification of tumours soft tissue and bone tumours. 5th ed. Lyon: International Agency for Research on Cancer; 2020. p. 290–3.
5. Baroudi MR, Ferguson PC, Wunder JS, Isler MH, Mottard S, Werier JA, Turcotte RE. Forearm soft tissue sarcoma: tumors characteristics and oncologic outcomes following limb salvage surgery. J Surg Oncol. 2014;110(6):676–81. https://doi.org/10.1002/jso.23686.
6. Post J, Houdek M, Folpe AL, Kakar SK, Wilke BK. A retrospective case series of synovial sarcoma of the upper extremity. Sarcoma. 2019;2019:8704936. https://doi.org/10.1155/2019/8704936.
7. Adani R, Delcroix L, Innocenti M, Marcoccio I, Tarallo L, Celli A, Ceruso M. Reconstruction of large posttraumatic skeletal defects of the forearm by vascularized free fibular graft. Microsurgery. 2004;24(6):423–9. https://doi.org/10.1002/micr.20067.
8. Gebert C, Hillmann A, Schwappach A, Hoffmann C, Hardes J, Kleinheinz J, Gosheger G. Free vascularized fibular grafting for reconstruction after tumor resection in the upper extremity. J Surg Oncol. 2006;94(2):114–27. https://doi.org/10.1002/jso.20326.
9. Houdek MT, Wagner ER, Wyles CC, Nanos GP, Moran SL. New options for vascularized bone reconstruction in the upper extremity. Semin Plast Surg. 2015;29(1):20–9). Thieme Medical Publishers, Inc. https://doi.org/10.1055/s-0035-1544167.
10. NCCN clinical practice guidelines in oncology (NCCN guidelines®) soft tissue sarcoma version 2.2021—April 28, 2021. http://nccn.ir/Guidelines/Summary/sarcoma.html#pf23. Accessed 11 May 2023.

30 Synovial Sarcoma of the Paravertebral Region with Osseous Involvement

Harzem Özger, Fatih Dikici, and Buğra Alpan

30.1 Introduction

Synovial sarcoma (SS) is a well-defined soft tissue neoplasm often located in the extremities. However, 5–15% of these neoplasms can arise in the trunk, and paravertebral localization is even rarer [1–4]. An important clinical feature is a slow-growing, well-bordered, tender soft tissue tumor, which is sometimes accompanied by significant long-standing local pain and minor limitation of motion. Most lesions are firmly attached to adjacent structures. The indolent behavior and well-circumscribed appearance are commonly misleading toward a benign clinical diagnosis. While it is most prevalent between ages 15 and 40, it can also be seen in older patients, with less than 5% in patients older than 50.

In most cases, the preoperative duration of symptoms ranges from 2 to 4 years, with tumor-related symptoms starting from even 20 years before surgery reported in the literature. In histopathologic examination, poorly differentiated areas are more commonly encountered in elderly patients and might resemble small round cell neoplasms such as Ewing's Sarcoma. The presence of a translocation between chromosomes X and 18 [t(X;18)] is pathognomonic but not mandatory for the diagnosis of SS. Young age, tumor size smaller than 5 cm, distal extremity location, and low tumor grade (absence of poorly differentiated areas) are good prognostic factors. Adequate surgical excision is the primary treatment modality, while radiotherapy is an essential adjunct for improved local control. Although the routine use of chemotherapy in uncomplicated localized disease is not supported by evidence, SS is a chemosensitive tumor, and chemotherapy has been shown to improve overall survival in high-risk patients [2, 5–10]. Posterior vertebral column resection is an extensive surgical procedure mainly used for correcting severe spinal deformities and is accompanied by instrumentation and fusion [11].

H. Özger (✉)
Department of Orthopedics and Traumatology, Istanbul University, Istanbul Medical Faculty, Istanbul, Türkiye
e-mail: harzemo@yahoo.com

F. Dikici · B. Alpan
Department of Orthopedics and Traumatology, Acıbadem Mehmet Ali Aydınlar University, School of Medicine, Istanbul, Türkiye
e-mail: bugra.alpan@acibadem.edu.tr

30.2 Brief Clinical History

A 50-year-old male patient presented with a soft tissue mass in his left thoracolumbar paravertebral region. The mass had first been detected incidentally 8 years ago during a PET-CT scan performed to investigate a nonspecific pulmonary nodule. The lesion had been presumed to be a benign soft tissue tumor due to low metabolic activity, and no imaging follow-up had been done. However, the patient and his family had noticed a gradual growth of the mass over the years. The patient had eventually been diagnosed with Ewing's sarcoma of the soft tissues upon a trucut biopsy in an elsewhere institution 7 months before presenting to our clinic. He had received seven cycles of chemotherapy (first a combination of gemcitabine and docetaxel, then a combination of etoposide and cisplatin due to lack of response with the former) as well as radiotherapy (a total dose of 50 Gy), which had been administered in 25 fractions and completed 2 months before presentation to our clinic. The patient was then told that surgery was required. However, the tumor was inoperable due to inadequate response.

Upon presentation to our clinic, he had no significant complaints besides occasional back pain and a slightly restricted thoracolumbar range of motion. Physical examination revealed a wide area of hyperpigmentation due to radiotherapy in his left thoracolumbar region with a non-tender paravertebral mass with indistinct borders underneath the irradiated skin area. Neurological examination was unremarkable. Imaging studies revealed that the left paravertebral mass measured approximately 21 × 8 × 4 cm, extended from the level of thoracic seventh to lumbar second vertebra in the soft tissues, and involved the posterior vertebral elements between T8 and L2 with substantial destruction of multiple spinous processes.

H. Özger et al. (eds.), *Diagnosis and Treatment of Soft Tissue Tumors*, https://doi.org/10.1007/978-3-031-77061-6_30

Compared with imaging before neoadjuvant treatment, a slight regression was observed regarding tumor size; however, diffuse contrast enhancement was still present. The previous biopsy specimen was consulted with our dedicated musculoskeletal pathologist to yield a possible corrected diagnosis of synovial sarcoma. Neither staging at the prior institution nor re-staging at presentation to our clinic showed any distant metastasis. A curative resection followed by possible spinal instrumentation and soft tissue reconstruction was planned.

30.3 Preoperative Local Imaging

See Figs. 30.1, 30.2, and 30.3.

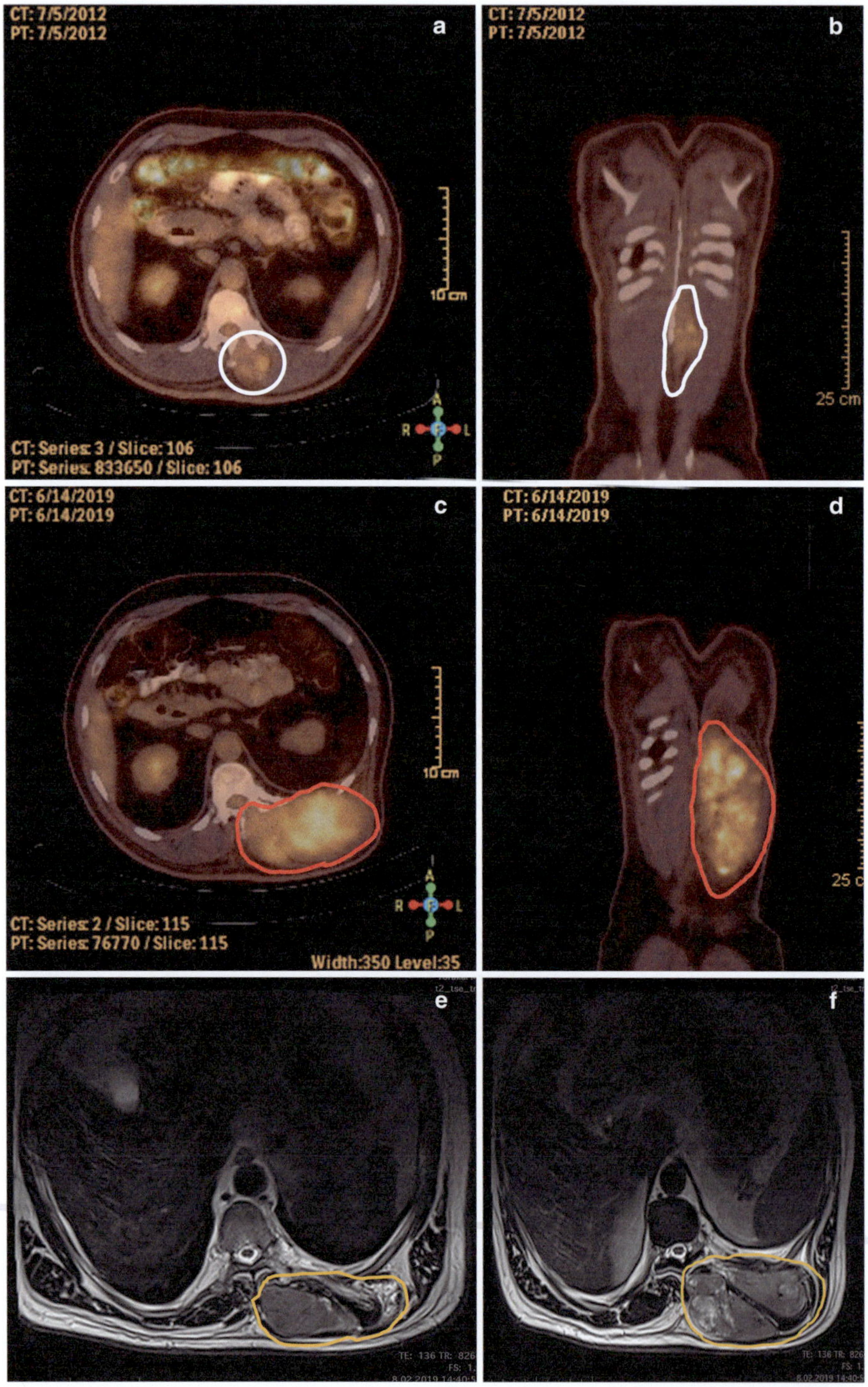

Fig. 30.1 Axial (**a**) and coronal (**b**) PET-CT fusion images show the low metabolic activity and relatively small size of the paravertebral soft tissue mass (white-dashed freeform) when it was initially discovered as an incidental lesion. A follow-up PET-CT scan, which was performed 7 years later due to the patient's complaint of growing mass, demonstrates a high metabolic activity consistent with malignancy and a marked increase in tumor size (red-dashed free forms in (**c** and **d**)). Axial T2-weighted MR images in (**e**) through (**h**) demonstrate the paravertebral soft tissue mass (yellow-dashed free forms) before neoadjuvant treatment

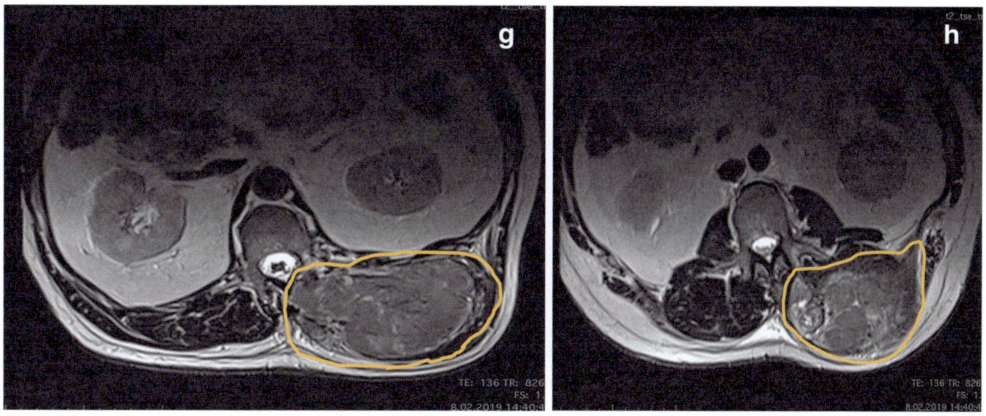

Fig. 30.1 (continued)

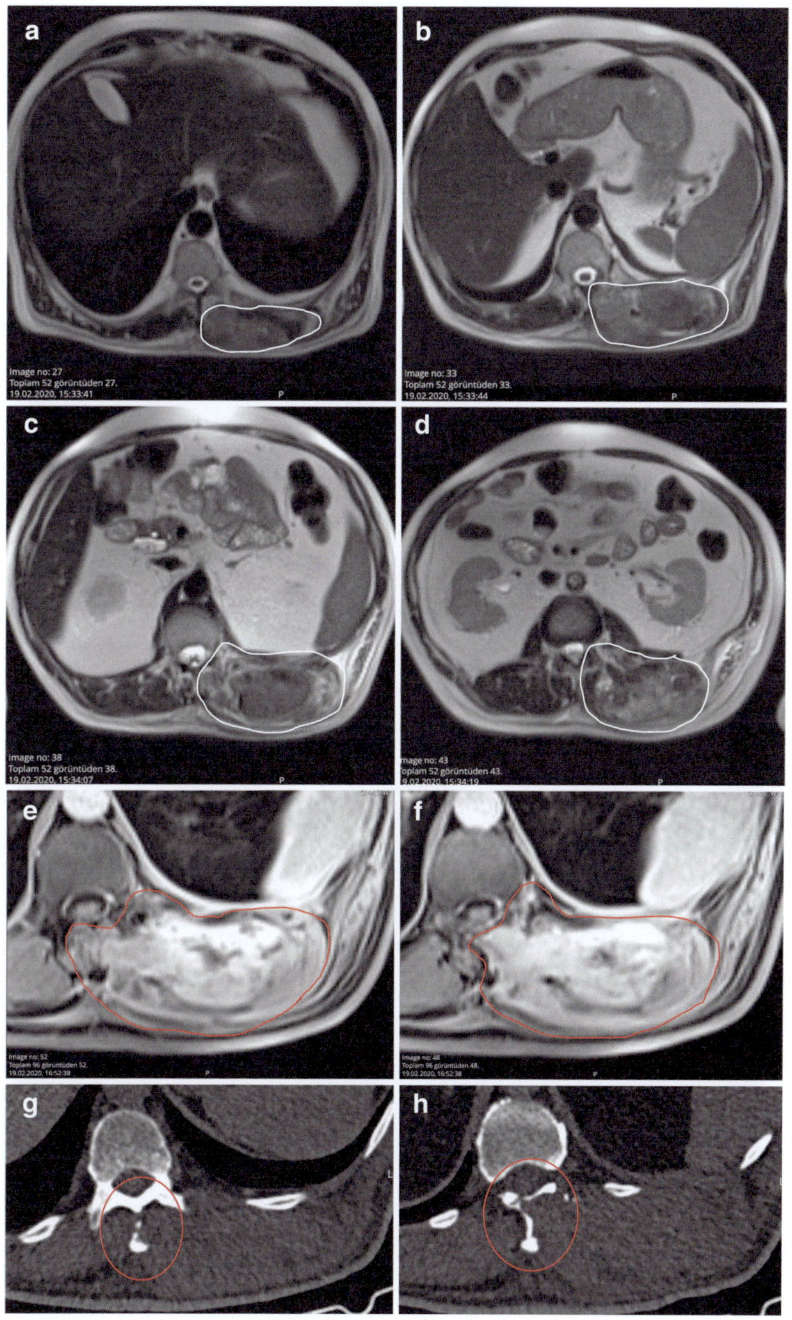

Fig. 30.2 Axial T2-weighted MR images in (**a**) through (**d**) show the left paravertebral soft tissue tumor (white-dashed freeforms) at presentation to our clinic following neoadjuvant treatment elsewhere. Axial T1 vibe-dixon contrast-enhanced images (red-dashed freeforms in (**e** and **f**)) and axial CT scans (red-dashed ellipses in (**g** and **h**)) demonstrate the osseous involvement of the posterior vertebral elements by the soft tissue tumor

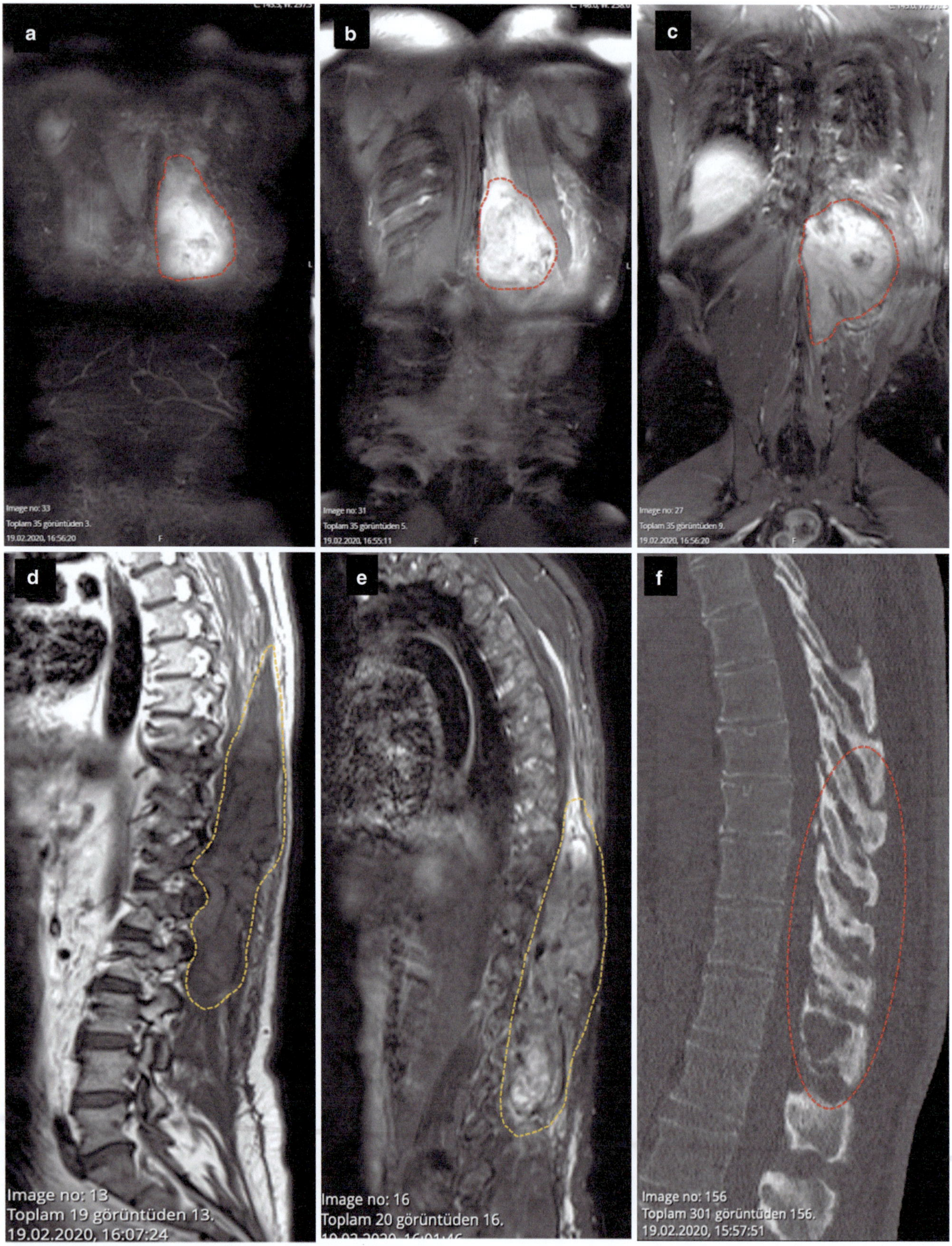

Fig. 30.3 Coronal T1 fat-suppressed contrast-enhanced MR images in (**a**) through (**c**) show the left paravertebral soft tissue tumor (red-dashed freeforms) at presentation to our clinic following neoadjuvant treatment elsewhere. Sagittal T1-weighted and STIR MR images show the longitudinal extent of the lesion (yellow-dashed free forms in (**d** and **e**)). The sagittal CT section in (**f**) demonstrates the erosion of the spinous processes by the tumor (red-dashed ellipse)

30.4 Preoperative Problem List

(a) The paravertebral lesion had a long history, increasing the risk of microscopic metastasis, even though systemic imaging did not reveal any macroscopic finding.
(b) The diagnosis was not definite despite a detailed immunohistochemistry panel and FISH study in a previous institution where the trucut biopsy specimen had been consulted. A diagnosis of Ewing's Sarcoma of the soft tissues must be assessed with precaution since small round cell histology might be encountered in various tumors [5, 7, 10]. Even so, a change in diagnosis was considered unlikely to alter the treatment strategy at this point. Neoadjuvant treatment had already been given, and the tumor response was inadequate.
(c) Surgical resection with adequate margins was the patient's only curative treatment option.
(d) A multi-level resection of posterior vertebral elements was required at the thoracolumbar region. Such an extensive resection could result in direct or indirect injury to the spinal cord and thus could lead to paraplegia and other neurologic complications [11].
(e) Even if acute neurologic complications could be avoided, resection of posterior spinal elements could lead to progressive kyphosis and progressive neurologic deterioration.
(f) The proposed surgical plan of posterior spinal instrumentation and fusion to prevent spinal deformity was complicated by an anticipated weak, soft tissue coverage following resection, exposing the patient to wound problems, deep infection, and even meningitis.
(g) The patient was middle aged (50 years old) and had a large tumor (>5 cm) with trunk and spine localization. These were all negative prognostic factors.

30.5 Treatment Strategy

(a) The main treatment objective was curative resection with safe margins since the patient had already received neoadjuvant treatment and had locally advanced disease at the time of presentation.
(b) The subsequent treatment objectives were to avoid neurologic and mechanical complications related to the spine.
(c) A multidisciplinary approach was essential for the best neurological, functional, and oncological outcomes.
(d) The patient and his family were informed in detail about the treatment goals, (lack of) meaningful alternative treatment strategies, and possible complications.

30.6 Basic Principles

(a) At the time of presentation to our clinic, detailed local and systemic imaging was performed for accurate re-staging and preoperative planning.
(b) The treatment strategy and possible complications were discussed thoroughly by the multidisciplinary team.
(c) The resection was planned together with the musculoskeletal radiologist in light of imaging findings before and after neoadjuvant treatment. Planned soft tissue margins included wide parts of the trapezius, latissimus dorsi, serratus posterior, longissimus thoracis, iliocostalis thoracis, and iliocostalis lumborum muscles, while planned osseous margins included posterior vertebral elements T8 through L2.
(d) Due to the spinal involvement, a spine surgeon who was experienced in spine tumors and had an excellent understanding of sarcoma surgery was included in the multidisciplinary team.
(e) The decision was to avoid spinal instrumentation if possible. However, implants were to be prepared in case unacceptable spinal instability was detected after resection.

30.7 Intraoperative Images

See Figs. 30.4 and 30.5.

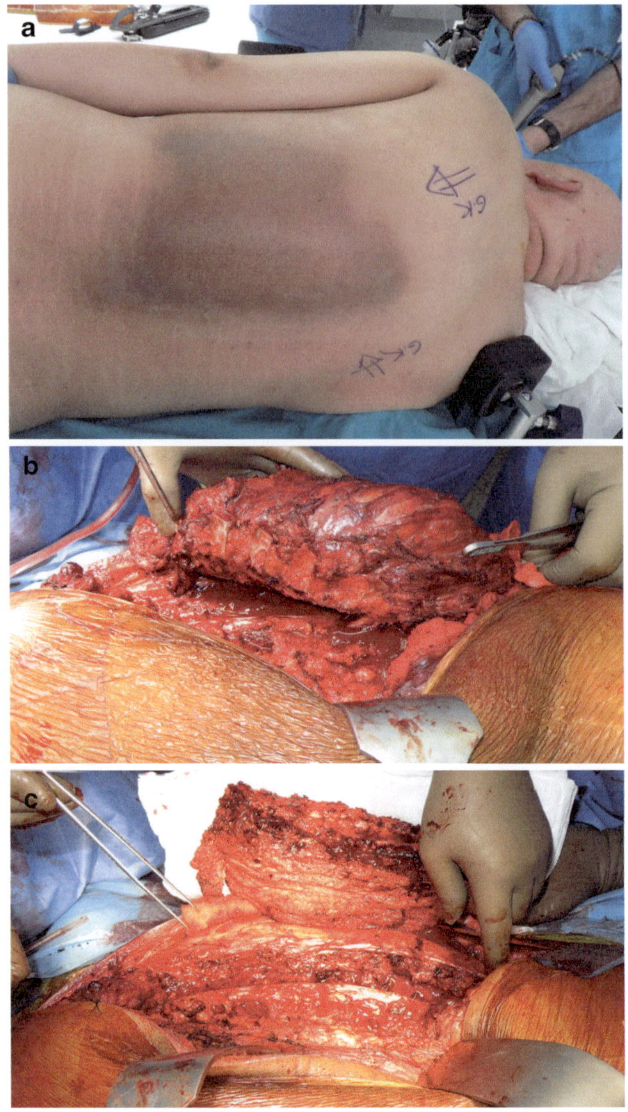

Fig. 30.4 In (**a**), the patient is shown positioned in a floppy right lateral decubitus position, which provides adequate soft tissue and spinal access for safe resection. The intraoperative photo in (**b**) shows that posterior vertebral elements (T8-L2) have been osteotomized on the opposite (right) side, and the tumor has been partially mobilized. In (**b**), it is also shown that the fasciocutaneous flap involving the irradiated skin area has been dissected and released from the superficial aspect of the tumor. In (**c**), the tumor mass is shown to be reflected toward the left flank region along its lateral border, exposing a long spinal cord segment

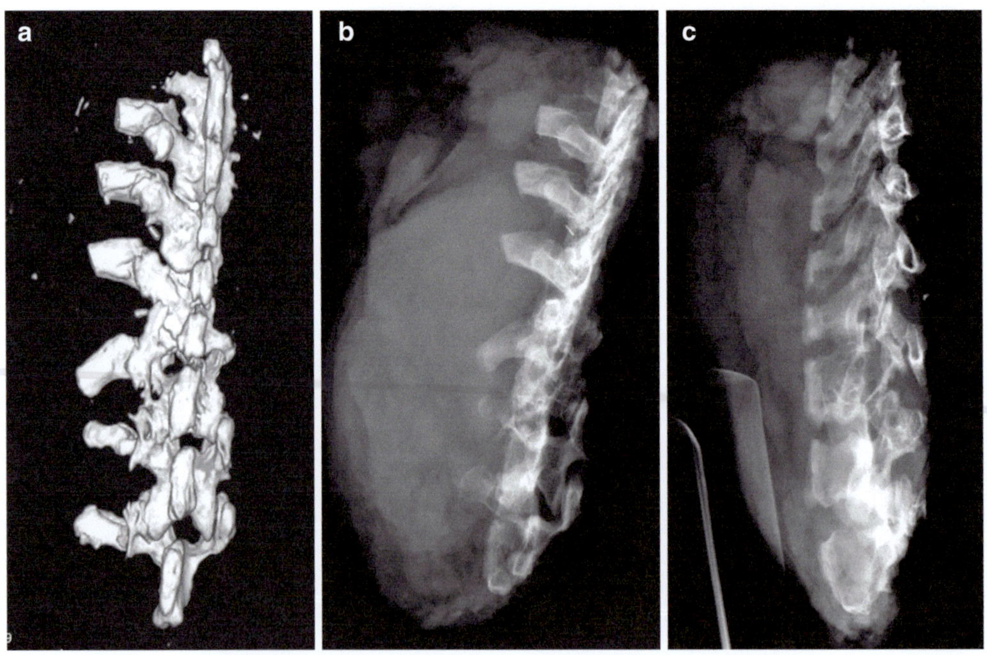

Fig. 30.5 In (**a**), the three-dimensional CT reconstruction of the osseous component of the resection specimen is shown, while radiographs in (**b** and **c**) show the whole specimen. The resected posterior elements include T7-L2 spinous processes, T12-L2 bilateral facet joints and laminae, T8-11 left hemilaminae, T9-12 left costotransverse junctions, and L1-2 left transverse processes

30.8 Technical Pearls

(a) The orthopedic oncologist and the spine surgeon should discuss their approaches and technical concerns, the patient's position, and intended surgical margins preoperatively. Virtual or actual 3D spine models can be utilized to plan the resection through posterior vertebral elements.
(b) While the resection is planned according to MR images obtained in a standard spine position, the dissection planes can change in the actual operation position due to gravity and depending on the tumor's mobility. In this case, the patient was positioned lateral decubitus, requiring the orthopedic oncologist and the spine surgeon to orient themselves accordingly.
(c) Dissecting the superficial, lateral, cranial, caudal, and deep aspects of the paravertebral tumor first and performing the spinal osteotomy last offers the advantage of being able to remove the tumor as soon as the spinal osteotomy is complete so that any possible epidural hemorrhage or dura injury can be dealt with swiftly and under total exposure.
(d) Muscle dissection technique is crucial to achieve adequate soft tissue margins. It should be kept in mind that muscle fibers are contractile (particularly with electrocautery use), and the muscle cuff can be easily stripped away during tumor manipulation if a scarce amount of marginal tissue is left.
(e) When dissecting the deep aspect of a paravertebral tumor with rib involvement, segmental resection of non-involved parts of ribs can be performed far laterally to improve exposure and to allow safe extrapleural dissection. The anesthesiology team should use a double-lumen endotracheal tube in cases involving thoracic wall resection so that the ipsilateral lung can be deflated independently to prevent lung parenchyma injury. If the dissection is extrapleural, as in this case, inserting a chest tube can be avoided.
(f) While the soft tissue dissection will guide the surgical team toward the involved spinal segments to a certain extent, fluoroscopic identification of vertebral levels is mandatory.
(g) The technique of posterior vertebral column resection is also crucial. The osseous dissection must start on the contralateral side of the paravertebral mass to achieve a safe approach from the tumor-free region. The operation table must be tilted anteriorly to the maximum. The patient, who is in a floppy lateral decubitus position, must also be rolled anteriorly to achieve an almost prone position. If the surgical team feels that adequate exposure cannot be achieved from the contralateral aspect of the spine by tilting the table and rolling the patient, then the soft tissue and bony resections can be planned in two stages with lateral decubitus position first and standard prone positioning next, by temporarily closing the wound and prepping and draping the patient again. Following entry into the spinal canal on the contralateral side with either laminectomy or facetectomy, the posterior epidural space must be dissected toward the tumor-involved side.
(h) The spinal cord must be mobilized adequately with ligation and transection of nerve roots on the tumor-involved side to complete the osteotomy of the posterior vertebral elements inside-out.
(i) Microscopic dissection with an operating microscope is essential during intraspinal dissection to obtain better visualization, achieve meticulous hemostasis, and prevent unnecessary neurologic morbidity.
(j) At the time of wound closure, the contralateral intact paravertebral musculature was rerouted to the midline as much as possible to fill the dead space caused by the posterior column resection and augment the soft tissue coverage over the spinal cord, which was devoid of posterior protection.

30.9 Outcome Radiographs and Images

See Figs. 30.6, 30.7, 30.8, and 30.9.

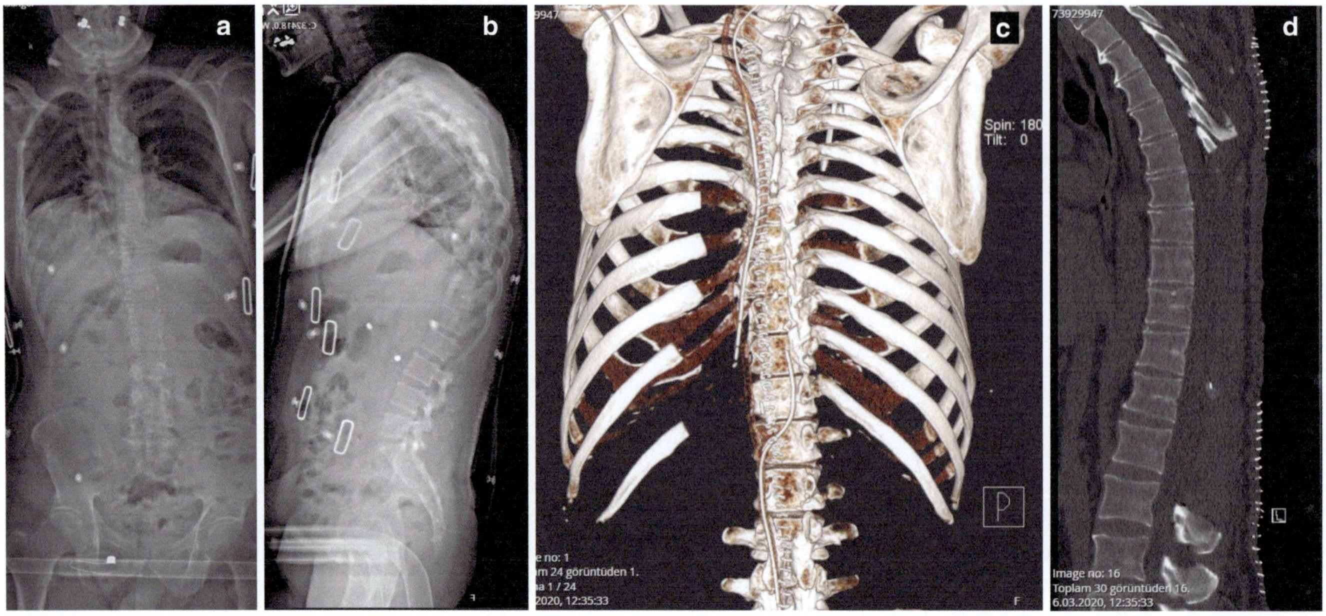

Fig. 30.6 Early postoperative AP and lateral standing radiographs of the whole vertebral column (**a** and **b**) show minimal spine deviation to the right side and slightly increased thoracic kyphosis. The posterior view of the operation site in a 3D-reconstructed CT image in (**c**) demonstrates the extent of bony resection, including the thoracic wall and spinal elements. In contrast, the midline sagittal CT image in (**d**) clearly shows the defect in the posterior vertebral column in the early postoperative period. No neurologic deficit was observed postoperatively

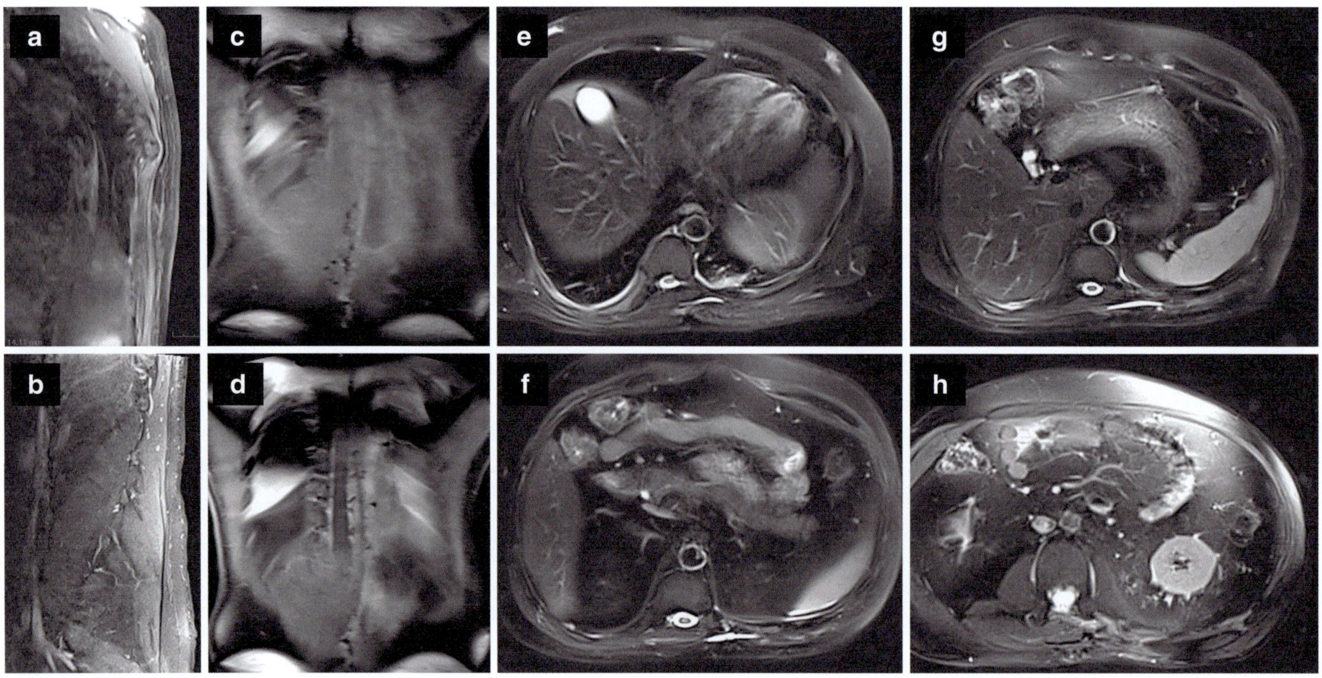

Fig. 30.7 The definitive diagnosis was reported as "synovial sarcoma with poorly differentiated areas." The surgical margins were negative, while tumor necrosis was poor. The patient received no additional oncological treatment and was scheduled for close surveillance. Sagittal (**a** and **b**), coronal (**c** and **d**), and transverse (**e–h**) MR images at postoperative 3.5 years show no evidence of local disease in the left paravertebral thoracolumbar region

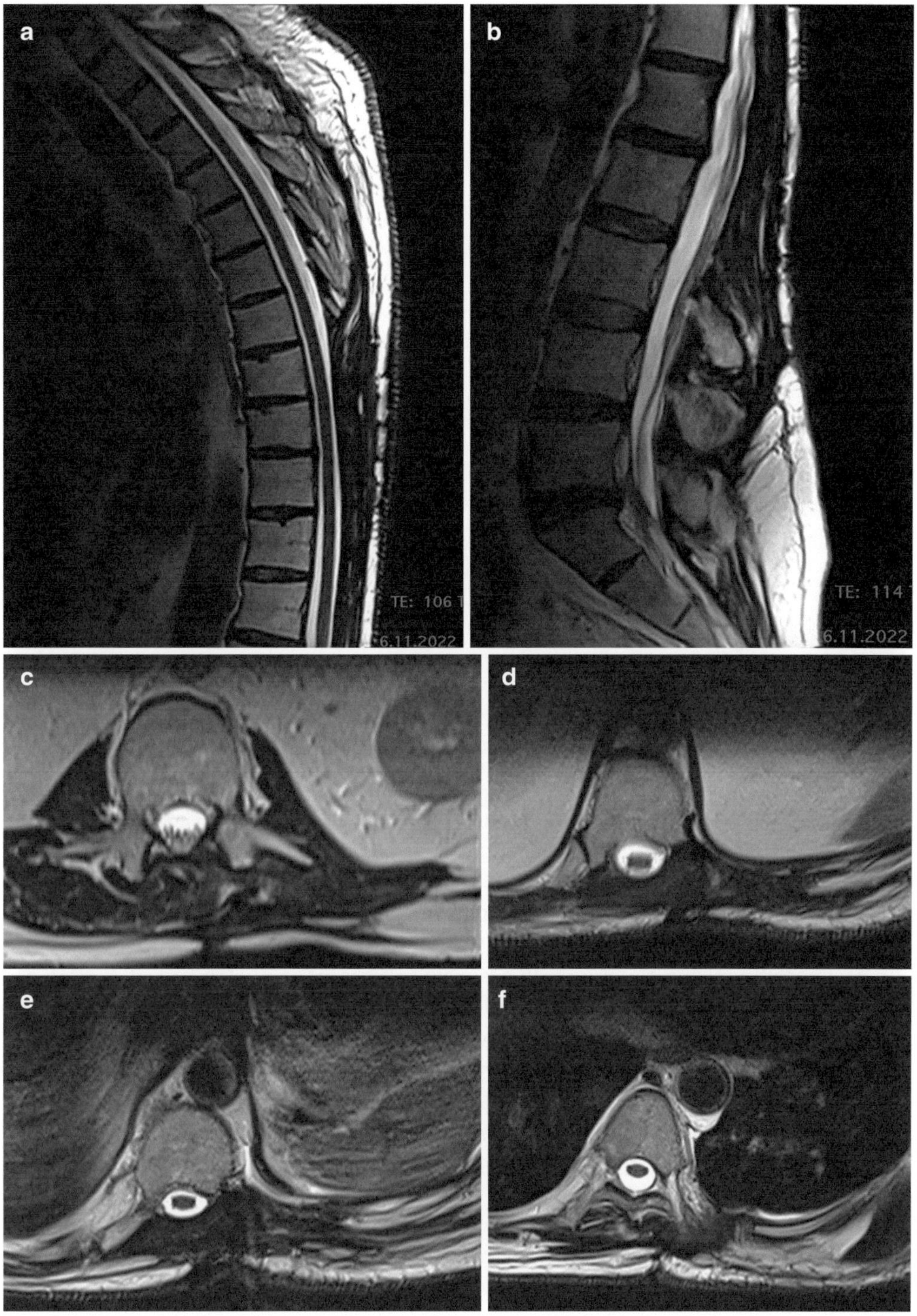

Fig. 30.8 Sagittal (**a** and **b**) and transverse (**c**–**f**) MR images at postoperative 3.5 years show no evidence of local disease in the thoracolumbar spine as well as no morphologic spinal cord abnormality despite slightly increased thoracic kyphosis

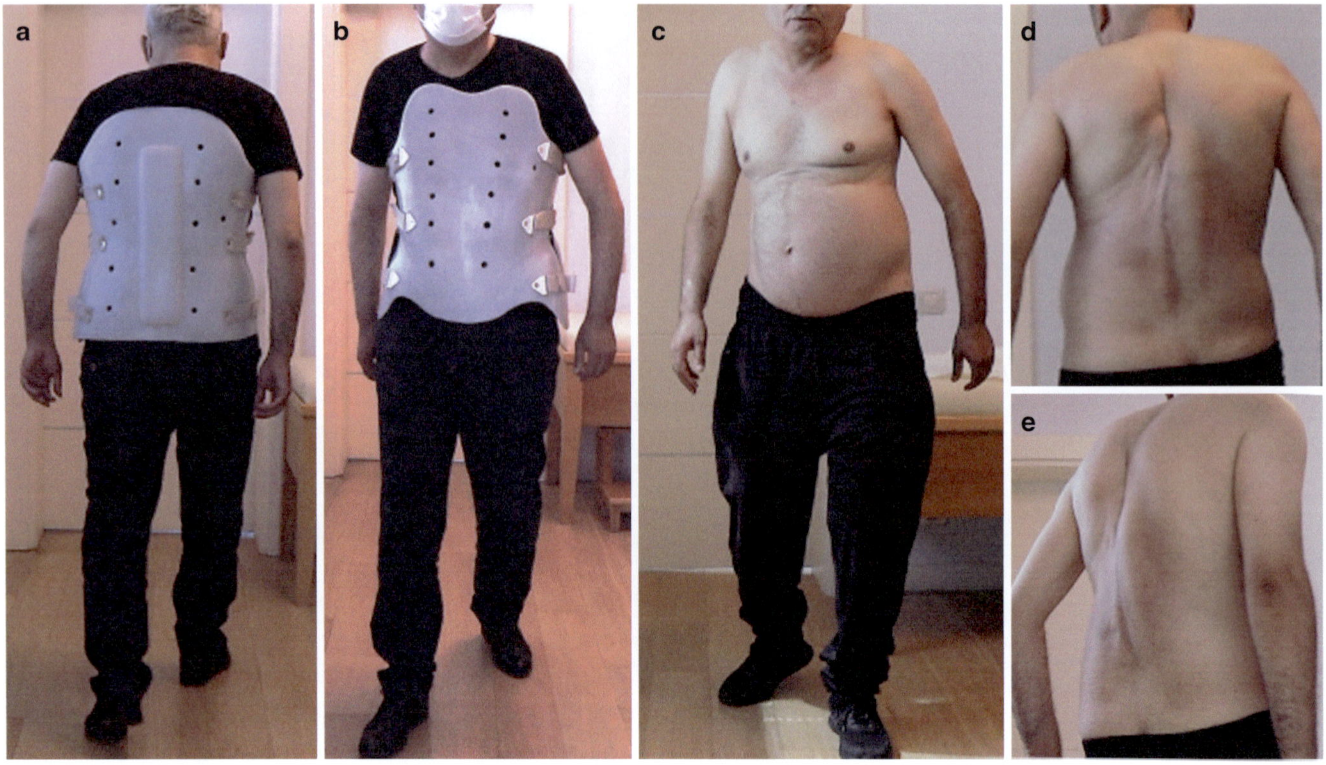

Fig. 30.9 Clinical images in (**a** and **b**) show the patient walking comfortably with a thoracolumbosacral orthosis (TLSO) brace at postoperative 3.5 years. The clinical image in (**c**) shows a slight right-sided trunk shift. Excellent soft tissue healing can be observed in (**d**). At the same time, the oblique clinical view from the right posterolateral aspect of the patient demonstrates the defective soft tissue appearance in the left posterolateral vertebral region. The patient had no neurological symptoms or findings at the last follow-up

30.10 Avoiding and Managing Problems

(a) An uncompromising resection with adequate soft tissue and bony margins was determined as the top priority since surgery was the patient's only curative treatment option. Inadequate local control was considered the ultimate failure in this localization since a salvage operation was unlikely compared to an extremity localization where amputation can be performed as a worst-case scenario in local recurrence.

(b) An incision through the irradiated skin area was avoided, and the resection was planned through an extended midline posterior approach to prevent wound problems. To achieve the planned soft tissue dissection, a wide fasciocutaneous flap was developed, including the irradiated skin and extending to the left flank.

(c) Patient and controlled osteotomy of the posterior vertebral elements, skilled dissection of the epidural space under microscopic visualization, and meticulous hemostasis were critical factors in avoiding intraoperative neurological (dura, nerve root) injury or postoperative neurological complications such as compression of the spinal cord by hematoma.

(d) Posterior vertebral column resection is a procedure mainly used to correct severe spinal deformities. However, it is often performed in shorter segments and is completed by spinal instrumentation and fusion [11]. In this case, the surgical team intraoperatively decided not to perform spinal instrumentation for two crucial reasons. Even if primary skin closure could be achieved over the implants, the soft tissue coverage would be weak due to neoadjuvant radiotherapy and resection. Wound problems, implant exposure, and deep infection were considered inevitable. Furthermore, presuming implants could be retained without any complication; the presence of implants would hinder the imaging quality in the follow-up.

(e) According to Denis' three-column theory, the posterior column is subjected to tension, while the middle and anterior columns have compression loads [12–14]. The loss of a significant portion of the posterior column in the thoracolumbar junction, including the supraspinous and interspinous ligaments and all skeletal structures, predisposes the patient to progressive kyphosis. The loss of facet joints also predisposes the spine to rotational instability. While some contribution to spinal stability might be expected from fibrotic changes in the postoperative period, this is probably negligible, and continuous external support is mandatory in the absence of fixation. The patient was made to wear a custom-made thoracolumbosacral orthosis (TLSO) in the immediate postoperative period as he was brought into the upright position. He was informed that he was obliged to wear his brace at all times, that he was ambulatory, and fervently avoided any trauma to his back.

(f) Due to progressive mechanical and neurological problems, spinal stabilization might still be required in the future. Since soft tissue coverage will still be a problem for posterior instrumentation and no fusion can be obtained even if instrumentation is successful, an alternative strategy can be anterior instrumentation and interbody fusion with thoracotomy.

(g) Seroma was observed in the operation site in the early postoperative period, and aspiration was performed, followed by compressive dressings. The patient was also made to wear a corset used by plastic surgeons in body-lifting procedures. It is imperative to take care not to injure the spinal cord during any aspiration procedure since it has no osseous protection.

(h) Postoperatively, the initial diagnosis of Ewing's sarcoma of soft tissues was definitively ruled out, and the diagnosis of "synovial sarcoma with poorly differentiated areas" was confirmed through histology and immunochemistry. Although the FISH analysis was negative for SS18-SSX translocation, the diagnosis of synovial sarcoma was retained, which was not considered prognostically significant. The surgical margins were clear. The tumor necrosis was poor despite neoadjuvant chemotherapy and radiotherapy. While the patient was designated as a "high-risk" patient due to the presence of multiple negative prognostic factors (middle-aged, large tumor, trunk localization, and poor tumor response), the consensus of the multidisciplinary team was that adjuvant chemotherapy was not predicted to provide any survival advantage. On the other hand, chemotherapy-related unnecessary complications could be anticipated. Consequently, adjuvant chemotherapy was avoided, and instead, the patient was scheduled for close local and systemic surveillance [2, 5–10].

References

1. Koehler SM, Beasley MB, Chin CS, Wittig JC, Hecht AC, Qureshi SA. Synovial sarcoma of the thoracic spine. Spine Journal. 2009;9(12):e1. https://doi.org/10.1016/j.spinee.2009.08.448.
2. Palmerini E, Staals EL, Alberghini M, Zanella L, Ferrari C, Benassi MS, Picci P, Mercuri M, Bacci G, Ferrari S. Synovial sarcoma: retrospective analysis of 250 patients treated at a single institution. Cancer. 2009;115(13):2988–98. https://doi.org/10.1002/cncr.24370.
3. Puffer R, Daniels D, Giannini C, Pichelmann M, Rose P, Clarke M. Synovial sarcoma of the spine: a report of three cases and literature review. Surg Neurol Int. 2011;2(1):18. https://doi.org/10.4103/2152-7806.76939.
4. Yang M, Zhong N, Zhao C, Xu W, He S, Zhao J, Yang X, Xiao J. Surgical management and outcome of synovial sarcoma in the spine. World J Surg Oncol. 2018;16(1):175. https://doi.org/10.1186/s12957-018-1471-x.
5. Blay JY, von Mehren M, Jones RL, Martin-Broto J, Stacchiotti S, Bauer S, Gelderblom H, Orbach D, Hindi N, Dei Tos A, Nathenson M. Synovial sarcoma: characteristics, challenges, and evolving therapeutic strategies. ESMO Open. 2023;8(5):101618. Elsevier B.V. https://doi.org/10.1016/j.esmoop.2023.101618.
6. Gambarotti M. Synovial Sarcoma. In: Picci P, Manfrini M, Fabbri N, Gambarotti M, Vanel D, editors. Atlas of musculoskeletal tumors and Tumorlike lesions. Springer; 2014. p. 359–64. https://doi.org/10.1007/978-3-319-01748-8.
7. Goldblum JR, Folpe AL, Weiss SW. Other malignant soft tissue tumors, including those of uncertain type. In: Goldblum JR, Folpe AL, Weiss SW, editors. Enzinger and Weiss's soft tissue tumors. 7th ed. Elsevier; 2020. p. 1175–268.
8. NCCN clinical practice guidelines in oncology (NCCN guidelines®) soft tissue sarcoma version 2.2021—April 28, 2021. http://nccn.ir/Guidelines/Summary/sarcoma.html#pf23. Accessed 11 May 2023.
9. Pasquali S, Pizzamiglio S, Touati N, Litiere S, Marreaud S, Kasper B, Gelderblom H, Stacchiotti S, Judson I, Dei Tos AP, Verderio P, Casali PG, Woll PJ, Gronchi A. The impact of chemotherapy on survival of patients with extremity and trunk wall soft tissue sarcoma: revisiting the results of the EORTC-STBSG 62931 randomized trial. Eur J Cancer. 2019;109:51–60. https://doi.org/10.1016/j.ejca.2018.12.009.
10. Suurmeijer AJH, Ladanyi M, Nielsen TO. Synovial sarcoma. In: WHO Classification of Tumours Editorial Board, editor. WHO classification of tumours soft tissue and bone tumours. 5th ed. Lyon: International Agency for Research on Cancer; 2020. p. 290–3.
11. Yang C, Zheng Z, Liu H, Wang J, Kim YJ, Cho S. Posterior vertebral column resection in spinal deformity: a systematic review. Eur Spine J. 2016;25(8):2368–75). Springer. https://doi.org/10.1007/s00586-015-3767-7.
12. Haher TR, Tozzi JM, Lospinuso MF, Devlin V, O'brien M, Tenant R, Ahulad J, Valenza J, Parrish S. The contribution of the three columns of the spine to spinal stability: a biomechanical model. Paraplegia. 1989;27:432–9. https://doi.org/10.1038/sc.1989.69.
13. Silva JAM, Ayala AR, Buitimea CJV, Salguero EL, Beltran MCV. Finite element analysis of thoracic vertebral stability supported by the fourth spine. Coluna/Columna. 2022;21(4) https://doi.org/10.1590/S1808-185120222104266858.
14. Widmer J, Cornaz F, Scheibler G, Spirig JM, Snedeker JG, Farshad M. Biomechanical contribution of spinal structures to lumbar spine stability—novel biomechanical insights. Spine J. 2020;20(10):1705–16. https://doi.org/10.1016/j.spinee.2020.05.541.

Metastatic Mixed-Type Liposarcoma of the Popliteal Fossa: Multimodal Treatment

31

Buğra Alpan, Melih Civan, İpek G. Eralp, Yesim Eralp, and Levent Eralp

31.1 Introduction

Liposarcomas (LPS) are soft tissue sarcomas (STS) arising from the adipocytic tissue. Epidemiologic data from large-scale registry studies have shown that liposarcomas constitute one of the most frequently diagnosed STS, comprising up to 11–13% of all soft tissue malignant tumors [1]. Along with gastrointestinal stromal sarcoma (GIST), leiomyosarcomas and undifferentiated sarcomas, the incidence of yearly LPS exceeds $10/10^6$ [2, 3]. While the fourth edition of the World Health Organization Classification of Soft Tissue and Bone classified LPS into four separate pathologic categories, there are three clinically recognized subgroups based on distinct clinical and molecular features [4, 5]. The well-differentiated/de-differentiated (WD/DD) LPS comprise the most frequent subtype, followed by the myxoid/round cell (MRC) and pleomorphic (Pl) subtypes [6]. Liposarcomas often present as painless masses which most frequently arise from the extremities or retroperitoneum. Surgical excision remains the only curative modality in localized disease [7–9]. However, there exists extensive heterogeneity in pathologic subtypes and clinical presentation, which mandates a personalized approach in management [6, 10, 11].

The case described below provides a perfect example of the pathological heterogeneity of LPS, the inherent complexity of management and the significance of targeting the biology of the tumor rather than a one-size-fits-for-all approach.

B. Alpan
Department of Orthopedics and Traumatology, Acıbadem Mehmet Ali Aydınlar University, School of Medicine, Istanbul, Türkiye
e-mail: bugra.alpan@acibadem.edu.tr

M. Civan (✉)
Department of Orthopedics and Traumatology, Başakşehir Çam ve Sakura City Hospital, Istanbul, Türkiye
e-mail: melihcivan@gmail.com

İ. G. Eralp
Rutgers University, Robert Wood Johnson Medical School, New Brunswick, NJ, USA
e-mail: ige8@rwjms.rutgers.edu

Y. Eralp
Department of Medical Oncology, Acıbadem Mehmet Ali Aydınlar University, School of Medicine, Istanbul, Türkiye
e-mail: Yesim.Eralp@acibadem.edu.tr

L. Eralp
Department of Orthopedics and Traumatology, Istanbul University, Istanbul Medical Faculty, Istanbul, Türkiye
e-mail: drleventeralp@gmail.com

31.2 Brief Clinical History

A 46-year-old female patient presented to the clinic with complaints of right leg and back pain which worsened over the last couple of months before admission in October 2018. Diagnostic evaluation with a contrast-enhanced MRI revealed an abdominal mass measuring 13 × 8 cm and a 15 × 8 cm left popliteal mass in addition to multiple lytic skeletal lesions, the largest of which were detected in the L4 vertebral body and the right femur (Figs. 31.1, 31.2, 31.3, 31.4, and 31.5).

The pathologic evaluation of a core-needle biopsy obtained from the popliteal mass was consistent with myxoid liposarcoma without any round cell, pleomorphic or de-differentiated components. She then underwent three cycles of combination chemotherapy consisting of doxorubicin and ifosfamide and a subsequent response assessment revealed partial regression of all the lesions. With these findings further treatment options were discussed at a comprehensive tumor board and a decision was made to remove the soft tissue masses following irradiation to the active skeletal lesions and popliteal mass. An en bloc wide resection of both masses was carried out during the same session with no major surgical complications (Figs. 31.6 and 31.7).

The pathologic evaluation of the excised intra-abdominal mass revealed a 13 × 10 cm mixed liposarcoma consisting of 30% de-differentiated and 70% myxoid components with a high mitotic rate and extensive necrosis, whereas the 4 × 5 cm retro-popliteal mass was diagnosed as pure myxoid liposarcoma without necrosis or co-existing components.

H. Özger et al. (eds.), *Diagnosis and Treatment of Soft Tissue Tumors*, https://doi.org/10.1007/978-3-031-77061-6_31

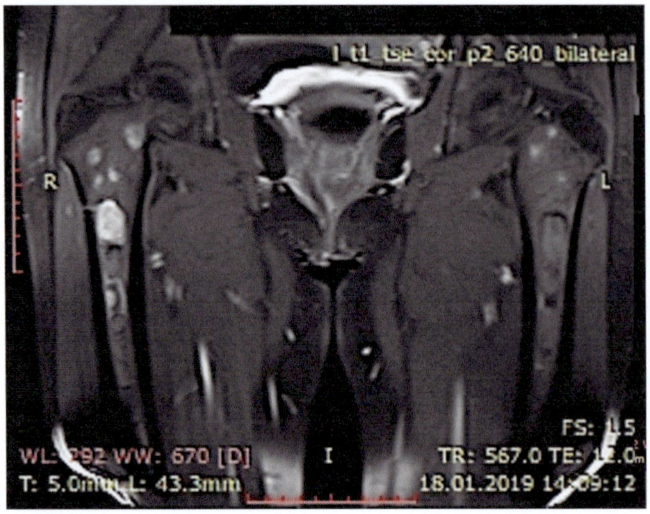

Fig. 31.1 MRI shows multiple lytic skeletal lesions on the right proximal femur

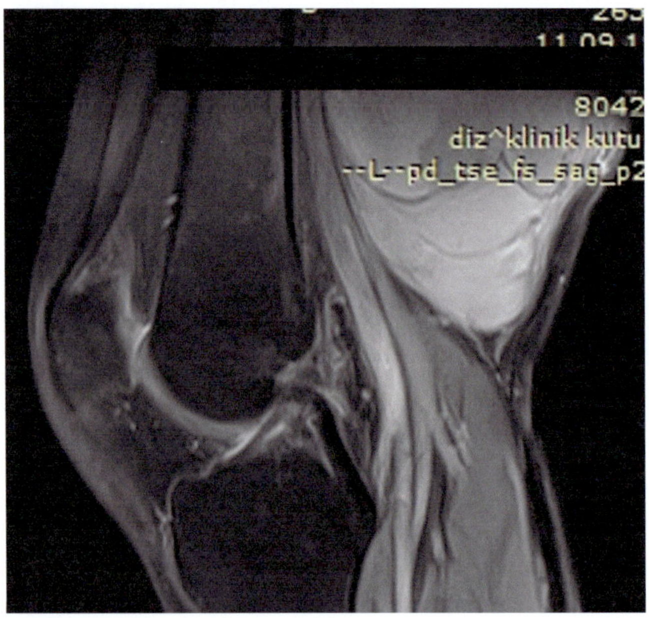

Fig. 31.2 Sagittal plane views of the contrast-enhanced MRI show left popliteal mass

Post-operatively, the patient received adjuvant radiotherapy to the left popliteal surgical area, while continuing chemotherapy for three more cycles which were completed in May 2019. Subsequent response assessment by a PET-MRI failed to show any active FDG avid lesions, whereas there were multiple skeletal lesions with heterogeneous contrast uptake indicating residual involvement. Therefore, we decided to continue the systemic treatment with a switch maintenance strategy comprising of a multikinase inhibitor. She received pazopanib 800 mg daily until March 2020 when progression of metastatic involvement within the left humerus was noted, in addition to a new metastatic lesion appearing within the right trapezius muscle.

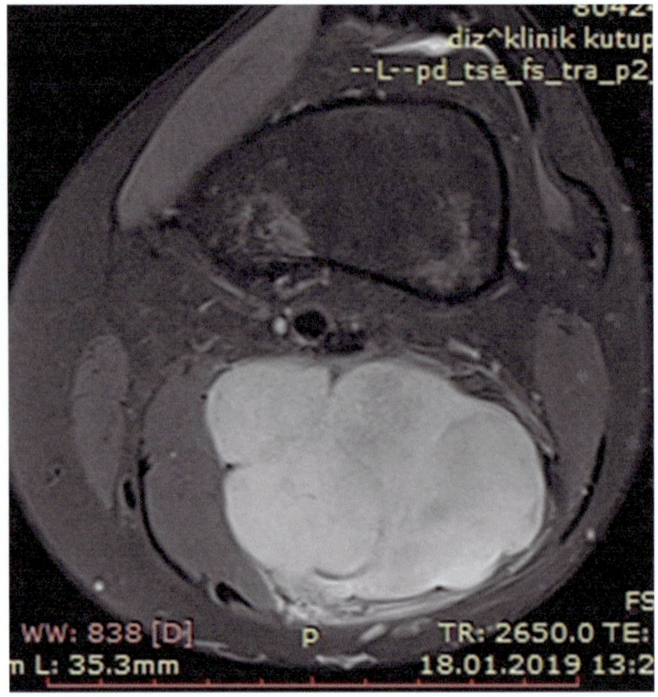

Fig. 31.3 Axial view of the contrast-enhanced MRI at the level of the largest width of the tumor in the left popliteal fossa

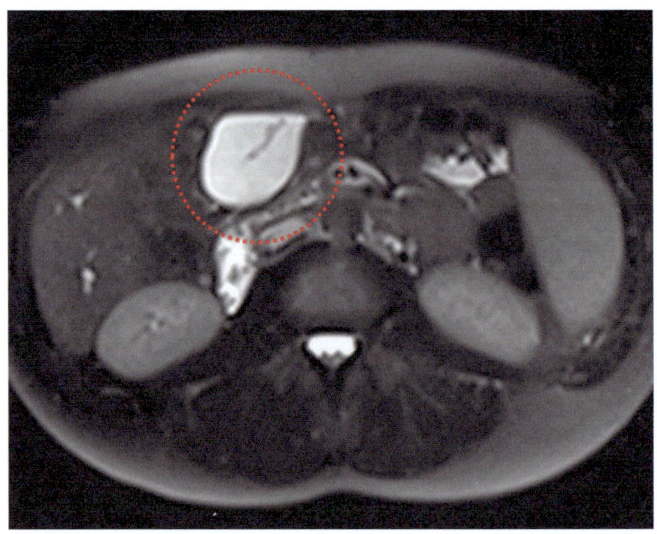

Fig. 31.4 Contrast-enhanced MRI shows abdominal mass

She then underwent an en bloc wide excisional resection of the mass, which confirmed the diagnosis as myxoid liposarcoma with round cell components. A subsequent genomic analysis of the tumor revealed a FUS-DDIT fusion, as well as genomic alterations in the PIK3CA E545K and PTEN genes. Based on accumulating data on the efficacy of trabectedin and olaparib for "translocation sarcomas," she was recommended to receive postoperative systemic therapy with this combination following irradiation of the left humeral metastasis. After six cycles of chemotherapy, imaging studies denied any active lesions, and we set up a follow-up plan

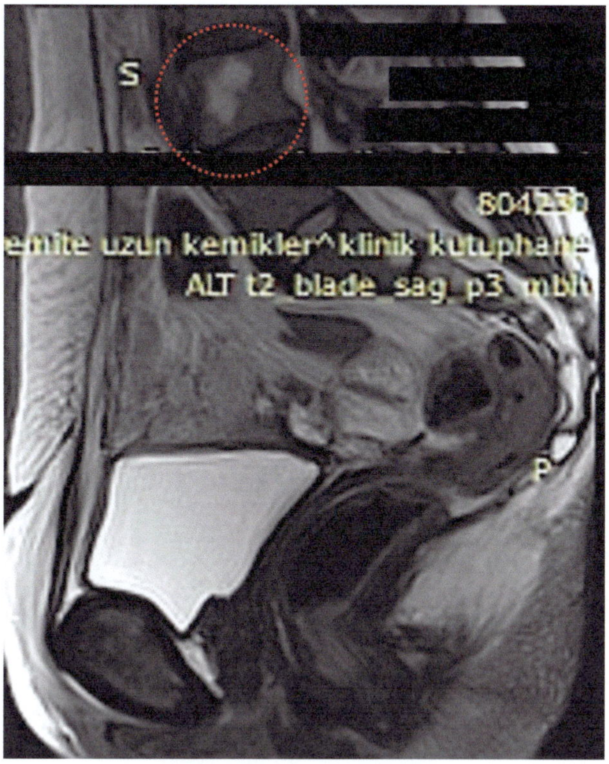

Fig. 31.5 Contrast-enhanced MRI reveals lytic skeletal lesion on L4 vertebral body

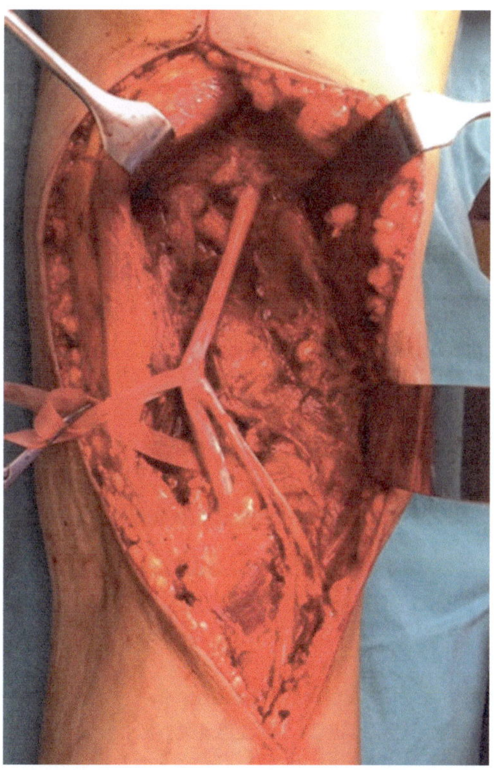

Fig. 31.6 Intraoperative photo of the surgical site after resection of the popliteal mass. Major anatomical structures were protected. No complications were encountered

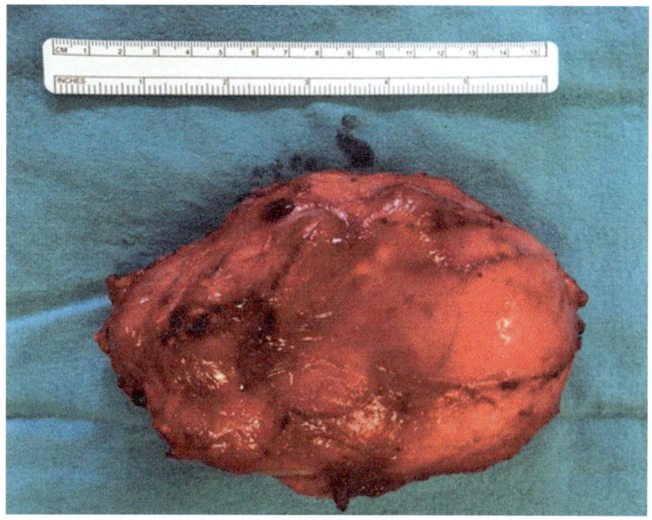

Fig. 31.7 Macroscopic view of the excised popliteal mass

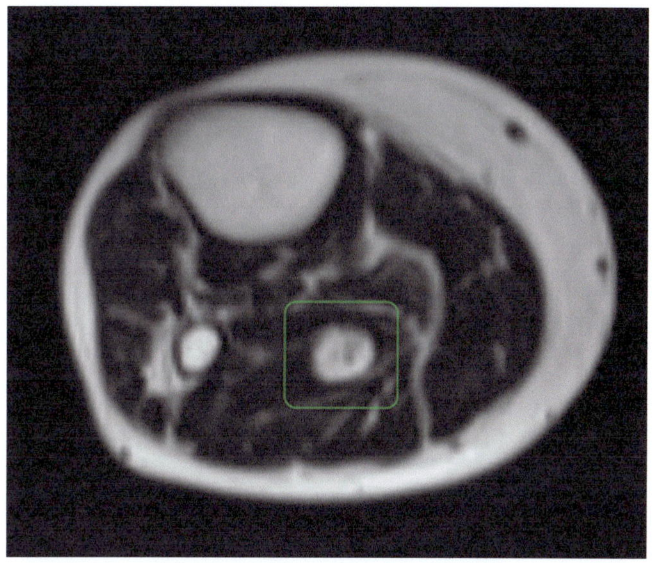

Fig. 31.8 Axial view of the metastatic lesion which is located in the right soleus muscle

whereby she remained on maintenance olaparib for 4 months until February 2021 when she developed a new metastatic lesion within the right soleus muscle (Fig. 31.8).

Following total excision of the mass, which was evaluated as a low grade myxoid liposarcoma, she was not recommended further systemic therapy. Unfortunately, routine imaging studies by MRI at her first follow-up visit in June 2021 revealed recurrent multicompartmental lesions in the left humerus and the right soleus muscle with invasion of the vascular structures and nerve bundles in juxtaposition with the tumor (Figs. 31.9, 31.10, 31.11, and 31.12).

Since a surgical excision would pose significant complications and morbidity, she was referred to the radiation oncology department, where she received 35 Gy irradiation

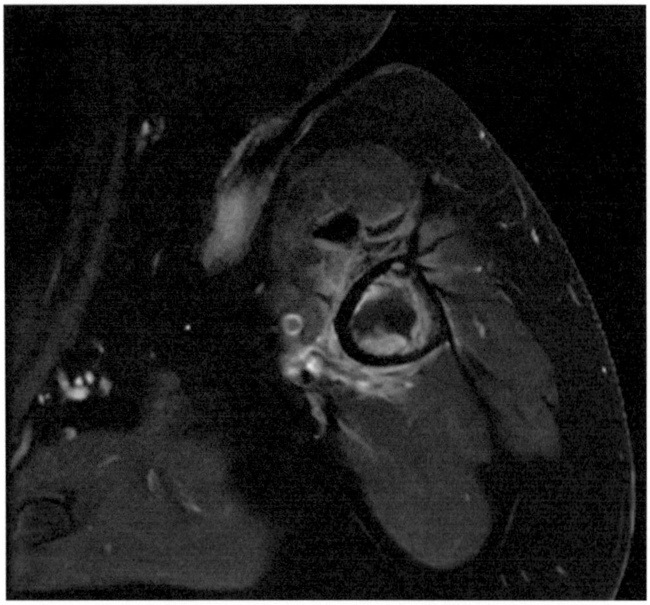

Fig. 31.9 Contrast-enhanced MRI of the patient shows lytic lesion on the left humerus

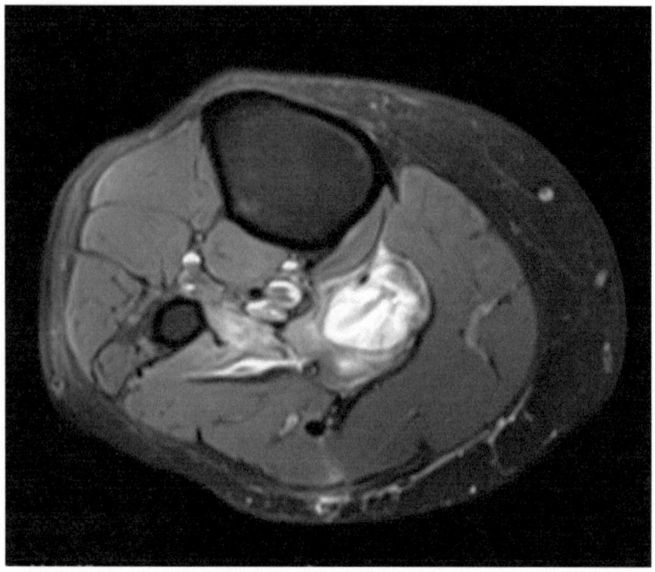

Fig. 31.11 A contrast-enhanced MRI shows multicompartmental soleus mass with invasion to the adjacent major anatomical structures

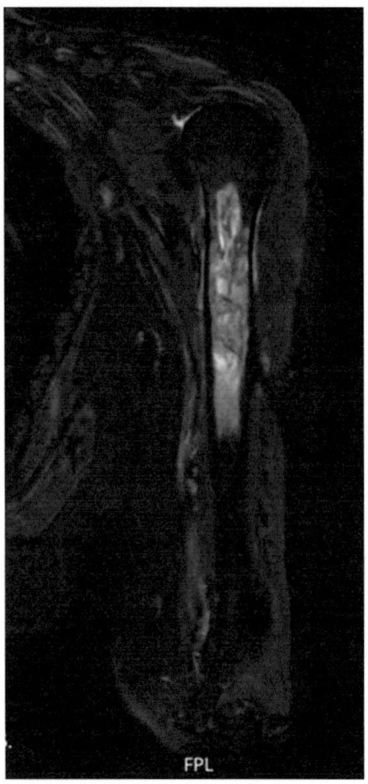

Fig. 31.10 Coronal view of the same lesion in previous figure shows osseous involvement

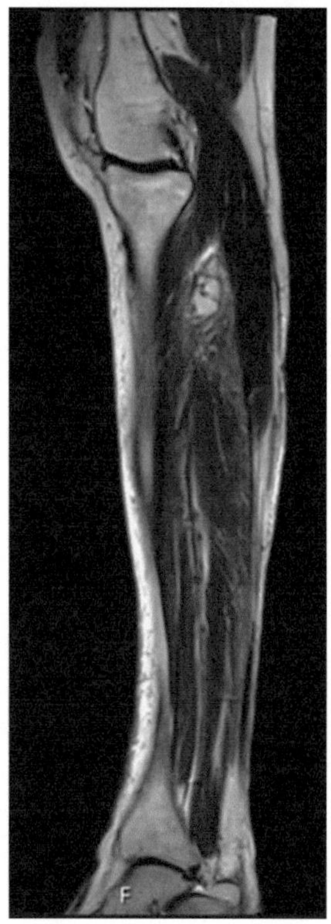

Fig. 31.12 Sagittal view of the same MRI of the previous figure

in 10 fractions to the tumors within the right posterior crural area and the left humeral shaft. Based on the previous genomic test results, she was recommended systemic treatment with alpelisib 300 mg daily, which has been used until February 2023 when a progression was noted within the left humerus. At her last follow-up, approximately 1.5 years after the continuum of alpelisib treatment, a whole-body MRI demonstrated continuous total regression of all lesions and significant progression of the metastatic lesion in the left humerus which had previously showed findings suspicious of radionecrosis (Fig. 31.13). Since additional radiotherapy to the involved area is not possible due to the large dose

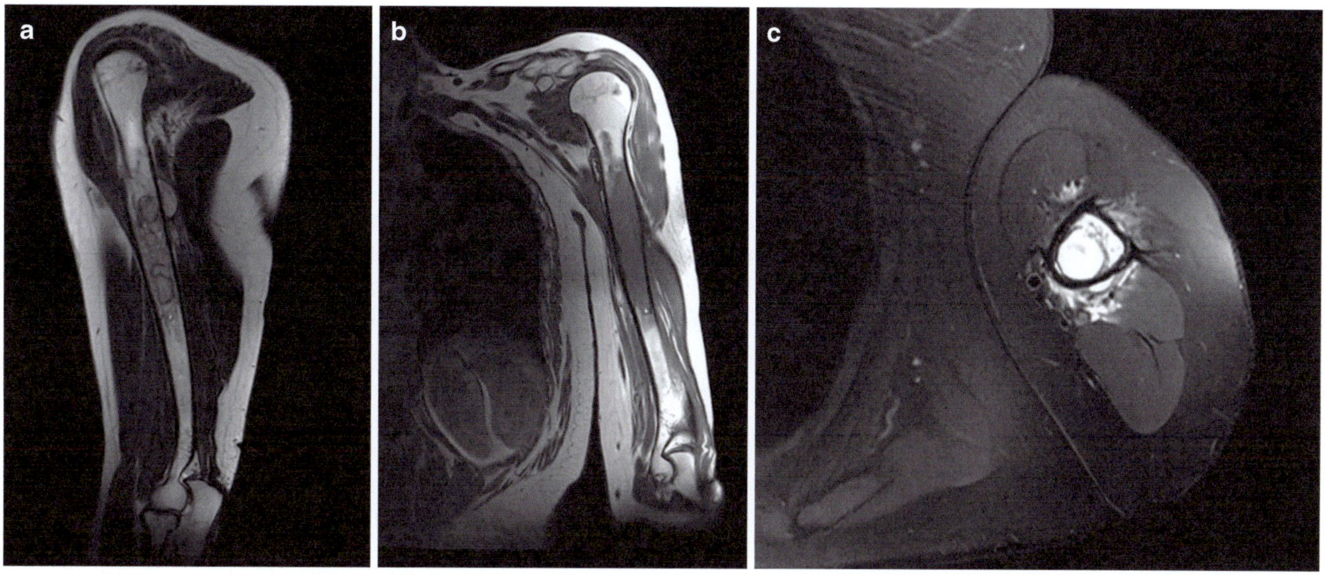

Fig. 31.13 Sagittal T1 (**a**), coronal T2 (**b**) and axial (**c**) view of the left humerus after 1.5-year alpelisib treatment shows significant progression of the metastatic lesion

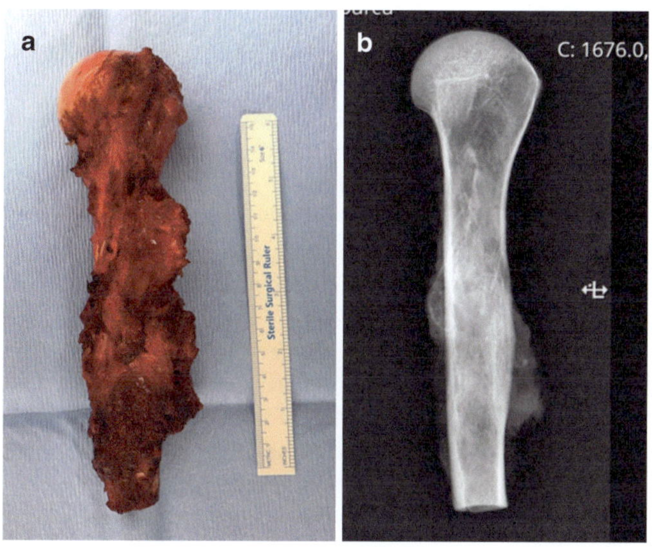

Fig. 31.14 Macroscopic (**a**) and radiological (**b**) view of the resection material of the left humeral metastatic lesion

received previously, she is under evaluation for the possibility of a radical surgical resection (Fig. 31.14).

31.3 Discussion

The case described above carries most of the clinical characteristics that have been associated with metastatic myxoid LPS. Multiple skeletal metastases with a predilection in the spine have been previously reported in a single center cohort study comprising 56% of all metastatic events in a cohort of 230 patients [12]. In addition, dissemination within the abdominal cavity is in concordance with the tendency for unconventional metastatic presentation of myxoid LPS in areas such as abdominal wall, retroperitoneum or serosal sites [13]. Since our main intention was to achieve a rapid and high tumor shrinkage, she received first line chemotherapy with the adriamycin ifosfamide combination, despite the lack of overall survival advantage with the combination as compared to single agent doxorubicin [14].

In line with clinical evidence indicating chemosensitivity of myxoid LPS, there was a major response attained with the combination [15]. Although surgery is not the mainstay of treatment for metastatic disease and is generally not considered as a favorable approach by several guidelines, it should be highlighted that survival of metastatic sarcoma with chemotherapy as the sole treatment modality remains poor, ranging between 13 and 21 months as shown in a European multicenter retrospective registry study including 805 patients [16–18]. Therefore, a multidisciplinary decision was undertaken to add locoregional therapies to all residual lesions with the intention to improve the outcome through employing a multimodal treatment in a responsive patient, deemed as a reasonable approach by several others [13, 16, 19]. Similarly, the decision to deliver adjuvant irradiation to the resected popliteal area reflects our radical management strategy. For localized extremity LPS, our practice involves irradiating large and deep tumors irrespective of margin status, which contradicts general consensus to defer irradiation for completely resected tumors [20]. In this case, neoadjuvant radiotherapy was not preferred, since she was diagnosed at an advanced stage and an apparent survival benefit with this approach was not demonstrated in the only randomized trial involving patients with localized retroperitoneal LPS [21].

Following completion of postoperative radiotherapy and chemotherapy, a switch maintenance strategy with pazopanib was undertaken due to imaging studies suspicious for microscopic residual disease. Pazopanib is a multikinase inhibitor against VEGF and KIT, which are demonstrated as key molecular targets driving angiogenesis and cellular proliferation in LPS xenografts [22]. Although pazopanib was excluded from LPS trials due to inefficacy shown in the EORTC 62043 study, there exists evidence on the potential role of pazopanib in treating intermediate and high grade LPS [23–25]. In fact, the time to progression of 10 months exceeds all outcomes attained by pazopanib in clinical trials. This discrepancy may be related to the intratumoral heterogeneity, which has been observed in our case over the course of her disease. Pathological evidence of de-differentiated, well-differentiated and round cell components reflect clonal selection due to pressure from previous therapies, as well as the temporal and spatial evolution of a wide array of genomic alterations, which has been implicated as a potential contributing factor in the contradictory results yielded by pazopanib against LPS [26].

The molecular heterogeneity of the described case is evident by the NGS genomic analysis of the recurrent tumor showing a FUS-DDIT fusion, in addition to several genomic alterations involving the PIK3CA and PTEN genes. Myxoid LPS which contains round cell components display a high-grade variant with an increased metastatic potential and poor prognosis [27]. Approximately 90–95% of the myxoid round cell LPS are characterized by the FUS-DDIT fusion, which results from the translocation t(12;16)(q13;p11) or less frequently the EWSR1-DDIT3 fusion caused by t(12;22)(q13;q12). This molecular alteration, which underpins the biology of myxoid/round cell LPS, acts as an aberrant transcription factor that interacts with lipoblastic transformation and DNA repair mechanisms [28–30]. Mutations and upregulation in PIK3CA gene as detected in our case, as well as those involving the MET and RET genes are reported in up to 18% of myxoid LPS, indicating a potential role for specific pathway inhibitors [31–35]. Furthermore, data from preclinical studies have shown a potential interaction with the FUS-DDIT fusion and several intracellular oncogenic pathways by upregulation of the PIK3/AKT genes through IGF2 activation [36]. Aberrant activation of the IGF pathway and overexpression of IGF receptor-1 by the FUS-DDIT translocation has been implicated to regulate the oncogenic transformation of myxoid/round cell LPS [34, 37]. These studies provide further proof that targeting these alterations may have a potential role in treating translocation-associated LPS.

Furthermore, there exists biologic evidence suggesting that DNA damaging agents, such as trabectedin may specifically target myxoid/round cell LPS through interaction with the fusion protein, leading to inhibition of cellular proliferation and restoration of normal lipoblast function [38]. In fact, a pooled analysis of two phase-II trials evaluating the efficacy of trabectedin have demonstrated a significant advantage favoring the myxoid/round cell subtype, yielding a median PFS of 7.4 months, ranging between 5.6 and 11.1 months [39–43].

Based on the mechanistic activity of trabectedin leading to irreversible DNA damage which in turn induces DNA repair pathways, it has been postulated that agents which interact with DNA repair systems may augment antitumor activity. There exists preclinical evidence that that PARP inhibitors may act synergistically through suppression of PARP1 activity, which is activated by trabectedin, leading to enhanced tumor cell killing [44]. A subsequent phase Ib trial including previously treated 50 sarcoma patients has shown encouraging activity with the combination, yielding antitumor response in 7 patients (14%) with a median duration of response of 7 months [45]. Based on the genomic findings and supporting early clinical data we treated the patient with a combination of trabectedin and olaparib at the recommended doses of trabectedin given at 1.1 mg/m^2 d1 and Olaparib 150 mg BID every 3 weeks. Following completion of 6 cycles, the treatment was continued with single agent Olaparib, yielding a total progression-free period of 9 months, consistent with previous clinical data.

Management of inoperable recurrent disease in our case included radiotherapy, which resulted in a substantial regression in tumor size, consistent with previous reports confirming the high activity of irradiation in myxoid LPS [46, 47]. In order to provide further anti-tumor activity where effective options have been exhausted, we decided to deliver systemic treatment with a targeted approach consisting of alpelisib which is a selective PIK3CA inhibitor. The off-label treatment with this agent provided complete disease control with a prolonged response duration reaching 18 months, exceeding clinical activity of any systemic agent evaluated against LPS in the advanced pre-treated setting until this date. To our knowledge, this is the first clinical evidence on the activity of alpelisib in PIK3Ca-mutated myxoid LPS. This observation provides further proof that even within the same histologic type, each tumor presents with a unique biology based on temporal evolution of genomic alterations through pressure from previous therapies with potentially different responses to targeted agents. Undeniably, identification of these molecular features is an unmet need to develop effective treatment combinations which will eventually lead to improved outcomes. Although understanding of the biology underpinning sarcomas have shown a slow progress over time, we are beginning to decipher the codes of each unique subtype, which may eventually fill our knowledge gaps.

As advent of molecular diagnostic methods and novel agents over the last couple of decades have caused a significant shift in cancer care with major improvements in outcome for numerous tumor types, we're hopeful that future perspectives of LPS treatment will include several dimensions of optimized management strategies. As shown in the case report, implementation of a multidisciplinary approach with a personalized biology-driven treatment is essential to improve survival of patients with advanced LPS.

31.4 Preoperative Imaging

Figures 31.1, 31.2, 31.3, 31.4, and 31.5.

31.5 Preoperative Problem List

- Extensive heterogeneity in pathologic subtypes and clinical presentation of the tumor.
- Multiple skeletal metastatic lesions during treatment which some of them shows invasion of the major anatomical structures.
- Tendency for unconventional metastatic presentation such as abdominal wall and trapezius muscle.

31.6 Treatment Strategy

- Is to achieve a rapid and high tumor shrinkage
- Is to consider surgical options to empower the systemic treatment
- Is to maintain multimodal treatment due to favorable response

31.7 Basic Principles

- Targeting the biology of the tumor
- En bloc wide resection of the masses when surgically available

31.8 Imaging During Treatment

Figures 31.6 and 31.7.

31.9 Technical Pearls

- Management of inoperable recurrent disease included radiotherapy resulted in a substantial regression in tumor size.
- Adapting biological treatment to the evolving genetic profile of the tumor often leads to improvements in survival rates.

31.10 Outcome Imaging

Figures 31.8, 31.9, 31.10, 31.11, 31.12, 31.13, and 31.14.

31.11 Avoiding and Managing Problems

- Always follow the fundamental principles of tumor resection.
- Administer biological drugs with regular and meticulous monitoring, accounting for both anticipated and unpredictable side effect profiles.
- Periodic PET scans are essential for tracking the biological activity of metastases.

References

1. Henze J, Bauer S. Liposarcomas. Hematol Oncol Clin North Am. 2013;27:939–55.
2. de Pinieux G, Karanian M, Le Loarer F, Le Guellec S, Chabaud S, Terrier P, Bouvier C, Batistella M, Neuville A, Robin YM, Emile JF, Moreau A, Larousserie F, Leroux A, Stock N, Lae M, Collin F, Weinbreck N, Aubert S, Mishellany F, Charon-Barra C, Croce S, Doucet L, Quintin-Rouet I, Chateau MC, Bazille C, Valo I, Chetaille B, Ortonne N, Brouchet A, Rochaix P, Demuret A, Ghnassia JP, Mescam L, Macagno N, Birtwisle-Peyrottes I, Delfour C, Angot E, Pommepuy I, Ranchere D, Chemin-Airiau C, Jean-Denis M, Fayet Y, Courrèges JB, Mesli N, Berchoud J, Toulmonde M, Italiano A, Le Cesne A, Penel N, Ducimetiere F, Gouin F, Coindre JM, Blay JY, NetSarc/RePPS/ResSos and French Sarcoma Group- Groupe d'Etude des Tumeurs Osseuses (GSF-GETO) networks. Nationwide incidence of sarcomas and connective tissue tumors of intermediate malignancy over four years using an expert pathology review network. PLoS One. 2021;16(2):e0246958.
3. Amadeo B, Penel N, Coindre JM, Ray-Coquard I, Ligier K, Delafosse P, Bouvier AM, Plouvier S, Gallet J, Lacourt A, Coureau G, Monnereau A, Mathoulin-Pélissier S, Desandes E. Incidence and time trends of sarcoma (2000-2013): results from the French network of cancer registries (FRANCIM). BMC Cancer. 2020;20(1):190.
4. Jo VY, Fletcher CD. WHO classification of soft tissue tumours: an update based on the 2013 (4th) edition. Pathology. 2014;46(2):95–104.
5. Dei Tos AP. Liposarcoma: new entities and evolving concepts. Ann Diagn Pathol. 2000;4(4):252–66.
6. Amer KM, Congiusta DV, Thomson JE, Elsamna S, Chaudhry I, Bozzo A, Amer R, Siracuse B, Ghert M, Beebe KS. Epidemiology and survival of liposarcoma and its subtypes: a dual database analysis. J Clin Orthop Trauma. 2020;11(Suppl 4):S479–84.
7. El Ouni F, Jemni H, Trabelsi A, et al. Liposarcoma of the extremities: MR imaging features and their correlation with pathologic data. Orthop Traumatol Surg Res. 2010;96:876–83.

8. Tseng W, Martinez SR, Tamurian RM, Borys D, Canter RJ. Histologic type predicts survival in patients with retroperitoneal soft tissue sarcoma. J Surg Res. 2012;172:123–30.
9. Ng VY, Scharschmidt TJ, Mayerson JL, Fisher JL. Incidence and survival in sarcoma in the United States: a focus on musculoskeletal lesions. Anticancer Res. 2013;33:2597–604.
10. de Vreeze RS, de Jong D, Koops W, Nederlof PM, Ariaens A, Haas RL, van Coevorden F. Oncogenesis and classification of mixed-type liposarcoma: a radiological, histopathological and molecular biological analysis. Int J Cancer. 2011;128(4):778–86.
11. Engström K, Bergh P, Gustafson P, Hultborn R, Johansson H, Löfvenberg R, Zaikova O, Trovik C, Wahlström O, Bauer HC. Liposarcoma: outcome based on the Scandinavian Sarcoma Group register. Cancer. 2008;113(7):1649–56.
12. Schwab JH, Boland P, Guo T, Brennan MF, Singer S, Healey JH, Antonescu CR. Skeletal metastases in myxoid liposarcoma: an unusual pattern of distant spread. Ann Surg Oncol. 2007;14(4):1507–14.
13. Dürr HR, Rauh J, Baur-Melnyk A, Knösel T, Lindner L, Roeder F, Jansson V, Klein A. Myxoid liposarcoma: local relapse and metastatic pattern in 43 patients. BMC Cancer. 2018;18(1):304.
14. Judson I, Verweij J, Gelderblom H, Hartmann JT, Schöffski P, Blay JY, Kerst JM, Sufliarsky J, Whelan J, Hohenberger P, Krarup-Hansen A, Alcindor T, Marreaud S, Litière S, Hermans C, Fisher C, Hogendoorn PC, dei Tos AP, van der Graaf WT, European Organisation and Treatment of Cancer Soft Tissue and Bone Sarcoma Group. Doxorubicin alone versus intensified doxorubicin plus ifosfamide for first-line treatment of advanced or metastatic soft-tissue sarcoma: a randomised controlled phase 3 trial. Lancet Oncol. 2014;15(4):415–23.
15. Jones RL, Fisher C, Al-Muderis O, Judson IR. Differential sensitivity of liposarcoma subtypes to chemotherapy. Eur J Cancer. 2005;41(18):2853–60.
16. Dangoor A, Seddon B, Gerrand C, Grimer R, Whelan J, Judson I. UK guidelines for the management of soft tissue sarcomas. Clin Sarcoma Res. 2016;6:20.
17. MacNeill AJ, van Houdt WJ, Swallow CJ, Gronchi A. Management of metastatic retroperitoneal sarcoma: a consensus approach from the Trans-Atlantic Retroperitoneal Sarcoma Working Group (TARPSWG). Ann Oncol. 2018;29(4):857–71.
18. Nagar SP, Mytelka DS, Candrilli SD, D'yachkova Y, Lorenzo M, Kasper B, Lopez-Martin JA, Kaye JA. Treatment patterns and survival among adult patients with advanced soft tissue sarcoma: a retrospective medical record review in the United Kingdom, Spain, Germany, and France. Sarcoma. 2018;2018:5467057.
19. Haddox CL, Riedel RF. Recent advances in the understanding and management of liposarcoma. Fac Rev. 2021;10:1.
20. Crago AM, Dickson MA. Liposarcoma: multimodality management and future targeted therapies. Surg Oncol Clin N Am. 2016;25(4):761–73.
21. Bonvalot S, Gronchi A, Le Péchoux C, Swallow CJ, Strauss D, Meeus P, van Coevorden F, Stoldt S, Stoeckle E, Rutkowski P, Rastrelli M, Raut CP, Hompes D, De Paoli A, Sangalli C, Honoré C, Chung P, Miah A, Blay JY, Fiore M, Stelmes JJ, Dei Tos AP, Baldini EH, Litière S, Marreaud S, Gelderblom H, Haas RL. Preoperative radiotherapy plus surgery versus surgery alone for patients with primary retroperitoneal sarcoma (EORTC-62092: STRASS): a multicentre, open-label, randomised, phase 3 trial. Lancet Oncol. 2020;21(10):1366–77.
22. Li H, Wozniak A, Sciot R, Cornillie J, Wellens J, Van Looy T, Vanleeuw U, Stas M, Hompes D, Debiec-Rychter M, Schöffski P. Pazopanib, a receptor tyrosine kinase inhibitor, suppresses tumor growth through angiogenesis in dedifferentiated liposarcoma xenograft models. Transl Oncol. 2014;7(6):665–71.
23. Sleijfer S, Ray-Coquard I, Papai Z, Le Cesne A, Scurr M, Schöffski P, Collin F, Pandite L, Marreaud S, De Brauwer A, van Glabbeke M, Verweij J, Blay JY. Pazopanib, a multikinase angiogenesis inhibitor, in patients with relapsed or refractory advanced soft tissue sarcoma: a phase II study from the European organisation for research and treatment of cancer-soft tissue and bone sarcoma group (EORTC study 62043). J Clin Oncol. 2009;27(19):3126–32.
24. Samuels BL, Chawla SP, Somaiah N, Staddon AP, Skubitz KM, Milhem MM, Kaiser PE, Portnoy DC, Priebat DA, Walker MS, Stepanski EJ. Results of a prospective phase 2 study of pazopanib in patients with advanced intermediate-grade or high-grade liposarcoma. Cancer. 2017;123(23):4640–7.
25. Morales CMV, Serra AF, Ramírez-Calvo M, Lopez-Martin JA, Romagosa C, Carrasco JA, Bauer S, Trufero JM, Jurado JC, Reichardt P, Serrano C, Grünwald V, Fra PL, Persiva O, Varona D, Morales-Barrera R, Kasper B, Broto JM, Ruiz-Sauri A, Lopez-Guerrero JA. Translational study associated to a phase II study evaluating the activity of pazopanib in patients (pts) with advanced/metastatic liposarcoma (LPS): a joint Spanish Sarcoma Group (GEIS) and German Interdisciplinary Sarcoma Group (GISG) study. J Clin Oncol. 2019;37(15_suppl):–11067.
26. Chamberlain FE, Wilding C, Jones RL, Huang P. Pazopanib in patients with advanced intermediate-grade or high-grade liposarcoma. Expert Opin Investig Drugs. 2019;28(6):505–11.
27. Creytens D. What's new in adipocytic neoplasia? Virchows Arch. 2020;476(1):29–39.
28. Fletcher CD. The evolving classification of soft tissue tumours—an update based on the new 2013 WHO classification. Histopathology. 2014;64(1):2–11.
29. Knight JC, Renwick PJ, Dal Cin P, Van den Berghe H, Fletcher CD. Translocation t(12;16)(q13;p11) in myxoid liposarcoma and round cell liposarcoma: molecular and cytogenetic analysis. Cancer Res. 1995;55(1):24–7.
30. Meis-Kindblom JM, Sjögren H, Kindblom LG, Peydró-Mellquist A, Röijer E, Aman P, Stenman G. Cytogenetic and molecular genetic analyses of liposarcoma and its soft tissue simulators: recognition of new variants and differential diagnosis. Virchows Arch. 2001;439(2):141–51.
31. Negri T, Virdis E, Brich S, Bozzi F, Tamborini E, Tarantino E, Jocollè G, Cassinelli G, Grosso F, Sanfilippo R, Casalini P, Greco A, Pierotti MA, Pilotti S. Functional mapping of receptor tyrosine kinases in myxoid liposarcoma. Clin Cancer Res. 2010;16(14):3581–93.
32. Demicco EG, Torres KE, Ghadimi MP, Colombo C, Bolshakov S, Hoffman A, Peng T, Bovée JV, Wang WL, Lev D, Lazar AJ. Involvement of the PI3K/Akt pathway in myxoid/round cell liposarcoma. Mod Pathol. 2012;25(2):212–21.
33. Tyler R, Wanigasooriya K, Taniere P, Almond M, Ford S, Desai A, Beggs A. A review of retroperitoneal liposarcoma genomics. Cancer Treat Rev. 2020;86:102013.
34. Sanfilippo R, Dei Tos AP, Casali PG. Myxoid liposarcoma and the mammalian target of rapamycin pathway. Curr Opin Oncol. 2013;25(4):379–83.
35. Damodaran S, Zhao F, Deming DA, Mitchell EP, Wright JJ, Gray RJ, Wang V, McShane LM, Rubinstein LV, Patton DR, Williams PM, Hamilton SR, Suga JM, Conley BA, Arteaga CL, Harris LN, O'Dwyer PJ, Chen AP, Flaherty KT. Phase II study of copanlisib in patients with tumors with *PIK3CA* mutations: results from the NCI-MATCH ECOG-ACRIN trial (EAY131) subprotocol Z1F. J Clin Oncol. 2022;40(14):1552–61.
36. Trautmann M, Menzel J, Bertling C, Cyra M, Isfort I, Steinestel K, Elges S, Grünewald I, Altvater B, Rossig C, Fröhling S, Hafner S, Simmet T, Åman P, Wardelmann E, Huss S, Hartmann W. FUS-DDIT3 fusion protein-driven IGF-IR signaling is a therapeutic target in myxoid liposarcoma. Clin Cancer Res. 2017;23(20):6227–38.
37. Yu JSE, Colborne S, Hughes CS, Morin GB, Nielsen TO. The FUS-DDIT3 interactome in myxoid liposarcoma. Neoplasia. 2019;21(8):740–51.

38. Forni C, Minuzzo M, Virdis E, Tamborini E, Simone M, Tavecchio M, Erba E, Grosso F, Gronchi A, Aman P, Casali P, D'Incalci M, Pilotti S, Mantovani R. Trabectedin (ET-743) promotes differentiation in myxoid liposarcoma tumors. Mol Cancer Ther. 2009;8(2):449–57.
39. Takahashi M, Takahashi S, Araki N, Sugiura H, Ueda T, Yonemoto T, Morioka H, Hiraga H, Hiruma T, Kunisada T, Matsumine A, Shimura M, Kawai A. Efficacy of trabectedin in patients with advanced translocation-related sarcomas: pooled analysis of two phase II studies. Oncologist. 2017;22(8):979–88.
40. Demetri GD, Chawla SP, von Mehren M, Ritch P, Baker LH, Blay JY, Hande KR, Keohan ML, Samuels BL, Schuetze S, Lebedinsky C, Elsayed YA, Izquierdo MA, Gómez J, Park YC, Le Cesne A. Efficacy and safety of trabectedin in patients with advanced or metastatic liposarcoma or leiomyosarcoma after failure of prior anthracyclines and ifosfamide: results of a randomized phase II study of two different schedules. J Clin Oncol. 2009;27(25):4188–96.
41. Kawai A, Araki N, Sugiura H, Ueda T, Yonemoto T, Takahashi M, Morioka H, Hiraga H, Hiruma T, Kunisada T, Matsumine A, Tanase T, Hasegawa T, Takahashi S. Trabectedin monotherapy after standard chemotherapy versus best supportive care in patients with advanced, translocation-related sarcoma: a randomised, open-label, phase 2 study. Lancet Oncol. 2015;16(4):406–16.
42. Blay JY, Leahy MG, Nguyen BB, Patel SR, Hohenberger P, Santoro A, Staddon AP, Penel N, Piperno-Neumann S, Hendifar A, Lardelli P, Nieto A, Alfaro V, Chawla SP. Randomised phase III trial of trabectedin versus doxorubicin-based chemotherapy as first-line therapy in translocation-related sarcomas. Eur J Cancer. 2014;50(6):1137–47.
43. Assi T, Kattan J, El Rassy E, Honore C, Dumont S, Mir O, Le Cesne A. A comprehensive review of the current evidence for trabectedin in advanced myxoid liposarcoma. Cancer Treat Rev. 2019;72:37–44.
44. Pignochino Y, Capozzi F, D'Ambrosio L, Dell'Aglio C, Basiricò M, Canta M, Lorenzato A, Vignolo Lutati F, Aliberti S, Palesandro E, Boccone P, Galizia D, Miano S, Chiabotto G, Napione L, Gammaitoni L, Sangiolo D, Benassi MS, Pasini B, Chiorino G, Aglietta M, Grignani G. PARP1 expression drives the synergistic antitumor activity of trabectedin and PARP1 inhibitors in sarcoma preclinical models. Mol Cancer. 2017;16(1):86.
45. Grignani G, D'Ambrosio L, Pignochino Y, Palmerini E, Zucchetti M, Boccone P, Aliberti S, Stacchiotti S, Bertulli R, Piana R, Miano S, Tolomeo F, Chiabotto G, Sangiolo D, Pisacane A, Dei Tos AP, Novara L, Bartolini A, Marchesi E, D'Incalci M, Bardelli A, Picci P, Ferrari S, Aglietta M. Trabectedin and olaparib in patients with advanced and non-resectable bone and soft-tissue sarcomas (TOMAS): an open-label, phase 1b study from the Italian Sarcoma Group. Lancet Oncol. 2018;19(10):1360–71.
46. Pitson G, Robinson P, Wilke D, Kandel RA, White L, Griffin AM, Bell RS, Catton CN, Wunder JS, O'Sullivan B. Radiation response: an additional unique signature of myxoid liposarcoma. Int J Radiat Oncol Biol Phys. 2004;60(2):522–6.
47. Betgen A, Haas RL, Sonke JJ. Volume changes in soft tissue sarcomas during preoperative radiotherapy of extremities evaluated using cone-beam CT. J Radiat Oncol. 2013;2(1):55–62.

Tenosynovial Giant Cell Tumour of the Foot with Osseous Involvement

32

Angus Crombie, Philip Rowell, James Bennett, Thomas Lloyd, Rino Olivotto, and Peter Steadman

32.1 Introduction

Tenosynovial giant cell tumour (TGCT), formally known as pigmented villonodular synovitis (PVNS), arises from the synovium of joints, tendon sheaths, and bursae [1–4]. Although once postulated to be an inflammatory process, TGCT is now considered a true neoplastic disease [4]. It is typically a benign lesion, which has been described to have the capacity to erode cartilage or bone as the disease progresses. They tend to affect individuals in the third to fifth decades of life, with a female preponderance of 2:1 [1, 5, 6]. Translocation of colony-stimulating factor (CSF) gene is frequently involved in this tumour, responsible for proliferation and recruitment of macrophages, which are a predominant cell type seen in TGCT [3, 5, 7].

A. Crombie · P. Rowell
Queensland bone and soft tissue tumour service, The Princess Alexandra Hospital, Woolloongabba, QLD, Australia

University of Queensland, Brisbane, QLD, Australia

J. Bennett
Queensland bone and soft tissue tumour service, The Princess Alexandra Hospital, Woolloongabba, QLD, Australia
e-mail: James_bennett2@snp.com.au

T. Lloyd
Department of Radiology, Princess Alexandra Hospital, Woolloongabba, QLD, Australia

Breast Screen Queensland, Chermside, QLD, Australia
e-mail: thomas.lloyd@health.qld.gov.au

R. Olivotto
Department of Radiology, Princess Alexandra Hospital, Woolloongabba, QLD, Australia

University of Queensland, Brisbane, QLD, Australia
e-mail: rino.olivotto@health.qld.gov.au

P. Steadman (✉)
Queensland bone and soft tissue tumour service, The Princess Alexandra Hospital, Woolloongabba, QLD, Australia

University of Queensland, Brisbane, QLD, Australia

Steadman Orthopaedics, South Brisbane, QLD, Australia
e-mail: clinic@steadman.com.au

Patients with TGCT classically present with vague symptoms, characterised by a slow-growing mass, usually painless, with the potential for associated joint effusions or haemarthroses causing stiffness. On occasion, TGCT loose bodies can lead to locking or mechanical symptoms upon presentation. Superficial lesions in the lower extremities can cause footwear discomfort. Mass effects on adjacent peripheral nerves may also cause symptoms such as paraesthesia [3, 6, 11].

As per the World Health Organisation classification, two subtypes of TGCT exist dependent on pattern of growth—localised (LTGCT) and diffuse (DTGCT) [1, 2, 4].

LTGCT are well-defined, solitary lesions arising from the synovium and are typically small. They classically affect the small joints of the digits and are more commonly extra-articular [1, 2].

DTGCT are generally large and firm, with a villous pattern in intra-articular and a multinodular appearance in extra-articular tumours [1]. They are most commonly seen in the knee [1, 2, 8], and are more technically challenging to surgically treat than LTGCT [8, 9].

In extremely rare circumstances, malignant TGCT (MTGCT) can develop, behaving similarly to soft tissue sarcoma. They can arise de novo or from multiple recurrences of a benign TGCT. Typical metastases appear in lymph nodes and the lungs [2, 5, 9, 10].

32.2 Clinical History

An otherwise healthy 32-year-old man developed atraumatic right foot pain. Three months after the onset of pain, he saw his General Practitioner, who suspected a traumatic injury. An ultrasound of the ankle was arranged and demonstrated no abnormality. The patient had persisting pain and eventually underwent an MRI of the foot, 6 months post onset of initial symptoms.

H. Özger et al. (eds.), *Diagnosis and Treatment of Soft Tissue Tumors*, https://doi.org/10.1007/978-3-031-77061-6_32

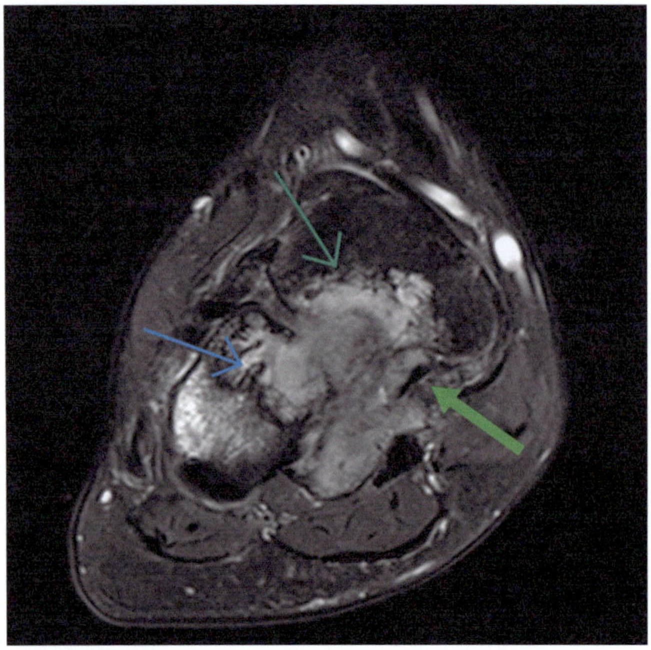

Fig. 32.1 Coronal T2 FS image shows a lesion of intermediate to low signal intensity at the plantar surface of the foot partially encasing and likely arising from the distal aspect of the tibialis posterior tendon sheath (Thick Green Arrow), deep to the crossing tendons of FHL and FDL. The lesion extends contiguously to involve the navicular bone (Thin Green Arrow) and cuboid (Blue Arrow) in this image. At the osseous margins there is a clear demarcation of lesion to adjacent bone with a low signal rim, suggesting haemosiderin. Reactive oedema in the lateral cuboid is also present

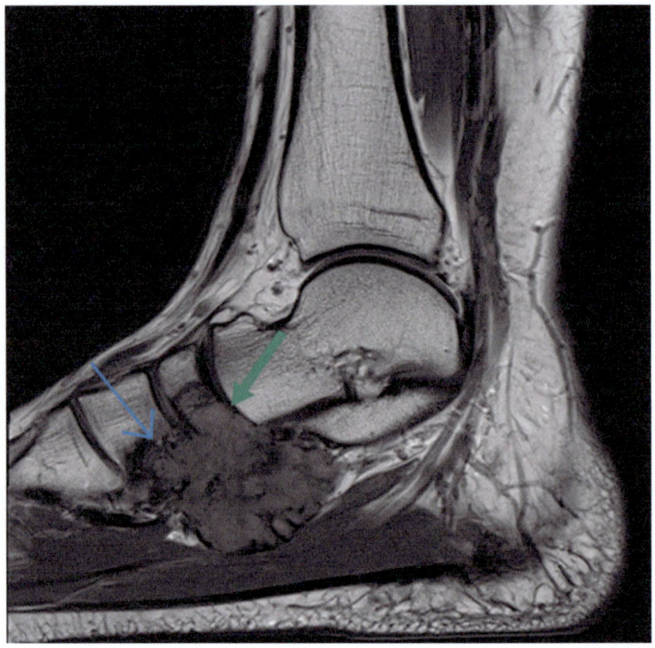

Fig. 32.2 Sagittal PD image shows the lesion with both intra and extraosseous components with extension into the navicular bone (green arrow) and intermediate cuneiform (blue arrow). A low signal rim is again evident around the lesion

32.3 Pre-operative Imaging

MRI remains the benchmark for evaluating TGCT. Classical appearance of DTGCT demonstrates infiltrative intra-articular diffuse thickening of synovium with villous, finger-like projections [8]. Outside of the large joints, LTGCT are typically a single, extra-articular mass with a capsule, closely related to a tendon and show a pushing rather than an infiltrative margin to adjacent muscle and bone [13]. Both subtypes are low intensity on T1 and T2 from haemosiderin deposition. T1 studies with gadolinium contrast exhibit moderate enhancement, while gradient echo sequences reveal low signal and blooming artefact [13, 14]. Associated joint effusions will typically demonstrate low T1 and high T2 signal intensity [2].

For this patient, Magnetic Resonance Imaging (MRI) demonstrated a heterogeneous lesion in the plantar aspect of the midfoot. The images were unusual in that they revealed plantar erosion of the tarsometatarsal bones (Figs. 32.1, 32.2 and 32.3).

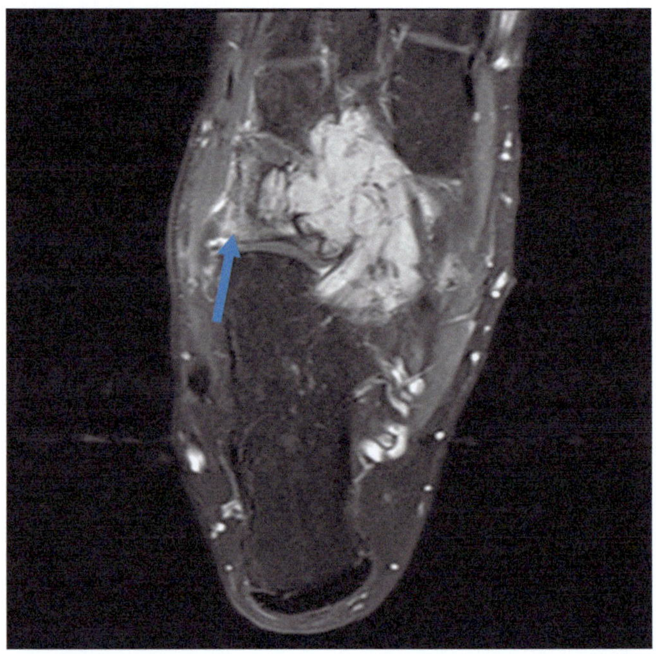

Fig. 32.3 Axial post-contrast FS T1 shows the lesion demonstrating marked uniform enhancement with mild reactive enhancement within the lateral most aspect of the imaged cuboid (blue arrow)

Our patient also underwent a Computed Tomography (CT) scan, which revealed a sclerotic rim at the junction of the bony erosion (Fig. 32.4). CT typically has limited value due to poor soft tissue contrast resolution. Synovial thickening and haemosiderin deposition in TGCT results in slightly higher attenuation than muscle, and low attenuation joint effusions may also be present. Bone erosion from mass effect may also be characterised with CT [2], which was helpful in this case.

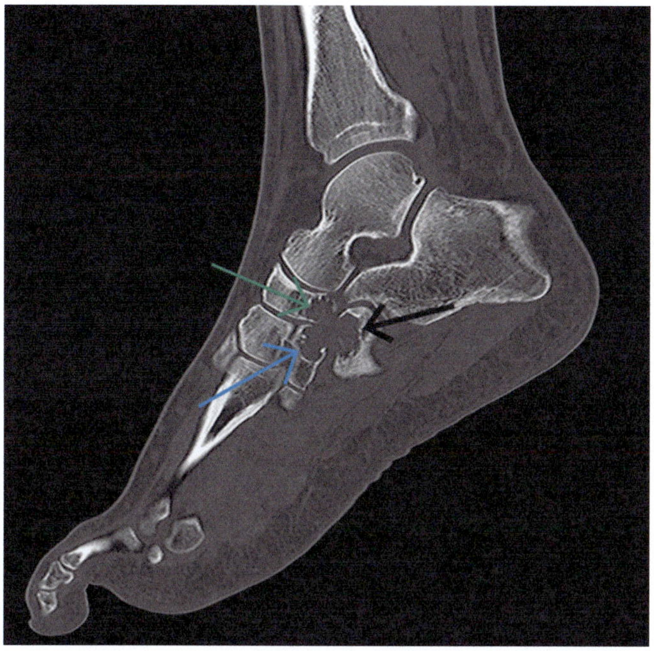

Fig. 32.4 Sagittal CT image in bone windows shows bone loss of the plantar aspect of the navicular (green arrow), cuboid (black arrow), and intermediate cuneiform (blue arrow) bones with a sharply demarcated and partially sclerotic rim at the bone/lesion interface, implying a pushing rather than an infiltrative margin

Alternative imaging, which were non-contributory pre-operatively for this case, include plain X-ray and ultrasound.

Imaging features of TGCT on plain radiographs include soft tissue density masses in peri-articular locations. Associated pressure erosion on adjacent bone is described on occasion. Calcification or periosteal reaction are uncommon findings [11].

Ultrasound is sometimes useful in demonstrating the relationship of a lesion to surrounding structures, with intimate association to a tendon sheath being the most diagnostically valuable sign. Most tumours will be homogenously hypoechoic, and will have some internal vascularity [12].

32.4 Pre-operative Problem List

1. Soft tissue lesion with mass effect on adjacent bone without definitive diagnosis.
2. Requirement to reconstruct bony defect for midfoot stability.

32.5 Treatment Strategy

1. Obtain tissue diagnosis.
2. Surgical resection.
3. Reconstruction of bony defect.
4. Confirm histopathology.

The patient underwent an image-guided core biopsy, which demonstrated a predominantly mononuclear stromal cell infiltrate, focal haemosiderin deposition, and no cytological atypia—compatible with a TGCT. Treatment options were discussed with the patient, and he was subsequently booked for surgery at seven months post first presentation of symptoms.

During his procedure, a medial approach to the midfoot was performed. A subperiosteal plane was utilised and the lesion readily identified. It became apparent that the mass easily separated from the bone, and using gentle blunt curette, a plane was developed between the soft tissue mass and the adjacent bone with an obvious encapsulation of the tumour. It was not possible to identify the plantar ligaments of the proximal tarsal bones and hindfoot separately. Following removal of the soft tissue mass *en bloc* (as opposed to piecemeal), the bony defect was noted in the plantar aspect of the tarsus. A synthetic bone substitute was inserted into the defect.

To prevent post-operative midfoot collapse, the patient was permitted to partial weight bear in a moon boot with a medial arch support. He was gradually returned to full weight-bearing and subsequently returned to normal footwear at three months post-operatively.

32.6 Histopathology

While history, examination, and imaging findings are often highly suggestive of TGCT, biopsy remains necessary to confirm the diagnosis in some cases. For smaller lesions in easily accessible locations such as the digits, excisional biopsy is generally sufficient. For larger, more infiltrative, or lesions involving critical structures such as neurovascular bundles, an image-guided core biopsy may be indicated to confirm the diagnosis before planning further treatment [9].

On macroscopic assessment, the haemosiderin deposition in TGCT gives the tumour a typical rust-coloured appearance [2, 5, 8].

Microscopic examination of DTGCT and LTGCT are nearly indistinguishable, comprising a population of neoplastic mononuclear cells, admixed with variable numbers of non-neoplastic inflammatory cells including monocytes, osteoclast-like giant cells, lymphocytes and foamy histiocytes. These cells are set within a hyalinised fibrous stroma, which almost always shows at least focal haemosiderin pigment deposition (Figs. 32.5,32.6, 32.7, 32.8, 32.9 and 32.10) [2, 4, 5, 8, 10].

The constituent neoplastic mononuclear cells in TGCT typically only represent a small proportion of the overall tumour mass [10]. These neoplastic cells most often show rearrangement of the CSF1 gene, resulting in increased production of CSF1 protein [4]. The neoplastic cells are thought to recruit and induce the proliferation of larger numbers of

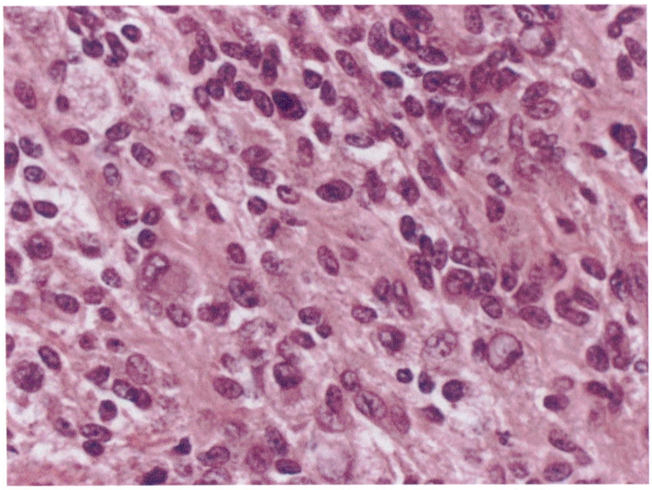

Fig. 32.5 Constituent mononuclear cells of TGCT. The majority of the cells in this image are small and histiocyte-like; however, several larger epithelioid cells are evident in the lower half of the image

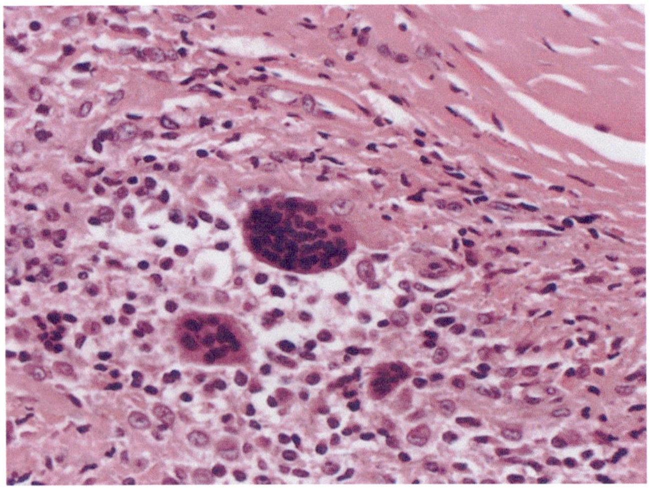

Fig. 32.6 Osteoclast-like giant cells may vary significantly—both in size and overall number

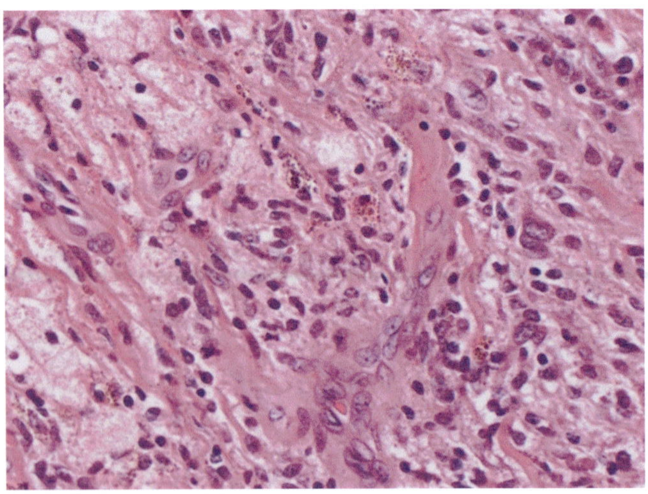

Fig. 32.7 Mononuclear cells are present on the right side of the image. Granular brown haemosiderin pigment is seen centrally. The ill-defined pale cells on the left side are foamy histiocytes

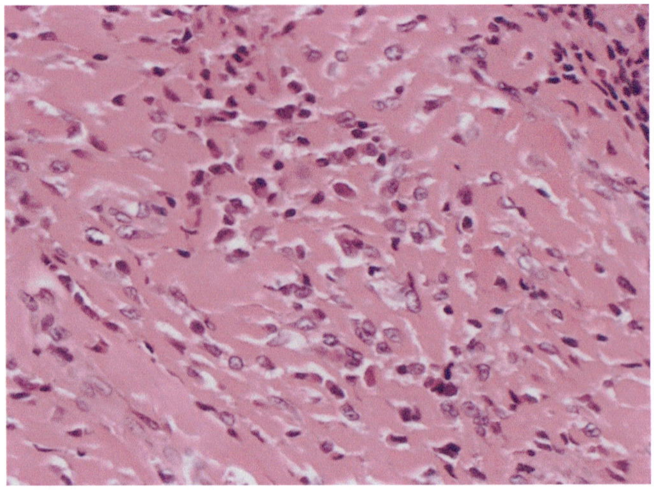

Fig. 32.8 Densely hyalinised background fibrous stroma is a common feature

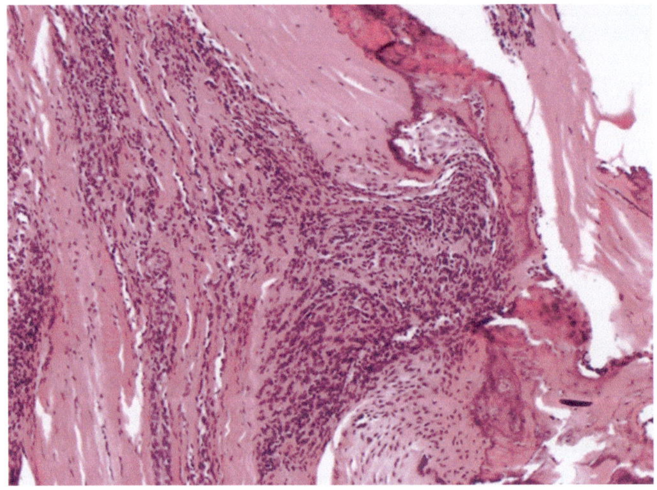

Fig. 32.9 A nodule of tumour cells is seen eroding into bone tissue at the right side of the image

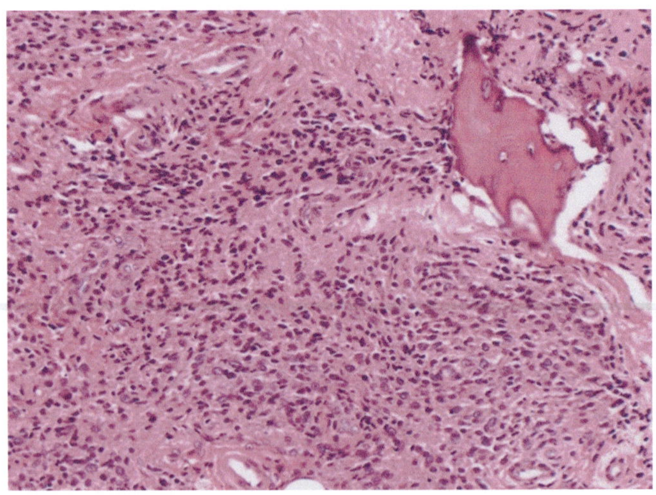

Fig. 32.10 High power image showing mononuclear cells surrounding a spicule of native eroded bone

non-neoplastic monocyte-macrophage lineage cells [10]. The mononuclear cells show a range of morphology—from small histiocyte-like cells, to larger epithelioid cells [4]. A spindled appearance can also be seen—which rarely may predominate, altering the typical microscopic picture. The number of admixed non-neoplastic osteoclast-like giant cells varies considerably from case to case, but most often these are conspicuous. Background lymphocytes and foamy histiocytes are a relatively consistent finding. Mitotic activity can be prominent; however, atypical mitotic figures should not be seen. Associated haemorrhage and occasional necrosis may be present [10]. Uncommonly, there is erosion into adjacent bone [4].

With appropriate clinical history, the histological diagnosis is usually straightforward. A predominant mononuclear spindle cell morphology, or a paucity of giant cells, may occasionally obscure the diagnosis—particularly on core biopsy specimens. In a small number of cases—at the appropriate site—the differential diagnoses could also include malignant entities such as epithelioid sarcoma, rhabdomyosarcoma, clear cell sarcoma, or melanoma [4, 5, 10]. A limited panel of immunohistochemical stains will readily exclude these entities. Intra-articular examples may occasionally be subtle, and can be overlooked as a non-specific chronic synovitis.

Although TGCT are almost always benign neoplasms, local recurrence is not uncommon. Unsurprisingly, recurrence is higher in the diffuse subtype (23–72%) [4, 9]. Distant metastases to the lung or lymph nodes occur in a very small number of cases [2, 5, 9, 10]. Malignant TGCT have been reported but are very rare. MTGCT typically comprises sheets of enlarged and pleomorphic mononuclear cells, resembling high-grade sarcoma. Mitotic activity is increased and includes atypical mitoses. Necrosis is often present [5].

32.7 Basic Principles

A patient-centred decision balancing the benign, potentially indolent course of TGCT versus the possible curative impact, potential for local recurrence, and associated treatment risks must be considered [9, 15]. Active surveillance may be more suitable than active treatment in some cases.

Multidisciplinary team discussion in a designated sarcoma centre may be of benefit for DTGCT, particularly in the setting of recurrent disease [9, 16].

Surgical management with marginal excision in LTGCT is typically sufficient, whereas extensive synovectomy for involved joints of tendon sheaths is necessary in DTGCT [9]. This can be technically challenging. Open synovectomy has been shown to have lower recurrence rate, although stiffness and reduced functional outcomes are a concern [8, 17]. In the knee, anterior arthroscopic and open posterior excisions have been shown to have acceptable recurrence rates with less morbidity [18, 19].

Open synovectomy of hip, although associated with a low rate of local recurrence, portends high osteochondral destruction risk and arthroscopic treatment can be safely considered to optimise function [20–22].

Specific to the foot and ankle, open synovectomy remains the mainstay of treatment given the high rate of extra-articular disease [23].

Arthroplasty can be effectively utilised to address joint-related pain and deformity, particularly in the hip and knee; however, it demonstrates a high local recurrence rate. Amputation can be reserved as a treatment of last resort for functional or unremitting pain indications [9, 15, 21].

Radiotherapy currently has insufficient high-quality, prospective randomised controlled trial data to be safely recommended. TGCT patients are typically young with non-life-threatening disease. Long-term complications of radiotherapy such as poor wound healing, pathological fracture, malignant transformation, and arthrofibrosis are of significant concern [9, 24], and the potential benefit of radiotherapy must be carefully balanced with the potential for significant morbidity.

Cryotherapy also has insufficient high-quality evidence supporting its use in treatment of TGCT [9, 25, 26].

Systemic therapy targeted against CSFR1 with tyrosine kinase inhibitors (pexidartinib, imatinib, nilotinib, and vimseltinib) or monoclonal antibodies (emactuzumab and cabiralizumab) have all shown varying levels of positive outcomes [9, 15, 27]. They are not currently widely available, although many countries have clinical trials or potential for off-label usage. In the United States, the only agent with Food and Drug Administration (FDA) approval is pexidartinib. The patient must have symptomatic TGCT with severe disease or functional limitation, and not be amenable to improvement with surgical intervention [16]. In those patients with symptomatic disease, significant functional impairment, and/or high risk of surgical morbidity, systemic therapy may be beneficial [9].

32.8 Prognosis

LTGCT and DTGCT can cause significant morbidity but are not fatal. Local recurrence rates are lower in LTGCT (9–12%) than in DTGCT (23–72%). Local recurrence rates are known to be reduced if patients are treated at a specialist centre (44% vs. 92%) [9, 16].

Local recurrence rates of DTGCT have also been shown to be higher with incomplete excisions [28–30], as well as cases present in the knee or large joints [31, 32]. Most recurrence occurs with the first 2 years [1]. Secondary osteochondral destruction and resultant arthritis are frequent and have been suggested to be more common in the hip [33].

Malignant TGCT is exceedingly rare, with incidence of <1/1,000,000/year. Of the limited case reports available in the literature, the metastatic rate is ~50% (commonly to lymph nodes and lungs), and mortality rate is 30% [2, 9]. MTGCT should be treated as soft tissue sarcoma, with management by a specialised sarcoma multidisciplinary team.

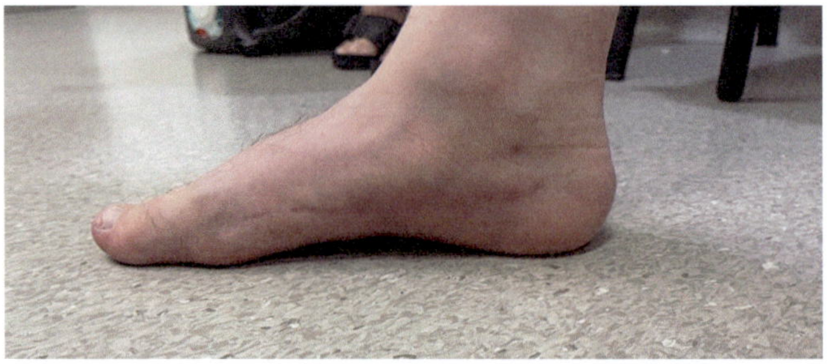

Fig. 32.11 Weight-bearing clinical photograph demonstrating maintained medial longitudinal arch 9 months post-operatively

32.9 Technical Pearls

1. Developing a plane between the tumour and bone in order to resect the mass *en bloc* is likely to reduce recurrence rate compared to intralesional resection. If the soft tissue mass is encased without being invasive as in this case, the soft tissue margin lifts away.
2. Putty-like synthetic bone graft is more likely to stay in the placed location and fill the irregular uneven bony defect cavity effectively than granular or milled graft.
3. Consider fusion of joints which have been significantly affected by the lesion.
4. Meticulous haemostasis will reduce post-operative haematoma and thereby infection risk.

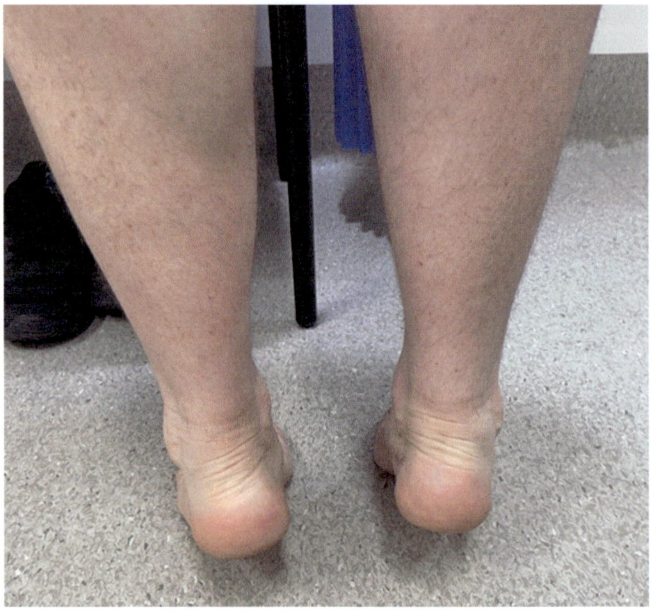

Fig. 32.12 Functional clinical photograph demonstrating stable midfoot with satisfactory alignment 9 months post-operatively

32.10 Outcome Radiographs and Images

At most recent review twenty four months post-surgery, his medial longitudinal arch is maintained (Figs. 32.11 and 32.12), and his foot pain resolved. An MRI was performed and shows no evidence of local recurrence, and post-operative radiographs demonstrate incorporation of bone graft (Fig. 32.13). He has returned to normal activities.

32.11 Avoiding and Managing Problems

1. Post-operative seroma formation can occur if large dead spaces are not filled with graft (bony defects) or managed with suction drains (soft tissue defects). This increases the risk of infection, particularly in the foot and ankle, and needs to be monitored during recovery.
2. Suitable prophylactic antibiotics given the need to implant foreign material into the defect.
3. Choosing an incision at the junction of the dorsal and plantar skin limits scar hypersensitivity or discomfort with weight-bearing areas.
4. Weight-bearing restrictions are advised in the early post-operative period to protect the wound and prevent bony foot collapse until the graft is able to incorporate and provide skeletal stability.
5. Orthotics such as Moon boot followed by medial arch supports can assist in allowing earlier weight-bearing and prevent loss of normal foot architecture.

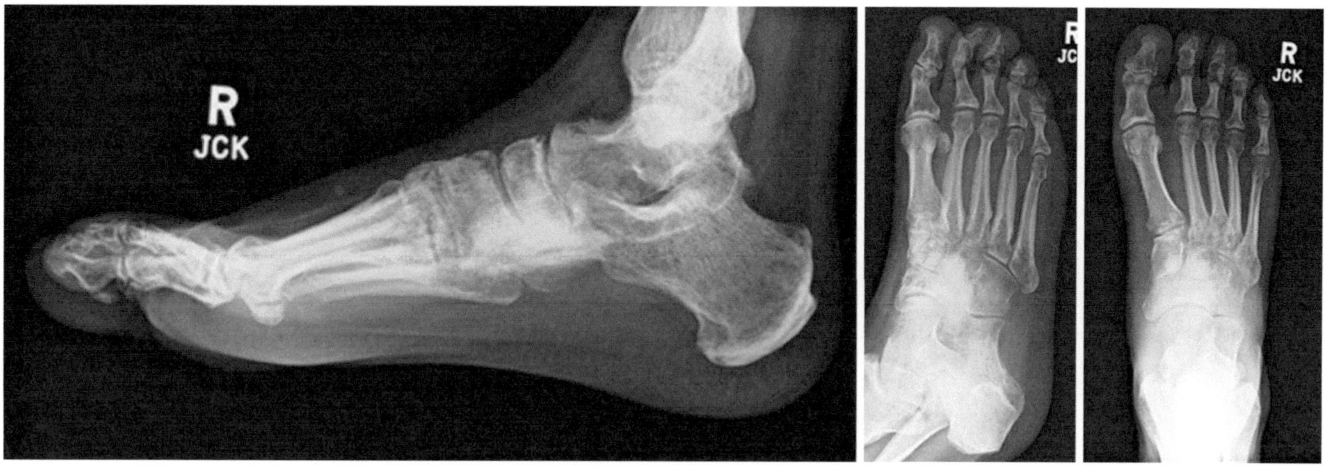

Fig. 32.13 Radiographs demonstrating incorporation of synthetic bone graft 9 months post-surgery

32.12 Summary

TGCT is the current nomenclature for a group of common benign tumours that occurs in many anatomical locations. They have a common histological appearance and were previously known under multiple pseudonyms.

Diagnosis is best confirmed with clinical history and examination, MRI imaging, core biopsy, or excisional biopsy depending on the lesion size and location.

At operative intervention, it has the classic appearance of a rust-coloured mass from haemosiderin deposition.

TGCT can cause significant morbidity, and treatment risks need to be balanced with the potential for high recurrence rate if surgery is intralesional. Marginal resection is generally satisfactory with a low local recurrence rate.

Each patient needs to be considered on a case-by-case basis, and as demonstrated in the example above, individualised care demands will involve surgical and other treatment nuances that must be aligned with the patient's wishes. For those patients with refractory DTGCT, multidisciplinary care at a specialist centre is likely to improve outcomes. New systemic therapies are becoming available for inoperable presentations, and fortunately malignant transformation rates are very low.

This case was unusual due to the bony erosion and joint destruction from an extra-articular location arising in the plantar foot soft tissues. Given that this TGCT lesion is now described as the same histological diagnosis throughout the body, it is more commonly seen pushing onto the bone. This case did not have the sclerotic moulded edge often seen with long-standing bony pressure changes seen in the fingers. It is also different to late DTGCT in and around the knee that 'punches' holes in the bone. In this case it was more infiltrative through the thin tarsal bone shell and 'pushed' into cancellous bone and joint spaces.

There were no adverse findings on histopathology examination. In the longer term, due to the marginal resection the deep ligaments of the mid and hindfoot remained intact. Fortunately, we have been able to preserve the normal foot arch and architecture, without evidence of early local recurrence.

References

1. Siegel M, Bode L, Südkamp N, Kühle J, Zwingmann J, Schmal H, et al. Treatment, recurrence rates and follow-up of Tenosynovial Giant Cell Tumor (TGCT) of the foot and ankle-A systematic review and meta-analysis. PloS One. 2021;16(12):e0260795.
2. Chen EL, de Castro CM, Hendzel KD, Iwaz S, Kim MA, Valeshabad AK, et al. Histologically benign metastasizing tenosynovial giant cell tumor mimicking metastatic malignancy: a case report and review of literature. Radiol Case Rep. 2019;14(8):934–40.
3. Healey JH, Bernthal NM, van de Sande M. Management of tenosynovial giant cell tumor: a neoplastic and inflammatory disease. J Am Acad Orthop Surg Glob Res Rev. 2020;4(11):e20.00028.
4. Board TWCoTE, editor. WHO classification of tumours soft tissue and bone tumours. 5th ed. Lyon: IARC Press; 2020.
5. Wang JC. Tenosynovial giant cell tumor. Pathology Outlines; 2023. https://www.pathologyoutlines.com/topic/softtissuegctlocal.html.
6. Gouin F, Noailles T. Localized and diffuse forms of tenosynovial giant cell tumor (formerly giant cell tumor of the tendon sheath and pigmented villonodular synovitis). Orthop Traumatol Surg Res. 2017;103(1s):S91–s7.
7. Robert M, Farese H, Miossec P. Update on tenosynovial giant cell tumor, an inflammatory arthritis with neoplastic features. Front Immunol. 2022;13:820046.
8. Chandra AA, Agarwal S, Donahue A, Handorf E, Abraham JA. Arthroscopic versus open management of diffuse-type tenosynovial giant cell tumor of the knee: a meta-analysis of retrospective cohort studies. J Am Acad Orthop Surg Glob Res Rev. 2021;4(12)
9. Stacchiotti S, Dürr HR, Schaefer I-M, Woertler K, Haas R, Trama A, et al. Best clinical management of tenosynovial giant cell tumour (TGCT): a consensus paper from the community of experts. Cancer Treat Rev. 2023;112:102491.
10. Liegl-Atzwanger B, Hornick JL. 11—giant cell–rich tumors. In: Hornick JL, editor. Practical soft tissue pathology: a diagnostic approach. 2nd ed. Philadelphia: Elsevier; 2019. p. 297–310.
11. Wang C-S, Duan Q, Xue Y-J, Huang X-M, Wang L-L, Chen Z-Y, et al. Giant cell tumour of tendon sheath with bone invasion in

extremities: analysis of clinical and imaging findings. Radiol Med. 2015;120(8):745–52.
12. Middleton WD, Patel V, Teefey SA, Boyer MI. Giant cell tumors of the tendon sheath: analysis of sonographic findings. AJR Am J Roentgenol. 2004;183(2):337–9.
13. Jeong HS, Lee SK, Kim JY, Yoo C, Joo MW, Kim JH. Tenosynovial giant cell tumors of digits: MRI differentiation between localized types and diffuse types with pathology correlation. Skeletal Radiol. 2023;52(3):593–603.
14. Bassetti E, Candreva R, Santucci E. Giant cell tumor of the flexor tendon of the wrist: US and MRI evaluation. Case report. J Ultrasound. 2011;14(1):37–9.
15. Burton TM, Ye X, Parker ED, Bancroft T, Healey J. Burden of illness associated with tenosynovial giant cell tumors. Clin Ther. 2018;40(4):593–602.e1.
16. Bernthal NM, Healey JH, Palmerini E, Bauer S, Schreuder H, Leithner A, et al. A prospective real-world study of the diffuse-type tenosynovial giant cell tumor patient journey: a 2-year observational analysis. J Surg Oncol. 2022;126(8):1520–32.
17. Quaresma MB, Portela J, Soares do Brito J. Open versus arthroscopic surgery for diffuse tenosynovial giant-cell tumours of the knee: a systematic review. EFORT Open Rev. 2020;5(6):339–46.
18. Colman MW, Ye J, Weiss KR, Goodman MA, McGough RL 3rd. Does combined open and arthroscopic synovectomy for diffuse PVNS of the knee improve recurrence rates? Clin Orthop Relat Res. 2013;471(3):883–90.
19. Heijden L, Mastboom MJL, Dijkstra PDS, Sande MAJ. Functional outcome and quality of life after the surgical treatment for diffuse-type giant-cell tumour around the knee. Bone Joint J. 2014;96-B(8):1111–8
20. Levy DM, Haughom BD, Nho SJ, Gitelis S. Pigmented villonodular synovitis of the hip: a systematic review. Am J Orthop (Belle Mead NJ). 2016;45(1):23–8.
21. Steinmetz S, Rougemont AL, Peter R. Pigmented villonodular synovitis of the hip. EFORT Open Rev. 2016;1(6):260–6.
22. Vastel L, Lambert P, De Pinieux G, Charrois O, Kerboull M, Courpied JP. Surgical treatment of pigmented villonodular synovitis of the hip. J Bone Joint Surg Am. 2005;87(5):1019–24.
23. Li X, Xu Y, Zhu Y, Xu X. Surgical treatment for diffused-type giant cell tumor (pigmented villonodular synovitis) about the ankle joint. BMC Musculoskelet Disord. 2017;18(1):450.
24. Lo SS, Sahgal A, Chang EL, Mayr NA, Teh BS, Huang Z, et al. Serious complications associated with stereotactic ablative radiotherapy and strategies to mitigate the risk. Clin Oncol (R Coll Radiol). 2013;25(6):378–87.
25. Verspoor FG, Scholte A, van der Geest IC, Hannink G, Schreuder HW. Cryosurgery as Additional Treatment in Tenosynovial Giant Cell Tumors. Sarcoma. 2016;2016:3072135.
26. Mohler DG, Kessler BD. Open synovectomy with cryosurgical adjuvant for treatment of diffuse pigmented villonodular synovitis of the knee. Bull Hosp Jt Dis. 2000;59(2):99–105.
27. Caldwell TM, Ahn YM, Bulfer SL, Leary CB, Hood MM, Lu WP, et al. Discovery of vimseltinib (DCC-3014), a highly selective CSF1R switch-control kinase inhibitor, in clinical development for the treatment of Tenosynovial Giant Cell Tumor (TGCT). Bioorg Med Chem Lett. 2022;74:128928.
28. Ogilvie-Harris D, McLean J, Zarnett M. Pigmented villonodular synovitis of the knee. The results of total arthroscopic synovectomy, partial arthroscopic synovectomy, and arthroscopic local excision. J Bone Joint Surg Am. 1992;74:119–23.
29. de Visser E, Veth RP, Pruszczynski M, Wobbes T, Van de Putte LB. Diffuse and localized pigmented villonodular synovitis: evaluation of treatment of 38 patients. Arch Orthop Trauma Surg. 1999;119(7–8):401–4.
30. Chiari C, Pirich C, Brannath W, Kotz R, Trieb K. What affects the recurrence and clinical outcome of pigmented villonodular synovitis? Clin Orthop Relat Res. 2006;450:172–8.
31. Ottaviani S, Ayral X, Dougados M, Gossec L. Pigmented villonodular synovitis: a retrospective single-center study of 122 cases and review of the literature. Semin Arthritis Rheum. 2011;40(6):539–46.
32. Schwartz H, Unni K, Pritchard D. Pigmented villonodular synovitis: a retrospective review of affected large joints. Clin Orthop Relat Res. 1989;247:243–55.
33. Ota T, Urakawa H, Kozawa E, Ikuta K, Hamada S, Tsukushi S, et al. Expression of colony-stimulating factor 1 is associated with occurrence of osteochondral change in pigmented villonodular synovitis. Tumor Biol. 2015;36(7):5361–7.

Visualization of Soft Tissue Sarcoma Margins Utilizing Indocyanine Green Fluorescence Angiography (ICGFA)

33

Matthew F. Gong and Kurt R. Weiss

33.1 Introduction

Soft tissue sarcomas are rare, and aggressive mesenchymal tumors comprise around 1% of adult malignancies and 7–15% of pediatric malignancies [2, 9] Around 60–80% of soft tissue sarcomas originate from the extremities, and more than 50 different histological subtypes have been identified [4]. Surgical resection is the foundation of soft tissue sarcoma treatment, with radiation therapy serving as an important adjuvant [9]. Chemotherapy also has a role as an adjuvant treatment but is more efficacious in specific subtypes including rhabdomyosarcoma and synovial sarcoma. During soft tissue sarcoma surgical resection, obtaining negative margins while maintaining a functional limb is the guiding principle of limb salvage surgery. Local recurrence is a devastating complication associated with greater likelihood of metastasis and death, with rates reaching as high as 50% in the setting of a positive surgical margin [3, 5, 7]. Techniques such as indocyanine green fluorescence angiography (ICGFA) are emerging as investigational tools for intraoperative margin assessment, which may assist the sarcoma surgeon in real time to obtain negative surgical margins and minimize the risk of local recurrence.

33.2 Case 1: Brief Clinical History

A 69-year-old female returned 2 years after she underwent radical excision of a right thigh myxofibrosarcoma with a recurrent enlarging mass in her right thigh. Originally, she presented with a right thigh mass and MRI obtained at that time demonstrating a heterogeneous T2-enhancing lesion within the vastus intermedius of her right thigh. A CT-guided biopsy was performed and demonstrated a high-grade myxofibrosarcoma. She subsequently underwent excision with a focally positive deep margin on final pathology. Her treatment included adjuvant radiation therapy, chemotherapy, as well as surgical resection of metastatic pulmonary nodules performed by the Thoracic Surgery service with negative margins achieved. Following radiation therapy, the patient also sustained a femoral shaft stress fracture, which was treated via operative fixation with an intramedullary nail.

Eighteen months after the patient's index procedure, an MRI scan was obtained that demonstrated recurrence of a soft tissue lesion involving her anterolateral thigh in the previous surgical field. Figures 33.1 and 33.2 demonstrate the T1 and T2 axial MRI, respectively, where the lesion can be appreciated superficial to the femur. Figure 33.3 demonstrates the T2 coronal MRI showing the proximal extent of the lesion, indicated by the yellow arrow. These findings were concerning for local recurrence of her previous myxofibrosarcoma, which was confirmed on CT-guided biopsy. No evidence of metastatic disease was found on CT scan of the chest, abdomen, and pelvis.

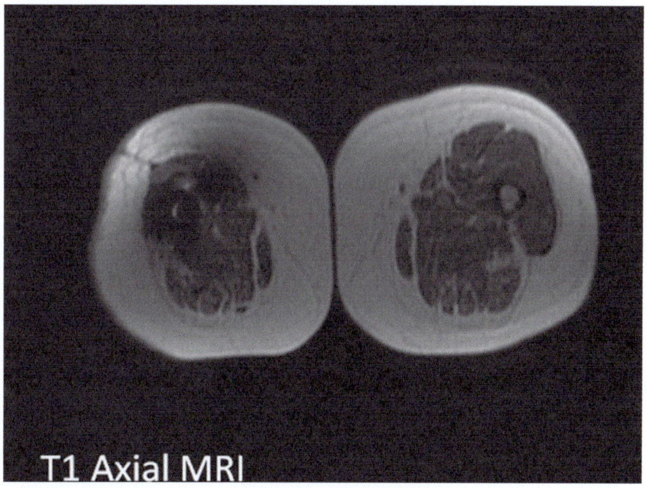

Fig. 33.1 Locally recurrent myxofibrosarcoma

M. F. Gong
Department of Orthopaedic Surgery, University of Pittsburgh Medical Center, Pittsburgh, PA, USA

K. R. Weiss (✉)
Department of Orthopaedic Surgery, Division of Musculoskeletal Oncology, University of Pittsburgh Medical Center, Pittsburgh, PA, USA
e-mail: weiskr@upmc.edu

H. Özger et al. (eds.), *Diagnosis and Treatment of Soft Tissue Tumors*, https://doi.org/10.1007/978-3-031-77061-6_33

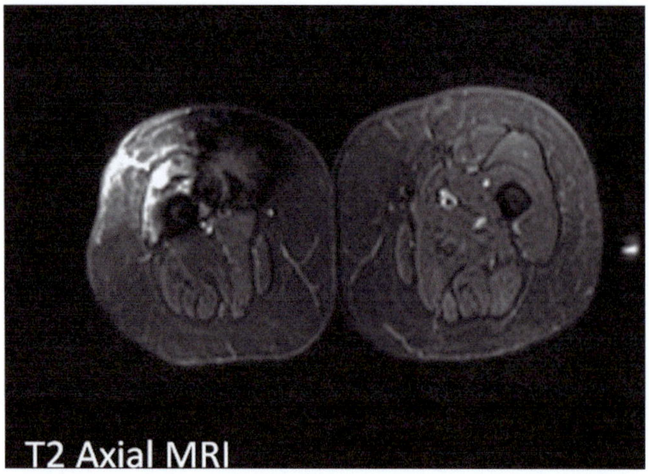

Fig. 33.2 Locally recurrent myxofibrosarcoma

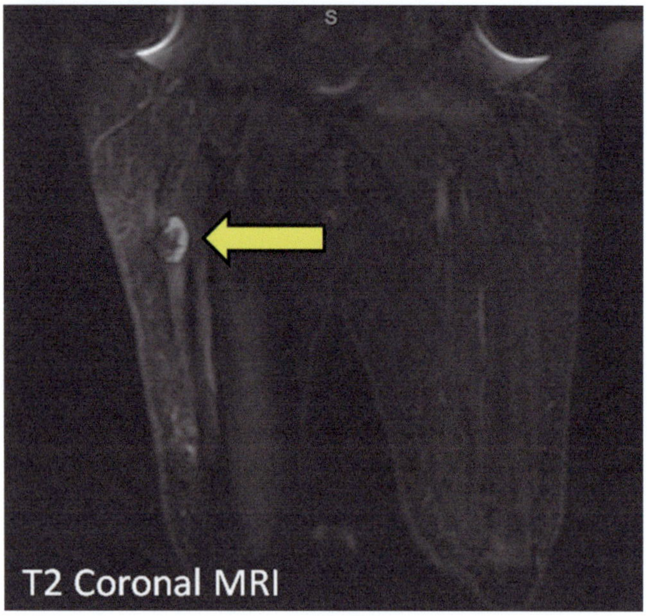

Fig. 33.3 Locally recurrent myxofibrosarcoma

33.3 Case 1: Preoperative Problem List

- Local recurrence of a high-grade soft tissue sarcoma of the anterolateral thigh within the prior surgical resection bed.
- Preservation of limb function while performing wide excision with the goal of obtaining negative margins.

33.4 Case 1: Treatment Strategy

- *Surgical Excision*: The primary goal of treatment for this case was to perform a surgical re-excision to obtain negative margins. At the time of recurrence, the patient did not demonstrate any evidence of metastatic disease.
- *Intraoperative Margin Assessment*: Final pathology is considered the definitive method to determine margin status after the excision of soft tissue sarcomas. In the intraoperative setting, frozen pathology can also be sent as an attempt to verify margin status when there is concern for tumor involvement. This enables the surgeon to perform a wider excision if the intraoperative frozen section is positive and enables sparing of non-cancerous tissue if margins are not involved. ICGFA is a technique to evaluate surgical margins intraoperatively in real-time, which may help to guide the surgeon to perform a precise excision while achieving negative margins and thus decreasing local recurrence.
- *Radiation Therapy*: In the setting of primary soft tissue extremity sarcoma, neoadjuvant or adjuvant radiation is typically used. In this case, the patient had already received radiation to the affected site.

33.5 Case 1: Basic Principles

- Careful preoperative planning is critical. Plain radiographs and MRI were obtained to evaluate the extent of the lesion. The relationship of the tumor to surrounding vital structures was determined to decide if limb salvage was feasible or not. The decision was made to perform a limb-sparing excision.
- In order to perform ICGFA to assist with intraoperative margin assessment, a preoperative infusion of ICG was performed. The patient was instructed to arrive 3 h prior to the time of their scheduled operation, such that a weight-based dose of 2.0 mg/kg of ICG could be infused in the preoperative holding area.
- As in the excision of a primary sarcoma, preserving a layer of non-cancerous tissue around the tumor is the guiding principle of surgery. The excision of a recurrent soft tissue sarcoma can be affected by postoperative and post-radiation fibrosis of the tissues surrounding the tumor. Meticulous dissection, understanding of the anatomy, and appreciation of the tumor's location enable the surgeon to maintain a wide margin.
- During this case, the prior surgical incision was exploited. A layer of irradiated tissue was maintained around the recurrent sarcoma. To evaluate the deep (femoral) margin, a frozen section was sent and read as negative.
- At this time, intraoperative margin assessment was performed with ICGFA. Based on literature in the surgical management of breast, lung, and gastrointestinal cancers, ICGFA is performed with a threshold of $\geq 77\%$ of fluorescence corresponding to a positive margin [6, 8], where the percentage value of 100% is calibrated to the brightest region of the excised tumor. During this evaluation, the surgeon was blinded to ICGFA results. In this

case, ICGFA suggested a positive margin near the superficial margin of the surgical bed.

- After tumor excision was completed, irrigation was performed and meticulous hemostasis of the tumor resection bed was obtained. The wound was then closed in layers. Negative suction drains can be utilized at this stage to reduce postoperative edema. In this instance, the patient was discharged immediately postoperatively without a drain.
- In the postoperative period, the patient was encouraged to mobilize as tolerated and advised to elevate the limb to reduce postoperative edema. A follow-up appointment in 2–4 weeks was planned.
- On final permanent pathology, the superficial margin of the performed resection was positive. Serial interval surveillance studies to evaluate the presence of local recurrence and/or metastasis were planned.

33.6 Case 1: Intraoperative Indocyanine Green Fluorescent Angiography (ICGFA) Margin Evaluation

- Utilizing the SPY-PHI near-infrared camera (Stryker Endoscopy, Kalamazoo, MI), fluorescence emitted from indocyanine green can be detected. The ability to visualize areas of ICG deposition in regions of tumor is thought to occur based on the Enhanced Permeability and Retention principle [1], wherein ICG is retained in sites of aberrant tumor vasculature while quickly dissipating in regions of intact vasculature.
- ICGFA implementation begins with calibration of the SPY-PHI camera for that specific case. The region of brightest fluorescence detected after a complete scan of the excised sarcoma is calibrated to 100%. While performing the complete scan of the resected tumor, areas of higher fluorescence may be encountered which will need to be re-calibrated to 100%, as indicated in Fig. 33.4. Calibration is complete when all remaining regions of the resected tumor are now measured with a percentage below 100%, with Figs. 33.5 and 33.6 demonstrate the completion scan of the excised tumor with different image filters.
- After calibration is completed, the SPY-PHI camera is then brought to the operative field to image the resected tumor bed. The camera should be held 1–2 feet away from the tissue being imaged. A threshold of fluorescence percentage ≥77% indicates a positive margin. In Fig. 33.7, the resected tumor bed is being imaged near the superficial margin, with a fluorescence of 93% suggestive of a positive margin. After final pathology was reviewed, a positive margin was found to involve the superficial margin, located in the same region identified intraoperatively with ICGFA.

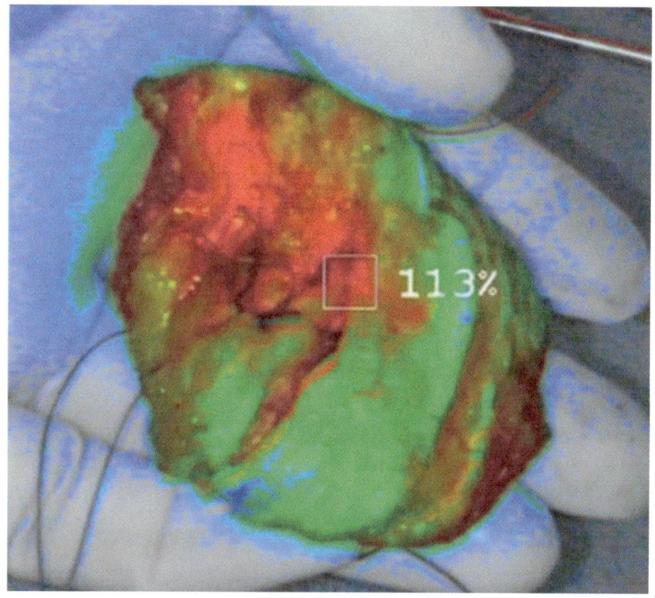

Fig. 33.4 Fluorescence is measured using the SPY-PHI camera of the resected tumor. This region, where 113%, is measured compared to an arbitrary calibrated value must be re-calibrated and set to 100% on the arbitrary percentage scale

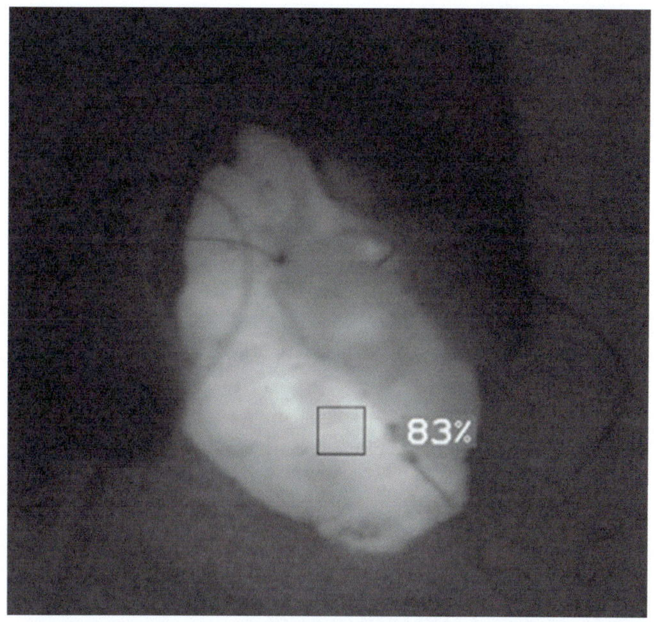

Fig. 33.5 Scanning to confirm calibration to highest fluorescent region of tumor utilizing the gray-scale filter. 83% indicates this region does not exceed the brightest portion of the tumor calibrated to 100%

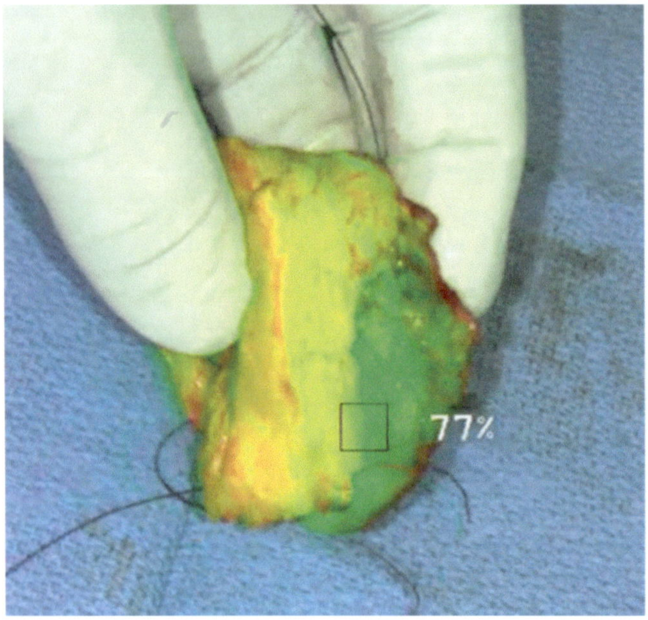

Fig. 33.6 Additional calibration of fluorescent percentage to resected tumor. 77% indicates this region is less fluorescent than the brightest region of tumor calibrated to 100%

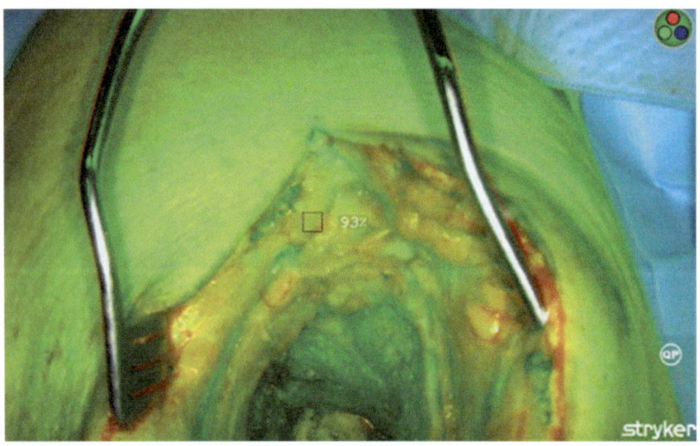

Fig. 33.7 Intra-operative evaluation of resected tumor bed using ICGFA. Fluorescence of 93% calibrated to the brightest portion of resected tumor was detected near the superficial margin of the resection bed, denoting a positive margin (≥77%)

33.7 Case 1: Technical Pearls

- In the setting of primary or local recurrent soft tissue sarcomas, maintaining a normal cuff of tissue during excision can be optimized with utilization of intraoperative margin assessment tools including frozen section pathology or ICGFA. During implementation of ICGFA, we found that meticulous calibration of the SPY-PHI camera to the brightest region of tumor required a complete evaluation of the entire excised specimen. Inadequate calibration may record a lower baseline fluorescence when imaging the wound bed, which could abnormally elevate readings obtained from the tumor bed, increasing risk of a surgeon potentially unnecessarily excising uninvolved tissue. Holding the camera approximately 1–2 feet away from the region of tissue being imaged provided the most consistent measurements of fluorescence. While performing calibration or imaging the excised tumor bed, utilizing the different filters which can be toggled on the SPY-PHI software allowed for the best ability to observe which regions of tissue were most fluorescent.

33.8 Case 1: Outcome

- In this case, final pathology noted a positive margin along the superficial margin of the excised tumor bed. The patient was advised to weight bear as tolerated, elevate the limb to reduce postoperative edema, strengthen the quadriceps, and perform manual massage maneuvers to prevent scar tissue related pain and maintain overall function while recovering in the postoperative setting. The patient was evaluated by radiation oncology and medical oncology with plans to continue surveillance to monitor for local recurrence and metastases.

33.9 Case 1: Avoiding and Managing Problems

- An unexpected positive margin is a possibility in surgery performed for any primary or recurrent soft tissue sarcoma, and minimizing this complication may be improved with utilization of intraoperative margin assessment techniques such as ICGFA. The utility of ICGFA to augment an experienced surgeon's eyes and hands is an area of active investigation with the hope that the development of this technology may reduce local recurrence rates.

References

1. Chan CD, Brookes MJ, Tanwani R, et al. Investigating the mechanisms of indocyanine green (ICG) cellular uptake in sarcoma. BioRxiv. 2021; https://doi.org/10.1101/2021.04.05.438013.
2. Greenlee RT, Hill-Harmon MB, Murray T, Thun M. Cancer statistics, 2001. CA Cancer J Clin. 2001;51:15–36. https://doi.org/10.3322/canjclin.51.1.15.
3. Gronchi A, Ferrari S, Quagliuolo V, et al. Histotype-tailored neoadjuvant chemotherapy versus standard chemotherapy in patients with high-risk soft-tissue sarcomas (ISG-STS 1001): an international, open-label, randomised, controlled, phase 3, multicentre trial. Lancet Oncol. 2017;18:812–22. https://doi.org/10.1016/S1470-2045(17)30334-0.
4. Morrison BA. Soft tissue sarcomas of the extremities. Proc (Bayl Univ Med Cent). 2003;16:285–90. https://doi.org/10.1080/08998280.2003.11927915.

5. O'Donnell PW, Griffin AM, Eward WC, et al. The effect of the setting of a positive surgical margin in soft tissue sarcoma. Cancer. 2014;120:2866–75. https://doi.org/10.1002/cncr.28793.
6. Pop F-C, Veys I, Vankerckhove S, et al. Absence of residual fluorescence in the surgical bed at near-infrared fluorescence imaging predicts negative margins at final pathology in patients treated with breast-conserving surgery for breast cancer. Eur J Surg Oncol. 2021;47:269–75. https://doi.org/10.1016/j.ejso.2020.09.036.
7. Stojadinovic A, Leung DHY, Hoos A, et al. Analysis of the prognostic significance of microscopic margins in 2,084 localized primary adult soft tissue sarcomas. Ann Surg. 2002;235:424–34. https://doi.org/10.1097/00000658-200203000-00015.
8. Veys I, Pop C-F, Barbieux R, et al. ICG fluorescence imaging as a new tool for optimization of pathological evaluation in breast cancer tumors after neoadjuvant chemotherapy. PLoS One. 2018;13:e0197857. https://doi.org/10.1371/journal.pone.0197857.
9. von Mehren M, Kane JM, Agulnik M, et al. Soft tissue sarcoma, version 2.2022, NCCN clinical practice guidelines in oncology. J Natl Compr Cancer Netw. 2022;20:815–33. https://doi.org/10.6004/jnccn.2022.0035.

34 Undifferentiated Pleomorphic Sarcoma of the Thigh: Diagnostic Pitfalls and Complex Reconstruction

Korhan Özkan, Erhan Okay, and Enes Kanay

34.1 Introduction

Soft tissue sarcomas (STS) constitute an uncommon and heterogeneous group of tumors of mesenchymal origin, with an estimated incidence of five cases/per 100,000 inhabitants/year in Europe [1]. They comprise approximately 1% of malignant tumors. There are more than 50 subtypes that need radiological and pathological correlation [2]. The diagnostic pathway should always start with thorough patient history documentation. Lumps that have not changed in size or shape over the years are most likely benign, whereas recently noticed, constantly enlarging may be malignant.

Early identification of patients with possible soft tissue sarcoma and prompt referral to a sarcoma center is essential to avoid unnecessary diagnosis delays and ensure optimal multidisciplinary treatment. While traumatic soft tissue swellings are usually painful, even relatively large STSs may be indolent.

A recent database indicated that these tumors are generally smaller than 5 cm with superficial localization, and preoperative imaging is not performed [3]. This fact explains why soft tissue sarcomas can be mistaken for benign lesions.

When sarcomas undergo unplanned excision, its treatment becomes more complicated. As a result, the local recurrence rate increases due to residual tumor after inadequate removal. In this scenario, surgical bed re-excision includes a more aggressive surgery with reconstructive techniques than a wide excision for a primary tumor. Also, the risk of amputation is higher compared to primary procedure [4].

If a soft tissue is suspected after multidisciplinary discussion including orthopedic oncologist and musculoskeletal radiologist, biopsy should be done compatible with oncologic principles. These are (a) contaminating only the compartment of the tumoral tissue, (b) taking care of not violating neurovascular structures or joint space, and (c) placing the biopsy tract and drains in line with the subsequent surgical incision. When these rules are not followed, there is a high risk of tumoral contamination of normal tissue planes. Hematoma is another misdiagnosis in soft tissue sarcomas. Herein, we present a soft tissue sarcoma case that previously had undergone repeated debridements in another institution which had been considered as traumatic soft tissue hematoma.

34.2 Brief Clinical History

Male patient aged 65 years old who had gradual swelling and pain in adductor region for the last 4 months administered to the orthopedics policlinic in another clinic. The patient had an unclear history of a muscle stain during sports activity, and hematoma was suspected. He had then undergone debridement under general anesthesia with a preliminary diagnosis of hematoma in the adductor region without any tomographic or MRI imaging. Neither biopsy nor microbiological sampling was performed before or during the operation. The lesion and the patients' symptoms resolved for a brief period of 1 month after the operation; however, the lesion started to get enlarged again. This time MRI was ordered, and the result was interpreted as a likely diagnosis of hematoma again with a little suspicion of soft tissue sarcoma. Again debridement was done without any tissue sampling before the surgery. However, samples were taken during the operation for pathological examination this time. Postoperative pathology report revealed undifferentiated pleomorphic sarcoma, and the patient was recommended for hip disarticulation in that institution.

After admission to our hospital, pathology slides from the referring hospital were rechecked by our hospital's musculoskeletal pathologists with confirmation of the results.

K. Özkan (✉) · E. Kanay
Department of Orthopedics and Traumatology, Acıbadem Ataşehir Hospital, Istanbul, Türkiye
e-mail: korhan.ozkan@acibadem.com

E. Okay
Department of Orthopedics and Traumatology, Göztepe Prof. Dr. Süleyman Yalçın City Hospital, Istanbul, Türkiye
e-mail: enes.kanay@acibadem.com

H. Özger et al. (eds.), *Diagnosis and Treatment of Soft Tissue Tumors*, https://doi.org/10.1007/978-3-031-77061-6_34

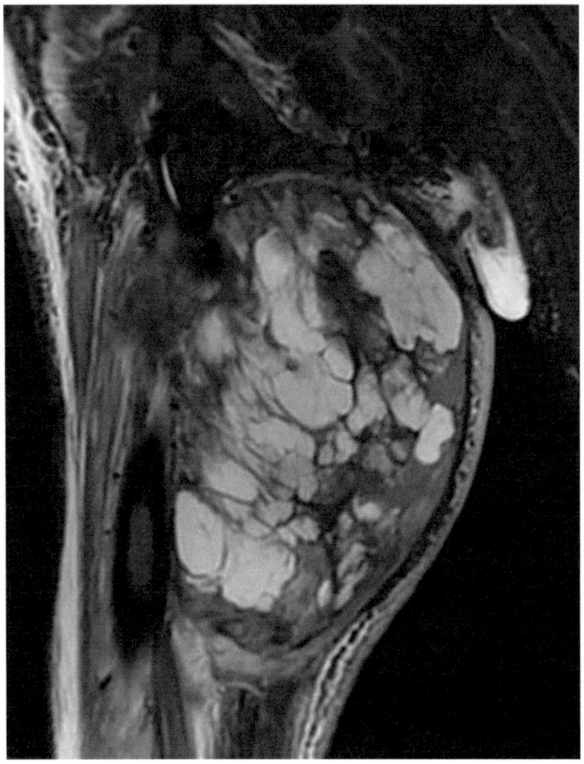

Fig. 34.1 T2 sequence displaying hemorrhagic cystic lesions within the tumoral mass

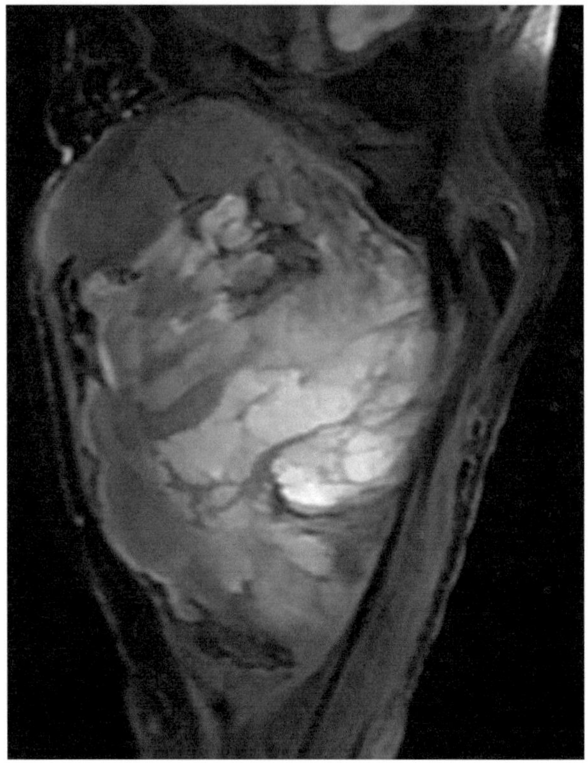

Fig. 34.2 T1 contrast-enhanced MRI sequence

A new contrast-enhanced thigh and pelvic MRI with PET-CT was ordered for local and distant staging. In the new MRI examination of the patient, close bony proximity of the giant soft tissue mass and extensive contamination of the tissue planes were evident (Figs. 34.1 and 34.2). Limb salvage surgery was offered, but the patient was also informed about the risk of amputation in the form of external hemipelvectomy during or after the procedure. Informed consent for amputation was also obtained from the patient. In this context, a short course preoperative radiotherapy was done. CT-angiography was requested to evaluate vascular involvement before surgery.

Since the tumor tissue extended to the subcutaneous tissue in a large area comprising proximal and medial of the thigh, surgical planning was performed in such a way that the incision line, which was previously done for debridement, would be the center, and an extensive skin tissue would be left on the mass to be excised. While the femoral neurovascular bundle was explored from the pelvic rim to the middle of the thigh in the anterior aspect, the sciatic nerve was dissected posteriorly. Soft tissue resection, including the type 3 pelvis and proximal femur bone resection, was done to obtain negative surgical margins. Resection was aimed at the widest possible margins during surgery, and no complications were encountered during the surgery. Utmost importance was given for hemostasis during the surgery. Bipolar cautery was used for hemostasis in the vicinity of the sciatic nerve. Since the tumoral lesion was closely adjacent to the proximal femur and ramus pubis superior and ramus pubis inferior, type 3 pelvic resection was also performed in addition to proximal femur resection (Figs. 34.3, 34.4, 34.5, and 34.6). Subsequently, a proximal femoral modular endoprosthesis was implanted from the medial thigh. (Fig. 34.7). The resulting defect was reconstructed from the opposite side using a rotational rectus abdominis flap for the soft tissue defect coverage over the adductor region (Fig. 34.8). Postoperative radiograph was adequate stability (Fig. 34.9).

In the early postoperative period, purulent discharge developed in the adductor area of the wound. Culture was consistent with Acinetobacter infection. Serial debridements with silver coated vacuum-assisted closure treatments were applied. The patient was discharged 1 month after surgery. Our multidisciplinary team evaluated the patient, and adjuvant chemotherapy was given. The patient is alive 1.5 years after the operation.

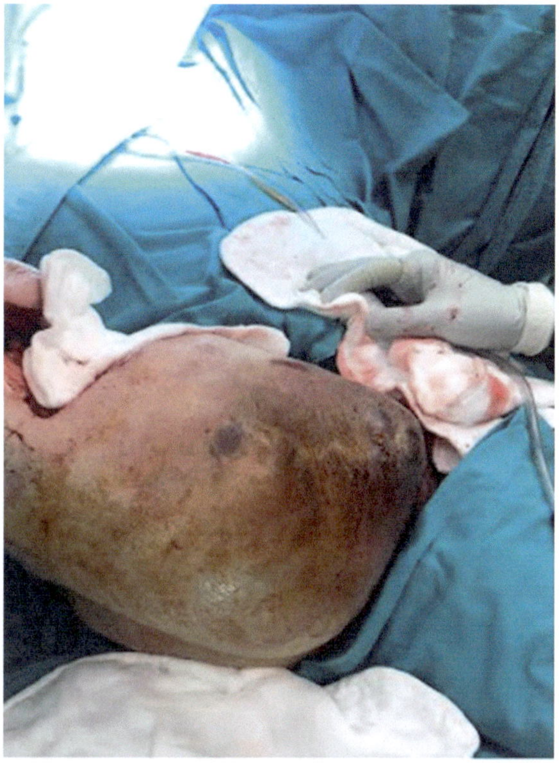

Fig. 34.3 Preoperative view of the lesion with previous incision scar

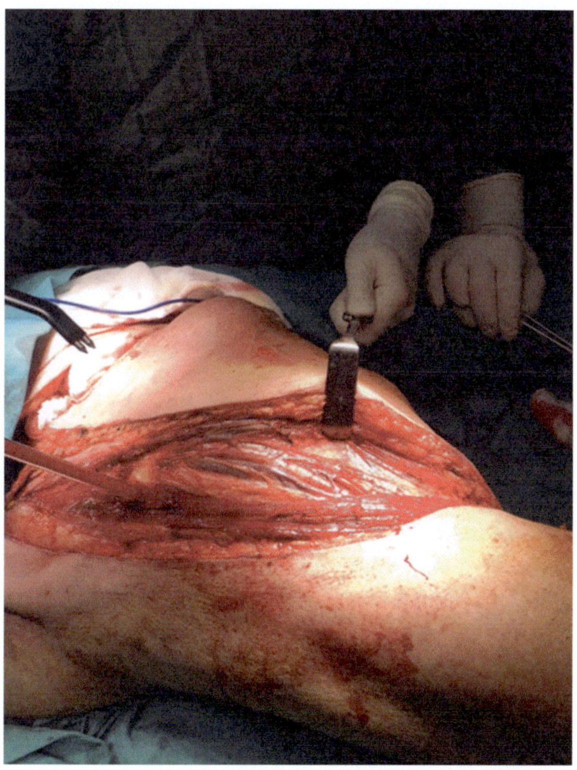

Fig. 34.4 Intraoperative view of the lesion during exposure, anterior and posterior flaps were made leaving the contaminated skin tissue on the mass

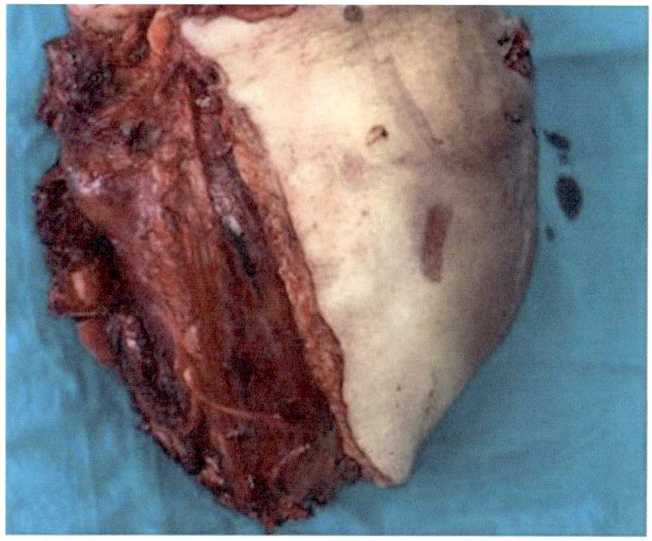

Fig. 34.5 The resected tumoral lesion with possible wide margins

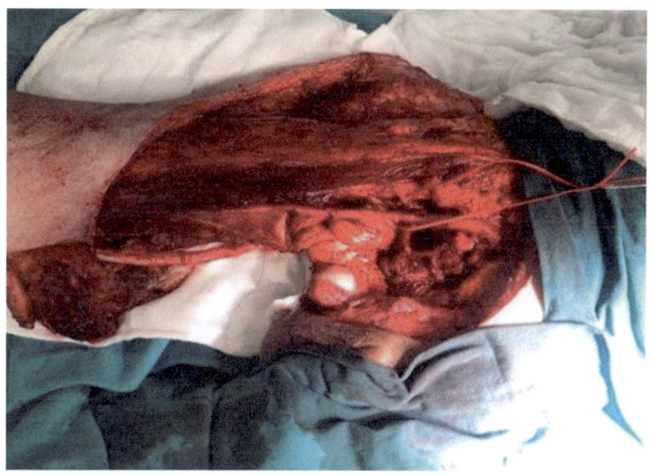

Fig. 34.6 Soft tissue defect after resection

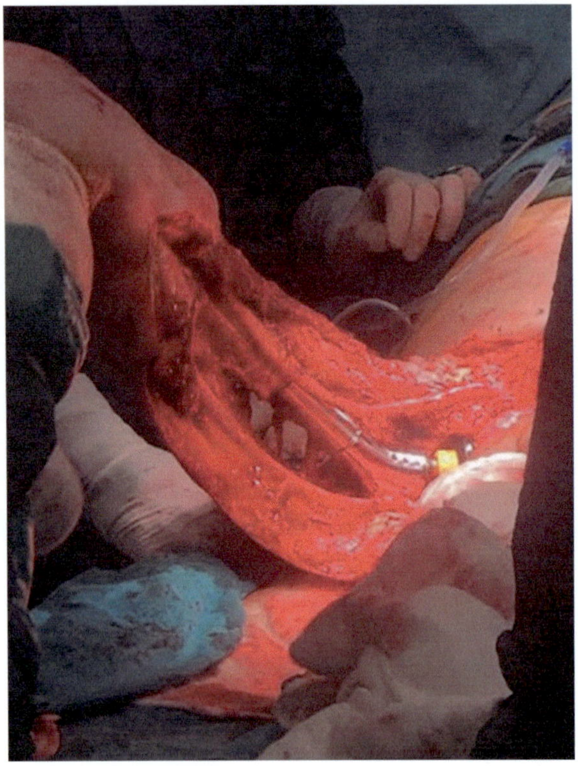

Fig. 34.7 Prosthetic reconstruction was also done

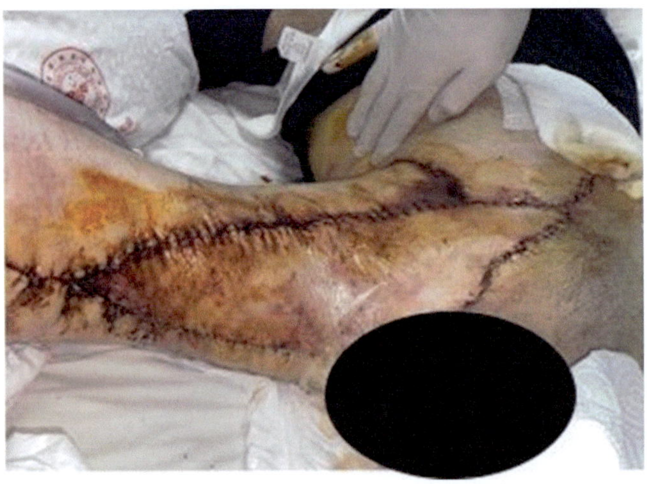

Fig. 34.8 Soft tissue defect was reconstructed with vertical rotational rectus abdominus flap

34.3 Preoperative Clinical Photos and Radiographs

34.4 Preoperative Problem List

(a) Contamination of the compartment in the location of the residual tumor.

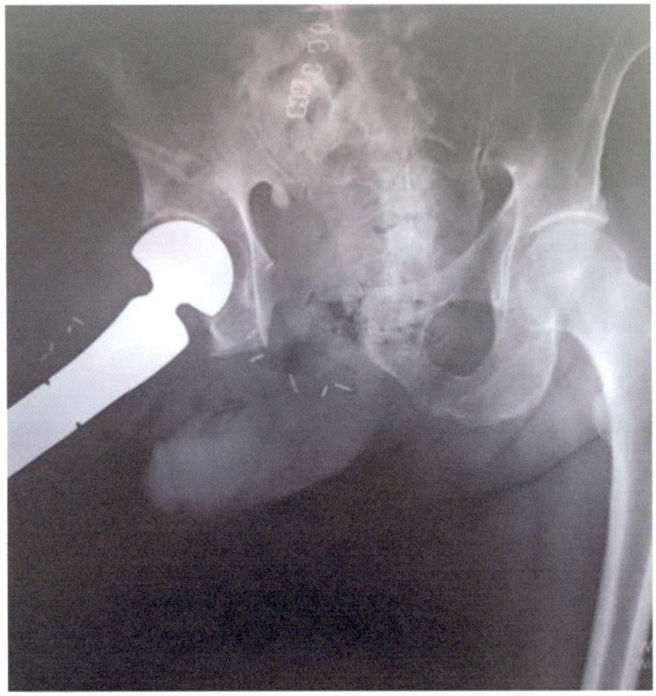

Fig. 34.9 Postoperative X-ray of the patient

(b) Postoperative edema which makes it difficult to accurately estimate the extent of the tumor. Moreover, fibrotic changes, loss of anatomical planes, and a big mass lesion complicate the extent of resection. Accurate evaluation and preoperative planning may not possible using contrast-enhanced MRI due to previous surgeries.
(c) Fibrotic changes after primary excision also challenge the accurate identification of neurovascular structures.
(d) The pathology report from other non-sarcoma centers can be questionable.

34.5 Treatment Strategy

(a) Previous histological slides should be obtained from the referring hospital to verify or modify the pathology results by a pathologist experienced in bone and soft tissue tumors.
(b) The optimum timing to require MRI is advised to be between 4 and 8 weeks after unplanned excision to minimize confounding postoperative changes although these changes do not disappear completely [5].
(c) Neoadjuvant radiotherapy may be useful to achieve local control and decreased morbidity thanks to tumor shrinkage and possible sterilization of the surgical bed before re-excision [6].
(d) To note, one recent study indicated increased disease-free survival in patients receiving neoadjuvant radiotherapy before re-excision. Our neoadjuvant radiotherapy

regimen includes 28 Gy in 8 fractions according to a recent study in our country. The proposed mechanism of neoadjuvant radiotherapy is to induce tumor shrinkage and possible sterilization of the surgical, which was extensively contaminated due to unplanned excisions and debridements [7].

(e) Wide surgical margins should be obtained at all costs.
(f) Reconstructive surgeries for tissue defects reconstruction and to decrease the likelihood of infections include vascularized or rotational local flap coverage and skin grafts.
(g) Vacuum-assisted closure (VAC) has been used to manage nearly every type of wound seen in orthopedic field [8].
(h) Chemotherapy may be given according to the grade and size of the tumor. The decision is made based on a multidisciplinary team meeting.

34.6 Basic Principles

(a) The plane of dissection is established based on MRI views obtained both before and after preoperative radiotherapy.
(b) Unfortunately, there is no highly reliable preoperative tool to specify the real extent of the surgical margin and contaminated area. The timing of the MRI is important; carried out too early following the IE it will show postoperative oedema/hemorrhage, and carried out too late it may delay re-excision. The optimum timing is thus probably between 4 and 8 weeks following the IE.
(c) The anatomical barriers have a critical role to guide the extent of the resection. We tend to include anatomical barriers like fascia, periosteum, capsule, ligaments, and even bone to the re-excision specimen when deemed necessary to achieve clean and wide surgical margins [5].
(d) Reconstruction should preserve the optimal postoperative function but should not deter the surgeon from achieving wide surgical margins.
(e) Feeling and gentle palpation of the tumor is crucial to disruption of the integrity of the pseudo capsule of the residual tumor.
(f) During re-excision, evaluation of the surgical margins should be evaluated repeatedly. Oedematous, reactive, or degenerative changes can modify the surgical planes. During any suspicion, repeated frozen pathology examination is advised.
(g) Tumor resection with clear margins increases the value of the resection giving "1" point. Preserving limb makes "10," functional limb "100," and good cosmetic view makes it "1000." If we fail to obtain negative margins, all the job means "0" points that makes waste all the previous reconstruction efforts as stated by Özger et al. [9].

34.7 Intraoperative Images

34.8 Technical Pearls

(a) There should be no compromise to achieve wide margins. Otherwise, amputation should be done.
(b) Soft tissue coverage is of utmost importance for prevention of infection and optimal clinical outcome.
(c) Multidisciplinary planning is very important for both medical and surgical treatments of the patients.

34.9 Avoiding and Managing Problems

(a) Increased awareness among orthopedic surgeons about unplanned excision of mass lesions which turn out to be sarcomas will likely decrease the need for re-excisions and their added morbidity.
(b) The pathology results at outside the sarcoma referral centers can be misleading due to lack of experience. Histological slides need to be reevaluated by an experienced musculoskeletal pathologist.
(c) In unplanned excision, radiotherapy alone is not sufficient to achieve local control and decrease local recurrence.
(d) MRI has moderate sensitivity and fairly high specificity in showing residual suggested by a recent meta-analysis [10].
(e) Inadvertent excision of lumps which turn out to be sarcomas is not uncommon.
(f) Imaging has a limited role in detecting microscopic residual disease but can show the extent of the previous surgical field.
(g) Standard treatment is wide re-excision, usually combined with radiotherapy.
(h) Residual tumor is found in an average of 50% of reported cases.
(i) The presence of residual disease is an adverse prognostic factor.
(j) All lumps bigger than a golf ball should have a diagnosis prior to excision [5].

References

1. Stiller CA, Trama A, Brewster DH, Verne J, Bouchardy C, Navarro C, Chirlaque MD, Marcos-Gragera R, Visser O, Serraino D, Weiderpass E, Dei Tos AP, Ascoli V, RARECARE Working Group. Descriptive epidemiology of Kaposi sarcoma in Europe. Report from the RARECARE project. Cancer Epidemiol. 2014;38(6):670–8. https://doi.org/10.1016/j.canep.2014.09.009. Epub 2014 Oct 22. PMID: 25454979.

2. Katz D, Palmerini E, Pollack SM. More than 50 subtypes of soft tissue sarcoma: paving the path for histology-driven treatments. Am Soc Clin Oncol Educ Book. 2018;38:925–38. https://doi.org/10.1200/EDBK_205423. PMID: 30231352
3. Melis AS, Vos M, Schuurman MS, van Dalen T, van Houdt WJ, van der Hage JA, Schrage YM, Been LB, Bonenkamp JB, Bemelmans MHA, Grünhagen DJ, Verhoef C, VKY H, Dutch Sarcoma Group (DSG). Incidence of unplanned excisions of soft tissue sarcomas in The Netherlands: a population-based study. Eur J Surg Oncol. 2022;48(5):994–1000. https://doi.org/10.1016/j.ejso.2021.11.123. Epub 2021 Nov 19. PMID: 34848102.
4. Traub F, Griffin AM, Wunder JS, Ferguson PC. Influence of unplanned excisions on the outcomes of patients with stage III extremity soft-tissue sarcoma. Cancer. 2018;124(19):3868–75. https://doi.org/10.1002/cncr.31648. Epub 2018 Oct 15. PMID: 30321451.
5. Grimer R, Parry M, James S. Inadvertent excision of malignant soft tissue tumours. EFORT Open Rev. 2019;4(6):321–9. https://doi.org/10.1302/2058-5241.4.180060. PMID: 31312520; PMCID: PMC6598609.
6. Levy A, Honoré C, Dumont S, Bourdais R, Cavalcanti A, Faron M, Ngo C, Haddag-Miliani L, Le Cesne A, Mir O, Le Péchoux C. Radiothérapie préopératoire versus postopératoire dans les sarcomes des tissus mous: état des lieux et perspectives [Preoperative versus postoperative radiotherapy in soft tissue sarcomas: state of the art and perspectives]. Bull Cancer. 2021;108(9):868–76. https://doi.org/10.1016/j.bulcan.2021.03.012. French. Epub 2021 Jul 8. PMID: 34246458.
7. Salduz A, Alpan B, Valiyev N, Özmen E, İribaş A, Ağaoğlu F, Bayram A, Bilgiç B, Özger H. Neoadjuvant radiotherapy for myxoid liposarcomas: Oncologic outcomes and histopathologic correlations. Acta Orthop Traumatol Turc. 2017;51(5):355–61. https://doi.org/10.1016/j.aott.2017.03.009. Epub 2017 Aug 30. PMID: 28869066; PMCID: PMC6197565.
8. Fourman MS, Ramsey DC, Kleiner J, Daud A, Newman ET, Schwab JH, Chen YL, DeLaney TF, Mullen JT, Raskin KA, Lozano-Calderón SA. Temporizing wound VAC dressing until final negative margins are achieved reduces myxofibrosarcoma local recurrence. Ann Surg Oncol. 2021;28(13):9171–6. https://doi.org/10.1245/s10434-021-10242-4. Epub 2021 Jun 18. PMID: 34143336.
9. Özger H, Alpan B. When and why biological/implant reconstruction? In: Özger H, Sim FH, Puri A, Eralp L, editors. Orthopedic surgical oncology for bone tumors. Cham: Springer; 2022. https://doi.org/10.1007/978-3-030-73327-8_1.
10. Kwee RM, Kwee TC. Diagnostic performance of MRI in detecting residual soft tissue sarcoma after unplanned excision: systematic review and meta-analysis. Eur J Radiol. 2021;145:110049. https://doi.org/10.1016/j.ejrad.2021.110049. Epub 2021 Nov 16. PMID: 34801876.

Undifferentiated Pleomorphic Sarcoma: Management of Recurrent Chest Wall Mass

35

Claire Park, Yazan Kadkoy, Joseph Ippolito, Edward Lee, and Joseph Benevenia

35.1 Introduction

Undifferentiated pleomorphic sarcoma (UPS) is a malignant soft tissue neoplasm; while originally named malignant fibrous histiocytoma, UPS was reclassified in 2002 by the WHO due to histopathological determinations [1, 2]. While this tumor can be found anywhere in the body, it has a high predilection for the extremities followed by the trunk and usually presents clinically as a large, painless solid mass. These malignant lesions generally feature a pseudocapsule covering internal areas of hemorrhage or necrosis. UPS carries a high risk for recurrence or metastases with about one-third of resected masses experiencing such complications in a 5-year period [3]. Initial management consists of appropriate staging with imaging and biopsy to confirm diagnosis, followed by wide resection with or without systemic chemotherapy. With over one-third of UPS tumors recurring or metastasizing within 5 years, UPS is treated with wide surgical excision in combination with radiation therapy [4]. The addition of chemotherapy is used in selected cases.

35.2 Brief Clinical History

A 59-year-old male initially presented with a nontender, firm, left posterior flank mass with a well-defined edge distal to his left scapula for 1 month. MRI revealed an 8 × 8 × 5-cm heterogenous mass surrounded by edema deep to the latissimus dorsi. PET-CT indicated no evidence of metastatic lesions. The patient was neurovascularly intact and exhibited a full range of motion without any complaints of pain. Biopsy identified the mass as a high-grade pleomorphic undifferentiated sarcoma with myxoid features.

Initial surgical management consisted of wide surgical resection with confirmed negative margins, as well as adjuvant brachytherapy. At his 7-month post-operative follow up, imaging identified a recurrent mass (4 × 2.2 × 1.1-cm) of his left flank and chest wall with involvement of the adjacent intercostal musculature and no evidence of rib invasion. Biopsy confirmed this mass was a recurrent lesion. This was managed initially with neoadjuvant chemotherapy and wide resection of the left chest wall with portions of the seventh, eighth, and ninth ribs. Reconstruction was performed with musculoskeletal oncology, cardiothoracic surgery, and plastic surgery. At the 10-year follow-up, the patient had no evidence of disease.

35.3 Preoperative Local Imaging

PET/CT depicting recurrent mass in left lateral lower chest wall (Fig. 35.1).

Axial (Figs. 35.2 and 35.3) and Coronal (Fig. 35.4) MRI showing recurrent mass in left chest wall.

C. Park
Rutgers New Jersey Medical School, Newark, NJ, USA
e-mail: cp906@njms.rutgers.edu

Y. Kadkoy · J. Ippolito · J. Benevenia (✉)
Department of Orthopaedics, Rutgers New Jersey Medical School, Newark, NJ, USA
e-mail: yk399@njms.rutgers.edu; ippolija@njms.rutgers.edu; benevejo@njms.rutgers.edu

E. Lee
Department of Plastic Surgery, Rutgers New Jersey Medical School, Newark, NJ, USA
e-mail: leee9@njms.rutgers.edu

H. Özger et al. (eds.), *Diagnosis and Treatment of Soft Tissue Tumors*, https://doi.org/10.1007/978-3-031-77061-6_35

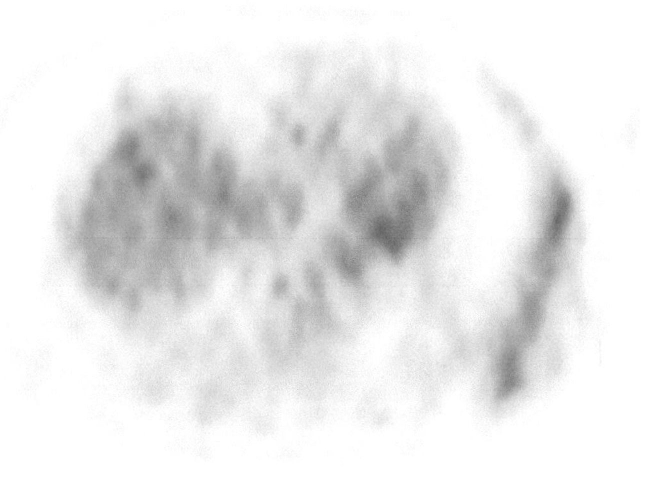

Fig. 35.1 PET/CT. The PET/CT scan shows a recurrent mass located in the left lateral lower chest wall

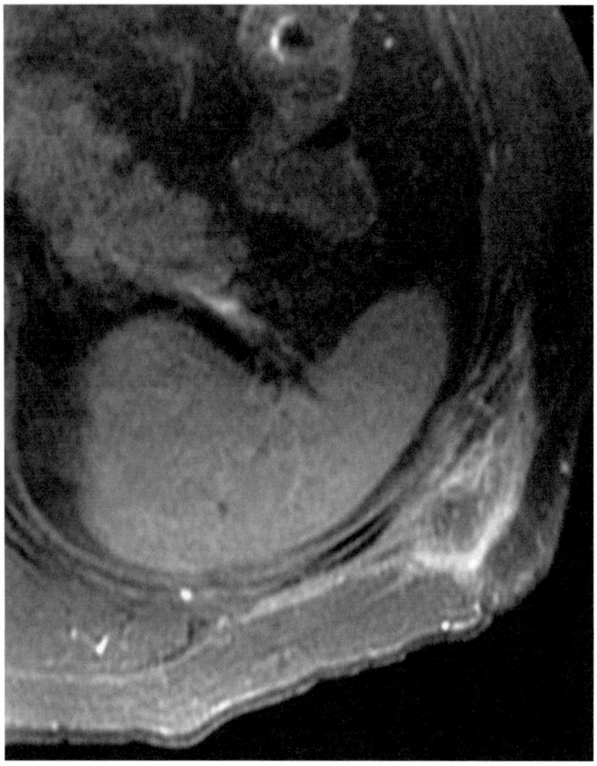

Fig. 35.2 Axial MRI. This axial MRI image illustrates the presence of a recurrent mass in the left chest wall

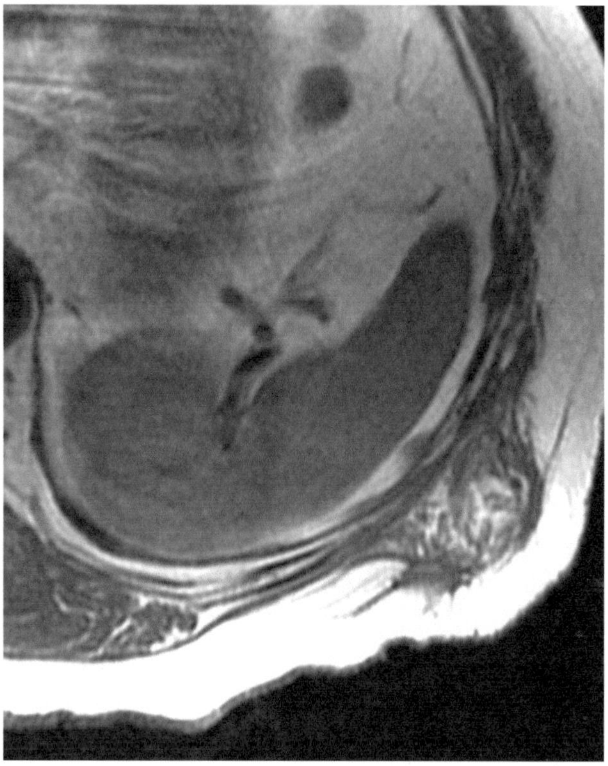

Fig. 35.3 Axial MRI. Another axial MRI image highlighting the recurrent mass in the left chest wall

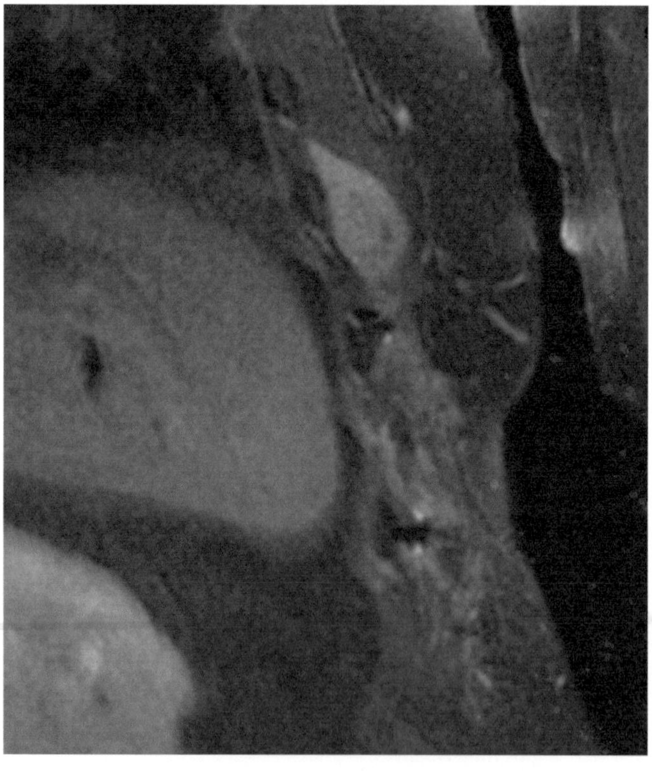

Fig. 35.4 Coronal MRI. This coronal MRI offers a different plane of visualization, displaying the recurrent mass in the left chest wall

35.4 Preoperative Problem List

- Recurrent undifferentiated pleomorphic sarcoma of the left flank and chest wall 1 year after treatment with wide resection, latissimus dorsi flap, and adjuvant brachytherapy.
- Complicated presentation due to involvement of contiguous intercostal muscles requiring rib resection and subsequent chest wall reconstruction.
- Proximity of left lung and hemithorax requiring thoracic surgical and anesthetic expertise.

35.5 Treatment Strategy

- Preoperative imaging is necessary in guiding optimal treatment strategy.
  - Local MRI and CT imaging delineate the extent of regional soft tissue and bony involvement (skip lesions), respectively.
  - Whole-body PET/CT evaluates the presence of regional and distant metastases, which in this case there were none.
- En bloc surgical resection with wide margins (2–5 cm) is the mainstay treatment modality of UPS with local control being the primary goal of management.
- Adjuvant radiation therapy is indicated with intermediate and high-grade tumors (II–III) or those with positive surgical margins (R1–R2), given the tumor's high propensity to locally recur.
  - Decision to employ systemic chemotherapy and local radiation involves (1) the tumor's anatomic location, including its proximity to vital neurovascular structures and organs and (2) consideration of whether the tumor is primary or recurrent.
  - In initial management, radiotherapy was given after successful wide resection with negative margins due to the tumor's high-grade (III). Adjuvant local brachytherapy was selected as the best option for this patient due to the tumor's localized nature, negative surgical margins, and proximity to the lungs. Given the risk of UPS recurrence, interstitial radiotherapy avoided the risk of pneumonitis and pulmonary fibrosis associated with external beam radiotherapy.
  - Despite negative margins after wide surgical resection with adjuvant brachytherapy, there was a local recurrence 7 months later, necessitating more extensive treatment with external beam radiation therapy.
- Neoadjuvant chemotherapy for UPS is reserved for specific cases (e.g., surgically unresectable, metastases, recurrent).
  - Due to the recurrent and locally aggressive nature of this tumor, the patient received three cycles of Adriamycin-based chemo prior to surgical resection.
- Reconstruction for wound coverage and structural stability depends on the extent of resection.
  - Multidisciplinary collaboration with cardiothoracic and plastic surgery is essential in complicated reconstructions of the chest wall to ensure optimal chest wall stabilization and adequate soft tissue coverage.
  - Initially, a latissimus dorsi bipedicle flap provided full-thickness coverage as part of the soft tissue reconstruction of the index surgery. However, preoperative imaging of the recurrent mass demonstrated that the tumor extended into the remaining latissimus dorsi as well as the undersurface of the eighth rib. To appropriately achieve wide enough margins, the remaining latissimus dorsi had to be resected with the posterolateral portions of the seventh, eighth, and ninth ribs.
  - Extensive chest wall resection of three adjacent ribs required utilizing osteosynthesis rib plating, biologic mesh, as well as serratus and external oblique muscle flaps for appropriate reconstruction.

35.6 Basic Principles

- Preoperative planning with imaging studies is crucial in (1) identifying the need for neoadjuvant or adjuvant treatments and (2) determining the best surgical approach. Surgical resection involves an amalgamation of variables including avoidance of vital neurovascular structures and organs, complete excision of the biopsy tract, wide margins, and adequate soft tissue coverage. In this patient, infiltration of the chest wall required especially careful attention to adequately prepare for reconstruction.
- For this case, an oval-shaped, oblique incision over the left flank was made to include the site of the original brachy catheters and biopsy tract.
- At the time of en bloc resection, margins are evaluated by frozen section. Following confirmation of negative margins, reconstruction can be initiated.
- Chest wall reconstruction aims at achieving sufficient chest wall stability without respiratory impairment while providing adequate tissue coverage. This is usually accomplished with mesh (prosthetic or biologic) and/or myocutaneous flaps. With a larger than 5-cm resection of at least two adjacent ribs or lateral rib resection, further structural support such as with rib plating becomes necessary for further support and to avoid paradoxical chest movement [5, 6].
- To minimize postoperative wound complications, the resected area is thoroughly irrigated with antibiotics in addition to maintaining intraoperative IV antibiotics.
- Pedicled muscle flaps provide optimal soft tissue coverage of the titanium rib plating.

  - In this patient, the latissimus dorsi had to be resected so the serratus and external oblique muscles were chosen to fully cover the rib plates.
- Adequate hemostasis must be achieved followed by JP drain placement and multilayered skin closure.
- Early mobilization is recommended in patients after surgery.

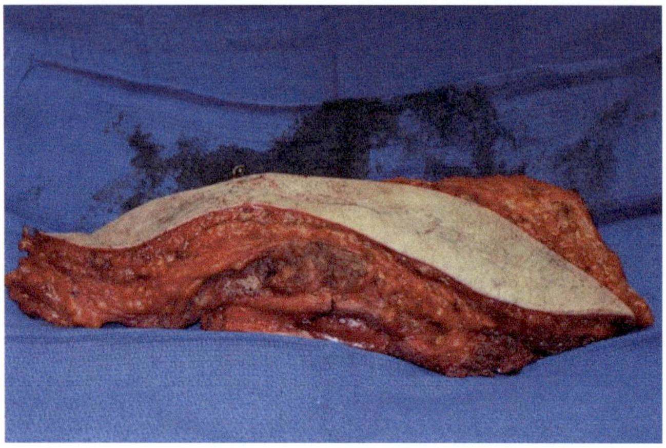

Fig. 35.5 Recurrent en bloc tumor resection. The surgical specimen includes a recurrent tumor mass resected en bloc along with sections of the seventh to ninth ribs, demonstrating the extent of involvement and the necessity for comprehensive surgical margins to ensure complete removal of malignant tissue

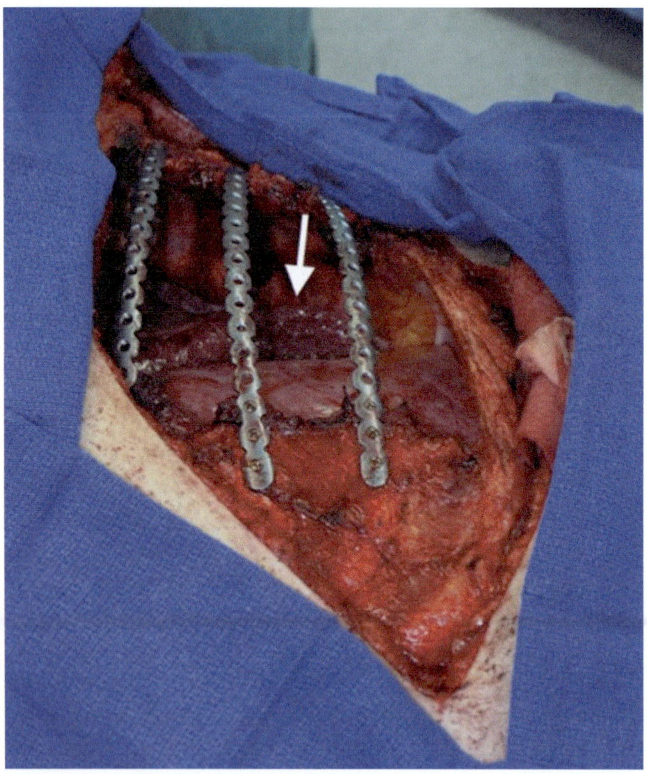

Fig. 35.6 Subsequent chest wall reconstruction with rib plating and deflated lung. The image shows the chest wall reconstruction process using rib plating. The white arrow indicates the deflated lung, highlighting the critical steps in ensuring structural integrity and lung protection during the procedure

35.7 Intraoperative Image

The recurrent en bloc tumor resection with attached portions of the seventh to ninth ribs (Fig. 35.5).

The subsequent chest wall reconstruction with rib plating (with deflated lung in Fig. 35.6 white arrow, with mesh in Fig. 35.7).

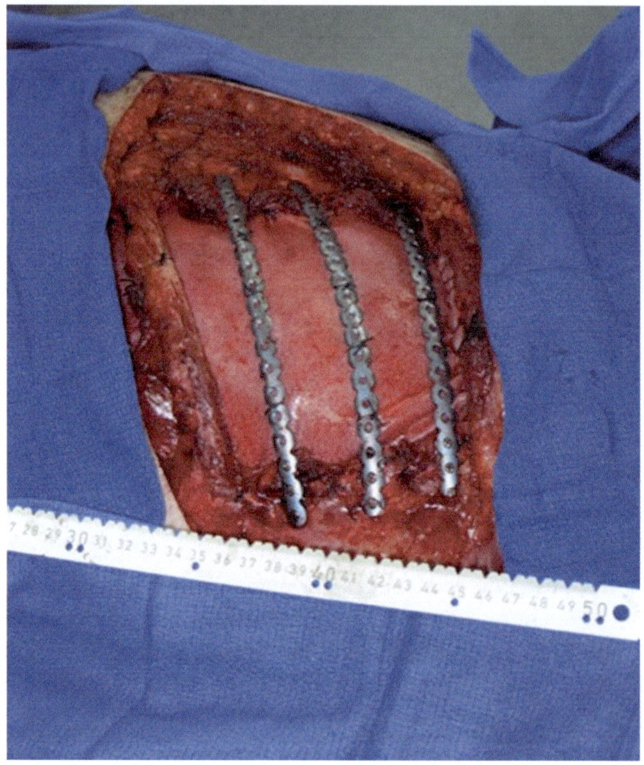

Fig. 35.7 Subsequent chest wall reconstruction with mesh. This figure demonstrates the use of mesh in the chest wall reconstruction process, providing additional support and stability to the reconstructed area following extensive tumor resection and rib plating

35.8 Technical Pearls

- Undifferentiated pleomorphic sarcoma has high rates of local recurrence (25–75%) and metastases making en bloc surgical resection with wide margins the main treatment method [7–15].
- In the event of contaminated margins or unrecognized microscopically positive margins, adjuvant radiotherapy has been shown to be beneficial at minimizing the rate of local recurrence. It is imperative to be judicious when selecting the type of radiotherapy—taking into consideration the tumor's anatomic location and surrounding structures and metastases.
  - In locally aggressive tumor presentations such as this where local recurrence is known to be highly likely, radiotherapy selection should also anticipate a future complication and need for additional treatment. In such cases, preference should be given to more localized forms of radiation like brachytherapy to minimize the extent of soft tissue and organ damage associated with systemic radiotherapy.
- When approaching resection of a chest wall sarcoma, it is imperative to prepare for possible intraoperative or postoperative complications due to the proximity of the lungs. In cases such as this where the mass has invaded intercostal muscles, lung isolation utilizing a double-lumen endotracheal tube is required to visualize margins and safely access the tumor. By creating better access, potential complications such as pneumothorax can be avoided.
- Large thoracic masses require thoughtful multidisciplinary surgical planning to ensure appropriate chest wall stabilization. Involvement of the thoracic team is often necessary.
  - Thoracostomy is placed to reestablish negative pressure in the pleural cavity and avoid pulmonary complications (e.g., hemothorax and pneumothorax).
- Even with wide resection and local radiotherapy, local recurrence can still be seen at a rate of 18–32%, usually within 18–24 months [8, 15–19]. The recurrence risk of UPS is significantly associated with masses greater than 5 cm, deeper than subcutaneous fat, higher grades, and when presented at older ages [14, 15]. Therefore, despite appropriate surgical and medical management, follow-up visits with imaging studies in stage II–IV tumors are essential to detect local recurrences as soon as possible.

35.9 Outcome Radiographs and Images

X-ray showing radical resection of recurrent chest wall sarcoma with excision of portions of the seventh to ninth left ribs followed by plate reconstruction (Fig. 35.8—AP; Fig. 35.9—Lateral).

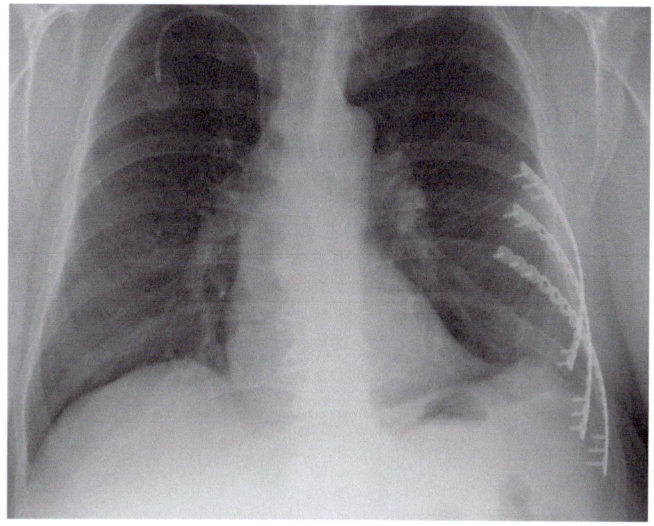

Fig. 35.8 Anteroposterior (AP) X-ray. The postoperative AP X-ray image illustrates the extensive surgical resection of a recurrent chest wall sarcoma, including the excision of portions of the seventh to ninth left ribs, and the subsequent plate reconstruction to restore structural integrity

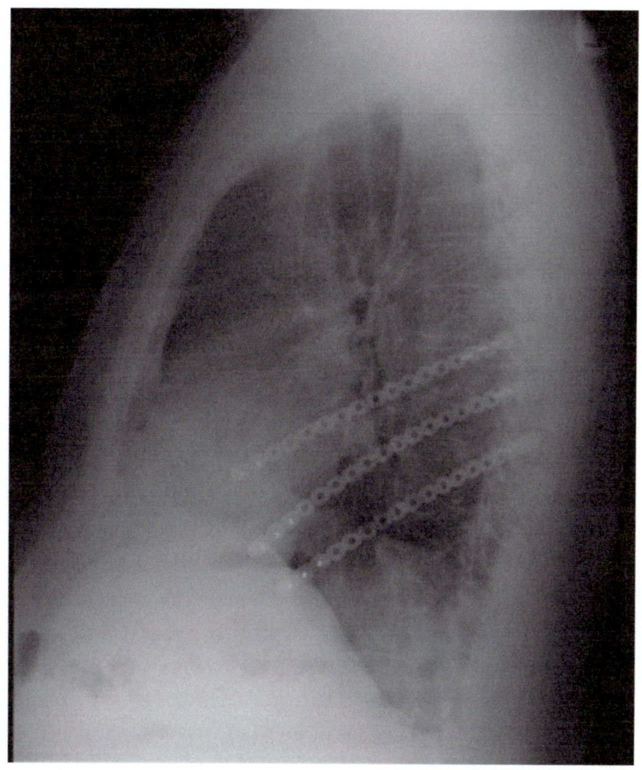

Fig. 35.9 Lateral X-ray. The postoperative lateral X-ray image provides a side view of the radical resection and reconstruction, highlighting the spatial arrangement and positioning of the plates used

35.10 Avoiding and Managing Problems

- Judicious use of flaps and skin grafts helps prevent wound complications such as skin necrosis and infection.
- To minimize risk of infection and promote granulation tissue production, vacuum-assisted closure is a useful method for postoperative wound management.
- Soft tissue sarcomas generally have a high potential for tumor seeding, especially in cases with locally aggressive tumors such as UPS. Careful postoperative surveillance of the thoracic cavity is recommended.
  - To minimize risk of local recurrence, precautionary measures to prevent intraoperative tumor spillage must be taken, and adjuvant radiation should be highly considered [18].
  - The location of the mass, size (>5 cm), depth of tumor invasion, tumor grade, and presence of narrow or positive surgical margins have been shown to be significant prognostic factors in cases of recurrence or metastases [14, 15].
- With aggressive tumors that may invade adjacent ribs, interdisciplinary involvement with cardiothoracic surgery can help avoid complications such as a pneumothorax or lung hernia by preparing for possible need for lung isolation to gain adequate surgical access and proper planning for optimal chest wall reconstruction when indicated.
- Most major complications with chest wall reconstruction include infection, respiratory deficits, restricted shoulder range of motion, and inadequate chest wall rigidity (e.g., hernias) [20–22]. Steps can be taken to mitigate complication development, including timely intraoperative debridement, coverage of major structural deficits with flaps and/or grafts, and chest stabilization. This patient initially experienced mild left shoulder stiffness at their 10-month postoperative visit, likely secondary to capsular contracture. With appropriate physical therapy and shoulder-strengthening exercises, the patient recovered with full range of motion. At their 16-month postoperative visit, patient complained of an intermittent pain in the anterior aspect of their left chest that improved over time.
- Similar to postoperative care after other major thoracic surgeries, patients should be encouraged to mobilize early and utilize respiratory treatments (e.g., incentive spirometry) to avoid atelectasis and other pulmonary complications [23].
- Pharmacologic or mechanical interventions for anticoagulation should be implemented to avoid the risk of venous thromboembolism.

References

1. Fletcher CD. The evolving classification of soft tissue tumours: an update based on the new WHO classification. Histopathology. 2006;48(1):3–12.
2. Choi JH, Ro JY. The 2020 WHO classification of tumors of soft tissue: selected changes and new entities. Adv Anat Pathol. 2021;28(1):44–58.
3. Chen S, Huang W, Luo P, Cai W, Yang L, Sun Z, et al. Undifferentiated pleomorphic sarcoma: long-term follow-up from a large institution. Cancer Manag Res. 2019;11:10001–9.
4. von Mehren M, Kane JM, Bui MM, Choy E, Connelly M, Dry S, et al. NCCN guidelines insights: soft tissue sarcoma, version 1.2021. J Natl Compr Cancer Netw. 2020;18(12):1604–12.
5. Weyant MJ, Bains MS, Venkatraman E, Downey RJ, Park BJ, Flores RM, et al. Results of chest wall resection and reconstruction with and without rigid prosthesis. Ann Thorac Surg. 2006;81(1):279–85.
6. Aghajanzadeh M, Alavy A, Taskindost M, Pourrasouly Z, Aghajanzadeh G, Massahnia S. Results of chest wall resection and reconstruction in 162 patients with benign and malignant chest wall disease. J Thorac Dis. 2010;2(2):81–5.
7. Weiss SW, Enzinger FM. Malignant fibrous histiocytoma: an analysis of 200 cases. Cancer. 1978;41(6):2250–66.
8. Belal A, Kandil A, Allam A, Khafaga Y, El-Husseiny G, El-Enbaby A, et al. Malignant fibrous histiocytoma: a retrospective study of 109 cases. Am J Clin Oncol. 2002;25(1):16–22.
9. Delisca GO, Mesko NW, Alamanda VK, Archer KR, Song Y, Halpern JL, et al. MFH and high-grade undifferentiated pleomorphic sarcoma-what's in a name? J Surg Oncol. 2015;111(2):173–7.
10. Vodanovich DA, Spelman T, May D, Slavin J, Choong PFM. Predicting the prognosis of undifferentiated pleomorphic soft tissue sarcoma: a 20-year experience of 266 cases. ANZ J Surg. 2019;89(9):1045–50.
11. Wang Z, Liu J, Han J, Yang Z, Wang Q. Analysis of prognostic factors of undifferentiated pleomorphic sarcoma and construction and validation of a prediction nomogram based on SEER database. Eur J Med Res. 2022;27(1):179.
12. Henderson MT, Hollmig ST. Malignant fibrous histiocytoma: changing perceptions and management challenges. J Am Acad Dermatol. 2012;67(6):1335–41.
13. Eckert H. Demonstration of phospholipids (including surfactant lipids) by light microscopy. Z Erkr Atmungsorgane. 1991;176(2–3):164.
14. Zhang S, Zhang X, Zhao Z, Xu L, Xu S, Liu T, et al. Undifferentiated pleomorphic sarcoma of the extremity and trunk: a retrospective cohort study of 166 cases in a large institution. Transl Cancer Res. 2022;11(4):678–88.
15. Winchester D, Lehman J, Tello T, Chimato N, Hocker T, Kim S, et al. Undifferentiated pleomorphic sarcoma: factors predictive of adverse outcomes. J Am Acad Dermatol. 2018;79(5):853–9.
16. Pisters PW, Harrison LB, Leung DH, Woodruff JM, Casper ES, Brennan MF. Long-term results of a prospective randomized trial of adjuvant brachytherapy in soft tissue sarcoma. J Clin Oncol. 1996;14(3):859–68.
17. Hsu HC, Huang EY, Wang CJ. Treatment results and prognostic factors in patients with malignant fibrous histiocytoma. Acta Oncol. 2004;43(6):530–5.

18. Goertz O, Pieper A, Lohe LV, Stricker I, Dadras M, Behr B, et al. The impact of surgical margins and adjuvant radiotherapy in patients with undifferentiated pleomorphic sarcomas of the extremities: a single-institutional analysis of 192 patients. Cancers (Basel). 2020;12(2):362.
19. Bleckman RF, Acem I, van Praag VM, Dorleijn DMJ, Verhoef C, Schrage YM, et al. Multimodality treatment of undifferentiated pleomorphic soft tissue sarcoma of the extremity (eUPS) in the elderly. Eur J Surg Oncol. 2022;48(5):985–93.
20. Netscher DT, Izaddoost S, Sandvall B. Complications, pitfalls, and outcomes after chest wall reconstruction. Semin Plast Surg. 2011;25(1):86–97.
21. D'Amico G, Manfredi R, Nita G, Poletti P, Milesi L, Livraghi L, et al. Reconstruction of the thoracic wall with biologic mesh after resection for chest wall tumors: a presentation of a case series and original technique. Surg Innov. 2018;25(1):28–36.
22. Khullar OV, Fernandez FG. Prosthetic reconstruction of the chest wall. Thorac Surg Clin. 2017;27(2):201–8.
23. Fowler TT, Taylor BC, Bellino MJ, Althausen PL. Surgical treatment of flail chest and rib fractures. J Am Acad Orthop Surg. 2014;22(12):751–60.

Nonsurgical Management of Desmoid-Type Fibromatosis

36

Hiroyuki Tsuchiya and Akihiko Takeuchi

36.1 Brief Clinical History

Case 1. A 61-year-old female noticed a soft tissue mass around her right shoulder without any known cause. MRI revealed a heterogeneous and irregular margin soft tissue tumor in the trapezius muscle. Needle biopsy proven desmoid-type fibromatosis.

Case 2. A 52-year-old male noticed a soft tissue mass at his left buttock with pain. MRI revealed a heterogeneous and irregular margin soft tissue tumor in the subcutaneous tissue. The tumor invaded to gluteus and erector spinae muscle. Needle biopsy proven desmoid-type fibromatosis.

36.2 Preoperative Radiographs

See Figs. 36.1 and 36.2.

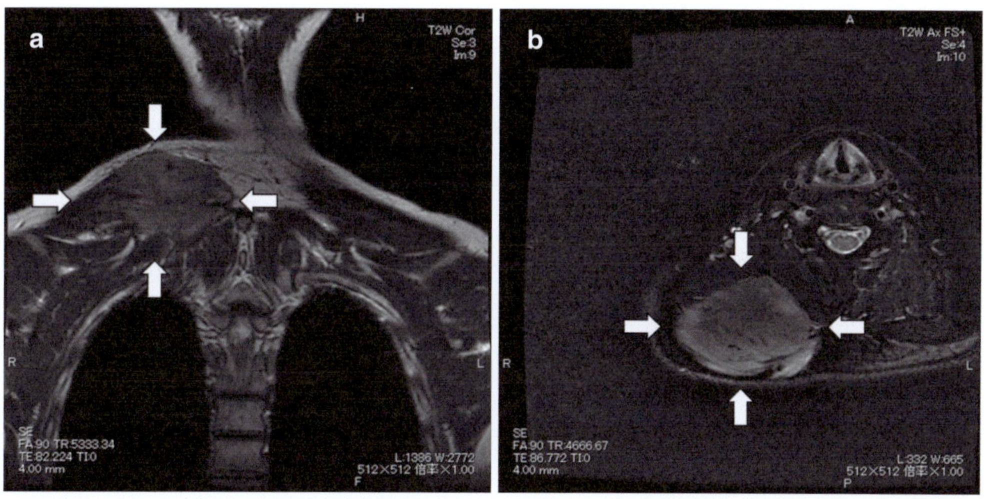

Fig. 36.1 MRI of case 1. Coronal T2-weighted (**a**) and axial short tau inversion recovery (STIR) (**b**) images showed heterogenous high-signal large and irregular margin tumor in her right trapezius muscle

H. Tsuchiya (✉) · A. Takeuchi
Department of Orthopaedic Surgery, Graduate School of Medical Science, Kanazawa University, Kanazawa, Ishikawa, Japan
e-mail: tsuchi@med.kanazawa-u.ac.jp

H. Özger et al. (eds.), *Diagnosis and Treatment of Soft Tissue Tumors*, https://doi.org/10.1007/978-3-031-77061-6_36

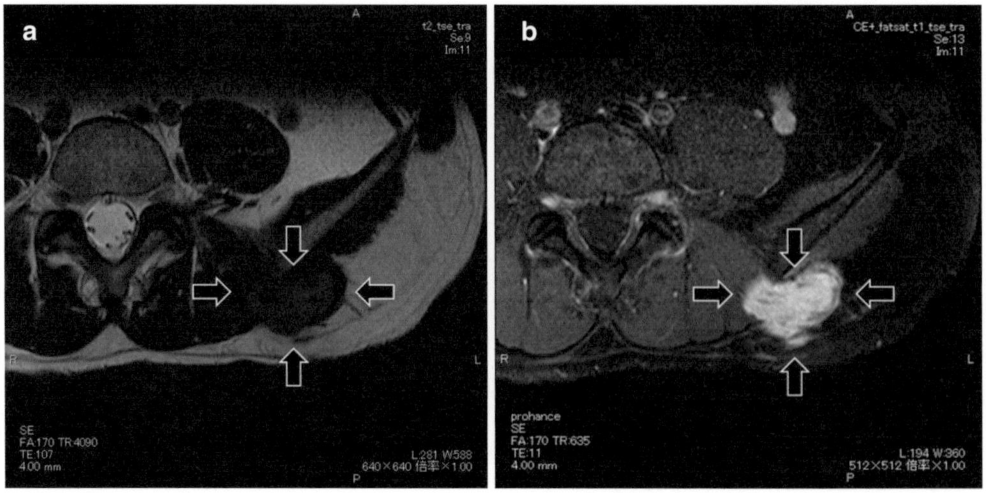

Fig. 36.2 MRI of case 2. Axial T2-weighted (**a**) image showed a heterogenous and slightly high-signal tumor with irregular margins, located on the superficial aspect of posterosuperior iliac spine and between the gluteus maximus and iliocostalis lumborum muscles. Axial contrast-enhanced fat-saturated T1-weighted image (**b**) showed diffuse contrast enhancement and marked irregularity of the borders

36.3 Preoperative Problem List

Case 1. Desmoid-type fibromatosis developed in trapezius muscle without pain.

Case 2. Desmoid-type fibromatosis developed in subcutaneous tissue of buttock with pain.

36.4 Treatment Strategy

Case 1. Active surveillance.

Case 2. Low-dose methotrexate plus vinblastine chemotherapy.

36.5 Basic Principles

Case 1 MRI every 3 months.

Case 2 VBL 6 mg/m^2 and MTX 30 mg/m^2 biweekly.

36.6 Images During Treatment

See Figs. 36.3 and 36.4.

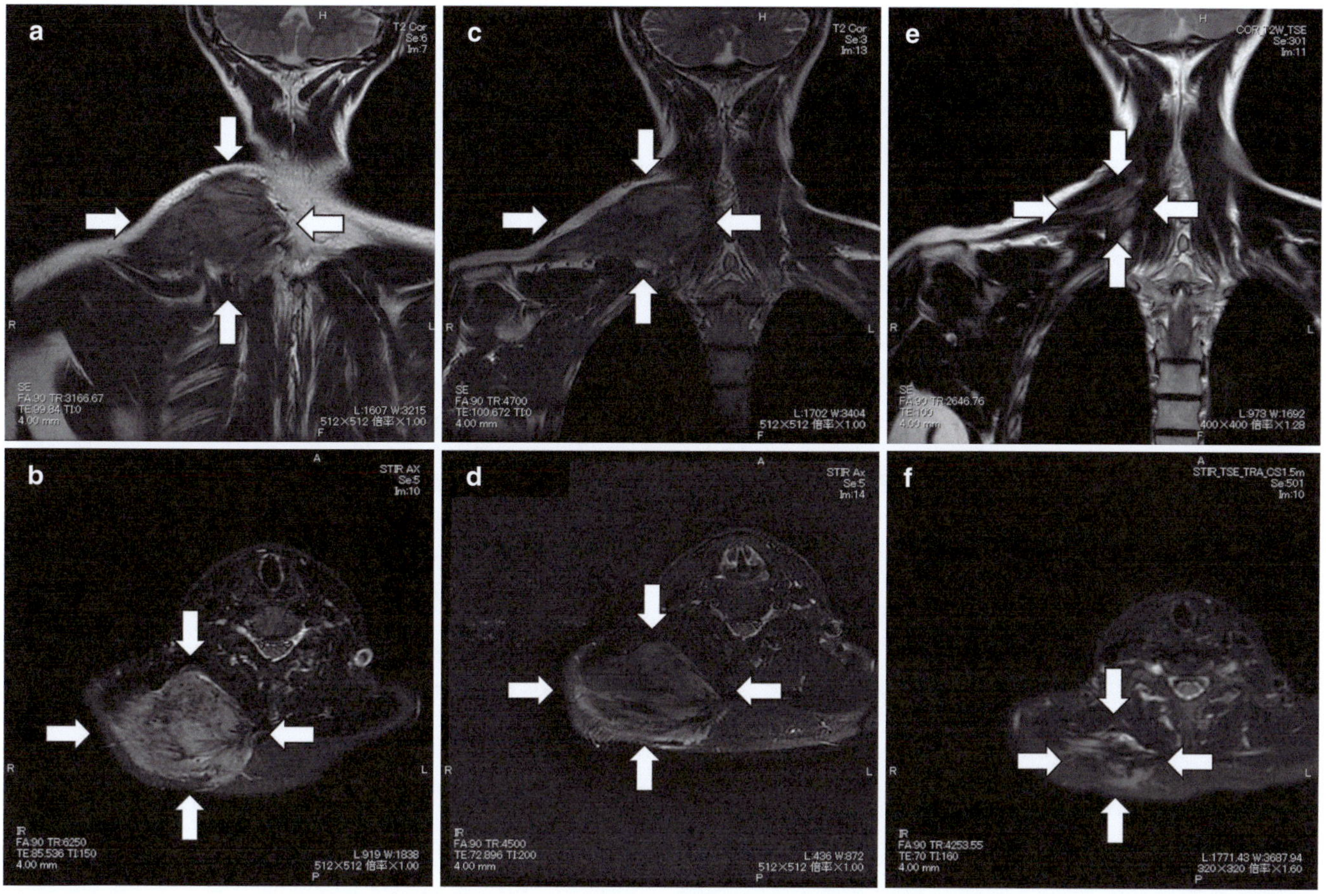

Fig. 36.3 Case 1. Coronal T2-weighted (**a**) and axial STIR (**b**) images in 8 months showed the enlargement of the tumor. Same condition images in 22 months (**c**, **d**) and 43 months (**e**, **f**) showed gradually shrinkage

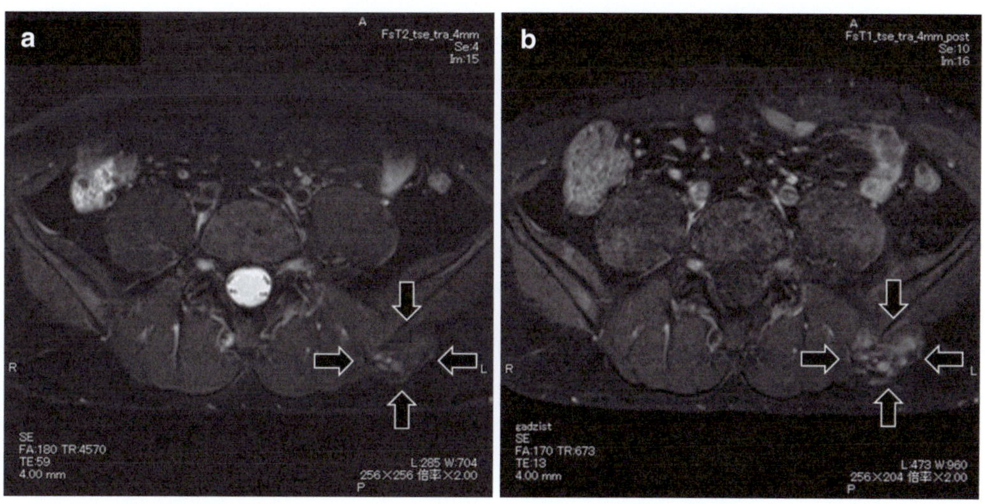

Fig. 36.4 Case 2. Axial STIR (**a**) image in 18 months (after 18 courses of chemotherapy) showed slight shrinkage of the tumor. Gd-enhanced T1-weighted (**b**) images showed markedly decrease of enhancement

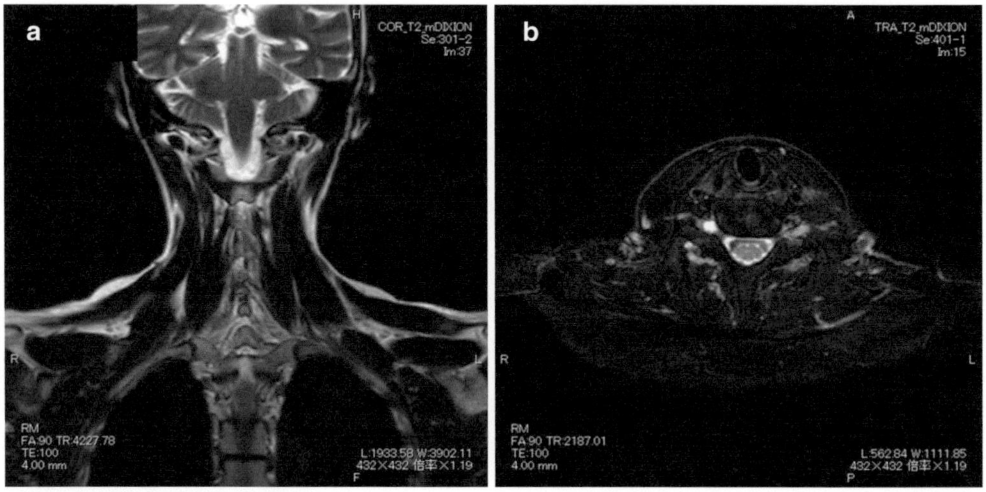

Fig. 36.5 Case 1. Coronal T2-weighted (**a**) and axial STIR (**b**) images in 67 months revealed the disappearance of the tumor

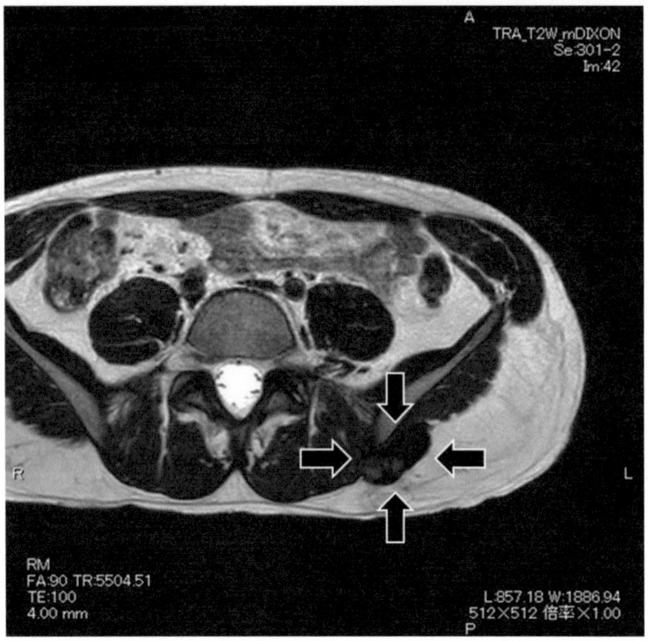

Fig. 36.6 Case 2. Axial T2-weighted image the keeping the size

36.7 Outcome Radiographs

See Figs. 36.5 and 36.6.

36.8 Avoiding and Managing Problems

Active surveillance (Case 1): MRI will be taken within 1–2 months and then extend to 3–6 months intervals. When the tumor enlarges in continuous three examinations, the result will be considered progressive disease based on the RECIST criteria. And the treatment plan will be changed to an active treatment.

Low-dose methotrexate plus vinblastine chemotherapy (Case 2): Adverse effects including liver enzyme elevation (alanine aminotransferase, aspartate aminotransferase, etc) and neutropenia needs to be assessed by a routine blood test [4]. If the patient is unable to tolerate the side effects, the treatment interval needs to be extended. Biweekly administration was reported that the rate of adverse effect was less compared to weekly interval, although the time to obtain a measurable response was longer in biweekly regimen compared to weekly regimen [5].

References

1. Fletcher CDM, Bridge JA, Hogendoorn P, Mertens F. WHO classification of tumours editorial board. Soft tissue and bone tumours. 5th ed. Lyon: IARC Press; 2020. p. 93–5.
2. Desmoid Tumor Working Group. The management of desmoid tumours: a joint global consensus-based guideline approach for adult and paediatric patients. Eur J Cancer. 2020;127:96–107. https://doi.org/10.1016/j.ejca.2019.11.013.
3. Smith K, Desai J, Lazarakis S, Gyorki D. Systematic review of clinical outcomes following various treatment options for patients with extraabdominal desmoid tumors. Ann Surg Oncol. 2018;25(6):1544–54. https://doi.org/10.1245/s10434-018-6408-7. Epub 2018 Apr 11. PMID: 29644533.
4. Toulmonde M, Pulido M, Ray-Coquard I, Andre T, Isambert N, Chevreau C, Penel N, Bompas E, Saada E, Bertucci F, Lebbe C, Le Cesne A, Soulie P, Piperno-Neumann S, Sweet S, Cecchi F, Hembrough T, Bellera C, Kind M, Crombe A, Lucchesi C, Le Loarer F, Blay JY, Italiano A. Pazopanib or methotrexate-vinblastine combination chemotherapy in adult patients with progressive desmoid tumours (DESMOPAZ): a non-comparative, randomised, open-label, multicentre, phase 2 study. Lancet Oncol. 2019;20(9):1263–72. https://doi.org/10.1016/S1470-2045(19)30276-1. Epub 2019 Jul 19. PMID: 31331699.
5. Nishida Y, Hamada S, Urakawa H, Ikuta K, Sakai T, Koike H, Ito K, Emoto R, Ando Y, Matsui S. Desmoid with biweekly methotrexate and vinblastine shows similar effects to weekly administration: a phase II clinical trial. Cancer Sci. 2020;111(11):4187–94. https://doi.org/10.1111/cas.14626. Epub 2020 Sep 5. Erratum in: Cancer Sci. 2021 Aug;112(8):3402. PMID: 32816351; PMCID: PMC7648024.

Wide Excision of a Large Sarcoma of the Pubic Region: Orthoplasty Reconstruction

37

Giuseppe Bianchi and Laura Campanacci

37.1 Introduction

Soft-tissue sarcomas are rare malignant tumors and account for about 2% of all malignancies. Surgery and radiotherapy are the standard treatments and in case of superficial and large neoplasm, a combined ortho-plastic surgical approach may improve oncologic outcomes with better local control and lower incidence of wound complication. We report about a soft tissue sarcoma case with a bulky tumor of the pubic area where combined ortho-plastic surgical approach was successful.

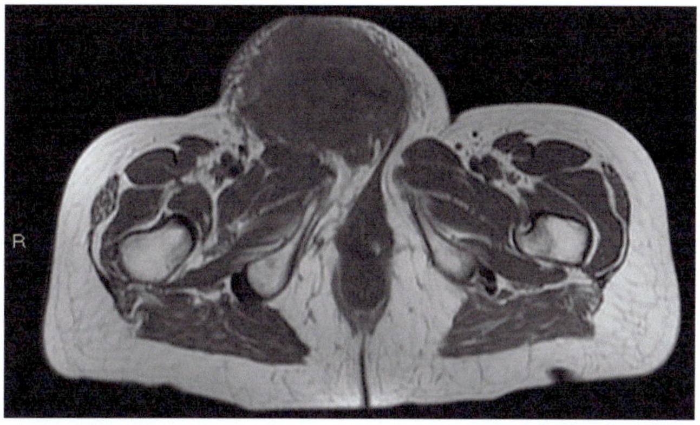

Fig. 37.1 T1-weighted axial MRI—solid subcutaneous mass, low-density signal

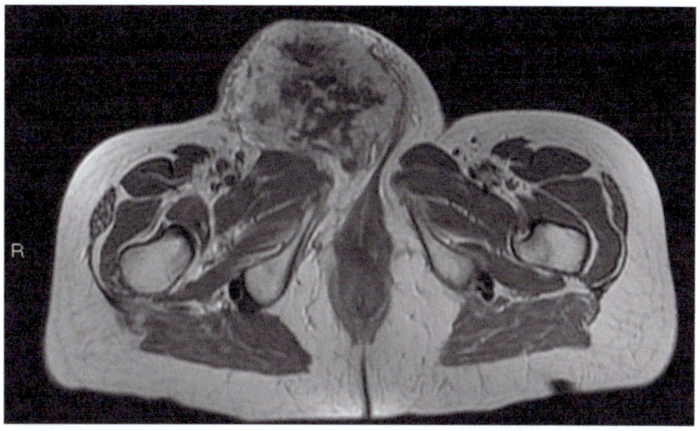

Fig. 37.2 T1-weighted axial MRI + C—solid subcutaneous mass, peripheral increase in density with contrast enhancement and central necrotic area

37.2 Basic Clinical History

A 68-year-old patient presented with a 12 months history of a painless lump of the pubic region with left extension to the right outer labia. No involvement of vaginal entrance or external urethral meatus. No significant disorders in past medical history were reported.

37.3 Preoperative/Pretreatment Clinical and Radiological Images

After a gadolinium-enhanced 1.5 T pelvic MRI (Figs. 37.1, 37.2, and 37.3), showing a necrotic soft tissue mass of 7 × 14 × 10 cm with disomogeneus contrast enhancement, a 14-gauge Tru-cut® needle biopsy was performed; pathologist reported the diagnosis of "proximal large cell type epithelioid sarcoma (SMARCB1-deficient vulvar variant)" [1]. Staging was completed with chest–abdomen–pelvis CT and 18-FDG PET scan (Fig. 37.4) with no local lymph nodes or distant metastases reported [AJCC 8th T3N0M0, Stage IIIB).

G. Bianchi · L. Campanacci (✉)
Oncologic Orthopaedic Clinic, IRCCS Istituto Ortopedico Rizzoli, Bologna, Italy
e-mail: giuseppe.bianchi@ior.it; laura.campanacci@ior.it

H. Özger et al. (eds.), *Diagnosis and Treatment of Soft Tissue Tumors*, https://doi.org/10.1007/978-3-031-77061-6_37

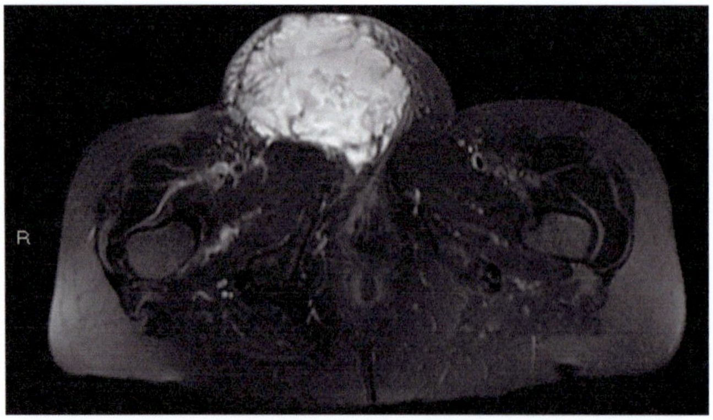

Fig. 37.3 T2 fat sat axial MRI—homogeneous increase of density

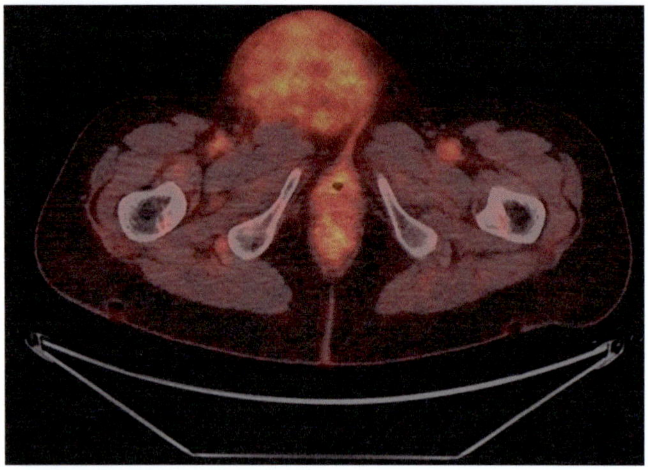

Fig. 37.4 18F-FDG PET/CT showing homogenous increase of 18 fluoro-deoxy-glucose (SUV 8.2)

37.4 Problem List

(a) High-grade localized soft tissue sarcoma with unpredictable course.
(b) Adverse prognostic factors: proximal type epithelioid sarcoma, large size, older age; estimated 5-year overall survival of 65% [2, 3].
(c) Extended en bloc surgical excision, vaginal wall, and external urethral meatus proximity.
(d) Soft tissue coverage and abdominal wall reconstruction.
(e) Toilet hygiene problems: temporary diverting colostomy.

37.5 Treatment Strategy

Systemic chemotherapy provides satisfactory palliation, but response is of short duration and relapse rates remain high despite multimodal therapy [4].

Wide surgical excision in combination with radiotherapy remains the mainstay of treatment [5].

Since the unpredictable response to systemic treatment and the evidence of localized disease, a multidisciplinary surgical team was set up including orthopaedic oncologist, plastic surgeon, and gynecologist. Postoperative radiation was preferred due to the concern of possible skin toxicity and wound-related complication.

37.6 Basic Principles

Patient was placed in supine position given a standard prep and draped free in the usual sterile manner. Lower limbs, external vaginal meatus, and bladder catheter were included in the surgical field.

A circumferential skin incision with 2 cm macroscopic tumor margin, where feasible, was carried out. On the right side, the neurovascular bundle was isolated with saphenous vein ligation at femoral vein junction (Fig. 37.5). Abdominal wall (external obliques, transversus abdominis, internal obliques, rectus abdominis, and pyramidalis) partial resection, subcutaneous dissection of the outer labia, and partial disinsertion of the clitoris were carried out with elevation of the surgical specimen from the right pubic rami after subperiosteal dissection. In the groin, pectineus was sacrificed as inferior tumor-safe margin. A synthetic Gore Dual Mesh® patch was prepared and fixed with nonabsorbable suture to remaining soft tissue to prevent bowel herniation (Fig. 37.6).

A fasciocutaneous anterolateral-thigh (ALT) propeller flap was prepared after subfascial dissection distal and proximal to the ALT harvest area, identifying perforators originating from either the deep femoral system or transverse branch of the lateral circumflex. The pedicled flap was "tunneled" under the superficial fascia of the thigh and rotated freely to cover the groin defect. Abdominoplasty completed the plastic reconstruction with complete coverage of the postsurgical defect (Figs. 37.7 and 37.8).

Pathological reports assessed wide margin excision. After complete wound healing, the patient received postoperative radiotherapy (66 Gy in 33 fr).

37.7 Photos and Imaging During Treatment

See Figs. 37.5, 37.6, 37.7, and 37.8.

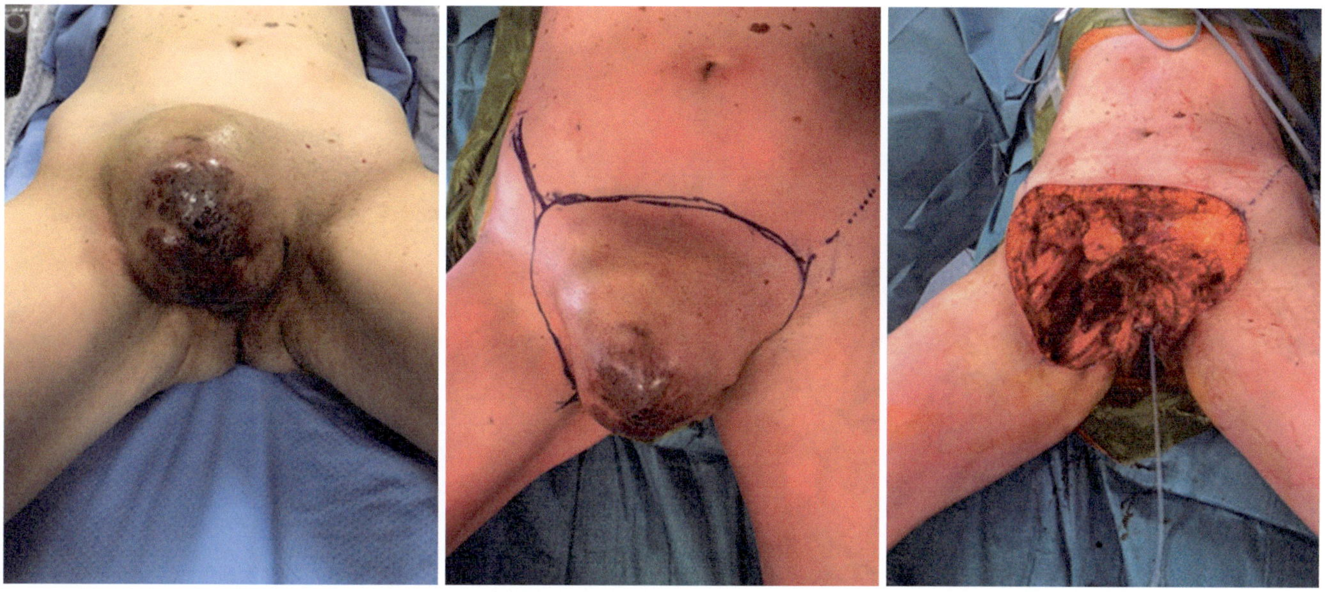

Fig. 37.5 Clinical presentation, skin incision, and surgical bed after tumour excision

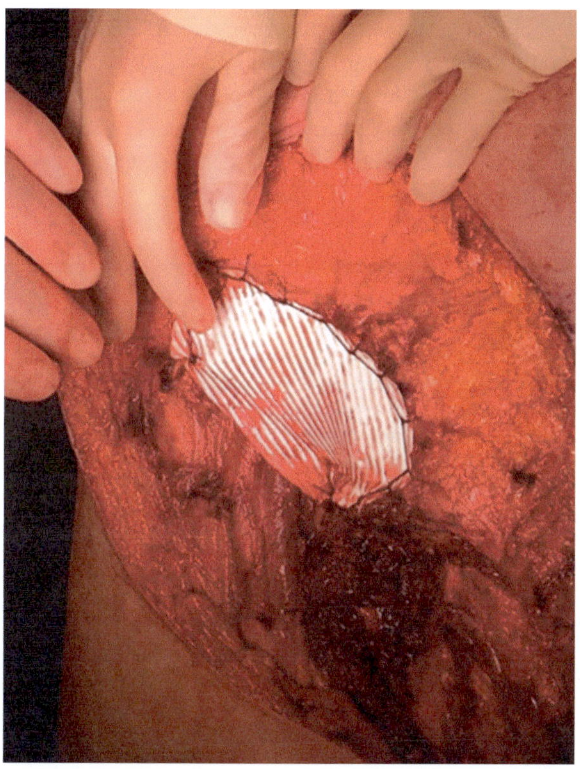

Fig. 37.6 Left abdominal wall repair with synthetic Gore Dual Mesh®

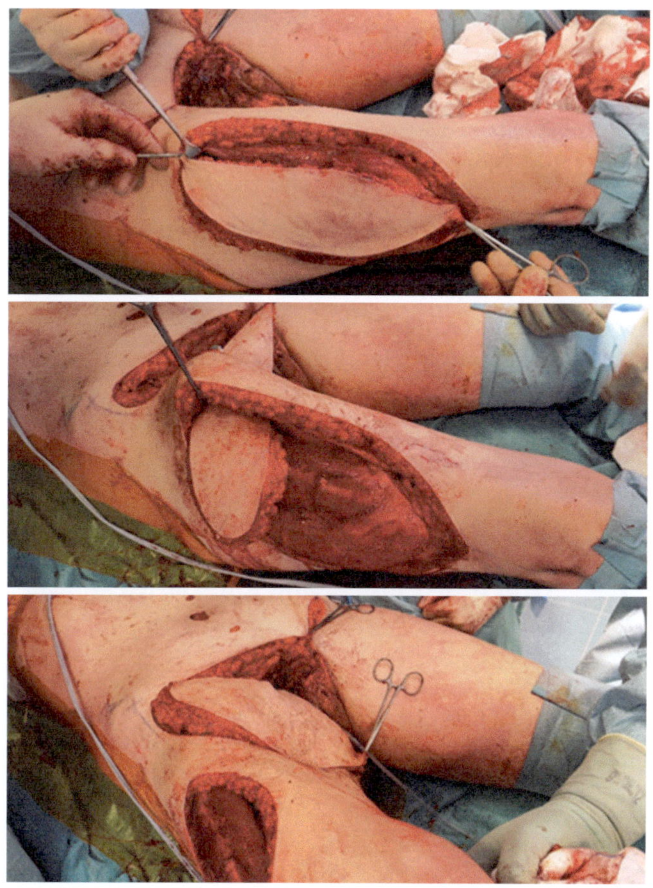

Fig. 37.7 Fasciocutaneous anterolateral-thigh (ALT) propeller flap

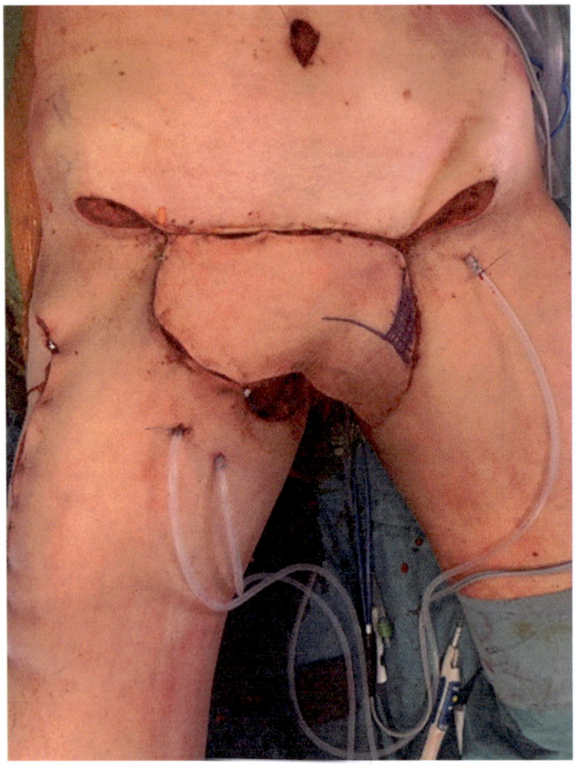

Fig. 37.8 Abdominoplasty

37.8 Technical Pearls

The propeller flap, based on a single vascular pedicle supplying a fasciocutaneous island of skin, is a very useful technique to **reconstruct soft tissue defects** and has wide applications throughout the body.

Precautional temporary diverting colostomy for toilet hygiene problems may be an option; nevertheless such additional surgery might be necessary with potential disadvantages in abdominoplastic procedure and was not considered in this case.

37.9 Outcome Clinical and Radiological Images

At 2 years' follow-up, the patient is continuosly disease free. Late Gore Dual Mesh® infection required minor surgery for partial mesh removal at 18 months (Fig. 37.9).

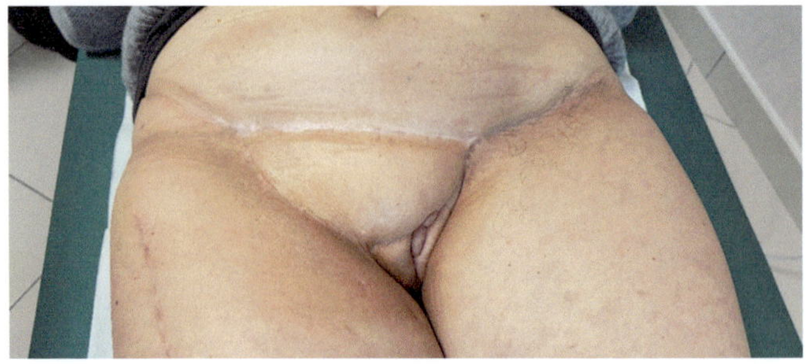

Fig. 37.9 Clinical result at 2 years of follow-up

37.10 Avoiding and Managing Complications

Pelvic girdle and groin soft tissue tumors may imply higher risk of complications due to anatomical site (proximity to GI and GU tracts) and possible extended surgery in case of huge masses. Postoperative lymphedema may occur and increase risk of wound dehiscence.

Preoperative radiotherapy may increase as well the risk of wound complications and postoperative RT should be preferred in case of vascular bypass or pedicled/free flaps.

Synthetic meshes are a good option for abdominal wall reconstruction but risk of infection, even late, may be possible particularly if surgical treatment is associated with radiotherapy.

References

1. Tajima S, et al. A SMARCB1-deficient vulvar neoplasm with prominent myxoid stroma: report of a case showing ERG and FLI1 expression. Int J Clin Exp Pathol. 2015;8(6):7526–32.
2. Hasegawa T, Matsuno Y, Shimoda T, Umeda T, Yokoyama R, Hirohashi S. Proximal-type epithelioid sarcoma: a clinicopathologic study of 20 cases. Mod Pathol. 2001;14(7):655–63. https://doi.org/10.1038/modpathol.3880368. PMID: 11454997.
3. https://www.pathologyoutlines.com/topic/softtissueepithelioidsarcoma.html
4. Thway K, Jones RL, Noujaim J, Fisher C. Epithelioid sarcoma: diagnostic features and genetics. Adv Anat Pathol. 2016;23(1):41–9. https://doi.org/10.1097/PAP.0000000000000102. PMID: 26645461.
5. Wolf PS, Flum DR, Tanas MR, Rubin BP, Mann GN. Epithelioid sarcoma: the University of Washington experience. Am J Surg. 2008;196(3):407–12. https://doi.org/10.1016/j.amjsurg.2007.07.029. Epub 2008 Apr 24. PMID: 18436180.

Limb Salvage with Isolated Limb Perfusion in Soft Tissue Sarcoma

38

Lars Erik Podleska, Arne Streitbürger, and Jendrik Hardes

38.1 Introduction

Soft tissue sarcomas (STS) represent a mixed group of malignancies that are characterized by their mesodermal origin. The most common location of STS is found in the extremities (59%). Resection of the tumor with adequate safety margins remains standard treatment whenever possible. High-grade STS can grow asymptomatically as a painless lump; therefore, deep-seated STSs often tend to be large, locally advanced tumors at the time of diagnosis. In tumors that are considered nonresectable—meaning that adequate safety margins are impossible to achieve without amputation or severe mutilation—a multimodal approach is currently considered standard treatment. Hyperthermic-isolated limb perfusion with TNF-alpha and Melphalan (TM-ILP) is a useful tool in a multidisciplinary treatment regime and is increasingly implemented for the treatment of locally advanced STS in otherwise unsalvageable limbs [1–3]. ILP is often used in a primarily curative intention, if applicable. In these cases, the subsequent resection of the devitalized and residual tumor is an integral part of the treatment concept. Response rates of TM-ILP are reported to range between 60% and 80%, resulting in limb salvage rates above 80%.

38.2 Brief Clinical History

A 67-year-old female presented with a giant, painless swelling in the left thigh. The swelling had been growing in the quadriceps muscle for a few months. The skin over the lesion was slightly reddened. The magnetic resonance imaging (MRI) (see Fig. 38.1) demonstrated a large tissue mass in the quadriceps muscle with inhomogenous contrast enhancement. The lesion had close contact with the ventral part of the femur. The patient did not suffer from any neurovascular deficits and did not show any general symptoms such as weight loss, or clinically apparent signs of infection, except for very high leucocyte counts (50–60/nL) and an elevation of C-reactive protein (CRP) around 12–15 mg/dL. Medical history revealed that the patient had been treated for a chronic myeloid leukemia for about 1 year with Imatinib and Hydroxycarbamide. Additionally, a pulmonary adenocarcinoma of the left lower lobe had been resected (R0-resection) 7 months earlier.

A core-needle biopsy diagnosed the soft tissue mass as a high-grade dedifferentiated liposarcoma with a significant inflammatory component. Staging investigations were negative for distant spread (cT2b N0 M0 G (high-grade)).

The interdisciplinary tumor board suggested a multimodal approach with an initial TNF-alpha and Melphalan-based isolated limb perfusion (TM-ILP), followed by a resection of the residual tumor after 6 weeks and postoperative radiation therapy. After a pre-ILP FDG-PET/CT (Fig. 38.1), the patient received TM-ILP as planned (hospital stay of 15 days). Much to our surprise the leucocyte count and the CRP normalized completely within the first week after TM-ILP. The 6 weeks PET/CT follow-up revealed a good response to ILP with almost complete necrosis of the tumor (Fig. 38.3) so that the resection of the residual tumor was performed 7 weeks after TM-ILP. Pathology revealed a successful R0-resection with close, but intact margins and confirmed the tumor's good response to TM-ILP pretreatment: more than 99% of tumor were devitalized by TM-ILP. After a 2-week stay in the hospital, the patient could be discharged in good general condition, independently mobile. She was advised in detail about the advantages and disadvantages of postoperative radiotherapy, finally decided in favor of it and subsequently received a radiation therapy of the thigh with 60Gy. In the follow-up, she did not develop a local recurrence of the soft tissue sarcoma, but unfortunately, about 3 years after the resection of the residual tumor, she developed a recurrence of her pulmo-

L. E. Podleska · A. Streitbürger · J. Hardes (✉)
Department of Orthopaedic Oncology, Essen University Hospital, Essen, Germany
e-mail: lars.podleska@uk-essen.de; arne.streitbuerger@uk-essen.de; Jendrik.hardes@uk-essen.de

H. Özger et al. (eds.), *Diagnosis and Treatment of Soft Tissue Tumors*, https://doi.org/10.1007/978-3-031-77061-6_38

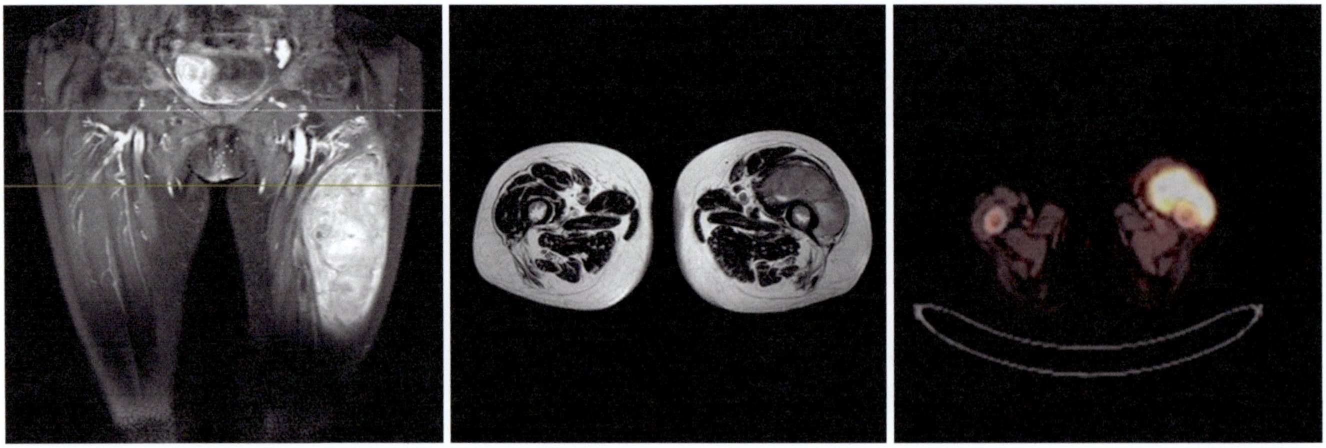

Fig. 38.1 Pre-ILP MRI- and FDG-PET/CT scans of the patient's left thigh. Left: T1 with fat saturation and contrast medium enhancement, middle: T2 in transversal plane, right: Fusion-image of CT and FDG-PET image information. Note the high contrast medium uptake and the high FDG-turnover of the tumor in the thigh's extensor compartment (SUVmax 18.4). Note also that the tumor is surrounding the entire ventral circumference of the femur

nary adenocarcinoma with diffuse metastasis in the lung and pleura, which rapidly lead to palliative treatment.

38.3 Preoperative Problem List

(a) A soft tissue sarcoma with an extensive infiltration of the quadriceps muscle including the extensor apparatus.
(b) Poor functional results can be expected after wide resection.
(c) Broad contact of the sarcoma to the femoral bone. Does the femoral bone have to be partially resected?
(d) Difficult muscle coverage of the femoral bone.
(e) Due to the age and comorbidities of the patient no neoadjuvant chemotherapy is possible.
(f) Close contact to the vessels without surrounding them.

38.4 Treatment Strategy

(a) Interdisciplinary tumor board discussion.
(b) Surgical resection mandatory—with the possibility of a partial resection of the corticalis or even a segmental resection of bone. The decision can often only be made intraoperatively, depending on whether the tumor can be removed from the bone.
(c) Chemotherapy—no benefit of (neo-) adjuvant chemotherapy due to the patient's age and comorbidities.
(d) Radiation therapy—our center's treatment concepts favor adjuvant radiation therapy. In cases of neoadjuvant radiation therapy, we do observe higher rates of disturbance in wound healing.
(e) Isolated limb perfusion with TNF-alpha and Melphalan (TM-ILP) offers the advantage of downstaging the tumor, allowing a better surgical margin to the vessels and especially the bone. Possibly there is no need of a partial or segmental bony resection after ILP.

38.5 Basic Principles

(a) R0-resection is the key factor for local recurrence-free survival. Careful examination of the MRI is necessary to receive information about the possible resection margin. Importantly, osseous involvement can be excluded by MRI. However, as in this case, it is uncertain whether the tumor can be resected with the periosteum as a valid oncological margin. This decision can only be made intraoperatively.
(b) The periosteum could—if it was resectable from the bone intact—serve as an anatomical barrier thus making a close margin tolerable.
(c) A partial bone resection often makes an additional plating or nailing necessary. Thus, in the long term implant failure is a possible complication, especially after additional radiation therapy.
(d) In the case of a segmental resection, the defect reconstruction is often challenging. Regardless of the method chosen for reconstruction (e.g., compound osteosynthesis, intercalary tumor prosthesis), it is associated with a high failure rate (infection, aseptic loosening, and implant failure). Furthermore, we observe a high rate of functional impairment in these patients.
(e) Muscle tissue should be spared to cover the deperiostized bone and to improve leg function (knee extension) as much as oncologically justifiable.
(f) In the present case, a possible downstaging of the tumor would aid to reduce damage or resection of the surrounding muscles and bone.

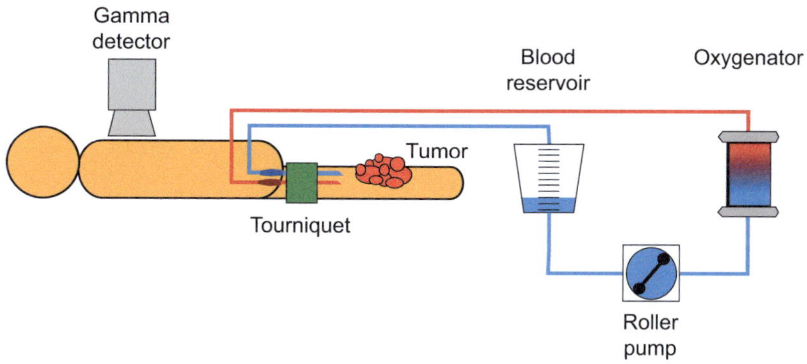

Fig. 38.2 Introperative setup of TM-ILP with a tumor located on the lower extremity, proximal tourniquet, arterial and venous catheters, and the heart-lung machine connected. Note the precordial gamma-detector, which is mandatory for all TNF-based isolated limb perfusions in order to detect any significant leakage from the extremity-circulation

38.6 Intraoperative Images

See Fig. 38.2 for the intraoperative setup of TM-ILP. We use a standard heart-lung-machine with a child-size tubing-system and oxygenator in order to reflect the rather low flow rates of blood (typically between 250 and 450 ml per minute) and keep the dead space volume of the system as low as possible.

38.7 Technical Pearls

(a) Isolated limb perfusion with TNF-alpha and Melphalan (TM-ILP) with mild hyperthermia (39 °C) is performed in general anesthesia in a suitable operating room as follows (see Fig. 38.2):
   1. Vascular access is established above the tumor by cannulation of the artery and vein supplying the extremities using two catheters.
   2. A rubber tourniquet or tourniquet cuff is applied around the extremity proximal to the catheter ends.
   3. Proximally, the catheters are connected to a heart-lung machine.
   4. For the duration of the procedure, the limb is now supplied only by the circulation of the heart-lung machine consisting of a reservoir, pump, and oxygenator.
   5. Installation of a continuous leak rate monitoring (gamma-detector) with Tc-99m applied into the extremity circulation and confirmation of no relevant leakage.
   6. TNF-alpha is applied in a dosage of 1–2 mg into the limb circulation.
   7. After 10–20 min, Melphalan is added to the circulation in a dose of 11–13 mg/L of limb volume.
   8. Perfusion with TNF and Melphalan is maintained for approximately 1 h.
   9. Then the blood, TNF-Melphalan perfusate is washed out from the extremity with 2–6 L of ringer solution.
   10. The tourniquet and the catheters are removed, the vessels and the incision are closed and the patient is transferred to an ICU for a 12-h monitoring period.

(b) TM-ILP facilitates resection of large and non-resectable high-grade soft tissue sarcoma [4].

(c) Response rates to TM-ILP are high and have been repeatedly reported to be above 60%, while limb salvage rates mostly exceed 80% [5].

(d) Although TM-ILP does not primarily result in much tumor shrinkage [6], it appears that TM-ILP can facilitate subsequent tumor resection by stabilizing future resection margins by widening of the fibrous capsule and the reactive zone around the tumor [7].

(e) Quality of life (QoL) after TM-ILP and subsequent tumor resection seems to be rather beneficial. Patients do have some functional impairments, depending on the type of resection, but their overall QoL is comparable to the normal population [8].

(f) Isolated limb perfusion is a rather complex procedure that requires a high expenditure of hospital resources, that is, 4–6 h of operating room time, extensive support from a nuclear medicine department, a heart-lung machine, or a suitable perfusion device. Because of this resource intensity and potential side effects, TM-ILP should be reserved exclusively for patients who would require amputation or severely mutilating tumor resections. These include, for example, resection of bone, large vessels, nerves, or large portions of functionally significant muscle groups. The latter two reasons are of particular importance in forearm tumors. It is precisely for the above reasons that TM-ILP is available in only a few specialized oncology centers.

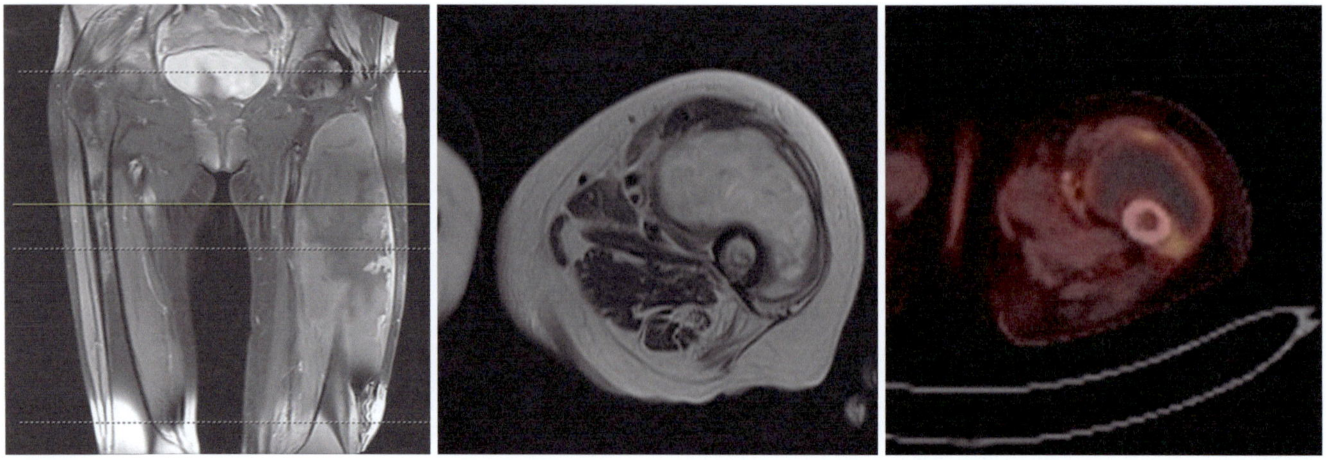

Fig. 38.3 Six weeks post-ILP MRI- and FDG-PET/CT scans. Left: T1 with fat saturation and contrast medium enhancement, middle: T2 in transversal plane, right: Fusion-image of CT and FDG-PET image information. In contrast to the pre-ILP MRI- and PET/CT images note the almost complete disappearance of MRI-contrast medium enhancement (left image) and strong decrease in FDG turnover (right image). SUVmax values decreased from initially 18.8 (before ILP) to 7.9 after ILP. The residual tumor was resected (R0 with close margins). Pathology confirmed the tumor's good response to TM-ILP pretreatment: more than 99% of devitalized tumor

38.8 Outcome Radiographs and Images

38.8.1 FDG-PET/CT Before and After TM-ILP

See Fig. 38.3.

38.9 Avoiding and Managing Problems

Table 38.1 Regional toxicity of TM-ILP according to Wieberdink [9] and Taeger [10]

Grade	Range (%)	Symptom
I	10–20	No reaction
II	60–75	Mild edema, hyperemia
III	5–12	Severe edema, blistering
IV	2–6	Epidermolysis, compartment syndrome
V	0.5–2	Tissue necrosis, amputation

Severe side effects after TM-ILP are extremely rare. The loss of limb/amputation due to ILP-induced complications is below 0.5% in our own patient group of more than 450 TM-ILP over the last 20 years.

Minor side effects such as reddening, swelling, and sensory impairment of the extremity are common (Table 38.1, Grades I–II) after TM-ILP but mostly temporary and usually vanish after 4–8 weeks. Patient's length of hospital stay after TM-ILP typically ranges between 5 and 10 days.

The swelling of the limb can be effectively treated by elevation and local cooling with cool packs. Severe side effects such as massive swelling of the extremity often associated with a compartment syndrome are rather rare (2–6%), but they do have to be treated quickly. The onset is mostly in the first hour after TM-ILP, or within the following 24 h and necessitates a complete fasciotomy of the lower leg or the lower arm. When covered with a vacuum-sponge system for 5–7 days, the swelling quickly recedes making secondary closure of the fasciotomy possible in almost all cases. Fortunately, also the long-term impairment of the limb function by a compartment syndrome that has been treated swiftly is very mild.

Systemic leakage of TNF-alpha is described as a possibly, and potentially harmful side effect, but fortunately, the occurrence of relevant systemic leakage is rare. In these cases, the isolation of the limb is insufficient, and relevant amounts TNF-alpha (usually more than 5% of the applied amount of TNF-alpha) leak into the systemic circulation, leading to sepsis-like conditions in varying grades of severity. We have experienced one case of an older patient with preexisting renal insufficiency who has developed circulatory failure requiring catecholamines and renal failure requiring dialysis over the course of 2 weeks. Fortunately, the patient recovered completely and could be discharged from hospital 4 weeks after ILP. As mentioned, these cases of relevant systemic leakage are very rare (<1% in our own group of patients). Light cases occur occasionally. They show only slight fever, slight tachycardia, and a general feeling of illness for a couple of days after TM-ILP. They are easily treated with Paracetamol.

Conversely, the question arises whether we can avoid radiotherapy and its complications in selected cases. Deroose and coauthors have analyzed their patient cohort retrospectively in this respect and found that patients who had a good response to TM-ILP (<50% of vital tumor), a successful R0-resection (narrow margins) and no radiation therapy had no significant increase in local recurrence rates compared to patients who had TM-ILP combined with postoperative radiation therapy [11].

References

1. Olofsson R, et al. Long-term outcome of isolated limb perfusion in advanced soft tissue sarcoma of the extremity. Ann Surg Oncol. 2012;19:1800–7.
2. Grunhagen DJ, et al. Isolated limb perfusion with tumor necrosis factor and melphalan prevents amputation in patients with multiple sarcomas in arm or leg. Ann Surg Oncol. 2005;12:473–9.
3. Smith HG, Hayes AJ. The role of regional chemotherapy in the management of extremity soft tissue malignancies. Eur J Surg Oncol. 2016;42:7–17.
4. Eggermont AM, et al. Isolated limb perfusion with tumor necrosis factor and melphalan for limb salvage in 186 patients with locally advanced soft tissue extremity sarcomas. The cumulative multicenter European experience. Ann Surg. 1996;224:756–64; discussion 764–755.
5. Jakob J, Hohenberger P. Role of isolated limb perfusion with recombinant human tumor necrosis factor alpha and melphalan in locally advanced extremity soft tissue sarcoma. Cancer. 2016;122:2624–32.
6. Grabellus F, et al. Size-based clinical response evaluation is insufficient to assess clinical response of sarcomas treated with isolated limb perfusion with TNF-alpha and melphalan. Ann Surg Oncol. 2012;19:3375–85.
7. Grabellus F, et al. Neoadjuvant treatment improves capsular integrity and the width of the fibrous capsule of high-grade soft-tissue sarcomas. Eur J Surg Oncol. 2012;39:61–7.
8. Podleska LE, et al. Lower limb function and quality of life after ILP for soft-tissue sarcoma. World J Surg Oncol. 2017;15:84.
9. Wieberdink J, Benckhuysen C, Braat RP, van Slooten EA, Olthuis GA. Dosimetry in isolation perfusion of the limbs by assessment of perfused tissue volume and grading of toxic tissue reactions. Eur J Cancer Clin Oncol. 1982;18:905–10.
10. Taeger G, Grabellus F, Podleska LE, Muller S, Ruchholtz S. Effectiveness of regional chemotherapy with TNF-alpha/melphalan in advanced soft tissue sarcoma of the extremities. Int J Hyperth. 2008;24:193–203.
11. Deroose JP, et al. Radiotherapy for soft tissue sarcomas after isolated limb perfusion and surgical resection: essential for local control in all patients? Ann Surg Oncol. 2011;18:321–7.

39 Synovial Sarcoma of the Foot

Panayiotis J. Papagelopoulos, Ioannis Trikoupis, and Panayiotis Gavriil

39.1 Introduction

Synovial sarcoma (SS) is a relatively common neoplasm accounting for 5–10% of all soft tissue sarcomas, typically occurring in younger patients between 15 and 35 years, predominately near the large joints of the extremities (60–70% in the lower extremity). Contrary to its name, SS does not originate from the synovial cell, and although it arises from within the joint in less than 5% of all cases, it is considered to have the highest incidence among primary intra-articular malignancies. The exact cell of origin remains unknown. This disease is relatively rare, accounting for approximately 5–10% of all soft tissue sarcomas, and typically affects adolescents and young adults. Synovial sarcoma is often characterized by a specific chromosomal translocation (t(X;18)(p11;q11)), which results in the formation of an abnormal fusion gene, SS18-SSX. This gene is believed to play a critical role in the development of the disease, although the exact mechanisms are not yet fully understood. The fusion gene leads to abnormal cell growth and division, resulting in the formation of a tumor. It typically presents as a slow-growing mass that may be indolent, and it is the most common sarcoma of the foot. Imaging may show a soft tissue mass with sometimes presence of calcification, and on T2 magnetic resonance imaging (MRI) sequence, there is typically a heterogeneous "triple-signal" (i.e., high, intermediate, and low intensity). Histologically, it presents most frequently as a biphasic form containing both a spindle cell and epithelioid components but it may also occur as monophasic, i.e., spindle cell pattern only. Surgery is usually the first-line treatment, aiming to remove the entire tumor along with a margin of healthy tissue. Therefore, adjuvant therapies, such as radiation therapy and chemotherapy, are often used to enhance the effectiveness of surgery and reduce the risk of recurrence. Factors that influence the prognosis include the size and location of the tumor, the patient's age and general health, and the extent of tumor spread at the time of diagnosis. The 5-year survival rate is reported to range from 30% to 74% [1–8].

39.2 Brief Clinical History

An 11-year-old boy presented with discomfort during walking, started 2 months previously. The clinical examination revealed swelling and a palpable mass at the plantar surface of the right foot (Fig. 39.1). No neurological deficits or major functional impairments were noticed.

P. J. Papagelopoulos (✉) · I. Trikoupis · P. Gavriil
First Department of Orthopaedic Surgery, School of Medicine, National and Kapodistrian University of Athens, Attikon University General Hospital, Athens, Greece

H. Özger et al. (eds.), *Diagnosis and Treatment of Soft Tissue Tumors*, https://doi.org/10.1007/978-3-031-77061-6_39

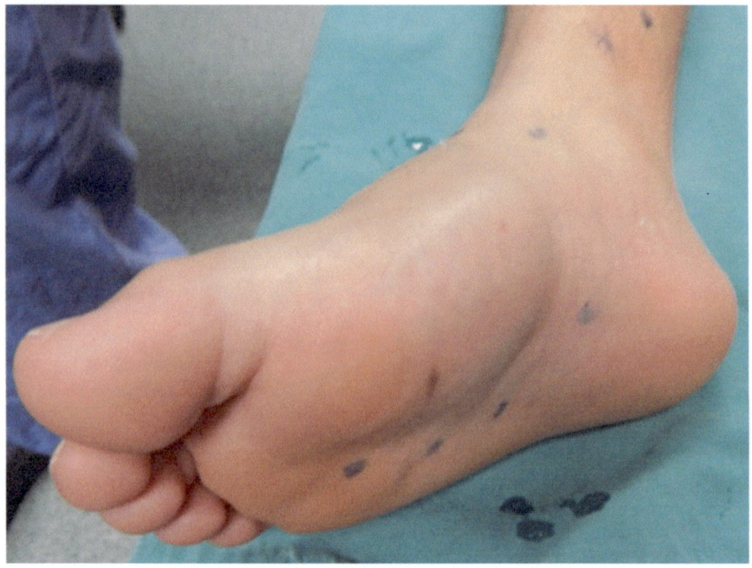

Fig. 39.1 A soft tissue mass is noted on the medial planar surface of the foot

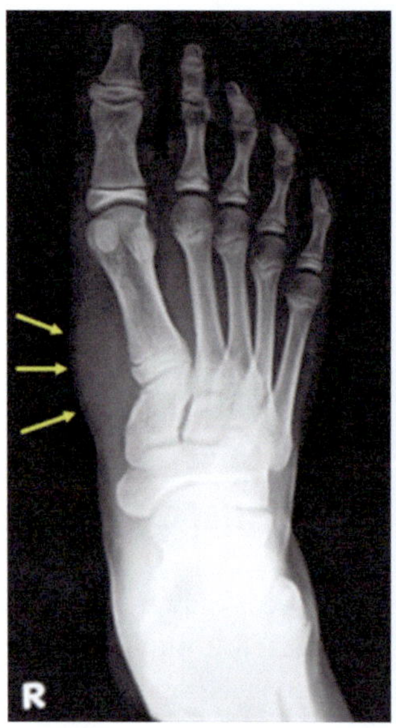

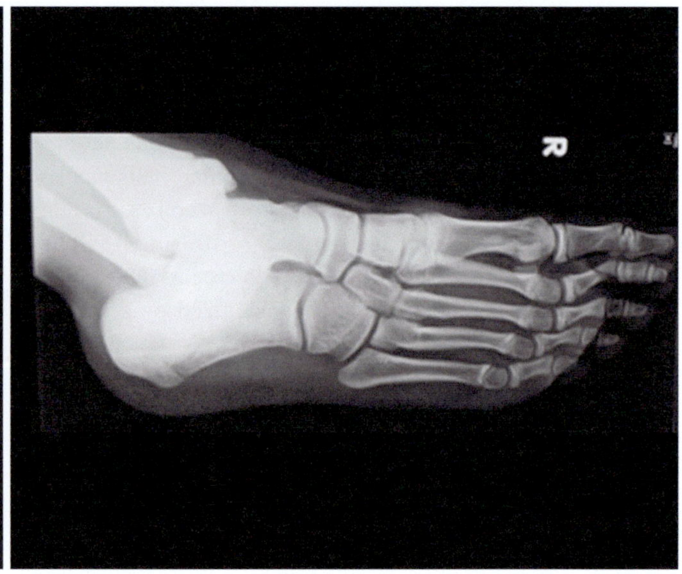

Fig. 39.2 Plain radiograph of the foot revealed the mass

39.3 Preoperative Images

Plain radiographs revealed a soft tissue mass in the region, without any specific characteristic (Figs. 39.2 and 39.3).

The MRI showed a mass, sized 3 cm × 2.5 cm × 5.5 cm, located on the plantar surface of the medial foot. The tumor is attached to the medial cuneiform and the first metatarsal, without any cortical or intramedullary involvement of the bone (Figs. 39.3 and 39.4). The staging imaging was negative for any distant metastasis.

39.3.1 Biopsy

The patient underwent a core needle biopsy and the histological findings confirmed the diagnosis of a monophasic synovial sarcoma (Fig. 39.5).

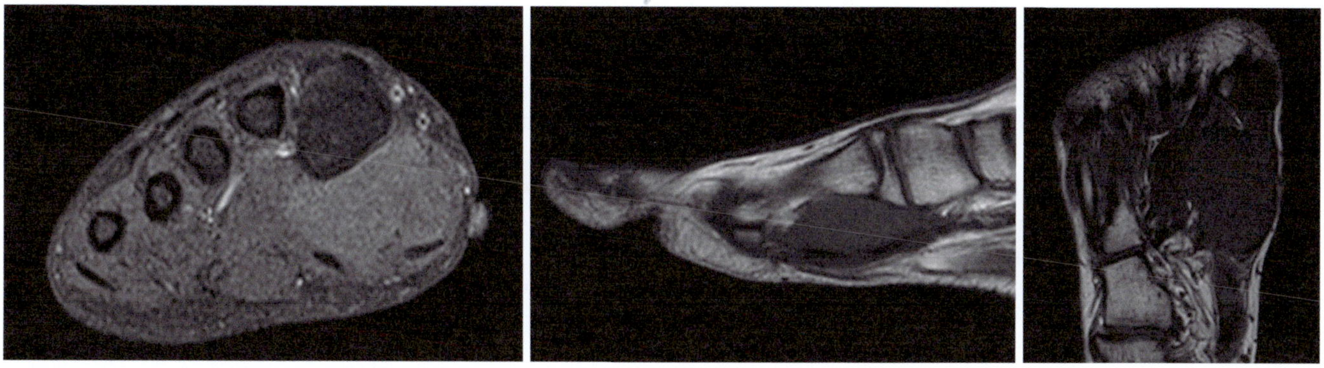

Fig. 39.3 T1 sequence revealed the location of the mass

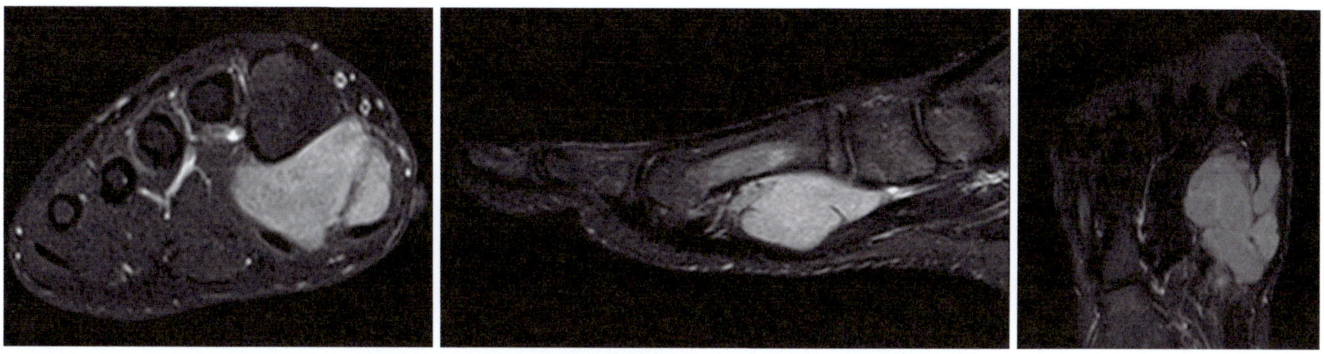

Fig. 39.4 No cortical or intramedullary involvement was detected on T2 sequence

Fig. 39.5 Histological features consistent with monophasic synovial sarcoma

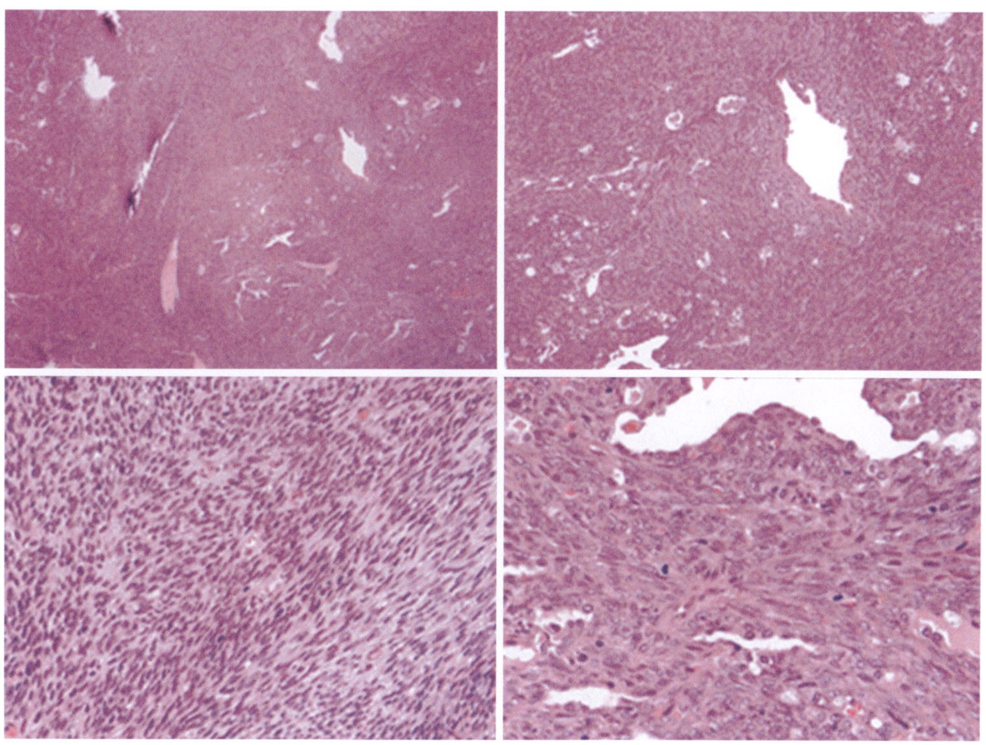

39.4 Preoperative Problem List

(a) Synovial sarcoma is a rare type of malignancy that primarily affects the soft tissues around the joints, such as tendons, ligaments, and bursae.
(b) Diagnosis is often challenging due to the nonspecific symptoms and the rarity of the disease.
(c) Due to the often deep-seated location of these tumors, complete surgical resection can be difficult to perform.

39.5 Treatment Strategy

After multidisciplinary oncological board review, the patient was decided to undergo neoadjuvant chemotherapy followed by limb salvage surgery and adjuvant chemotherapy.

39.6 Basic Principles

(a) Under general anesthesia, through a medial approach, the incision was carried out to the first metatarsal and medial cuneiform bone.
(b) A sagittal osteotomy of the first metatarsal and medial cuneiform bone, including abductor hallucis, was performed.
(c) A medial plantar artery perforator flap was used to reconstruct the soft tissue deficit (Fig. 39.6).
(d) There was satisfactory wound healing (Fig. 39.7).

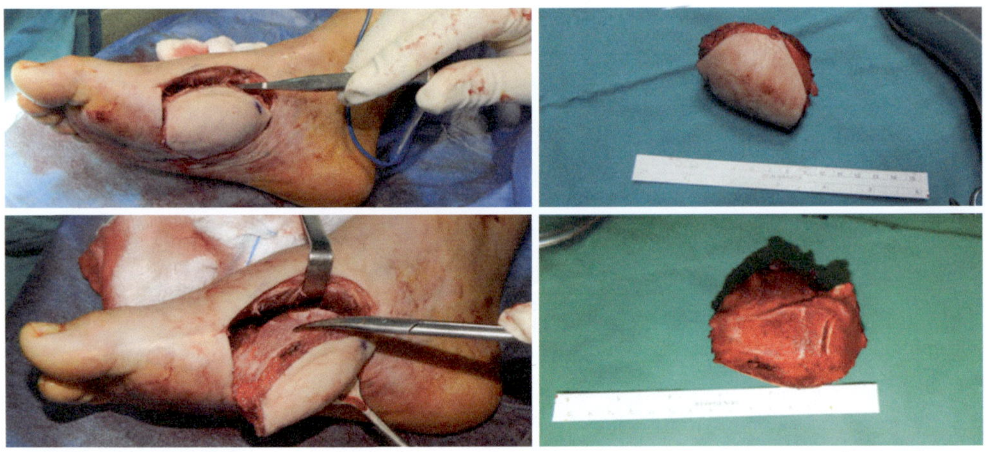

Fig. 39.6 Surgical approach and tumor excision

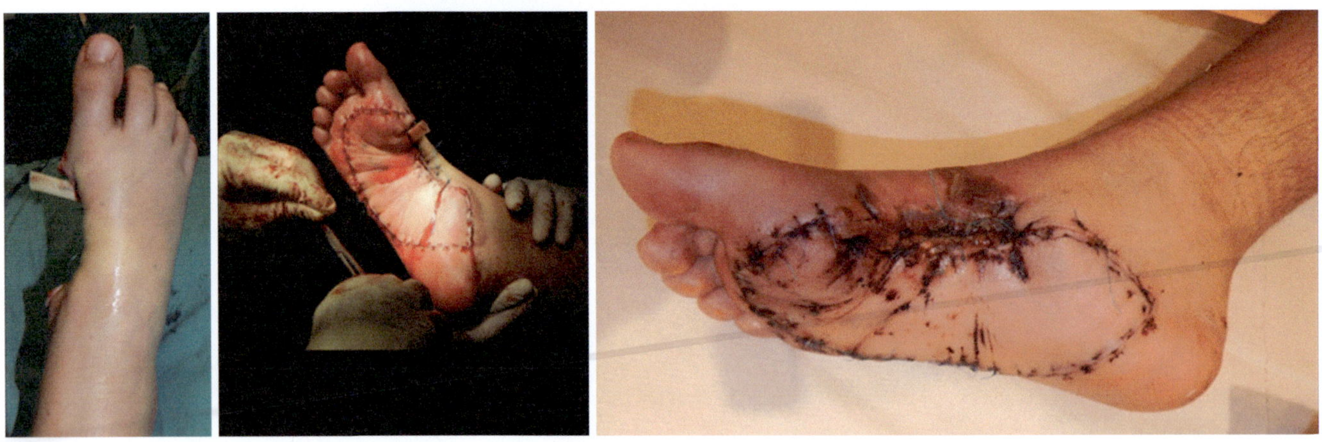

Fig. 39.7 Flap reconstruction and wound healing

39.7 Intraoperative Images

At 3 weeks postoperatively, the patient started adjuvant chemotherapy.

39.8 Outcome Images

At the 5-year follow up, MRI showed no evidence of local recurrence (Fig. 39.8). The patient has no evidence of distant metastases.

There is mild valgus deformity of the great toe. The patient is using a silicone plantar pad insert.

There is no daily activity restriction, and he resumes sport activities with any limitation (Fig. 39.9).

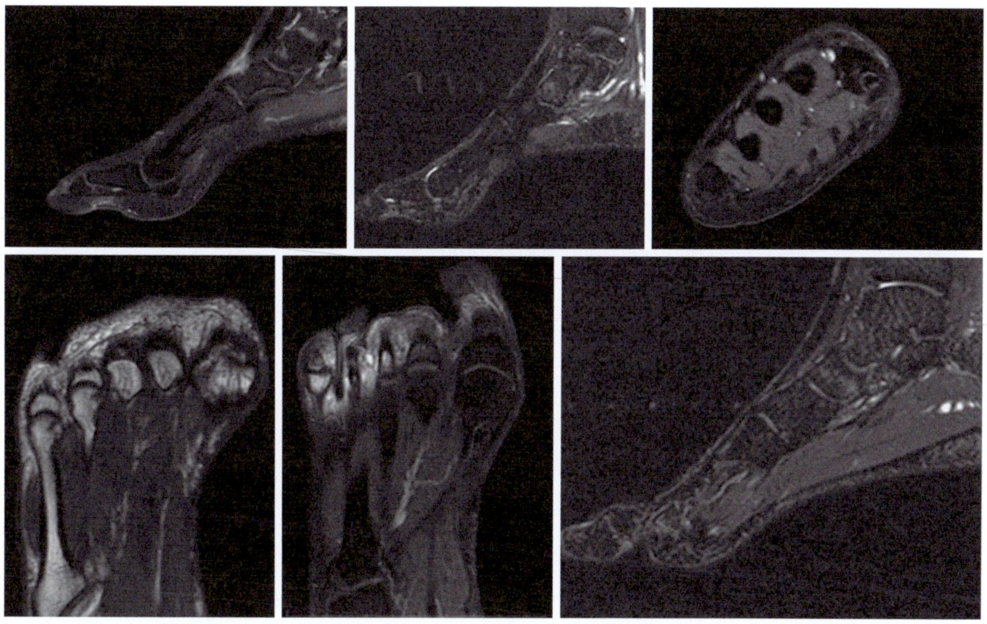

Fig. 39.8 MRI imaging, at 5-year follow-up

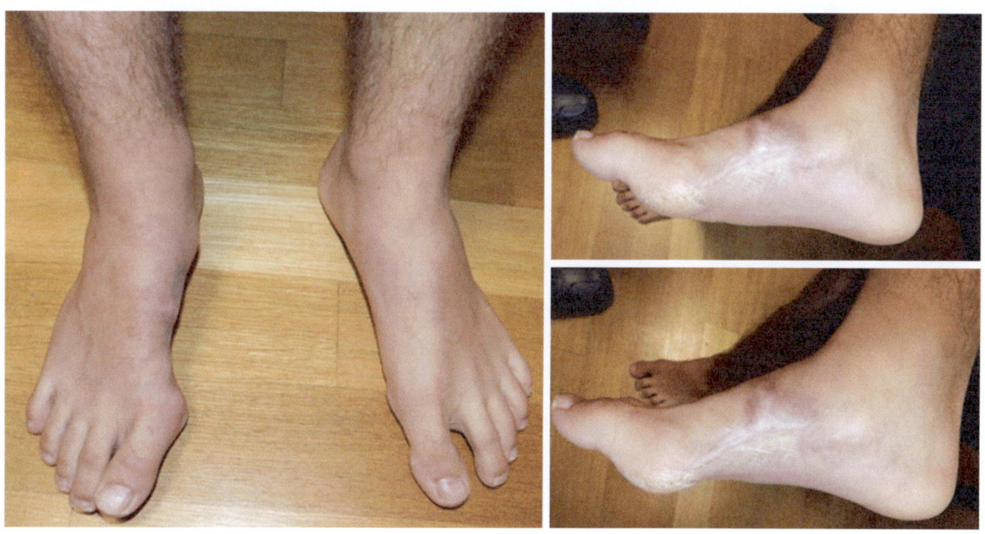

Fig. 39.9 Clinical examination at the latest follow-up

39.9 Avoiding and Managing Problems

(a) Despite aggressive treatment, synovial sarcoma has a relatively poor prognosis, with a 5-year survival rate of approximately 50–60% [8].
(b) The disease often spreads (metastasizes) to other parts of the body, most commonly the lungs, which significantly worsens the prognosis [8].
(c) Molecular targeted therapies, which aim to block the growth and spread of cancer by interfering with specific molecules involved in tumor growth and progression, are currently being investigated. Immunotherapy, which uses the body's immune system to fight cancer, is another promising area of research.

References

1. Karaca MO, Başarır K, Merter A, Acar E, Özbek EA, Özyıldıran M, Yıldız HY. Malignant tumors of the foot and ankle. Foot Ankle Int. 2022;43(9):1232–41. https://doi.org/10.1177/10711007221097654. Epub 2022 Jun 13. PMID: 35695294; PMCID: PMC9465811.
2. Özger H, Alpan B, Aycan OE, Valiyev N, Kir MÇ, Ağaoğlu F. Management of primary malignant bone and soft tissue tumors of foot and ankle: is it worth salvaging? J Surg Oncol. 2018;117(2):307–20. https://doi.org/10.1002/jso.24817. Epub 2017 Sep 6. PMID: 28876452.
3. Ebeid WA, Abo-Senna WG, Hasan BZ, Badr IT, Mesregah MK. Functional and oncological outcomes of limb-salvage surgery for foot and ankle tumors. Foot (Edinb). 2019;41:34–8. https://doi.org/10.1016/j.foot.2019.06.007. Epub 2019 Jun 27. PMID: 31678860.
4. Latt LD, Turcotte RE, Isler MH, Wong C. Case series. Soft-tissue sarcoma of the foot. Can J Surg. 2010;53(6):424–31. PMID: 21092437; PMCID: PMC2993038.
5. Gross E, Rao BN, Bowman L, Michalkiewicz E, Pappo A, Santana V, Kaste S, Greenwald C, Pratt C. Outcome of treatment for pediatric sarcoma of the foot: a retrospective review over a 20-year period. J Pediatr Surg. 1997;32(8):1181–4. https://doi.org/10.1016/s0022-3468(97)90678-3. PMID: 9269966.
6. Savvidou OD, Chloros GD, Koutsouradis P, Megaloikonomos PD, Skarpidi E, Papagelopoulos PJ. Synovial sarcoma complicating total knee arthroplasty. Clin Orthop Surg. 2017;9(4):547–52. https://doi.org/10.4055/cios.2017.9.4.547. Epub 2017 Nov 10. PMID: 29201311; PMCID: PMC5705317.
7. Friedman MV, Kyriakos M, Matava MJ, McDonald DJ, Jennings JW, Wessell DE. Intra-articular synovial sarcoma. Skeletal Radiol. 2013;42(6):859–67. https://doi.org/10.1007/s00256-013-1589-4. Epub 2013 Mar 1. PMID: 23455705.
8. van der Heide HJ, Veth RP, Pruszczynski M, Wobbes T, van Hoesel QG, Lemmens JA. Synovial sarcoma: oncological and functional results. Eur J Surg Oncol. 1998;24(2):114–9. https://doi.org/10.1016/s0748-7983(98)91433-0. PMID: 9591026.

40 Multimodal Treatment and Functional Soft Tissue Reconstruction in Giant Liposarcoma of the Thigh

Panayiotis J. Papagelopoulos, Dimitra Melissaridou, and Ioannis Trikoupis

40.1 Introduction

Myxoid liposarcoma is one of the most common types of liposarcoma. When it occurs in the thigh, it can cause symptoms like a noticeable lump, swelling, pain, or discomfort. However, in some cases, there might not be any symptoms until the tumor has grown quite large. The exact cause of myxoid liposarcoma is unknown, but it is thought to be related to certain genetic changes. It is more common in adults between the ages of 30 and 60, and it tends to affect men more often than women. Diagnosis of myxoid liposarcoma typically involves a combination of imaging tests, such as X-rays, CT scans, and MRI scans, as well as a biopsy to confirm the presence of cancerous cells. Once the diagnosis is confirmed, further tests may be conducted to determine the extent of the disease and whether it has spread to other parts of the body. Treatment for myxoid liposarcoma typically involves tumor resection and perioperative radiation therapy for the optimal local control of the disease. Chemotherapy may also be used, especially in patients with metastatic disease. The prognosis for myxoid liposarcoma varies depending on several factors, including the size and location of the tumor, the stage, and the patient's overall health. However, myxoid liposarcoma tends to be less aggressive than some other types of sarcomas, and many patients can achieve a good outcome with appropriate treatment [1–7].

40.2 Brief Case Presentation

A 52-year-old male presented with an enlarging painless left thigh mass (Fig. 40.1) for over 1 year. Family and past medical history were negative.

P. J. Papagelopoulos (✉) · D. Melissaridou · I. Trikoupis
First Department of Orthopaedic Surgery, School of Medicine, National and Kapodistrian University of Athens, Attikon University General Hospital, Athens, Greece

H. Özger et al. (eds.), *Diagnosis and Treatment of Soft Tissue Tumors*, https://doi.org/10.1007/978-3-031-77061-6_40

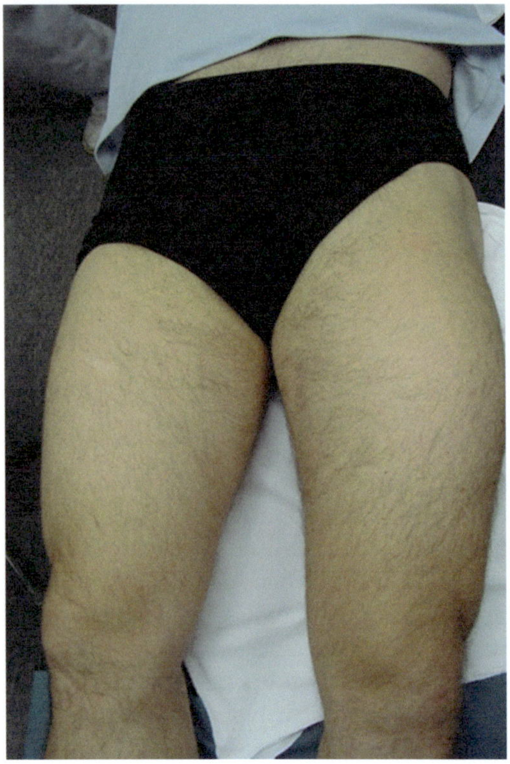

Fig. 40.1 Clinical presentation with a large palpable mass on the left thigh

40.3 Preoperative Images

Preoperative computed tomography (CT) scan showed a soft tissue mass in the anterior compartment of the thigh attached to the anterolateral cortex of the femur (Figs. 40.2 and 40.3).

Magnetic resonance imaging (T1,T2,STIR) showed a heterogenous mass (Fig. 40.4) with dimensions: 19 × 13 cm (Fig. 40.5). Bone scintigram showed increased uptake at the thigh soft tissues without periosteal involvement. Staging with Chest CT-scan and abdomen CT-scan showed no evidence of distant metastases.

40.3.1 Biopsy

A core needle biopsy was performed. Histological examination was consistent with myxoid liposarcoma (Fig. 40.6).

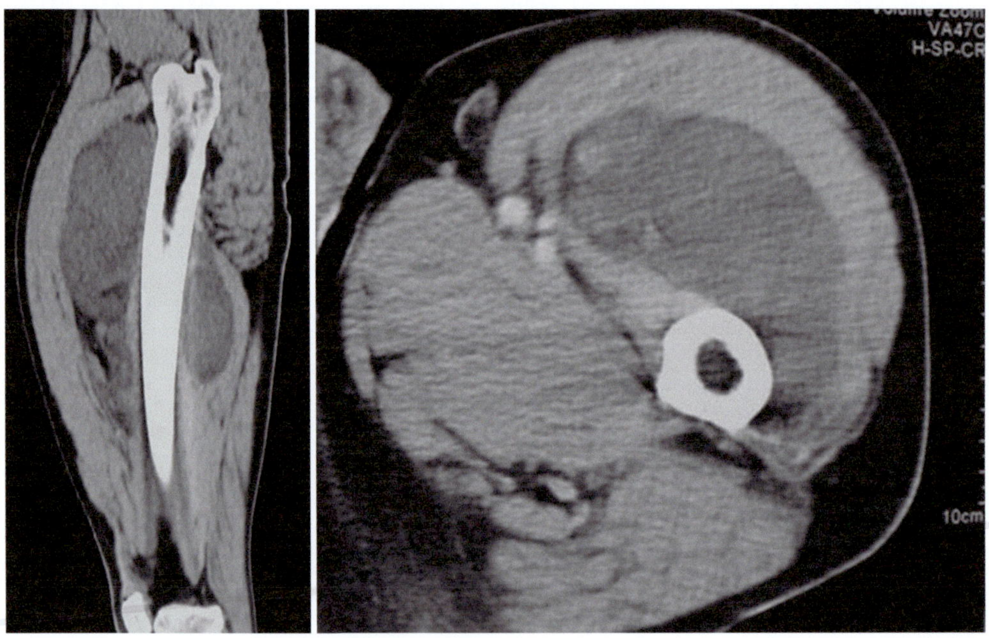

Figs. 40.2 and 40.3 Sagittal and axial view of preoperative CT scan revealed a soft tissue mass of the anterior thigh

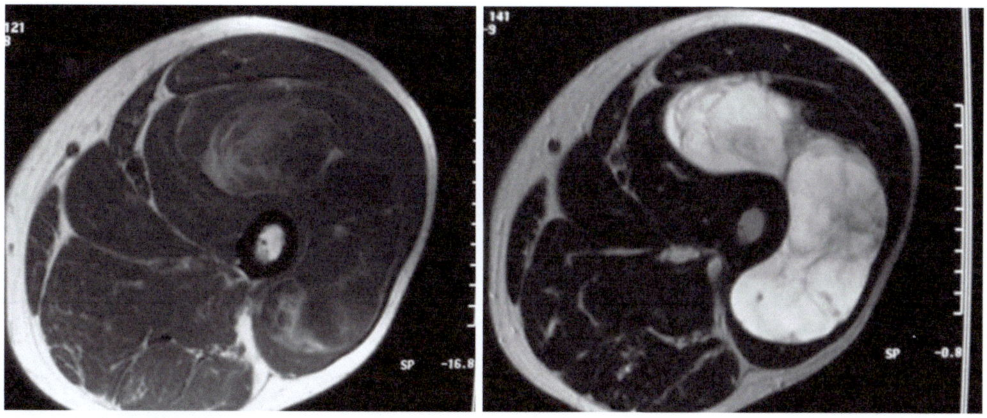

Fig. 40.4 Transverse MRI T1 (left) and T2 (right) images revealed heterogenicity of the mass consistent with liposarcoma

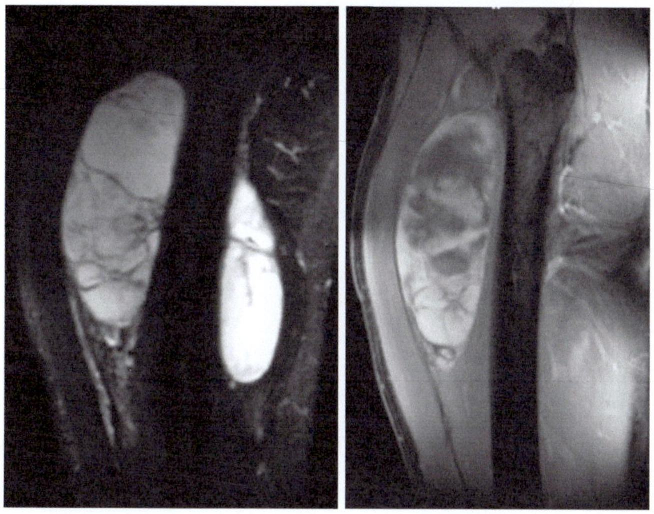

Fig. 40.5 MRI STIR images showed heterogeneous mass engulfing the femoral diaphysis

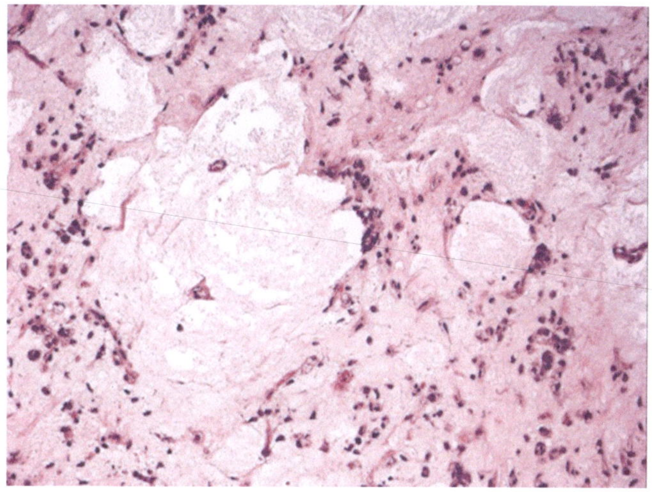

Fig. 40.6 Histological photograph showing spindle and stellate cells within a myxoid matrix, consistent with myxoid liposarcoma

40.4 Preoperative Problem List

(a) Early detection and intervention are crucial for improving the prognosis and survival rates of patients.
(b) In some cases, amputation may be necessary, especially if the tumor is large or has spread extensively.

40.5 Treatment Strategy

After multidisciplinary board discussion, the patient had external beam radiation therapy of 50 Gy followed by limb salvage surgery. The post-radiation MRI showed moderate shrinkage of the tumor (Fig. 40.7).

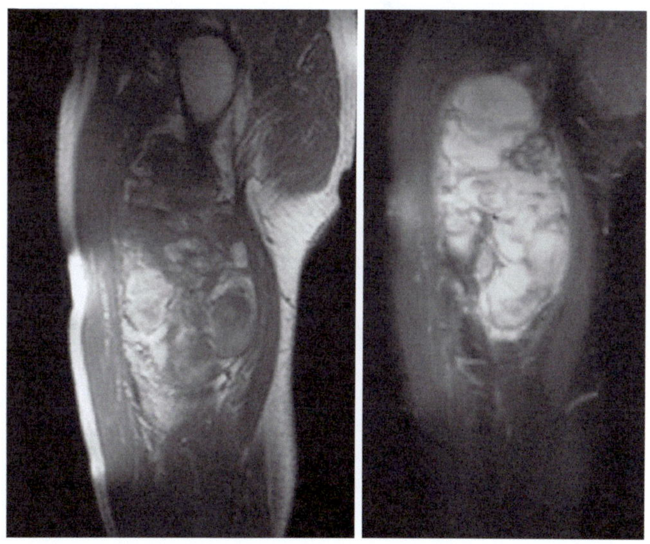

Fig. 40.7 Post-radiation MRI in sagittal and coronal view. The tumor size is moderately reduced

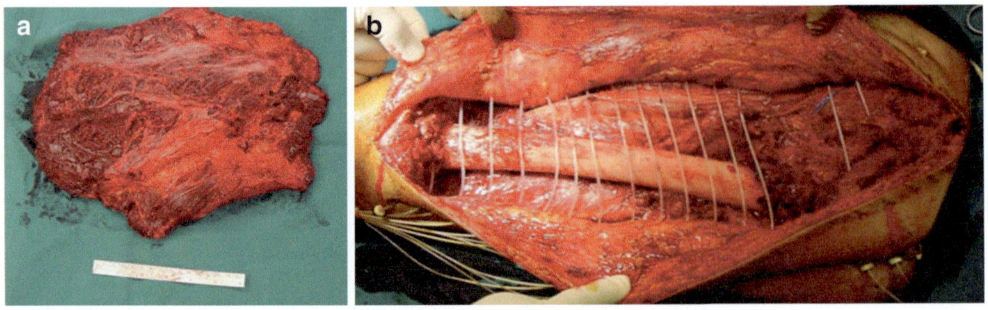

Fig. 40.8 (**a**, **b**) Macroscopic appearance of the resected specimen. After resection, brachytherapy tubes were inserted for supplementary radiation therapy

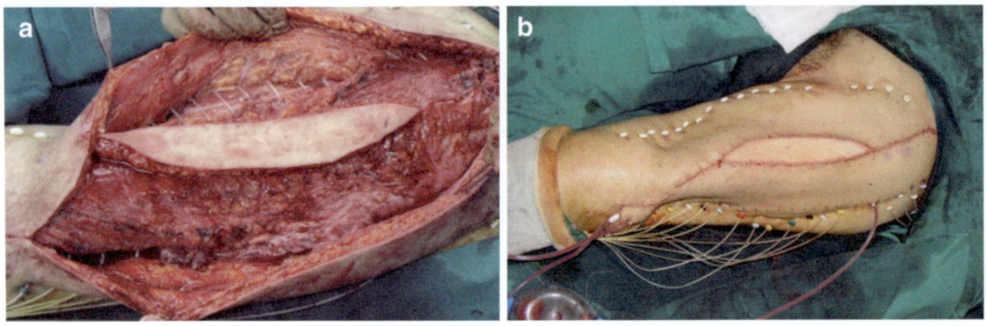

Fig. 40.9 (**a**, **b**) The free vascularized and innervated latissimus dorsi musculocutaneous flap was placed to cover the soft tissue defect

40.6 Basic Principles

(a) En bloc resection of the tumor was performed including the vastus lateralis and intermedius femoris and stripping of the periosteum of the femur bone (Fig. 40.8a, b).
(b) Rectus femoris and adductors muscle were preserved.
(c) Supplementary brachytherapy of 12Gy was performed (Fig. 40.9a, b).
(d) The soft tissue reconstruction was done using a free dorsi latissimus innervated muscle flap (Fig. 40.10a, b).

40.7 Intraoperative Images

See Figs. 40.8 and 40.9.

40.8 Outcome Images

Postoperative course was uncomplicated and the patient after a year had satisfactory ambulation without any aid (Fig. 40.10). The patient had no local recurrence. He developed distant lung and bone metastases and died 15 years postoperatively.

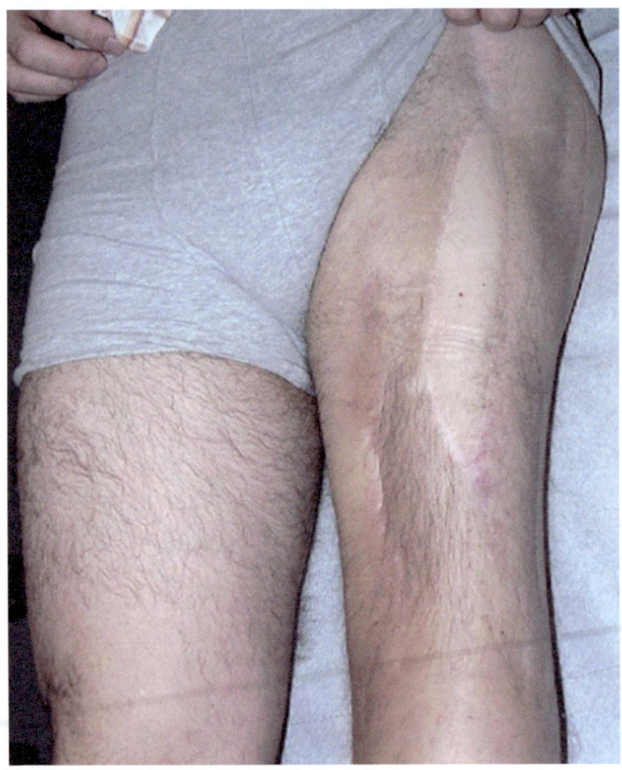

Fig. 40.10 Clinical presentation at the latest follow-up shows satisfactory wound healing at the left thigh

40.9 Avoiding and Managing Problems

(a) The symptoms of myxoid liposarcoma can vary depending on the location and size of the tumor. In some cases, the tumor may be painless and slow growing, leading to a delay in diagnosis [1, 4].
(b) The risk of recurrence remains a concern, and regular follow-up appointments and monitoring are essential [1–4].
(c) Radiation therapy is often used to reduce the risk of local recurrence [1, 5–7].
(d) Chemotherapy may also be used to address systemic metastases [1, 3].

References

1. Tfayli Y, Baydoun A, Naja AS, Saghieh S. Management of myxoid liposarcoma of the extremity. Oncol Lett. 2021;22(2):596. https://doi.org/10.3892/ol.2021.12857. Epub 2021 Jun 9. PMID: 34188698; PMCID: PMC8228380.
2. Vos M, Koseła-Paterczyk H, Rutkowski P, van Leenders GJLH, Normantowicz M, Lecyk A, Sleijfer S, Verhoef C, Grünhagen DJ. Differences in recurrence and survival of extremity liposarcoma subtypes. Eur J Surg Oncol. 2018;44(9):1391–7. https://doi.org/10.1016/j.ejso.2018.03.028. Epub 2018 Apr 6. PMID: 29673808.
3. Moreau LC, Turcotte R, Ferguson P, Wunder J, Clarkson P, Masri B, Isler M, Dion N, Werier J, Ghert M, Deheshi B, Canadian Orthopaedic Oncology Society (CANOOS). Myxoid\round cell liposarcoma (MRCLS) revisited: an analysis of 418 primarily managed cases. Ann Surg Oncol. 2012;19(4):1081–8. https://doi.org/10.1245/s10434-011-2127-z. Epub 2011 Nov 4. PMID: 22052112.
4. Nishida Y, Tsukushi S, Nakashima H, Ishiguro N. Clinicopathologic prognostic factors of pure myxoid liposarcoma of the extremities and trunk wall. Clin Orthop Relat Res. 2010;468(11):3041–6. https://doi.org/10.1007/s11999-010-1396-3. PMID: 20499293; PMCID: PMC2947684.
5. Lansu J, Bovée JVMG, Braam P, van Boven H, Flucke U, Bonenkamp JJ, Miah AB, Zaidi SH, Thway K, Bruland ØS, Baldini EH, Jebsen NL, Scholten AN, van den Ende PLA, Krol ADG, Ubbels JF, van der Hage JA, van Werkhoven E, Klomp HM, van der Graaf WTA, van Coevorden F, Schrage Y, van Houdt WJ, Haas RL. Dose reduction of preoperative radiotherapy in myxoid liposarcoma: a nonrandomized controlled trial. JAMA Oncol. 2021;7(1):e205865. https://doi.org/10.1001/jamaoncol.2020.5865. Epub 2021 Jan 21. PMID: 33180100; PMCID: PMC7662477.
6. Fiore M, Ford S, Callegaro D, Sangalli C, Colombo C, Radaelli S, Frezza AM, Renne SL, Casali PG, Gronchi A. Adequate local control in high-risk soft tissue sarcoma of the extremity treated with surgery alone at a reference centre: should radiotherapy still be a standard? Ann Surg Oncol. 2018;25(6):1536–43. https://doi.org/10.1245/s10434-018-6393-x. Epub 2018 Feb 22. PMID: 29470819.
7. Pisters PW, Harrison LB, Leung DH, Woodruff JM, Casper ES, Brennan MF. Long-term results of a prospective randomized trial of adjuvant brachytherapy in soft tissue sarcoma. J Clin Oncol. 1996;14(3):859–68. https://doi.org/10.1200/JCO.1996.14.3.859. PMID: 8622034.

Alternative to Extra-Articular Resection in Synovial Sarcoma of the Knee

41

Harzem Özger and Buğra Alpan

41.1 Introduction

Synovial sarcoma (SS) is a well-defined soft tissue neoplasm, which is often located para-articularly and often, paradoxically, unrelated to any synovial tissue, both in origin and differentiation. Rarely (<5%), SS can be encountered as a true intra-articular tumor. The knee is a common site of involvement. An important clinical feature is a slow-growing, well-bordered, tender soft tissue tumor, which is sometimes accompanied by significant long-standing local pain and minor limitation of motion. Most lesions are firmly attached to adjacent structures. The indolent behavior and well-circumscribed appearance are commonly misleading toward a benign clinical diagnosis. While it is most prevalent between ages 15 and 40, it can also be seen in children younger than 10.

In most cases, the preoperative duration of symptoms ranges from 2 to 4 years. Adequate surgical excision is the primary treatment modality, while radiotherapy is an essential adjunct for improved local control. Excision of regional lymph nodes might be indicated. Local recurrence commonly develops within the first 2 years. 5-year overall survival rates range from 56% to 76%. Late metastases and long periods of survival after metastasis are not infrequent. Young age, tumor size smaller than 5 cm, distal extremity location, and low tumor grade (absence of poorly differentiated areas) are good prognostic factors, while the significance of histologic subtype (biphasic/monophasic) is unclear. While SS is chemosensitive, routine use of chemotherapy in uncomplicated localized disease is not supported by evidence. However, chemotherapy and targeted therapies can offer significant survival benefits in selected cases such as locally recurring, locally advanced, or metastatic disease [1–3].

The differential diagnosis of intra-articular tumors of the knee includes pigmented villonodular synovitis, synovial chondromatosis, lipoma arborescens, synovial hemangioma, and very rarely primary sarcoma (synovial sarcoma being the most common) [4]. While some of these entities may be identified solely based on imaging studies, there is a small but real risk of resecting an intra-articular sarcoma if surgical treatment is performed directly [5–7]. Arthroscopic biopsy or excision of these lesions is not recommended from an orthopedic oncologic perspective due to the risk of spreading tumor cells intra-articularly and beyond the joint cavity with saline insufflation [7]. The diagnostic difficulties associated with intra-articular malignant neoplasms such as synovial sarcoma are also directly related to the therapeutic difficulties since the contamination of the joint cavity theoretically necessitates an extra-articular resection (EAR) and megaprosthetic reconstruction if limb salvage is intended. While the functional outcomes are usually worse with EAR when compared to intra-articular resections, a secondary amputation is also highly probable with EAR in the long term due to a high rate of complications [8, 9]. Surgical margin modification with radiotherapy might be utilized in specialized centers with an individualized approach to avoid an EAR and associated limb salvage complications, especially in a pediatric patient. However, the surgeon must be prepared to manage complications caused by radiotherapy of the knee region in a skeletally immature patient [10, 11].

41.2 Brief Clinical History

A 10-year-old male patient was brought to our clinic following an intra-articular soft tissue mass resection from his right knee with arthrotomy in an elsewhere hospital. The patient described a slowly increasing knee swelling with marked tenderness in the suprapatellar region throughout 1 year preceding the surgery. A preoperative MR imaging of

H. Özger (✉)
Department of Orthopedics and Traumatology, Istanbul University, Istanbul Medical Faculty, Istanbul, Türkiye
e-mail: harzemo@yahoo.com

B. Alpan
Department of Orthopedics and Traumatology, Acıbadem Mehmet Ali Aydınlar University, School of Medicine, Istanbul, Türkiye
e-mail: bugra.alpan@acibadem.edu.tr

H. Özger et al. (eds.), *Diagnosis and Treatment of Soft Tissue Tumors*, https://doi.org/10.1007/978-3-031-77061-6_41

the knee revealed a well-circumscribed contrast-enhancing soft tissue lesion occupying the suprapatellar recess. The lesion had been presumed benign clinically and radiologically. However, following the excision, the pathology result had been reported as biphasic synovial sarcoma, and the surgical margins had been described as "adjacent to the dyed margins at some places while mostly covered with a thin pseudocapsule." A follow-up MRI, Thorax CT scan, and PET-CT scan had been performed upon obtaining the pathology result to reveal postoperative changes in the knee with no apparent macroscopic residual tumor and no distant metastasis. An extra-articular resection with tumor prosthesis reconstruction had been proposed to the family due to intra-articular contamination of the knee joint. At this point, the family had decided to seek a second opinion. Upon presentation to our clinic, the pathology specimens were consulted with the musculoskeletal pathologist of our multidisciplinary team, and the diagnosis of "biphasic synovial sarcoma" was confirmed. A physical examination of the patient was performed. Preoperative and postoperative imaging studies were reviewed together with the musculoskeletal radiologist of our multidisciplinary team to demonstrate there was no macroscopic residue and no distant metastasis. A detailed discussion was held with the family to explain treatment alternatives and to involve the family in decision-making. A treatment strategy of watchful waiting was chosen instead of immediately intervening with a high-morbidity treatment protocol. Local recurrence was detected after a follow-up period of 8 months. Then, a knee joint preserving wide local excision was performed following preoperative radiotherapy. He also received postoperative chemotherapy. He underwent two major and two minor surgeries for knee deformity and leg length discrepancy in the follow-up. At postoperative 9 years, he is disease-free with excellent functional outcome.

41.3 Preoperative Local Imaging

See Figs. 41.1, 41.2, 41.3 and 41.4.

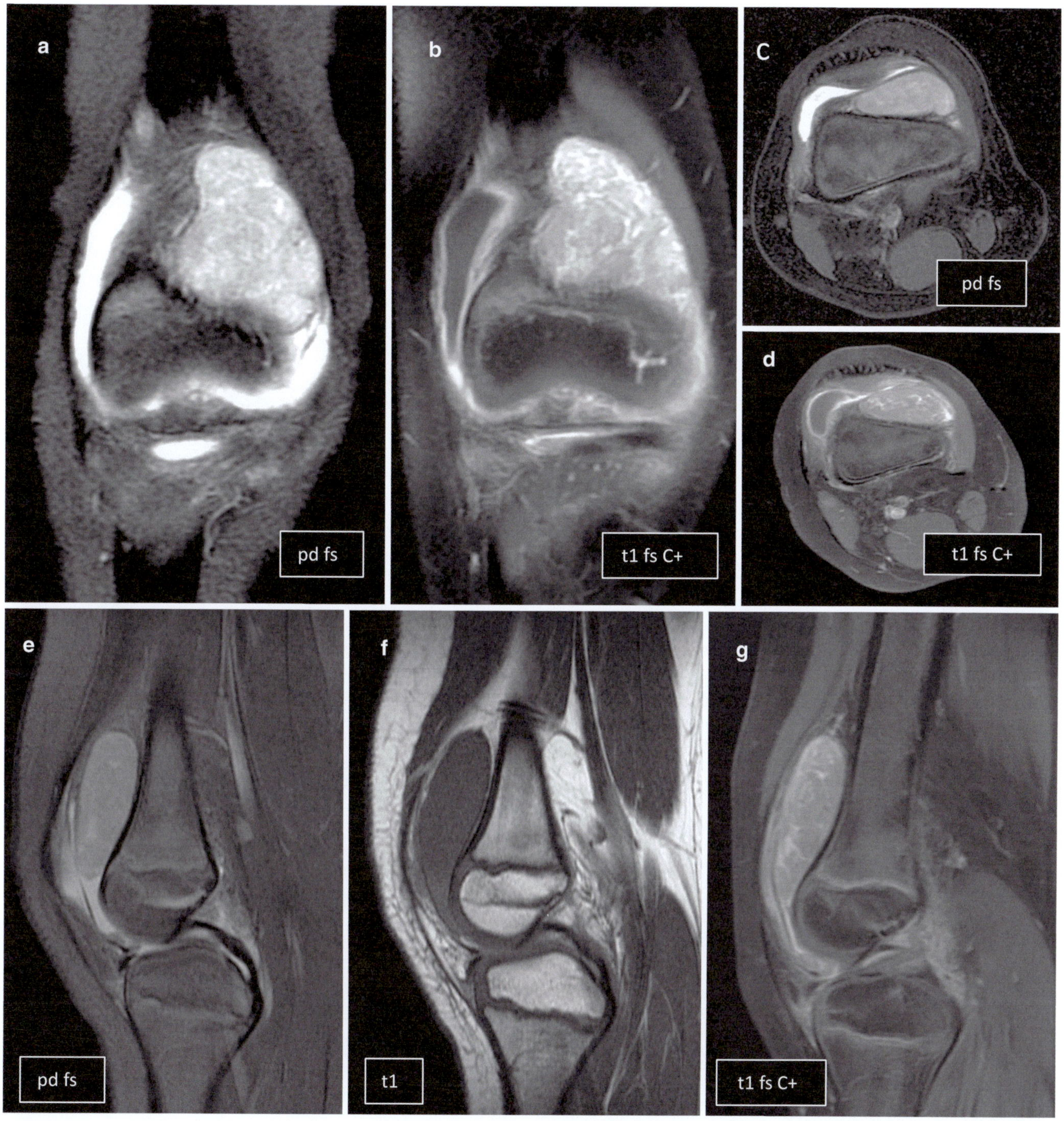

Fig. 41.1 MRI images in (**a**)–(**g**) demonstrate the intra-articular soft tissue mass of the right knee at the time of presentation to elsewhere hospital. The tumor can be seen arising from the medial aspect of the suprapatellar recess

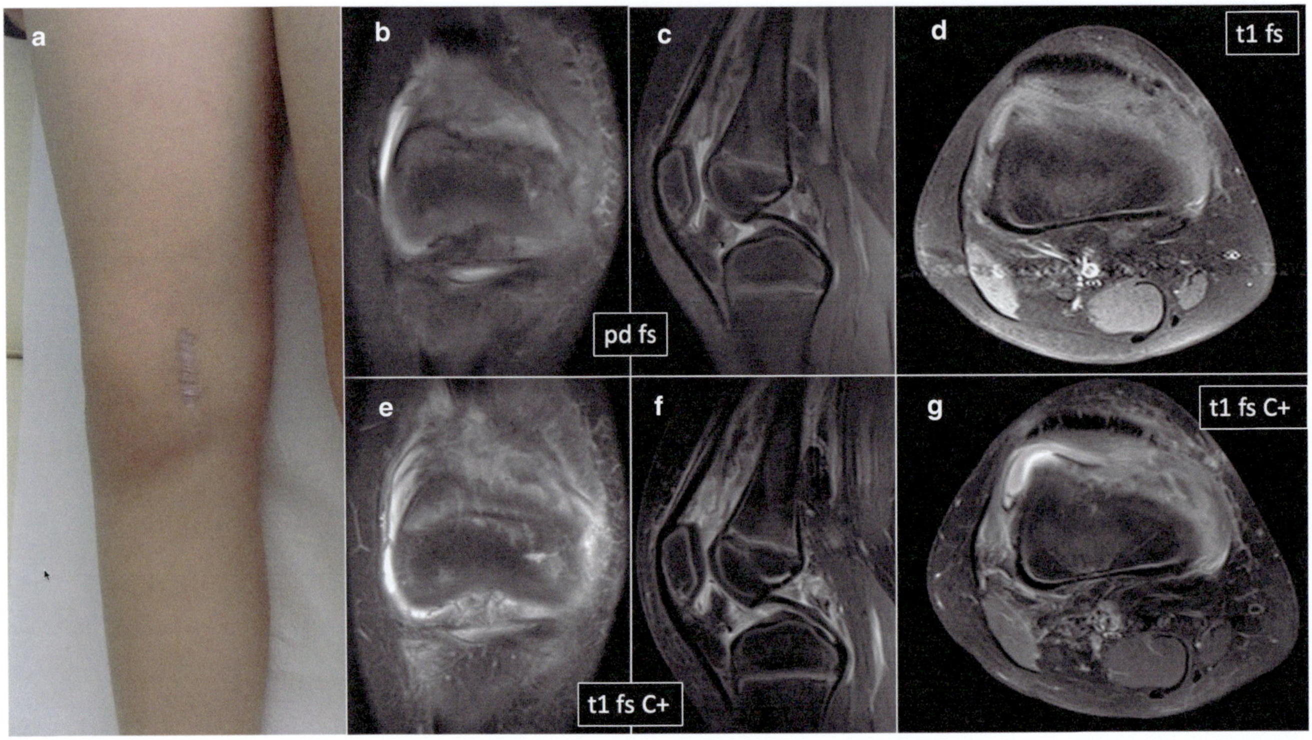

Fig. 41.2 The clinical image in (**a**) demonstrates the healed medial parapatellar incision scar at the time of presentation to our clinic. MR images in (**b**)–(**g**) reveal postoperative changes. However, no apparent residual or recurrent tumor can be observed

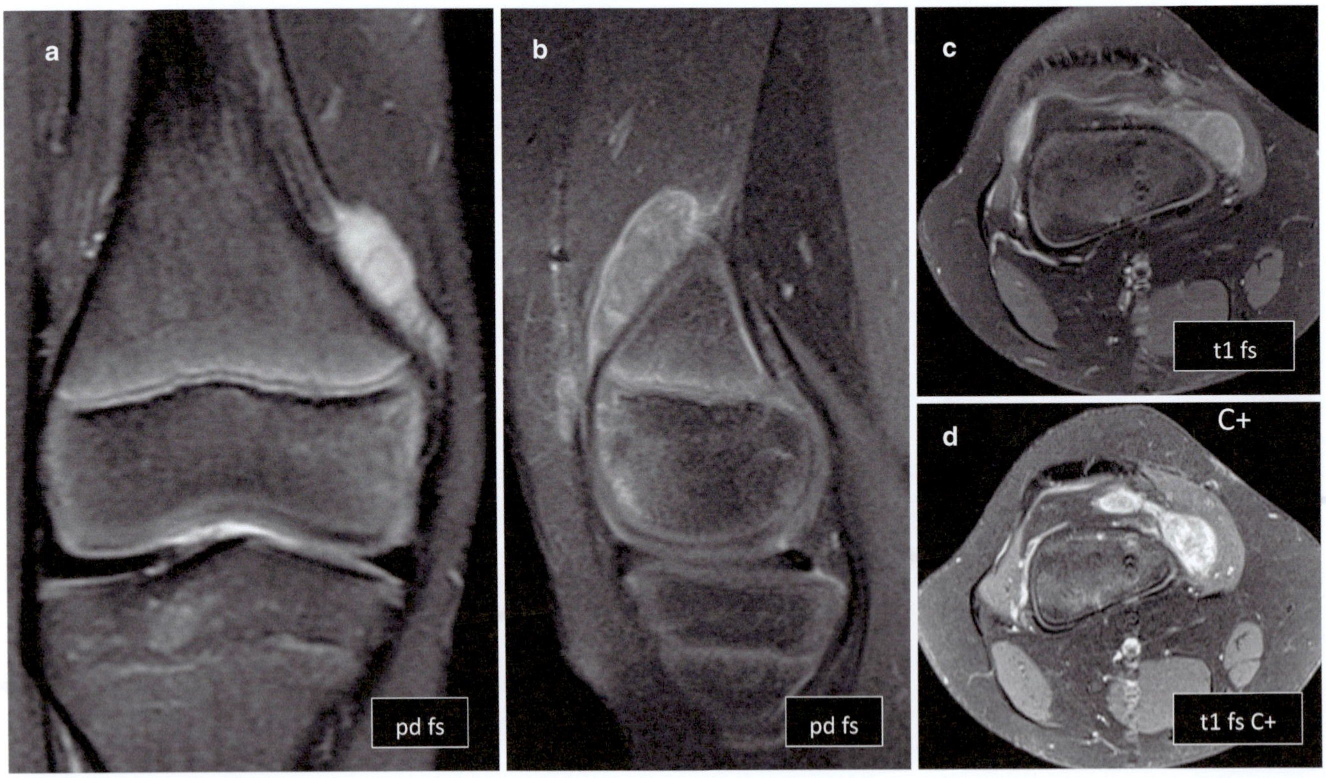

Fig. 41.3 MR images in (**a**)–(**d**) show the locally recurrent tumor detected at postoperative 8 months

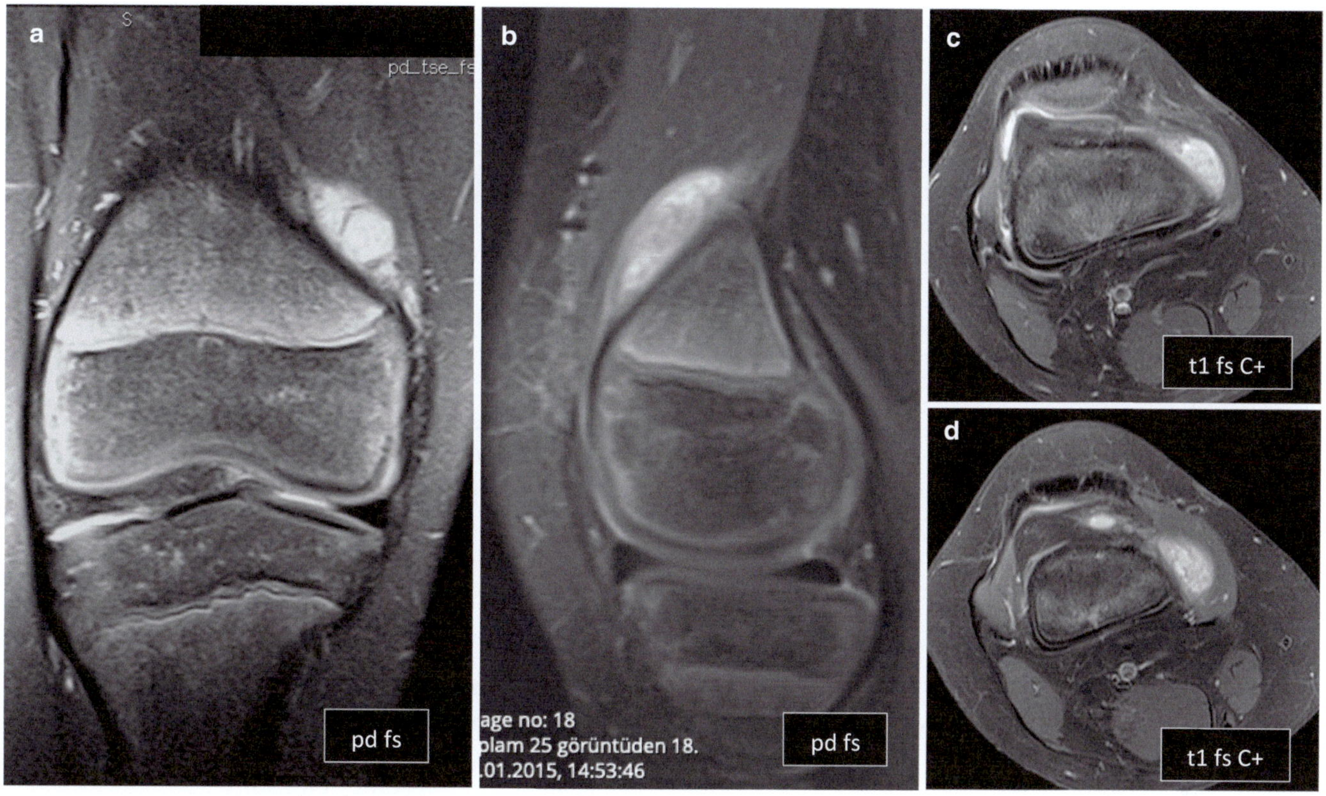

Fig. 41.4 MR images in (**a**)–(**d**) show the locally recurrent tumor following neoadjuvant radiotherapy. While there is a slight decrease in tumor size, diffuse contrast enhancement can still be observed

41.4 Preoperative Problem List

(a) The patient presented following an unplanned resection of a high-grade intra-articular soft tissue sarcoma. Surgical margins can be accepted as R1 based on the initial pathology report, which stated that the tumor was adjacent to the dyed margin in some parts, denoting a <1-mm margin.

(b) The incision tract and the whole knee joint cavity must be presumed contaminated. Depending on the intraoperative handling of tissues and management of postoperative hematoma, peri-articular tissues and the underlying bone might be contaminated. The extent of actual contamination is difficult to assess. Any limb salvage procedure will be complicated by significant tissue loss due to the resection of the contaminated volume.

(c) The patient is skeletally immature, with a significant amount of growth remaining. The site involved is the knee region, where most lower extremity growth occurs. This is concerning for two reasons:

  (i) An extra-articular knee resection followed by tumor prosthesis reconstruction will result in the loss of both the distal femoral and proximal tibial physeal plates, leading to a significant limb length discrepancy (LLD).

  (ii) A joint-preserving resection might be attempted with the use of preoperative radiotherapy to modify surgical margins. However, radiation damage to the physeal plates, particularly in the distal femur, should also be anticipated with the use of radiotherapy. This might also lead to LLD or angular deformities.

(d) Since the patient is a pediatric patient, there is a high functional expectation for any proposed limb salvage procedure.

(e) The conventional method of limb salvage in such a case is an extra-articular resection followed by tumor-prosthesis reconstruction. However, the functional outcome and longevity of the limb salvage are questionable due to the anticipated significant loss of tissue and long-term complications of the prosthesis.

41.5 Treatment Strategy

(a) Limb salvage surgery is the main treatment objective and resection with safe margins is the most crucial aspect of LSS.

(b) A multidisciplinary approach is essential for the best functional and oncological outcome. The multidisciplinary board should discuss thoroughly whether adjuvant treatment modalities are indicated and the timing of these possible interventions to facilitate safe resection, improve systemic disease control, and minimize complications [12].

(c) Preserving the knee extensor mechanism (the quadriceps muscle and tendon, the patella, and the patellar tendon) and the knee joint is desirable for the best functional outcome.

(d) Avoiding a high-morbidity limb salvage procedure, such as an extra-articular resection and a tumor-prosthesis reconstruction, in this skeletally immature patient is a priority.

(e) Although debatable in the setting of an unplanned resection with R1 margins in a high-grade soft tissue sarcoma, close monitoring for a highly probable local recurrence instead of any immediate intervention and reserving any adjuvant treatment for a confirmed recurrence might be a valid strategy to best address the concerns and priorities mentioned above.

41.6 Basic Principles

(a) Since the initial procedure was done elsewhere, the pathology specimen must be consulted with the pathologist in the multidisciplinary team to confirm or correct the diagnosis. The pathologist's assessment of whether the tumor will benefit from adjuvant treatment is crucial.

(b) High-quality and detailed local MR imaging must be performed immediately to assess the route of surgical exposure and the contaminated surgical planes. With an intra-articular sarcoma of the knee, major pathoanatomical concerns are whether the contamination is limited inside the joint capsule or there is extravasation (especially toward popliteal neurovascular structures), whether intra-articular structures such as cruciate ligaments and articular cartilages show tumor invasion, whether there is osseous involvement and whether the physeal plates and the epiphyses are spared in skeletally immature patients. The study must be examined by the radiologist in the multidisciplinary team to distinguish postoperative changes and possible recurrent/residual lesions.

(c) Systemic and pulmonary imaging must also be performed at the time of presentation to complete staging.

(d) The conventional approach in the unplanned resection of a high-grade lesion with R1 margins should be prompt re-excision with wide margins. While radiotherapy is imperative in this scenario, the timing (pre-/postoperative) will depend on surgeon preference and institutional policy. While high-grade tumors might also benefit from chemotherapy, the use and the timing of chemotherapy (neoadjuvant, adjuvant, both) are to be decided by the multidisciplinary team, depending on patient characteristics and the specific tumor histology.

(e) The biopsy tract needs to be removed en bloc with the tumor.

(f) It must be remembered that articular cartilage is a strong tumor barrier. While a subchondral osseous tumor or a longstanding intra-articular soft tissue mass resting against the articular cartilage are more likely to penetrate the articular cartilage, it is relatively implausible for tumor cells, which were dispersed into the joint cavity due to an unplanned resection, to penetrate and invade an intact articular surface. Thus, it is highly unlikely that normal-appearing cartilage surfaces on MRI will harbor tumor foci.

(g) The capsule, ligaments, and tendons also have good tumor barrier properties on their outer surfaces, while they are more vulnerable to tumor invasion through their osseous insertion sites and conveyance via intrasubstantial route.

(h) Osseous involvement is an indication for osseous resection and reconstruction in STSs. However, if the bone is not invaded or completely (360°) engulfed by the tumor, then the bone can be spared with "bone tangential resection," provided that necessary adjuvant treatment(s) and adequate surgical skill have been applied to modify the margins.

(i) Preserving active knee range of motion is the key to an excellent functional outcome in lower extremity tumors.

(j) The patient's and the family's expectations must be well understood, and they must be well informed about the advantages and disadvantages of various treatment strategies, particularly about debatable, high-risk treatment strategies.

41.7 Intraoperative Images

See Figs. 41.5 and 41.6.

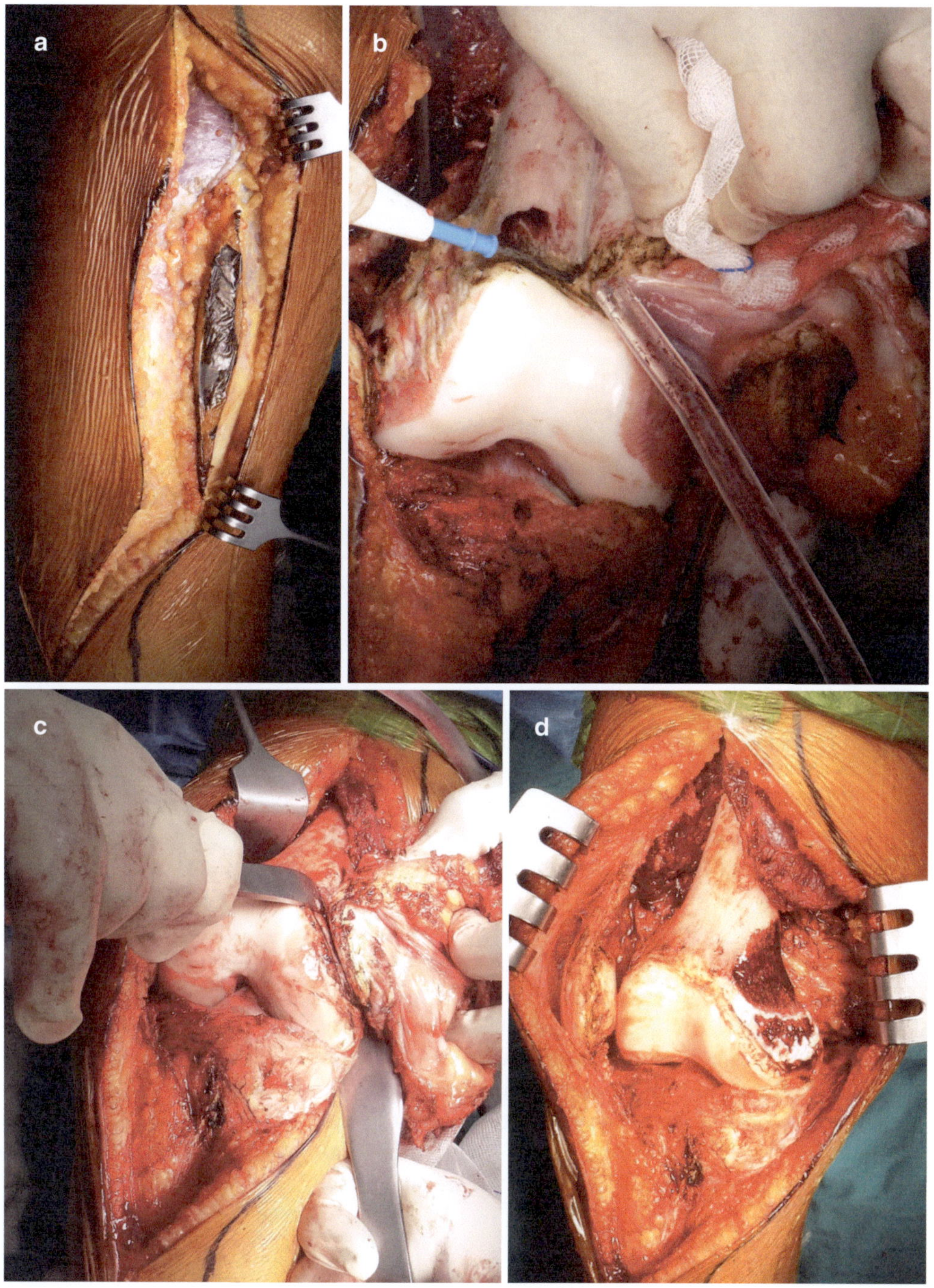

Fig. 41.5 The extended medial parapatellar incision, including the previous scar in fish-mouth fashion, can be seen in (**a**). (**b**) shows the resection of the suprapatellar recess and synovia off the anterior supracondylar femoral cortex with electrocautery dissection. (**c**) shows how the tangential osteotomy is completed with an osteotome following a controlled corticotomy with a reciprocating powered microsaw. The bone resection site and the medial aspect of the physeal plate are exposed in (**d**) after the resection is complete. All synovia and the Hoffa's fat pad have also been removed en bloc. The extensor mechanism has been preserved

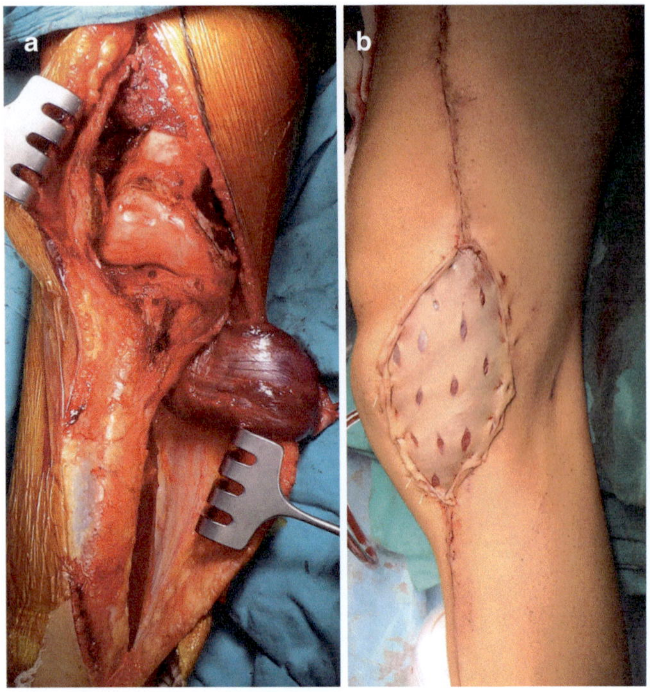

Fig. 41.6 (**a**) shows the preparation of the medial gastrocnemius flap. (**b**) demonstrates the completed soft tissue reconstruction with split-thickness skin grafting over the medial gastrocnemius flap. The pathology report revealed that the soft tissue and bony margins were clear, while tumor necrosis was less than 10%

41.8 Technical Pearls

(a) Operating under a tourniquet is essential due to the delicate nature of the resection and the need for clear visibility in the field.

(b) While not a true and conventional knee extra-articular resection, a modified extra-articular knee resection might be feasible in the setting of an intra-articular soft tissue sarcoma if there is no osseous invasion, the tumor is localized in detailed, high-quality preoperative imaging and necessary neoadjuvant treatment has been applied.

(c) The modified extra-articular resection must be performed en bloc and must include the following components:
   (i) A meticulous synovectomy.
   (ii) The removal of Hoffa's fat pad.
   (iii) The resection of the incision scar and the primarily contaminated soft tissues en route to the tumor from the previous unplanned resection (in this case, medial retinaculum, and a significant portion of the vastus medialis muscle), and.
   (iv) The "tangential" resection of the cortical bone, where the tumor is in contact with but not invading the bone.

(d) Stripping the soft tissues from intra-articular and peri-articular surfaces should preferably be done with electrocautery.

(e) The tangential cortical resection must be performed very carefully so as not to remove unnecessary bone in terms of depth or not to penetrate the deep aspect of the tumor lying on the cortex. Concerning this, the extent of the tangential resection will be determined by the contact area between the tumor and the cortex. A reciprocating powered microsaw can be used for precise and safe corticotomy, while the osteotomy through cancellous bone can be completed with an osteotome of appropriate size and curvature.

(f) While this modified approach allows sparing of the osteoarticular structures and thus a less morbid resection than a conventional knee extra-articular resection, soft tissue reconstruction can still be challenging. A medial gastrocnemius rotational flap was more suitable in this case, as the soft tissue defect was on the anteromedial aspect of the knee. Split-thickness skin grafting was also necessary due to the removal of the previous incision scar.

41.9 Outcome Radiographs and Images

See Figs. 41.7 and 41.8.

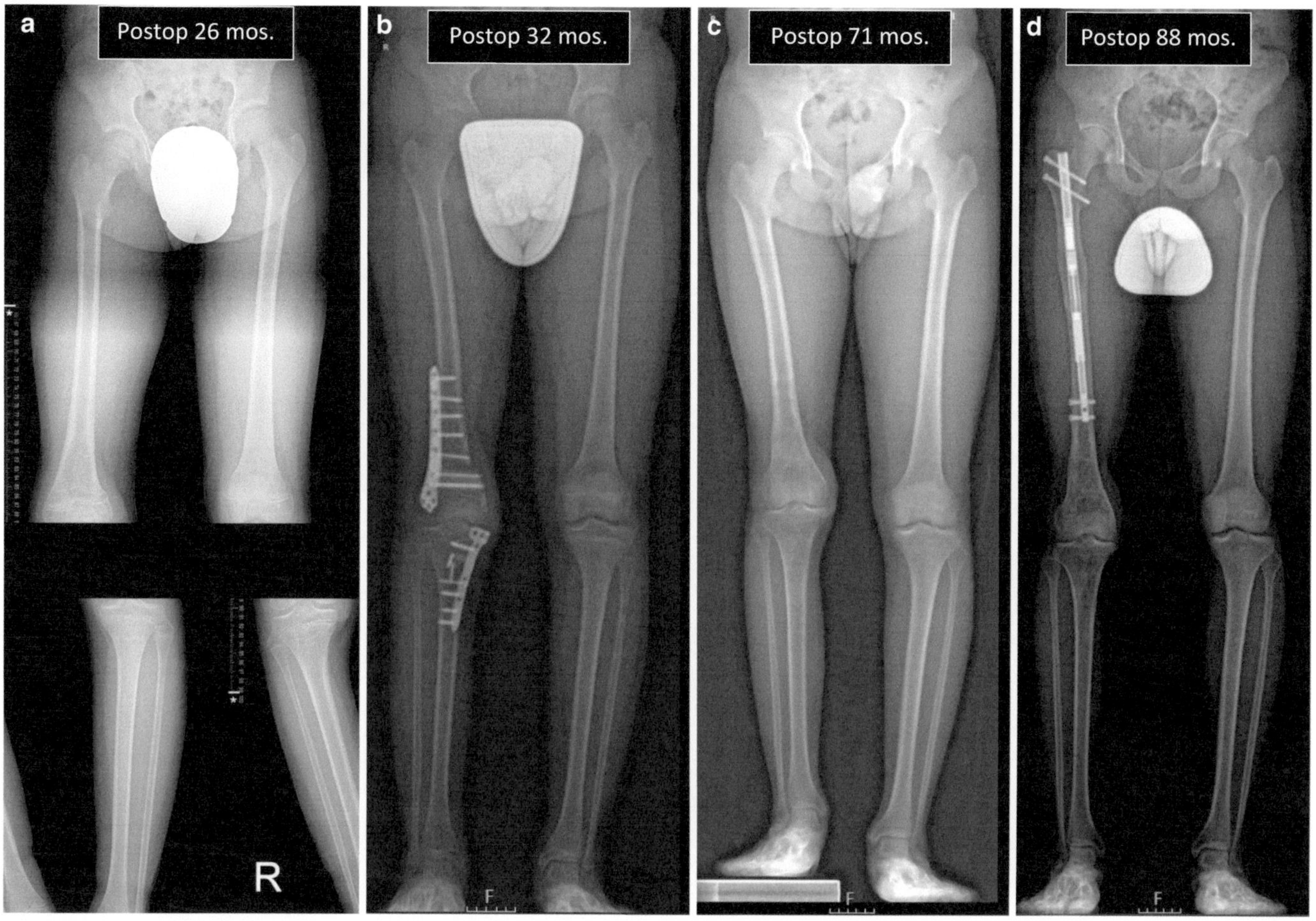

Fig. 41.7 The orthoroentgenogram at postoperative 26 months in (**a**) shows varus deformity of the right knee because of physeal injury precipitated by surgical resection and preoperative irradiation. Distal femoral and proximal tibial corrective osteotomies were performed subsequently to reveal corrected alignment at postoperative 32 months in (**b**). The orthoroentgenogram at postoperative 71 months in (**c**) demonstrates shortness of 4 cm in the right lower extremity. Follow-up orthoroentgenogram at postoperative 88 months shows the management of leg length discrepancy with an intramedullary magnetic nail

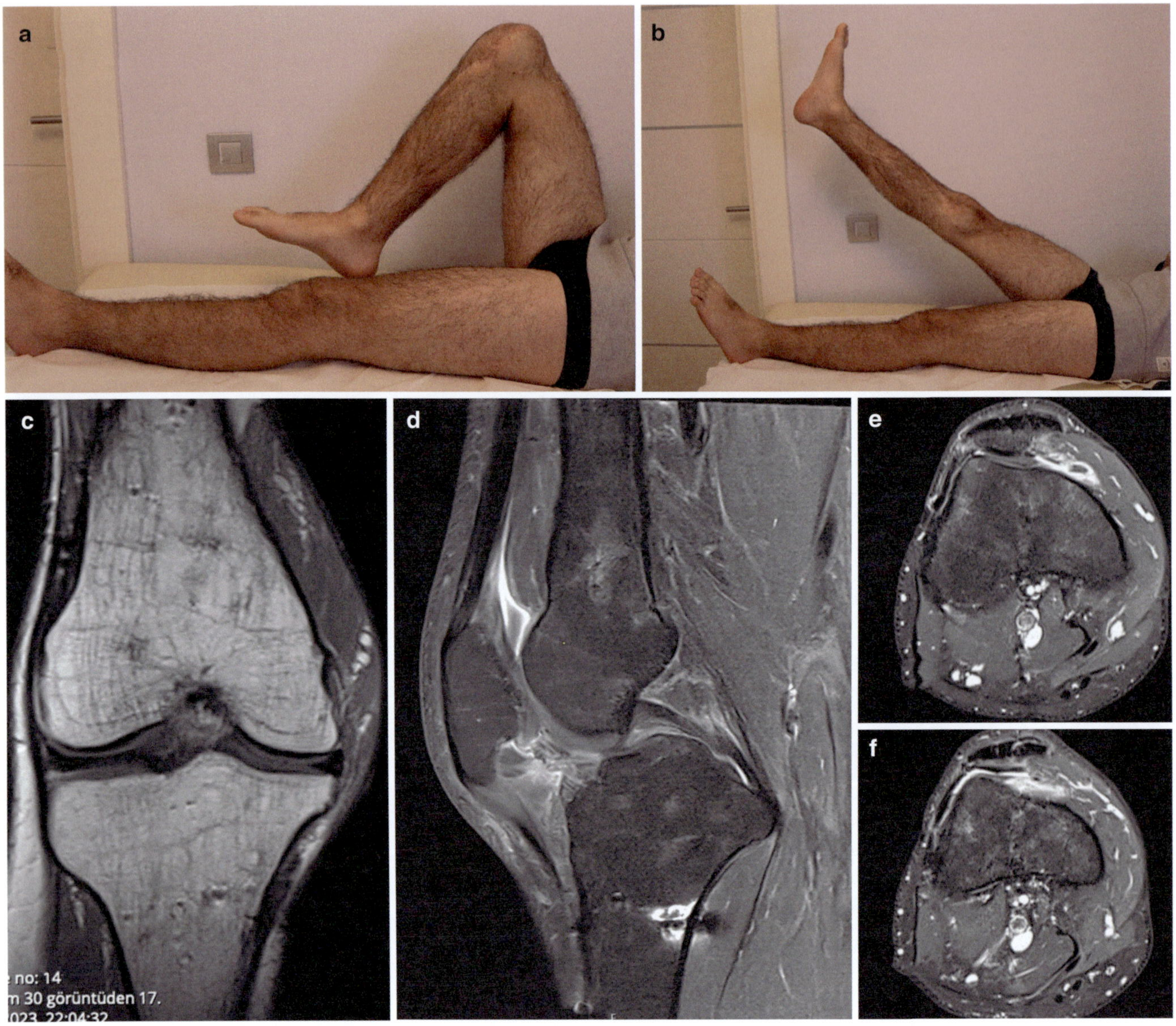

Fig. 41.8 Clinical images in (**a**) and (**b**) show excellent knee function at postoperative 8 years, while MR images in (**c**)–(**f**) demonstrate no local recurrence with preserved knee joint. The patient is metastasis-free by the last follow-up at postoperative 8 years

41.10 Avoiding and Managing Problems

(a) The orthopedic team should regularly check the patient during the neoadjuvant radiotherapy and the following waiting period until surgery to detect complications like tumor progression under treatment, severe radiation dermatitis, skin breakdown, and tumor necrosis-related abscess formation and exulceration to avoid unpleasant surprises at the anticipated time of surgery. Timely detection of such complications might impact limb salvage surgery planning, such as preparation for a free flap or implant reconstruction. It might even change the indication from LSS to immediate amputation.

(b) While a true total synovectomy might not be achieved, the widest possible synovectomy must be attempted, including the suprapatellar recess, synovial lining of the medial and lateral gutters, and synovia covering the cruciate ligaments.

(c) Healthy soft tissue coverage of stripped osteoarticular surfaces is crucial to prevent wound problems and periarticular deep infection. A pedicled or free muscle flap is essential for extensive defects. A primary, tight skin closure must be avoided, particularly in the setting of neoadjuvant radiotherapy. Delayed wound closure with negative pressure wound treatment can be preferred since some degree of unpredictable skin necrosis might develop over the first few postoperative days. If delayed primary closure is not possible after the edema subsides, skin grafting can be performed over a healthy muscle flap.

(d) Due to the increased risk of joint contracture, starting physiotherapy as soon as adequate soft tissue healing is observed is especially critical in a joint-sparing resection preceded by radiotherapy and completed by flap reconstruction.

(e) Adjuvant chemotherapy should be strongly considered in a locally recurring high-grade soft tissue sarcoma, even if the patient is free of distant metastasis in re-staging.

(f) Skeletally immature patients undergoing radiotherapy or surgery involving the physeal plates should be closely monitored for leg length discrepancy and deformity. Conservative management (e.g., shoe lift, protective brace) should be the treatment of choice in the short term since most local recurrences occur within the first two postoperative years. However, considering the oncologic outcome, surgical intervention (e.g., corrective osteotomy, lengthening) might be necessary in the medium to long term.

References

1. Gambarotti M. Synovial Sarcoma. In: Picci P, Manfrini M, Fabbri N, Gambarotti M, Vanel D, editors. Atlas of musculoskeletal tumors and tumorlike lesions. Springer; 2014. p. 359–64. https://doi.org/10.1007/978-3-319-01748-8.
2. Goldblum JR, Folpe AL, Weiss SW. Other malignant soft tissue tumors, including those of uncertain type. In: Goldblum JR, Folpe AL, Weiss SW, editors. Enzinger and Weiss's soft tissue tumors. 7th ed. New York: Elsevier; 2020. p. 1175–268.
3. Suurmeijer AJH, Ladanyi M, Nielsen TO. Synovial sarcoma. In: WHO Classification of Tumours Editorial Board, editor. WHO classification of tumours soft tissue and bone tumours. 5th ed. International Agency for Research on Cancer; 2020. p. 290–3.
4. Auran RL, Martin JR, Duran MD, de Comas AM, Jacofsky DJ. Evaluation and management of intra-articular tumors of the knee. J Knee Surg. 2022;35(06):597–606. https://doi.org/10.1055/s-0042-1743223.
5. Friedman MV, Kyriakos M, Matava MJ, McDonald DJ, Jennings JW, Wessell DE. Intra-articular synovial sarcoma. Skeletal Radiol. 2013;42(6):859–67. https://doi.org/10.1007/s00256-013-1589-4.
6. Justin EH, Ryan PF, Austin H, Joshua S, Nathan D, Michael F, Travis H. Primary intra-articular synovial sarcoma of the knee: a report of two cases and review of the literature. Int J Radiol Imag Technol. 2018;4(1):31. https://doi.org/10.23937/2572-3235.1510031.
7. Rougraff BT, Aboulafia A, Biermann JS, Healey J. Biopsy of soft tissue masses: evidence-based medicine for the musculoskeletal tumor society. Clin Orthop Relat Res. 2009;467(11):2783–91. https://doi.org/10.1007/s11999-009-0965-9.
8. Nottrott M, Streitbürger A, Gosheger G, Guder W, Hauschild G, Hardes J. Intra-articular soft-tissue sarcoma of the knee: is extra-articular resection and tumor endoprosthetic reconstruction the solution? A retrospective report on eight cases. Orthop Rev. 2019;11(1):6–8. https://doi.org/10.4081/or.2019.7764.
9. Shahid M, Albergo N, Purvis T, Heron K, Gaston L, Carter S, Grimer R, Jeys L. Management of sarcomas possibly involving the knee joint when to perform extra-articular resection of the knee joint and is it safe? Eur J Surg Oncol. 2017;43(1):175–80. https://doi.org/10.1016/j.ejso.2016.05.018.
10. Ozger H, Bulbul M, Eralp L. Complications of limb salvage surgery in childhood tumors and recommended solutions. Strateg Trauma Limb Reconstr. 2010;5(1):11–5. https://doi.org/10.1007/s11751-009-0075-y.
11. Paulino AC. Late effects of radiotherapy for pediatric extremity sarcomas. Int J Radiation Oncol Biol Phys. 2004;60(1):265–74. https://doi.org/10.1016/j.ijrobp.2004.02.001.
12. NCCN Clinical Practice Guidelines in Oncology (NCCN guidelines®) soft tissue sarcoma. Version 2.2021 – April 28, 2021. (n.d.). Retrieved May 11, 2023, from http://nccn.ir/Guidelines/Summary/sarcoma.html#pf23.

42 Limb Salvage Made Possible Through Neoadjuvant Treatment in Inoperable Infantile Fibrosarcoma

İnci Ayan, Harzem Özger, and Buğra Alpan

42.1 Introduction

Infantile Fibrosarcoma is a malignant fibroblastic tumor that has a locally aggressive behavior and is rarely metastatic. It is considered a separate entity from its adult counterpart due to its more favorable clinical behavior and distinctive molecular features, such as *ETV6-NTRK3* fusion. It is usually encountered as a non-tender, painless mass. One-third of cases are found at birth, while 14% are detected in utero with ultrasonography. Most cases are diagnosed within the first year of life, and the most involved sites are the extremities, especially the regions of the foot, ankle, lower leg, hand, wrist, and forearm. Tumors can reach huge sizes, eventually involving or even replacing the whole extremity part. The tumor borders are usually infiltrative with entrapment of fat, muscle, and other surrounding tissues. Rhabdomyosarcoma must be considered in differential diagnosis. Staging is not clinically relevant. Despite aggressive histology, wide local excision is the treatment of choice. Preoperative chemotherapy has an essential role in tumors, for which straightforward excision is not feasible, and the limb salvage outcome might benefit from tumor shrinkage. Although the role of adjuvant chemotherapy is less well defined, it is indicated when the surgical margins are positive. The 10-year survival rate is approximately 90% with standard treatment protocols, while local recurrence rates can be as high as 25–40%, especially with incomplete resection [1, 2].

İ. Ayan
Department of Pediatric Oncology, Acıbadem Maslak Hospital, Istanbul, Türkiye

H. Özger (✉)
Department of Orthopedics and Traumatology, Istanbul University, Istanbul Medical Faculty, Istanbul, Türkiye
e-mail: harzemo@yahoo.com

B. Alpan
Department of Orthopedics and Traumatology, Acıbadem Mehmet Ali Aydınlar University, School of Medicine, Istanbul, Türkiye
e-mail: bugra.alpan@acibadem.edu.tr

42.2 Brief Clinical History

A female newborn, who had been under our surveillance since the last trimester due to a right lower extremity mass diagnosed with prenatal ultrasonography, underwent a core needle biopsy immediately after birth with Caesarean section at 37 weeks of gestation without any incident. The physical examination revealed a large soft tissue mass involving the entire right calf. The distal circulation was unremarkable, while the motor examination of the ankle and toes was suboptimal. Active motion was not observed in the distal extremity despite the presence of a passive range of motion. An abdominal ultrasound was also performed on the same day to rule out any intraabdominal pathology. The patient was admitted to the neonatal intensive care unit. A lower extremity contrast-enhanced MRI and a contrast-enhanced Thorax CT scan were performed under general anesthesia (sedation) the next day to demonstrate a 12.5 × 11 × 9 cm soft tissue tumor with heterogeneous but significant contrast enhancement and no pulmonary involvement. The tumor involved all crural compartments diffusely and engulfed both the tibia and the fibula, causing bone remodeling. The major neurovascular structures were not distinguishable from the surrounding tumoral mass. The pathology was reported as congenital/infantile fibrosarcoma. A pediatric oncology consultation was done. Upon informing the parents about the diagnosis, the natural history of the disease, and the treatment options and risks, they stressed their desire for their child to be saved together with her leg.

42.3 Preoperative Local Imaging

See Figs. 42.1 and 42.2.

H. Özger et al. (eds.), *Diagnosis and Treatment of Soft Tissue Tumors*, https://doi.org/10.1007/978-3-031-77061-6_42

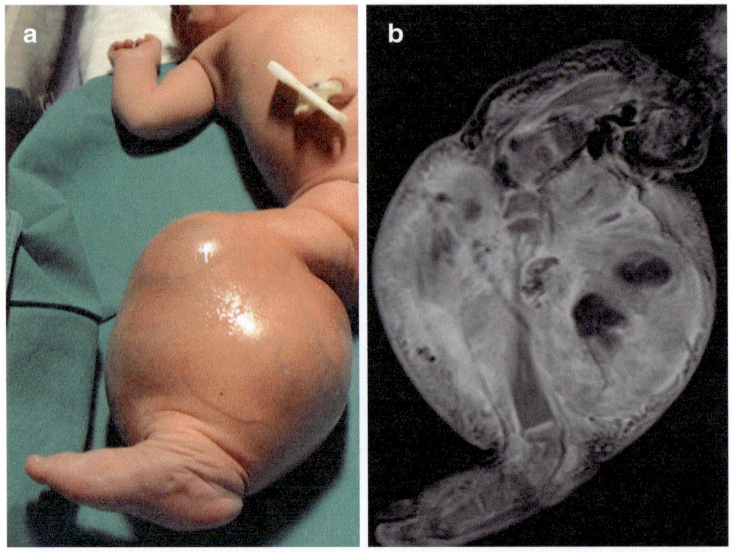

Fig. 42.1 (**a**) Demonstrates the clinical image of the tumor involving the right lower leg right after C/S birth. The stretched skin and superficial varicose veins can be seen over the tumor. A trucut needle biopsy was performed immediately after birth. The sagittal MRI section of the leg in (**b**) shows that all musculature has either been infiltrated or stretched/compressed beyond recognition by the tumor. The needle biopsy tract can also be observed in the MR image, crossing diagonally from upper left to lower right

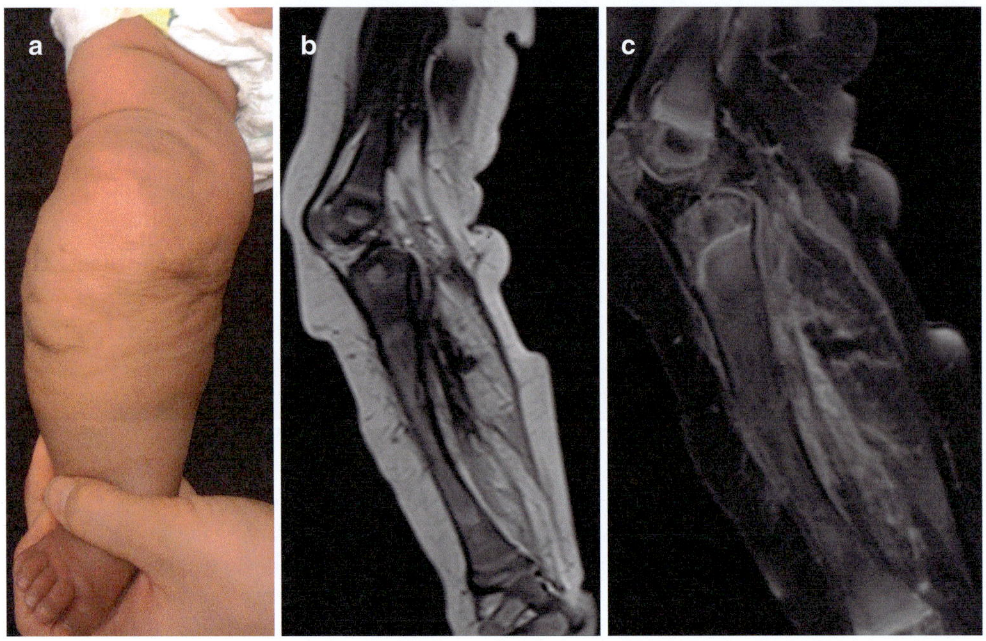

Fig. 42.2 (**a**) Shows the dramatic clinical response following 8 months of neoadjuvant chemotherapy. The extreme swelling has subsided, and the skin has softened with wrinkles appearing. Sagittal MR images in (**b**) and (**c**) show the dramatic radiologic response with total regression of the tumoral mass. Muscles of the lower leg, however, show marked atrophy. There is residual fibrotic tissue in the deep posterior compartment adjacent to the posterior neurovascular bundle

42.4 Preoperative Problem List

(a) Although, for this case, the large tumor did not cause any intrauterine or birth-related complications, intrauterine rupture of a prenatally diagnosed congenital/infantile sarcoma is a reported fatal complication [3].
(b) While the diagnosis of a malignant tumor in a child always leads to a considerable psychological burden for the family, such a diagnosis in a newborn is extra devastating and understandably complex to cope with. The sensitive nature of the situation might make it difficult for the medical team to explain the treatment strategy and the risks involved.
(c) Imaging studies, particularly MRI, require anesthesia, which can be challenging. However, imaging studies of shorter duration might be performed during natural sleep.
(d) Due to the extensive tumor involvement of all muscle compartments and the inability to visualize the neurovascular bundle clearly, the tumor is inoperable at the time of diagnosis.
(e) Whether the limb is surgically salvageable depends on the neoadjuvant treatment response.
(f) The recovery of motor deficit in the distal extremity is ambiguous.
(g) The bone remodeling due to compression by the tumor raises the question of whether bone invasion might be present.

(h) Increased vascularity of the large tumor might lead to ipsilateral increased growth in the affected limb segment. At the same time, the possible involvement of the physeal plates might impair growth in the affected segment.
(i) The patient must start neoadjuvant chemotherapy in the newborn stage when she is in a very vulnerable period in terms of risk of infection and growth impairment.
(j) Since the tumor involvement is too extensive at the beginning of the treatment, the pathoanatomical changes, even after a complete response to neoadjuvant therapy, are hard to predict. The exact site or compartment where the tumor originated might not be identifiable at all. A difficult tumor bed dissection through diffuse fibrosis around neurovascular structures in a minute anatomy can be anticipated.

42.5 Treatment Strategy

(a) A multidisciplinary approach is essential for the best functional and oncological outcome. The multidisciplinary board should discuss thoroughly whether adjuvant treatment modalities are indicated, and the timing of these possible interventions to facilitate safe resection, improve systemic disease control, and minimize complications [4].
(b) While the inoperable clinical and radiological appearance of the tumor at presentation combined with the diagnosis of fibrosarcoma might lead one to consider an immediate amputation at first evaluation, neoadjuvant chemotherapy must be the first line of treatment, and the surgical indication should be postponed until seeing the response to the first 2–3 cycles of neoadjuvant chemotherapy. Amputation should be reserved for nonresponders.
(c) Despite the patient's neonatal status, neoadjuvant treatment must be started as soon as possible (e.g., depending on the nutritional status, presence of any neonatal infection, and cardiologic examinations).
(d) If the treatment response is good, limb salvage surgery will be applied. The surgery should focus on the identification and release of major neurovascular structures, the release of muscle compartments, and the resection of residual tumoral, necrotic, or fibrotic tissues [5].

42.6 Basic Principles

(a) If a straightforward wide local excision is not feasible for a non-metastatic patient with high-grade soft tissue sarcoma, resectability must be re-evaluated following neoadjuvant treatment. For specific pathologies such as non-pleomorphic rhabdomyosarcoma and infantile fibrosarcoma, resectability must be re-evaluated following neoadjuvant chemotherapy [4, 6].
(b) While the conventional goal of limb salvage is resection with wide (adequate) margins, marginal margins might be accepted or required following neoadjuvant treatment for extreme limb salvage in the setting of such inoperable tumors [5].
(c) High-quality and detailed local MR imaging must be performed at the time of diagnosis and after the completion of the neoadjuvant treatment. The study must be examined by the radiologist in the multidisciplinary team to interpret treatment response and to guide the surgeon in a heavily traumatized anatomic site.
(d) Following neoadjuvant treatment, the pathoanatomy must be assessed as that of a limb segment that underwent compartment syndrome and is now in the process of healing.

42.7 Intraoperative Images

See Fig. 42.3.

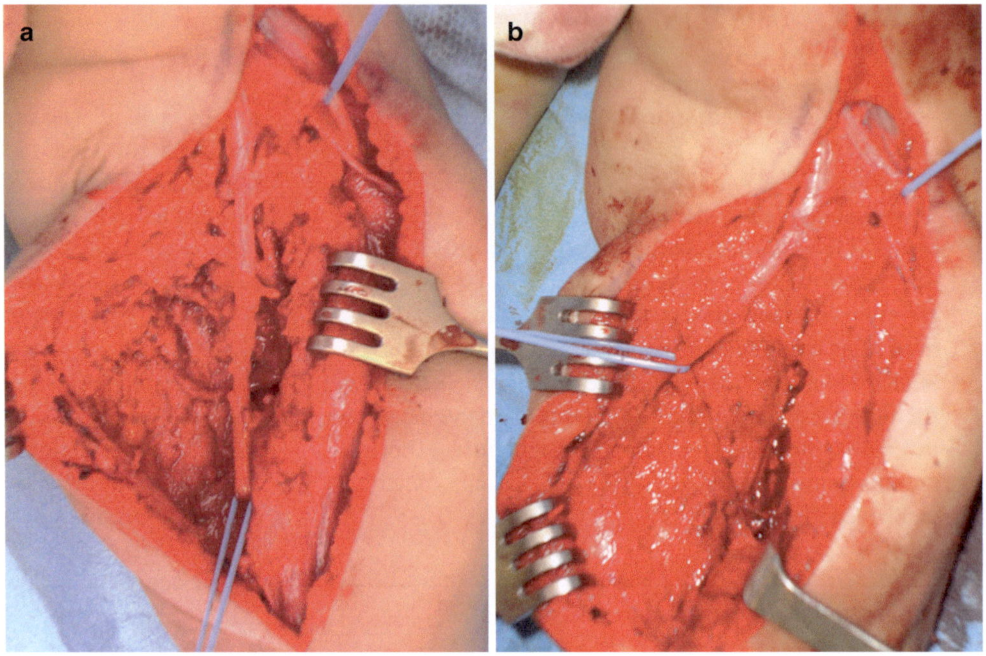

Fig. 42.3 (**a** and **b**) Show the posterior aspect of the right knee and proximal calf intraoperatively. The tibial and fibular nerves have been identified and dissected for decompression (neurolysis). The fibrotic sheath removed during dissection was sent to pathology to reveal complete tumor necrosis

42.8 Technical Pearls

(a) Taking into consideration the excellent chemotherapy response with regressive, fibrotic-appearing residual tissues confined to the deep posterior compartment of the calf in the MRI, the dissection and resection of these fibrotic tissue sheath or band are indicated to ensure local tumor control and to release the main nerves and vessels, which were severely compressed by the tumor for a long time.

(b) An excellent dissection technique and knowledge of crural anatomy are essential. All soft tissues must be handled delicately and carefully.

(c) Extensive exposure relative to the child's size might be necessary. While a tourniquet could help create a clearer surgical field and prevent blood loss, it can only be used if appropriately sized for such a small infant.

42.9 Outcome Radiographs and Images

See Fig. 42.4.

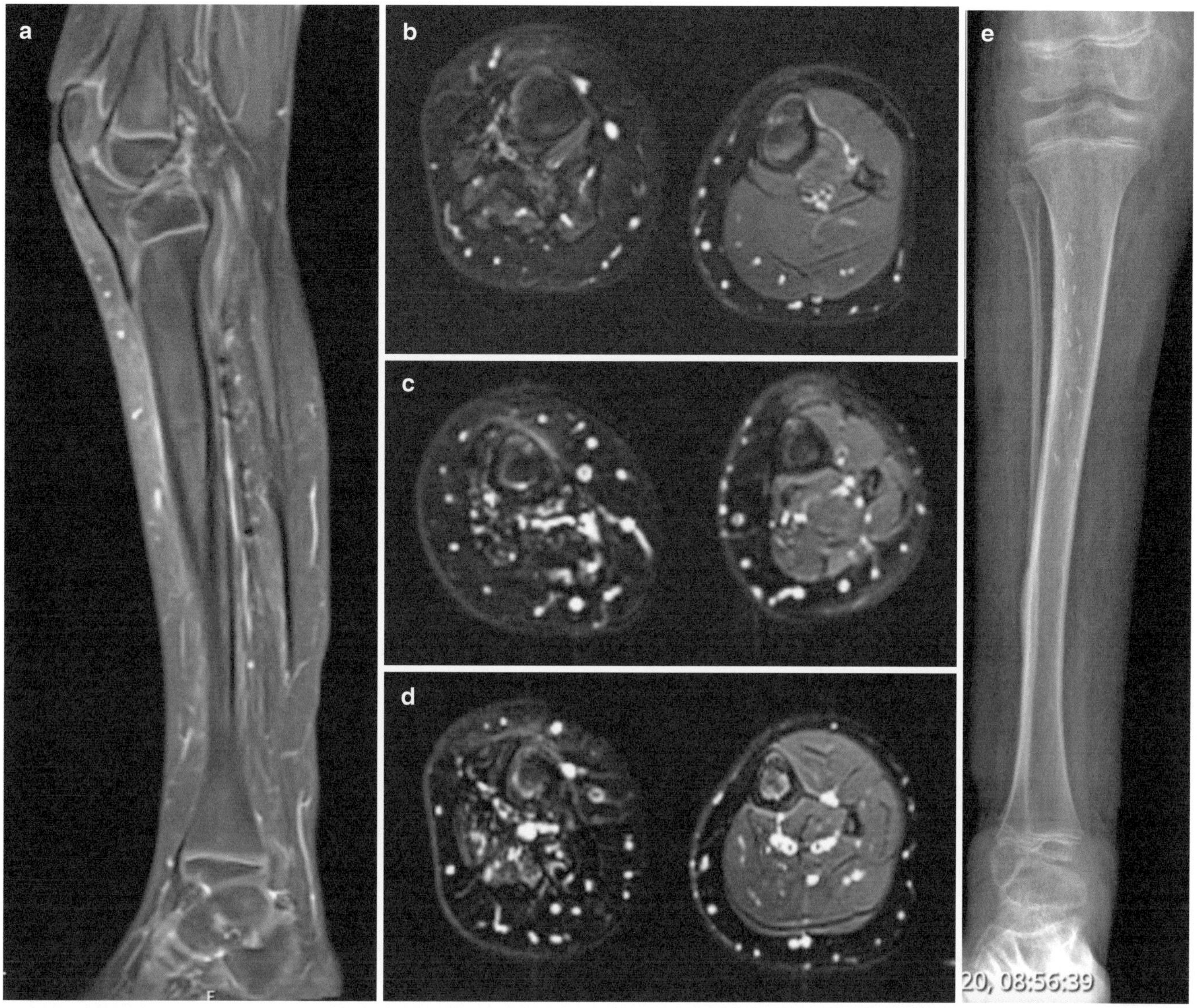

Fig. 42.4 The MR images at postoperative 7 years follow-up in (**a**–**d**) show that the lower leg is free of local disease. The radiograph in (**e**) reveals numerous hemoclips superposed with the proximal half of the tibia, showing extensive neurovascular dissection previously. Clinical images in (**f**–**h**) demonstrate a good functional outcome at postoperative 10 years. She can be seen weight-bearing in a plantigrade fashion following Achilloplasty due to equine deformity. A knee flexion contracture of 10° was accepted as a sequela. The patient was advised to compensate for one-centimeter extra length in her right lower extremity (the operated side) with a shoe lift on the contralateral side

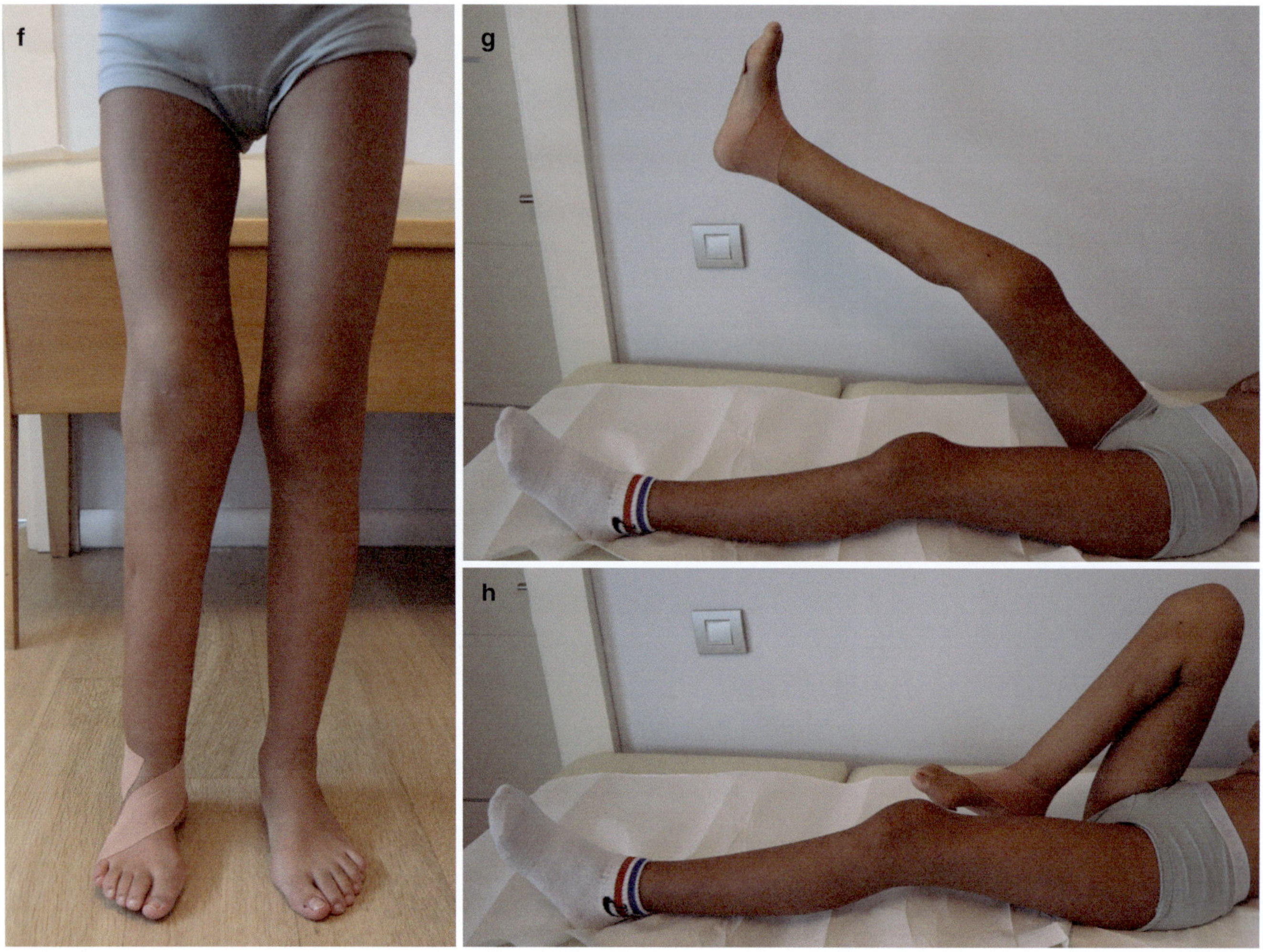

Fig. 42.4 (continued)

42.10 Avoiding and Managing Problems

(a) The orthopedic team should regularly check the patient during the neoadjuvant chemotherapy period to detect complications like tumor progression under treatment, skin breakdown, or tumor-necrosis-related abscess formation, and exulceration to avoid unpleasant surprises at the anticipated time of surgery. Timely detection of such complications might impact the planning of limb salvage surgery and even change the indication from LSS to immediate amputation.

(b) Rapid tumor necrosis might also lead to a sepsis-like condition, which is mainly in the scope of pediatric oncologists. However, such a complication during neoadjuvant treatment might necessitate emergency amputation.

(c) Unnecessary resection of fibrotic/atrophic-appearing muscle tissues should be avoided. Due to the patient's very young age, the soft tissues might exhibit significant plasticity and healing potential.

(d) Due to the increased risk of joint contracture, starting physiotherapy as soon as adequate soft tissue healing is observed is especially critical.

(e) Apart from close oncological surveillance for 10 years postoperatively, the patient must be followed up until skeletal maturity due to the risk of contractures, deformity, gait abnormalities, and leg length discrepancy.

References

1. Weiss SW. Borderline and malignant fibroblastic/myofibroblastic tumors. In: Goldblum JR, Folpe A, editors. Enzinger and Weiss's soft tissue tumors. 7th ed. Elsevier; 2020. p. 306–74.
2. Davis JL, Antonescu CR, Bahrami A. Infantile fibrosarcoma. In: WHO Classification of Tumours Editorial Board, editor. WHO classification of tumours soft tissue and bone tumours. 5th ed. International Agency for Research on Cancer; 2020. p. 119–21.
3. Dumont C, Monforte M, Flandrin A, Couture A, Tichit R, Boulot P. Prenatal management of congenital infantile fibrosarcoma: unexpected outcome. Ultrasound Obstet Gynecol. 2011;37(6):733–5. https://doi.org/10.1002/uog.8878.

4. NCCN clinical practice guidelines in oncology (NCCN guidelines®) soft tissue sarcoma version 2.2021—April 28, 2021. http://nccn.ir/Guidelines/Summary/sarcoma.html#pf23. Accesed 11 May 2023.
5. Sulkowski JP, Raval MV, Browne M. Margin status and multimodal therapy in infantile fibrosarcoma. Pediatr Surg Int. 2013;29(8):771–6. https://doi.org/10.1007/s00383-013-3318-4.
6. Gronchi A, Colombo C, Raut CP. Surgical management of localized soft tissue tumors. Cancer. 2014;120(17):2638–48. Wiley. https://doi.org/10.1002/cncr.28715.

43 Extensive Periosteum-Stripping Resection Without Prophylactic Femur Fixation in Thigh Tumors

Harzem Özger and Buğra Alpan

43.1 Introduction

Pleomorphic sarcomas are high-grade soft tissue sarcomas (STSs), which can be histologically classified as undifferentiated pleomorphic sarcomas (previously designated as "*malignant fibrous histiocytoma*") or pleomorphic sarcomas with a specific line of differentiation (e.g., *pleomorphic liposarcoma, pleomorphic rhabdomyosarcoma*). The clinical behavior is mostly similar for all these tumors with a rapidly growing soft tissue mass, which might be superficially or deeply located [1–3]. The main treatment components are radiotherapy and surgery, as in other high-grade STSs [4]. Chemotherapy might be utilized depending on the extent of the disease and with an individualized treatment approach [4]. While the histological subtype of STSs dictates the role of adjuvant treatment(s) and the rules for the oncological safety of surgical resection, the complication profile of limb salvage surgery (LSS) is closely related to the anatomical location of the tumor. Lower extremities, especially the thigh, constitute a common localization for STSs.

43.2 Brief Clinical History

A 31-year-old male patient presented with a soft tissue mass in his right thigh in March 2018. The patient had noticed the swelling in October 2017 and had associated it with a recent sports injury. Upon progression of the swelling, the patient had sought medical attention in January 2018 and had been followed up with the presumption of hematoma for one more month, after which magnetic resonance imaging had demonstrated that the mass was consistent with a soft tissue sarcoma. An open biopsy was performed in another institution in February 2018, and the patient was offered amputation upon a diagnosis of leiomyosarcoma. The patient, who refused amputation, then presented to our clinic for a second opinion. Local and systemic imaging studies were updated, and the previous pathological specimen was consulted with our dedicated musculoskeletal pathologist. Considering the morphology and the diffuse positivity of SMA, it was concluded that the tumor was a pleomorphic sarcoma with leiomyosarcomatous differentiation (FNCLCC grade III). He was non-metastatic at presentation, with the tumor located in the lateral aspect of the vastus intermedius muscle and measuring 25 × 11 × 8 cm. Neoadjuvant chemoradiotherapy followed by limb salvage surgery was planned. The patient received a total dose of 45 Gray radiation concurrently with Ifosfamide and Etoposide chemotherapy regimen over 5 weeks. After the neoadjuvant treatment, the tumoral mass showed significant softening with clinical examination and marked loss of contrast enhancement with cystic changes in MRI. Femur-sparing wide resection with modified margins was performed, followed by adjuvant chemotherapy. He used a pair of crutches while weight-bearing as tolerated and received physiotherapy for 12 months after the operation. At postoperative 5 years, the patient is disease-free and has normal ambulation with good knee function.

43.3 Preoperative Local Imaging

See Figs. 43.1, 43.2, 43.3, 43.4, and 43.5.

H. Özger (✉)
Department of Orthopedics and Traumatology, Istanbul University, Istanbul Medical Faculty, Istanbul, Türkiye
e-mail: harzemo@yahoo.com

B. Alpan
Department of Orthopedics and Traumatology, Acıbadem Mehmet Ali Aydınlar University, School of Medicine, Istanbul, Türkiye
e-mail: bugra.alpan@acibadem.edu.tr

H. Özger et al. (eds.), *Diagnosis and Treatment of Soft Tissue Tumors*, https://doi.org/10.1007/978-3-031-77061-6_43

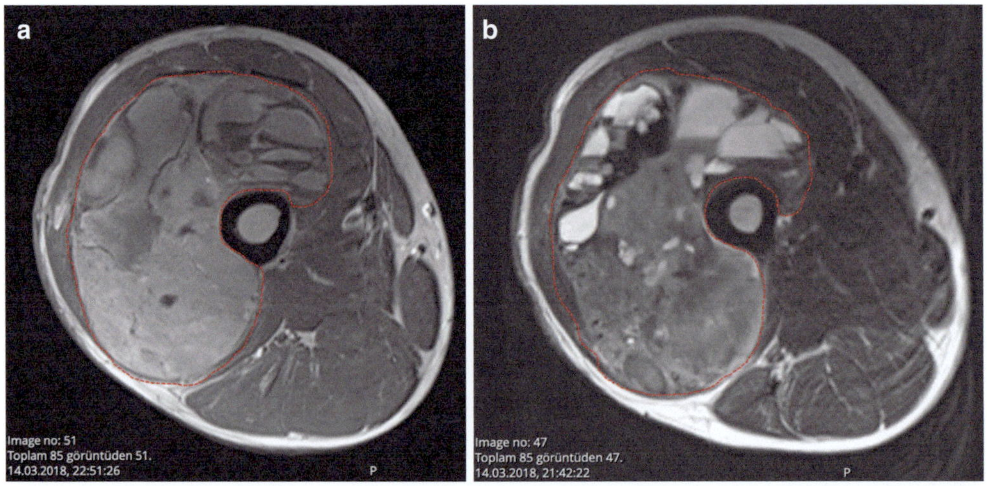

Fig. 43.1 (**a** and **b**) Transverse T1 FS MRI images at presentation. Red-dashed freeform delineates the deep-seated thigh tumor, which surrounds the femur 270° in the anterior compartment

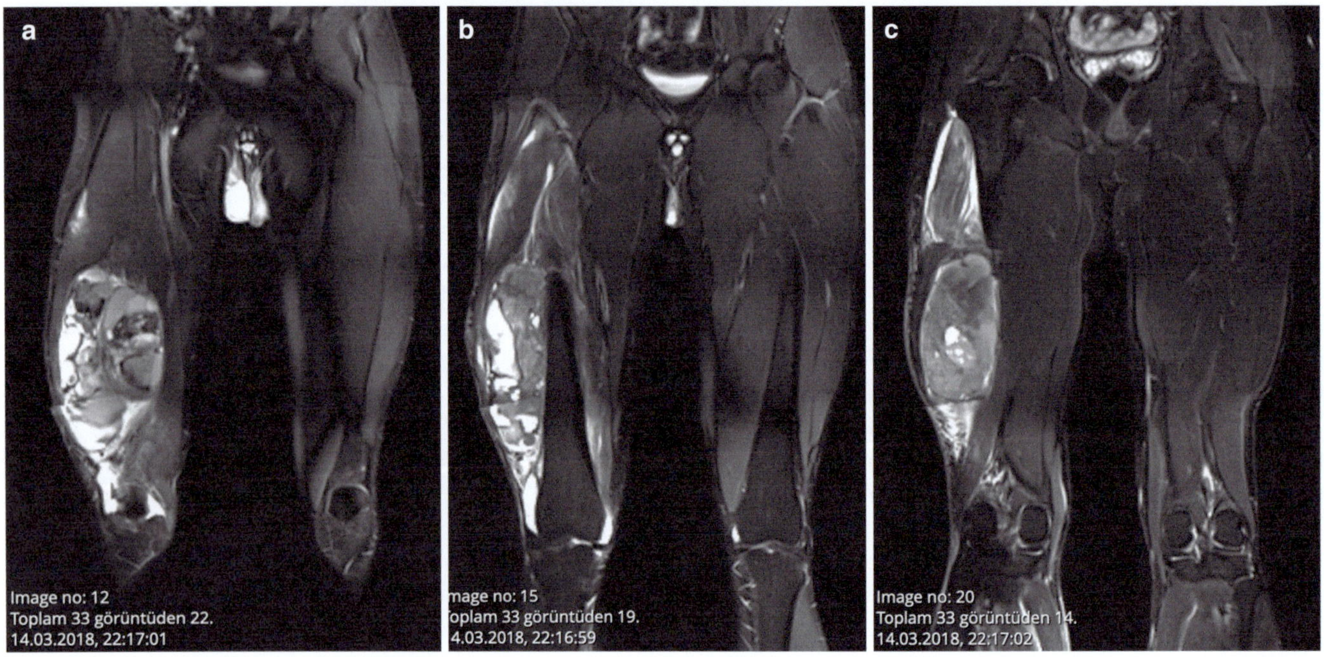

Fig. 43.2 (**a**–**c**) Coronal STIR MRI images at presentation. The tumor extends from the proximal to distal ends of the lateral part of the anterior compartment. The patient was offered amputation in an elsewhere institution after a delayed diagnosis of leiomyosarcoma

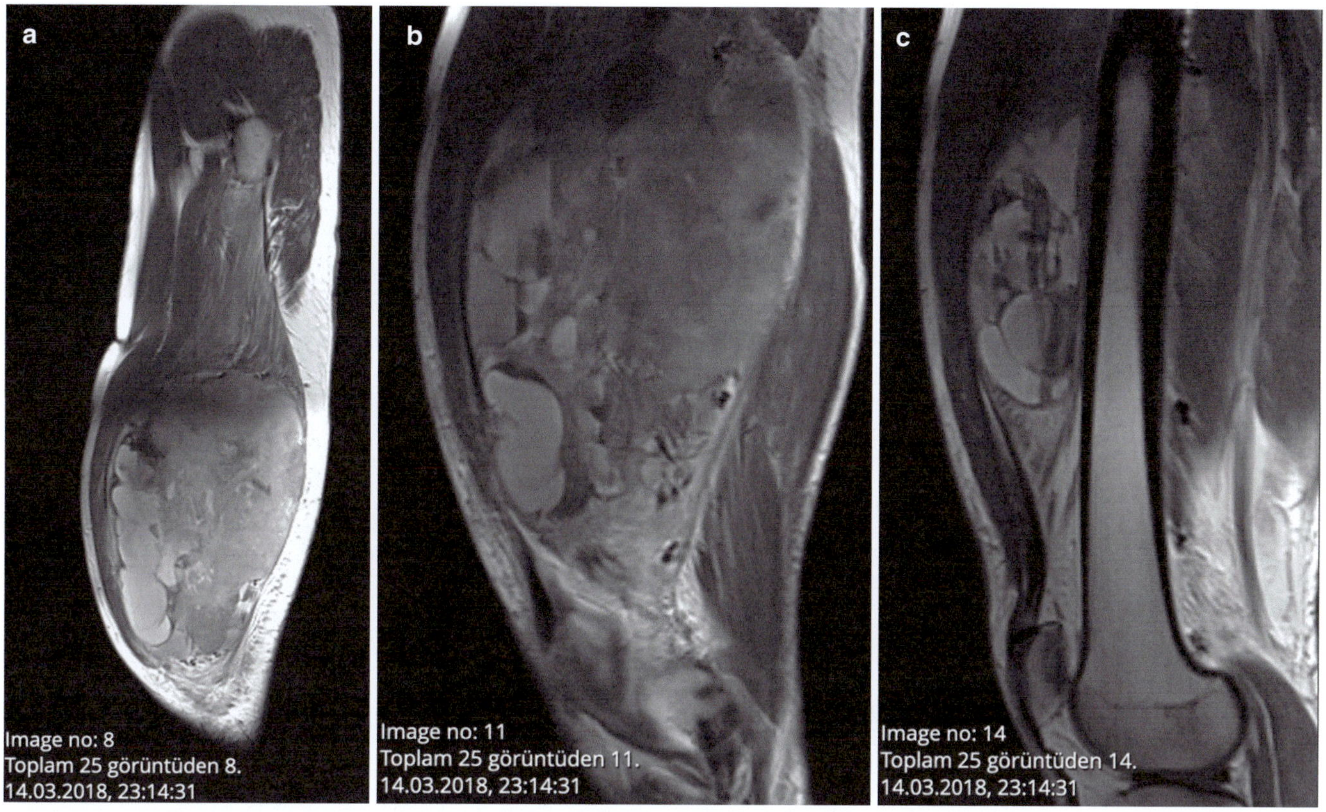

Fig. 43.3 T2 MR images in (**a**–**c**) demonstrate the extensive involvement of the quadriceps muscle in the sagittal plane at presentation

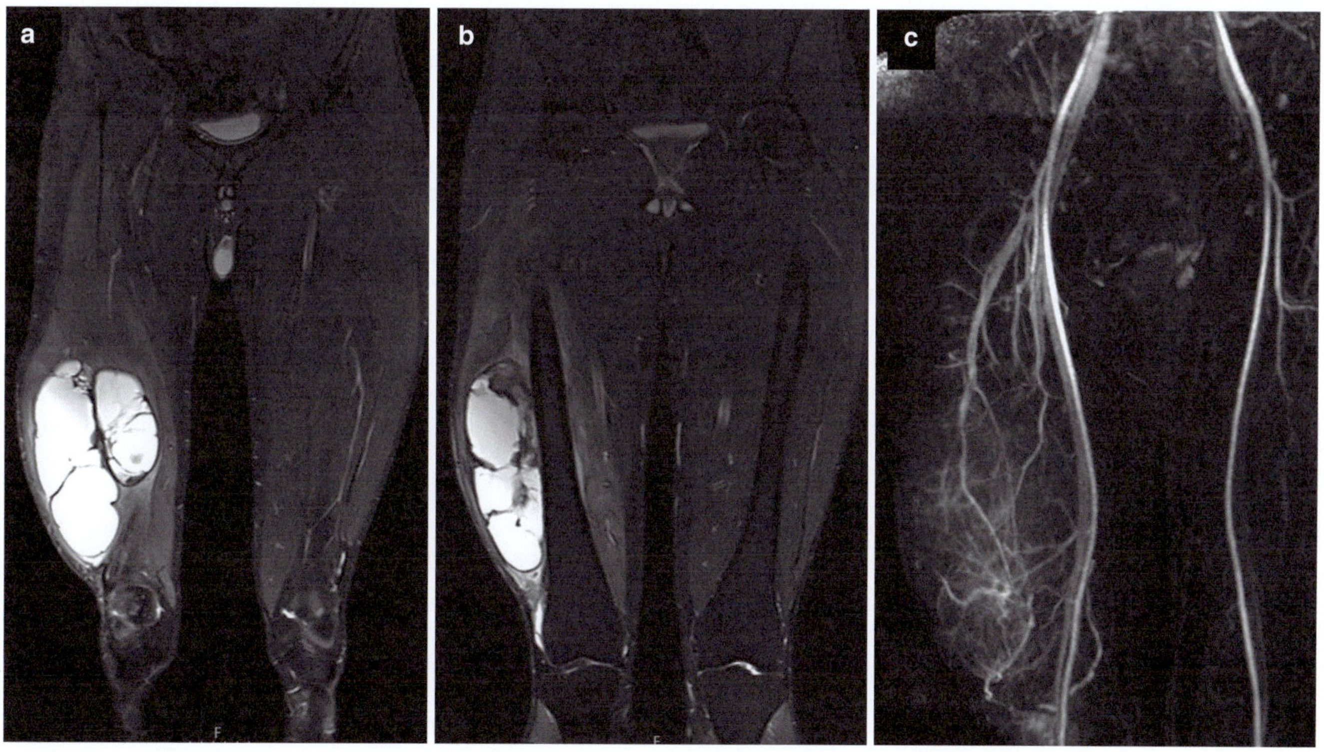

Fig. 43.4 Coronal TRIM MR images in (**a** and **b**) demonstrate tumor consolidation and moderate shrinkage after neoadjuvant treatment. Coronal image from the angio-twist sequence (**c**) shows significant vascularization of the tumor despite neoadjuvant treatment

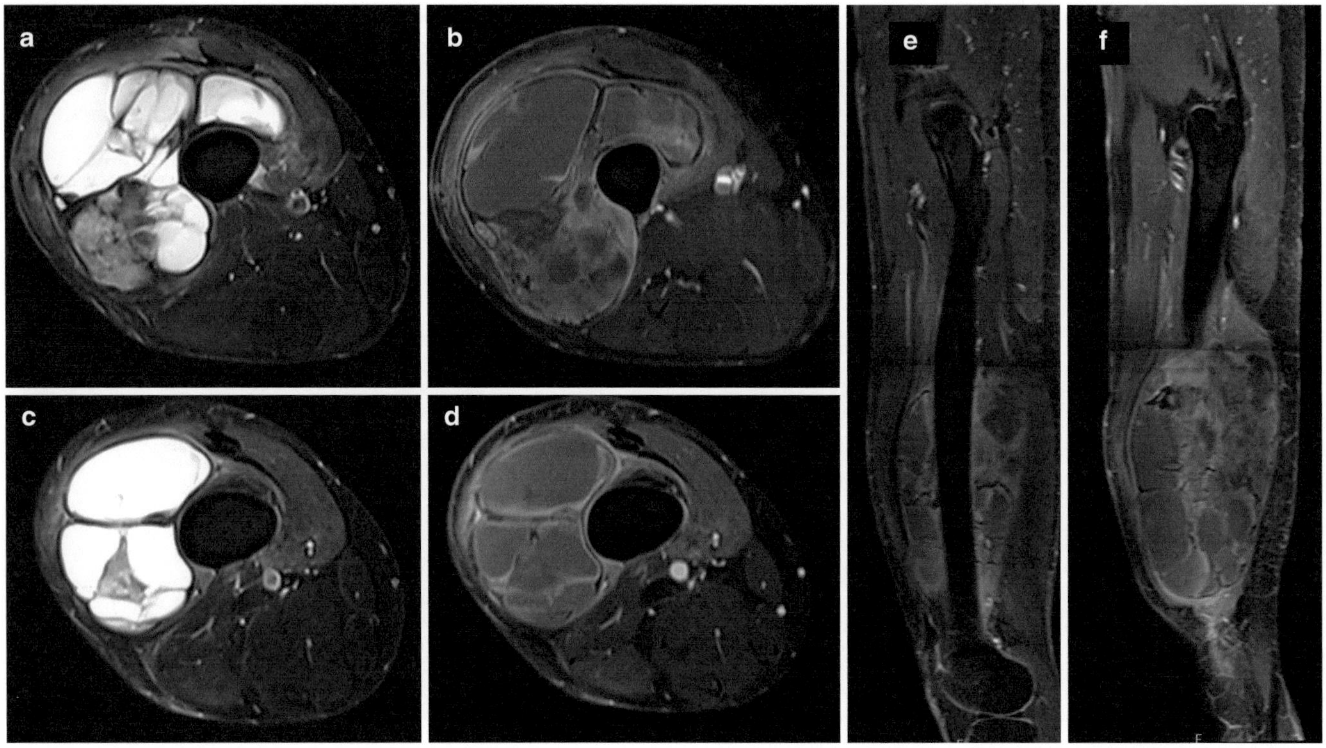

Fig. 43.5 Transverse TRIM and contrast-enhanced T1 FS MR images in (**a**–**d**) demonstrate tumor consolidation and moderate shrinkage after neoadjuvant treatment. However, the tumor shows significant necrosis, with only peripheral contrast-enhancing cystic spaces predominating the mass. Contrast-enhanced sagittal T1 FS MR images in (**e** and **f**) demonstrate marked tumor necrosis

43.4 Preoperative Problem List

(a) The tumor has a large volume, which causes multiple potential problems regarding systemic disease, oncologically safe resection, preserving function, and avoiding complications:
   1. Even though the patient is non-metastatic, according to systemic evaluation at presentation, the large tumor size increases the probability of microscopic metastasis.
   2. While the tumor seems to arise from and be constrained within the vastus intermedius muscle, it is unclear how much of the quadriceps muscle can be spared and whether a functional extensor mechanism can be preserved.
   3. The tumor's distal-most projections extend to the knee joint's vicinity.
   4. The proximal-most tail-like projections of the tumor extend between the muscle fibers without a definitive border.
   5. A large dead space, which is prone to seroma and hematoma formation, is inevitable following the removal of such a large mass.

(b) The tumor is in direct contact with the femur's lateral, anterior, and anteromedial aspects and surrounds it 210° in the transverse plane.
   1. While osseous resection might as well be considered to achieve wide resection, even if the bone is spared, extensive periosteal stripping is inevitable, and the vascular supply of the bone is very likely to be compromised.
   2. The possible use of radiotherapy for local control might further compromise the vitality of the bone, leading to osteonecrosis and pathological/iatrogenic fracture [5–7].
   3. Intramedullary prophylactic nailing of the femur will cause imaging difficulties in the follow-up period.

(c) The cystic–necrotic changes seen after the neoadjuvant make the mass prone to rupture and tumor spill during resection.

43.5 Treatment Strategy

(a) Limb salvage surgery is the main treatment objective and resection with safe margins is the most crucial aspect of LSS.

(b) A multidisciplinary approach is essential for the best functional and oncological outcome. The multidisciplinary board should discuss thoroughly whether adjuvant treatment modalities are indicated and the timing of these possible interventions to facilitate safe resection, improve systemic disease control, and minimize complications [4].

(c) In this case, preservation of the knee extensor mechanism (the quadriceps muscle and tendon) is desirable for the best ambulatory function.

(d) Avoiding an osseous resection, which will dramatically increase the treatment morbidity, is also a priority.

43.6 Basic Principles

(a) If the biopsy was done elsewhere, either the pathology specimen must be consulted with the pathologist in the multidisciplinary team or the biopsy must be repeated to confirm or correct the diagnosis.

(b) Excision with safe margins is the primary treatment method for high-grade STSs if the excision is possible with acceptable morbidity. Radiotherapy is particularly beneficial for local control in high-grade tumors. The timing of radiotherapy (pre-/postoperative) will depend on surgeon preference and institutional policy [4].

(c) On the other hand, if excision with safe margins is not feasible at presentation for a high-grade STS, resectability must be re-evaluated following radiotherapy. Radiotherapy and chemotherapy can be used concurrently in the neoadjuvant setting to facilitate resection with safe margins, especially in large, deeply seated tumors, for which local control is questionable, and the patient is at increased risk of metastasis during the neoadjuvant treatment period [4].

(d) The biopsy tract needs to be removed en bloc with the tumor.

(e) Osseous involvement is an indication for osseous resection and reconstruction in STSs. However, if the bone is not invaded or completely (360°) engulfed by the tumor, the bone can be spared, provided that necessary adjuvant treatment(s) and adequate surgical skill have been applied to modify the margins.

(f) While "bone tangential resection," "periosteal stripping," and the application of "radiotherapy" are risk factors for osteonecrosis and pathological/iatrogenic fracture in the involved bone segment, prophylactic fixation has disadvantages, such as impairing MR imaging, increasing the risk of tumor contamination of the bone, and increasing operation time and blood loss [6].

(g) Preserving active knee range of motion is the key to an excellent functional outcome in lower extremity tumors.

43.7 Intraoperative Images

See Fig. 43.6.

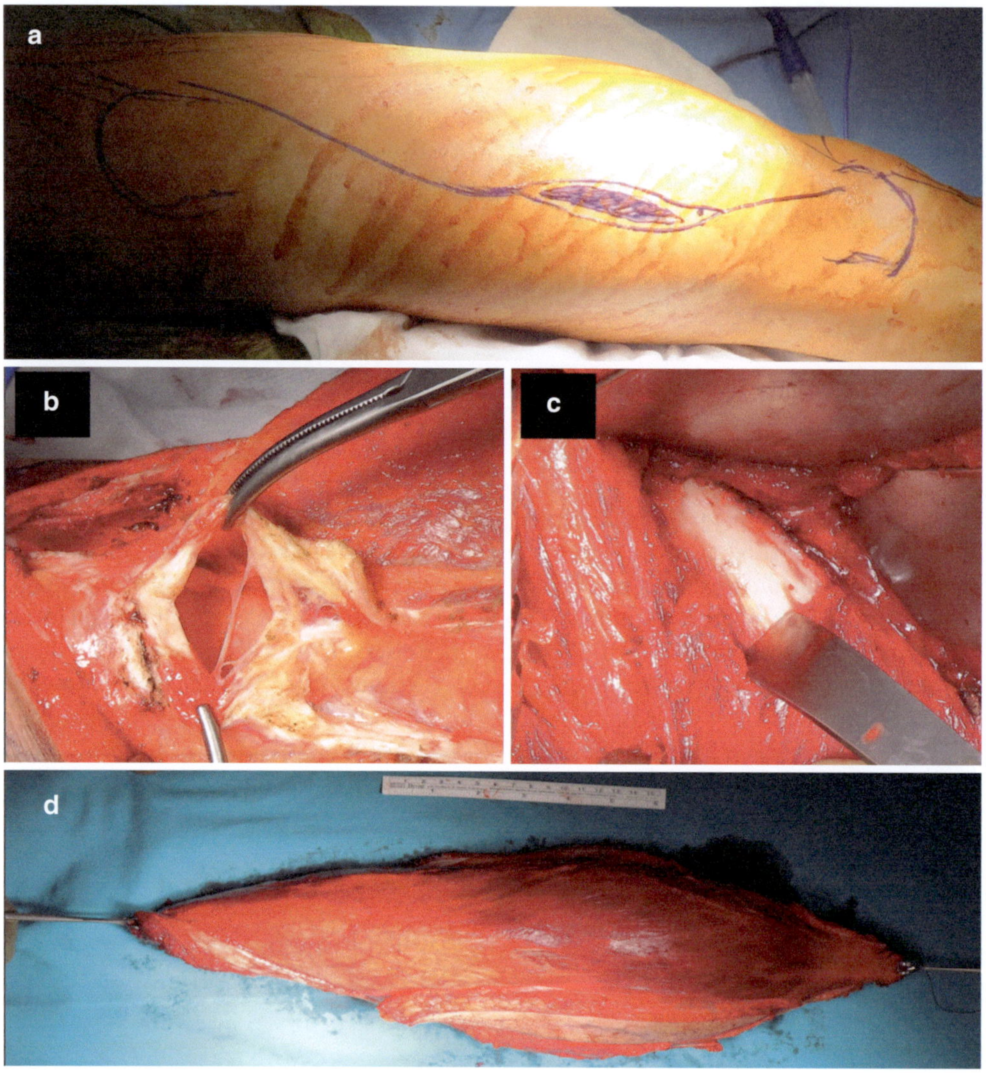

Fig. 43.6 The intraoperative image in (**a**) shows the lateral aspect of the right thigh and knee, with the planned incision including the previous open biopsy scar. (**b**) Shows the separation of the quadriceps tendon through the portions coming from the rectus femoris and vastus intermedius. The deeper portion of the tendon from the v. intermedius will be resected together with the tumor as a barrier, while the superficial portion will be preserved for the integrity of the extensor apparatus. (**c**) Shows the subperiosteal dissection of the vastus intermedius from the femur, a measure that was made possible and encouraged by good response to neoadjuvant concurrent chemoradiotherapy. (**d**) Shows the widely resected specimen, which includes a significant portion of the anterior compartment musculature. (**e**) Demonstrates the resection lodge with more than 25 cm of the femur exposed, with only linea aspera muscle attachments preserved. (**f**) Shows that the biceps femoris has been transferred to the rectus femoris to augment the extensor apparatus, cover the naked femur segment (at least partially), and decrease the dead space. No wound problem was observed postoperatively, and the pathology report revealed 95% necrosis with clear margins

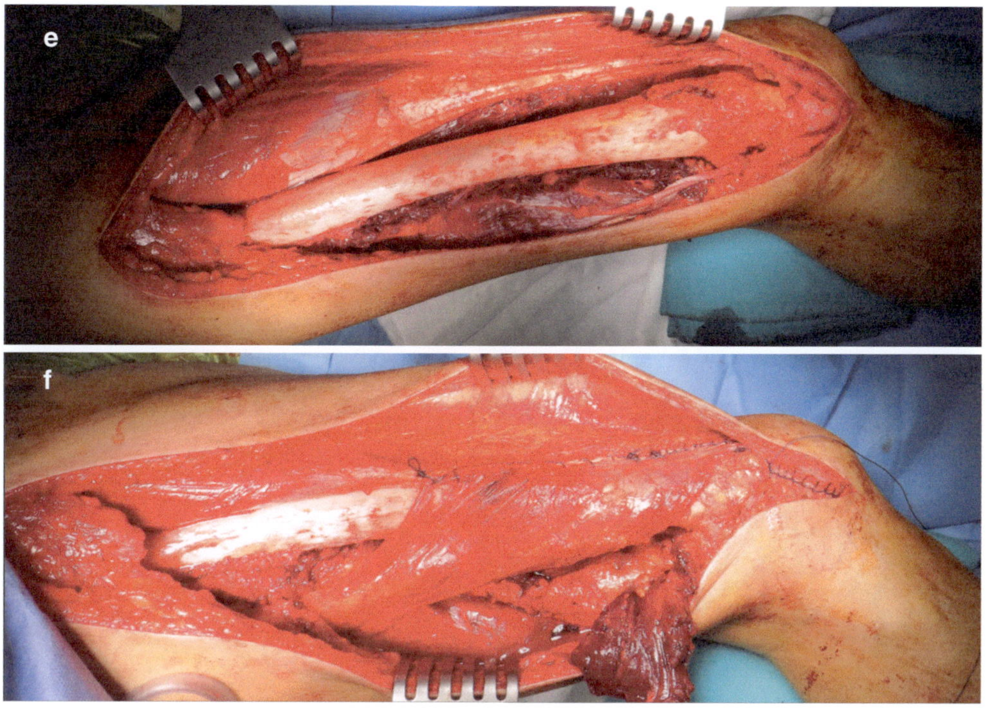

Fig. 43.6 (continued)

43.8 Technical Pearls

(a) While a significant volume of the quadriceps muscle needs to be sacrificed to achieve oncologically safe surgical margins, every effort must be made to preserve the integrity of the extensor mechanism. Even sparing a thin bundle of the rectus femoris muscle and keeping the superficial portion of the quadriceps tendon will be important assets in ambulatory function.

(b) Resection with proper wide margins is imperative in the distal and proximal poles of the tumoral mass, which has a fusiform morphology and suspicious extensions along muscle fibers in the distal and proximal ends.

(c) If the surgeon considers that the neoadjuvant treatment has been effective, "bone tangential resection" of the tumor can be performed with subperiosteal and extracortical dissection, preferably with electrocautery, taking care to preserve the integrity of the periosteum which will act as a modified barrier.

(d) The mass must be handled gently all through the operation to prevent rupture of the cystic–necrotic spaces inside the tumor.

43.9 Outcome Radiographs and Images

See Fig. 43.7.

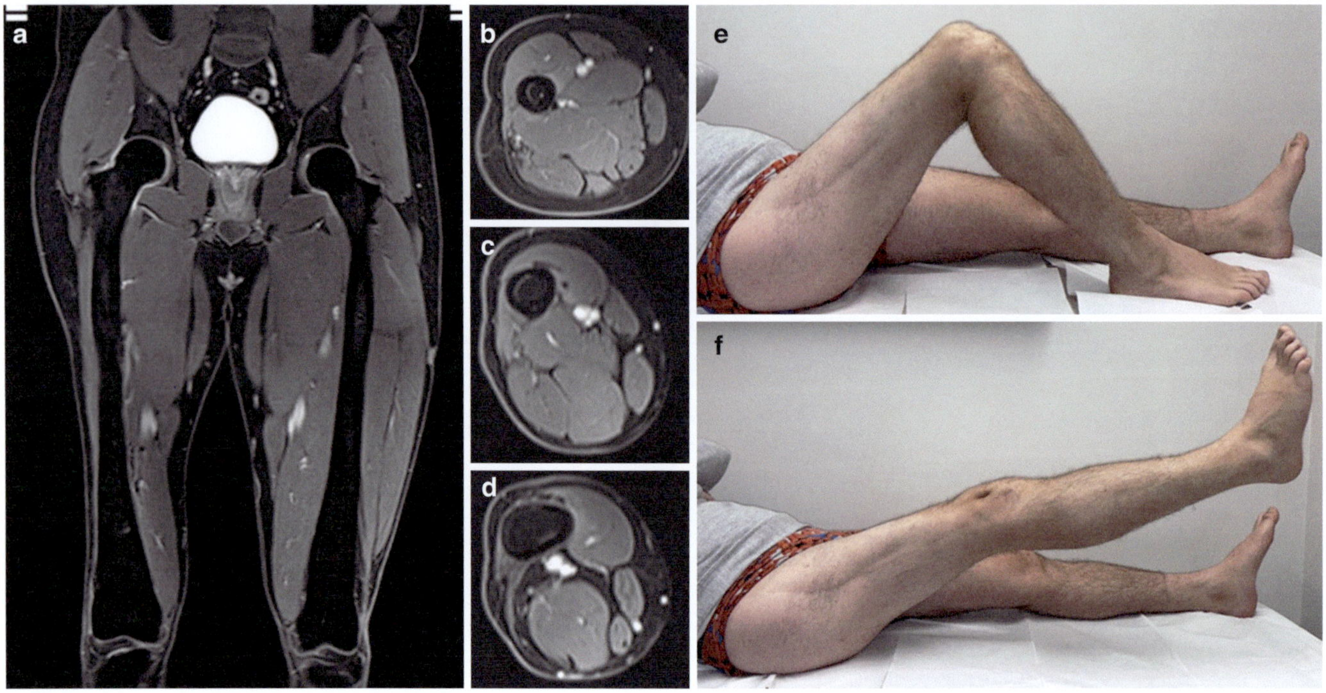

Fig. 43.7 Contrast-enhanced coronal (**a**) and transverse (**b–d**) MRI images at 51 months postoperatively show no residual disease, local recurrence, or abnormal bone signal associated with bone edema or insufficiency fracture. Clinical images in (**e** and **f**) show very good knee function at postoperative 5 years. The patient was non-metastatic at the time of the last follow-up visit

43.10 Avoiding and Managing Problems

(a) To minimize the risk of local recurrence, margin modification with neoadjuvant radiotherapy is crucial in the local management of high-grade STSs if proper wide resection is not possible with acceptable morbidity. While adjuvant radiotherapy can be preferred in some centers due to institutional or surgeon preference, postoperative radiotherapy is not used as a margin-modifying modality but rather as a second-line treatment for possible residual microscopic disease. Although neoadjuvant radiotherapy is more favorable for its margin-modifying effect and improving the safety of resection, it also brings together the increased risk of postoperative wound complications. Therefore, the surgical team must be able to prevent or treat soft tissue failures in the setting of neoadjuvant radiotherapy. Radiotherapy must be given by a radiation oncology team that is experienced in sarcoma treatment to maximize tumor necrosis and minimize local complications.

(b) When neoadjuvant radiotherapy alone is deemed inadequate to facilitate safe resection for limb salvage surgery, concurrent chemoradiotherapy might be administered to boost local control and simultaneously provide systemic protection against metastasis. This approach is helpful in extreme limb salvage cases that present with large and exulcerated tumors. The medical oncology team must be familiar with concurrent treatment to maximize the tumoricidal effect and manage the toxicity.

(c) The orthopedic team should regularly check the patient during the neoadjuvant treatment and the following waiting period until surgery to detect complications like tumor progression under treatment, severe radiation dermatitis, skin breakdown, and tumor-necrosis-related abscess formation and exulceration to avoid unpleasant surprises at the anticipated time of surgery. Timely detection of such complications might impact the preparations for LSS, such as planning for a free flap or implant reconstruction. It might even change the indication from LSS to immediate amputation.

(d) Multiple suction drains are recommended to prevent hematoma and seroma formation in ample post-resection dead space. Delayed wound closure with negative pressure wound treatment systems (e.g., vacuum-assisted closure "VAC" device) might also be considered to manage the dead space and prevent wound necrosis associated with preoperative radiotherapy.

(e) Extensive "periosteal stripping," "bone tangential resection," and "radiotherapy" predispose to pathological/iatrogenic fracture in lower extremity STSs, and it is very difficult to obtain bone healing, especially if pathologic fracture occurs in the setting of radiotherapy.

Due to an increased risk of unmanageable complications, some surgeons prefer prophylactic fixation at the time of resection. On the other hand, prophylactic fixation impairs high-quality MR imaging in the follow-up. The pros and cons of not performing prophylactic fixation must be explained and discussed with the patient. While the fracture risk cannot be eliminated completely, protracted partial weight-bearing with assistive devices can be recommended when fixation has not been performed. The cortical surface carries a significant risk of local recurrence in cases where periosteal stripping was performed. Therefore, the involved bone and its vicinity must be visualized in detail without metal artifacts during the follow-up. In addition to impairment of postoperative imaging, fixation extends the operation time and thus contributes to increased blood loss and risk of infection. Besides, intramedullary prophylactic fixation impedes the endosteal blood flow, although temporarily in theory, and further weakens the bone, which has already lost its periosteal blood supply. Alternative reasonable strategies include:

1. Elective (staged) fixation in the ensuing months after careful clinical and radiological observation with intervention performed in patients with pain or imaging evidence of developing insufficiency fracture,
2. Fixation using non-ferromagnetic implants to minimize interference with MRI imaging.

(f) Physiotherapy must be initiated in the early postoperative period to gain maximum knee extension power from the remaining quadriceps muscle and to prevent knee arthrofibrosis and adhesion of quadriceps muscle to the femur.

References

1. Gambarotti M. General principles of bone pathology. In: Picci P, Manfrini M, Fabbri N, Gambarotti M, Vanel D, editors. Atlas of musculoskeletal tumors and tumorlike lesions. Cham: Springer; 2014. p. 351–3.
2. Dei Tos AP, Mertens F, Pillay N. Undifferentiated sarcoma. In: WHO Classification of Tumours Editorial Board, editor. WHO classification of tumours soft tissue and bone tumours. 5th ed. Lyon: International Agency for Research on Cancer; 2020. p. 318–20.
3. Weiss SW. Undifferentiated pleomorphic sarcoma. In: Goldblum JR, Folpe A, editors. Enzinger and Weiss's soft tissue tumors. 7th ed. Philadelphia: Elsevier; 2020. p. 452–75.
4. NCCN clinical practice guidelines in oncology (NCCN guidelines®) soft tissue sarcoma version 2.2021—April 28, 2021. [cited 2023 May 11]. http://nccn.ir/Guidelines/Summary/sarcoma.html#pf23.
5. Pak D, Vineberg KA, Griffith KA, Sabolch A, Chugh R, Ben-Josef E, et al. Dose-effect relationships for femoral fractures after multimodality limb-sparing therapy of soft-tissue sarcomas of the proximal lower extremity. Int J Radiat Oncol Biol Phys. 2012;83(4):1257–63.
6. Sambri A, Gardini L, Dalla Rosa M, Zavatta G, Keskinbora M, Ferrari C, et al. Femoral fracture in primary soft-tissue sarcoma of the thigh treated with radiation therapy: indications for prophylactic intramedullary nail. Arch Orthop Trauma Surg. 2021;141(8):1277–82.
7. Elswick SM, Curiel DA, Wu P, Akhavan A, Molinar VE, Mohan AT, et al. Complications after thigh sarcoma resection. J Surg Oncol. 2020;121(6):945–51.

44 Exulcerated Angiosarcoma of the Head and Neck Treated with Neoadjuvant Chemoradiotherapy and Flap Reconstruction

Fulya Ağaoğlu, Harzem Özger, Mehmet Veli Karaaltın, and Buğra Alpan

44.1 Introduction

Angiosarcomas are rare malignant soft tissue neoplasms commonly involving the skin and superficial soft tissues. The histology might vary from highly differentiated tumors resembling a hemangioma to anaplastic lesions resembling poorly differentiated carcinoma or pleomorphic sarcoma. Surrounding tissues are often infiltrated destructively. They can be distinguished from other sarcomas by overexpression of genes related to angiogenesis. The most common clinical form is "primary cutaneous angiosarcoma," which arises in the absence of underlying factors such as radiation or lymphedema. The head, neck, and face are common areas of involvement. The lesions can be protuberant, nodular, and exulcerated. The infiltrative nature of the borders makes it difficult to determine the tumor extent and complicates surgical excision with clean margins. Staging of angiosarcomas is not relevant due to the aggressive behavior. Survival beyond 1 year from diagnosis is less than 50%. Death usually occurs due to lung, liver, and lymph node metastases. Younger patients with tumors less than 5 cm in diameter and negative surgical margins have better prognoses, while patients older than 50 years, patients with larger tumors, positive surgical margins, and epithelioid morphology show worse outcomes. Complete surgical excision is the main treatment modality [1–6]. Radiotherapy is an essential adjuvant modality to facilitate surgery and minimize the risk of local recurrence in locally advanced tumors [7, 8]. Cytotoxic chemotherapy and targeted therapies can also be used for both systemic and local control [8]. Pedicled trapezius flaps, on the other hand, are important tools in the reconstruction of soft tissue defects around the posterior cranium and the neck [9–11].

44.2 Brief Clinical History

A 26-year-old male patient presented to our clinic with a fungating soft tissue tumor of the head and neck region. His history revealed that he had undergone an unplanned excision of an MRI-documented superficial soft tissue mass (3 × 2 × 2 cm) from the left posterior aspect of his head and neck, 3 months ago, in an elsewhere hospital. The lesion had been excised with the presumption of lipoma. However, the postoperative pathology had been reported as a malignant mesenchymal tumor. MRI-documented local recurrence had been observed within 2 months. According to intraoperative photos obtained from the patient, a relatively wider re-excision of the rapidly growing and exulcerating recurrent mass (12 × 6 × 6 cm) was performed. While a major part of the left occipital bone had been exposed following resection, the scalp defect had been reduced significantly with purse-string suturing, and the remaining defect had been closed with split-thickness skin grafting. However, the tumor had aggressively recurred a second time just after 1 month and had become hemorrhagic on the surface.

Upon presentation to our clinic, his physical examination yielded a dark red to purple colored, painless, exophytic, lobular, and hemorrhagic soft tissue mass protruding from the left occipitocervical region. Tumor dimensions were 14 × 9 × 5 cm. The neck range of motion was preserved, and the neurologic examination was unremarkable. He was mildly anemic due to recent frequent bleeding episodes. A new open biopsy was performed as an office procedure, and

F. Ağaoğlu
Department of Radiation Oncology, Acıbadem Atakent Hospital, Istanbul, Türkiye
e-mail: fulya.agaoglu@acibadem.com

H. Özger (✉)
Department of Orthopedics and Traumatology, Istanbul University, Istanbul Medical Faculty, Istanbul, Türkiye
e-mail: harzemo@yahoo.com

M. V. Karaaltın
Department of Plastic and Reconstructive Surgery, Acıbadem Taksim Hospital, Istanbul, Türkiye

B. Alpan
Department of Orthopedics and Traumatology, Acıbadem Mehmet Ali Aydınlar University, School of Medicine, Istanbul, Türkiye
e-mail: bugra.alpan@acibadem.edu.tr

H. Özger et al. (eds.), *Diagnosis and Treatment of Soft Tissue Tumors*, https://doi.org/10.1007/978-3-031-77061-6_44

the previous pathology specimens were also consulted with our multidisciplinary team's musculoskeletal pathologist. His serological tests were negative for HIV and HHV8. Taking into consideration the histopathology and the serological parameters, Kaposi sarcoma was ruled out and the diagnosis was specified as "cutaneous angiosarcoma." Pulmonary metastatic nodules were positive at presentation. The patient described severe anxiety and discomfort due to the relentless recurrence and progression of the tumor as well as the easily bleeding fragile nature of the lesion, which required frequent wound dressing changes.

44.3 Preoperative Local Imaging

See Fig. 44.1.

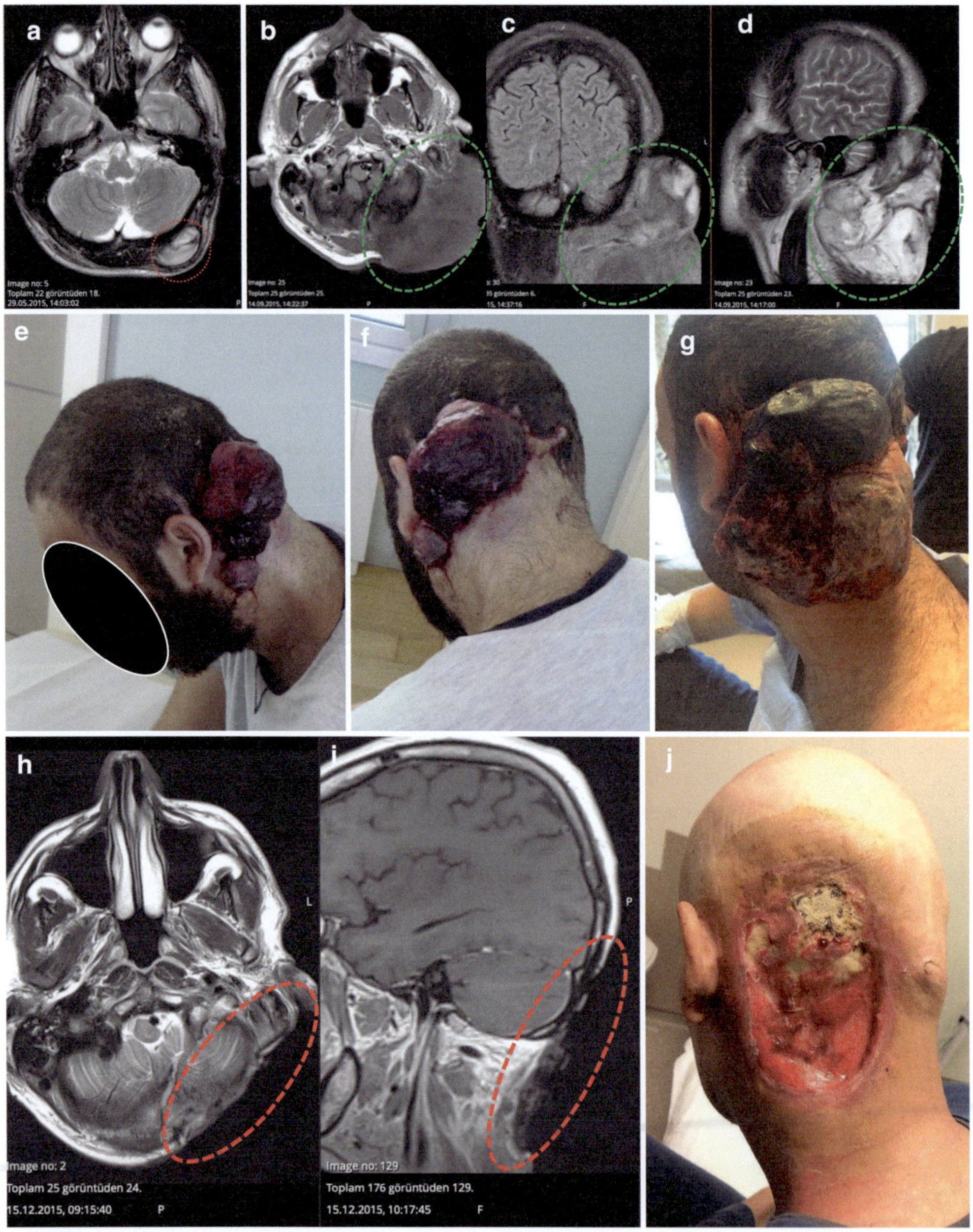

Fig. 44.1 Transverse cranial MR image in (**a**) shows the extracranial tumoral mass (red-dashed circle) adjacent to the left occipital bone at first presentation to elsewhere hospital. Transverse, coronal, and sagittal cranial MR images in (**b–d**) show the large exophytic recurrent tumor (green-dashed ellipse) at presentation to our clinic, after two failed surgeries elsewhere. Clinical images in (**e**, **f**) show the exophytic, and hemorrhagic soft tissue mass protruding from the left occipitocervical region at presentation to our clinic. While neoadjuvant radiotherapy was started immediately, the clinical image in (**g**) shows tumor progression under radiotherapy 1 week after presentation, leading to a treatment change. Following concurrent chemoradiotherapy, the exophytic tumor showed a dramatic radiological and clinical response. Transverse and sagittal cranial MR images in (**h** and **i**) demonstrate the complete disappearance of the tumoral mass (red-dashed ellipse), while the clinical image in (**j**) shows the partially granulated tumor base and exposed occipital bone after neoadjuvant treatment

44.4 Preoperative Problem List

(a) Due to the tumor's aggressive behavior, pathology specimens consisted of mainly necrotic tissue, causing a major diagnostic challenge for the pathologist.
(b) The main treatment for angiosarcoma is an "absolute wide resection." In the most extreme scenarios involving tumors of the limbs, this can be achieved with amputation or in other words an "ablative surgery." However, ablative surgery was not applicable in this location.
(c) An adequately wide local excision was not a realistic goal without neoadjuvant treatment.
(d) The patient was started on radiotherapy immediately upon presentation to control bleeding and to facilitate shrinkage. However, the tumor was clinically observed to progress even under radiotherapy.
(e) A significant impact on local control is highly unlikely with the use of chemotherapy alone.
(f) The exophytic and fragile nature of the tumor poses a significant risk of profuse bleeding, which can even be life threatening or can cause susceptibility to infection further compromising conditions for surgery.
(g) Soft tissue coverage after tumor resection is highly challenging since a large scalp defect can be expected.
(h) The base of the tumor rests on the occipital bone in close contact with the transverse sinus, which complicates a highly probable tangential osseous resection. Venous sinuses lying inside the cranium are practically considered inoperable due to the impossibility of hemostasis.
(i) The presence of pulmonary metastases is a very unfavorable prognostic factor in angiosarcoma, which is mainly expected to benefit from surgery, and chemotherapy and radiotherapy are usually only palliative.

44.5 Treatment Strategy

(a) A multidisciplinary approach is essential for local and systemic control in such a high-grade soft tissue sarcoma. Even if the planned surgery for the primary tumor aims for palliation and not cure, every weapon must be utilized to minimize the risk of local recurrence, which will have a devastating effect on patient comfort and ultimately survival outcome.
(b) Since the patient did not benefit from radiotherapy alone, concomitant chemoradiotherapy can be employed for a superior tumoricidal effect and to facilitate surgical resection.
(c) The effectiveness of neoadjuvant treatment is also very crucial to prevent tumor ulceration and hemorrhage.
(d) Wide local resection following effective margin-modifying adjuvant treatment is the most crucial aspect of surgical intervention.
(e) A preoperative neurosurgery consultation is advisable in this case due to the critical anatomic location, which is highly likely to necessitate an osseous cranial (the outer table) resection to achieve safe margins.
(f) Just like limb salvage procedures, an extensive resection in the head and neck region will also require sophisticated soft tissue reconstruction. A preoperative consultation with a plastic surgeon experienced in head and neck flap reconstruction is mandatory.

44.6 Basic Principles

(a) If the biopsy was done elsewhere, either the pathology specimen must be consulted with the pathologist in the multidisciplinary team, or the biopsy must be repeated to confirm or correct the diagnosis. Both options were performed for this patient due to the high necrosis rate in the tumor.
(b) Excision with safe margins is the primary treatment method for high-grade STSs if the excision is possible with acceptable morbidity. Radiotherapy is particularly beneficial for local control in high-grade tumors. The timing of radiotherapy (pre-/postoperative) will depend on surgeon preference and/or institutional policy. However, the tumor in this case showed progression under neoadjuvant radiotherapy.
(c) Radiotherapy and chemotherapy can be used concurrently in the neoadjuvant setting to facilitate resection with safe margins, especially in large, fungating tumors, for which local control is questionable and the patient is at increased risk of metastasis during the neoadjuvant treatment period.
(d) Osseous involvement requires an osseous resection: In this case, a "bone tangential resection" of the left occipital bone must be implemented.
(e) Soft tissue reconstruction must be planned in detail preoperatively.

44.7 Intraoperative Images

See Fig. 44.2.

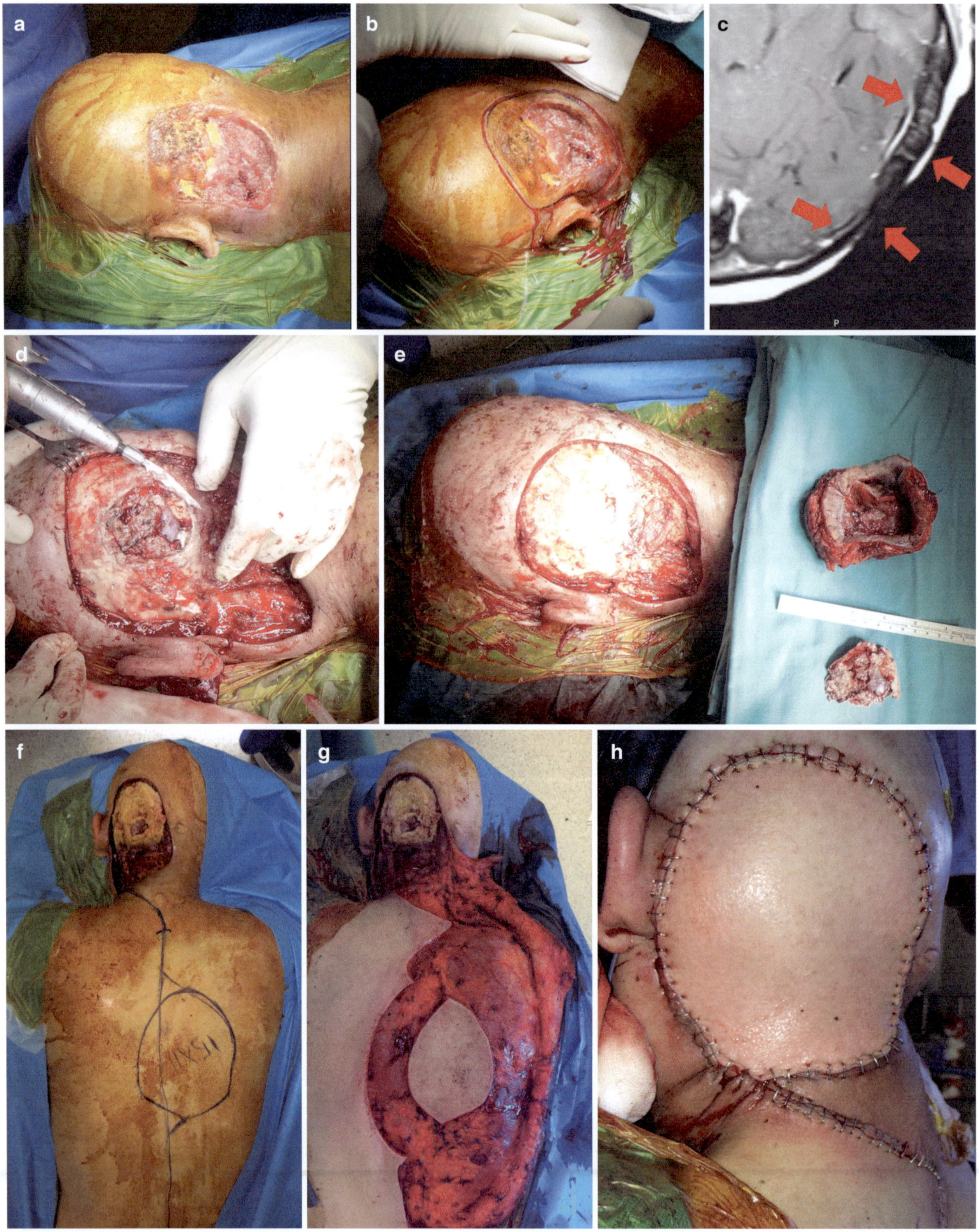

Fig. 44.2 (**a**) Shows the intraoperative preparation with prone positioning, while the peripheral incision with safe margins around the tumor base can be seen in (**b**). The cranial MR image in (**c**) shows the transverse sinus adjacent to the tumor base (red arrows) involving the occipital bone. (**d**) Demonstrates a controlled high-risk tangential osteotomy through the outer table of the cranium using a reciprocating powered microsaw. It should be noted that the osteotomy was performed by the orthopedic surgeon in the attendance of a neurosurgeon. Although this is a very extreme case involving an uncommon localization, the authors believe that such critical resections must nevertheless be performed by the orthopedic oncologist so as not to compromise surgical margins. (**e**) Shows the scalp defect, the soft tissue specimen, and the osseous specimen following resection. While marked tumor necrosis was already evident clinically before the operation, the scalp and neck soft tissue margins and the occipital bone osseous margins were also found to be clear in the postoperative pathological examination. The planning, harvesting, and transfer of the extended distal trapezius myocutaneous island flap for soft tissue reconstruction can be observed in (**f–h**)

44.8 Technical Pearls

(a) Peripheral soft tissue margins must include an adequate amount of scalp around the base of the necrotic tumor. Depth-wise, the resection must include the cranial periosteum and the outer table.

(b) The tangential cortical resection must be performed very carefully so as not to remove unnecessary bone in terms of depth or not to penetrate the inner table of the cranium. If the inner cortex is penetrated, the transverse sinus might be exposed, and fatal bleeding or brain injury might occur. A reciprocating powered microsaw can be used for precise and safe corticotomy, while the osteotomy through cancellous bone can be completed with an osteotome of appropriate size and curvature.

(c) The extended distal trapezius myocutaneous island flap is an excellent tool for covering the scalp and posterior neck defects. It is a thin and pliable flap with a very long constant pedicle, a wide arc of rotation, and minor donor-site morbidity, permitting a safe flap elevation.

44.9 Outcome Radiographs and Images

See Fig. 44.3.

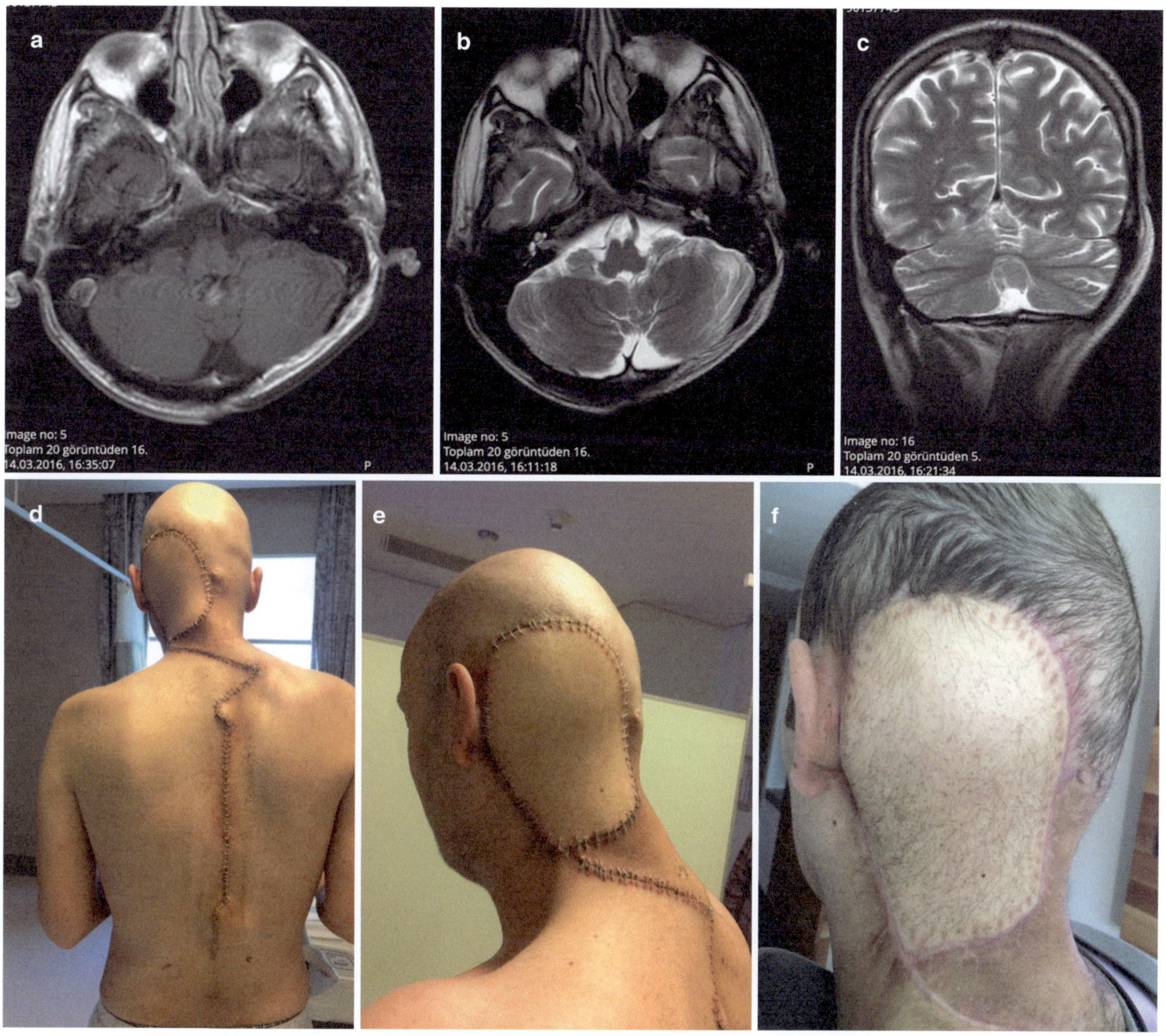

Fig. 44.3 Cranial MR images at postoperative 3 months in (**a**–**c**) demonstrate no local recurrence with healed flap over the tangential occipital defect. Early postoperative clinical photos in (**d** and **e**) show no wound complication, while the clinical image in (**f**) shows a completely healed flap at postoperative 3 months. Unfortunately, the patient was lost due to systemic metastases without local recurrence at postoperative 6 months

44.10 Avoiding and Managing Problems

(a) The osseous resection is essential to minimize the risk of local recurrence. However, the osteotomy technique required to achieve this depends on surgical skill, experience, and fine surgical tools.
(b) Trapezius flap reconstruction is an essential part of surgical treatment since this resection cannot be performed without adequate soft tissue reconstruction.
(c) The patient must be kept under close oncologic surveillance postoperatively due to the high risk of rapidly emerging metastases and local recurrence as well.

References

1. Breakey RWF, Crowley TP, Anderson IB, Milner RH, Ragbir M. The surgical management of head and neck sarcoma: the Newcastle experience. J Plast Reconstr Aesthet Surg. 2017;70(1):78–84. https://doi.org/10.1016/j.bjps.2016.09.026.
2. Gambarotti M. Vascular tumors: hemangioma, epithelioid hemangioendothelioma, and angiosarcoma. In: Picci P, Manfrini M, Fabbri N, Gambarotti M, Vanel D, editors. Atlas of musculoskeletal tumors and tumorlike lesions. Cham: Springer; 2014. p. 321–7. https://doi.org/10.1007/978-3-319-01748-8.
3. Goldblum JR. Malignant vascular tumors. In: Goldblum JR, Folpe AL, Weiss SW, editors. Enzinger and Weiss's soft tissue tumors. 7th ed. Philadelphia: Elsevier; 2020. p. 785–816.
4. Oashi K, Namikawa K, Tsutsumida A, Takahashi A, Itami J, Igaki H, Inaba K, Yamazaki N. Surgery with curative intent is associated with prolonged survival in patients with cutaneous angiosarcoma of the scalp and face—a retrospective study of 38 untreated cases in the Japanese population. Eur J Surg Oncol. 2018;44(6):823–9. https://doi.org/10.1016/j.ejso.2018.02.246.
5. Singh RP, Grimer RJ, Bhujel N, Carter SR, Tillman RM, Abudu A. Adult head and neck soft tissue sarcomas: treatment and outcome. Sarcoma. 2008;2008:654987. https://doi.org/10.1155/2008/654987.
6. Thway K, Billings SD. Angiosarcoma. In: WHO Classification of Tumours Editorial Board, editor. WHO classification of tumours soft tissue and bone tumours. 5th ed. Lyon: International Agency for Research on Cancer; 2020. p. 176–8.
7. Katano A, Yamashita H, Nakagawa K. Radical radiotherapy for localized cutaneous angiosarcoma of the scalp. Mol Clin Oncol. 2021;15(3):195. https://doi.org/10.3892/MCO.2021.2357.
8. NCCN clinical practice guidelines in oncology (NCCN guidelines®) soft tissue sarcoma version 2.2021—April 28, 2021. http://nccn.ir/Guidelines/Summary/sarcoma.html#pf23. Accessed 11 May 2023.
9. Mathes SJ, Stevenson TR. Reconstruction of posterior neck and skull with vertical trapezius musculocutaneous flap. Am J Surg. 1988;156(4):248–51. https://doi.org/10.1016/S0002-9610(88)80284-8.
10. Ou KL, Dai YH, Wang HJ, Chen TM, Dai NT, Chang SC, Deng SC, Tzeng YS, Wang CH, Chen SG. The lower trapezius musculocutaneous flap for head and neck reconstruction: two decades of clinical experience. Ann Plast Surg. 2013;71(Suppl 1):S48. https://doi.org/10.1097/SAP.0000000000000036.
11. Uğurlu K, Özçelik D, Hüthüt I, Yildiz K, Kilinç L, Baş L. Extended vertical trapezius myocutaneous flap in head and neck reconstruction as a salvage procedure. Plast Reconstr Surg. 2004;114(2):339–50. https://doi.org/10.1097/01.PRS.0000131984.55825.9D.

Soft Tissue Sarcoma of the Foot and Ankle: Wide Resection and Free Gracilis Flap

45

Philipp T. Funovics and Oskar Aszmann

45.1 Brief Clinical History

This chapter entails three case scenarios of a soft tissue sarcoma of the foot and ankle region in order to present slightly different treatment approaches in the use of a free gracilis muscle flap for soft tissue reconstruction.

Case 1 The first case is an otherwise healthy and active 55-year-old male patient who complained about a slowly growing mass of 3.5 cm in diameter on the sole of his left foot, which he initially has observed over 3 months (see Fig. 45.1). Due to increasing pain during barefoot ambulation he presented to the outpatient clinic where a core needle biopsy under local anesthesia revealed a clear cell sarcoma of the soft tissues with EWSR1-ATF1 fusion. Staging showed no evidence of metastatic disease, the multidisciplinary team (MDT) decided against neo-adjuvant therapy. The patient underwent primary wide tumor resection and reconstruction by an ipsilateral free vascularized gracilis flap with split skin graft of the defect to the planta pedis (see Fig. 45.4). There were no complications. Due to tumor size, distant and superficial location, as well as a high risk of radiation-induced infection, the MDT decided against any adjuvant treatment. There were no complications. The patient was mobilized non-weight-bearing in an aircast-walker for 8 weeks after surgery, returning to full weight-bearing thereafter. Three years after surgery the patient showed unrestricted function with no evidence of disease (see Fig. 45.7).

Case 2 The second case is a 59-year-old male patient with a history of high risk b-cell acute lymphoblastic leukemia (ALL) presenting with a growing, increasingly painful and nearly fungating lesion of 2 cm in diameter to his right dorsal heel which he has first noticed 6 weeks before (see Fig. 45.2). An open incisional biopsy was already performed at an outside institution and established the diagnosis of a clear cell sarcoma of the soft tissues without further metastases. According to MDT decision, the patient underwent no neo-adjuvant treatment. Primary wide resection of the tumor and defect reconstruction was performed by use of an ipsilateral free vascularized gracilis flap with split skin graft. The skin graft of the flap for the weight-bearing part of the heel was glabrous skin harvested from the inner planta pedis, while the rest of the flap and the dermal defect of the inner planta were covered by a skin graft harvested from the medial thigh in the area of the gracilis flap (see Fig. 45.5). The MDT indicated no further treatment due to his extensive previous therapy of ALL. The patient showed a prolonged wound dehiscence in the proximal area of the flap around the Achilles tendon and consequently underwent revision by debridement and secondary closure 4 months later, while being mobilized by partial weight-bearing in an aircast-walker. Six months after surgery the patient presented with full skin closure and unrestricted ambulatory ability (see Fig. 45.8). One year after resection there was no evidence of disease.

Case 3 The third case presents an otherwise healthy 66-year-old male patient with an indolent, yet slowly growing mass of 9 cm in diameter around the medial right ankle, which he has observed for 15 months, before seeking consultation (see Fig. 45.3). A core needle biopsy revealed a leiomyosarcoma G2, and staging was free of metastatic disease. Due to tumor size, the patient underwent preoperative radiotherapy according to the MDT decision. Six weeks after radiotherapy, however, the tumor showed only insignificant change in size. The patient underwent wide resection and reconstruction by an ipsilateral free vascularized gracilis flap with split skin graft of the medial ankle (see Fig. 45.6) without complications. Four cycles of doxorubicin monotherapy were indicated as adjuvant treatment. The patient was non-weight-bearing in

P. T. Funovics (✉)
Department of Orthopaedics and Trauma Surgery, Medical University of Vienna, Vienna General Hospital, Vienna, Austria
e-mail: philipp.funovics@meduniwien.ac.at

O. Aszmann
Department of Plastic and Reconstructive Surgery, Medical University of Vienna, Vienna General Hospital, Vienna, Austria
e-mail: oskar.aszmann@meduniwien.ac.at

H. Özger et al. (eds.), *Diagnosis and Treatment of Soft Tissue Tumors*, https://doi.org/10.1007/978-3-031-77061-6_45

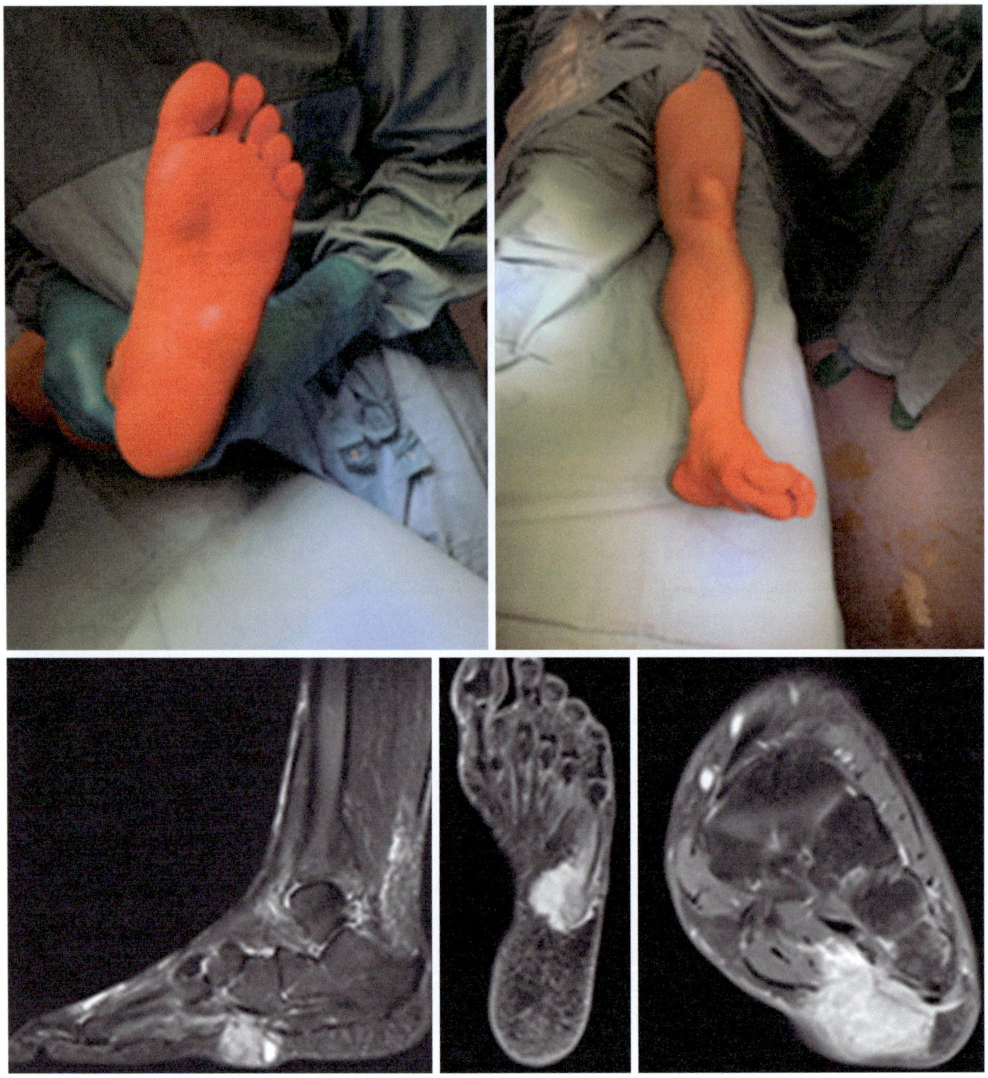

Fig. 45.1 Preoperative imaging of case 1. Clinical appearance (upper row) and preoperative MRI scans (lower row) of a 55-year-old male patient with clear cell sarcoma of the sole of the left foot

an aircast walker for 8 weeks and fully ambulatory thereafter. Nine months postoperatively the patient showed unrestricted function and no evidence of disease (see Fig. 45.9).

These three cases are intended to represent the surgical flexibility in the use of a free pedicled gracilis muscle transfer to the foot and ankle region after wide resection of a soft tissue sarcoma to both (a) restore the resulting soft tissue defect thereby providing a vital cover for adequate wound closure and (b) achieve sufficient stability for the reconstruction of the weight-bearing soft tissues in the foot.

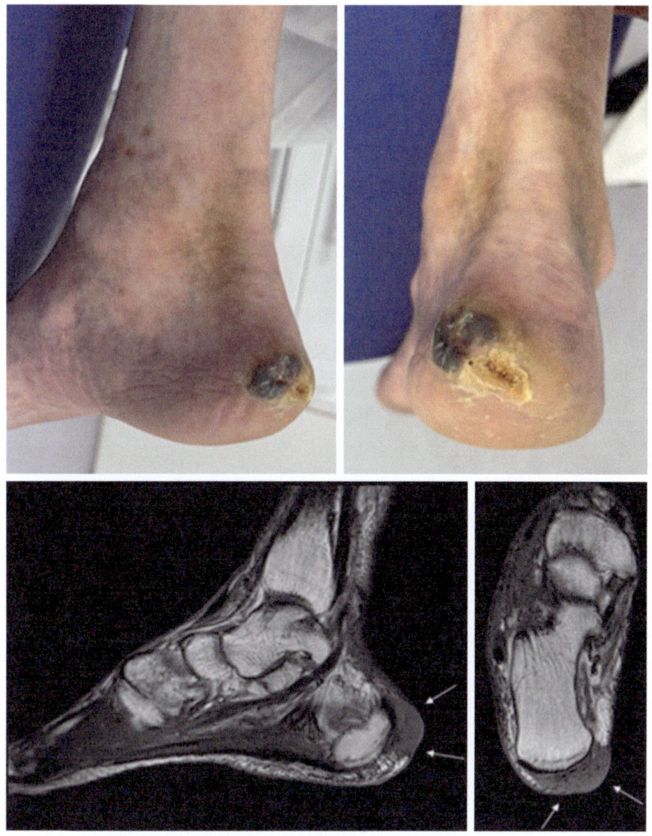

Fig. 45.2 Preoperative imaging of case 2. Clinical appearance (upper row) and preoperative MRI scans (lower row, tumor marked by white arrows) of a 59-year-old male patient with clear cell sarcoma of the right heel. The scar of the open biopsy is visible in the center of the nearly fungating tumor

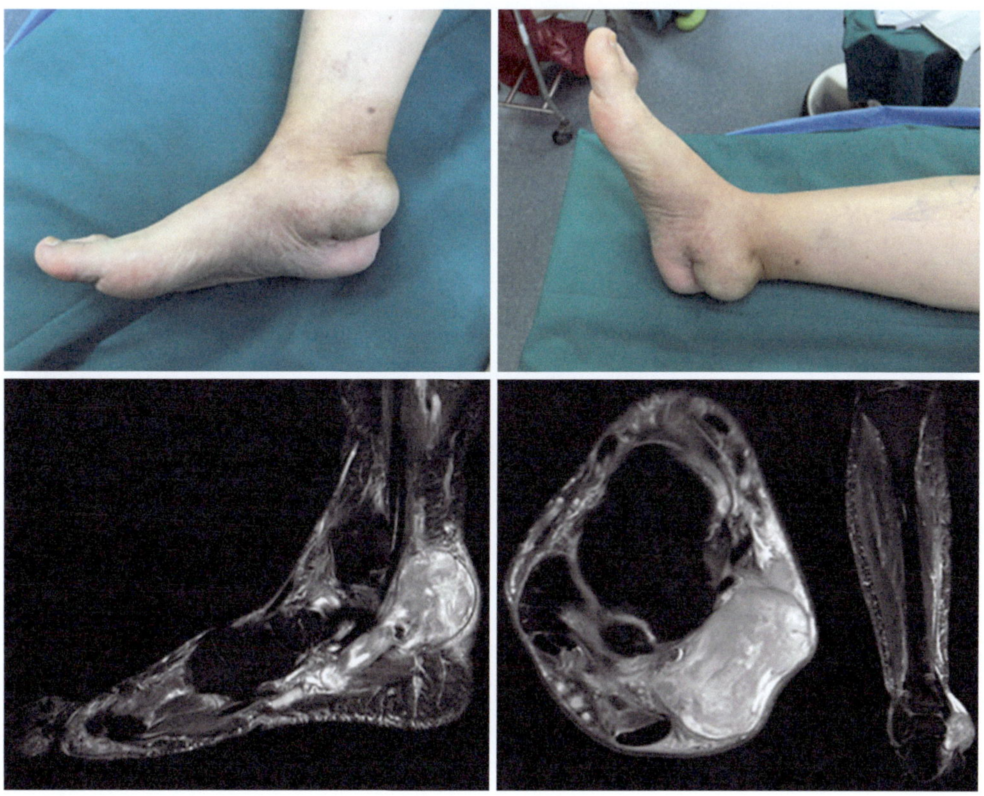

Fig. 45.3 Preoperative imaging of case 3. Clinical appearance (upper row) and preoperative MRI scans (lower row) of a 66-year-old male patient with leiomyosarcoma G2 of the right medial ankle. An additional MRI sequence of the full lower leg is performed to rule out local skip metastases

45.2 Preoperative Photos and Radiographs

See Figs. 45.1, 45.2, and 45.3.

45.3 Preoperative Problem List

(a) Low incidence of tumors of the foot and ankle accounting for 4–5% of all musculoskeletal tumors with a quarter of them being malignant [1–3]; high risk of diagnostic delays in primary tumors and especially metastases [4]; requirement of concise preoperative planning and diagnostic work-up [5]; indication of limb salvage surgery, evaluation of alternate treatment options (e.g., radiotherapy, systemic treatment, isolated limb perfusion) or ablative surgery;
(b) Ultimately limited soft tissue envelope in the foot and ankle region, requirement of tissue transfer after wide tumor resection;
(c) General and vascular patient status, ability to perform free flap transfer, metabolic disease, nicotine consumption, requirement of preoperative vascular investigation like angiography, CT-angiography, or MRI-angiography of the lower extremity to rule out vascular abnormalities;
(d) Anatomical feasibility of wide tumor resection by limb salvage surgery versus amputation, tumor size and site, evaluation of bone affection and neurovascular involvement, requirement of additional arthrodesis after concomitant bone resection;
(e) Sufficient soft tissue transfer for defect reconstruction, choice of muscle flap and size (e.g., gracilis versus latissimus dorsi or anterolateral thigh flap), restoration of the planta pedis as weight-bearing soft tissue cover of the foot, skin graft by glabrous versus hairy skin [6, 7];
(f) Technical equipment for microsurgical tissue transfer, intraoperative microscope;
(g) Postoperative care and mobilization, patient ability of non-weight-bearing;
(h) Timing and sequencing of adjuvant treatment, pre- versus postoperative radiotherapy;

45.4 Treatment Strategy

(a) Preoperative planning should entail adequate diagnostics of the lesion and exact histological work-up including molecular pathology when indicated. Indication for limb salvage surgery has to respect the general status of the patient, the ability to follow postoperative rehabilitation and (neo-)adjuvant treatments, stage of disease, tumor size and site. Alternate treatment options may include amputation, especially when limb salvage entails a high risk to result in positive margins. Wide tumor resection of soft tissue sarcoma of the foot and ankle will almost always require soft tissue reconstruction using a free muscle transfer due to ultimately limited local soft tissue to cover of bony structures and tendons. Accordingly, biopsies of foot tumors should preferably be performed by use of core needle systems instead of incisional techniques, to keep resulting defects from biopsy tract removal as minimal as possible.
(b) Wide tumor resection is intended to achieve clear margins to avoid recurrence. Hence, doubtful tumor invasion into neurovascular structures may require further preoperative diagnostics such as angiographic investigations of blood vessels or MRI fiber tracking of neural structures. T1-weighed MRI-sequences of the whole lower leg or a PET-CT are helpful in ruling out skip lesions or lymphatic tumor propagation. In case of neurovascular involvement, options of segmental vascular and/or neural repair, like sural nerve interposition, should remain at hand during surgery and patients should be consented accordingly. Ultimately, in doubtful resections patients must be informed of the potential need to switch to ablative surgery.
(c) Likewise, any affection of the skeleton of the foot may require additional resection of bony structures and consequently may result in partial or pan-arthrodesis of instable joints. The hardware used for these reconstructions will add another reason to provide a sufficient soft tissue cover by a free flap to minimize the risk of implant infection. Massive bone defects may even call for larger reconstructions by a free vascularized bone graft like a fibula and or auto/homologous bone grafts. In this case the concomitant soft tissue cover might change from a free flap to a combined osteo-myo-cutaneous tissue transfer (e.g., vascularized fibula autograft including muscle and skin). Accordingly, the surgical planning should always involve a multidisciplinary team from the start to define the right surgical procedure.
(d) Since the physiological soft tissue cover around the bony structure of the foot and ankle are scarce, infection rates are higher than with many other sites, especially in the case of extensive soft tissue components or even fungating tumors. Adequate (even preoperative) antibiotic prophylaxis and/or treatment should be provided.
(e) Consequently, the preoperative resection plan will allow to define the exact extent of the defect size to be expected from an oncologically adequate resection. This will facilitate to decide between different options of soft tissue transfer including the latissimus dorsi, anterolateral thigh or gracilis as the most frequently used flaps. The latter provides the advantage of an easy accessible site in the proximal (mostly ipsilateral) thigh, a predictable vascular pedicle, and the ability to apply the muscle as a

broad yet not too thick fillet-like cover, which is ideal for the anatomy of the foot and its requirement to fit in a shoe. Finally, its harvest does not inflict with the use of crutches like the latissimus dorsi, which is especially favorable in case of secondary amputation for any complication. The decision of adequate flap choice will, however, also include patient status, metabolic or vascular disease potentially affecting local vessels for the micro-anastomosis and therefore, might imply further angiographic work-up. Finally, the length of the vascular pedicle of the flap may also be an important parameter in flap choice, as the next available donor vessels may be out of reach for some flaps, i.e., the gracilis muscle flap only provides a very small pedicle (5 cm), whereas the ALT can have a pedicle of up to 10 cm.

(f) Inclusion of the biopsy tract often requires the use of an additional split skin graft to allow a tension-free skin closure. Mostly, the skin is taken from the ipsilateral lateral thigh, which should be prepared accordingly when draping the patient. Defect reconstructions of the planta pedis, the medial or lateral foot will be required to withstand full weight-bearing after consolidation. In this case it might be helpful to use skin grafts by glabrous skin to cover the region exposed to mechanical stress. This skin graft can be harvested from the medial inner planta pedis while the resulting dermal defect in this area (which is usually not exposed to weight-bearing) can be covered by a standard hairy skin graft taken from the lateral thigh (see Fig. 45.5).

(g) The availability of the adequate surgical and anesthesiologic technical equipment required for a successful free soft tissue transfer and management of intraoperative complications needs to be reassured.

(h) Postoperative surveillance should establish adequate blood pressure management as well as optimization of microcirculation and rheology. Regular flap controls will identify early vascular complications and allow indication of revision surgery. Finally, patients always need to be informed that ultimately secondary amputation might be the consequence of unsuccessful soft tissue defect management.

(i) Postoperative care and mobilization is mainly oriented towards full healing of the soft tissue reconstruction. Hence, immobilization in an orthosis is advisable over a period of 6 weeks in combination with increased partial weight-bearing according to the defect. Patients with limited functional ability are preferably immobilized by casting.

(j) (Neo-)Adjuvant treatment is based on a multidisciplinary decision. Whenever possible, its indication and timing should consider an elevated risk of infection without compromising the overall oncological outcome.

45.5 Basic Principles

(a) Multidisciplinary preoperative planning is essential and should entail all of the afore mentioned considerations. Diagnostic work-up should include all necessary investigations to allow wide resection and safe reconstruction. The resection plan will define the extent of the resection and if a free gracilis flap is the adequate choice for reconstruction [8].

(b) The surgery is performed in supine position. Draping and preparation of the patient should include the whole affected extremity to allow anatomical access to the foot as the area of resection and reconstruction and the thigh as the area of muscle and skin harvest. Due to reasons of oncological safety, these areas should be surgically managed completely independent from each other regarding surgical teams and instruments to avoid potential tumor propagation from the foot to the thigh. In general, once a wide resection and limb salvage surgery is established, the microsurgical team can start harvesting the gracilis flap (see Fig. 45.4).

(c) Incision and approach for tumor resection are mainly dependent from tumor site and extension, including incision during biopsy. In this context, core needle biopsies are facilitating less soft tissue loss during resection. Biopsy at the center of later resection should be advocated. Incision and approach for harvesting the pedicled gracilis muscle as a free flap follow its anatomy in the thigh. A tourniquet can be used according to preference, but in this context is not recommended by us for potential complications.

(d) When wide tumor resection with macroscopically clear margins and all required bone and joint reconstructions are performed and therefore limb salvage is accomplished, the area of the defect is anatomically screened for adequate vessels for microsurgical anastomosis. Only thereafter the gracilis free flap should be harvested and dissected from its pedicle to keep ischemia as short as possible. Also, once the resection is established the full size of the defect including potential hardware to be covered will be measurable to decide about according flap size.

(e) After the resection, the microsurgical team will set the gracilis free flap into the defect of the foot and perform the microsurgical anastomosis, usually starting with the artery. Once a physiological blood flow is established the flap is then fixed by sutures into the surrounding soft tissues and should provide a complete closure of bony structures and all hardware.

(f) Depending on tumor location and resulting defect size, skin closure may require further split skin grafts or alternatively the free gracilis flap is transplanted together with a cutaneous soft tissue spindle from the thigh to facilitate

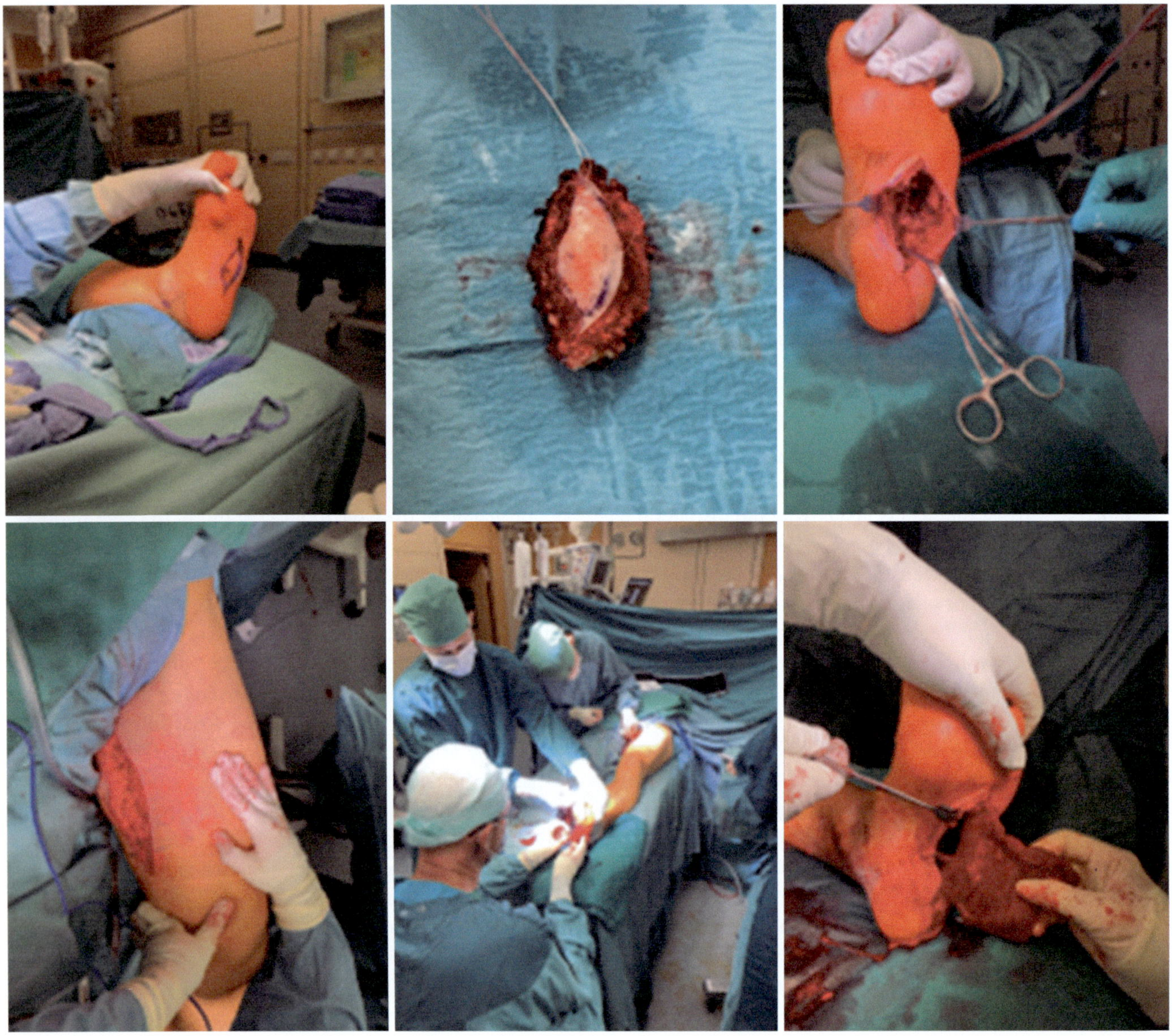

Fig. 45.4 Intraoperative imaging of case 1. The incision lines for the planned wide resection of the tumor on the sole of the left foot are marked (upper row, left). The resected specimen is marked by sutures for orientation during histopathological analysis (upper row, middle). Vessels for micro-anastomosis are identified in the area of the defect after resection (upper row, right). Once limb salvage by a successful resection is confirmed, the gracilis flap can be harvested from the ipsilateral thigh by a second team, working independently from the site of tumor resection (lower row, left and middle). The free gracilis flap is then transplanted into the defect and micro-anastomosis is performed (lower row, right)

dermal closure. In areas of expected weight-bearing through ambulation skin grafts should consist of glabrous skin taken from the inner medial area of the planta pedis to provide better mechanical resistance.

(g) Postoperative rehabilitation and temporary immobilization are recommended with regard to the aforementioned regimen. Thrombo-embolic, rheological, and antibiotic management is performed accordingly. Regular postoperative clinical flap controls over at least 24 hours are recommended to detect vascular complications in an early stage amenable to revision surgery. Postoperative cortisone will provide edema control as does positioning of the extremity on a pillow. Dangling of the extremity usually starts at the third day and non-weight-bearing ambulation on the fifth day for no more than 30 minutes three times per day. If the bony reconstruction is adequate, full weight-bearing ambulation is allowed after 7 days with compressive garment to prevent edema of the flap.

45.6 Photos and Imaging During Treatment

See Figs. 45.4, 45.5, and 45.6.

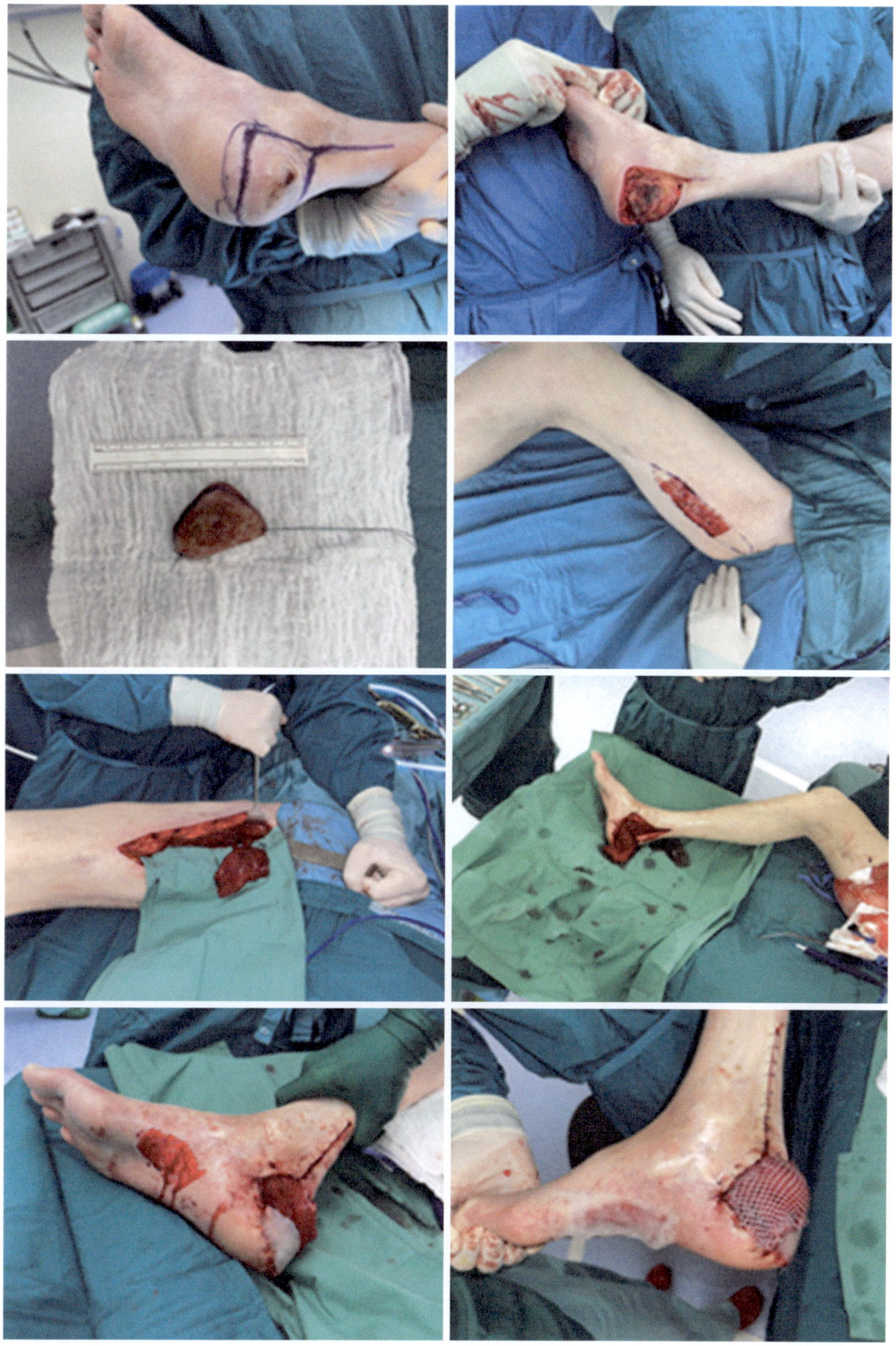

Fig. 45.5 Intraoperative imaging of case 2. The incision lines for the planned wide resection of the tumor on the heel of the right foot are marked (upper row, left). The tumor was dissected off the calcaneal bone together with the periosteum, the cauterization of the bone is visible as a dark area in the center of the defect (upper row, right). The resected specimen is marked by sutures for orientation during histopathological analysis (second row, left). A split skin graft is harvested from the ipsilateral medial thigh in the area of the gracilis flap for later coverage (second row, right). The gracilis flap is harvested out of the medial thigh and the pedicle is identified, while the flap is left in the circulation until its transplantation to keep ischemic time at a minimum (third row, left). Once the vessels for micro-anastomosis are identified in the area of the defect, the flap is then transplanted (third row, right). Where the flap is exposed to mechanical stress in the shoe, it is covered by glabrous skin, taken from the medial foot (lower row, left; the glabrous skin to be identified in the picture as the white area on top of the flap), whereas the rest of the flap and the site of skin harvest in the medial foot are covered with the skin graft from the thigh (lower row, right)

45.7 Technical Pearls

(a) Oncological: intraoperative tumor contamination, especially in radiologically undetected vascular tumor invasion or cystic tumor components with the risk of rupture and spill out during preparation;

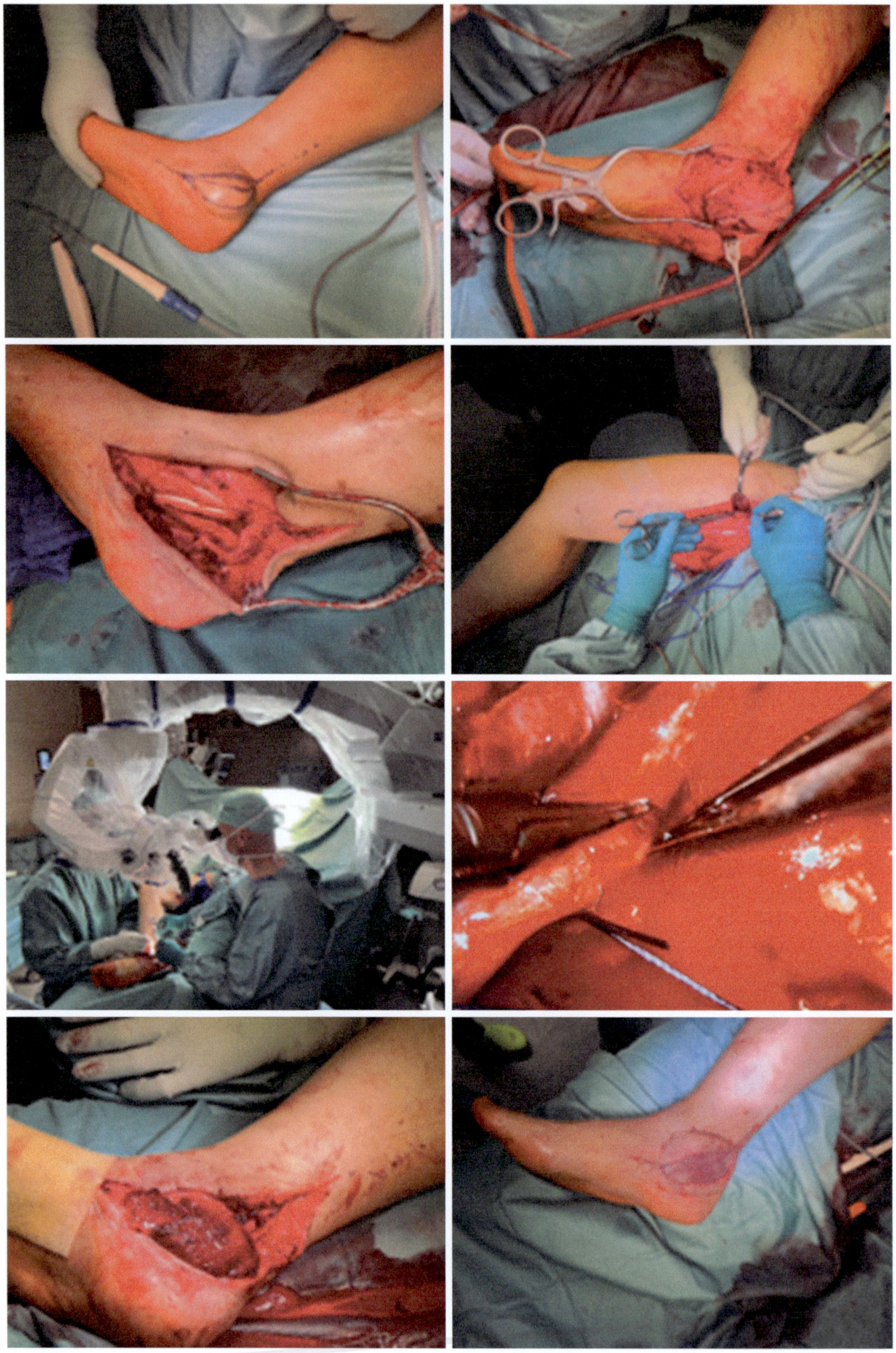

Fig. 45.6 Intraoperative imaging of case 3. The incision lines for the planned wide resection of the tumor on the right ankle are marked (upper row, left). The tumor is mobilized against neurovascular structures and tendons (upper row, right). After resection vessels for micro-anastomosis are easily accessible in the area of the dorsal tibial artery (second row, right). Once the vessels are identified, the flap is harvested (second row, right). The flap is transplanted and the vascular anastomosis is performed under the microscope (third row, left and right). The flap is then fixed into the defect by sutures (lower row, left) and covered by a split skin graft taken from the thigh (lower row, right)

(b) Neurovascular: lesions to the posterior tibial neurovascular structures, bleeding, complications of the micro-anastomosis, lesion of the pedicle, thrombo-embolism, vasospasm in pediatric patients with small vascular diameter, peroneal palsy due to iatrogenic trauma, insufficient neurolysis, delayed compression due to hematoma, compartment syndrome, neural compression syndrome through bandage, tight casting or wrong post-operative bedding of the patient, especially when using pain catheters, bleeding in the gracilis compartment of the thigh;

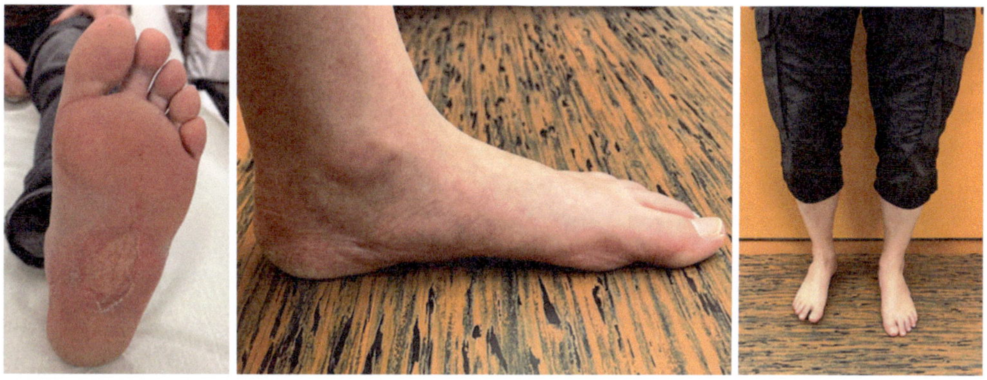

Fig. 45.7 Postoperative imaging of case 1. Clinical appearance 3 years after gracilis transfer to the sole of the foot, with the flap and skin graft fully ingrown and thinned out to the level of the planta pedis allowing the patient to walk normally barefoot

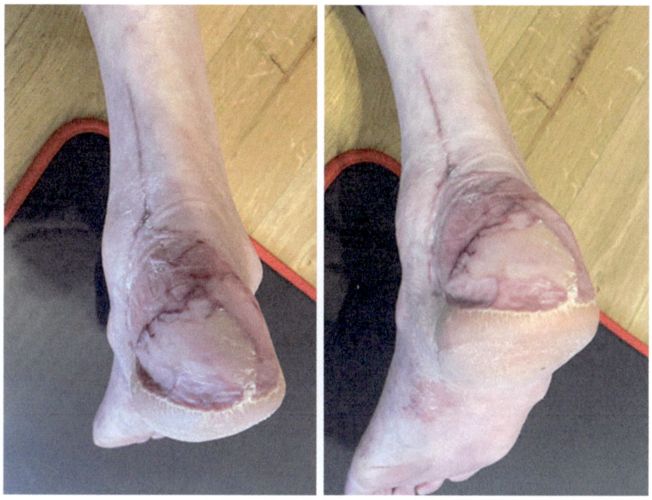

Fig. 45.8 Postoperative imaging of case 2. Clinical appearance 6 months after gracilis transfer to the heel of the foot with the flap and the glabrous and hairy skin graft fully ingrown allowing the patient to wear normal shoes

(c) Orthopedic: iatrogenic fracture during preparation or implantation of hardware, ligamentous instability after resection, subluxation, local osteoporosis and chronic regional pain syndrome due to prolonged immobilization, chronic lymphedema;

(d) Septic: wound healing disturbance, intraoperative contamination, insufficient soft tissue cover, deep hardware infection, inadequate skin closure, necrosis of flap or skin graft, donor site complications after skin harvest;

45.8 Outcome Photos and Imaging

See Figs. 45.7, 45.8, and 45.9.

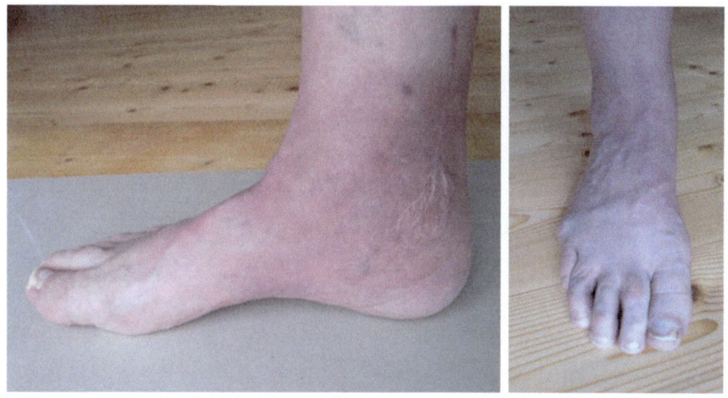

Fig. 45.9 Postoperative imaging of case 3. Clinical appearance 9 months after gracilis transfer to the medial ankle with the flap and skin graft fully consolidated

45.9 Avoiding and Managing Complications

(a) Intraoperative complications: Resection and reconstruction of tumors of the foot can be challenging due to limited soft tissue cover and the complex anatomy. This implies a high risk for infection ad tumor recurrence. Hence, preoperative planning and preparation of the patient are essential. An interdisciplinary surgical team should be included from the planning and beginning of the surgery. The whole leg should remain accessible for the management of complications during surgery.

(b) Infection: Infection still constitutes one of the most frequent yet disastrous complications, with a high risk of secondary amputation. Prolonged antibiosis may be administered in selected primary cases. Most cases of infection will require early and repeated revisions to obtain the most favorable result. In case of implants their removal is highly advocated to resolve deep infection.

(c) Tumor recurrence: Local recurrence is severely compromising the overall outcome. Concise preoperative diagnostics to identify tumor extension and potential skip lesions and thorough preparation during surgery are essential. In addition conventional or CT-based intraoperative navigation have shown to raise surgical precision during resection and should be advocated in complex cases of bone tumors of the foot and ankle. In soft tissue tumors fluorescence-guided surgical techniques may be considered for improved intraoperative visualization.
(d) Microsurgical and soft tissue management: Exact neurovascular preparation has to be performed preferably by an experienced and technically well-equipped microsurgical team, especially in pediatric patients due to small and fragile structures. A concise preoperative plan will help to match defect size and its reconstruction by the gracilis flap.
(e) Secondary amputation: In case of postoperative complications that require repeated revisions with questionable outcome, patients need to be informed early about the possibilities of amputation and the expected functional outcomes. Results of limb salvage surgery around the foot and ankle may be superior to amputation [9] However, especially when oncological outcomes are at risk or already have been compromised before by inadvertant surgery, tumors of the foot and ankle will allow safe below-knee amputation with rapid recovery and excellent function as a viable alternative to complex and demanding limb salvage procedures [10].

References

1. Angelini A, Biz C, Cerchiaro M, Longhi V, Ruggieri P. Malignant bone and soft tissue lesions of the foot. J Clin Med. 2023;12(8):3038.
2. Rammelt S, Fritzsche H, Hofbauer C, Schaser KD. Malignant tumours of the foot and ankle. Foot Ankle Surg. 2020;26(4):363–70.
3. Ruggieri P, Angelini A, Jorge FD, Maraldi M, Giannini S. Review of foot tumors seen in a university tumor institute. J Foot Ankle Surg. 2014;53(3):282–5.
4. Evans S, Ramasamy A, Jeys L, Grimer R. Delayed diagnosis in metastatic lesions of the foot. Ann R Coll Surg Engl. 2014;96(7):536–8.
5. Singer AD, Datir A, Tresley J, Langley T, Clifford PD, Jose J, Subhawong TK. Benign and malignant tumors of the foot and ankle. Skeletal Radiol. 2016;45(3):287–305.
6. Gould JS, Shi SM. Free vascularized soft tissue flaps for coverage of the foot and ankle. Clin Orthop Relat Res. 1995;314:26–36.
7. Kozusko SD, Liu X, Riccio CA, Chang J, Boyd LC, Kokkalis Z, Konofaos P. Selecting a free flap for soft tissue coverage in lower extremity reconstruction. Injury. 2019;50(Suppl 5):S32–9.
8. DeGroot H 3rd. Approach to the management of soft tissue tumors of the foot and ankle. Foot Ankle Spec. 2008;1(3):168–76.
9. Smolle MA, Leithner A, Kapper M, Demmer G, Trost C, Bergovec M, Windhager R, Hobusch GM. Complications, mobility, and quality of life in ankle sarcoma patients. Bone Joint J. 2021;103-B(3):553–61.
10. Yang P, Evans S, Bali N, Ramasamy A, Evans R, Stevenson J, Jeys L, Grimer R. Malignant bone tumours of the foot. Ann R Coll Surg Engl. 2017;99(7):568–72.

Synovial Sarcoma of the Foot Treated with Recycled Bone Graft and Soft Tissue Reconstruction

46

Abigail R. Tud, Kuan-Lin Chen, Chao-Ming Chen, and Wei Ming Chen

46.1 Basic Clinical History

A 40-year-old female with no contributory history noted a coin-sized, painless mass on her left foot dorsum. No apparent increase in size was observed over a period of 4 years; however, due to its persistence, the patient sought a consultation with a practitioner of traditional Chinese medicine. After a series of massages, gradual swelling accompanied by intermittent pain developed, prompting consult at a local hospital. The initial impression was a ganglion cyst and fluid aspiration was performed, with inconclusive results. Subsequent magnetic resonance imaging (MRI) showed a lobulated, hyperintense mass at the first webspace of the left foot. This prompted referral to orthopedic oncology, where ultrasound-guided biopsy confirmed the mass as synovial sarcoma. Metastatic workup revealed two non-specific, subcentimeter subpleural nodules at the right upper and left upper lung lobes but was otherwise unremarkable.

46.2 Preoperative/Pretreatment Clinical and Radiologic Images

While plain radiographs have little role in determining appropriate surgical margins for excision, intralesional mineralization has been documented in as much 40% of cases. X-rays may also reveal evidence of bone remodeling or invasion, which has been associated with poor prognosis. Magnetic resonance imaging is the diagnostic modality of choice to define the extent of soft tissue and bone involvement. Synovial sarcoma appears as a hypointense lesion relative to muscle on T1-weighted imaging, and heterogenous on T2 imaging due to intralesional hemorrhage and necrosis [1, 2] (Figs. 46.1 and 46.2).

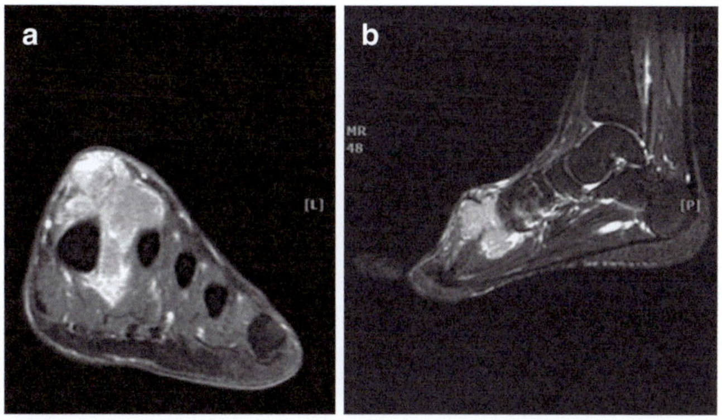

Fig. 46.1 T2-weighted coronal (**a**) and sagittal (**b**) images revealed a contrast-enhancing, multi-lobulated soft tissue mass located at the first intermetatarsal space of the left foot, measuring 3.3 cm × 4.0 cm × 4.2 cm

A. R. Tud · K.-L. Chen · C.-M. Chen · W. M. Chen (✉)
Department of Orthopedics and Traumatology, Taipei Veterans General Hospital, Taipei, Taiwan
e-mail: wmchen@vghtpe.gov.tw

H. Özger et al. (eds.), *Diagnosis and Treatment of Soft Tissue Tumors*, https://doi.org/10.1007/978-3-031-77061-6_46

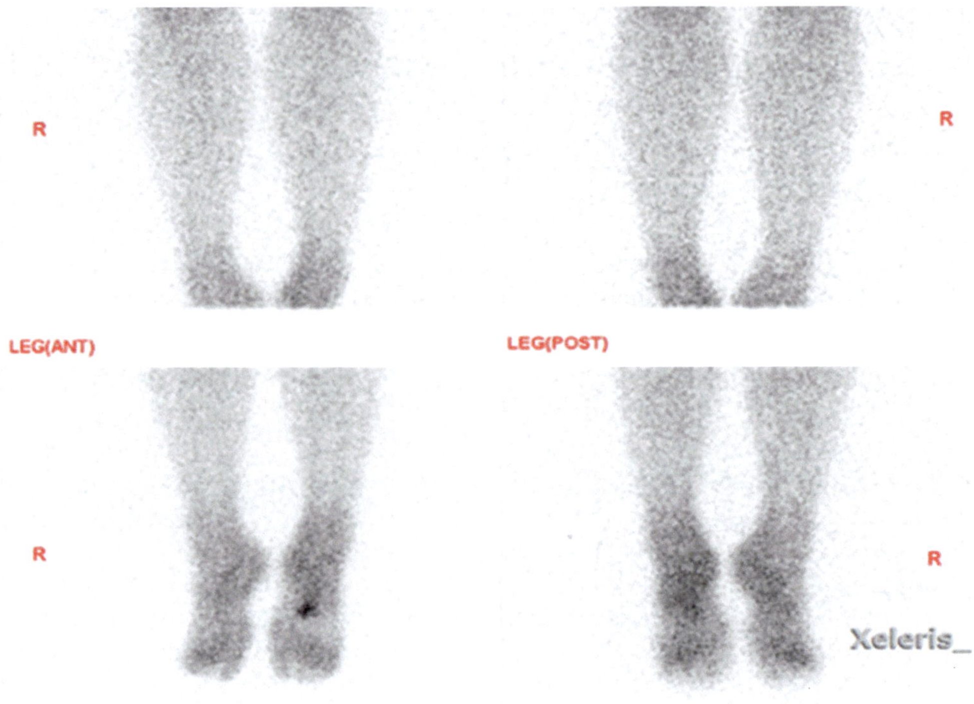

Fig. 46.2 Whole-body bone scans showed increased uptake over the first intermetatarsal space of the left foot, but otherwise no evidence of distant bone metastases

46.3 Problem List

1. Biopsy confirmed soft tissue sarcoma with extension to the first and second rays of the foot
2. Manipulation of mass prior to diagnosis
3. Evidence of possible distant metastases
4. Soft tissue coverage

46.4 Treatment Strategy

The standard approach to localized extremity soft tissue sarcomas is surgical excision, with or without radiotherapy. Chemotherapy may be recommended for patients who present with or subsequently develop metastatic disease after surgery. It may also be an option for unresectable lesions. Overall, the treatment goals are local tumor control, management or prevention of systemic disease, and preservation of function [3].

Radiation therapy is prescribed for cases wherein excision is expected to achieve less than wide surgical margins. There is still no consensus regarding the timing of radiotherapy relative to surgery [3, 4].

In contrast to most soft tissue sarcomas, synovial sarcoma is known to be chemo-sensitive. Neoadjuvant chemotherapy with Ifosfamide and Doxorubicin was initiated for the patient with the aim of downsizing the tumor prior to surgery and decreasing the risk of metastatic disease. Radiation therapy was planned postoperatively if margins were less than wide.

After two cycles, wide excision of the mass was performed. Reconstruction was completed by using a structural bone allograft, followed by dual metatarsal plate fixation. Adequate soft tissue coverage was achieved using a bi-pedicled transposition flap. Histopathologic assessment of the resected specimen was compatible with initial biopsy, and all margins were free from tumor involvement.

Following surgical resection, remaining chemotherapy cycles were completed and surveillance monitoring conducted at regular intervals. At 9 years post-surgery, the patient continues to weight-bear fully on the left foot with normal gait and remains disease-free, without signs of local recurrence.

46.5 Basic Principles

Synovial sarcoma is a type of high-grade soft tissue sarcoma with predilection for the lower extremities, commonly affecting adults within the first four decades. It is the most common sarcoma of the foot, with incidence ranging from 45% to 56%. Its nonspecific presentation often leads to misdiagnosis and consequently, diagnostic as well as treatment delays [1].

Time between symptom onset and diagnosis as well as histologic grade has been reported to have a significant effect on prognosis. A painless mass with insidious pattern of growth is the usual reason for consult. Patients with a longer duration of symptoms have been found to have less aggressive biologic activity, lower histologic grade, and thus better prognosis. Conversely, patients with rapidly enlarging tumors typically have higher histologic grade, with an increased risk for early metastasis even with prompt diagnosis [1].

Even with early detection and adequate surgical margins, synovial sarcomas have a high propensity for local recurrence as well as distal metastasis, including lymph node involvement. As much as 75% of cases have been found to have extra-compartmental invasion by the time of diagnosis. Overall survival at 10 years has been reported at 53% [1, 2].

46.6 Photos and Imaging During Treatment

See Fig. 46.3.

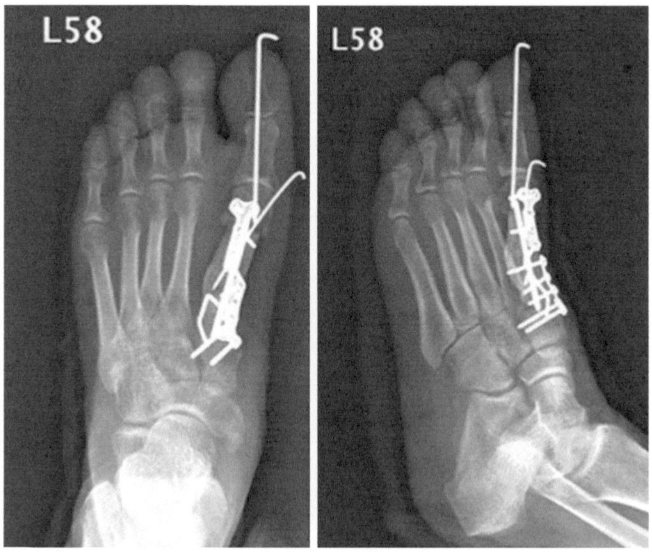

Fig. 46.3 Immediate postoperative radiographs of the left foot. Anteroposterior and oblique (AP/O) views show the structural allograft and implants, augmented with Kirschner wires

46.7 Technical Pearls

Wide surgical margins are recommended to minimize local recurrence of synovial sarcoma. This may leave a sizeable soft tissue defect considered unsuitable for primary closure. Soft tissue reconstruction in such cases adheres to the orthoplastic reconstructive principles described by Levin in 1993 [4, 5].

Exposure of deeper structures such as nerves, blood vessels, tendons, bone, and/or hardware necessitates the use of a flap. The surgical team must consider that significant alterations to the local milieu in terms of vascular perfusion, scarring, and viable bone and soft tissue attachments can create significant challenges both during and after the procedure. Intraoperative surgical dissection may also affect the area at risk for local recurrence or for subsequent radiation therapy [4–6].

While a variety of flap options are available, local flaps remain preferable due to their simplicity. A bipedicled fasciocutaneous flap can provide adequate coverage and durability for dorsal foot defects while obviating the need for microsurgery.

46.8 Outcome: Clinical and Radiological Images

See Fig. 46.4.

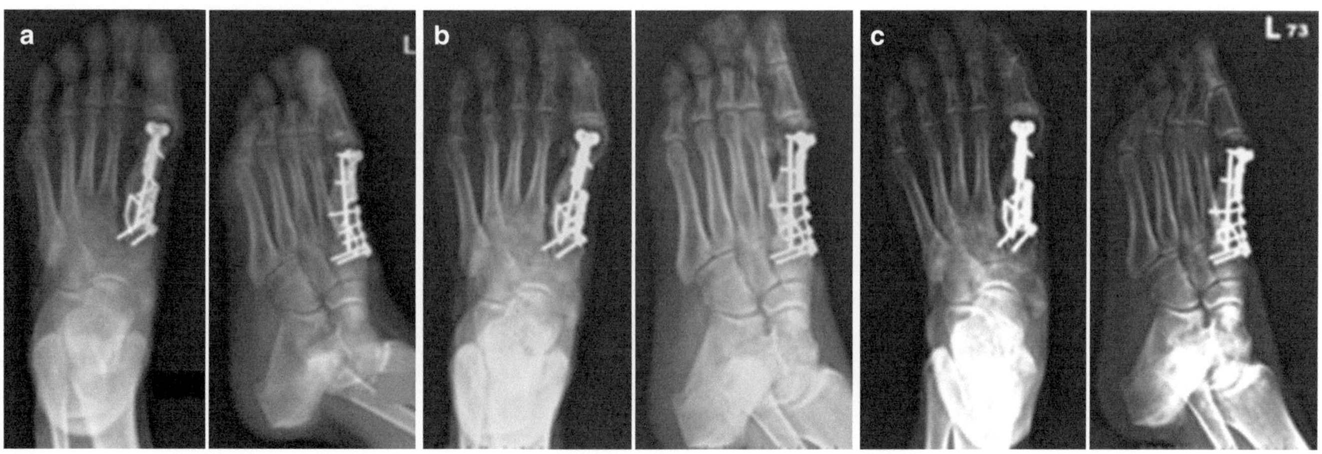

Fig. 46.4 Follow-up AP/O radiographs of the left foot at 1 year (**a**), 4 years (**b**), and 9 years (**c**) post-surgery. Osteopenic changes and valgus alignment of the left hallux can be observed. Allograft has fully consolidated, and implants remain well positioned

46.9 Avoiding and Managing Complications

Determining the local extent of the tumor, histologic grade and presence of metastases are essential to improving outcomes and decreasing postoperative complications [2, 3].

The strongest predictor of local recurrence after resection of synovial sarcoma is a positive surgical margin. This emphasizes the importance of reliable diagnostic imaging prior to surgery, which serves as the guide to the extent of resection as well as possible issues with soft tissue closure. Magnetic resonance scans allow for accurate delineation of soft tissue extension as well as the presence of any bone involvement [1–3].

Preoperative radiation has been found to reduce tumor volume and induce fibrotic changes in the pseudocapsule, leading to better anatomic delineation and easier dissection from neighboring structures. However, it has also been associated with higher wound complication rate. These risks can be mitigated by performing surgery once radiation-induced hyperemia and edema have resolved [2, 3]. At present most authors recommend a 2–4 week interval between the last session of preoperative radiotherapy and definitive surgery [2, 3, 5].

References

1. Scully SP, Temple HT, Harrelson JM. Synovial sarcoma of the foot and ankle. Clin Orthop Rel Res. 1999;36(4):220–6.
2. Cockshott S, Hayward K, Grimer R. Synovial sarcoma of the foot. Orthop Proc. 2018;93-B(Supp III):315–6. British Orthopaedic Association.
3. Ramu EM, Houdek MT, Isaac CE, Dickie CI, Ferguson PC, Wunder JS. Management of soft-tissue sarcomas; treatment strategies, staging, and outcomes. SICOT J. 2017;3:20.
4. Levin LS. The reconstructive ladder. An orthoplastic approach. Orthop Clin North Am. 1993;24(3):393–409.
5. Dickie CI, Catton CN, Chung PWM, Ferguson PC, Wunder JS, O'Sullivan B. The influence of time interval between preoperative radiation and surgical resection on the development of wound healing complications in extremity soft tissue sarcoma. Ann Surg Oncol. 2015;22(9):2824–30.
6. Serletti JM, Moran SL. Soft tissue coverage options for dorsal foot wounds. Foot Ankle Clin. 2001;6(4):839–51.

47 Recurrent Pleomorphic Sarcoma of the Thigh Treated with Radiotherapy and Total Femur Prosthesis

Abigail R. Tud, Kuan-Lin Chen, Chao-Ming Chen, and Wei Ming Chen

47.1 Basic Clinical History

A 51-year-old female was referred for orthopedic consult due to a low-energy fracture of the left femoral shaft. She fractured her left femur due to a simple sprain at her ipsilateral ankle and foot when walking. Relevant history included a diagnosis of poorly differentiated cervical squamous cell carcinoma, International Federation of Gynecology and Obstetrics (FIGO) Stage IB1 2 years prior, for which she had undergone total abdominal hysterectomy with bilateral salpingo-oopherectomy and 28 fractions of radiotherapy. Based on her preexisting condition, a metastatic pathological fracture at left femur was impressed and open reduction, intramedullary nailing was performed at a local hospital. Specimens were then sent for histopathologic analysis.

However, pathology findings were inconsistent with metastasis and found to have sarcomatous features. This together with persistent pain at the previous fracture site prompted an orthopedic oncology referral. Subsequent slide review confirmed the diagnosis of undifferentiated pleomorphic sarcoma with a secondary pathological fracture.

MRI scans revealed a heterogenous, contrast-enhancing lobulated mass around the previous fracture site and intramedullary nail, with surrounding soft tissue inflammation. Additional metastatic workup showed increased uptake at the ipsilateral knee and ankle joints attributed to immobility and postoperative change (knee joint) as well as previous sprain injury at her ipsilateral ankle and foot joints. Her chest CT showed a single nonspecific sub-centimeter opacity at the left lower lobe, but otherwise no distant metastases were found.

47.2 Preoperative/Pretreatment Clinical and Radiologic Images

A thorough pre-operative assessment is necessary to review appropriate surgical margins in relation to pertinent anatomic structures, identify indications and contraindications to the proposed surgery, and anticipate possible issues with soft tissue closure particularly in the setting of neoadjuvant radiotherapy or revision surgery.

Plain radiographs are the simplest, most economical way to visualize the femur and extent of tumor involvement, as well as guide selection of appropriate implant sizes and possible modular modifications [1, 2].

Nuclear imaging with whole-body bone scans assist in identifying systematic bone involvement by the tumor. The uptakes at tibia and ankle joints should be well discussed with radiologists to rule out the possibilities of distant metastasis of the tumor [1, 2] (Figs. 47.1, 47.2, 47.3, and 47.4).

A. R. Tud · K.-L. Chen · C.-M. Chen · W. M. Chen (✉)
Department of Orthopedics and Traumatology,
Taipei Veterans General Hospital, Taipei, Taiwan
e-mail: wmchen@vghtpe.gov.tw

H. Özger et al. (eds.), *Diagnosis and Treatment of Soft Tissue Tumors*, https://doi.org/10.1007/978-3-031-77061-6_47

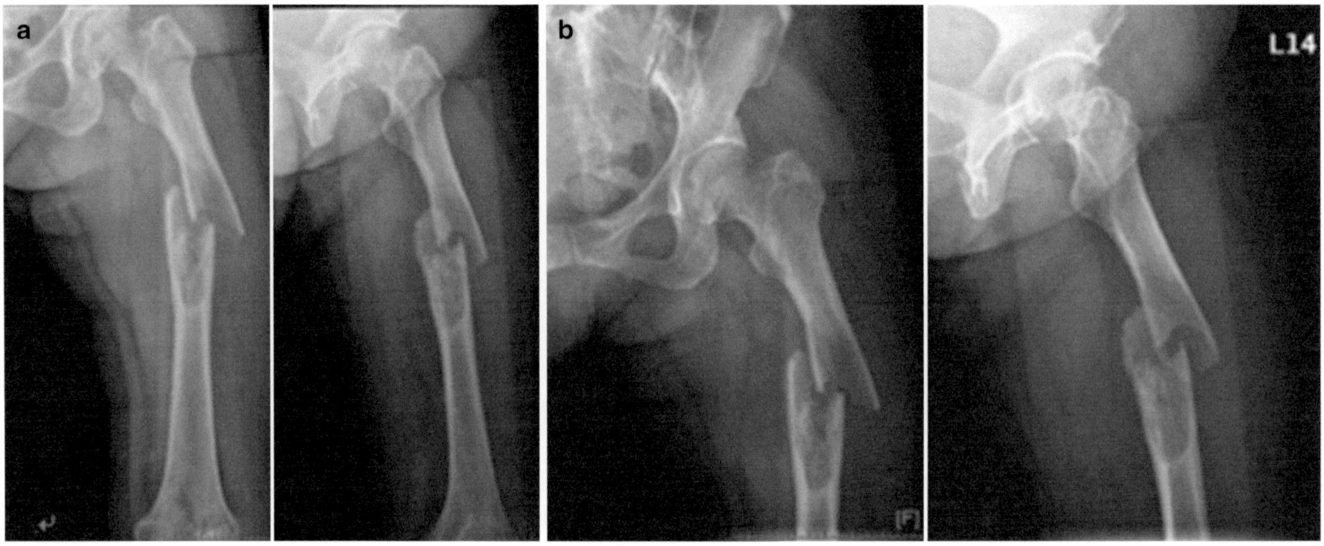

Fig. 47.1 Radiographs showing AP and lateral (L) views of the left femur (**a**) and hip (**b**) show a pathologic fracture through an expansile lytic lesion at the proximal third of the diaphysis

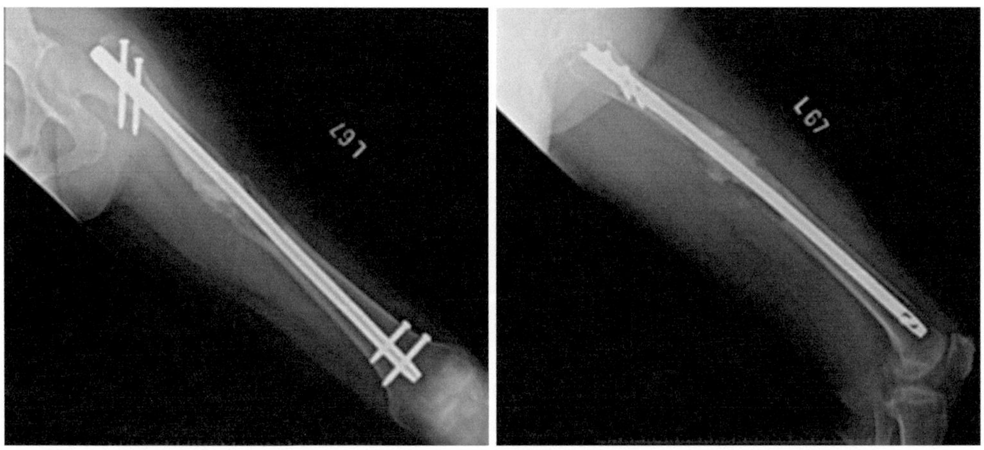

Fig. 47.2 AP/L radiographs of the left femur showing the intramedullary nail in place

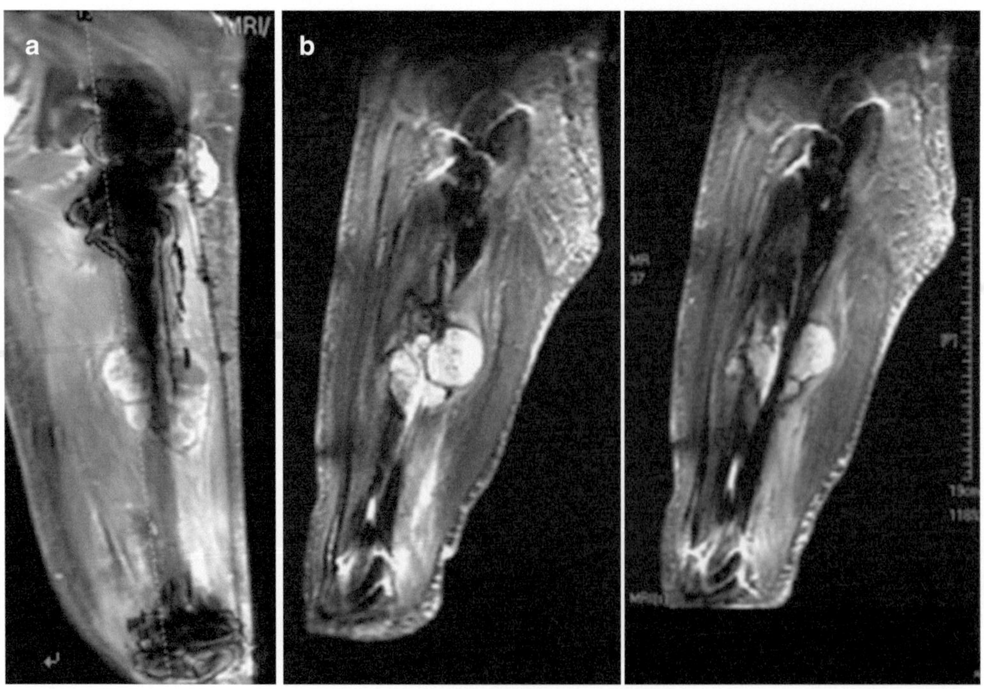

Fig. 47.3 T2-weighted coronal (**a**) and sagittal (**b**) images post-intramedullary nailing show a contrast-enhancing, multi-lobulated soft tissue mass surrounding the previous fracture site, measuring 6.2 cm × 7.0 cm × 8.4 cm

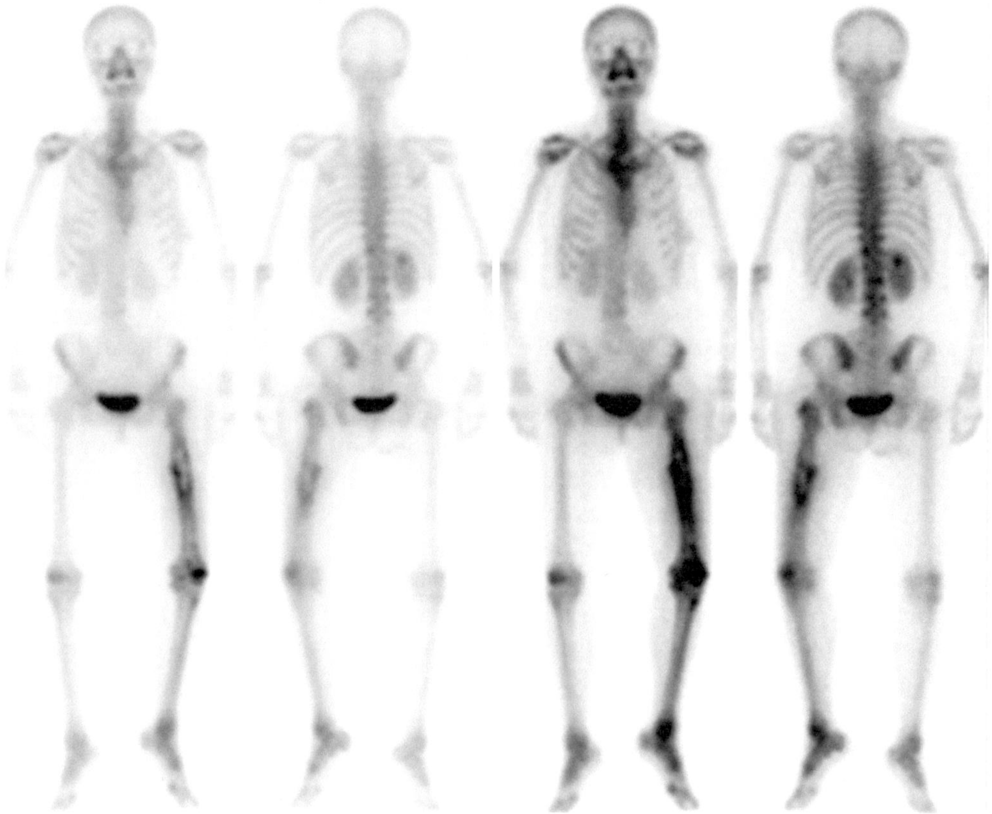

Fig. 47.4 Whole-body bone scan (WBBS) shows increased uptake over the left femur, ipsilateral knee, and ankle joints. After discussion with radiologist, the uptake over the knee may be resulted from postoperative changes after intramedullary nailing. The uptake at her ipsilateral foot and ankle joints may be related to the sprain when she fell

47.3 Problem List

1. Initial misdiagnosis and inadvertent intramedullary reaming and nailing of a sarcoma-affecting bone would result in severe contamination and increase risk of distant metastasis.
2. Double primary cancer may affect decision making.
3. Complications secondary to prolonged immobility
4. Risk for infection

47.4 Treatment Strategy

Chemotherapy prior to definitive surgery was initiated. After two cycles of Ifosfamide and Epirubicin, wide excision of the entire left femur and soft tissue component was performed, followed by total femoral replacement. Final histopathologic analysis confirmed the diagnosis as pleomorphic liposarcoma.

The patient completed her remaining chemotherapy cycles unremarkably, and subsequent metastatic workup showed resolution of the previously reported lesions on both WBBS and chest computed tomography (CT) scan. Surveillance monitoring was conducted at regular intervals, with close attention given to the previous soft tissue component location. At 9 years post-surgery the patient remains disease-free, without evidence of local recurrence or distant metastases.

47.5 Basic Principles

Cervical cancer is the second most common malignancy among women, with a relatively high 10-year survival rate of over 65%. Bone metastases secondary to hematogenous spread is relatively rare, accounting for 0.8–23% of all cases. The majority of patients with metastatic bone disease present within the first year of treatment completion, with relatively poor prognosis. Lesions over the long bones may cause debilitating pain, pathologic fracture, and significant disability. However, physical exam and diagnostic imaging findings are nonspecific, emphasizing the need for thorough assessment and characterization, especially with solitary metastases. Radiation therapy plays a key role in the treatment of locally advanced disease but has been associated with increased risk of secondary cancers on long-term follow-up particularly for heavily irradiated sites such as the small and large intestine, female genito-urinary tract, and bones [2, 3].

The proximal femur and femoral diaphysis are frequent sites for primary bone lesions. Advances in chemotherapy, radiation modalities, and joint prostheses have increased survival rates while improving local disease control as well as postoperative function. However, extensive primary or secondary tumor involvement may lead to insufficient residual bone for stable fixation using standard implants. In addition, the possibility of progression in the setting of metastatic bone disease underlines the need for a durable reconstruction [1, 2].

Indications for total femoral replacement include diaphyseal tumors with both proximal and distal involvement, distal or proximally located tumors extending to or beyond 130 mm of the opposite articular surfaces, and extensive metastatic bone involvement. Total femoral replacement may also be the only option for patients with significant contamination of the intramedullary canal following fixation of a primary bone or soft tissue malignancy. This may or may not be complicated by the presence of a pathologic fracture [1, 4].

Total femur resection is not recommended for patients with primary malignancies where achieving appropriate oncologic margins may not be possible, either due to tumor contamination or a sizeable soft tissue component. It is also contraindicated for patients with documented metastases from sarcoma, or widespread systemic and/or local infection. Relative contraindications include femoral nerve palsy, which may compromise postoperative hip stability and function, tumor involvement requiring concomitant total quadriceps resection, which would lead to loss of extension support on attempted weight-bearing, and femoral vessel compromise [1].

47.6 Photos and Imaging During Treatment

See Fig. 47.5.

47.7 Technical Pearls

The minimum length of residual bone required for adequate fixation of a tumor endoprosthesis at the proximal femur is 130 mm. When tumors extend from the proximal femur to an area beyond the distal meta-diaphyseal junction, or a primarily diaphyseal tumor presents with concomitant lesions involving the proximal or distal femur, total femoral resection should be considered [1].

Hip stability is a major determinant of postoperative return to function. Hip abductors should therefore be preserved whenever possible. If the greater trochanter is not involved, a transtrochanteric approach may be used to facilitate reattachment of the abductor muscles to the total femoral prosthesis. This can be completed using cables or wires. Performing a capsulotomy is also recommended with the goal of preserving the native hip capsule, thus affording additional stability. The ensuing repair may be augmented by suturing to any remaining muscles around the joint [1].

The length of the construct determines soft tissue tension. Overlengthening is a common technique employed during limb salvage to address decrease in soft tissue tension. This may, however, lead to patellofemoral dysfunction and decrease range of motion post-surgery. It is recommended to use contralateral knee and hip radiographs as a guide to approximate the native joint line and patellar position. To determine if the soft tissue tension is appropriate, the patella should be positioned over the proximal half of the anterior distal femoral component [1].

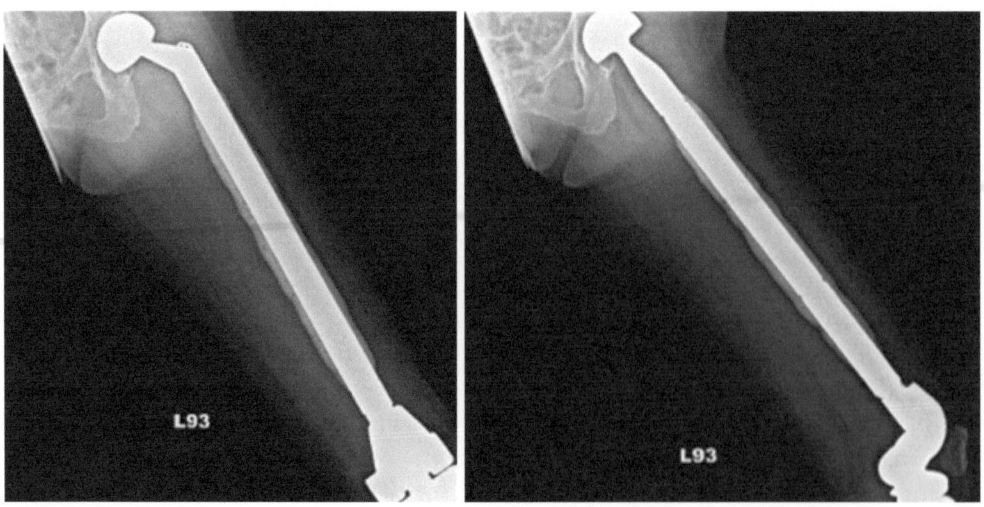

Fig. 47.5 AP/L radiographs of the left femur after wide tumor excision and total femoral replacement

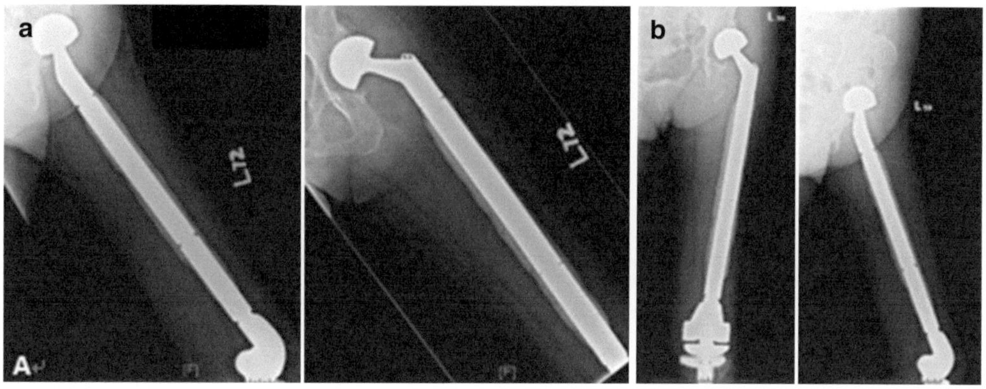

Fig. 47.6 Follow-up AP/L radiographs of the left femur foot at 1 year (**a**) and 5 years (**b**) post-surgery. Implants remain well positioned without evidence of acetabular lysis or protrusion

47.8 Outcome—Clinical and Radiological Images

See Fig. 47.6.

47.9 Avoiding and Managing Complications

A thorough preoperative assessment is necessary to review appropriate surgical margins in relation to pertinent anatomic structures, identify indications and contraindications to the proposed surgery, and anticipate possible issues with soft tissue closure particularly in the setting of neoadjuvant radiotherapy or revision surgery.

Among the most common complications encountered after total femoral resection and replacement are instability about the hip joint, inadequate soft tissue tension, and increased risk of infection [1].

The hip capsule and abductor musculature should be preserved as much as possible. Overlengthening is often performed during limb salvage to mitigate decreased soft tissue tension after tumor resection; however, this may result in nerve palsy. Assessing patients for femoral nerve palsy prior to and after surgery must be emphasized. Overlengthening may also lead to patellofemoral dysfunction and decrease range of motion post-surgery. It is, therefore, imperative to review contralateral knee and hip radiographs to determine the relationship between the contralateral fibula and proximal tibia and use this as a guide to approximate the native joint line and patellar positioning [1].

References

1. Sim FH, Choong PFM, Weber KL. Orthopedic oncology and complex reconstruction. 1st ed. Philadelphia: Lippincott Williams and Wilkins; 2011.
2. Chaturvedi AK, Engeles EA, et al. Second cancers among 104760 survivors of cervical cancer: evaluation of long-term risk. J Natl Cancer Inst. 2007;2007(99):1634–43.
3. Eulo V, Lesmana H, Doyle LA, Nichiles KE, Hirbe AC. Secondary sarcomas: biology, presentation, and clinical care. Am Soc Clin Oncol Educ Book. 2020;40:1–12.
4. Thanapprapasr D, Nartthanarung A, Likittanasombut P, Na Ayudhya NI, Charakorn C, Udomsubpayakul U, et al. Bone metastasis in cervical cancer patients over a 10-year period. Int J Gynecol Cancer. 2010;2010(20):373–8.

Treating the Soft Tissue Tumor of the Hand

48

Wan Faisham Nu'man Wan Ismail
and Arman Zaharil Mat Saad

48.1 Introduction

The function of the hand is to grip, grasp, and do precise movements. The thumb along with the four fingers form four oblique arches, of which the arch of the index finger functionally is the most important especially for precision grip. The arch of the little finger contributes an important locking mechanism for power grip. The basic function of the hand is complex and must be considered during evaluation and reconstruction for surgery in hand tumors.

Hand tumors are common entities, and most are benign. Familiarity with the most frequent lesions allows clinicians to accurately diagnose these disorders, but one must stay vigilant to avoid missing the rare malignant disease. Features suggestive of malignant disease include rapid growth, pain at rest, size greater than 5 cm, and radiographic signs of invasion into local tissues. For most benign lesions, surgery alone is the preferred mode of treatment [1–3].

The principle of treatment for hand sarcomas is to achieve oncological clearance with preservation of maximum function and cosmesis. This strategy may include radiotherapy or chemotherapy on an adjuvant or neo-adjuvant basis. Marginal resection is not suitable due to high local recurrence. The decision to opt for limb sparing surgery or amputation is based on many factors, which include the compartment involved and the ability to obtain R0 resection with anticipated functional outcome. Basic 'tripod function' of the finger and key pincer motion together with integrity of long tendon and hand arch should be maintain for optimum function. Wide margin surgery of the hand always requires reconstruction for wound closure and to have flexible tissue for optimum hand function. Reconstruction of a defect in the hand needs to be tailored to maintain the dexterity and mobility of the hand. A robust reconstruction should withstand early mobilization and local radiation [4–6].

The authors share their experience in the management of several cases of hand lesions; both, benign and malignant to show the variability and options available for surgical management and reconstruction.

48.2 Case 1: Dermatofibrosarcoma Protuberance of Thumb

A 36-year-old gentleman left hand dominant presented with a rapidly growing mass over the dorsum of the right thumb following an excision biopsy and primary closure (Fig. 48.1a, b). Histopathology evaluation confirmed the diagnosis of dermatofibrosarcoma protuberance (DPSP). MRI demonstrated a tumor infiltrating the entire skin and subcutaneous fat almost three quarters circumferentially around the thumb with infiltration of the extensor tendon. The periosteum, bone, and both digital neurovascular structures were free (Fig. 48.1c–e).

48.2.1 Problem List

(a) DPSP has high potential for local recurrence and needs wide resection with adequate margins for local control [7].
(b) Extensive skin loss that needs a good flexible tissue closure for thumb function.
(c) Need for primary reconstruction of extensor tendon for function.

W. F. N. Wan Ismail (✉)
Orthopaedic Oncology Reconstructive Unit,
Prince Court Medical Centre, Kuala Lumpur, Malaysia

Orthopaedic Oncology reconstructive Unit,
School of Medical Sciences, Universiti Sains Malaysia,
Kubang Kerian, Kelantan, Malaysia
e-mail: faisham@usm.my

A. Z. Mat Saad
Plastic Reconstructive Hand and Microsurgery,
MSU Medical Centre, Management and Science University,
Shah Alam, Selangor, Malaysia

H. Özger et al. (eds.), *Diagnosis and Treatment of Soft Tissue Tumors*, https://doi.org/10.1007/978-3-031-77061-6_48

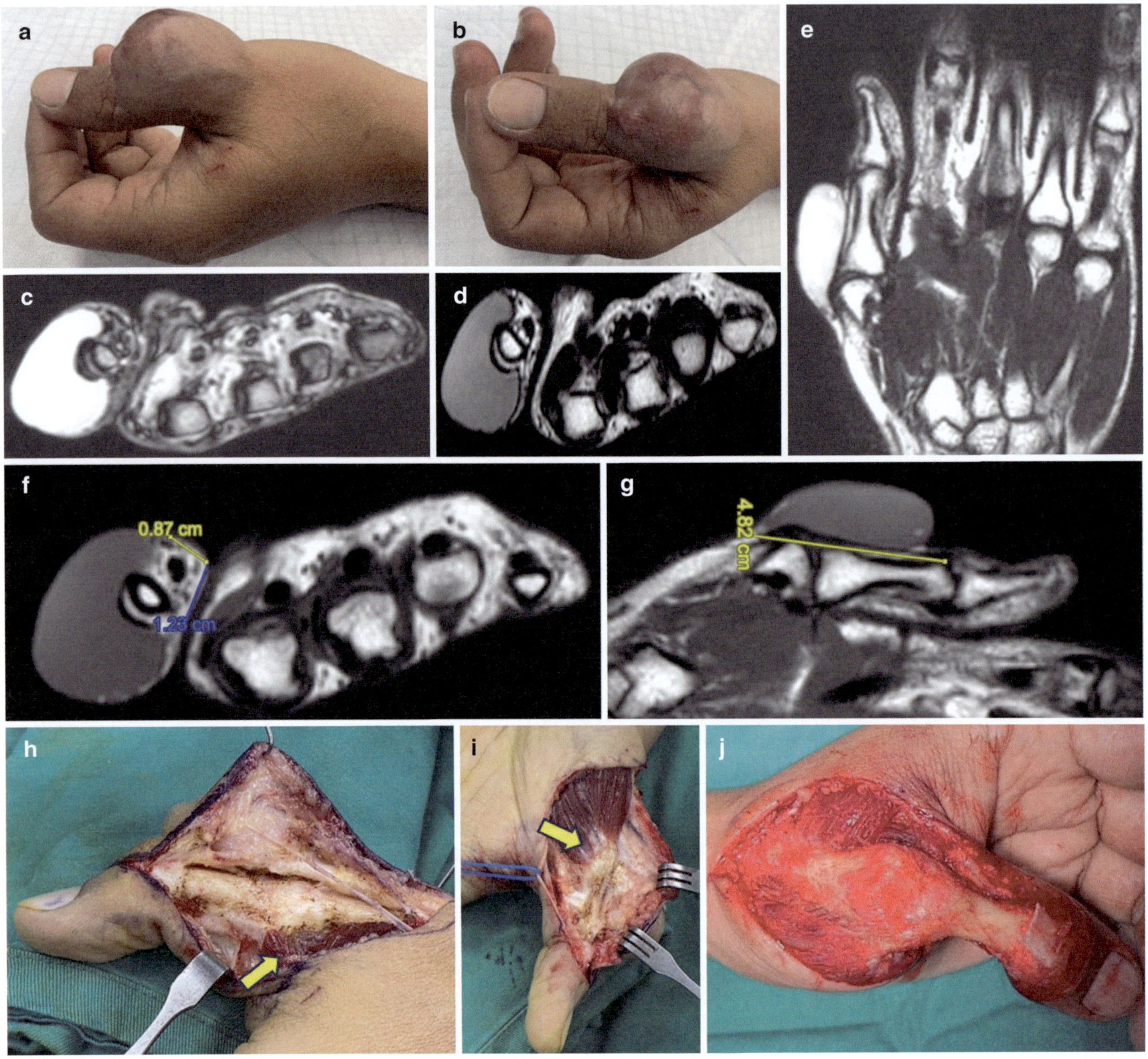

Fig. 48.1 (**a**, **b**) Swelling dorsum right thumb. (**c–e**) Axial and sagital image of MRI to show tumor extension. (**f**, **g**) Surgical planning and extent of resection on MRI. (**h–j**) Intraoperative procedures and resection margin. (**h**) Opponens pollicis. (**i**) Abductor pollicis. (**k**) Pedicle radial forearm flap with split skin grafting over donor sites. (**l–n**) Functional outcome

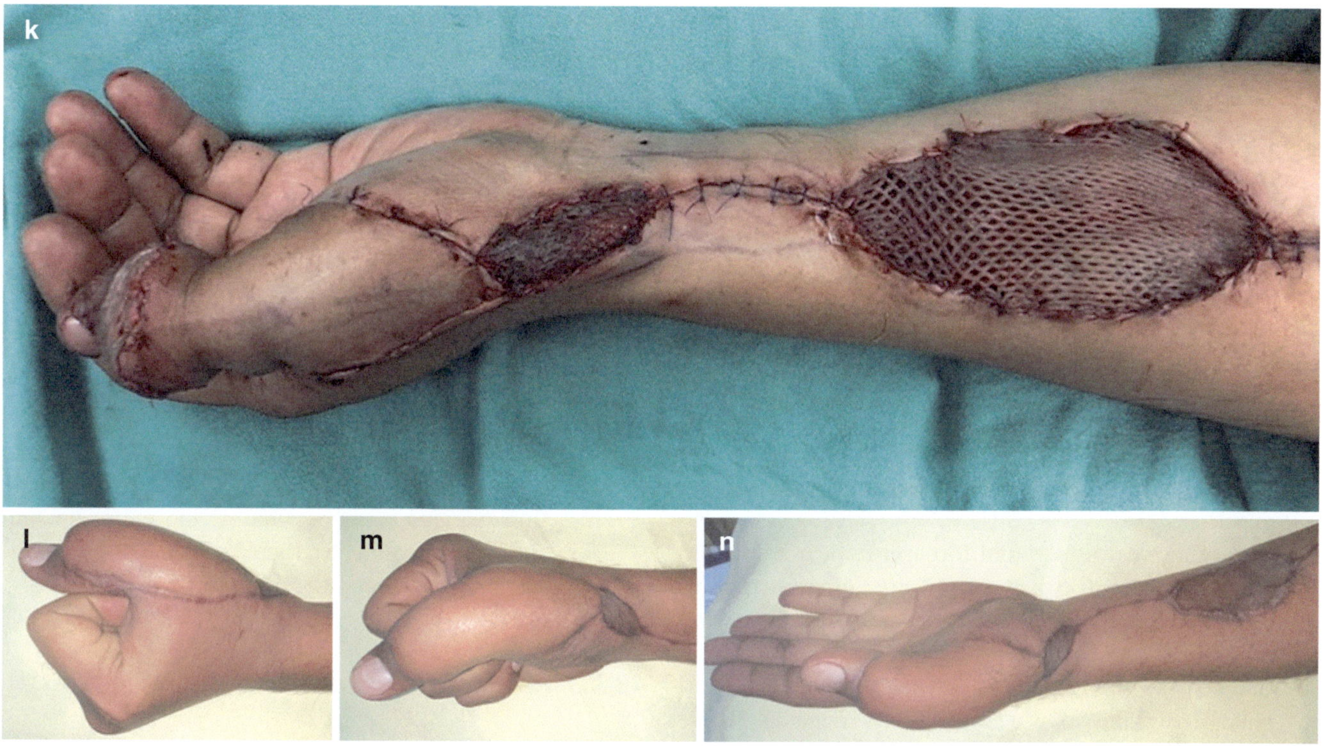

Fig. 48.1 (continued)

48.2.2 Treatment Strategy

(a) Multidisciplinary treatment includes wide margin surgery, flexible vascular tissue reconstruction, and tendon graft.
(b) Planning of skin and subcutaneous tissue resection based on MRI for surgical guidance is important to prevent violation of margins and ensure adequate oncological margins.
(c) The extensor tendon of the thumb is included in the resection because the tumor was found abutting it and contaminated by previous resection.
(d) Preoperative planning with the plastic reconstructive surgeon for flexible closure is mandatory. The final reconstruction of the defect must be resilient (in case postoperative radiotherapy is indicated); robust and flexible for early mobilization to ensure optimum function of the thumb.
(e) Various options for reconstruction of soft tissue defect include: [6]
   - Regional flaps like a radial forearm flap, ulnar artery flap, and posterior interosseous artery flap offer a simpler reconstructive option. Tendon graft can be hcs during flap exposure [8, 5].
   - Free flap requires technical expertise in microsurgery; able to customize the flap and can include a vascularized tendon graft as part of the soft tissue composite flap.
   - Distant flaps such as groin flap, abdominal, and chest wall flap are an option, but it necessitates a staged surgery, presents a potential risk of tumor contamination, and does not permit satisfactory mobilization.

48.2.3 Surgical Steps

(a) Preoperative planning of skin margins based on MRI evaluation is a crucial part of ensuring adequate resection margins (Fig. 48.1f, g).
(b) Exploration and preservation of the digital neurovascular bundle for distal vascularity and sensory of the thumb (Fig. 48.1h).
(c) Preservation of opponens and abductor tendon attachment, as these are not involved by the tumor (Fig. 48.1i).
(d) Resection of the entire extensor tendon till the periosteum to get R0 margins (Fig. 48.1j).

Reconstruction with radial forearm flap is a versatile option for large skin and tissue defects at the dorsum of the thumb. The vascularized fasciocutaneous flap provides flexible tissue and tension-free closure for early rehabilitation.

The procedure does not require advanced microvascular techniques.

48.2.4 Reconstruction of the Defect

(a) The aim is to replace missing tissue as closely as possible. In this case, the ideal reconstruction needs a thin pliable tissue with a tendon component than can withstand early mobilization for rehabilitation purpose.
(b) Reversed flow pedicled radial forearm flap is used in this patient due to its easy access; being in the same surgical field/exposure and offering a simple option for reconstruction that does not require microvascular expertise.
(c) Before harvesting a radial forearm flap, it is mandatory to assess the patency of the ulnar artery to ensure the hand is adequately perfused by using Allen's test.
(d) The defect size is measured and can be planned & centered along the axis of the radial artery anywhere between the wrist crease and cubital fossa after ascertaining the flap's reach from its pivot point.
(e) As this is a reversed flow flap, it is important to carefully dissect both vena comitantes and their communicating branch to facilitate venous outflow; some may include subcutaneous pedicle for this purpose, but this increases the pedicle volume and bulkiness.
(f) The donor site of the skin flap and part of the turnover pedicle are covered by split thickness skin graft (Fig. 48.1k).

Functional outcome after completed local radiotherapy (Fig. 48.1l–n).

48.3 Case 2: Dermatofibrosarcoma Protuberance of Ring Finger

This is another case of dermatofibrosarcoma protuberance (DFSP). A 30-year-old lady, right-hand dominant presented with a lesion on the ring finger over the dorsal aspect of the distal phalanx, which she noted for 3 months and grew slowly over time (Fig. 48.2a, b).

48.3.1 Problem List

(a) This case highlighted that tumor extension on MRI was beyond skin infiltration and need to be excised for clear margin (Fig. 48.2c–e).
(b) Local flap options are limited in this area, and free tissue transfer is not suitable in a very small defect with a small recipient for microvascular reconstruction.

48.3.2 Surgical Steps

(a) Preoperative planning of margins based on MRI evaluation is a crucial part of ensuring adequate resection margins.
(b) Extensor tendon was not involved on MRI, and this was reconfirmed intraoperatively by visualizing a good fatty layer below the tumor (Fig. 48.2f–g).
(c) The defect measured 3 cm long × 2 cm wide, with the bare extensor tendon exposed (Fig. 48.2h). Adequate resection margins were possible as the entire dorsum skin of the finger could be resected with the mass including 3–5 mm peripheral margin.

48.3.3 Reconstruction of Tissue Defect

(a) The ideal reconstruction would be a thin pliable skin flap; however, the position of the defect was overlying the distal and middle phalanx (very distal) leaving very limited reconstructive options from adjacent skin.
(b) Being a relatively "young" patient, postoperative stiffness was unlikely to be a major issue. Hence, we opted for an adipofascial cross-finger flap (to give a good bulk of tissue with overlying full thickness skin graft for good quality coverage of the wound and optimum aesthetic outcome (Fig. 48.2i–m).
(c) A neighboring long finger (middle) adipofascial flap was used.
(d) A finger tourniquet was used. First, we elevated a thin flap (later used for closing the donor defect) that turns away from the defect (Fig. 48.2j). Subsequently the adipofascial flap of the appropriate defect size was elevated and turned to the defect side and inset on the defect (Fig. 48.2k). Post finger tourniquet release demonstrated good bleeding from the flap (Fig. 48.2l), and a full-thickness skin graft was used to resurface the raw area with the two fingers stitched together for 18 days (normally range between 2 and 3 weeks) till neovascularization of the flap from the wound bed was achieved.

Postoperative histo-pathological examination (HPE) confirmed adequate surgical margins; peripheral skin of 3 mm and a deep margin of 2 mm. The functional and aesthetic outcome was good with early rehabilitation (Fig. 48.2n–o). No radiotherapy was given postoperatively 2 years postoperatively she is well controlled with no local recurrence.

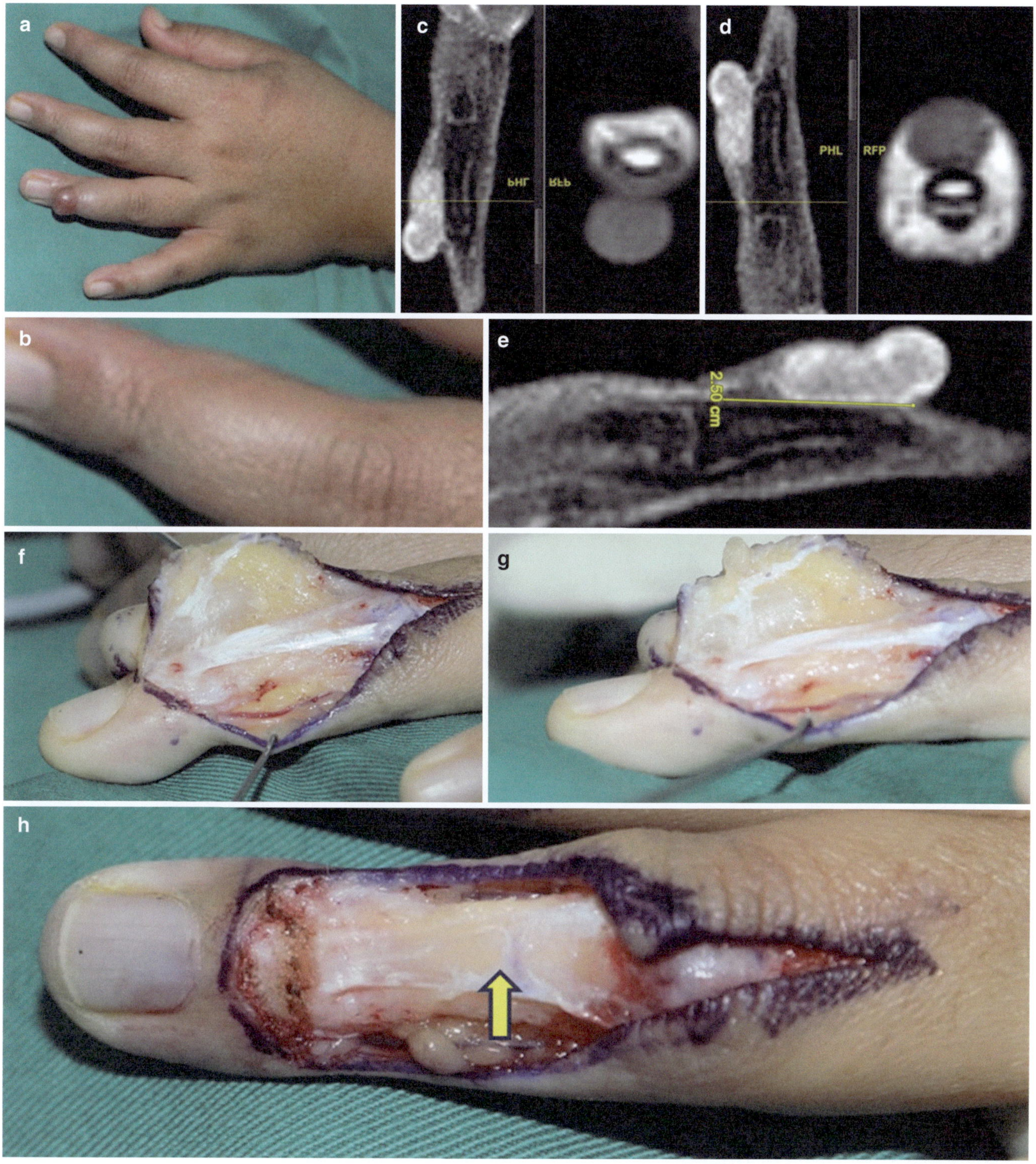

Fig. 48.2 (**a**, **b**) Dermatofibrosarcoma protuberance dorsum ring finger. (**c**–**e**) MRI findings and surgical planning. (**f**–**h**) Resection margin with preservation of extensor tendon. (**i**–**m**) Step-by-step surgical technique of adipofascial cross finger flap. (**n**, **o**) Functional outcome at 2 years

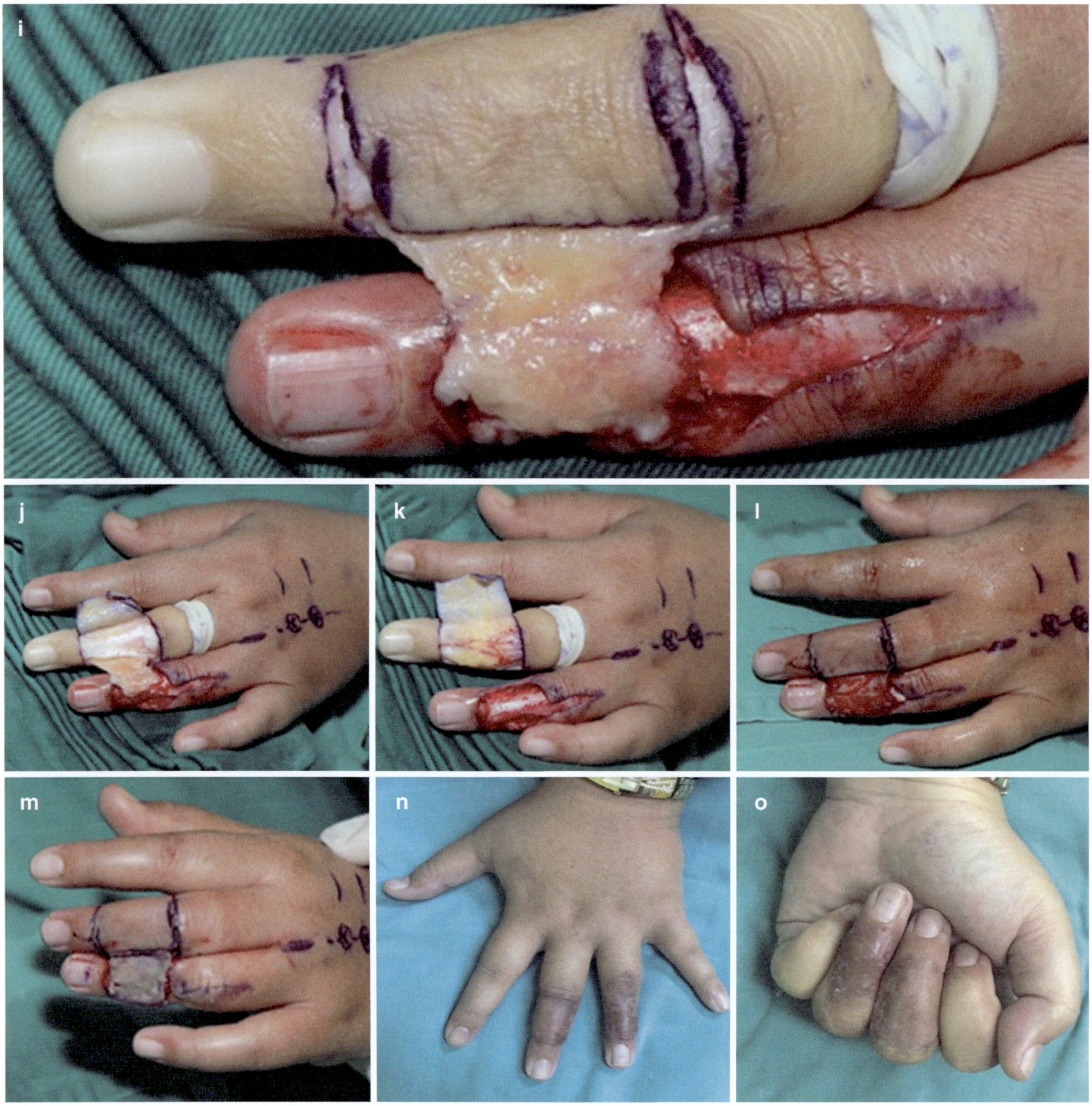

Fig. 48.2 (continued)

48.4 Case 3: Sarcoma of Thumb

A 70-year-old gentleman, right-hand dominant, presented with swelling over the dorsum of his left thumb over the distal phalanx of 3 months duration. MRI showed pulp of the thumb to be free of local infiltration (Fig. 48.3a–d). Biopsy confirmed pleomorphic sarcoma involving nail bed and abutting the tip of the distal phalanx bone.

48.4.1 Problem List

(a) Resection of entire dorsum of the thumb including nail bed, and bone was necessary to achieve complete R0 surgical resection.
(b) Preservation of the pulp of the thumb and remaining half of the bone would significantly retain the thumb length and function.

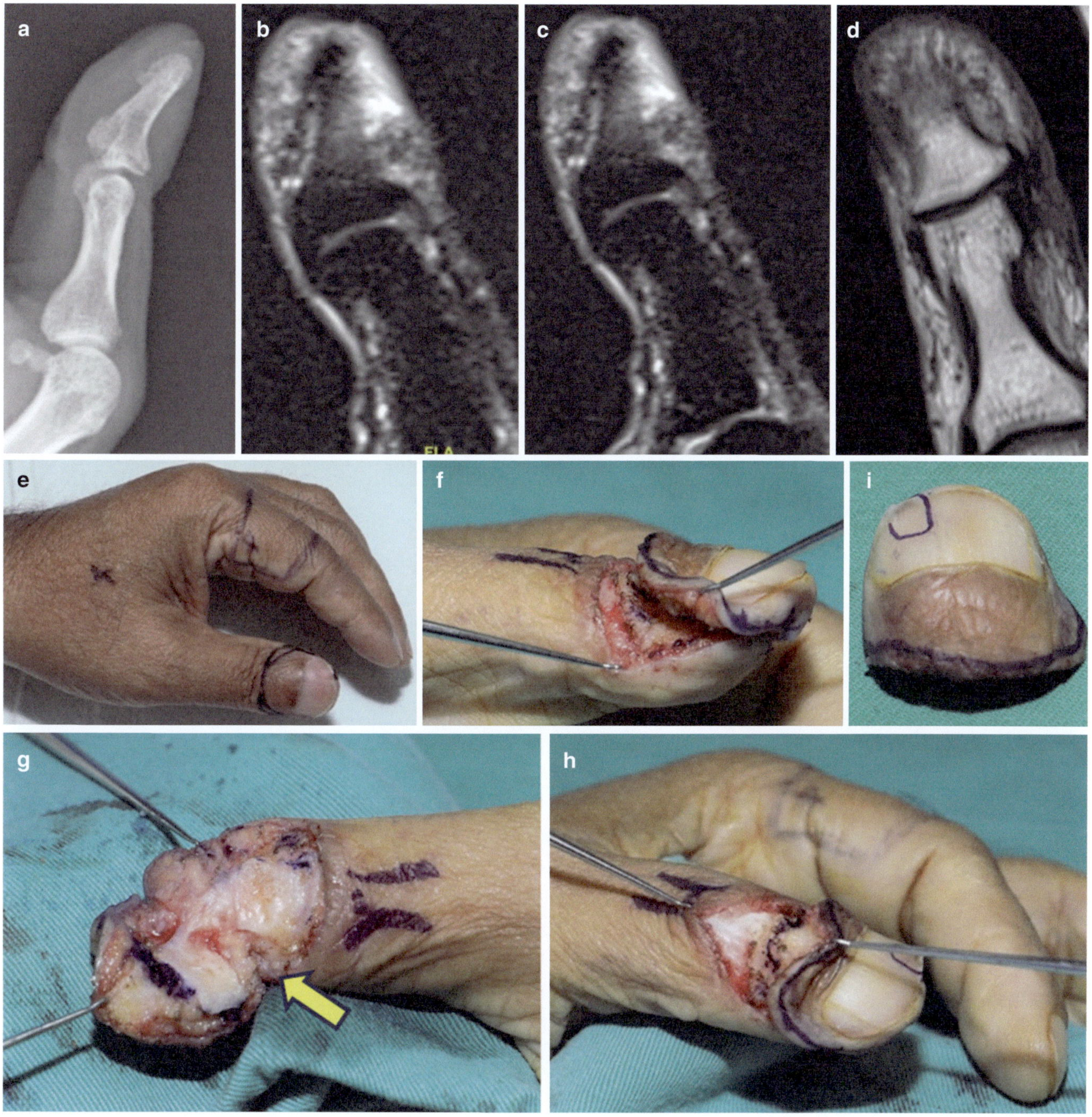

Fig. 48.3 (**a–d**) Radiograph and MRI image showed sarcoma over dorsum of thumb without bony involvement. (**e–i**) Surgical step of resection dorsum of skin with nail bed and tip of distal phalanx. (**j–m**) Surgical technique of first dorsal metacarpal artery flap. (**n**, **o**) Functional outcome

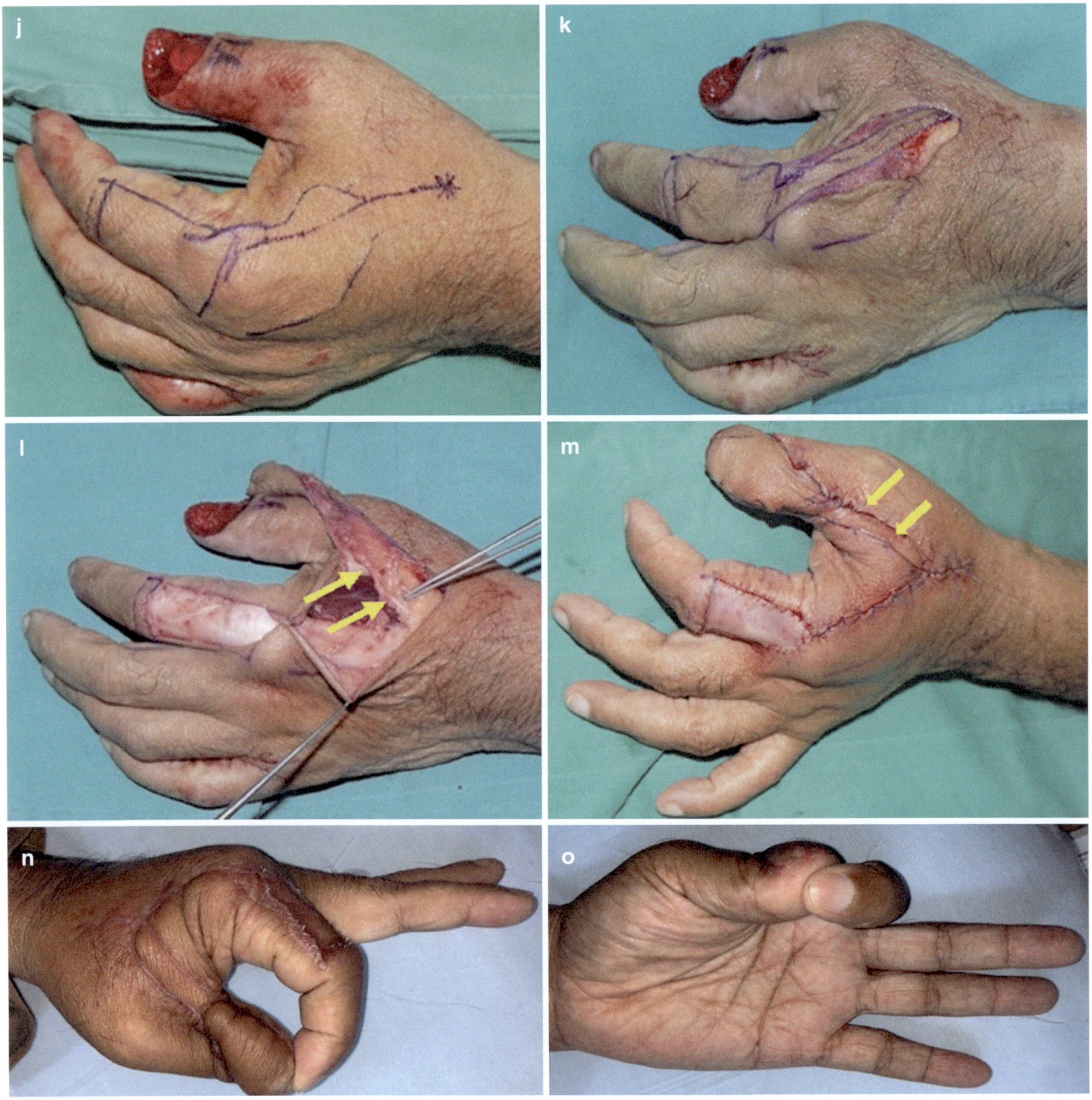

Fig. 48.3 (continued)

48.4.2 Surgical Steps

(a) Elevation of skin from superior margin proximal to the nail bed (Fig. 48.3e, f, h).
(b) The resection margin includes the nail bed and part of bone tip of the thumb (Fig. 48.3i).
(c) Part of distal pulp was removed for clear margins leaving more than half of the thumb pulp tissue for better sensation, length, function, and cosmesis.
(d) Retained the attachment of thumb extensor and flexor for function at the base of distal phalanx for better function and movement (Fig. 48.3g).

48.4.3 Reconstruction Option [9]

(a) First dorsal metacarpal artery flap is designed to cover the entire raw area and to keep the length of thumb and the pulp surface for better function (Fig. 48.3j).
(b) The course of the first dorsal metacarpal artery was marked preoperatively with pencil Doppler, and the skin flap was designed over the dorsum of the index finger proximal phalanx (Fig. 48.3j).
(c) This is a neurovascular islanded flap which will give good sensation to the reconstructed tip of the thumb. See yellow arrow—dorsal digital nerve (Fig. 48.3l).

(d) Note that there is an extension of the skin flap which looks like a "tadpole" design—a modification frequently used to avoid pedicle compression from tunneling. An ulnar mid axial incision is made to inset the flap and position the "tail" part of the flap (Fig. 48.3k, m).
(e) The donor site is partially closed primarily, and full-thickness skin graft used for the remaining area (Fig. 48.3m).

Long-term follow-up after 3 years shows no recurrence, good functional outcome with good sensation over the flap, and remaining thumb pulp (Fig. 48.3n, o).

48.5 Case 4: Sarcoma Hand

A 36-year-old lady presented with 5-month history of aggressive swelling over her right-dominant hand. It was painless with limited loss of hand function and there are no constitutional symptoms (Fig. 48.4a, b). Biopsy confirmed the diagnosis of synovial sarcoma.

MRI showed sarcoma involving fourth and third interosseous muscle and abutting on the third metacarpal. Resection amputation of fourth and fifth rays and clearance of third interossei muscle would result in soft tissue loss and need a reliable soft tissue cover for brachytherapy (Fig. 48.4c–f).

48.5.1 Problem List

(a) Sarcomas over the dorsum/palm of the hand commonly involve interosseous muscles with the metacarpal neurovascular structures course lying within this compartment.
(b) Resection margin for salvaging the finger is narrow, and sometimes oncological clearance is not optimal.
(c) In an ulnar-located lesion, a careful dissection of ulnar artery/vein while maintaining their continuity to the palmar arches is necessary to enable regional flap options for reconstruction.

48.5.2 Treatment Strategy

(a) Resection with ray amputations planned to achieve wider margin, while retaining maximum possible function of the hand is the main aim for palmar hand sarcomas.
(b) Resection amputation of fourth and fifth rays and clearance of third interossei muscle leave soft tissue loss and need a reliable soft tissue cover for brachytherapy.
(c) Soft tissue coverage with robust and pliable flap to allow adjunct brachytherapy and rehabilitation for hand function.
(d) Localized specific brachytherapy is an option to deliver high dose radiation postoperatively and minimize complications of wider external beam radiation to the remaining hand.

48.5.3 Surgical Steps

(a) Dorsal approach includes mobilization of skin with good margin and frees the extensor tendon to the middle finger (Fig. 48.4g, h).
(b) Palmar exploration includes maintaining metacarpal artery to the middle and all radial fingers from superficial palmar arch (Fig. 48.4i, j).
(c) Ulnar nerve exploration and preserving radial branch to the thenar and remaining interossei is important to maintain remaining optimum hand function.
(d) Periosteum of the middle finger is removed in total together with the third interossei muscle.
(e) The final resection amputation aims for good oncological margin, vascularity to the remaining finger, and optimum motor and sensory nerve function.
(f) Brachytherapy is an option in this case for delivering early high dose radiation to improve local control as wide margin is not possible for the small hand compartment. These brachytherapy tubes are placed during the surgery prior to flap inset.
(g) It is important to maintain the superficial arch and deep arch to the hand and finger to avoid the need of free tissue transfer/flap. A reversed flow radial forearm fasciocutaneous flap can be used for reconstruction (Fig. 48.4k).

Figure Legend (Fig. 48.4k–m)

- Brachytherapy tubes/rods were placed directly onto the tumor bed.
- Dorsal/ulnar view of completed reversed radial forearm flap with brachytherapy tubes in-situ.
- Intra-operative view of reversed flow radial forearm flap elevations. Green arrows show skin perforators. Yellow arrows show the main pedicle-radial artery with its vena comitantes.

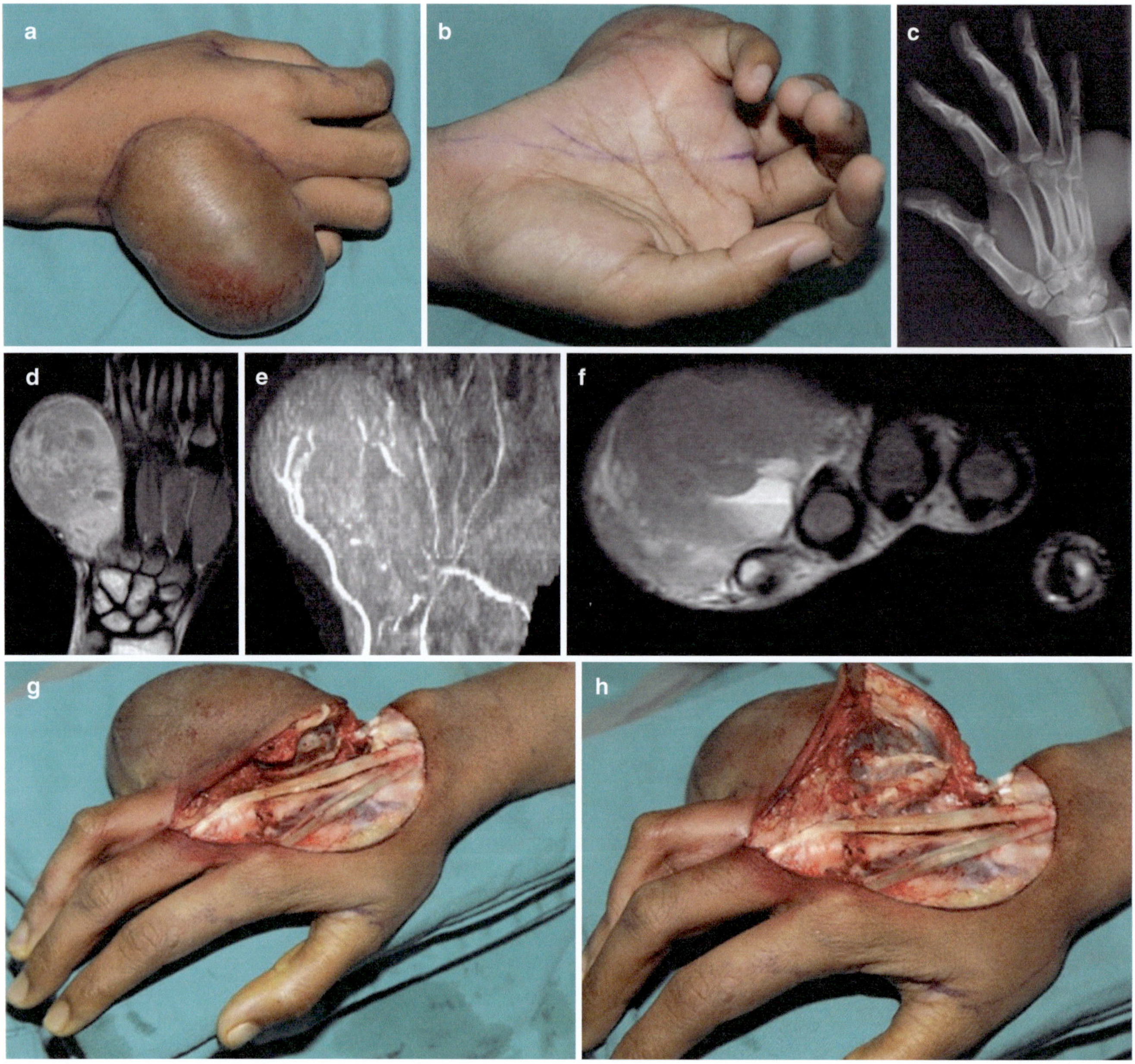

Fig. 48.4 (**a**–**f**) Clinical presentation, radiograph, and MRI evaluation of aggressive sarcoma right hand. (**g**–**j**) Step-by-step surgical approach resection of sarcoma with lateral two rays' amputation and arrows: (1) Superficial palmar arch. (2) Ulnar nerve. (**k**–**m**) Radial forearm fasciocutaneous flap with brachytherapy tube insertion over the surgical bed. Arrows: (1) Radial artery and vein. (2) Fasciocutaneous perforator vessels

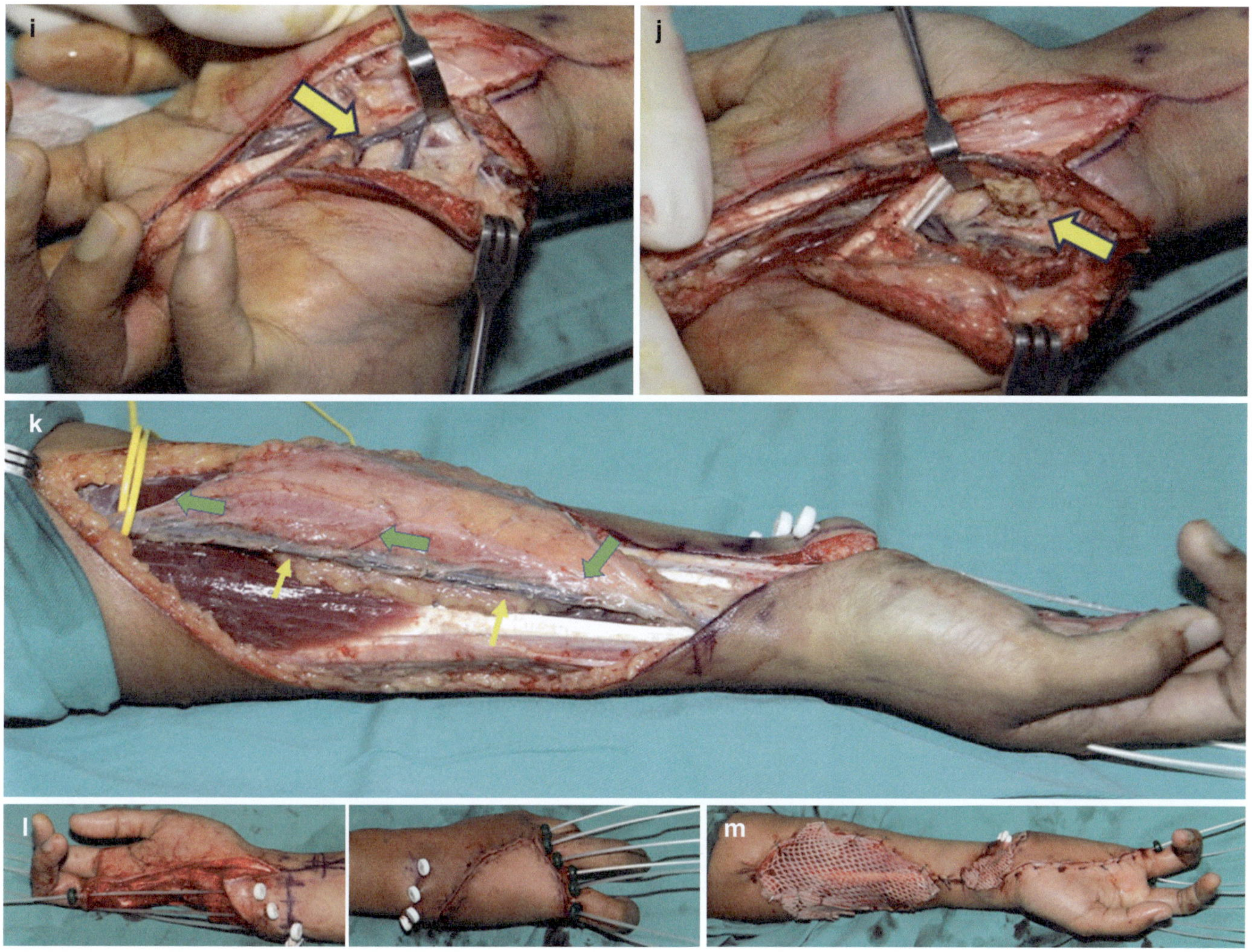

Fig. 48.4 (continued)

48.6 Case 5: Superficial Hemangioma Finger

A 6-year-old boy with a slow growing mass occupied the entire dorsum of proximal and middle ring finger and not responding to medical treatment and multiple treatment sessions with intralesional Nd-YAG laser. The lesion was growing slowly and causing recurrent punctate bleeding (Fig. 48.5a).

Photo showing the lesion over the dorsum of left ring finger with overlying skin changes. The dorsal metacarpal artery perforators are marked with red marker identified using doppler. MRI showed cavernous type of hemangioma involving the entire dermis with preservation of the extensor tendon (Fig. 48.5b–d).

48.6.1 Treatment Strategy

(a) Resection of entire hemangioma with good margins is important to minimize intraoperative bleeding and prevention of recurrence.
(b) To ensure adequate soft tissue cover for flexible mobility and optimum function of the finger, a distally based metacarpal artery perforator flap was planned [9].

48.6.2 Surgical Steps Flaps

(a) The lesion was excised completely, utilizing an incision on the ulnar border onto the plane just above the extensor tendon.

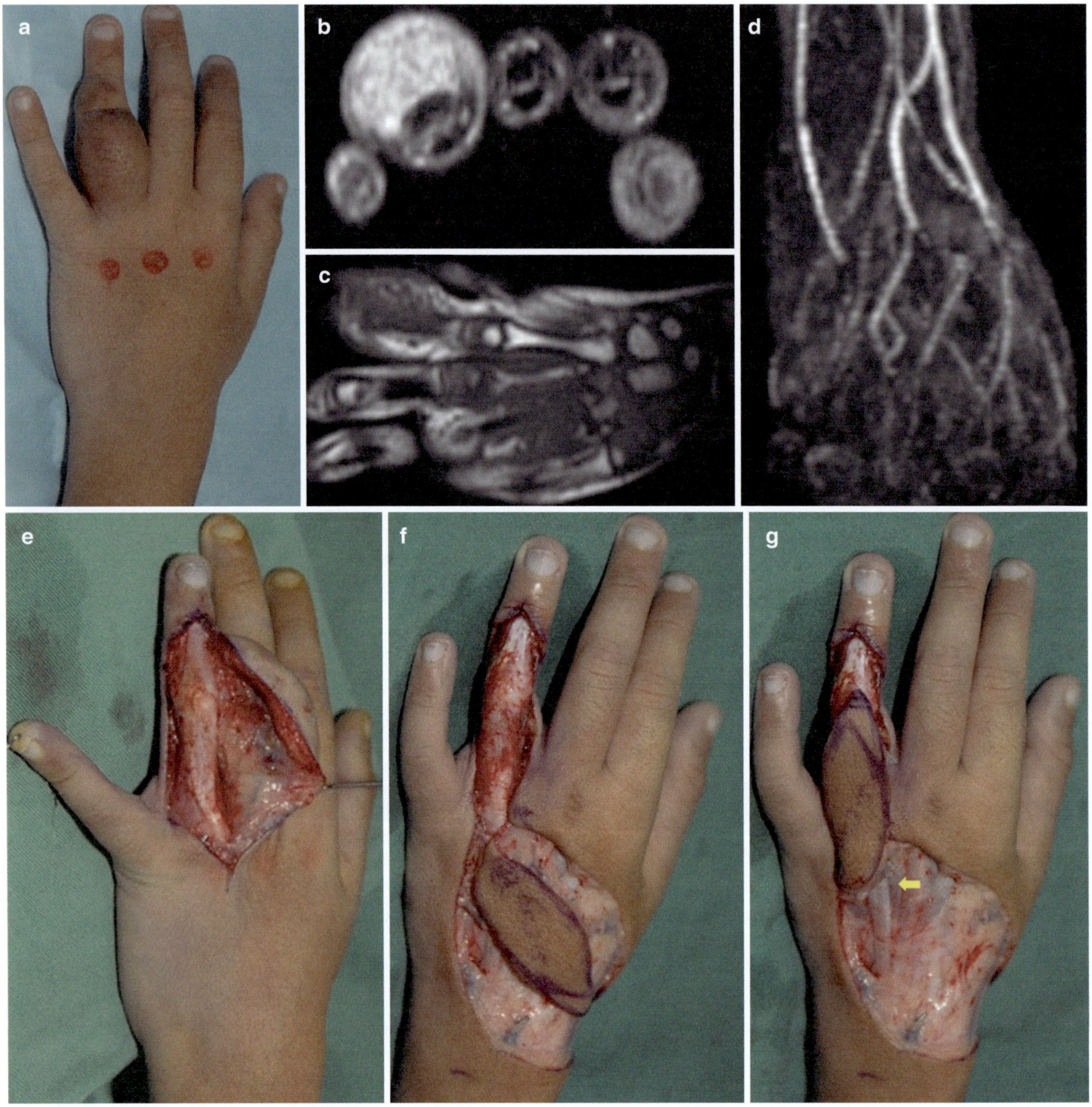

Fig. 48.5 (**a**–**d**) Clinical photo and MRI evaluation of superficial hemangioma of ring finger. (**e**–**g**) Resection of hemangioma with preservation of extensor tendon with island dorsal metacarpal artery perforator flap

(b) An elliptical skin flap was designed and raised based on third metacarpal artery perforator.
(c) The flap was positioned diagonally across the dorsum of the hand to maximize the length of the flap and to reduce the rotational angle (twisting of the perforating vessel on its axis).
(d) To facilitate primary closure, the scar was directed away so as not to limit the flexion of the fingers with resultant contractures.

Figure Legend

- The entire soft tissue and skin over dorsum of the proximal and middle phalanx was involved, but the extensor tendon remained intact (Fig. 48.5e).
- The Islanded dorsal metacarpal artery perforator flap is based on third web space palmar dorsal anastomosis at the metacarpal neck (Fig. 48.5f).
- The flap rotated at its perforator (yellow arrow) to cover the entire defect on the dorsum of the finger (Fig. 48.5g).

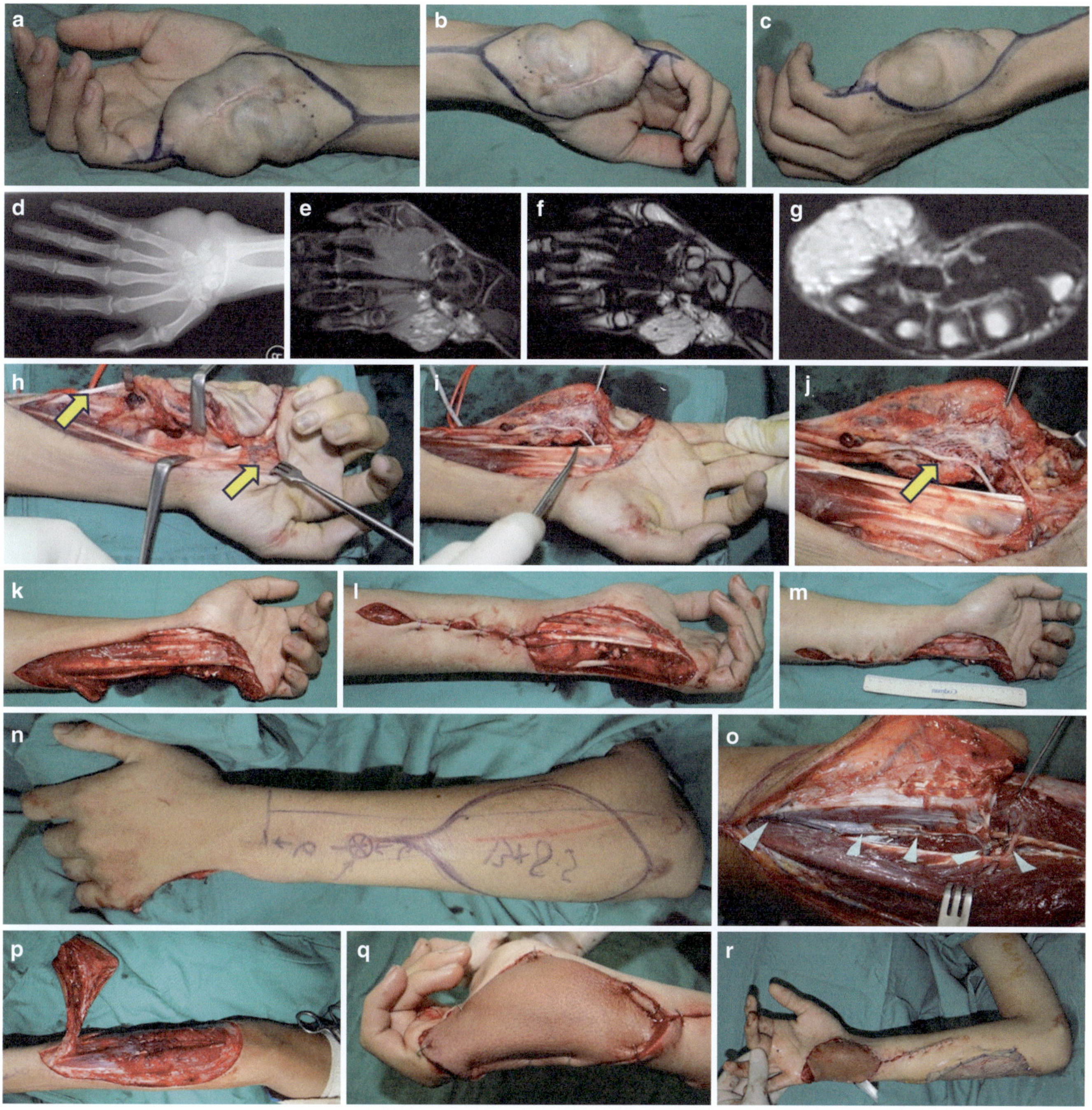

Fig. 48.6 (**a**–**g**) Clinical photo and MRI evaluation of hemangioma hypothenar eminence right hand. (**h**–**m**) Surgical steps of resection hypothenar eminence with partial preservation motor branch of ulnar nerve. Arrows: (1) Ulnar nerve. (2) Superficial palmar arch. (3) Branch of ulnar nerve to interossei and adductor pollicis. (**n**–**r**) Surgical steps posterior interosseous artery fasciocutaneous flap

48.7 Case 6: Deep Hemangioma of Hypothenar Eminence

An 18-year-old girl presented with a lesion over the hypothenar eminence of her right hand over 6 years. This was resected over 1 year ago but rapidly recurred, and she complained of chronic neuropathic pain over ulnar distributed fingers. The lesion continued to grow and increase in size and began to affect her daily activity and schooling (Fig. 48.6a–c).

MRI showed extensive involvement of the entire hypothenar muscle and superficial skin; however, the fourth web space does not involve. The ulnar vessels and its continuity to the deep palmar arch are involved within the hemangioma (Fig. 48.6d–g).

48.7.1 Problem List

(a) Massive skin and hemangioma resection leading to a major defect exposing major nerves, tendons, bones, and joints.
(b) Single vessel for palmar arch supply of the hand post resection (radial artery only).
(c) Enabling a flexible closure for optimum function.

48.7.2 Treatment Strategy

(a) Resection of hemangioma with free macroscopic margin would result in sacrifice of ulnar nerve (mainly sensory), hypothenar eminence and ulnar vessels that contribute to the palmar arch.
(b) Preserving part of ulnar motor branch for interossei muscle and adductor pollicis to retain optimum function.
(c) Radial forearm flap to be avoided as it would compromise the entire vascularity to the hand (Fig. 48.6h–m) [4, 5, 6].

48.7.3 Reconstructive Strategies

(a) A free flap or posterior interosseous artery (PIA) fasciocutaneous flap is an option. In this case, a PIA flap was chosen even though this flap is technically more tedious and difficult to raise/elevate [8, 10, 11].
(b) A skin island of flap was planned at the junction between proximal third and middle third of the forearm along its vascular axis, which lies between a line drawn from lateral epicondyle of humerus and ulnar styloid with the hand in full pronation.
(c) Due to its smaller caliber vessels and reverse flow in nature, a subcutaneous pedicle was designed to improve the venous outflow from the flap.
(d) The flap pedicle was then tunneled under a short skin bridge and inset into the defect—here the skin is loosely stitched at some area to allow exudate/blood to escape from the wound. Note that relatively dark skin due to minor congestion of the flap initially is expected in this flap.

Figure Legend

- Flap design and planning intra-operatively (Fig. 48.6n).
- The posterior interosseous artery (green arrows) in septum between extensor carpi ulnaris and extensor digiti minimi muscles (Fig. 48.6o).
- The flap is fully raised with its main pedicle and subcutaneous pedicle.
- Flap inset; Donor flap covered with split thickness skin graft (also note a slightly darker flap skin color due to minor congestion) (Fig. 48.6q).
- Long-term result show that there is no recurrence, flap healed well and no contracture (Fig. 48.6r).

48.8 Conclusions

Management of hand tumors should not be generalized. Each lesion should be assessed thoroughly via clinical history and examination to record the functional status for each component—movements, sensations, and appearance. The main goal of adequate oncological clearance is paramount. This must be achieved while enabling preservation or restoration of function with appropriate reconstruction choices. Various options for reconstructive closure with flaps significantly improve functional outcome.

Acknowledgement The authors thank Professor Zulmi Wan, Dr. Mohammad Paiman, Dr. Nor Azman Mat Zin, Dr. Syurahbil Abdul Halim, Professor Wan Azman Wan Sulaiman, and Professor Ahmad Sukari Halim for contribution to this chapter and team member managing all the patients.

References

1. Lans J, Yue KLC, Castelein RM, Suster DI. Benign hand tumours (part II): soft tissue tumors. Hand. 2020;17(3):519.
2. Lans J, Yue KLC, Castelein RM, Suster DI. Soft-tissue sarcoma of the hand: patient characteristics, treatment, and oncologic outcomes. JAAOS. 2021;29(6):297–307.
3. Puhaindran ME, Rohde RS, Chou J, Morris CD. Clinical outcomes for patients with soft tissue sarcoma of the hand. Cancer. 2011;1171:175–9.
4. Naalla R, Chauhan S, Dave A. Reconstruction of post-traumatic upper extremity soft tissue defects with pedicled flaps: an algorithmic approach to clinical decision making. Chin J Traumatol. 2018;21(6):338–51.
5. Sabapathy SR. Refinements of pedicle flaps for soft tissue cover in the upper limb. In: Venkataswami R, editor. Surgery of the injured hand. New Delhi: Jaypee Brothers; 2009. p. 131–8.
6. Tubiana R, Gilbert A, Masquelet AC. An atlas of surgical techniques of the hand and wrist. London: Martin Dunitz Ltd; 1999.
7. Roman M, Patel A. Dermatofibrosarcoma protuberans—an illustration of the reconstructive ladder for defects following Slow Mohs excision. Eur J Surg Oncol. 2022;48(1):E26.
8. Rab M, Prommersberger KJ. Distally pedicled posterior interosseous artery flap for the coverage of defects on the wrist and hand. Oper Orthop Traumatol. 2008;20:111–8.
9. Webster N, Saint-Cyr M. Flaps based on the dorsal metacarpal artery. Hand Clin. 2020;36(1):75–83.
10. Franchi A, Häfeli M, Scaglioni MF, Elliot D. The use of chimeric musculocutaneous posterior interosseous artery flaps for treatment of osteomyelitis and soft tissue defect in hand. Microsurgery. 2019;39(5):416–22.
11. Acharya AM, Bhat AK, Bhaskaranand K. The reverse posterior interosseous artery flap: technical considerations in raising an easier and more reliable flap. J Hand Surg Am. 2012;37(3):572–82.
12. Tang P, Hornicek FJ, Gebhardt MC, Cates J, Mankin HJ. Surgical treatment of hemangiomas of soft tissue. Clin Orthop Relat Res. 2002;(399):205–10.

Neoadjuvant Treatment Facilitating Surgery

49

E. J. Ortiz-Cruz, N. Bonsfills, M. Tapia-Viñé, B. Belinchon-Olmeda, A. Redondo, and J. J. Pozo-Kreilinger

49.1 Basic Clinical History

A 72-year-old male presented with a spontaneous soft tissue mass in his left arm. Initially, he was diagnosed with a hematoma from a possible rupture of the long head of the biceps brachii muscle by initial MRI.

Four months later, due to a rapid growth of the mass, the patient came to our sarcoma center. A new MRI was indicated, describing a tumor in the middle third of the anterior medial part of the left arm, with a size of 57 × 37 × 81 mm. After appropriate work-up of the mass, in which detectable metastases were ruled out, by thoracic CT and PET-CT, a percutaneous core Tru-Cut biopsy CNB performed under ultrasound guidance, and the final pathologic report was a high-grade undifferentiated pleomorphic sarcoma (UPS) grade 2 by Fédération Nationale des Centres de Lutte Contre Le Cancer (FNCLCC) and IIIA (G3 T2 N0 M0) by American Joint Committee on Cancer (AJCC).

49.2 Pretreatment Clinical and Radiological Images

See Figs. 49.1, 49.2, and 49.3.

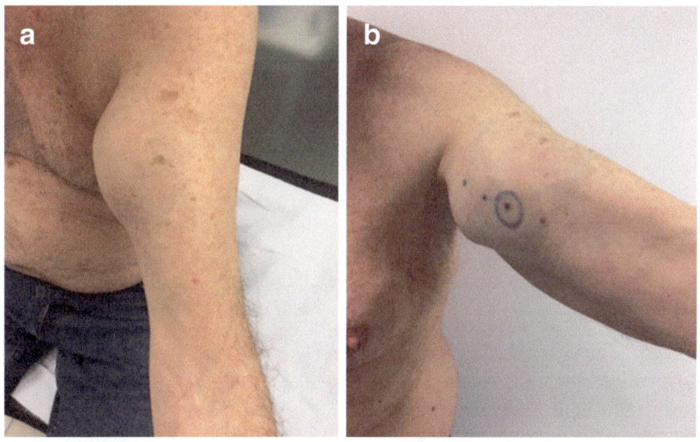

Fig. 49.1 Pretreatment clinical image of the mass at the time of diagnosis. (**a**) Soft tissue mass in the medial part of the left arm. (**b**) Planned incision and planned site of biopsy

E. J. Ortiz-Cruz (✉) · N. Bonsfills
Orthopaedic Oncology Section, Department of Orthopedics, Hospital Universitario La Paz, Madrid, Spain
e-mail: eduardojose.ortiz@salud.madrid.org

M. Tapia-Viñé
Musculoskeletal Radiology Section, Department of Radiology, Hospital Universitario La Paz, Madrid, Spain

B. Belinchon-Olmeda
Sarcoma Radiotherapy Section, Department of Radiation Oncology, Hospital Universitario La Paz, Madrid, Spain

A. Redondo
Sarcoma Unit, Department of Medical Oncology, Hospital Universitario La Paz, Madrid, Spain

J. J. Pozo-Kreilinger
Musculoskeletal Section, Department of Pathology, Hospital Universitario La Paz, Madrid, Spain

H. Özger et al. (eds.), *Diagnosis and Treatment of Soft Tissue Tumors*, https://doi.org/10.1007/978-3-031-77061-6_49

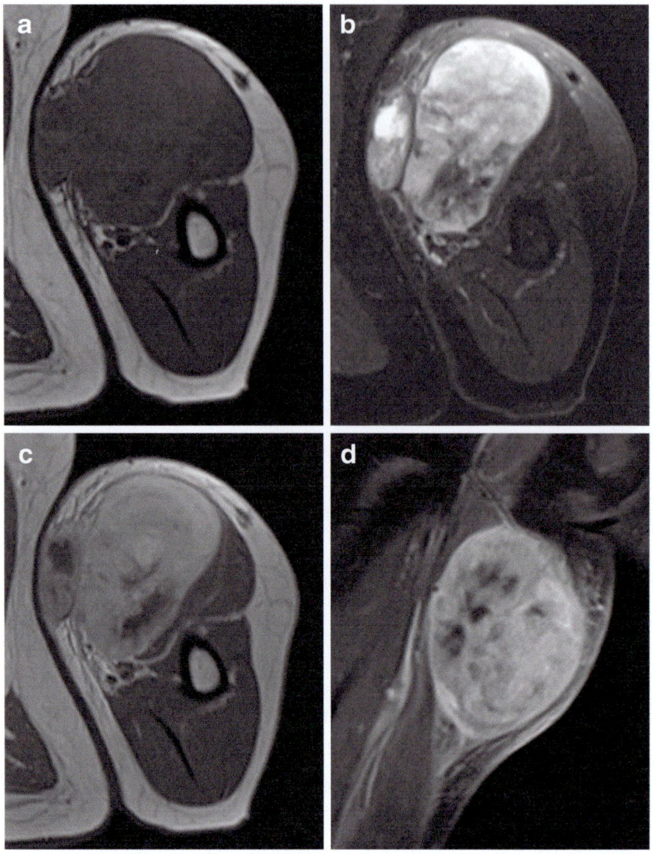

Fig. 49.2 Pretreatment MRI of the left arm showed a relatively well-circumscribed bilobated mass located in the biceps brachii muscle, with a signal isointense with the muscle on T1-weighted sequences (**a**) and heterogeneous, high signal intensity in fat-suppressed T2-weighted sequences, exerting a positive mass effect on surrounding structures due to their large size. It measured about 9 × 8.7 × 5.2 cm. No signs of invasion of the humerus (**b**). After the administration of paramagnetic contrast, the mass showed prominent enhancement of solid components and non-enhancing necrotic areas (**c**). Sagittal T1-weighted MRI and paramagnetic contrast: enhancing tail of tumor extending along the remaining portion of the muscle (**d**)

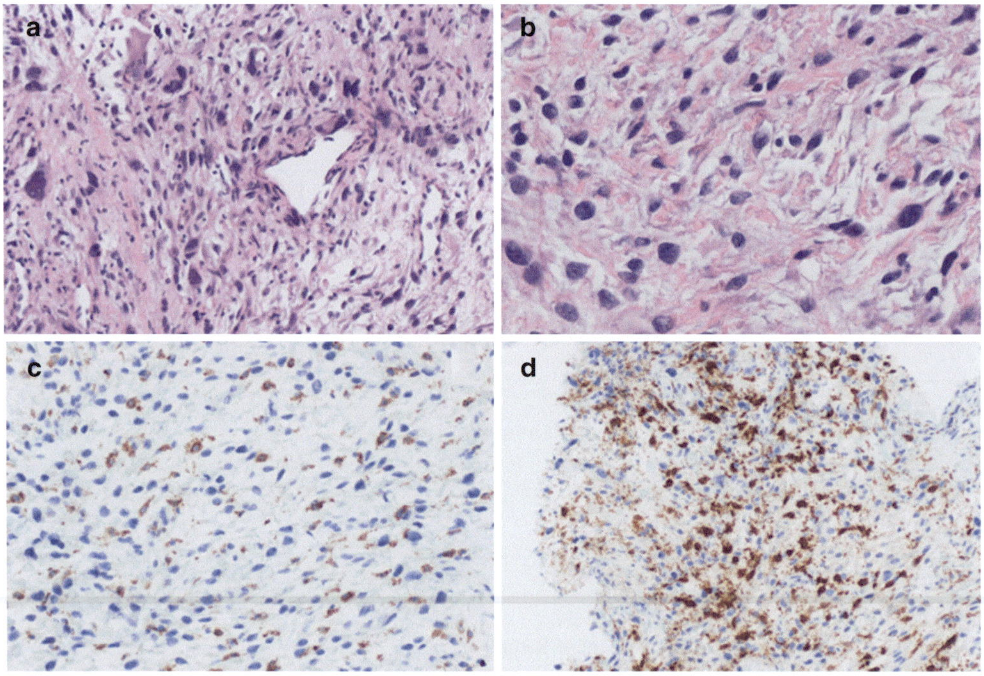

Fig. 49.3 Microscopic images of the percutaneous biopsy. There is a malignant fusocellular mesenchymal proliferation, high-grade pleomorphic, with evident cytologic atypia, presence of hyperchromatic variable in shape and size nuclei, occasional macronucleoli, and evident mitotic activity. Maximum cell proliferation index (Ki67) was 30%. (**a**) H&E staining, ×200. (**b**) H&E staining, ×400. Cells were immunoreactive to CD68 (**c**) and XIIIa factor (**d**), and negative to smooth muscle actine, desmin, caldesmon, S-100 protein, CD34, and STAT6

49.3 Problem List

(a) A soft tissue mass that can be clinically misdiagnosed as a benign pathology without an adequate medical history and a perfect physical exam.
(b) Attribute the radiological abnormality to a benign process (hematoma, traumatic, or orthopedic problem).
(c) Once diagnosed as a soft tissue sarcoma (STS), sometimes the surgeon needs to reduce the mass with neoadjuvant therapy to achieve oncological wide surgical margins with less functional impairment, or postoperative therapies that may imply complications in the follow-up.

49.4 Treatment Strategy

(a) Appropriate preoperative work-up (with history, physical exam, plain X-rays, ultrasound, CT, MRI, and bone scan, followed by percutaneous biopsy)
(b) Precise staging of the tumor and multidisciplinary committee decision about preoperative therapies
(c) Preoperative neoadjuvant treatment (radiotherapy and/or chemotherapy) prior to wide tumor resection surgery.
(d) Neoadjuvant chemotherapy with the regimen epirubicin + ifosfamide (x3 cycles). The last cycle was synchronous with the first sessions of radiotherapy
(e) Neoadjuvant radiotherapy included a radiation dose of 50 Gy (2 Gy/day) with 6 MV beam energy, for 5 weeks, with IMRT technique (intensity-modulated radiation therapy)
(f) Surgical oncological resection 6 weeks after the end of radiotherapy
(g) More functional resection with wide safe margins of the reduced mass and subsequent soft tissue reconstruction with local or free flaps

49.5 Basic Principles

1. Basic warning signs to make a referral to a sarcoma center:
   (a) Mass greater than 4 cm (subcutaneous or deeper)
   (b) Mass that has experienced recent growth
   (c) Pain is not a straightforward symptom of a soft tissue sarcoma, but together with any of the previous signs may reinforce the presumption of malignancy
   (d) Maintain appropriate level of suspicion
2. If the patient is going to be referred
   (a) Do not biopsy and, if necessary, avoid excisional biopsies
   (b) The biopsy tract must be planned with the surgeon.
   (c) Planning the biopsy site is essential and should be in the area of the incision.
   (d) The biopsy should be done after imaging studies are performed. It is the final part of the staging process.
3. Document every step with clinical and radiological images to assess the effect of therapies and the recurrence.
4. Neo/adjuvant chemotherapy has demonstrated to improve overall survival in patients with a high-grade STS of the extremities >5 cm (except in chemoresistant histotypes).
5. Radiotherapy in extremities STS increases local control and survival:
   (a) Advantages of preoperative radiotherapy compared to postoperative: lower radiation dose, smaller treatment volume, improved resectability, margin-negative resections, better oxygenation of tumor cells, fewer long-term toxicities.
   (b) Collaboration between surgeon and radiation oncologist is essential for the integration of local treatments and includes recurrence risk assessment, defining areas of concern for close or positive margins.
6. Surgery
   (a) Basic surgical principles
      - Safe wide oncological margin.
      - Resection overcomes reconstruction when defining surgical resection.
      - Adjuvant radiotherapy or chemotherapy does not compensate for an improper surgery.
      - Adequate soft tissue reconstruction.
   (b) Approach:
      - The scar and the biopsy track must be included en-bloc in the surgical procedure.
      - The incision must always be longitudinal in the extremities.
      - Careful oncologic dissection.
   (c) Resection
      - Resection overcomes reconstruction when defining surgical resection.
      - Ascertain safe oncological margins.
      - Make an intraoperative biopsy.
      - After resection of the tumor:
        – Change gloves and surgical instruments.
        – Very careful hemostasis must be ensured.
        – Bring personally the mass to the pathology laboratory.
        – The drains—if needed—should be placed in line with the scar.
        – Put clips in the surgical bed if postoperative radiotherapy is needed.
   (d) Adequate soft tissue reconstruction

49.6 Photos and Imaging During Treatment

See Figs. 49.4, 49.5, 49.6, 49.7, 49.8, 49.9, 49.10, and 49.11.

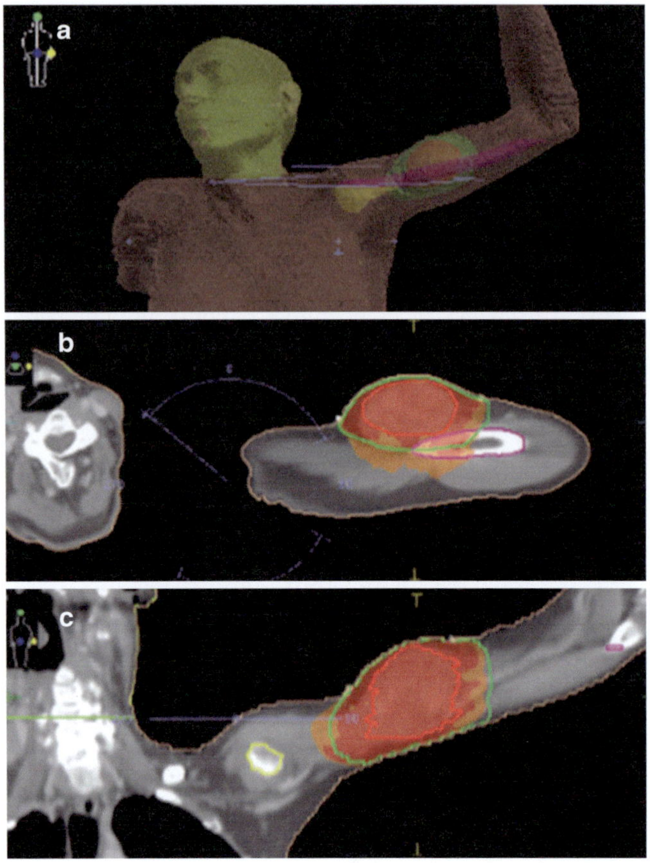

Fig. 49.4 Clinical and dosimetric images of the neoadjuvant radiotherapy. (**a**) 3D plan. (**b**) Axial section. (**c**) Coronal section

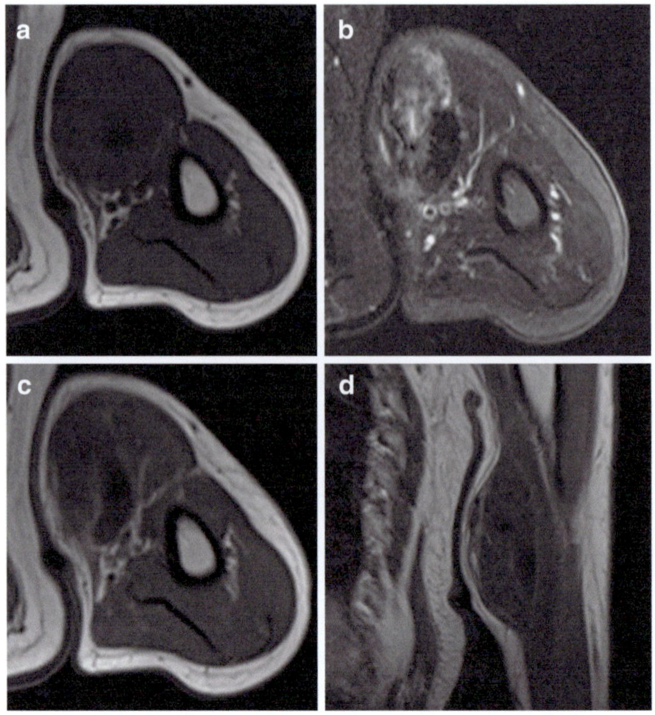

Fig. 49.6 MRI images after neoadjuvant treatment showed a clear reduction in the size—measured 7 × 5 × 2.1 cm—and a change in the characteristics of the mass with a hypointense foci on T1-weighted sequences (**a**) and fat-suppressed T2-weighted sequences corresponding to hemosiderin deposits secondary to bleeding. In these sequences, a decrease in the cellular component is also observed, which leads to a decrease in the mass signal (**b**). After the administration of paramagnetic contrast, the mass showed discrete enhancement (**c**). Sagittal T1-weighted MRI and paramagnetic contrast: the enhancing tails have disappeared (**d**). According to RECIST criteria, there was a partial response: >30% decrease in longest axis measurement, no new lesions

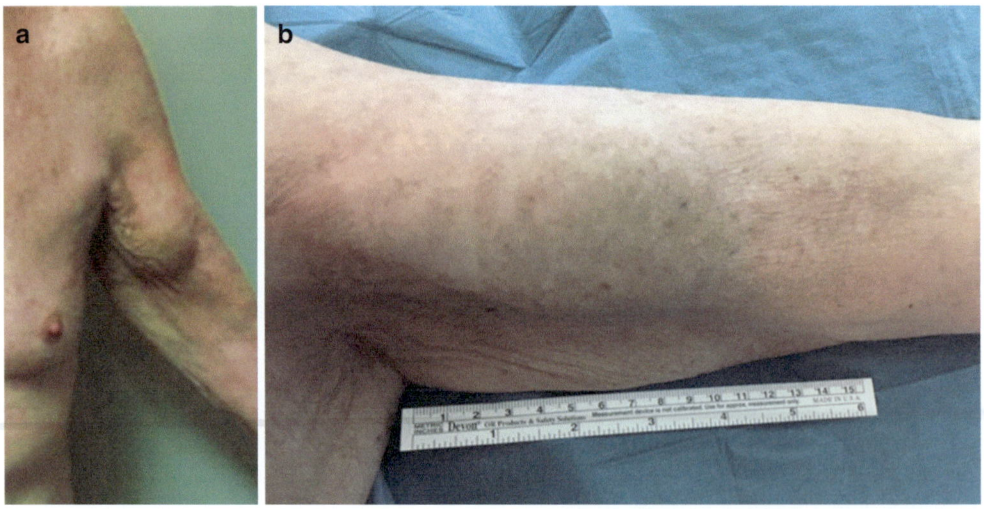

Fig. 49.5 Clinical images (**a**: frontal view with the patient standing and **b**: with the patient supine) at the end of the neoadjuvant treatment. A reduction of the size (and palpated consistency) can be observed in compared with Fig. 49.1

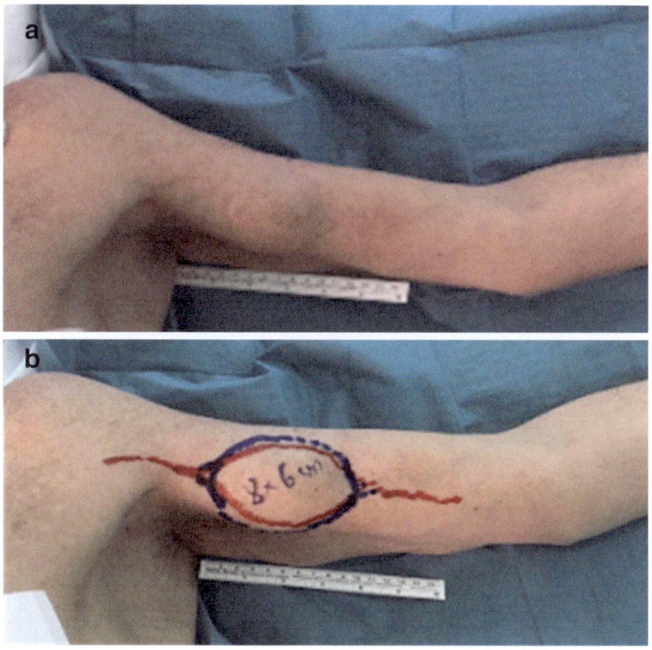

Fig. 49.7 Surgical approach. (**a**) Clinical picture before surgery. (**b**) Planned cutaneous resection along with the mass

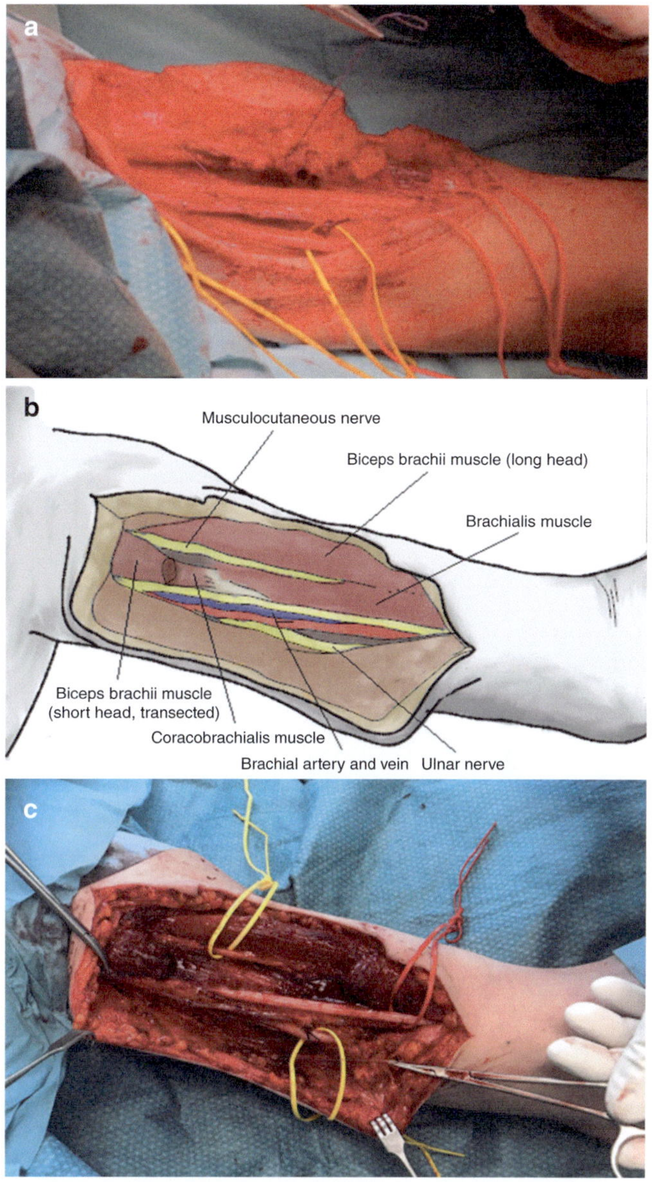

Fig. 49.8 Oncological surgical resection. (**a**) Mass dissected and elevated from its surgical bed. (**b**) Scheme of the surgical bed after the resection. (**c**) Photograph of the surgical bed after the resection

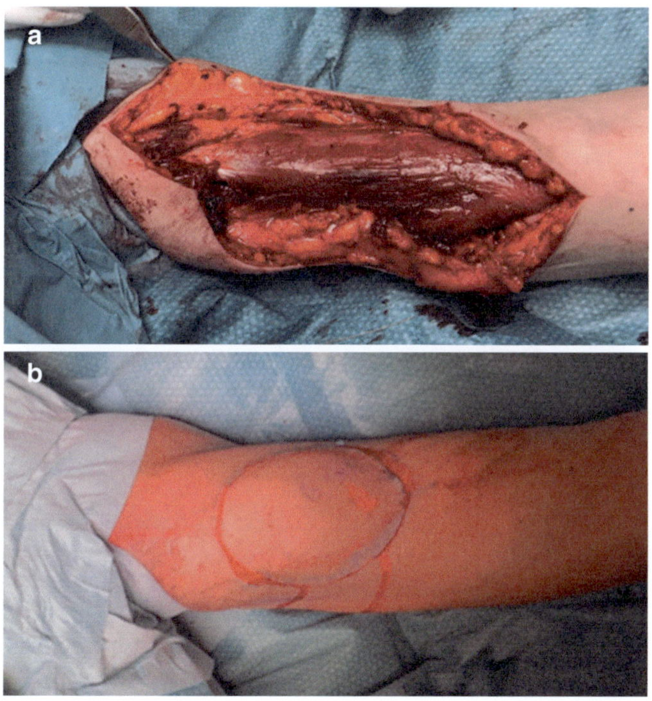

Fig. 49.9 Soft tissue reconstruction. (**a**) Biceps brachii is repositioned anteriorly, leaving the neurovascular bundle medial to its muscular mass. (**b**) The cutaneous defect is closed with a local flap

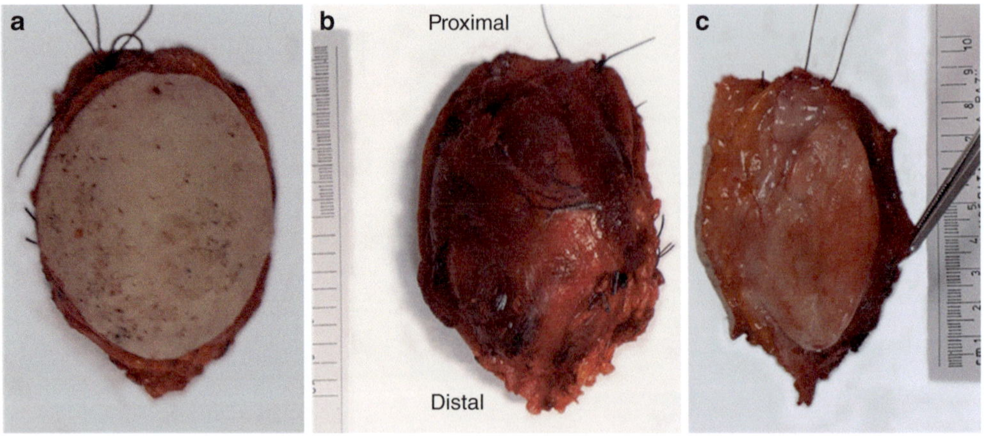

Fig. 49.10 Macroscopic images of the specimen. Size of the resected tissue was 7 × 4 × 3.2 cm. (**a**) Anterior superficial view. (**b**) Posterior deep view (with muscular belly of the short biceps brachii). (**c**) Longitudinal section. When sectioned, a well-delimited, oval-shaped, clear pink mass is seen, surrounded by skin in the surface and striated skeletal muscle in the depth. In both proximal and distal ends, there is lax grayish tissue that matches the tails seen in the MRI

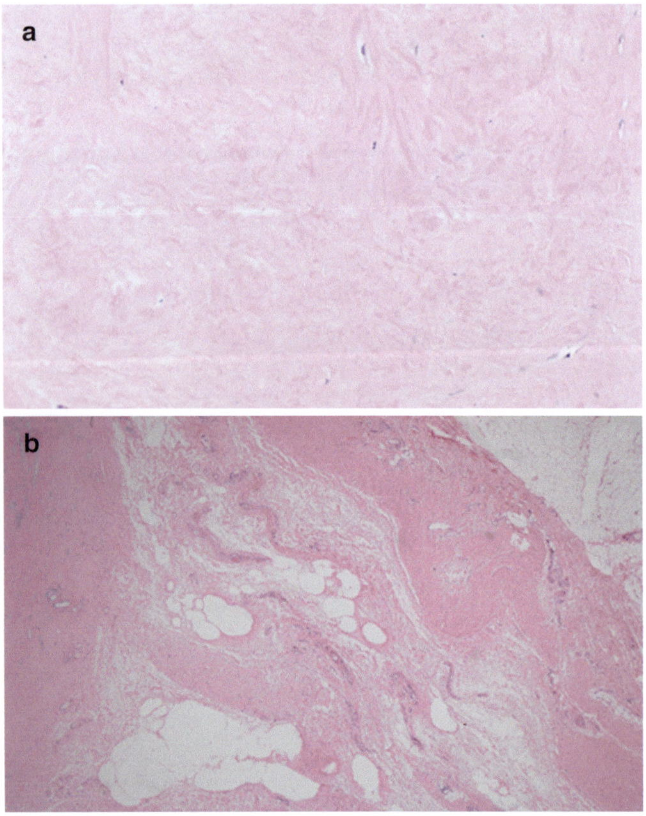

Fig. 49.11 Microscopic images of the specimen. H&E staining. The residual tumoral mass shows hyalinization and no signs of viability after chemotherapy and radiotherapy. (**a**) Fragment of the center of the mass, ×200. (**b**) Fragment of one of the tails, observing, from left to right: hyalinized no viable tumor, lax connective tissue of the tail, fascia, and subcutaneous cellular tissue

49.7 Technical Pearls

1. Neoadjuvant therapy
   (a) Chemotherapy according to first line protocols for UPS.
   (b) Radiotherapy focused on the size and grade of the tumor, thus avoiding extended postoperative irradiation of the surgical bed.
   (c) IMRT is better than 3D conformal radiotherapy because of the normal tissue sparing and increased local control.
2. Surgical resection
   (a) An adequate margin should consider:
      - Quantity margin width.
      - Quality margin—type of anatomical barrier
        - Close to nerves: Epineurium resection. In this case, no major nerves or branches were resected or transected, only medial cutaneous brachial nerve in the approach.
        - Close to vessels: Adventitia resection or vessels resection and by-pass. Adventitia was preserved (Fig. 49.6).
        - Close to bone (increased bone uptake or by MRI): Periosteum resection or bone resection. Although periosteum was seen after the resection of the short head of the biceps brachii muscle, it was not affected.
        - Close or adjacent skin: resection of the affected skin with wide margins, and skin graft, or free or local muscular flap.

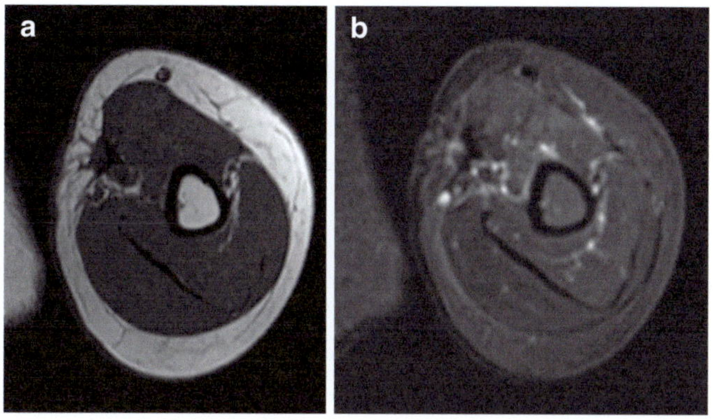

Fig. 49.12 MRI 3 years after surgery. Axial sections (**a**) T1 sequence. (**b**) T2 sequence. No signs of local recurrence are observed

(b) The quality of the surgery will be defined by its worst margin.
(c) Every attempt should be made to avoid positive microscopic surgical margins.
(d) A positive margin over an anatomical barrier was the worst surgical prognostic factor for local recurrence. This issue did not happen in the case presented.

49.8 Outcome Clinical and Radiological Images

From a clinical point of view, the patient is asymptomatic, with no signs of local recurrence, and no functional deficit.

MRI obtained 3 years after resection: no tumor or signal alterations are visualized, only areas of low signal in all the sequences that correspond to fibrosis. No distant disease is observed either (Fig. 49.12).

49.9 Avoiding and Managing Complications

(a) Drains should be placed at the incision line.
(b) Drains should be maintained, mainly in patients with preoperative radiotherapy, until the debit is less than 30–50 cc/24 h.
(c) Do not remove staples or stitches until the third week postoperative.
(d) Antibiotic therapy, while maintaining drainage or bladder catheter.
(e) Radiation is an adjunct, not a substitute, for poor surgical technique.
(f) Surgery preferably takes place 4–6 weeks after completion neoadjuvant radiotherapy in order to decrease the risk of wound complications.
(g) The surgeon must take the resected specimen to the pathology laboratory, to show the pathologist its orientation, and to assess high-risk areas with a positive or close margin.
(h) In case of doubt, an intraoperative biopsy should be performed.
(i) Soft tissue reconstruction should not be started until the intraoperative biopsy is reported to the surgical team.
(j) Processing may affect the difference between the margin reported and the margin you thought you delivered.
 1. Communicate with your pathologist.

Acknowledgments We want to thank our patient, J.A.G., for his collaboration to prepare and show his case. We also want to thank Ms. Marta Bodega, case coordinator nurse of the Sarcoma Unit and the Sarcoma Committee at Hospital Universitario La Paz, who takes care of the patient and coordinates all diagnostic and therapeutic appointments and plans.

Suggested Readings

American Joint Committee on Cancer. AJCC cancer staging manual. 8th ed. New York: American Joint Committee on Cancer; 2017.

Barrientos-Ruiz I, Ortiz-Cruz EJ, Serrano-Montilla J, Bernabeu-Taboada D, Pozo-Kreilinger JJ. Are biopsy tracts a concern for seeding and local recurrence in sarcomas? Clin Orthop Relat Res. 2017;475(2):511–8. https://doi.org/10.1007/s11999-016-5090-y. PubMed PMID: 27655183.

Gronchi A, Miah AB, Dei Tos AP, Abecassis N, Bajpai J, Bauer S, Biagini R, Bielack S, Blay JY, Bolle S, Bonvalot S, Boukovinas I, Bovee JVMG, Boye K, Brennan B, Brodowicz T, Buonadonna A, De Álava E, Del Muro XG, Dufresne A, Eriksson M, Fagioli F, Fedenko A, Ferraresi V, Ferrari A, Frezza AM, Gasperoni S, Gelderblom H, Gouin F, Grignani G, Haas R, Hassan AB, Hecker-Nolting S, Hindi N, Hohenberger P, Joensuu H, Jones RL, Jungels C, Jutte P, Kager L, Kasper B, Kawai A, Kopeckova K, Krákorová DA, Le Cesne A, Le Grange F, Legius E, Leithner A, Lopez-Pousa A, Martin-Broto J, Merimsky O, Messiou C, Mir O, Montemurro M, Morland B, Morosi C, Palmerini E, Pantaleo MA, Piana R, Piperno-Neumann S, Reichardt P, Rutkowski P, Safwat AA, Sangalli C, Sbaraglia M, Scheipl S, Schöffski P, Sleijfer S, Strauss D, Strauss S, Sundby Hall K, Trama A, Unk M, van de Sande MAJ, van der Graaf WTA, van Houdt WJ, Frebourg T, Casali PG, Stacchiotti S, ESMO Guidelines Committee, EURACAN and GENTURIS. Electronic address: clinicalguidelines@esmo.org. Soft tissue and visceral sarcomas: ESMO-EURACAN-GENTURIS clinical practice guidelines for diagnosis, treatment and follow-up☆. Ann Oncol. 2021;32(11):1348–65. https://doi.org/10.1016/j.annonc.2021.07.006. Epub 2021 Jul 22. PMID: 34303806.

Kwee RM, Kwee TC. Diagnostic performance of MRI in detecting locally recurrent soft tissue sarcoma: systematic review and meta-analysis. Eur Radiol. 2022;32(6):3915–30. https://doi.org/10.1007/s00330-021-08457-w. Epub 2022 Jan 12. PMID: 35020015.

Merino-Rueda LR, Barrientos-Ruiz I, Bernabeu-Taboada D, Pozo-Kreilinger JJ, Peleteiro-Pensado M, Cordero-García JM, Ortiz-Cruz EJ. Radiological and histopathological assessment of bone infiltration in soft tissue sarcomas. Eur J Orthop Surg Traumatol. 2022;32(4):631–9. https://doi.org/10.1007/s00590-021-03018-9. Epub 2021 May 31. PMID: 34057623.

Rodriguez JD, Selleck AM, Abdel Razek AAK, Huang BY. Update on MR imaging of soft tissue tumors of head and neck. Magn Reson Imaging Clin N Am. 2022;30(1):151–98. https://doi.org/10.1016/j.mric.2021.06.019. PMID: 34802577.

Rose PS. What's new in musculoskeletal tumor surgery. J Bone Joint Surg. 2021;103(24):2251–60. https://doi.org/10.2106/JBJS.21.00935.

Salerno KE. Radiation therapy for soft tissue sarcoma: indications, timing, benefits, and consequences. Surg Clin North Am. 2022;102(4):567–82. https://doi.org/10.1016/j.suc.2022.04.001. Epub 2022 Jun 24. PMID: 35952688; PMCID: PMC9372474.

von Mehren M, Kane JM, Agulnik M, Bui MM, Carr-Ascher J, Choy E, Connelly M, Dry S, Ganjoo KN, Gonzalez RJ, Holder A, Homsi J, Keedy V, Kelly CM, Kim E, Liebner D, McCarter M, McGarry SV, Mesko NW, Meyer C, Pappo AS, Parkes AM, Petersen IA, Pollack SM, Poppe M, Riedel RF, Schuetze S, Shabason J, Sicklick JK, Spraker MB, Zimel M, Hang LE, Sundar H, Bergman MA. Soft tissue sarcoma, version 2.2022, NCCN clinical practice guidelines in oncology. J Natl Compr Canc Netw. 2022;20(7):815–33. https://doi.org/10.6004/jnccn.2022.0035. PMID: 35830886.

WHO classification of tumours. 5th ed. Soft tissue and bone tumours. Editorial Board. Lyon: International Agency for Research on Cancer; 2020.

Biau DJ, Weiss KR, Bhumbra RS, Davidson D, Brown C, Griffin A, Wunder JS, Ferguson PC. Monitoring the adequacy of surgical margins after resection of bone and soft-tissue sarcoma. Ann Surg Oncol. 2013;20(6):1858–64. https://doi.org/10.1245/s10434-012-2863-8. Epub 2013 Jan 31. PMID: 23370669.

Blay JY, Hindi N, Bollard J, Aguiar S Jr, Angel M, Araya B, Badilla R, Bernabeu D, Campos F, Caro-Sánchez CHS, Carvajal B, Carvajal Montoya A, Casavilca-Zambrano S, Castro-Oliden V, Chacón M, Clara M, Collini P, Correa Genoroso R, Costa FD, Cuellar M, Dei Tos AP, Dominguez Malagon HR, Donati D, Dufresne A, Eriksson M, Farias-Loza M, Fernandez P, Frezza AM, Frisoni T, Garcia-Ortega DY, Gelderblom H, Gouin F, Gómez-Mateo MC, Gronchi A, Haro J, Huanca L, Jimenez N, Karanian M, Kasper B, Lopes David BB, Lopez-Pousa A, Lutter G, Martinez-Said H, Martinez-Tlahuel J, Mello CA, Morales Pérez JM, Moura David S, Nascimento AG, Ortiz-Cruz EJ, Palmerini E, Patel S, Pfluger Y, Provenzano S, Righi A, Rodriguez A, Salas R, Santos TTG, Scotlandi K, Soule T, Stacchiotti S, Valverde C, Waisberg F, Zamora Estrada E, Martin-Broto J. SELNET clinical practice guidelines for soft tissue sarcoma and GIST. Cancer Treat Rev. 2022;102:102312. https://doi.org/10.1016/j.ctrv.2021.102312. Epub 2021 Nov 14. PMID: 34798363.

Bilgeri A, Klein A, Lindner LH, Nachbichler S, Knösel T, Birkenmaier C, Jansson V, Baur-Melnyk A, Dürr HR. The effect of resection margin on local recurrence and survival in high grade soft tissue sarcoma of the extremities: how far is far enough? Cancers (Basel). 2020;12(9):2560. https://doi.org/10.3390/cancers12092560. PMID: 32911853; PMCID: PMC7563962.

Bonvalot S, Wunder J, Gronchi A, Broto JM, Turcotte R, Rastrelli M, Papai Z, Radaelli S, Lindner LH, Shumelinsky F, Cubillo A, Rutkowski P, Demaire C, Strens D, Nalbantov G. Complete pathological response to neoadjuvant treatment is associated with better survival outcomes in patients with soft tissue sarcoma: results of a retrospective multicenter study. Eur J Surg Oncol. 2021;47(8):2166–72. https://doi.org/10.1016/j.ejso.2021.02.024. Epub 2021 Feb 26. PMID: 33676792.

Garner HW, Kransdorf MJ, Bancroft LW, Peterson JJ, Berquist TH, Murphey MD. Benign and malignant soft-tissue tumors: posttreatment MR imaging. Radiographics. 2009;29(1):119–34. https://doi.org/10.1148/rg.291085131. PMID: 19168840.

Gronchi A. Surgery in soft tissue sarcoma: the thin line between a surgical or more conservative approach. Future Oncol. 2021;17(21s):3–6. https://doi.org/10.2217/fon-2021-0449. Epub 2021 Jun 10. PMID: 34107729.

Harati K, Lehnhardt M. The changing paradigm of resection margins in sarcoma resection. Innov Surg Sci. 2017;2(4):165–70. https://doi.org/10.1515/iss-2017-0043. PMID: 31579750; PMCID: PMC6754025.

Kransdorf MJ, Murphey MD. Imaging of soft tissue tumors. In: Kransdorf MJ, Murphey MD, editors. Imaging of soft tissue tumors. 2nd ed. Philadelphia: Lippincott Williams & Wilkins; 2006. p. 38–79.

Smolle MA, van de Sande M, Hayes A, Bergovec M, Smith HG, Liegl-Atzwanger B, Tunn PU, Niethard M, Windhager R, Szkandera J, Leithner A. Comparison of the 7th and 8th version of the AJCC classification system for soft tissue sarcomas of extremities and trunk in patients with localised, intermediate or high-grade disease treated at European tertiary sarcoma centres. Eur J Surg Oncol. 2021;47(8):2182–8. https://doi.org/10.1016/j.ejso.2021.03.252. Epub 2021 Mar 29. PMID: 33865657.

50 Soft Tissue Sarcoma in Contact with Bone: Is Bone Resection Indicated?

E. Pala, G. Trovarelli, M. C. Cerchiaro, and P. Ruggieri

50.1 Introduction

Treating soft tissue sarcoma of the extremities requires a multidisciplinary team in a referral sarcoma center. Combining chemotherapy, radiotherapy, and surgery is crucial in high-grade, deep, and large soft tissue tumors [1].

Limb salvage surgery with wide margins is the gold standard of surgical treatment. Indeed, although it is not wholly demonstrated, surgery with wide margins seems related to low local recurrence rates and high disease survival [2, 3].

Resection of nerves or vessels involved in the tumor is mandatory; however, resection of the bone in contact with the tumor is debated. If wide margins are not achievable, amputation could be necessary [3–6].

We present a case of a malignant peripheral nerve sheath tumor (MPNST) in the distal thigh leaning against the femur.

50.2 Clinical History and Radiological Images

Male, 25 years old, with left thigh swelling for 3 months. The Magnetic Resonance Imaging (MRI) showed an inhomogeneous mass in the left thigh adherent to the femoral cortex and a reactive lymph node in the popliteal fossa (Fig. 50.1).

An incisional biopsy (performed in another hospital) led to the histological diagnosis of a malignant peripheral nerve sheath tumor (MPNST) with heterologous rhabdomyoblastic and chondroblastic differentiation, Fédération Nationale des Centres de Lutte Contre le Cancer (FNCLCC) Grade 3 (histological re-evaluation at the Padua Hospital Institute of Pathological Anatomy).

The CT scan showed three small pulmonary nodules; the PET scan showed high uptake in the distal femoral cortex and surrounding soft tissue (Fig. 50.2).

E. Pala · G. Trovarelli · M. C. Cerchiaro · P. Ruggieri (✉)
Department of Orthopedics and Orthopedic Oncology, University of Padova, Padova, Italy
e-mail: elisa.pala@unipd.it; giulia.trovarelli@aopd.veneto.it; mariachiara.cerchiaro@unipd.it; pietro.ruggieri@unipd.it

H. Özger et al. (eds.), *Diagnosis and Treatment of Soft Tissue Tumors*, https://doi.org/10.1007/978-3-031-77061-6_50

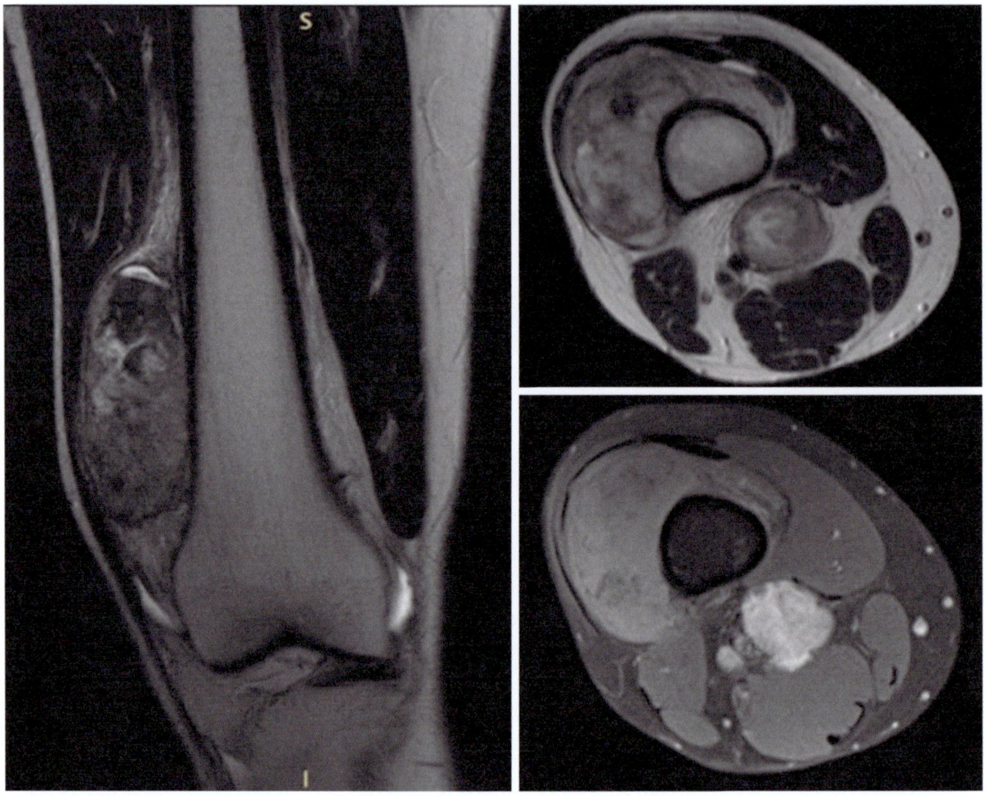

Fig. 50.1 MRI of the right knee shows the heterogeneous soft tissue mass surrounding the femur and a pathologic lymph node in the popliteal fossa

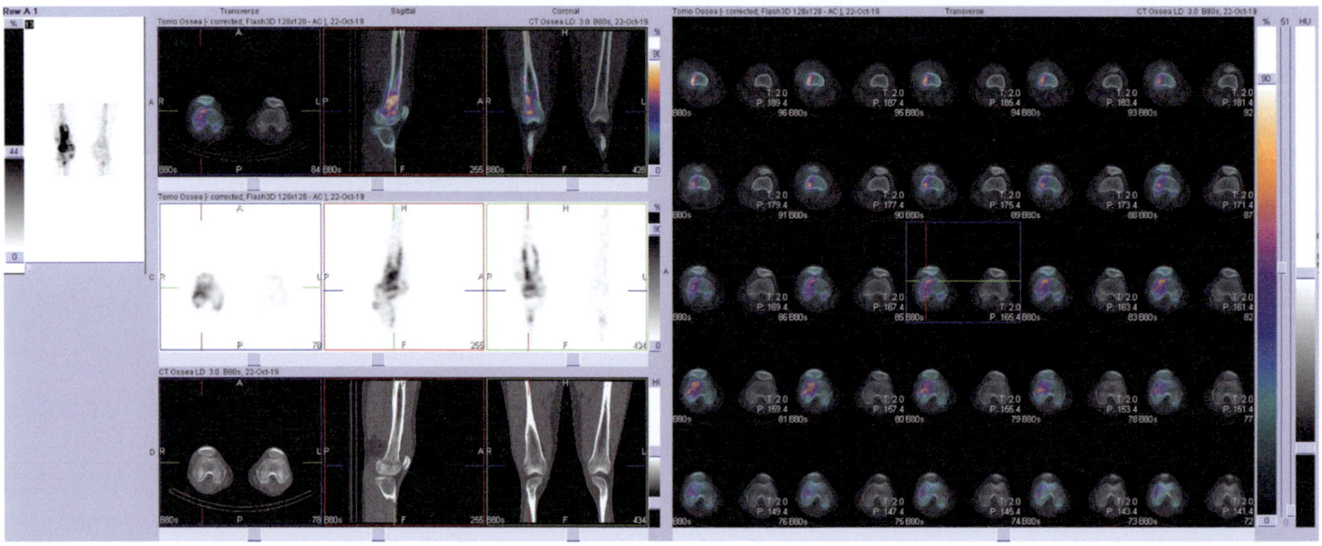

Fig. 50.2 PET scan shows high up-take in the distal lateral and anterior thigh (SUV 13.78), high up-take in a probable lymph node in the popliteal fossa (SUV 7.29), three nodules with high up-take in the lungs (SUV 3.39)

50.3 Challenges

1. High-grade soft tissue sarcoma (grade 3 MPNST)
2. Importance of obtaining wide margins
3. Femur involvement
4. Probably lung and lymph node metastases

50.4 Treatment Strategy

After multidisciplinary discussions, the patient started preoperative chemotherapy with three cycles of epirubicin and ifosfamide. After the multidisciplinary discussion, the radiotherapy was initially excluded due to the presence of two big nodules and the close relation with the vessels. It was decided to start with the chemotherapy and to do a restaging after the first cycle.

At the end of the chemotherapy, a re-staging showed a complete disappearance of lung nodules and a good local response (Fig. 50.3). The PET scan showed a good local response with the disappearance of intramedullary uptake in the femur (Fig. 50.4). Due to the good response and to avoid wound and vessel problems during the surgery, it was decided to wait the margins for radiotherapy.

Due to femur involvement and histology malignancy, we planned to remove the involved bone.

Consequently, the patient underwent soft tissue sarcoma excision contextually with the distal femur resection and reconstruction with tumor prosthesis.

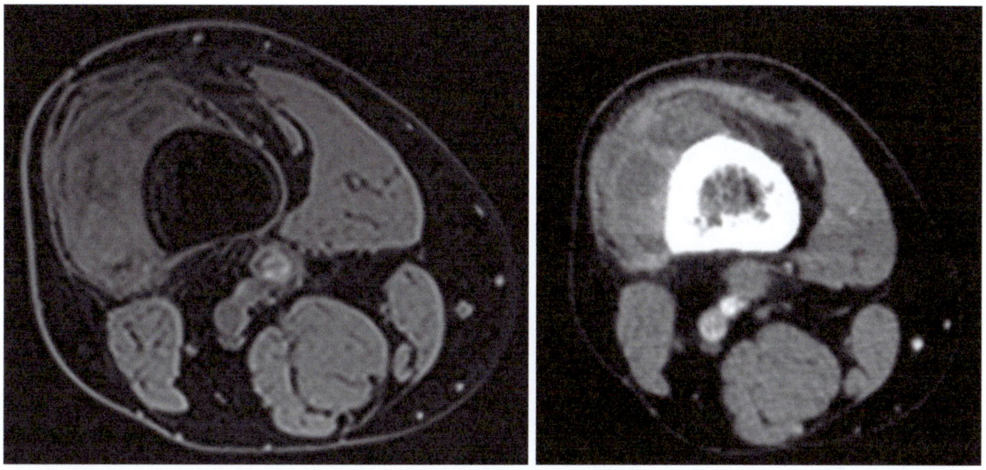

Fig. 50.3 MRI and CT scan of the right knee showed a reduction in the volume of the tumor and lymph node

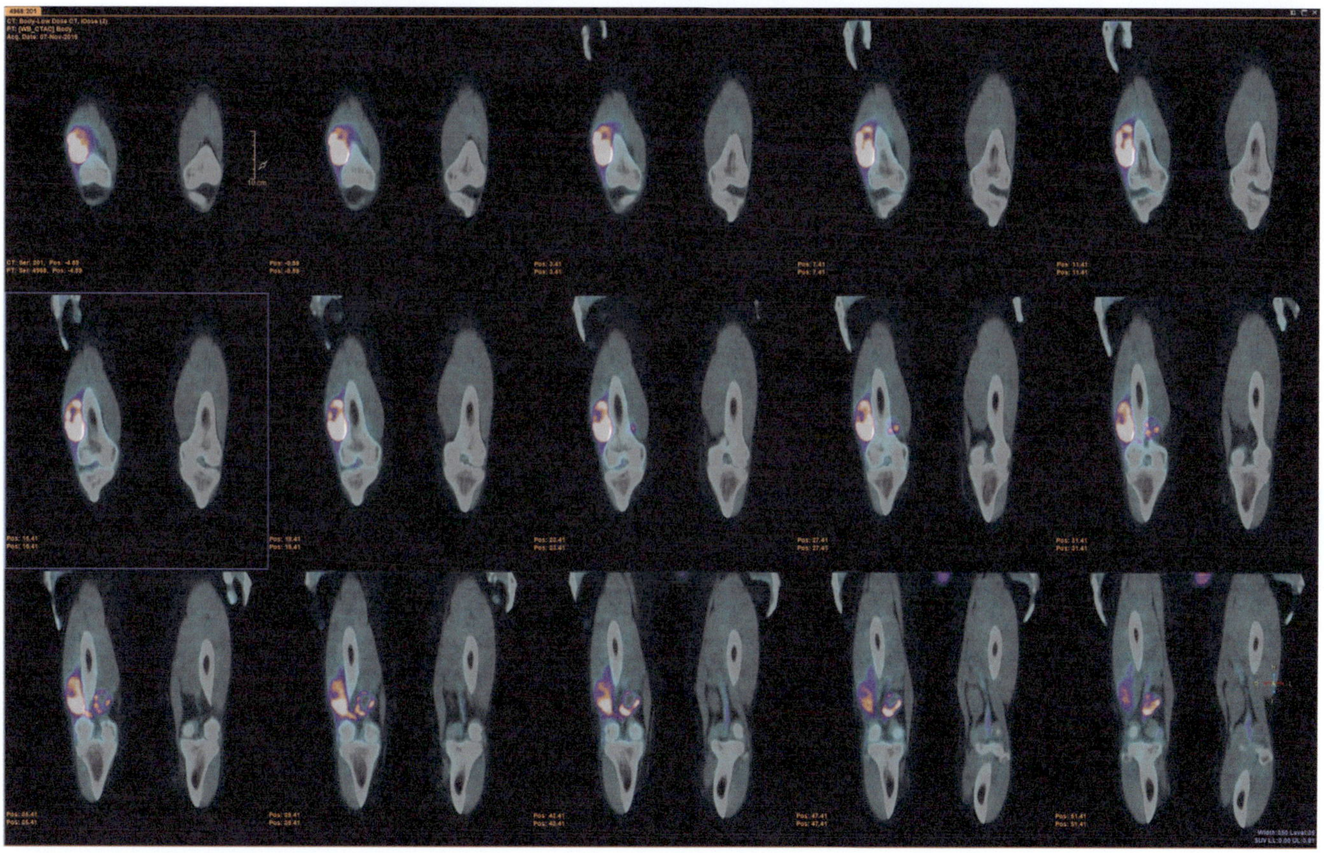

Fig. 50.4 PET scan shows lower up-take in the distal lateral and anterior thigh with no up-take in the femur

50.5 Basic Principles

Preoperative planning is mandatory to have wide margins. MRI is crucial to determine the extension of the tumor in the soft tissue, the involvement of the medullary canal, and the level of bone resection.

CT scan is essential to evaluate the proximity to the tumor of neurovascular bundles.

The incision included the biopsy scar (Fig. 50.5a).

Then the lesion was isolated, leaving a surrounding layer of healthy tissue (Fig. 50.5b).

The neurovascular bundle was identified, isolated, and protected.

The lesion was not detached from the femur to allow its complete excision with the involved bone.

The osteotomy of the femur was done 20 cm from the distal joint line (Fig. 50.5c).

The lymph node was removed after the tumor and distal femur excision.

After the correct preparation, a modular prosthesis was implanted (GMRS Stryker with press-fit femoral stem) (Fig. 50.6).

The final histology confirmed MPNST with 95% cell necrosis and wide margins (in bone and soft tissue). In addition, the histological examination documented that the tumor had invaded the bone cortex. The histology of the lymph node did not show neoplasm, but it was just inflammation.

The histological margins were wide so it was again decided to not proceed with radiotherapy.

After surgery, three postoperative cycles of chemotherapy were performed with the same regimen. Subsequently, oral chemotherapy with cyclophosphamide was administered for another 6 months.

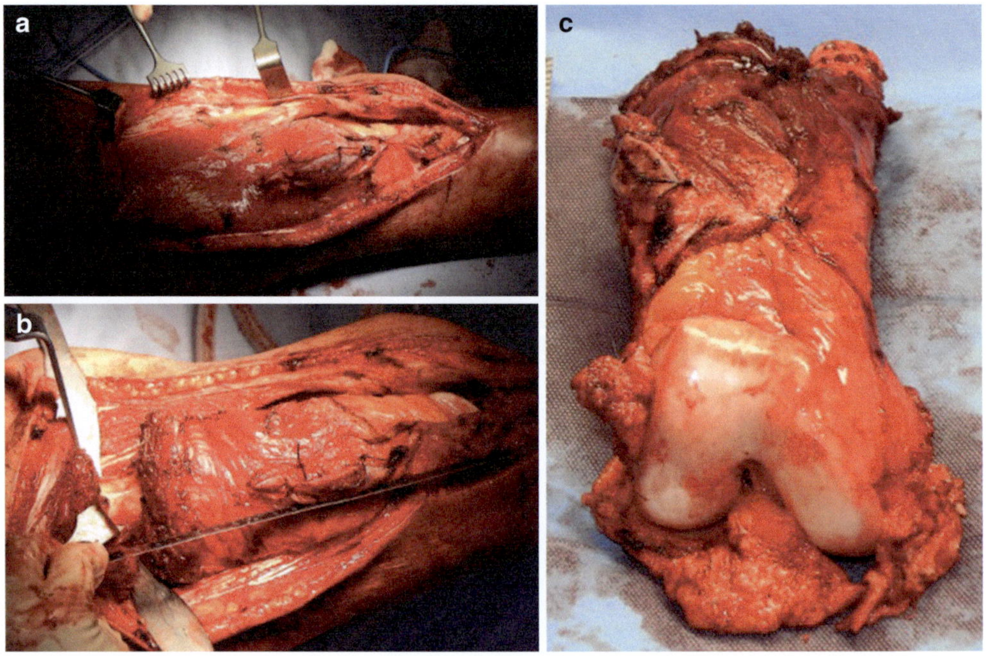

Fig. 50.5 Some photos during the surgery. (**a**) The biopsy scar has been excised with the tumor. (**b**) The complete isolation of the tumor that remained attached to the femur and the 20 cm planned resection level. (**c**) The femur and tumor were removed together

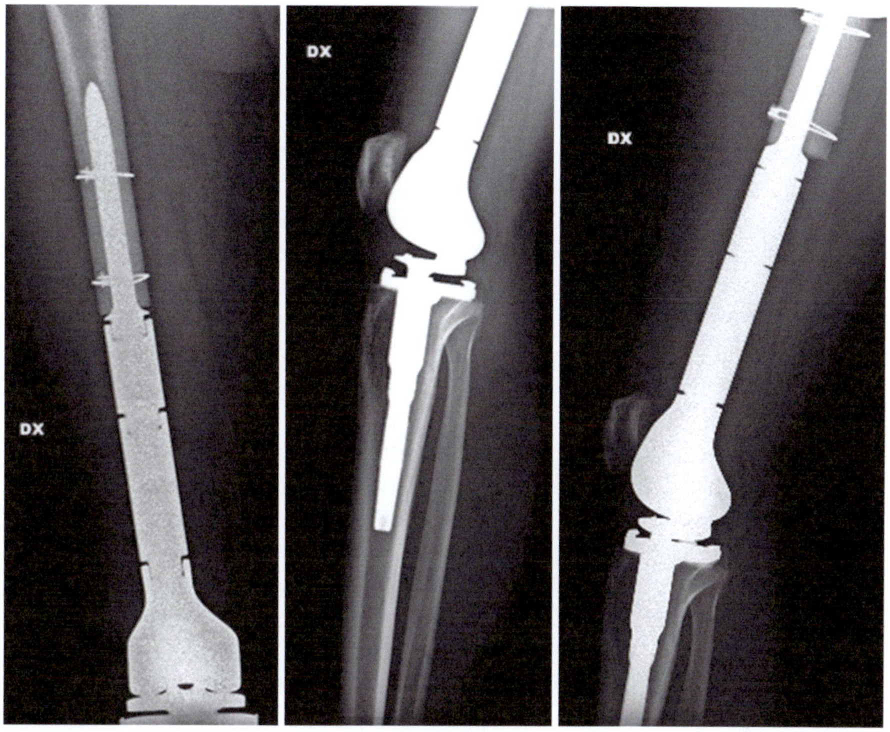

Fig. 50.6 Postoperative X-rays of the modular prostheses implanted

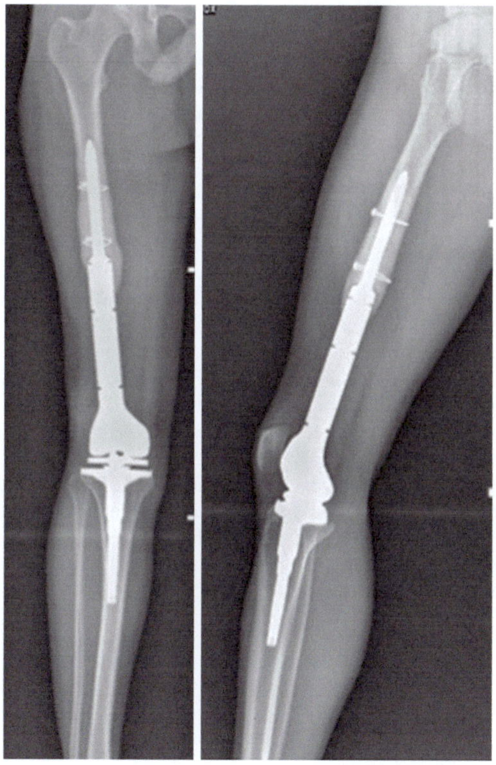

Fig. 50.7 X-rays at 3 years showing a good bone integration of the stem

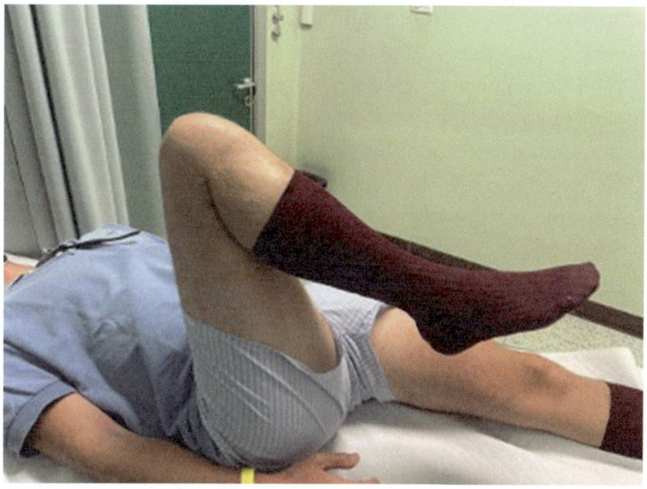

Fig. 50.8 Range of motion after 3 years with 120° knee flexion

50.6 Outcome Clinical and Radiological Images

During the follow-up, the patient underwent an X-ray of the prosthesis, thigh, and chest CT every 3 months. At the last follow-up, 3 years after surgery, the patient was continuously free of disease, the prosthesis had no complication, and the range of motion of the right knee was excellent (0–120°) without pain and aids (Figs. 50.7 and 50.8).

50.7 Discussion

MPNSTs are sporadic tumors derived from the Schwann cells or the pluripotent cells of the neural crest [7]. They comprise ~2% of all sarcomas, representing a small fraction of a group of cancers, with an incidence of 0.001% in the general population. Nevertheless, they can rise to 13% in NF1 patients, representing a frequent cause of death. Patients between 20 and 50 years of age are the most affected. This age group also presents a 40% rate of metastasis, most frequently to the lungs. The pathogenesis of MPNST is not well known, but it is established that an NF1 gene inactivation is crucial for tumor growth [8, 9].

The primary treatment for MPNST is wide tumor excision. The size and location of the defect, the exposure of vital structures, and the need for adjuvant RT will dictate the type of reconstruction. Limb salvage surgery as a treatment for soft tissue tumors, with neoadjuvant and adjuvant therapy, has become the treatment of choice for most patients [1, 10].

Our patient had no clinical signs of NF1, such as café au lait spots or multiple neurofibromas, nor a family history of the disease. After the biopsy, the patient was staged by a CT scan that revealed three pulmonary nodules, interpreted as possible metastasis of the thigh tumor. The PET/CT confirmed this. The subsequent CT scan performed after neoadjuvant chemotherapy showed a reduction of the mass and a disappearance of the pulmonary nodules.

It is debated in the literature whether it is necessary to scarify the bone in case of involvement by the tumor [6].

In our case, we decided to perform an excision, including the resection of the femur, to ensure wide margins. The tumor's malignancy justifies us being as aggressive as we can. The mid-term follow-up free of the disease confirms our decision.

In conclusion, the primary objective of the surgery in all malignant soft tissue tumors is to plan a "one shot" surgery. In our experience, the more aggressive the tumor is, the more radical the surgery must be, even including major surgeries, since removing only the periosteum is not enough to guarantee wide margins.

Even if debated in the treatment of soft tissue tumors, chemotherapy could produce cytoreduction of the tumor locally and in distant metastases, as in the presented case [10, 11]. For this reason, we suggest neoadjuvant chemotherapy every time possible to improve the chances of curing the patient.

References

1. Casali PG, Abecassis N, Aro HT, Bauer S, Biagini R, Bielack S, et al. Soft tissue and visceral sarcomas: ESMO-EURACAN clinical practice guidelines for diagnosis, treatment and follow-up. Ann Oncol. 2018;29(Suppl 4):iv51–67.
2. Brinkmann EJ, Ahmed SK, Houdek MT. Extremity soft tissue sarcoma: role of local control. Curr Treat Options in Oncol. 2020;21(2):13.
3. Dickinson IC, Whitwell DJ, Battistuta D, Thompson B, Strobel N, Duggal A, et al. Surgical margin and its influence on survival in soft tissue sarcoma. ANZ J Surg. 2006;76(3):104–9.
4. Bonvalot S, Levy A, Terrier P, Tzanis D, Bellefqih S, Le Cesne A, et al. Primary extremity soft tissue sarcomas: does local control impact survival? Ann Surg Oncol. 2017;24(1):194–201.
5. Novais EN, Demiralp B, Alderete J, Larson MC, Rose PS, Sim FH. Do surgical margin and local recurrence influence survival in soft tissue sarcomas? Clin Orthop Relat Res. 2010;468(11):3003–11.
6. Yan TQ, Zhou WH, Guo W, Yang RL, Dong S, Liang WM, Sun YF. Endoprosthetic reconstruction for large extremity soft-tissue sarcoma with juxta-articular bone involvement: functional and survival outcome. J Surg Res. 2014;187(1):142–9.
7. Jones KE, Patel A, Kunesh MG, Thuro BA. Malignant peripheral nerve sheath tumor of the orbit: a case report and review of the literature. Orbit. 2022;41(5):642–6.
8. Somatilaka BN, Sadek A, McKay RM, Le LQ. Malignant peripheral nerve sheath tumor: models, biology, and translation. Oncogene. 2022;41(17):2405–21.
9. Shimatani A, Aono M, Hoshi M, Oebisu N, Iwai T, Takada N, Nakamura H. Two case reports of fair lower limb function after sciatic nerve sacrifice for the treatment of a malignant peripheral nerve sheath tumor. Int Cancer Conf J. 2018;7(4):137–41.
10. Pervaiz N, Colterjohn N, Farrokhyar F, Tozer R, Figueredo A, Ghert M. A systematic meta-analysis of randomized controlled trials of adjuvant chemotherapy for localized resectable soft-tissue sarcoma. Cancer. 2008;113(3):573–81.
11. Gronchi A, Ferrari S, Quagliuolo V, Broto JM, Pousa AL, Grignani G, et al. Histotype-tailored neoadjuvant chemotherapy versus standard chemotherapy in patients with high-risk soft-tissue sarcomas (ISG-STS 1001): an intenational, open-label, randomised, controlled, phase 3, multicentre trial. Lancet Oncol. 2017;18(6):812–22.

Soft Tissue Sarcoma with Osseous Invasion

51

Yang-Guk Chung

51.1 Introduction

Soft tissue sarcomas (STSs) usually arise from extra-osseous sites and do not infiltrate bone. However, sometimes they abut on adjacent bone or infiltrate into the bone itself. Lin et al. reported that among 50 patients with STSs abutting bone, composite resection of bone and soft tissue were performed in 11 cases and three (6%) cases of true osseous invasion were verified pathologically [1]. In another series by Elias et al., out of 51 soft tissue tumor patients, 44 lesion sites showed bone abutment, and 11 sites (20%) showed osseous invasion on histopathological assessment [2].

Bone invasions of STSs can be well evaluated using magnetic resonance imaging (MRI) scans. Osseous abutment, defined as loss of a normal soft tissue interface between the tumor mass and osseous cortex on T1-weighted images, by tumor, cortical destruction, cortical and medullary signal intensity change on T1- and T2-weighted images are assessed. Findings of cortical destruction, cortical and medullary signal intensity change on T1- and T2-weighted images are also evaluated and they are sensitive and specific in the detection of osseous invasion by STSs [2]. In the equivocal cases, fixation to the underlying bone on physical examination and increased uptake of radioisotope on bone scan are also helpful to detect bone invasion.

For proper surgical excision of STSs with bone invasion, part of the bone should be resected together (composite resection) and an appropriate bone reconstruction will be necessary. On assessment of the extent of STSs abutting adjacent bone, a thorough preoperative evaluation of bone involvement status using physical examination and imaging studies are important.

A surgeon should consider these questions when planning surgical excision of a STS with suspicious bone abutment or invasion. What is the ideal soft tissue dissection plane to acquire an adequate surgical margin? Will any neoadjuvant treatment be helpful to obtain narrower safe margin? How much portion of bone will be included in composite resection (subperiosteal dissection only/resection of a hemicylinder of bone/resection of a whole segment of bone)? What kind of material will be used for bone reconstruction (tumor prosthesis/structural allograft/recycled autograft/vascularized fibular graft (VFG)/internal bone transport/combined)? What method will be used for stable internal bone fixation?

Y.-G. Chung (✉)
Department of Orthopedic Surgery, Seoul St. Mary's Hospital, College of Medicine, The Catholic University of Korea, Seoul, Republic of Korea
e-mail: ygchung@catholic.ac.kr

51.2 Clinical History and Preoperative Imaging

A 33-year-old female patient presented with about 10 cm sized slow-growing painless mass in the posteromedial thigh which was first recognized 3 months ago. On palpation there was no tenderness. The mass had solid consistency and was relatively fixed to the underlying bone.

Initial right femur anteroposterior (AP) and lateral radiographs showed no definite bone abnormality. However, close observation of lateral view revealed a focal bony erosion on posterior surface of femur at subtrochanteric portion (Fig. 51.1a, b).

MRI demonstrated an intramuscular soft tissue mass in medial compartment which was abutting the posteromedial surface of proximal femur (Fig. 51.2a–g). Contrast-enhanced fat-saturated (FS) T1-weighted MR images showed well enhancing soft tissue mass (Fig. 51.2b, d, g) and T2-weighted FS images revealed a hyperintense lesion with focal signal voids which suggested prominent tumor vasculature (Fig. 51.2f, black arrows). There were a couple of focal bony erosions on the posterior linea aspera femoris area, suggesting tumor infiltration (Fig. 51.2a–g, yellow allow). Osseous abutment, loss of a normal soft tissue interface between the tumor mass and osseous cortex, was also observed along the posterior surface of femur in the axial images (Fig. 51.2e–g, white arrow).

H. Özger et al. (eds.), *Diagnosis and Treatment of Soft Tissue Tumors*, https://doi.org/10.1007/978-3-031-77061-6_51

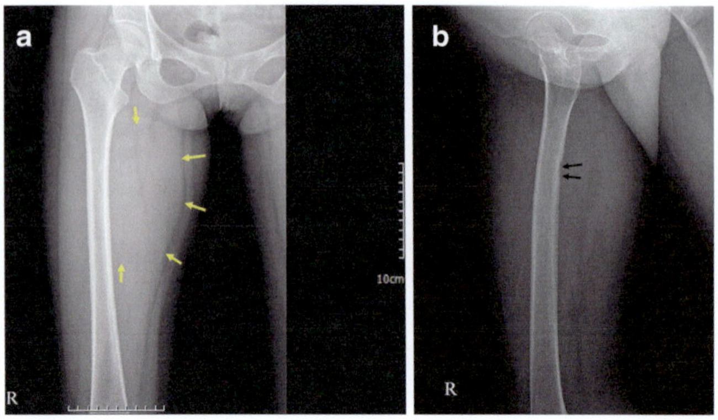

Fig. 51.1 Initial right femur anteroposterior (**a**) and lateral (**b**) radiographs showed soft tissue shadow (yellow arrows) and a focal bony erosion (black arrows) on posterior surface of femur at subtrochanteric portion

Incisional biopsy through a 4 cm length longitudinal incision on the medial aspect of thigh was performed. Intraoperative frozen section confirmed that proper tumor tissue was harvested. Pathological diagnosis was a low-grade solitary fibrous tumor. A three-variable risk model for the prediction of metastatic risk in solitary fibrous tumor revealed low intermediate risk (total 3 points) [age: <55 year (0 point), Mitosis/10 HPF: 2–3 (1 point), Tumor size: 10.2 cm (2 point)] [3]. Staging work-up including chest computed tomography (CT) and positron emission tomography (PET)-CT showed no regional or distant metastasis.

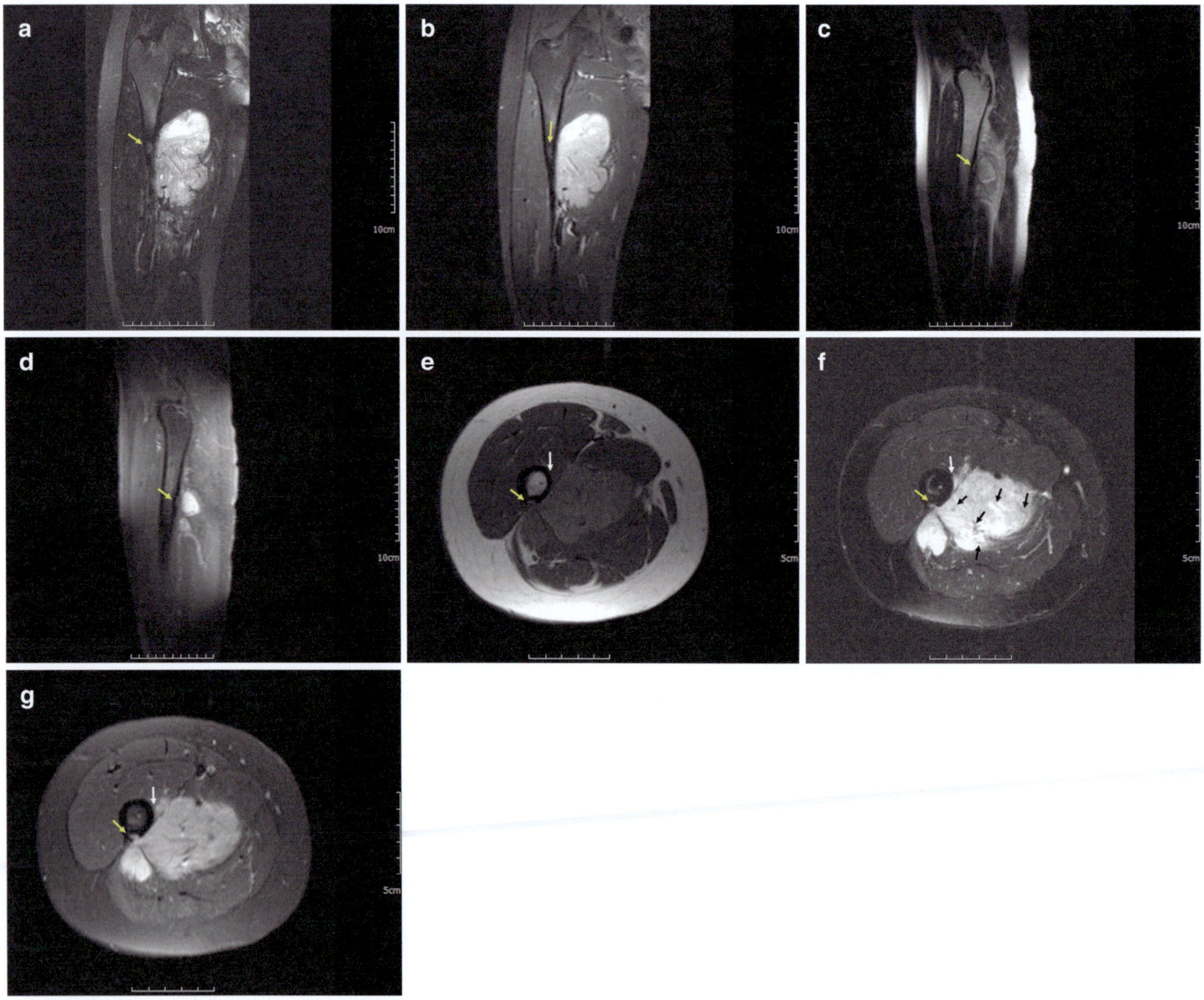

Fig. 51.2 MRI demonstrates an intramuscular soft tissue mass abutting the posteromedial surface of proximal femur in medial compartment of thigh. (**a**–**g**) Coronal T2-weighted FS (**a**), and contrast-enhanced T1-weighted FS (**b**) MR images show well-enhanced hyperintensity soft mass with focal cortical signal changes (yellow arrow). Sagittal T-weighted (**c**) and contrast-enhanced T1-weighted FS (**d**) MR images revealed focal cortical erosion on posterior surface of proximal femur. Axial T1-weighted (**e**), T2-weighted FS (**f**) and contrast-enhanced T1-weighted FS (**g**) MR images demonstrate focal osseous invasion on posterior cortex (yellow arrow) and prominent tumor vasculatures of signal voids (**f**, black arrows). The osseous abutment, loss of a normal soft tissue interface between the tumor mass and osseous cortex was observed along the posterior surface of bone on axial images (**e**–**g**, white arrow)

51.3 Preoperative Problem List

(a) A deep seated, 10.2 cm sized STS of thigh abutting the posteromedial surface of proximal femur.
(b) Presence of focal tumor invasion in posterior cortical bone at linear aspera femoris area.
(c) Need to resect a segment of the femur together and reconstruct the bone defect to restore structural stability.

51.4 Treatment Strategy

(a) A biopsy for deep-seated, 10.2 cm sized soft mass is mandatory to establish histologic type, subtype and grade.
   - Ultrasound-guided needle biopsy is preferred and advantageous for most of the STSs. It is minimally invasive and allows immediate neoadjuvant treatment if indicated.
   - Incisional biopsy is the standard procedure to obtain sufficient volume of tumor tissue for histologic diagnosis including hematoxylin and eosin (H&E) staining, immunohistochemistry and/or molecular studies.
   - Biopsy tract should be excised en block together with the main mass at the definitive surgery.
   - Thorough hemostasis is needed to prevent tumor cell spread through hematoma.
   - We performed an incisional biopsy. The tumor had much vasculature in the substance and was prone to bleeding through the core needle biopsy tract. During incisional biopsy, we made a waterproof pseudocapsular sutures to prevent hematoma formation at the outside of tumor mass.
   - We chose the biopsy route through the adductor muscle due to a short distance from the skin and apart from the major neurovascular structures.

(b) Consideration of neoadjuvant radiotherapy and/or chemotherapy: The tumor was a low-grade solitary fibrous tumor with a low intermediate risk for metastasis, and there was no evidence of distant metastasis on the staging work-up. Even though bone abutment and focal cortical bone invasion were detected, it was located far from the major neurovascular structures. We concluded a neoadjuvant radiotherapy or chemotherapy was not indicated.
(c) Surgical approach: It should allow an easy composite bone and soft tissue mass excision including the biopsy tract and stable internal fixation for bone reconstruction. We used medial transmuscular approach through adductor longus and brevis muscles.
(d) Planning of the surgical margin for low-grade STS: Intraoperatively soft tissue dissection was performed with about 5–10 mm margin distance to ensure at least 2 mm negative margin on histologic evaluation of resected formalin fixed specimen.
(e) Planning of bone resection:
   - A hemicylinderical bone resection together with the soft tissue tumor mass would carry little mechanical problem. However, there can be much difficulty in mobilization of the bone-soft tissue tumor composite as one block and it should be a technically demanding procedure.
   - A whole segment bone resection is easy to obtain safe bone and soft tissue margin targeted, and it is feasible to resect the composite tissue mass as one block due to much increased mobility after osteotomy.
   - A subperiosteal dissection combined with curettage and electric cautery at osseous invasion site might carry higher risk of contamination and local recurrence: not suitable for cases with true osseous invasion.
   - We chose to resect a whole segment of bone together with the soft tissue tumor.

(f) Bone reconstruction
   - Material: Among various options of intercalary tumor prosthesis, structural allograft, recycled autograft, VFG, internal bone transport and combinations, we chose recycled pasteurized autograft because the resected bone segment was still structurally sound without destruction, which would provide sufficient biomechanical strength. It also provided good match of size and shape to the original bone defect and no additional cost was necessary.
   - Method of internal fixation: we used long length intramedullary nail with static interlocking screws and short anti-rotation plate and screws at the distal junction.
   - Autologous cancellous bone graft at host bone-pasteurized bone junctions: helpful to obtain early bone healing.

51.5 Basic Principles for STSs with Osseous Invasion

(a) Decision making whether a part of bone should be resected with soft tissue tumor which is abutting or infiltrating adjacent bone is based on evaluations of the tumor extent. In addition to the finding of physical examination and plane radiographs, contrast-enhanced MRI and bone scintigraphy would give much information on the status of bone invasion.
   - If the soft tissue tumor is abutting the periosteum and is apart from the bone itself, a subperiosteal resection will be safe [1].

- In the case of true cortical bone destruction or medullary extension, a part of bone should be resected with the soft tissue tumor together as one block [1].
- In the case of bone contact without direct bone invasion, it may be dependent on the findings of physical examination or bone scintigraphy. Fixation to the underlying bone on physical examination or increased focal radioisotope uptake in bone scan suggest bone invasion, so composite resection of bone and soft tissue tumor is advisable.
- In this case of a low-grade solitary fibrous tumor abutting the bone surface with focal cortical invasions, at least a part of adjacent bone should be resected together as a composite.
- We preferred to resect a whole segment of bone and to reconstruct the intercalary bone defect by reimplantation of recycled pasteurized autobone. A rigid internal fixation with interlocking intramedullary (IM) nailing and adjuvant short plate fixation at distal junction for rotational stability were performed.

(b) Adequate surgical resection with appropriate bone and soft tissue margins is the cornerstone in the management of STS with osseous invasion. Both margin dimension and margin quality should be considered. Anatomic structures such as fascia, periosteum, joint capsule provide a strong barrier to tumor infiltration. Thin barriers such as perineurium, perivascular sheathes are equivalent to 2 cm thick conventional muscle or fat tissue dimension. And thick barriers such as fascia, articular cartilage in adults are equivalent to 3 cm thick conventional tissue dimension.

From the literature review, current recommendations for pathologically assessed surgical margin are as follows [4–7]:

- Low-grade STSs: more than 2 mm margin
- Non-infiltrative STSs: more than 5 mm margin
- Infiltrative STSs: more than 10 mm margin
- Less margin with fascia or periosteum: acceptable

So for this low-grade solitary fibrous tumor, more than 5 mm negative margin we obtained would be sufficient.

(c) Surgical approach from the side of maximum tumor volume, apart from major neurovascular structures, and in line with previous biopsy tract is recommended.

We approached through the medial aspect of proximal thigh which allowed feasible soft tissue tumor dissection with adequate wide margin and segmental bone resection and reconstruction. For IM nail entry to fix the intercalary pasteurized autobone, additional small incision from the tip of greater trochanter was used.

(d) During the dissection of soft tissue tumors including a layer of normal tissue around the tumor mass and entire biopsy tract, proximal and distal osteotomies enabled the maximum mobilization of bone-soft tissue tumor composite which would facilitated further dissection.

(e) Thorough hemostasis during dissection and after complete resection has a paramount importance to prevent massive bleeding and hematoma formation. Massive hematoma may increase the risk of postoperative infection and tumor cell spreading if surgical margin is contaminated.

(f) Favored bone reconstruction option: each method has advantages and disadvantages.

- Intercalary tumor prosthesis reconstruction will provide immediate structural stability and enable early full weight-bearing ambulation. Main drawbacks are loosening, breakage, stress shielding on long-term follow-up. Recently, 3D-printed patient-specific implant has become available, which can provide perfect match of size and shape, with high plasticity in implant design. However, high cost and time delay for manufacture are limitations.
- Structural allograft is one of the reliable option. With metallic implant fixation bridging the whole length of graft bone, structural intercalary allograft usually provides sufficient biomechanical stability and results in good functional outcome. Higher rate of complications of nonviable structural bone constructs, such as nonunion, infection, fracture, resorption, have been reported. It takes long time to get junctional bone union. Size and shape mismatch, possibility of immune reaction, cost and availability are additional issues.
- Recycled autograft has similar advantages and disadvantages to structural allograft as a nonviable bone construct. However, it has several additional advantages compared to allograft, i.e., perfect size and shape match, no cost, no immune reaction and immediately available. And pasteurized autograft still contains bioactive BMPs and show better bone healing [8].
- So, if destruction of the resected bone is minimal, recycled autograft is our center's preferred material for reconstruction of intercalary bone defects. We usually use pasteurization (treated at 65 °C, 30 min in hot water bath) to eradicate viable tumor cells. Irradiation and freezing/thawing with liquid nitrogen are also established methods of treatment for recycling.
- VFG provides viable bone construct, which has resistance to infection and has potential of hypertrophy in response to mechanical loading. But the small volume of fibula bone needs protection until sufficient hypertrophy occurs to avoid fracture. High technical demand is also a limiting factor.
- Internal bone transport (callotaxis) and junctional osteosynthesis can be applied for this intercalary bone defect. It can provide good structural bone

reconstruction. It will take a long time for bone formation and consolidation. Much discomfort should be endured during the progression.
  - Combinations of structural allograft and VFG or Recycled autograft and VFG will overcome some disadvantages of nonviable bone constructs even though it can be technically demanding.

(g) Stable internal fixation is pre-requite for early rehabilitation and functional recovery. Intramedullary nailing through the central axis of long bone in lower extremity provides excellent biomechanical stability. Intercalary segment has less rotational stability which requires a short plate and screw fixation at the host- and recycled bone junction. To overcome the difficulty of bicortical screw insertion due to intramedullary nail, unicortical screws and/or cables were used.

(h) Systematic and sophisticated rehabilitation program will be necessary. Junctional bone union between host bone and nonviable recycled bone will take several months. Protected timely weight bearing and ambulation according to the progression of bone union are recommended.

51.6 Surgical Procedures and Intraoperative Image

- We approached through the medial aspect of proximal thigh in line with the biopsy tract. During the dissection of the soft tissue tumors including a layer of normal tissue around the tumor mass and entire biopsy tract, we made proximal and distal osteotomies at preoperatively planned sites to mobilize the bone-soft tissue tumor composite. It facilitated further dissection.
- After composite resection of a segment of femur and soft tissue tumor (Fig. 51.3a), bone segment was separated from the composite (Fig. 51.3b) and pasteurized at 65 °C for 30 min by immersing into the hot water bath to eradicate the viable tumor cells (Fig. 51.3c).
- The heat-treated bone segment was put into in situ position and internal fixation using long intramedullary nail and static interlocking screws was proceeded. And a short low-profile plate and screw fixation using unicortical screws and a couple of cables was performed at the distal junctions.
- Autologous iliac cancellous bone chips were harvested and grafted at both proximal and distal junctions (Fig. 51.4a, b).
- Pathological assessment reported absent resection margin involvement with 0.5 cm free from the tumor (Fig. 51.5).

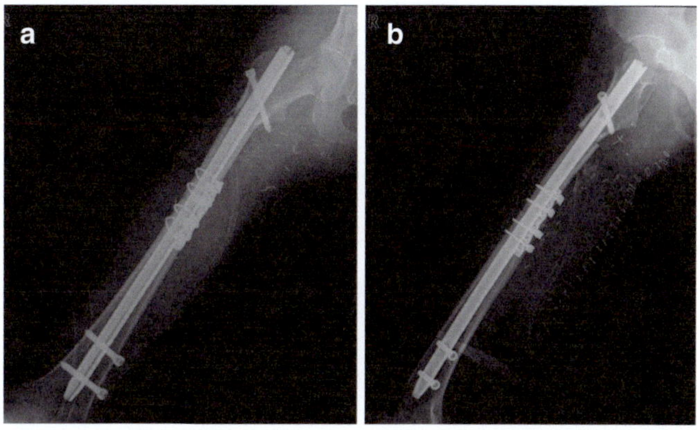

Fig. 51.4 Postoperative right femur AP (**a**) and lateral (**b**) radiographs showed well-fixated bone construct with static interlocking IM nail and an additional short plate at distal junction. Grafted cancellous bone chips at both proximal and distal junctions were seen also

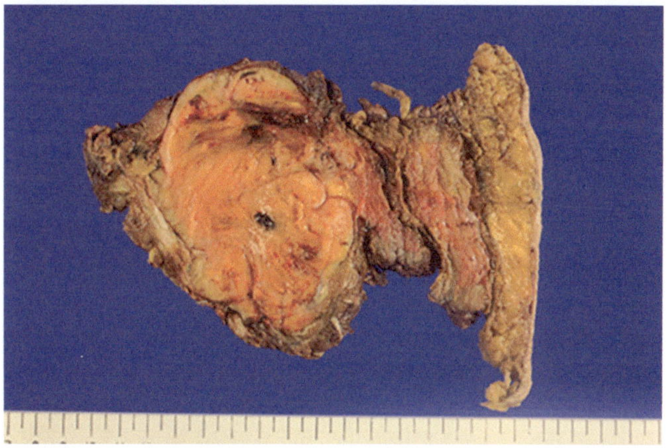

Fig. 51.5 Gross specimen photo shows soft tissue tumor mass with biopsy tract. Pathological assessment reported no resection margin involvement with 0.5 cm free from tumor

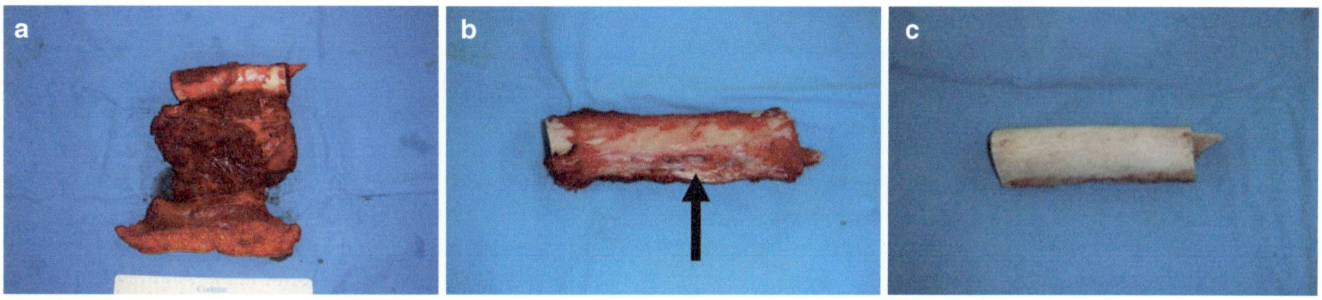

Fig. 51.3 Intraoperative clinical photographs show resected composite bone-soft tissue tumor mass including biopsy tract (**a**) and isolated bone segment (**b**), which reveals a couple of bony erosions (black arrow). The bone segment was blanched after pasteurization (**c**)

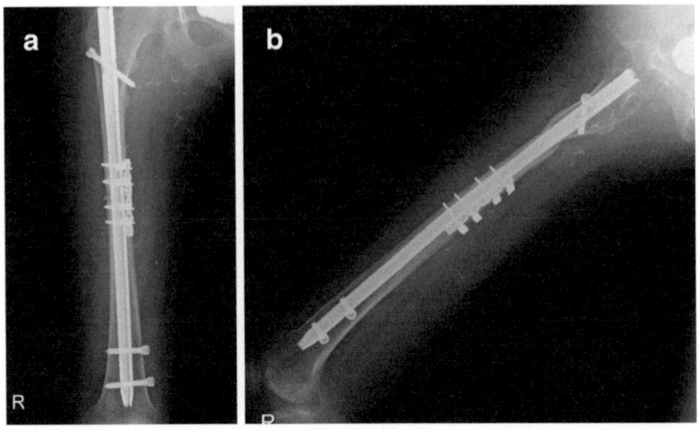

Fig. 51.6 At 8 months after surgery, solid bone unions were obtained at both proximal and distal host bone-recycled graft bone junctions (**a**, **b**)

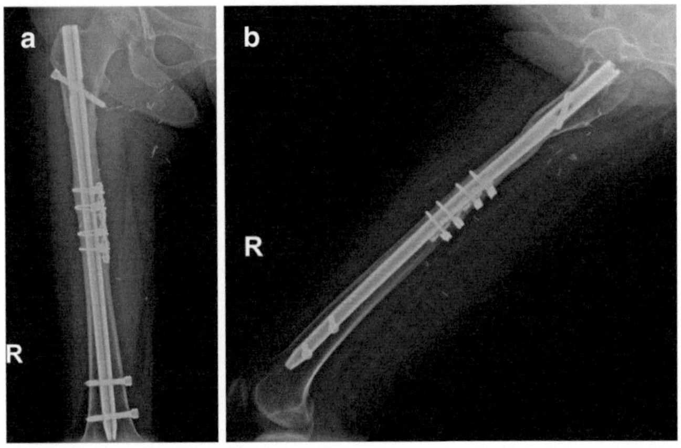

Fig. 51.7 POD 12 year follow-up radiographs (**a**, **b**) show stable bone construct with solid unions

51.7 Outcome (Radiographs and Images)

1. At POD 8 months, solid bone unions were obtained at both proximal and distal host bone-recycled graft bone junctions (Fig. 51.6a, b).
2. At POD 12 year follow-up, the patient showed continuous disease free status oncologically.
3. Final functional outcome according to ISOLS functional evaluation system was 100% function with emotional acceptance (Fig. 51.7a, b).

51.8 Technical Pearls

1. Identification and assessment of bone invasion

   In the case of STSs abutting the adjacent bone, thorough and detailed assessment of osseous invasion status is important. Presurgical assessment by contrast-enhanced MRI has been proven to be sensitive and specific to detect periosteal and osseous invasion [9, 10].

   - If there is a thin layer of normal soft tissue separating the lesion from the cortical bone, it is negative for true osseous abutment.
   - No soft tissue interface between the lesion and bone cortex means true osseous abutment.
   - If there is a signal intensity change in cortex adjacent to soft-tissue mass, it can be a finding of true osseous invasion. However, such signal intensity change may be a findings of reactive remodeling change of bone only. PET CT or diffusion-weighted images of MR will be helpful to differentiate true osseous invasion from false positive imaging findings.
   - Findings of cortical destruction are the definite sign of true osseous invasion.
   - Medullary signal intensity change associated with cortical penetration may represent the true medullary extension. However, medullary signal intensity change without cortical penetration may be a finding of hematopoiesis or radiation therapy-associated changes if radiation therapy was performed preoperatively.
2. Decision making on bone resection and reconstruction.
   - Composite bone and soft tissue tumor resection is indicated in the cases of true osseous invasion. How much portion of bone (a part of bone, hemocylinder or a whole segment of bone) should be resected is dependent on the extent of osseous invasion and feasibility of en -block composite tissue resection [1, 10] (Fig. 51.8a–g).
   - If there is no true osseous invasion, a subperiosteal dissection will be acceptable (Fig. 51.9a–h). An electrical cauterization of bone surface and a postoperative radiation therapy ensure local control [1, 10].
3. Stable internal fixation

   In the cases of composite bone/soft tissue lesion resection, restoration of mechanical osseous stability is paramount to get undelayed postoperative therapy and early functional recovery. In the lower extremity, intramedullary nail fixation located in the central axis of long bone is preferred. Securing of rotational stability is required for the intercalary bone segment, which will be obtained by short plate and screw fixation at least one junction of host bone-intercalary bone. Step cutting or chevron osteotomy will be helpful to get rotational stability.
4. Enhancing early bone union at host bone-recycled bone junctions

   Early bone union at junctions between host bone and intercalary bone will improve the patient's quality of life and minimize the possibility of adverse osseous complications such as delayed union or nonunion, metallic breakage, infection associated with multiple revision procedures if necessary.

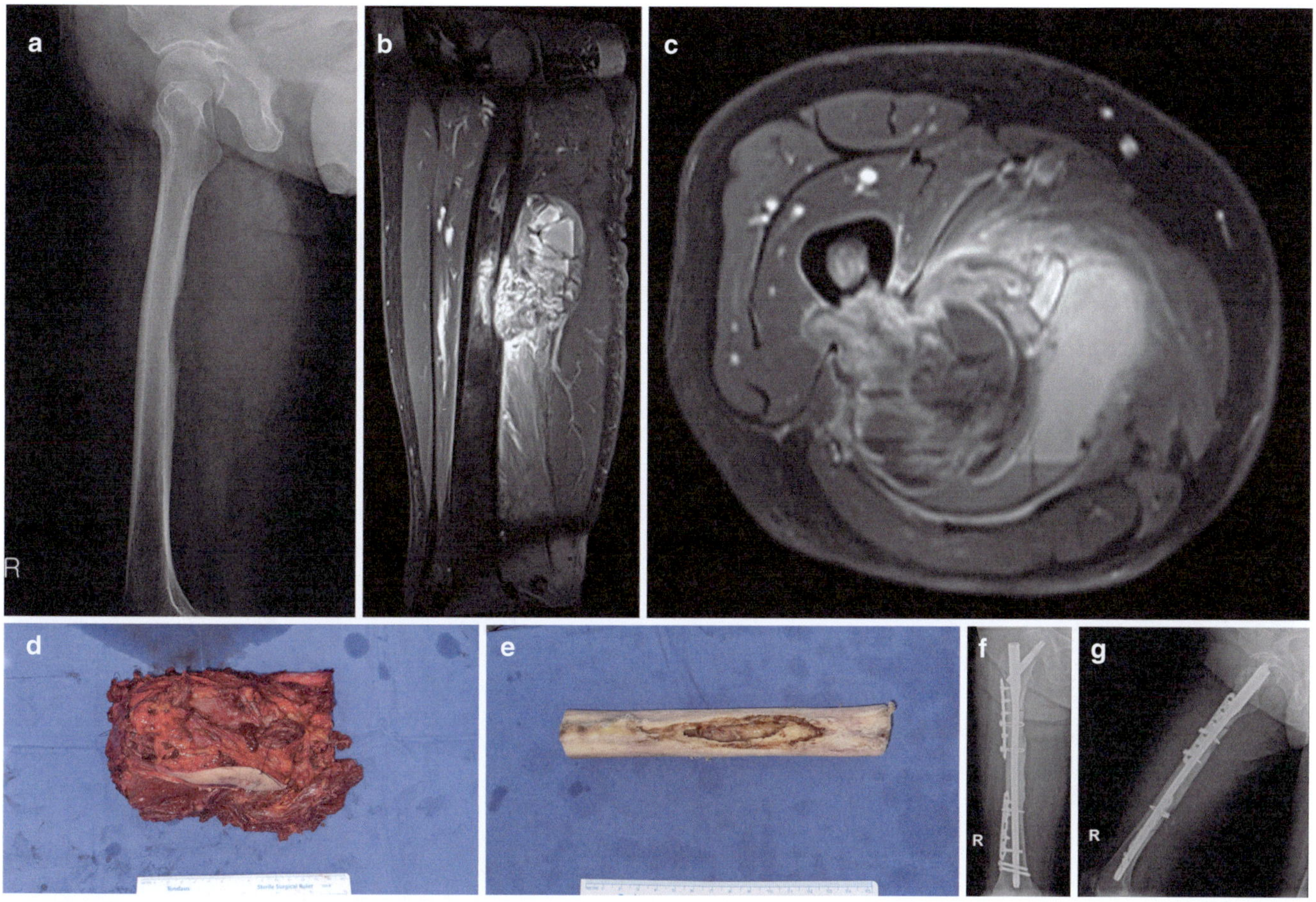

Fig. 51.8 A 64-year-old female patients with huge undifferentiated pleomorphic sarcoma in right posterior thigh. Right femur lateral radiograph (**a**) shows soft mass shadow with posterior cortical destruction. Contrast-enhanced T1-weighted FS MR images (**b**, **c**) reveal huge soft mass with osseous invasion and extension into the medullary space. After neoajduvant radiation therapy and chemotherapy, a segment femur bone was resected with soft tissue tumor together (**d**). The pasteurized bone segment (**e**) was put into the original site and fixed with static interlocking IM nail and two additional short plates at proximal and distal junctions. Autologous cancellous bone chips were grafted at both junctions (**f**, **g**). Pathological report was more than 95% of cell necrosis and negative resection margin involvement with minimum 2 mm distance

Mechanical stability is the prerequisite for early bone healing. Autologous iliac cancellous bone grafting is the gold standard to enhance bone union. If autobone grafting is not feasible, application of demineralized bone matrix or BMP will be alternatives.

5. Multidisciplinary team approach

Management of bone and soft tissue sarcomas is quite complicated and involves many subspeciality aspects. A multidisciplinary approach is the key strategy to obtain best oncologic and functional outcomes. It is more important in STSs with osseous invasion for accurate diagnosis, staging, evaluation of disease extent including osseous invasion, decision making on neoadjuvant and adjuvant treatment, pathologic assessment for surgical margin and/or treatment response, timely rehabilitation, and emotional and psychological support.

For this patient, all members of multidiscriplinary team actively participated and did their roles, which guaranteed the good result.

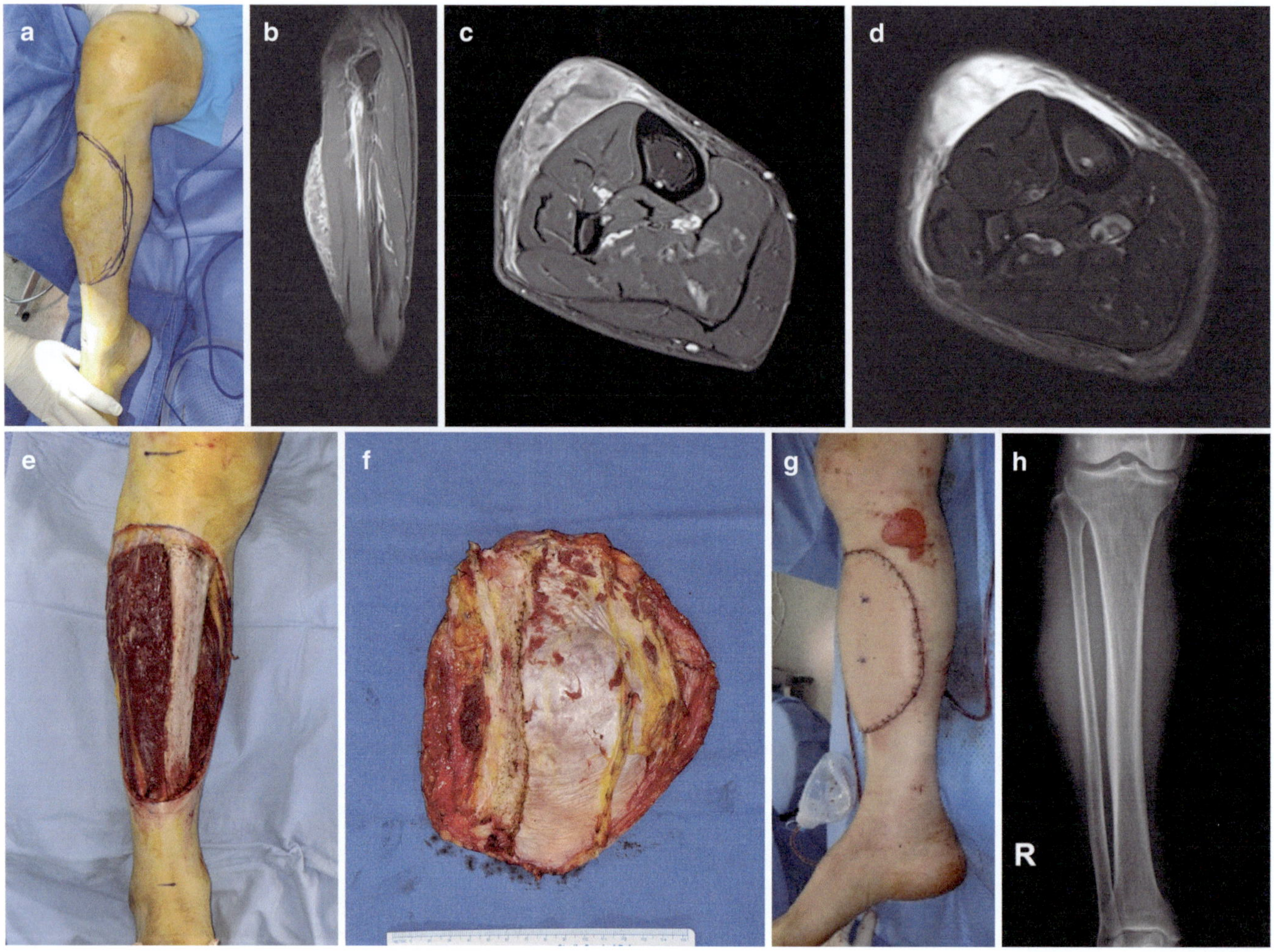

Fig. 51.9 A 79-year-old male patients with huge myxofibrosarcoma on anterolateral surface of right leg. A clinical photography (**a**) shows bulging soft tumor mass. Contrast-enhanced T1-weighted FS sagittal (**b**) and axial (**c**) MR images and T2-weighted FS axial MR image (**d**) reveal tumor extent. A thin periosteal sleeve was maintained on anterior surface of tibia. A subperiosteal dissection was performed (**e**, **f**). The soft tissue defect was covered with fasciocutaneous free flap from the anterolateral thigh (**g**). Postoperative radiogram reveals intact preserved tibia bone (**h**). Resection margin involvement was negative in pathological assessment

51.9 Avoiding and Managing Problems

1. Postoperative pain control: For emotional stabilization and early recovery, a proper postoperative pain management is an important issue.
   - Use patient-controlled analgesia (PCA) containing a cocktail of analgesics with booster dose button.
   - Additional PRN narcotics application in acute postoperative stage if PCA does not control the pain sufficiently (e.g., parenteral Tramadol/Pethidine HCl).
   - Switch on the oral analgesics as soon as possible to prevent dependency on narcotics (e.g., Celecoxib/Oxycodon).
2. Prevention of infection
   - Preoperative measures such as building up patient's general condition including nutritional support, hygiene care, and taking shower on the day before operation.
   - Parenteral preventive antibiotics 1 h before incision and every 2 h during surgery.
   - Thorough cleaning, scrubbing and painting on the surface of patient's body region before surgery in the operating room.
   - Double gloving of all participant in surgery.
   - Appropriate postoperative appropriate antibiotics coverage: broad spectrum parenteral antibiotics for about 1 week period and then oral antibiotics until wound healing in case of composite bone-soft tissue tumor excision and bone reconstruction with nonviable materials.
   - Negative pressure drainage bag is kept until the amount of draining blood decreases to less than 20 mL.

   - A close postoperative monitoring for any sign or symptom of infection including draining blood and/or draining bag line tip culture are helpful for early detection of low-grade infection and implementation of prompt measures to eradicate infection.
3. Prevention of nonunion at host bone-recycled graft bone junctions.
   - Stable internal fixation including restoration of rotational stability is the prerequisite of bone union.
   - Bone grafting at host bone-recycled graft bone junctions: autologous fresh iliac cancellous bone grafts provide osteoinductive, onteoconductive and osteogenic functions which enhance the junctional bone union. Application of demineralized bone matrix or BMP will be alternatives.
   - Protected ambulation using walking aids such as crutches or walker during progression of bone union is recommended.
4. Prevention of ankylosis
   - Compared to the joint resection-reconstruction, intercalary bone resection-reconstruction usually results in good range of motion at adjacent joints and excellent functional outcome.
   - General measures such as immediate encouraged bedside ROM exercise, early ambulation with walking aids, and timely protected staged weight bearing are necessary to ensure better functional recovery of operated limb.
5. Local recurrence and distant metastasis.
   - Consider adjuvant radiotherapy and/or chemotherapy: The tumor was low-grade solitary fibrous tumor with a low intermediate risk for metastasis and there was no evidence of distant metastasis. The surgical margin was negative. Only close monitoring would be necessary without any adjuvant radiotherapy or chemotherapy.
   - Follow-up examinations using standard protocol of postoperative oncologic monitoring for local recurrence and distant metastasis were performed regularly.

References

1. Lin PP, Pino ED, Normand AN, Deavers MT, Cannon CP, Ballo MT, et al. Periosteal margin in soft tissue sarcoma. Cancer. 2007;109:598–602.
2. Elias DA, White LM, Simpson DJ, Kandel RA, Tomlinson G, Bell RS, Wunder JS. Osseous invasion by soft-tissue sarcoma: assessment with MR imaging. Radiology. 2003;229:145–52.
3. Demicco EG, Park MS, Araujo DM, Fox PS, Bassett RL, Pollock RE, Lazar AJ, Wang WL. Solitary fibrous tumors. A clinicopathological study of 110 cases and proposed risk assessment model. Mod Pathol. 2012;25:1298–306.
4. Fujiwara T, Sumathi V, Parry M, Stevenson J, Tsuda Y, Kneuchi Y, Jeys L. The role of surgical margin quality in myxofibrosarcoma and undifferentiated pleomorphic sarcoma. Eur J Surg Oncol. 2020;47:1756–61.
5. Fujiwara T, Stevenson J, Parry M, Tsuda Y, Kneuchi Y, Jeys L. The adequacy of resection margin for non-infiltrative soft-tissue sarcomas. Eur J Surg Oncol. 2021;47:429–35.
6. Novais EN, Demiralp B, Alderete J, Larson MC, Rose PS, Sim FH. Do surgical margin and local recurrence influence survival in soft tissue sarcomas? Clin Orthop Relat Res. 2010;468:3003–11.
7. Sambri A, Caldari E, Fiore M, Zucchini R, Giannini C, Pirini MG, et al. Margin assessment if soft tissue sarcomas: review of the literature. Cancers. 2021;13:1687.
8. Manabe J, Ahmed AR, Kawaguchi N, Matsumoto S, Kuroda H. Pasteurized autologous bone graft in surgery for bone and soft tissue sarcoma. Clin Orthop Relat Res. 2004;419:258–66.
9. Panicek DM, Gatsonis C, Rosenthal DI, Seeger LL, Huvos AG, Moore SG, Caudry DJ, Palmer WE, Mcneil BJ. CT and MR imaging in the local staging of primary malignant musculoskeletal neoplasm: report of the Radiology Diagnostic Oncology Group. Radiology. 1997;202:237–46.
10. Mreino-Rueda LR, Barrientos-Ruiz IB, Bernabeu-Taboada D, Pozo-Kreilinger JJ, Peleteiro-Pensado M, Cordero-Garcia JM, Ortiz-Cruz EJ. Radiological and histological assessment of bone infiltration in soft tissue sarcomas. Eur J Orthop Surg Traumatol. 2022;32:631–9.

MIX
Papier aus verantwortungsvollen Quellen
Paper from responsible sources
FSC® C105338

If you have any concerns about our products,
you can contact us on
ProductSafety@springernature.com

In case Publisher is established outside the EU,
the EU authorized representative is:
Springer Nature Customer Service Center GmbH
Europaplatz 3, 69115 Heidelberg, Germany

Printed by Libri Plureos GmbH
in Hamburg, Germany